D0138705

Principles of RADIOGRAPHIC IMAGING

5th Edition

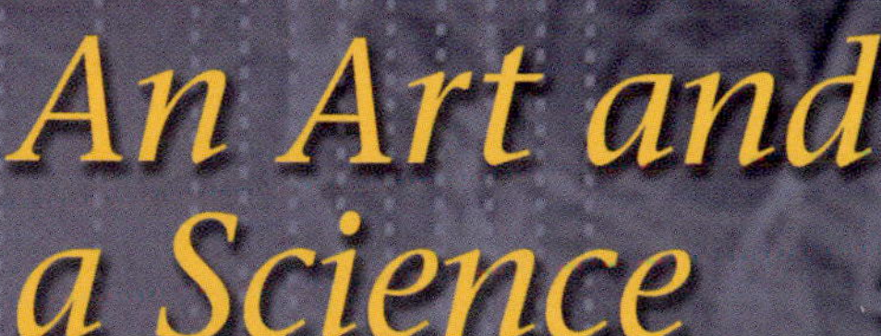

An Art and a Science

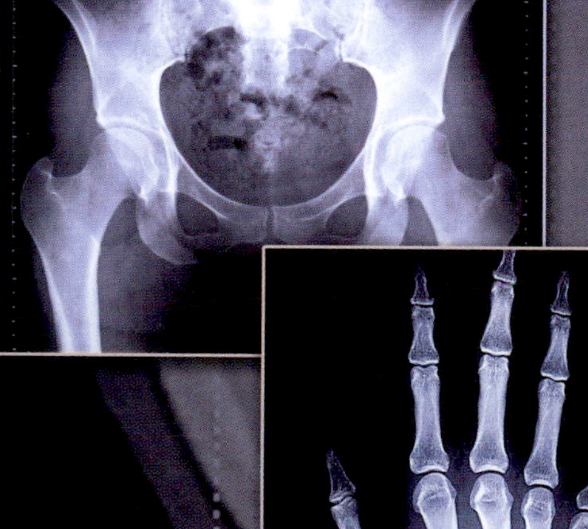

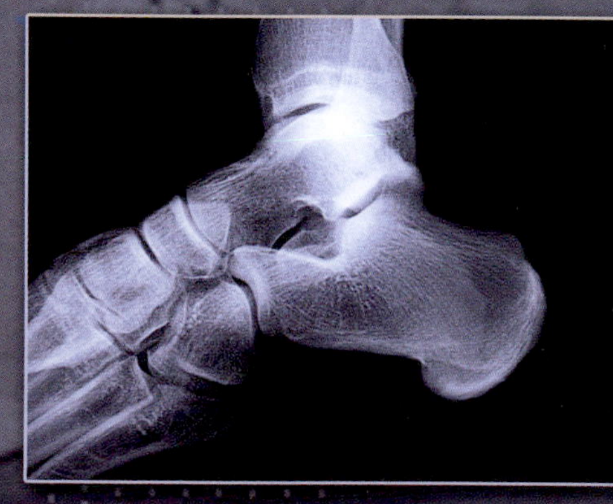

Principles of RADIOGRAPHIC IMAGING

5th Edition

An Art and a Science

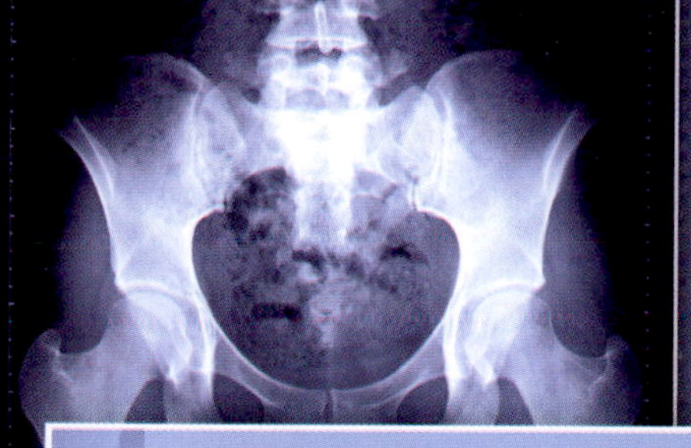

Richard R. Carlton, M.S., R.T.(R)(CV), FAEIRS
Associate Professor and Coordinator of Radiologic and Imaging Sciences
Grand Valley State University
Grand Rapids, Michigan

Arlene M. Adler, M.Ed., R.T.(R), FAEIRS
Professor and Director, Radiologic Sciences Programs
Indiana University Northwest
Gary, Indiana

Contributors
William Faulkner, Rick Hay, Julie Hollenbeck, Lisa King, Sharon Lakia,
Carolyn Kaut Roth, Barbara J. Smith, Christina Truluck

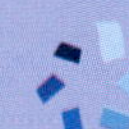
DELMAR
CENGAGE Learning

Australia • Brazil • Japan • Korea • Mexico • Singapore • Spain • United Kingdom • United States

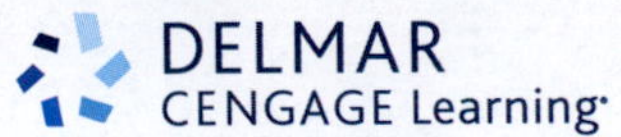

Principles of Radiographic Imaging: An Art and a Science, 5th Edition
Richard R. Carlton and Arlene M. Adler

Vice President, Editorial: Dave Garza

Director of Learning Solutions: Matthew Kane

Associate Acquisitions Editor: Christina Gifford

Managing Editor: Marah Bellegarde

Product Manager: Natalie Pashoukos

Media Editor: William Overocker

Editorial Assistant: Anthony Souza

Vice President, Marketing: Jennifer Baker

Marketing Director: Wendy Mapstone

Associate Marketing Manager: Jonathan Sheehan

Production Manager: Andrew Crouth

Senior Content Project Manager: Kenneth McGrath

Senior Art Director: David Arsenault

Technology Project Manager: Patti Allen

Library of Congress Control Number: 2011931912

ISBN-13: 978-1-4390-5872-5

ISBN-10: 1-4390-5872-5

Delmar
5 Maxwell Drive
Clifton Park, NY 12065-2919
USA

Cengage Learning is a leading provider of customized learning solutions with office locations around the globe, including Singapore, the United Kingdom, Australia, Mexico, Brazil, and Japan. Locate your local office at: **international.cengage.com/region**

Cengage Learning products are represented in Canada by Nelson Education, Ltd.

To learn more about Delmar, visit **www.cengage.com/delmar**

Purchase any of our products at your local college store or at our preferred online store **www.cengagebrain.com**

Printed in the United States of America
1 2 3 4 5 6 7 14 13 12 11

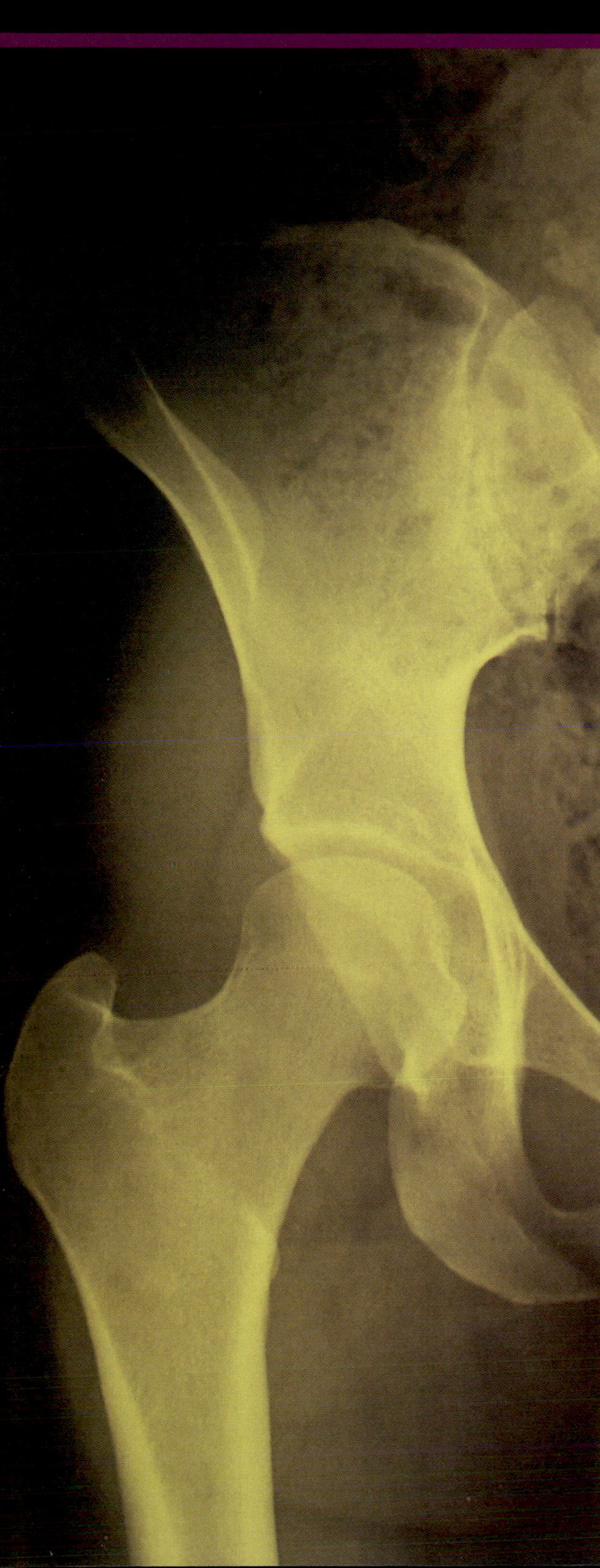

Dedication

*In memory of Raymond P. Rossi.
Our mentor, friend, teacher,
and coauthor. We miss you, Ray.
To Sidney Finkleman and Quentin
Garlets for teaching us to be
radiographers, to LaVerne Ramaeker,
Kay Shriver, and our students
for teaching us to be teachers,
and, most importantly,
to our families and friends
for sustaining us throughout.*

Contributors

William Faulkner, B.S., R.T.(R)(MR)(CT), FSMRT
William Faulkner and Associates

Rick Hay, Ph.D., M.D., FAHA
Adjunct Faculty in Radiologic and Imaging Sciences
Grand Valley State University

Julie Hollenbeck, B.S., R.T.(T)
Director, Radiation Therapy Program
University of Michigan-Flint

Lisa J. King, R.T.(R)(M)(BD), CBDT
Bone and Mineral Lab/JSC NASA
Wyle, Integrated Science and Engineering Group
Houston, Texas

Sharon Lakia, M.S., R.T.(R), RDMS, RVT
Director, Diagnostic Medical Sonography
Indiana University Northwest
Gary, Indiana

Carolyn Kaut Roth, R.T.(R)(MR)(CT)(M)(CV), FSMRT
CEO, Imaging Education Associates

Barbara J. Smith, M.S., R.T.(R)(QM)
Portland Community College
Radiological Sciences
Portland, Oregon

Christina A. Truluck, Ph.D., C.N.M.T., R.T.(N)
Assistant Professor and Program Director (NM, PET/CT)
Department of Radiologic Sciences
Thomas Jefferson University
Philadelphia, Pennsylvania

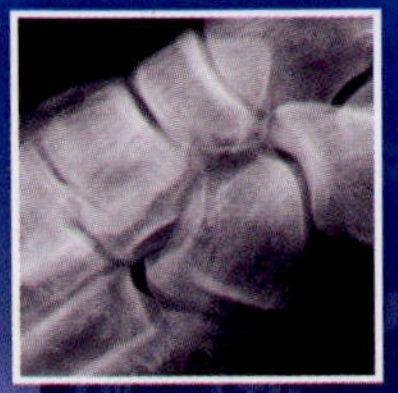
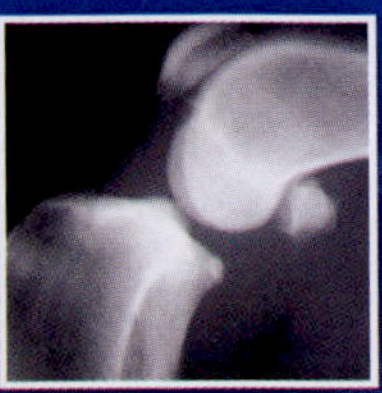
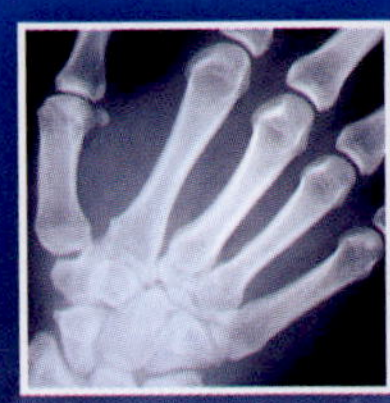

The Founders of Radiography

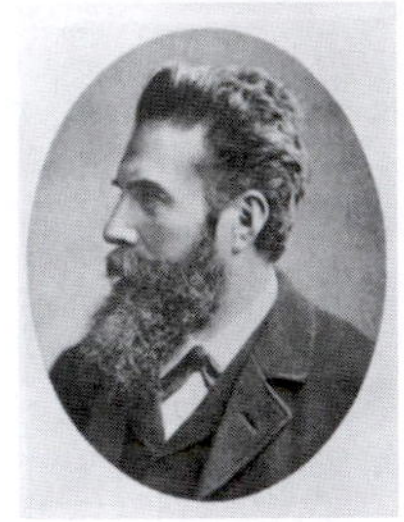

(Portrait courtesy of the American College of Radiology)

Wilhelm Conrad Röntgen (1845–1923)

Wilhelm Conrad Röntgen became the first radiographer when he discovered x-rays on November 8, 1895, in his laboratory at the University of Würzburg in Germany. His original paper *On a New Kind of Rays* is printed in Appendix A. For his discovery he received the first Nobel Prize in physics in 1901 and was decorated by Prussia, Bavaria, Great Britain, Austria, Mexico, Germany, France, the Netherlands, Sweden, Italy, Turkey, and the United States.

Eddy Clifford Jerman (1865–1936)

Ed C. Jerman is known as the "Father of Radiography" in the United States because he was the first teacher of radiography. He began teaching x-ray techniques in 1897; he founded the American Association of Radiological Technicians (now known as the American Society of Radiologic Technologists), and personally examined the first 1,000 members of the American Registry of X-Ray Technicians. He brought order to the principles of radiographic exposure technique by naming the qualities of the radiographic image: density, contrast, detail, and distortion. In 1928 he published *Modern X-Ray Technic*, the first book on radiographic principles.

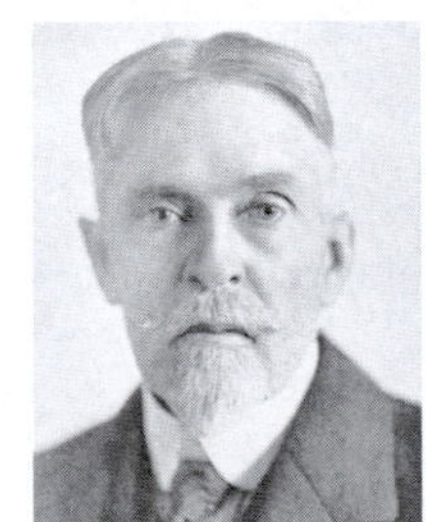

(Portrait courtesy of the American Society of Radiologic Technologists)

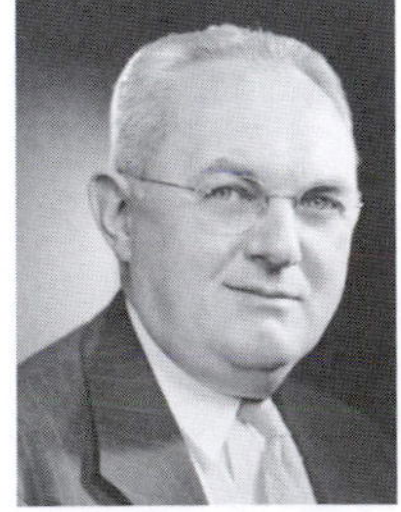

(Portrait courtesy of the family of Arthur Fuchs)

Arthur Wolfram Fuchs (1895–1962)

Arthur W. Fuchs is known as the inventor of the fixed kilovoltage technique of radiography. His father, Wolfram Fuchs, established the first x-ray laboratory in Chicago in 1896 but became one of the early martyrs of radiation, dying from excessive exposure. Arthur performed radiography for the United States Army in both World Wars I and II. During World War II he wrote the U.S. Army training manual *Principles of Radiographic Exposure*, in which he outlined his success with the optimal fixed kVp technique system. In 1955 he first published his book *Principles of Radiographic Exposure and Processing*.

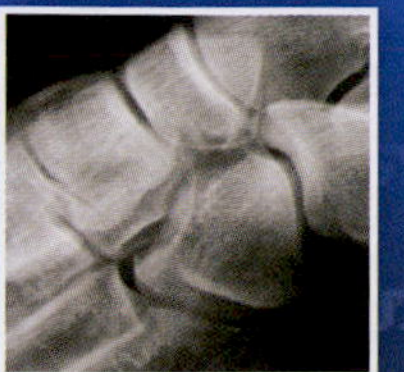
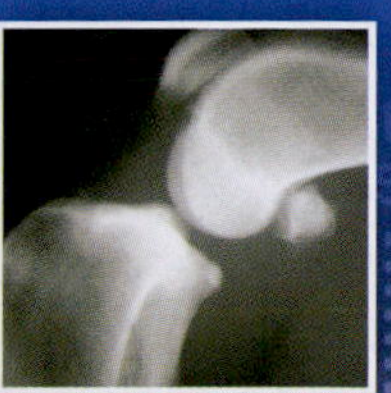
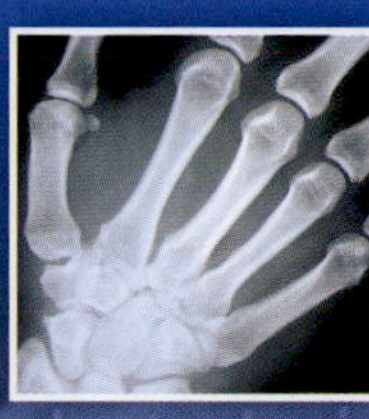

Contents

List of Tables xv
Foreword xix
Preface xx
About the Authors xxv
Acknowledgments xxvi
How to Use StudyWARE™ xxx

UNIT I CREATING THE BEAM

CHAPTER 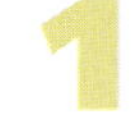

Basic Mathematics 2

Arithmetic / 3
Algebra / 8
Units of Measurement / 16

CHAPTER 

Radiation Concepts 20

Matter and Energy / 21
Atomic Theory / 24
Types of Energy / 32
Electromagnetic Spectrum / 33
The Discovery of X-Rays / 35
X-Ray Properties / 36

CHAPTER 3

Electricity 39

Electrostatics / 40
Electrodynamics / 45
Series and Parallel Circuits / 53

CHAPTER 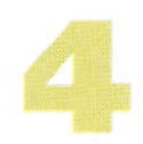

Electromagnetism 59

Magnetism / 60
Electromagnetism / 64
Solenoids and Electromagnets / 67
Controlling Electrical Current / 76
Rectification / 81

CHAPTER 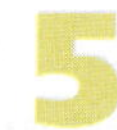

X-Ray Equipment 90

Types of X-Ray Equipment / 91
Power for X-Ray Generation / 94
A Basic X-Ray Circuit / 96
Generators / 99
Automatic Exposure Controls / 104

CHAPTER 6

The X-Ray Tube 108

The Cathode Assembly / 109
The Anode Assembly / 113
The Envelope / 120
Protective Housing / 121
Rating Charts and Cooling Curves / 123
Recommendations for Extending Tube Life / 126

CHAPTER 7

X-Ray Production 129

Conditions / 130
Target Interactions / 130
Emission Spectrum / 133

UNIT II
PROTECTING PATIENTS AND PERSONNEL

CHAPTER 8

Radiation Protection Concepts and Equipment 140

The Basics of Radiation Protection Principles and Practice / 141
Quantities and Units Relevant to Radiation Protection / 144
Detection and Measurement of Ionizing Radiation / 147

CHAPTER 9

Radiation Protection Procedures for Patients and Personnel 155

Advisory Groups and Regulatory Agencies / 156
Limiting Exposure to Ionizing Radiation / 156
Protection of Personnel / 159
Protection of the Patient / 161
Radiation Exposure and Pregnancy / 164

CHAPTER 10

Filtration 170

Measurement / 171
Types of Filtration / 172
Effect on Output / 175

CHAPTER 11

The Prime Factors 178

The Prime Factors / 179
Milliamperage-Second (mAs) / 179
Kilovoltage (kVp) / 183
Distance / 185
Image Quality Factors / 188

CHAPTER 12

X-Ray Interactions 191

X-Ray Interaction with Matter / 192
Photoelectric Absorption / 193
Coherent Scattering / 196
Compton Scattering / 197

Pair Production / 199
Photodisintegration / 199
Effect on Technical Factor Selection / 200

CHAPTER 13

Minimizing Patient Dose 204

Estimating Approximate Entrance Skin Exposure / 205
Typical Entrance Skin Exposure / 208
Reducing Patient Dose with Communication / 209
Reducing Patient Dose with Positioning / 209
Reducing Patient Dose with Technical Factors / 209
Discussing Radiation Risk Versus Benefit With Patients / 213

UNIT III CREATING THE IMAGE

CHAPTER 14

Vision and Perception 220

Image Perception / 221
Controlling the Image in Space / 226
Radiography as an Art Form / 227

CHAPTER 15

Beam Restriction 233

Controlling Scatter / 234
Beam Restrictors / 236
Ancillary Devices / 238

CHAPTER 16

The Patient as a Beam Emitter 240

Attenuation / 241
The Human Body as an Attenuator / 241
The Patient's Relationship to Image Quality / 243

CHAPTER 17

The Pathology Problem 246

Pathology and Radiation Absorption / 247
Increased Attenuation (Additive) Conditions / 250
Decreased Attenuation (Destructive) Conditions / 253

CHAPTER 18

The Grid 257

Purpose of the Grid / 258
Grid Construction / 259
Grid Patterns / 262
Grid Types / 262
Grid Uses / 263
Grid Selection/Conversions / 264
Grid Performance Evaluation / 265
Grid Errors / 265
An Alternate Scatter Reduction Method—The Air-Gap Technique / 269

CHAPTER 19

Radiographic Film 273

Construction / 274
Latent Image Formation / 278
Types of Film / 279
Film Storage and Handling / 280
Film Identification / 280

CHAPTER 20

Film Processing 283

Developing / 284
Fixing / 287
Archiving / 288
Automatic Processing / 288
Darkroom / 290
Silver Recovery Systems / 291

CHAPTER 21

Film Sensitometry 294

Sensitometric Equipment / 295
The D Log E Curve / 298
Film Characteristics / 299

CHAPTER 22

Intensifying Screens and Film/Screen Combinations 308

Construction / 309
Phosphors / 311
Characteristics / 312
Cassettes and Holders / 315
Care / 316
Emission Spectra / 316
Characteristics / 317

CHAPTER 23

Digital Radiography 323

Historical Development / 324
Digital Image Formation / 324
Image Processing Operations / 327
Digital Image Quality / 332
Exposure Indicators / 333
Computed Radiography (PSP) Systems / 339
Flat Panel Digital Radiography / 353
Digital Radiography Artifacts / 356

CHAPTER 24

Picture Archiving and Communications Systems (PACSs) 362

Informatics / 363
Image Acquisition / 365
Image Distribution / 365
Image Display / 366
Storage / 369

UNIT IV
ANALYZING THE IMAGE

CHAPTER 25

The Imaging Process 375

The Imaging Process / 376
Professional Imaging Standards / 380

The Analytical Process / 380
Acceptance Limits / 381

CHAPTER 26

Density/Image Receptor Exposure 386

Assessing Density/IR Exposure / 387
Effects on Image Appearance / 388
Factors Affecting Density/IR Exposure / 388

CHAPTER 27

Contrast 403

Assessing Contrast / 404
Image Contrast / 407
Evaluating Contrast / 411
Factors Affecting Contrast / 416

CHAPTER 28

Recorded Detail 424

Assessing Recorded Detail / 425
Effects on Image Appearance / 430
Factors Affecting Recorded Detail / 431

CHAPTER 29

Distortion 442

Assessing Distortion / 443
Factors Affecting Size Distortion / 443
Factors Affecting Shape Distortion / 448
Effect on Image Appearance / 453

CHAPTER 30

The Art of Image Critique 458

Implementing Imaging Standards / 459
Identifying an Imaging Problem / 459
An Effective Image Critique Method / 460
Applying the Image Critique Method / 463

CHAPTER 31

Quality Management 467

Quality Assurance and Quality Control / 468
Purchasing Equipment / 469
Monitoring Equipment Performance / 470
Ancillary Equipment / 476
PACS Systems / 478
Repeat-Image Studies / 478
Troubleshooting / 479

UNIT V COMPARING EXPOSURE SYSTEMS

CHAPTER 32

Exposure Systems 487

Exposure System Selection / 488
Establishing an Exposure System / 490
Establishing Fixed Kilovoltage Exposure Systems / 492
Establishing a Variable Kilovoltage Peak Exposure System / 496

CHAPTER 33

Automatic Exposure Controls 506

Ionization Chambers / 507
Positioning Skills / 509

CHAPTER 34

Exposure Conversion Problems 514

Standard Conversion Relationships and Tables / 515
Solving Complex Exposure Problems / 517

UNIT VI SPECIAL IMAGING SYSTEMS AND MODALITIES

CHAPTER 35

Mobile Radiography 523

Special Patient Considerations / 524
Special Radiation Protection Considerations / 527
Types of Equipment / 527
Special Technical Factor Selection Considerations / 528

CHAPTER 36

Fluoroscopy 533

Historical Development / 534
Fluoroscopic Uses / 534
Types of Equipment / 534
Fluoroscopic X-Ray Tubes / 535
Image Intensification Tubes / 536
Image Quality / 540
Video Viewing Systems / 541
Digital Fluoroscopy / 542
Recording the Fluoroscopic Image / 542
Mobile Fluoroscopic Equipment / 543
Radiation Protection During Fluoroscopy / 543

CHAPTER 37

Tomography and Digital Tomosynthesis 548

The Tomographic Principle / 549
Tomographic Quality / 551
Types of Motion / 554
Digital Tomosynthesis / 555
Tomographic Procedures / 556

CHAPTER 38

Mammography 561

Historical Development / 562
Generator Characteristics / 567
X-Ray Tube / 571
Accessories / 581
Resolution / 584
Digital Mammography / 584
Quality Control / 585

CHAPTER 39

Bone Densitometry 589

History and Overview / 590
Bone Science / 591
Osteoporosis / 592

WHO Diagnostic Criteria / 595
DXA Principles and Instrumentation / 596
Scan Acquision and Analysis / 596
Femur / 596
Spine / 598
Forearm / 600
Quality Control / 601
Radiation Safety and Protection / 601

CHAPTER 40

Vascular Imaging Equipment 604

History of Vascular Imaging / 605
Digital Image Acquisition / 607
Modes of Digital Image Acquisition / 609
Image Post-Processing / 610
C-Arm Assembly / 611
Angiographic Tables / 612
Contrast Medium Injection Devices / 613
Quality Control / 615

CHAPTER 41

Computed Tomography 617

The Invention of Computed Tomography / 619
Scanner Generations / 619
The Components of a CT Unit / 626
CT Numbers (Hounsfield Units) / 633
Image Reconstruction / 633
Image Quality / 638
Scanning Procedures / 639
Artifacts / 641
Radiation Protection / 643

CHAPTER 42

Magnetic Resonance Imaging 648

History / 649
Instrumentation / 649
MRI Physics / 653
MRI / 656
MR Safety / 666

CHAPTER 43

Nuclear Medicine and PET Scanning 671

Nuclear Physics / 672
Radioactive Decay / 672
Radiochemistry and Radiopharmaceuticals / 673
Imaging Instrumentation / 683
Positron Emission Tomography (PET) / 689
Hybrid SPECT/CT and PET/CT Imaging / 690
Nonimaging Instrumentation / 692
Radiation Protection / 693
Clinical Applications / 696

CHAPTER 44

Radiation Therapy 703

Historical Overview / 704
Consultation / 704
Treatment Planning / 706
Treatment / 711
Specialized Treatments and Units / 720

CHAPTER 45

Diagnostic Medical Sonography 724

Introduction / 725
Sound Waves / 726
Attenuation / 735
Range / 736
Field / 736
Doppler / 737
Harmonics / 737
Transducer and Components / 738
Instrumentation / 741

APPENDIX A

On a New Kind of Rays 745

APPENDIX B

Answers to Case Studies 750

APPENDIX C

Epigraph Sources and Credits 752

Glossary 754

Index 774

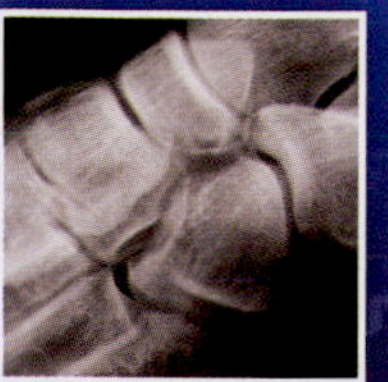
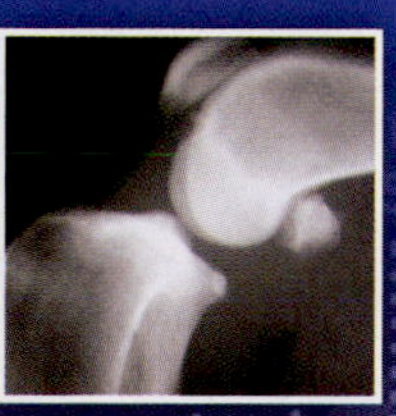
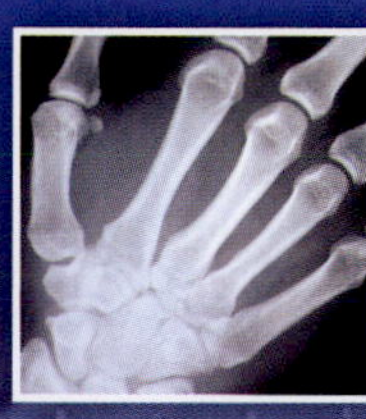

List of Tables

1-1.	Multiplication Notation	3
1-2.	SI Units of Measurement	17
1-3.	SI Unit Values	17
1-4.	Commonly Used SI Prefixes	18
2-1.	Atomic Particles	27
3-1.	Properties of Conducting Materials	47
3-2.	Effect of Circuit Type on Current, Potential Difference, and Resistance (with an example circuit of three resistances)	53
4-1.	Fleming's Hand Rules for Electromagnetic Relationships	66
5-1.	Common Diagnostic X-Ray Console Controls	99
6-1.	Heat Unit Rectification Constants	124
6-2.	Recommendations for Extending Tube Life	126
7-1.	Characteristic Photon Emissions from X-Ray Target Materials	133
8-1.	Comparison of Collective Effective Dose(S) and Effective Dose per Individual in the U.S. Population (E_{us}) as Reported in NCRP (1987a) and in This Report (annual values for percent are rounded to the nearest 1%)	144
8-2.	Conversions between Conventional and SI Units	145
8-3.	Comparison between SI and Conventional Units	147
9-1.	Effective Dose Limit Recommendations	157
9-2.	Occupational Dose Limits for Adults—NRC Regulation IOCFR20	158
10-1.	Minimum Half-Valve Layer (HVL) Requirements for X-Ray Systems in United States (Title 21 of 21 CFR 1020.30)	172
10-2.	Percent Attenuation of Monochromatic Radiation by Various Thicknesses of Aluminum Filtration	175
10-3.	Recommended Minimum Total Filtration Levels	175

10-4.	Comparison of Patient Exposure with Filtration	176
11-1.	Factors Affecting X-Ray Emission	179
12-1.	K-Shell Binding Energies of Radiologically Significant Elements	194
12-2.	Percentage of Photon Interactions, Attenuation, and Transmission Characteristics in Soft Tissue Based on Effective Photon Energies	195
13-1.	A Typical mR/mAs Chart	206
13-2.	Medical ESE Values for Selected Radiographic Exams	208
13-3.	Effects of Radiographic Exposure Variables on Patient Dose	210
13-4.	Comparison of Approximate Entrance Skin Exposures with Fixed and Variable kVp Technique Systems	210
13-5.	Gross Comparison of Relative Radiation Levels	215
13-6.	Estimated Loss of Life Expectancy Due to Various Causes	215
16-1.	Basic Substances Comprising the Human Body	241
17-1.	Summary of Pathology Problems	251
18-1.	Grids for Use in Digital Imaging	260
18-2.	Grid Conversion Factors	264
19-1.	Relationship of Film Crystal and Emulsion to Film Factors	277
19-2.	Standard Radiographic Film Sizes	278
20-1.	Automatic Radiographic Processing Chemicals and Their Functions	285
21-1.	Example Opacities, Optical Density Numbers, and Light Transmission Percentages	298
21-2.	Relationship between Contrast, Latitude, and Patient Dose	306
21-3.	Relationship between Speed and Patient Dose	306
22-1.	K-Shell Edges for Intensifying-Screen Phosphors	314
22-2.	Relationship between Relative Speed Number and Exposure Sensitivity	318
23-1.	Binary Code Numbers	325
23-2.	Typical Memory Requirements for Various Imaging Modalities	333
23-3.	Exposure Index Numbers Relative to Imaging Plate Exposure	335
23-4.	Suggested kVp Ranges for Digital Imaging Systems	339
24-1.	DICOM Information Classes	364
26-1.	Conversion Factors Effect of Generator ϕ on IR Exposure	393
26-2.	Projections That May Use the Anode Heel Effect to Advantage	394
26-3.	mAs Change Factors for Approximate Exposure Maintenance When Distance Changes	396
26-4.	Effect on Density/IR Exposure When Factors Are Changed	401
27-1.	Relationship between Terms Used to Describe Contrast	406

27-2.	Changes Necessary to Produce Visible Contrast Differences	415
27-3.	Effects of Changing Factors on Contrast	421
28-1.	Spatial Resolution Quality Measures	427
28-2.	Grayscale Bit Depth (Z-Axis)	427
28-3.	Effects of Intensifying-Screen Factors on Resolution	436
28-4.	Effects of Various Methods for Reducing Exposure Time to Avoid Motion	438
28-5.	Effect of Changing Factors on Recorded Detail	439
29-1.	SID Compensations for Common Tube Angulations	453
29-2.	Effect of Changing Factors on Distortion	455
31-1.	FOCUS-PDCA Method	468
31-2.	Causes of Repeated Image	478
31-3.	Retake Percentage by Room	479
31-4.	Retake Percentage by Technologist	479
32-1.	Average Adult Part Thickness by Region	489
32-2.	Common Optimal kVp Ranges for the Major Body Regions	495
32-3.	Fixed kVp Technique Chart	496
32-4.	2-kVp/cm Chart	499
32-5.	Variable Kilovoltage Scales	499
32-6.	Stepped Variable kVp Technique Chart	501
34-1.	Effects of Radiographic Exposure Variables on the Primary Factors	515
34-2.	Exposure Maintenance Rules	516
34-3.	Conversion Factors: Effect of Generator Phase on Exposure	516
34-4.	The 15 Percent Rule	516
34-5.	The mAs Formula	516
34-6.	The Exposure Maintenance Formula	516
34-7.	Recommended Compensation for Subject Part Thickness	516
34-8.	Grid Conversion Formula	516
34-9.	Grid Conversion Factors	517
34-10.	Relative Speed Formula	517
35-1.	Radiation Protection Rules for Mobile Radiography	527
36-1.	Typical Limiting Spatial Resolution in Fluoroscopy	540
38-1.	Technical Differences between Mammography and Conventional Radiography	568
38-2.	Characteristic X-Rays from Mammography X-Ray Targets	577
39-1.	Risk Factors Associated with Osteoporosis	594

39-2.	DXA Collimator/Detector Types	597
39-3.	Radiation Safety and Patient Dose	601
40-1.	Modes of Digital Image Acquisition	609
40-2.	Factors Affecting Flow Rate	614
40-3.	Safety Mechanisms for Contrast Medium Injectors	614
41-1.	Major Characteristics of CT Unit Generations	620
41-2.	Advantages and Disadvantages of Helical (Spiral) Computed Tomography	624
41-3.	CT Pitch Formulas	624
41-4.	Hounsfield Units (HUs) (CT Numbers) of Various Tissues	635
41-5.	Appropriate Computed Tomography Window Widths	638
43-1.	The Half-Lives, Gamma Energies, Production Methods, and Usages of Radionuclides Nuclear Medicine	675
43-2.	Technetium-99m–Labeled Radiopharmaceuticals and Their Uses	676
43-3.	Non–Tc-99m Radiopharmaceuticals and Their Uses	677
43-4.	Radiopharmaceuticals Used for Radionuclide Therapy	678
43-5.	Radiopharmaceutical Quality Control Tests	679
43-6.	Quality Control Testing of Imaging Instrumentation	691
43-7.	Highlights of NRC Regulations Pertaining to Operation of a Nuclear Medicine Facility; Title 10 of the Code of Federal Regulations, Part 20 Addresses Radiation Protection Requirements; Part 35 Addresses Medical Uses of Byproduct Material	694
45-1.	Appropriate Computed Tomography Window Widths	731

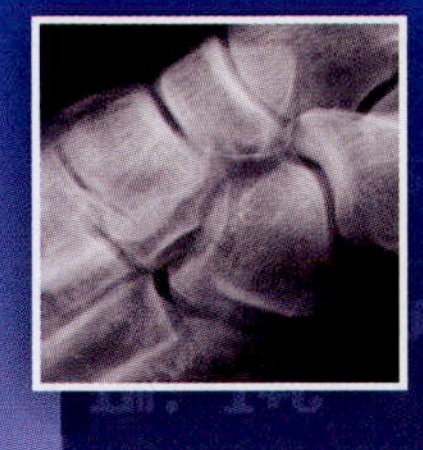
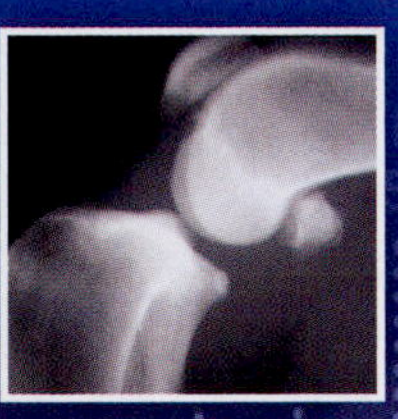
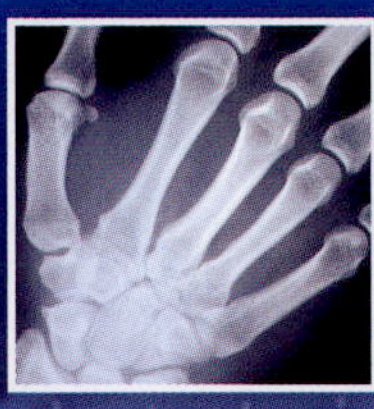

Foreword

What? Arlene Adler and Rick Carlton publishing another revision! I know it is hard to believe—again the two of them. How fortunate for medical imaging sciences professionals to have such hard-working, dedicated scholars, who, by their very nature, continually strive to provide the most comprehensive and practical text of relevant and essential principles for the medical imaging sciences professional community.

As one of the most popular imaging sciences texts on the market, this fifth edition of *Principles of Radiographic Imaging* includes the quality attributes and fundamentals of prior editions, preserving essential concepts and condensing and deleting older conventional content while addressing newer, more modern imaging principles.

Noteworthy to the fifth edition is a considerable rework and expansion of chapters on digital imaging principles containing solidified terminologies. Educators throughout our profession have hungered for reliable, comprehensive, and practical learning resources for digital imaging technologies, and Carlton and Adler's fifth edition has definitely delivered. Significant expansion of digital radiography content produced a need to revise nearly all, and in some cases, consolidate, principles chapters. Additional content areas address other newer imaging equipment, such as digital tomosynthesis and PACS.

As educators are keenly aware, visuals included in prior editions have always positively reinforced student learning. The new edition is no exception, as illustrative art throughout the text has been expanded and updated. Of course, the accompanying laboratory manual and instructor resources have undergone appropriate revisions to complement updates incorporated in the text.

The nationally recognized curriculum requires educators to support student learning in other related imaging modalities and disciplines. To this end, this fifth edition of *Principles of Radiographic Imaging* includes chapters that address essentials of imaging sciences instrumentation used in bone densitometry, nuclear medicine and PET scanning, radiation therapy, and diagnostic medical sonography.

As technologists writing for technologists, Mr. Carlton and Ms. Adler danced a delicate dance to determine what to condense, what to delete, and how to expand. They have, yet again, served up a respected authoritative teaching and learning resource for medical imaging sciences professionals—one that is concise yet thorough, and one that certainly broadens the scope of understanding of imaging principles for the entire profession.

Denise Moore, M.S., R.T.(R)
Professor Emeritus
Radiologic Technology
Sinclair Community College
Dayton, Ohio

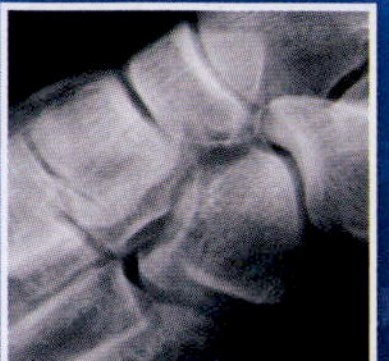
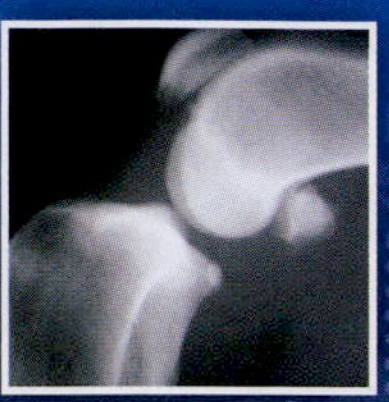
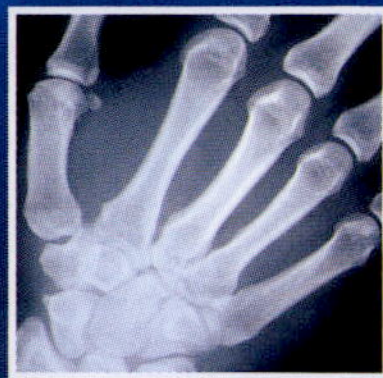

Preface

INTRODUCTION

As radiography educators, we designed this textbook with students and educators in mind: each chapter contains an outline, key terms, objectives, a summary, review questions, and a detailed bibliography. There is also a considerable number of ancillaries that faculty can access through their Delmar Cengage Learning representative (they can be reached through the website at www.cengage.com/delmar, or for product information and technology assistance, contact them at Cengage Learning Customer and Sales Support, 1-800-354-9706.). Although the order of the chapters is based on our experiences in reaching our students, most chapters stand alone and can be used in the order that is most appropriate within a given program.

We have made a special effort to represent our belief that professional development should be a prime objective of any radiography curriculum. This is best achieved through the demonstration of technical competence. This book is designed to assist students in developing this cornerstone of professionalism. Through technical competence and a professional demeanor students will be ready to assume their role as experts in the radiographic imaging process. In addition, we believe that true professionals take immense pride in their work to the extent that it becomes an art as well as a science.

There is a special focus on making sure digital imaging terminology and parameters are the primary orientation with references to conventional film-based imaging, as educators have made it clear that there are still facilities that utilize it, although we know they will cease in the near future. Special effort is made to emphasize both the technical information and the ethical importance of understanding the specifics of image receptor sensitivity in order to be able to reduce exposure to the patient.

References used extensively to assure both educators and students that we address all content expected for successful professional practice include the American Registry of Radiographic Technologists' *Content Specifications for the Examination in Radiography*, the *Radiography Curriculum* by the American Society of Radiologic Technologists, and various materials prepared by the Canadian Association of Medical Radiation Technologists.

CONTENT

A special attempt was made to provide an introduction to physics and the imaging modalities, as well as to explore the details of the principles of radiographic exposure techniques. Well-established image quality factors (density/image receptor exposure, contrast, recorded detail, and distortion) are incorporated into digital imaging while new considerations such as the difference between monitor brightness and density are added to the image production and viewing chain. Five phases of digitized image production are introduced: acquisition, processing, archiving, displaying, and analyzing. Each includes well-known radiographic imaging parameters but each is also enhanced by the addition of digital factors that now impact on all imaging decisions.

ORGANIZATION

The overall design of the book separates the 45 chapters into six units: Creating the Beam, Protecting Patients and Personnel, Creating the Image, Analyzing the Image, Comparing Exposure Systems, and Special Imaging Systems and Modalities. We are pleased to offer four new chapters that address the instrumentation for bone densitometry, nuclear medicine and PET scanning, radiation therapy, and diagnostic medical sonography. Along with the chapters on mammography, vascular imaging equipment, computed tomography, and magnetic resonance imaging, we now offer framework information on all radiologic and imaging sciences modalities and treatments. This design helps organize the content for students by following a logical progression from introductory physics through the production and control of the beam to advanced modality systems.

We remain extremely pleased that our book remains one of the resources listed in the Radiography Curriculum of the American Society of Radiologic Technologists, and we have long been pleased that this book continues to be recommended by the Canadian Association of Medical Radiation Technologists for preparation for its certification in Radiological Technology.

NEW TO THIS EDITION

The rapid changes in technology present a challenge to textbook authors who are committed to providing current information for learners. The authors and contributors to the fifth edition carefully reviewed all content to identify areas requiring updating or new topics. As a result, numerous changes were made. The more significant changes are as follows:

- Significant rewrite of digital radiography imaging principles with appropriate condensation of conventional radiography.
- New chapters on radiologic and imaging sciences instrumentation used for bone densitometry, nuclear medicine and PET scanning, radiation therapy, and diagnostic medical sonography.
- Updates on new imaging equipment such as digital tomosynthesis and PACS, as well as making sure information on modalities such as CT and MRI remain current.

FEATURES

In addition to the updated and new content, this new edition continues to feature the following learning aids and critical content:

- Physical concepts are clearly explained and illustrated with many high-quality figures.
- Effects of changing parameters on image quality are carefully described and illustrated with numerous images.
- Criteria for image analysis are presented to help learners develop analytical skills.
- High-quality radiographs are included throughout the text.
- Radiation protection concepts and procedures are emphasized for both patients and radiographic personnel.
- Chapter-end summaries provide a quick reference to critical concepts and developments in the science of radiography.
- Numerous troubleshooting tips are included to ensure quality radiographs.
- Extensive references and recommended readings provide a historical perspective and provide learners a means to expand their understanding of concepts and systems.
- Epigraphs and historical photos help trace the evolution of radiography to the present.
- Unique emphasis on the art versus the science of radiography illustrates the broad applications of the technology.

ADDITIONAL TEACHING/ LEARNING RESOURCES

StudyWARE

The StudyWARE software includes interactive quizzes and activities that provide additional practice, and fun, while learning. Activities include games such as concentration and hangman as well as flashcards, crossword puzzles, and image labeling exercises. See "How to Use the StudyWARE" on page xxx for details.

Workbook

(ISBN: 978-1-4390-5870-1)

The workbook was created as a series of activities, both laboratories and worksheets, to provide higher-level synthesis and analysis for each chapter in the textbook. There are a total of 99 exercises: 62 are laboratories and 37 are worksheets.

Premium Website (ISBN: 978-1-1337-0276-4)

A Premium Website is available to accompany the text that includes the StudyWARE™, slide presentations in PowerPoint®, and an image library.

Redeeming an Access Code:

1. GO TO: http://www.CengageBrain.com.
2. ENTER THE Access code in the Prepaid Code or Access Key field, **REDEEM.**
3. REGISTER as a new user or LOG IN as an existing user if you already have an account with Cengage Learning or CengageBrain.com.
4. SELECT **Go to MY Account.**
5. OPEN the product from the My Account page.

Also Available:

- Premium Website IAC to accompany *Principles of Radiographic Imaging: An Art and a Science*, Fifth Edition (ISBN: 978-1-1337-0275-7)

Instructor Resources CD-ROM (ISBN: 978-1-4390-5869-5)

The Instructor Resources CD-ROM is a robust computerized tool designed to meet your instructional needs. A must-have for all instructors, this comprehensive and convenient CD-ROM contains the following components.

Instructor's Manual

The Instructor's Manual includes answers to the review questions contained within the textbook. The review questions are designed to assess the students' accomplishment of the chapter objectives and may be useful as a homework assignment or simply as a self-assessment tool for the student. The manual also provides the instructor with additional student assignment ideas, which may be used to assess students' understanding of the content and/or help expand their knowledge of the content beyond the scope of the text.

Answers are also provided for the worksheets and laboratory exercises in the workbook, with the exception of laboratories in which the student answer determines the results.

PowerPoint® Presentations

More than 1,700 PowerPoint slides are designed to aid you in planning your class presentations. If a student misses a class, a printout of the slides for a lecture provides a helpful review page. Instructors, please feel free to add your own slides for additional topics you introduce to the class.

Computerized Test Bank in ExamView®

The test bank includes approximately 1,770 test questions. These include multiple-choice, short-answer, matching, and completion questions, as well as problems. Users can add their own questions. This software allows the user to create tests in less than 5 minutes, with the ability to print them out in a variety of layouts. It also has electronic "take-home testing" (put test on disk) and Internet-based testing capabilities.

Image Library

The image library includes more than 600 files containing images from the textbook.

Instructor Companion Site

An Instructor Companion Site is available that includes the Instructor Resources.

To access the Instructor Companion site, go to http://login.cengage.com.

- *If you have a Cengage SSO account:* Sign in with your e-mail address and password.
- *If you do not have a Cengage SSO account:* Click Create My Account and follow the prompts.

WebTUTOR™

(WebTUTOR™ on Blackboard ISBN: 978-1-4390-5867-1)

Designed to complement the textbook, WebTUTOR™ is a content-rich, Web-based teaching and learning aid that reinforces and clarifies complex concepts. The Blackboard™ platform also provides rich communication tools to instructors and students, including a course calendar, chat, email, and threaded discussions.

CourseMate

(CourseMate PAC (printed access card) ISBN: 978-1-1337-0273-3) (CourseMate IAC (instant access code) ISBN: 978-1-1337-0274-0)

Principles of Radiographic Imaging: An Art and a Science, Fifth Edition includes CourseMate, a complement to your textbook. CourseMate includes:

- An interactive eBook
- Interactive teaching and learning tools, including:
  - Quizzes
  - Flashcards
  - PowerPoint slides
  - Glossary
  - and more
- Engagement Tracker, a first-of-its-kind tool that monitors student engagement in the course

To access these materials online, visit http://login.cengage.com.

STATEMENT OF CONTENT ACCURACY

Although we assume full responsibility for any errors, including those that may be construed as arising from quoting other works out of context, we have made every effort to ensure the accuracy of the information. However, appropriate information sources should be consulted, especially for new or unfamiliar procedures. It is the responsibility of every practitioner to evaluate the appropriateness of a particular procedure in the context of actual clinical situations. Therefore, neither the authors nor the publisher take responsibility or accept any liability for the actions of persons applying the information contained herein in an unprofessional manner. This information is designed to supplement and enhance the instructional methodologies of educators in JRCERT (Joint Review Committee on Education in Radiologic Technologies [USA]) and CAMRT (Canada) approved radiography programs and should not be applied, especially to human subjects, without this background. In committing this book to print we fully realize that it is never finished, merely suspended for the time being.

Finally, as a reader your perceptions are important to us. We encourage you to communicate with us regarding facets of the book you appreciate or would like to see changed. We especially appreciate constructive comments and notice of errors. Our intention is to present the principles of radiography in an interesting format that provides a base from which true professionalism can develop. Any commentary readers care to make toward this end will be valued and welcomed.

Richard R. Carlton
Grand Valley State University
Radiologic and Imaging Sciences
Center for Health Sciences
Suite 455
301 Michigan St. NE
Grand Rapids, MI 49503
616-331-5600

Arlene M. Adler
Indiana University Northwest
3400 Broadway
Gary, IN 46408
1219-980-6540
aadler@iun.edu

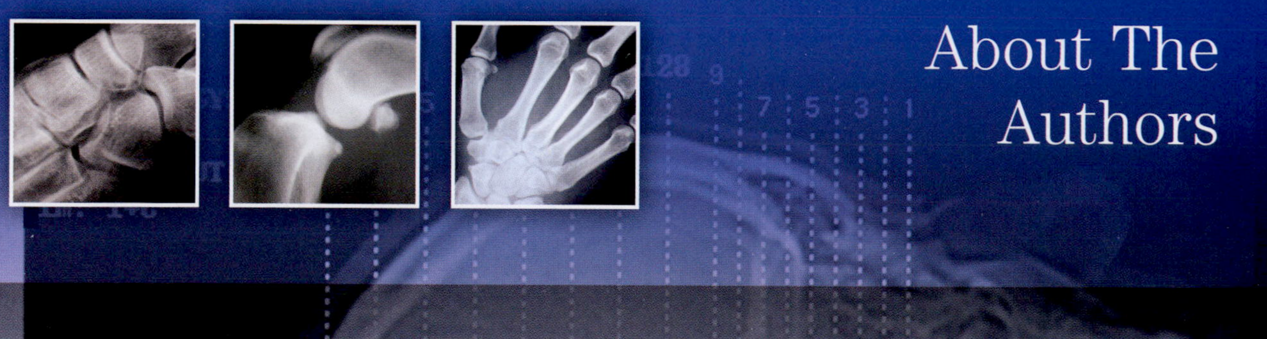

About The Authors

Richard R. Carlton is currently Associate Professor and Coordinator of Radiologic and Imaging Sciences at Grand Valley State University in Grand Rapids, Michigan. He is a past President and Chairman of the Board of the Association of Educators in Imaging and Radiologic Sciences. Rick co-founded the Michigan Radiologic and Imaging Sciences Consortium (a consortium of community colleges and a university that offers advanced clinical education), and established the Center for Medical Imaging in Bioanthropology (for field work x-raying mummies in Peru), Lambda Nu (the national honor society for the radiologic and imaging sciences), and The Sectional Anatomy Consortium. He has published more than 20 books, was the founding editor of two journals, and is a charter Fellow of the Association of Educators in Radiologic Sciences (AEIRS). Rick has been a JRCERT accreditation site visitor for more than 30 years, and was a Fulbright Scholarship alternate, as well as author of numerous journal articles. He has given more than 250 lectures in 36 states and 9 countries.

He holds an M.S. from National Louis University, B.S. in Radiologic Sciences from The Chicago Medical School, and an A.A.S. from Illinois Central College. He is ARRT certified in radiography and cardiovascular-interventional technology and has taught radiologic sciences for over 30 years in Chicago, Ohio, San Francisco, Arkansas, and Michigan. With Arlene Adler, he is the author of the best-selling radiographic physics textbook *Principles of Radiographic Imaging* as well as *Introduction to Radiography and Patient Care*, both now in fifth editions. Rick has also been the radiology section consultant to *Taber's Cyclopedia Medical Dictionary* for the past three editions.

Arlene Adler is a Full Professor and Director of the Radiologic Sciences Programs at Indiana University Northwest in Gary. She received her radiography education at Michael Reese Medical Center in Chicago. She has a B.S. degree in Radiologic Sciences from the University of Health Sciences/Chicago Medical School and a Master's Degree in Education from the University of Illinois at Urbana–Champaign. Arlene has been an active member of the American Society of Radiologic Technologist and the Association of Educators in Radiologic Sciences (AEIRS). For her service to AEIRS, she was awarded Fellow status. She has lectured across the country on numerous topics in radiologic sciences and, in particular, was a past Honors Lecturer for an AEIRS Annual Meeting and a past Keynote Speaker for the Associated Science Program at the Radiologic Society of North America (RSNA) annual meeting. For her service on the Indiana Radiation Control Advisory Commission, she received the Governor's Award, Sagamore of the Wabash.

In addition to her professional service, Arlene has authored numerous articles and, along with Rick Carlton, is coauthor of the text *Principles of Radiographic Imaging: An Art and a Science* and coeditor of the text *Introduction to Radiography and Patient Care.*

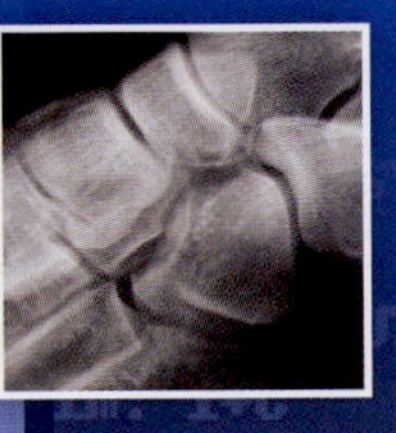
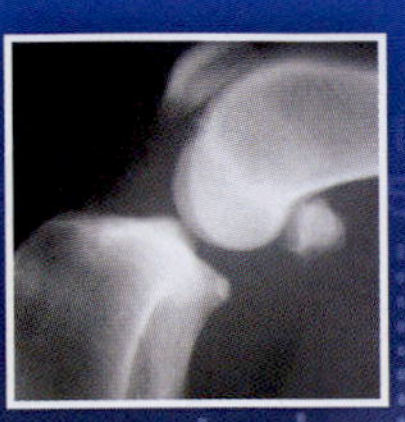
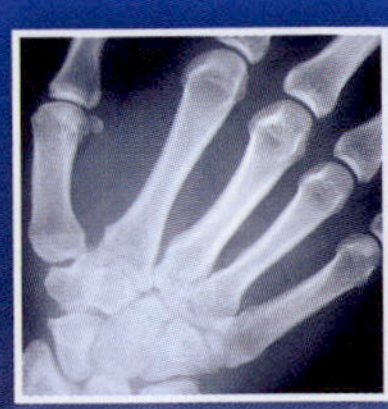

Acknowledgments

We wish to acknowledge the support provided by Dean Roy Olsson and Associate Dean Linda Goossen at Grand Valley State University in Grand Rapids, Michigan; Dean Patrick Bankston, Associate Dean Linda DeLunas, and the wonderful radiologic sciences faculty at Indiana University Northwest, including Robin Jones, Vesna Balac, Sharon Lakia, Dorothy Rytczak, Sue Woods, Julie Aguayo, Shannon Baimakovich, Helen Campbell, Char Gilpin, Susan Janosky, Heather Lane, Pat Lewis, Tiffany O'Day, Sheri Stremplewski, Becky Wantland, Sue Wilson, and Laura Zlamal.

The fifth edition has been produced by our most dedicated team at Delmar, Cengage Learning. It includes our editors, Natalie Pashoukos, Sherry Dickinson, and Christina Gifford, and our publishing mentor, Ken McGrath.

We are especially grateful to Joe Chovan, the most spectacular artist we have ever worked with. Joe's artistic skills are on exhibit throughout the last few editions of this book and we were pleased to be working with him again for the fifth edition, as he allows us to bring new insight into complex content through his sparkling and insightful illustrations.

We are indebted to the unstinting contributions from Barbara Smith of Portland Community College. A significant portion of the accuracy of the book derives from the constant inspection and contributions she has made as well as the constant input of Denise Moore, Professor Emeritus at Sinclair Community College in Dayton, Ohio, who has been our constant conscience from the first edition. Randy Griswold at Bellin College in Green Bay, Wisconsin has been an enthusiastic and regular contributor to this text for many years and his additions and updates have been greatly appreciated. We also cannot forget the contributions made to the first through fourth editions by Barry Burns of the University of North Carolina, who routinely went far beyond our wildest hopes in critiquing our text, producing films to illustrate his points, disproving old wives, tales in his laboratory, and generously sharing his results (and venison) with us. Much more than a friend, Barry has become a backbone of the technical aspects of this book. Eugene Frank, formerly of the Mayo Clinic and Riverland Community College in Minnesota, continued his persistent and knowledgeable critique of our efforts. We are grateful for Gene's unique contributions, especially his ability to never let nearly two decades of friendship come between us and a more accurate reworking of verbiage or the details of an illustration.

We acknowledge detailed contributions from John Skinner at Mid Michigan Community College; Jeff Lloyd at Spectrum Butterworth in Grand Rapids, Michigan; John Godisak at Grand Rapids Community College, Michigan; and Jennifer Lockhart from Saint Anthony Medical Center in Crown Point, Indiana.

The students, faculty, and staff at Arkansas State University played a major role in the third edition. Special thanks were due Dean Susan

Hanrahan for unremitting support and constant enthusiasm for what we are trying to accomplish in the radiologic sciences.

We thank the faculty and students who have found our work valuable in the process of radiography education and practice since the first edition was published. The success of this book and the invitation to produce a new edition are a direct result of the acceptance of our work by the radiography profession, which we gratefully acknowledge.

Our families once again deserve our thanks for their understanding. Don Adler and Lynn Carlton have both given countless hours that were rightfully theirs, for which we extend a peace offering of love. Much appreciation is also extended to Arlene's daughters Meri and Katie for their love and support. Rick's family now includes not only his children but his growing group of grandchildren: Nathan, Michael, Zach, Mercie-Marie, Maxwell, and the twins Addison and Paige, all of whom get their time, book or not.

Once again, we have been assisted in our work by a wide spectrum of colleagues in the radiologic sciences and related fields. In addition to those who assisted us during the earlier edition, we wish to add our colleague Euclid Seeram of British Columbia Institute of Technology, Irven Rule of the Siemens Training and Development Center in Cary, North Carolina; Alfred Hufnagl of the Northern Alberta Institute of Technology, Canada; Penelope Roberts of the Department of Medical Physics and Medical Engineering at Southampton University Hospitals, UK; Kathheryn Root of Holyoke Community College, Massachusetts; Dr. Appel and Kevin Sisak at DuPont; Garry Harris at Agfa; and Gregory Wheeler of Wheeler and Associates, San Francisco, California.

Our ability to devote the countless hours necessary to make this book what it has become is in great part due to the support we have received from our bosses, Robert Moon at Indiana University Northwest and Sam Bassitt at Lima Technical College. Our faculties have also made significant contributions through their consistent willingness to comment on the countless details we have explored with them over the years. Thank you, Jody Ellis, Sandy Piehl, Laura Richards, Marie Ross, Debra Sobota, Andy Shappell, and Deb Scroggins. Special thanks goes to Barb Hanna and Wil Reddinger, who provided us with their expertise in verifying laboratory results, producing new images, and refining our clumsy attempts to illustrate many concepts. Allen Lindmark from the Department of Chemistry at Indiana University Northwest, also needs our thanks for his review of our basic explanations of chemistry concepts.

And, finally, we thank those fellow educators who have taken the time to sit down with us at meetings, write letters, make phone calls, compose email, and fax their comments and suggestions to us. Although we are certain we have not remembered all of you (for which we apologize), these include Mike Madden of Hays State University; John Clouse of Owensboro Community College, Kentucky; Marianne Tortorici and Mike Mixdorf at the University of Nevada, Las Vegas; Bob Misiak, Orange County Community College, New York; Jack Thomas at Lakeland Community College, Ohio; Lisa Iacovelli at Crozer-Chester Medical Center, Pennsylvania; Max Grady at Kettering College of Medical Arts, Ohio; Donna Mitchell at John Peter Smith Hospital, Texas; Anita Slechta of California State University at Northridge; Elwin Tilson of Armstrong State College, Georgia; Shay Mercer at New Mexico State University; Judy Williams of Grady Memorial Hospital, Georgia; Marilyn Sinderbrand of Northern Virginia Community College; Bill Sykes of Shawnee State University, Ohio; Bart Schraa of Daniel Denhoed University, Rotterdam, Netherlands; Frank Porter at St. Vincent Infirmary Medical Center, Arkansas; Mitchell Bieber, University of Virginia Medical Center; Donna Foster at Northern New Mexico Community College; Bill May of Iatwamba Community College, Mississippi; Lorraine Henry of Orange Coast Community College, California; and Steve Dowd of the University of Alabama at Birmingham.

Appreciation is also expressed to the colleagues who reviewed the manuscripts for this edition. Their critical reviews helped to guide us in the preparation of the final manuscript.

Reviewers

Patricia Fair Wynne, B.S. Ed, R.T.(R)
Central Georgia Technical College
Macon, Georgia

Jeff Hamzeh, Ph.D., M.S.M.E., B.S.M.E
Keiser University
Longwood, Florida

John Skinner, B.A., M.Ed., M.S.A., R.T.(R)
Mid Michigan Community College
Harrison, Michigan

Cameron J. Vander Stel, M.B.A., B.S., R.T.(R)
Baker College of Muskegon
Muskegon, Michigan

Susyn Dees, M.S., R.T.(R)(CT)
Champlain College
Burlington, Vermont

Robert J. Slothus, R.T.(R), ARRT, M.S.
Pennsylvania College of Technology
Williamsport, Pennsylvania

George Pales, Ph.D., R.T.(R)(MR)(T)
University of Nevada, Las Vegas
Henderson, Nevada

Jeff L. Berry, M.S., R.T.(R)(CT)
University of Oklahoma
Oklahoma City, Oklahoma

William Faulkner, B.S., R.T.(R)(MR)(CT), FSMRT
William Faulkner and Associates
Chattanooga, Tennessee
Dennis Tan
Lawrenceville, New Jersey

Sherry Floerchinger, M.A., R.T.(R)(N)(QM)
Dixie State College of Utah
Saint George, Utah

Joy Menser, M.S.M., R.T.(R)(T)
Owensboro Community and Technical College
Madisonville, Kentucky

First Edition Acknowledgments

The production of this book would not have been possible without the support of our spouses, Don and Lynn. In addition, we gratefully acknowledge the role played by Delmar Cengage Learning; Indiana University Northwest; Lima Technical College; and St. Rita's Medical Center of Lima, Ohio. Special thanks are due Dr. LaVerne Ramaeker, Sam Bassitt, Marlene Ledbetter, and Dennis Spragg for their support. A major contribution to the accuracy of the information and illustrations was made by the consistent presence of Eugene Frank, formerly of the Mayo Clinic Foundation, throughout.

We are in the professional debt of many who inspired us, taught us, and collaborated with us throughout the years. Much of what is contained in this work is a direct result of these efforts. Those to whom we are especially indebted are Tracy Ahdel, Janice Akin, Judy Baron, Karen Brinkman, John Cortez, Marion Frank, Mick Jagger, Karen Jefferies, Robin Jones, Dr. George Koptik, Judy Koptik, Jon Lilly, Dr. Marzuto, Kathy Miller, Joe Mosqueda, Traci O'Donnell, LaVerne Ramaeker, Karen Schmidl, Kay Shriver, Tracy Thegze, Jean Widger, Rob Wilcoxen, and Sue Wilson. And of course our students at Indiana University Northwest, Lima Technical College, Wilbur Wright College, Malcolm X College, and Michael Reese Hospital and Medical Center.

Like our colleagues and students, we owe much to the institutions that contributed to our professional expertise. We wish to thank Indiana University Northwest, Lima Technical College, Michael Reese Hospital and Medical Center, Lutheran General Hospital, Mercy Hospital and Medical Center (Chicago), Northwestern Memorial Hospital (Chicago), Wilbur Wright College, Illinois Central College, Carl Sandburg College, Evanston Hospital, Methodist Medical Center (Peoria), and Community Memorial Hospital (Monmouth).

We owe special thanks to many people for sharing their personal expertise and material collections. One of the highest forms of professionalism, the willingness of radiologic technologists to freely give of their time and knowledge, was demonstrated again and again by everyone from whom we requested assistance in our compilation of the multitude of photographs, drawings, radiographs, and other illustrative materials in the text and those who assisted in the numerous reviews of our writing. Among these deserving special thanks are Gene Frank and Norlin Winkler of the Mayo Clinic Foundation and Ray Rossi of the University of Colorado for their commentary and technical assistance above and beyond the normal bonds of friendship; Philip W. Ballinger of the Ohio State University; Terry West of Toronto, Secretary-General of the International Society of Radiographers and Radiological Technicians; Stewart Bushong of Baylor College of Medicine; Terry Eastman of Dallas; Joe Fodor of the University of Cincinnati Medical Center; Nina Kowalczyk of Riverside Methodist Hospital, Columbus, Ohio; Denise Moore of Sinclair Community College, Dayton, Ohio; Bruce Long of Indiana University Medical Center; Marilyn Holland of the University of Iowa Hospitals and Clinics; Charles R. Griffith of FGHB Certified Radiation Physicists; Loren Garlets of Hays State University, Kansas; Pat Sharp of Gannon University, Erie, Pennsylvania; Tim Penning of Athens Regional Medical Center, Georgia; Seymour Sterling, FASRT, of Yardley, Pennsylvania; Jerome Taubel of the Mayo Clinic Foundation, Rochester, Minnesota; Bob Kobistek in Cleveland and Martin Ratner and Steve Szeglin in Carle Place, New York, both of Victoreen, Inc./Nuclear Associates; Terry Hanby of DuPont; Robert Trinkle, formerly of DuPont; Mike Wilsey of Agfa Matrix; Robert Lockery and Walter Weigl of Siemens Corporation; Robert Busic of General Electric Medical Systems; William Conklin of Orangeburg, SC; Rene Abgrall of Thoard, France; Toshinori Komba of Komazawa University, Tokyo, Japan; Angela Pickwick of Montgomery County Community College, Maryland; Jerry Conlogue of Gulf Coast Community College, Florida; Barb Imber of St. Rita's Medical Center, Lima, Ohio; Rick Halker of Lima Memorial Hospital, Ohio; The Radiology Department of Van Wert County Hospital, Van Wert, Ohio, John Stone of Emory University Medical School, Atlanta; Tom Beery and Will Wells of Lima Technical College; Judy Shaw of Lima Technical College; Doug Raver and Chris Innskeep of Lima Technical College for video and software graphics; and Jan Krietemeyer of Lima, Ohio, for bibliographic research.

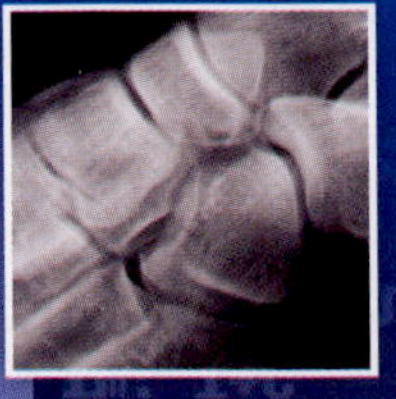

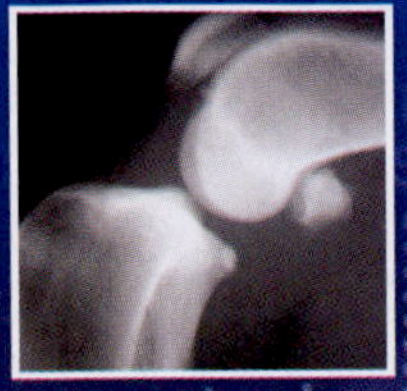

How to Use StudyWARE™ to Accompany Principles of Radiographic Imaging: An Art and a Science

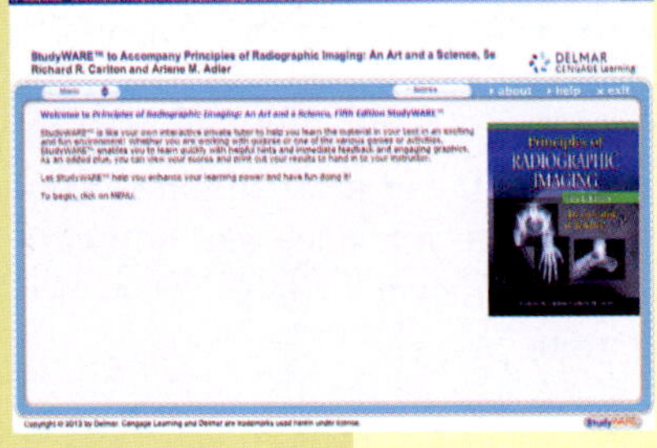

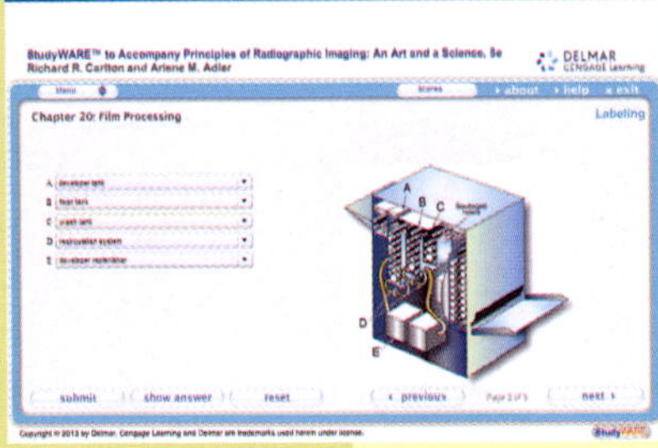

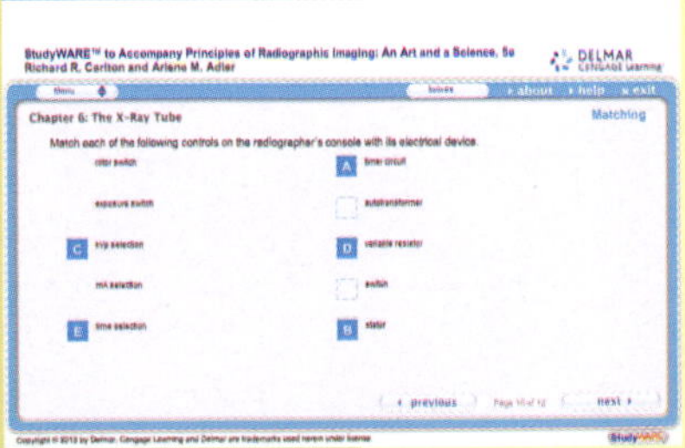

The StudyWARE™ software helps you learn terms and concepts in *Principles of Radiographic Imaging: An Art and a Science.* As you study each chapter in the text, be sure to explore the activities in the corresponding chapter in the software. Use StudyWARE™ as your own private tutor to help you learn the material in your *Principles of Radiographic Imaging: An Art and a Science* textbook.

Getting started is easy. Install the software by inserting the CD-ROM into your computer's CD-ROM drive and following the on-screen instructions. When you open the software, enter your name so the software can store your quiz results. Then choose a chapter from the menu to take a quiz or explore one of the activities.

Menus

You can access the menus from wherever you are in the program. The menus include Quizzes, Activities, and Scores.

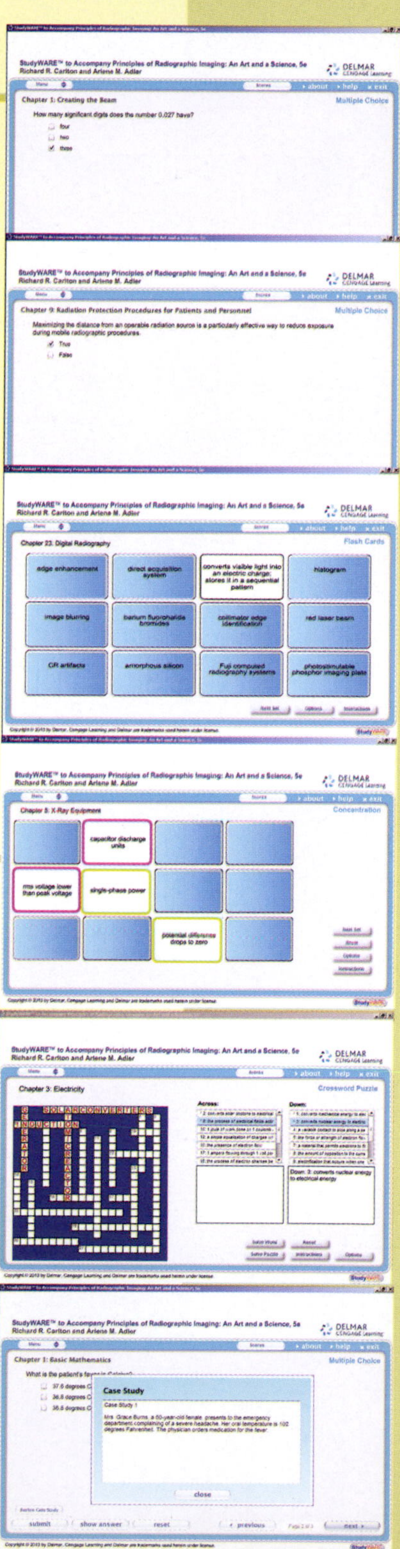

Quizzes

Quizzes include multiple-choice, true/false, fill-in-the-blank, and matching questions. You can take the quizzes in both Practice Mode and Quiz Mode. Use Practice Mode to improve your mastery of the material. You have multiple tries to get the answers correct. Instant feedback tells you whether you're right or wrong—and helps you learn quickly by explaining why an answer was correct or incorrect. Use Quiz Mode when you are ready to test yourself and keep a record of your scores. In Quiz Mode, you have one try to get the answers right, but you can take each quiz as many times as you want.

Activities

Activities include flashcards, concentration, hangman, crossword puzzles, and case studies. Have fun while increasing your knowledge!

Scores

You can view your last scores for each quiz and print your results to hand in to your instructor.

Unit I

Creating the Beam

1 Basic Mathematics / 2

2 Radiation Concepts / 20

3 Electricity / 39

4 Electromagnetism / 59

5 X-Ray Equipment / 90

6 The X-Ray Tube / 108

7 X-Ray Production / 129

An inherent quality of a professional is the possession of expertise regarding the technical aspects of a field far above that of a nonprofessional. Knowledge of the principles of radiographic image production is part of the technical expertise of the professional radiographer. Radiography programs provide students with classroom instruction, laboratory experience, and clinical practice in this subject. No other medical professional experiences as intensive or comprehensive a study of radiographic imaging. This unit is designed to provide the basics necessary for this knowledge by building a framework of information regarding the creation of the diagnostic x-ray beam.

The framework begins with an elementary review of **basic mathematics** and **radiation concepts**, including atomic theory, x-ray properties, and necessary units of measurement. Although this may be a review of previous science coursework for many readers, it is important to make sure everyone is on the same wavelength before using the information in the remainder of the book. **Electricity** and **electromagnetism** are large chapters that lay the foundation for understanding how to control the beam. **X-ray equipment**, **the x-ray tube**, and **x-ray production** provide an understanding of exactly how basic physics is used to create the x-ray beam.

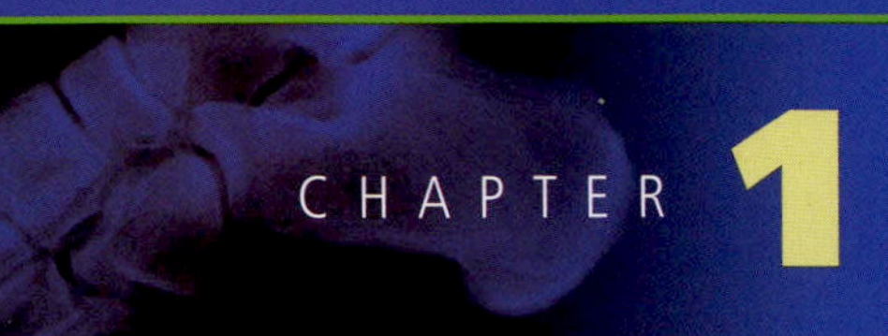

Basic Mathematics

KEY TERMS

absolute value
algebraic expression
coulomb per kilogram
direct variation
equation
equivalent equation
gray
identity
inverse variation
kilogram
like term
meter
open equation
second
sievert

> Do not worry about your difficulties in mathematics. I can assure you mine are still greater.
>
> *Attributed to Albert Einstein*

OBJECTIVES

Upon completion of this chapter, the student should be able to:

- Perform functions with fractions and decimals.
- Determine significant digits in a number.
- Perform calculations in scientific notation with signed numbers and exponents.
- Simplify algebraic expressions.
- Convert units within the SI system.

Mathematics is the language of science. Radiographers need to be able to speak this language. In order to quantify science, standard units of measurement were established. The fundamental units of measurement are mass, length, and time. Units of measurement were officially defined on an international level through the adoption of the SI unit system. The seven base SI units are mass, length, time, electric current, temperature, amount of substance, and luminous intensity. Radiologically important derived units are the coulomb per kilogram (C/kg), formerly the roentgen (R); the gray (Gy), formerly the rad (radiation absorbed dose); and the sievert (Sv), formerly the rem (radiation equivalent man). This review is intended to refresh essential skills in the use of math as well as appropriate units for the radiologic and imaging sciences.

ARITHMETIC

Fractions

Addition and Subtraction. To add or subtract two fractions with **like** denominators, add or subtract the numerators and keep the like denominator.

EXAMPLES:

$$\frac{3}{8}+\frac{2}{8}=\frac{5}{8}$$

$$\frac{7}{8}-\frac{4}{8}=\frac{3}{8}$$

$$\frac{a}{b}+\frac{c}{b}=\frac{a+c}{b}$$

$$\frac{a}{b}-\frac{c}{b}=\frac{a-c}{b}$$

To add or subtract two fractions with **unlike** denominators, rewrite each fraction with a like or common denominator. Then add or subtract the numerators and keep the like or common denominator.

EXAMPLES:

$$\frac{1}{4}+\frac{5}{6}=\frac{3}{12}+\frac{10}{12}=\frac{13}{12}$$

$$\frac{7}{5}-\frac{1}{3}=\frac{21}{15}-\frac{5}{15}=\frac{16}{15}$$

$$\frac{a}{b}+\frac{c}{d}=\frac{ad}{bd}+\frac{bc}{bd}=\frac{ad+bc}{bd}$$

$$\frac{a}{d}-\frac{c}{d}=\frac{ad}{bd}-\frac{bc}{bd}=\frac{ad-bc}{bd}$$

Multiplication. Multiplication can be written in several ways (Table 1-1). To multiply two fractions, multiply the numerators and multiply the denominators.

EXAMPLES:

$$\frac{2}{5}\times\frac{3}{7}=\frac{2\times 3}{5\times 7}=\frac{6}{35}$$

$$\frac{a}{b}\times\frac{c}{d}=\frac{a\times c}{b\times d}$$

Division. To divide two fractions, rewrite the division problem as a multiplication problem by multiplying the first fraction by the second fraction inverted.

TABLE 1-1. Multiplication Notation

Throughout this review the algebraic notation for multiplication will be used.

Example: 3×4 will be written as $3 \cdot 4$.

A · (dot) is used as a symbol for multiplication.

Example: $a \times b$ will be written as $a \cdot b$ or as ab.

When two letters are used the dot is usually omitted.

Example: $3 \times a$ will be written as 3a or as $3 \cdot a$.

Parentheses can also be used to represent multiplication.

Example: 3×4 can be written as (3)(4).

EXAMPLES:

$$\frac{2}{5} \div \frac{3}{7} = \frac{2}{5} \times \frac{7}{3} = \frac{2 \times 7}{5 \times 3} = \frac{14}{15}$$

$$\frac{a}{b} \div \frac{c}{d} = \frac{a}{b} \times \frac{d}{c} = \frac{a \times d}{b \times c}$$

Decimals

Decimal number place value (columns) is determined as shown in Figure 1-1.

Addition and Subtraction. To add or subtract two decimal numbers, line up the decimal points in each number, adding or subtracting as with whole numbers. Remember to add in zeros to fill out the decimal positions if necessary. The decimal point must remain in the same position.

EXAMPLES:

Add:	***Subtract:***	***Rewrite as:***
76.81	76.1	76.10
+ 384.1	− 2.96	−2.96
460.91		73.14

Multiplication. To multiply two decimal numbers, multiply the numbers as if they were whole numbers. Place the decimal point in the product so the number of places in the product equals the sum of the number of decimal places in each number.

EXAMPLES:

Multiply:

2.31	2 decimal positions
× 6.8	1 decimal position
1848	
1386	
15.708	3 decimal positions

Division. To divide two decimal numbers, set up as if doing whole number division. Move the decimal point in the divisor to the right to make the divisor a whole number. Move the decimal point in the dividend the same number of places to the right (as was done for the divisor). Add zeros if necessary to maintain the position of the decimal. Divide the numbers as if they were whole numbers. Place the decimal point in the quotient directly above the decimal point in the dividend. Add zeros if necessary to maintain the position of the decimal.

Decimal number place value (columns)

Millions	Hundred thousands	Ten thousands	Thousands	Hundreds	Tens	Units	Decimal point	Tenths	Hundredths	Thousandths	Ten-thousandths
1,000,000	100,000	10,000	1,000	100	10	1	•	$\frac{1}{10}$	$\frac{1}{100}$	$\frac{1}{1,000}$	$\frac{1}{10,000}$

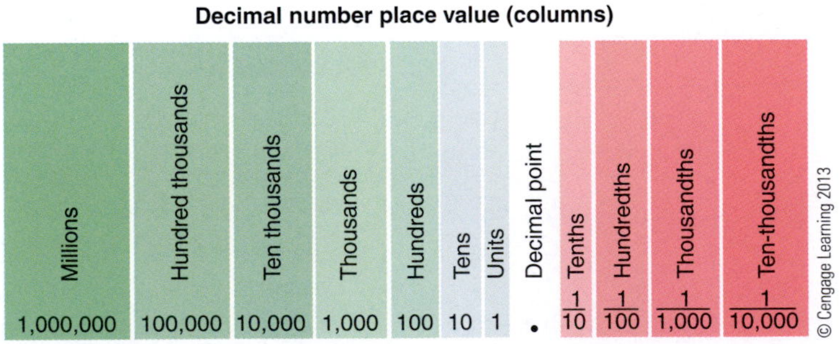

FIGURE 1-1. Decimal number place values.

> ***EXAMPLES:***
>
> $.25\overline{)1250}$
>
> $\begin{array}{r} 5000. \\ .25\overline{)125000.} \end{array}$
>
> $1.3\overline{)733.2}$
>
> $\begin{array}{r} 564. \\ 13.\overline{)7332.} \\ \underline{65} \\ 83 \\ \underline{78} \\ 52 \\ \underline{52} \\ 0 \end{array}$

Convert a Fraction into a Decimal Number. To convert a fraction into a decimal, divide the denominator into the numerator.

> ***EXAMPLE:*** Convert 7/8 into a decimal:
>
> $\begin{array}{r} .875 \\ 8\overline{)7.000} \\ \underline{64} \\ 60 \\ \underline{56} \\ 40 \\ \underline{40} \end{array}$

Convert a Percent to a Decimal. To convert a percent to a decimal, move the decimal point two places to the left.

> ***EXAMPLE:*** Convert 78.5% to a decimal:
>
> 78.5% = .785

Convert a Decimal to a Percent. To convert a decimal to a percent, move the decimal point two places to the right.

> ***EXAMPLE:*** Change .452 to a %:
>
> .452 = 45.2%

Computation with Values (Numbers)

Exact. Some numbers are exact values, like the counting numbers (1, 2, 3,...). For example, there are exactly four legs on a chair. Exact numbers in computations are as accurate or as precise as needed.

Significant Digits. Some values are obtained by measurement and are only as accurate as the measuring device. The last digit in the reading is usually estimated. **When dealing with these values in computations, the results will only be as accurate as the least accurate value.** This is the concept of significant digits.

To determine the number of significant digits in a value (number):

1. Count all nonzero digits.
2. Count all zeros between nonzero digits.
3. Count all zeros at the end of a decimal value.

The number of significant digits in a value is the sum of the numbers obtained in steps 1, 2, and 3.

> ***EXAMPLES:*** The following are measured values from a radiation dose meter (dosimeter).
>
> 7.14 mR has three significant digits.
>
> 90.104 mR has five significant digits.
>
> 0.048 mR has two significant digits.
>
> 7300 mR has two significant digits.
>
> 6.900 mR has four significant digits.

Precision. The precision of a value refers to the decimal position of the last significant digit.

EXAMPLE:

.0218 is precise to the ten-thousandths.

Rounding Off. To round a number the last digit to be retained is:

1. Left unchanged if the digit to the right of the last digit to be retained is less than 5.
2. Increased by one if the digit to the right of the last digit to be retained is 5 or greater.

EXAMPLES:

75.2581 rounded to 4 significant digits is 75.26.

6836.66 rounded to 2 significant digits is 6800.

0.0381 rounded to 2 significant digits is 0.038.

0.0299 rounded to 2 significant digits is 0.030.

Multiplication and Division of Approximate Values. When multiplying or dividing two or more approximate values, the number of significant digits in the final answer is no greater than the number of significant digits in the value with the least number of significant digits.

EXAMPLES: Using the calculator, $(103.81) \cdot (1.34) = 139.1054$. However, because 1.34 has only three significant digits, the answer should have only three significant digits. Therefore, 139.1054 needs to be rounded to three significant digits, making it 139.

Addition and Subtraction of Approximate Values. When adding or subtracting two or more approximate values, the final answer should be no more precise than the **least** precise of the values.

EXAMPLES: Add the following:

$$\begin{array}{r} 123.1 \\ 89.123 \\ +103.3456 \\ \hline 315.5686 \end{array}$$

Because the least precise number is 123.1, the answer should be rounded to 315.6.

Powers of 10

The decimal system is based on powers of 10, as is the metric system. These are very important systems to the radiographer. When a^n is written, a is called the base and n is the exponent. Integers are defined as the numbers $\ldots -3, -2, -1, 0, 1, 2, 3, \ldots$.

Positive Integer Exponents. Definition:

$$a^n = \underbrace{a \cdot a \cdot a \cdots a}_{\text{n times}} \text{ (multiply n times)}$$

EXAMPLES:

$10^1 = 10$

$10^2 = 10 \cdot 10 = 100$

$10^3 = 10 \cdot 10 \cdot 10 = 1000$

$10^n = 10 \cdot 10 \cdot 10 \cdots 10 = 100\ldots0$ (n zeros)

Negative Integer Exponents. Definition:

$$a^{-n} = \frac{1}{a^n} \text{(for } a \neq 0\text{)}$$

$$10^{-1} = \frac{1}{10} = .1$$

$$10^{-2} = \frac{1}{10^2} = .01$$

$$10^{-3} = \frac{1}{10^3} = .001$$

$$10^{-n} = \frac{1}{10^n} = .00\ldots001 \text{ (n − 1) zeros}$$

Zero Exponents. Definition: $a^0 = 1$ (for $a \neq 0$)

EXAMPLE:

$10^0 = 1$

Scientific Notation

A number written in scientific notation is written as the product of a number between 1 (including 1) and 10 times a power of 10. In other words, $N \times 10^p$, where $1 \le N < 10$ and p is an integer.

EXAMPLES:

7.15×10^4 is a number in scientific notation.

1.598×10^{-5} is a number in scientific notation.

7.58×10^0 is a number in scientific notation.

Converting Numbers from Ordinary to Scientific Notation. To write a number in scientific notation, the decimal point must be moved to the position following the first nonzero digit.

EXAMPLES:

$70.57 = 7.057 \times 10^1$ $(p = 1)$

$.00815 = 8.15 \times 10^{-3}$ $(p = -3)$

$7.58 = 7.58 \times 10^0$ $(p = 0)$

In the first example, the decimal point is moved one digit to the left, making the power of 10 (p), 1. In the second example, the decimal point is moved three digits to the right, making the power of 10, −3. In the third example, the decimal point is not moved and the power of 10 is 0.

In general, when moving the decimal point to the left, the power of 10 will be the number of positions moved. When moving the decimal point to the right, the power of 10 will be negative the number of positions moved. When the decimal point is not moved, the power of 10 will be zero.

Converting Numbers from Scientific to Ordinary Notation. To convert a number in scientific notation to ordinary notation, the decimal position is moved according to the following:

1. If the power of 10 is positive, move the decimal point to the right the number of positions in the exponent.
2. If the power of 10 is negative, move the decimal point to the left the number of positions in the exponent.
3. If the power of 10 is zero, the decimal remains in the same position.

In all of the above, once the decimal point has been moved, the 10 and its power are dropped. Zeros are added if necessary.

EXAMPLES:

$3.7 \times 10^4 = 37{,}000$

$5.56 \times 10^{-5} = .0000556$

$1.34 \times 10^0 = 1.34$

Dimensional Analysis

The concept of dimensional analysis is useful when converting from one set of units to another. The principle is based on fractions whose quotients are 1.

EXAMPLE:

$$\frac{12\text{ in}}{1\text{ ft}} = 1 \text{ or } \frac{1\text{ ft}}{12\text{ in}} = 1$$

Recall that multiplying a quantity by 1 does not change the value of the quantity. In order to convert from one set of units to another, algebraic operations are performed with units in the same way they are with algebraic symbols.

EXAMPLE: Convert 7.0 ft to inches.

$$7.0\text{ ft} = 7.0\ \cancel{\text{ft}} \cdot \frac{12\text{ in}}{1\ \cancel{\text{ft}}} = 7 \cdot 12\text{ in} = 84\text{ in}$$

Note that it is possible to "cancel" the feet unit, leaving the inches unit.

Convert 70.0 km/hr to m/s.

$$70.0\ \frac{\text{km}}{\text{hr}} =$$

$$70.0\frac{\cancel{\text{km}}}{\cancel{\text{hr}}} \cdot \frac{1000\text{ m}}{1\ \cancel{\text{km}}} \cdot \frac{1\ \cancel{\text{hr}}}{60\ \cancel{\text{min}}} \cdot \frac{1\ \cancel{\text{min}}}{60\text{ s}} =$$

$$70.0 \cdot 1000 \cdot \frac{1}{60} \cdot \frac{1\text{ m}}{60\text{ s}} = 19.4\ \frac{\text{m}}{\text{s}}$$

Recall that 1 km = 1000 m, 1 hr = 60 min, and 1 min = 60 s. Note that it is possible to "cancel" the km unit, the hr unit, and the min unit.

When converting cubic units or square units, extra attention needs to be given to the conversion factors. Study the following example carefully.

EXAMPLE: Convert 3.8000 ft³ (cubic feet) to cubic inches (in³).

$$3.8000\text{ ft}^3 = 3.8000\text{ ft}^3 \cdot \frac{12\text{ in}}{1\text{ ft}} \cdot \frac{12\text{ in}}{1\text{ ft}} \cdot \frac{12\text{ in}}{1\text{ ft}}$$

$$= 6566.4\text{ in}^3$$

or

$$3.8000\text{ ft}^3 = 3.8000\text{ ft}^3 \cdot \left(\frac{12\text{ in}}{1\text{ ft}}\right)^3 = 6566.4\text{ in}^3$$

EXAMPLE: Convert 10 roentgens per hour to roentgens per minute.

$$10.0\,\frac{\text{roentgens}}{\text{hour}} = 10.0\,\frac{\text{roentgens}}{\text{hour}} \cdot \frac{1\text{ hour}}{60\text{ m}}$$

$$= .167\,\frac{\text{roentgens}}{\text{minute}}$$

ALGEBRA

Signed Numbers

Numbers are not always positive. For example, the thermometer indicates that it is very cold at −20°F. Negative numbers can be illustrated by using a number line (Figure 1-2). Positive numbers are assigned to the right of the zero point and negative numbers to the left of the zero point. A statement that 7 is less than 10 (written as $7 < 10$) indicates that 7 is to the left of 10 on the number line. A statement that −5 is greater than −9 (written as $-5 \leq -9$) indicates that −5 is to the right of −9 on the number line.

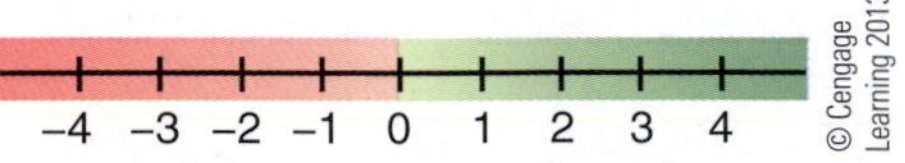

FIGURE 1-2. Number line.

Absolute Value. The **absolute value** of a number is the distance from 0 to that number on the number line. Because distance is the same number of units whether moving up or down the number line, that means that the absolute value of a number is always positive or zero. The notation used for absolute value is two vertical bars (| |).

EXAMPLES:

$|-2| = 2$ $|4| = 4$ $|0| = 0$

Because −2 is two units from zero on the number line, the absolute value is 2. Because 4 is four units from zero on the number line, the absolute value is 4. Because 0 is zero units from zero on the number line, the absolute value is 0.

Addition. To add two positive numbers, add their absolute values and attach a positive sign to the result. The positive sign is usually omitted.

EXAMPLE:

$(+7) + (+8) = +15$ $7 + 8 = 15$

To add two negative numbers, add their absolute values and attach a negative sign to the result.

EXAMPLE:

$(-7) + (-8) = -15$ $-7 + (-8) = -15$

To add two numbers with unlike signs, subtract the smaller in absolute value from the larger in absolute value and attach the sign of the larger in absolute value to the result.

EXAMPLES:

$(-10) + (3) = -7$ $4 + (-9) = -5$

$(8) + (-5) = 3$ $-3 + (7) = 4$

Negative of a Number. The negative of a number is the opposite of the number in sign.

EXAMPLES:

The negative of 7 is −7; the negative of −7 is 7.

If $b = 7$, then $-b = -7$.

If $b = -7$, then $-b = -(-7) = 7$.

Subtraction. Subtraction is rewritten as addition, as in $a - b = a + (-b)$.

EXAMPLES:

$8 - 10 = 8 + (-10) = -2$

$8 - (-10) = 8 + 10 = 18$

$-8 - 10 = -8 + (-10) = -18$

$-8 - (-10) = -8 + 10 = 2$

All of the above subtraction problems are rewritten as addition and then the rules for addition of signed numbers are used.

Multiplication. To multiply two numbers, multiply their absolute values. If both numbers are positive or both numbers are negative, attach a positive sign to the result. If the numbers are opposite in sign, attach a negative sign to the result.

EXAMPLES:

$(2)(3) = 6$

$(-2)(-3) = 6$

$(2)(-3) = -6$

$(-2)(3) = -6$

Division. To divide two numbers, divide their absolute values. If both numbers are positive or both numbers are negative, attach a positive sign to the result. If the numbers are opposite in sign, attach a negative sign to the result.

EXAMPLES:

$8 \div 2 = 4$

$-8 \div -2 = 4$

$8 \div (-2) = -4$

$-8 \div 2 = -4$

Order of Operation

Order-of-operation problems may occur when parentheses are not indicated. For example, evaluate $2 + 3 \cdot 4$. Depending on whether addition or multiplication is performed first the answer might be 20 or 14. The answer actually depends on the order of operation. Rules have been established that make the correct result 14.

The difference between the unary minus sign (−) and the subtraction sign (−) and the difference between the unary plus sign (+) and the addition sign (+) must be understood before order-of-operation rules can be learned.

A subtraction sign (−) is used between two numbers:

EXAMPLE:

7 − 8 (subtraction sign)

A unary minus sign − is used before one number.

EXAMPLE:

−7 (unary minus sign)

An expression can have both a subtraction sign and a unary minus sign.

EXAMPLE:

−7 − 8 (the first is a unary minus, the second a subtraction sign)

An addition sign (+) is used between two numbers:

EXAMPLE:

$8 + 10$ (addition sign)

A unary plus sign (+) is used before one number.

EXAMPLE:

$+8$

Rules for Order of Operation

1. Perform all operations inside grouping symbols (parentheses, radical symbols, fraction bar, brackets, etc.)
2. Exponentiation (raising to a power or roots)
3. Unary minus (−) or unary plus (+)
4. Multiplication and division
5. Addition and subtraction

Operations are performed from the lowest level (#1) to the largest level (#5). Operations on the same level are evaluated left to right.

EXAMPLES:

$2 + 3 \cdot 4$ (multiplication first)

$= 2 + 12$ (addition)

$= 14$

$8 \cdot 6 - 12 \div 2$ (multiplication and division first)

$= 48 - 6$ (subtraction)

$= 42$

$\frac{8+7}{2+3}$ (bar acts as grouping symbol)

$= \frac{15}{5}$ (add numerator and add denominator first)

$= 3$ (divide)

$(-2)^3$ (exponentiation first)

$= -8$

(continues)

(continued)

$-(2)^4$ (exponentiation first)

$= -(16)$ (unary minus sign)

$= -16$

$3(7 + 4)$ (add inside parenthesis first)

$= 3 \cdot 11$ (multiply)

$= 33$

$2(6 + 1)^2$ (add inside parenthesis first)

$= 2(7)^2$ (exponentiation next)

$= 2 \cdot 49$ (multiply)

$= 98$

Algebraic Expressions

Algebraic expressions are letters and/or numbers that are multiplied, divided, added, subtracted, or raised to a power.

EXAMPLES:

$3x^3 + 5x^2 - 7x = 8$

$\frac{x+5}{y-7}$

There are several rules for combining algebraic expressions.

Distributive Law. The statement of the distributive law is:

$$a(b + c) = a \cdot b + a \cdot c$$

EXAMPLES:

$7(x + y) = 7x + 7y$

$7(3 + 5) = 7 \cdot 3 + 7 \cdot 5 = 21 + 35 = 56$

$p(x + 4) = px + 4p$ (The numeral is normally written in front of the letter.)

If the addition sign were a subtraction sign, then:

$$a(b - c) = a \cdot b - a \cdot c$$

EXAMPLES:

$7(x - y) = 7x - 7y$

$7(3 - 5) = 7 \cdot 3 - 7 \cdot 5$

$= 21 - 35 = 21 + (-35) = -14$

$p(x - 4) = px - 4p$

Care needs to be taken when one or two negative signs are involved.

EXAMPLES:

$-7(x + y) = -7x + (-7y)$ [distributive law]

$= -7x - 7y$ (the reverse definition of subtraction)

$-7(x - y) = -7x - (-7y)$ (distributive law)

$= -7x + 7y$ (definition of subtraction)

$-7(-3 -8) = (-7)(-3) - (-7)(8)$ (distributive law)

$= 21 - (-56)$ (multiply)

$= 21 + 56$ (definition of subtraction)

$= 77$

Addition and Subtraction of Like Terms. Like terms are terms with identical literal factors. A literal factor is a factor denoted by a letter. Like terms may be added or subtracted.

EXAMPLE:

$7x + 3x = 10x$ (like terms)

EXAMPLE:

$7x + 3y = 7x + 3y$ (unlike terms may not be added)

EXAMPLE:

$7x - 3x = 4x$

EXAMPLE:

$-7x - 3x = -7x + (-3x)$ (definition of subtraction)

$= -10x$ (combine like terms)

EXAMPLE:

$-7x - (-3x) = -7x + 3x$ (definition of subtraction)

$= -4x$ (combine like terms)

Parentheses. When an algebraic expression involves parentheses, the parentheses need to be removed in order to simplify the expression.

EXAMPLE:

$7(x + y) + 4(x + y)$

$= 7x + 7y + 4x + 4y$ (distributive law)

$= 11x + 11y$ (combine like terms)

EXAMPLE:

$7(x + y) - 4(x + y)$

$= 7(x + y) + (-4)(x + y)$ (definition of subtraction)

$= 7x + 7y + (-4x) + (-4y)$ (distributive law)

$= 3x + 3y$ (combine like terms)

EXAMPLE:

$7(x - y) - 4(x - y)$

$= 7(x - y) + (-4)(x - y)$ (definition of subtraction)

$= 7x - 7y + (-4x) - (-4y)$ (distributive law)

$= 7x + (-7y) + (-4x) + (4y)$ (definition of subtraction)

$= 3x + (-3y)$ (combine like terms)

$= 3x - 3y$ (reverse of definition of subtraction)

EXAMPLE:

$$x - (y - x) = x + (-1)(y - x)$$
$$= x + (-y) - (-x)$$
$$= x + (-y) + x$$
$$2x - y$$

If an expression involves parentheses within parentheses, then it is simplified from the innermost parentheses out.

EXAMPLE:

$7 - [6x - (x - 4)]$

$= 7 - [6x - x + 4)]$ (remove innermost parentheses)

$= 7 - [5x + 4]$ (simplify within parentheses)

$= 7 - 5x - 4$ (remove parentheses [square bracket])

$= 3 - 5x$ (combine like terms)

Exponents. Definition:

$$a^n = \underbrace{a \cdot a \cdot a \cdots a}_{n \text{ times}}$$

where a is the base and n is the exponent.

EXAMPLE:

$$3^4 = 3 \cdot 3 \cdot 3 \cdot 3 = 81$$

Laws of Exponents

Law 1: $a^m \cdot a^n = a^{m+n}$

EXAMPLES:

$$a^4 \cdot a^3 = a^{4+3} = a^7$$
$$a \cdot a^5 = a^{1+5} = a^6$$

Law 2: $\dfrac{a^m}{a^n} = \begin{cases} a^{m-n} & \text{if } m \geq n \\ \dfrac{1}{a^{n-m}} & \text{if } n > m \end{cases} \quad a \neq 0$

EXAMPLES:

$$\frac{x^5}{x^2} = x^{5-2} = x^3$$
$$\frac{x^7}{x^{10}} = \frac{1}{x^{10-7}} = \frac{1}{x^3}$$

Law 3: $(ab)^m = a^m b^m$

EXAMPLE:

$$(ab)^4 = a^4 b^4$$

Law 4: $\left(\dfrac{a}{b}\right)^m = \dfrac{a^m}{a^m},\ b \neq 0$

EXAMPLE:

$$\left(\frac{a}{b}\right)^5 = \frac{a^5}{b^5}$$

Law 5: $(a^m)^n = a^{m \cdot n}$

EXAMPLE:

$$(a^4)^5 = a^{4 \cdot 5} = a^{20}$$

Definition: $a^0 = 1$ for $a \neq 0$

EXAMPLES:

$$5^0 = 1$$
$$x^0 = 1$$
$$(5x)^0 = 1$$
$$5x^0 = 5 \cdot 1 = 5$$

Definition: $a^{-n} = \dfrac{1}{a^n}$ for $a \neq 0$

EXAMPLES:

$$x^{-7} = \frac{1}{x^7}$$

(continues)

(continued)

$$2^{-3} = \frac{1}{2^3} = \frac{1}{8}$$

It can also be shown that:

$$\frac{1}{a^{-n}} = a^n \text{ for } a \neq 0.$$

EXAMPLES:

$$\frac{1}{5^{-2}} = 5^2 = 25$$

$$\frac{1}{x^{-5}} = x^5$$

Multiplying Numbers in Scientific Notation. When multiplying two numbers in scientific notation, the Ns are multiplied and the powers of 10 are added. This is simply using the rule of exponents when the bases are the same.

EXAMPLE:

$(2.4 \times 10^3)(3.8 \times 10^{11})$

$= (2.4 \cdot 3.8) \times 10^{3+11}$

$= 9.1 \times 10^{14}$

Dividing Numbers in Scientific Notation. When dividing two numbers in scientific notation, the Ns are divided and the exponents are subtracted. This is another example of using the rules of exponents.

EXAMPLE:

$(8.3 \times 10^4) \div (2.7 \times 10^{11})$

$= 8.3 \div 2.7 \times 10^{4-11}$

$= 3.1 \times 10^{-7}$

Evaluating Algebraic Expressions

To evaluate an algebraic expression, replace each unknown with the given value and then perform the indicated operations.

EXAMPLE: Evaluate $2a^2 + 5b$ for $a = 3$ and $b = 4$.

$2a^2 + 5b = 2(3)^2 + 5(4)$

$= 2 \cdot 9 + 20$

$= 18 + 20$

$= 38$

Formulae are examples of equations where algebraic expressions are evaluated.

EXAMPLE:

Convert 60.0°F to C.
The formula involved is $C = 5/9(F - 32°)$.
Determine C when $F = 60.0°$.

$C = 5/9(F - 32°)$
$C = 5/9(60.0° - 32°)$ (substitute 60.0° for F)
$C = 5/9(28°)$
$C = 15.6°C$

Convert 20.0°C to F.
The formula to use is $F = 9/5C + 32°$.
Determine F when $C = 20.0°$.

$F = 9/5(20°) + 32°$
$F = 36° + 32°$
$F = 68°$

Equations

An **equation** is a statement that contains an equal sign. For example, $A = B$ is an equation. An equation can be either a true or a false statement.

EXAMPLES:

$5 + 3 = 7$	(false statement)
$5 + 3 = 8$	(true statement)

Both of these statements are equations but only one is true.

An equation that contains at least one unknown (variable) is an **open equation**.

EXAMPLES:

$x + 5 = 7$

$3x + 5 = 7 - 2x$

An open statement becomes either true or false when the unknown (variable) is replaced (substituted) with a numeric value.

EXAMPLES:

In $x + 5 = 7$, replace x with 3.

$3 + 5 = 7$ is a false statement.

In $x + 5 = 7$, replace x with 2.

$2 + 5 = 7$ is a true statement.

The solution of an equation is that numeric value which, when substituted in the equation, gives a true statement. In the earlier example, 2 is the solution to the equation.

There may be many solutions to an equation. For example, in the equation $x + 5 = x + 5$, all numeric values for x will give a true statement. This type of equation is called an **identity**.

There may be no solutions to an equation. For example, in the equation $x + 5 = x + 6$, there are no numbers that, when substituted in the equation, give a true statement. Therefore, there are no solutions to the equation.

Equivalence Principles. The principles of equivalence are needed to solve equations. **Equivalent equations** are equations that have the same solutions.

Addition and Subtraction Principle. If the same number is added to each side or subtracted from each side of an equation, the equation remains equivalent.

EXAMPLE:

$x - 5 = 7$ (add 5 to both sides)

$x - 5 + 5 = 7 + 5$ (equivalent equation to

$x = 12$ $x - 5 = 7$)

EXAMPLE:

$x + 3 = 12$ (subtract 3 from both sides)

$x + 3 - 3 = 12 - 3$ (equivalent equation to

$x = 9$ $x + 3 = 12$)

Multiplication and Division Principle. If the same nonzero number is multiplied or divided by each side of the equation, the equation remains equivalent.

EXAMPLE:

$\frac{x}{5} = 6$ (multiply each side by 5)

$5 \cdot \frac{x}{5} = 5 \cdot 6$ (equivalent equation)

$x = 30$

EXAMPLE:

$3x = 12$ (divide each side by 3)

$\frac{3x}{3} = \frac{12}{3}$ (equivalent equation)

$x = 4$

To find a solution to an equation, the unknown (variable) must be isolated on one side of the equation.

EXAMPLE:

Solve: $x + 7 = 12$ for x

$x + 7 = 12$

$x + 7 - 7 = 12 - 7$ (subtract 7 from each side)

$x = 5$

Check:

$x + 7 = 12$

$5 + 7 = 12$ (substitute value for x)

$12 = 12$ (statement is true; therefore, 5 is solution to equation)

EXAMPLE:

Solve $\frac{x}{6} = 18$ for x

$\frac{x}{6} = 18$

$6 \cdot \frac{x}{6} = 6 \cdot 18$ (multiply both sides by 6)

$x = 108$

Check:

$\frac{x}{6} = 18$

$\frac{108}{6} = 18$ (substitute 108 to x)

$18 = 18$ (statement is true)

EXAMPLE:

Solve: $5a = 30$ for a

$5a = 30$

$\frac{5a}{5} = \frac{30}{5}$ (divide both sides by 5)

$a = 6$

Check:

$5a = 30$

$5(6) = 30$ (substitute 6 for a)

$30 = 30$ (statement is true)

EXAMPLE:

Solve: $7x - 5 = 3x + 7$ for x

$7x - 5 = 3x + 7$

$7x - 5 + 5 = 3x + 7 + 5$ (add 5 to both sides)

$7x = 3x + 12$

$7x - 3x = 3x + 12 - 3x$ (subtract 3x from both sides)

$4x = 12$

$\frac{4x}{4} = \frac{12}{4}$ (divide both sides by 4)

$x = 3$

(continues)

(continued)

Check:

$7x - 5 = 3x + 7$

$7(3) - 5 = 3(3) + 7$ (substitute 3 for x)

$21 - 5 = 9 + 7$

$16 = 16$ (statement is true)

To solve an equation with parentheses, the parentheses need to be eliminated using some correct procedure, usually the distributive law.

EXAMPLE:

Solve: $7(x + 6) = 21$ for x

$7(x + 6) = 21$ (distributive law)

$7x + 42 = 21$ (subtract 42 from each side)

$7x = -21$ (divide each side by 7)

$x = -3$

Check:

$7(x + 6) = 21$ (substitute −3 for x)

$7(-3 + 6) = 21$

$7(3) = 21$

$21 = 21$ (statement is true)

Sometimes a formula needs to be rearranged. This is just like solving an equation for an unknown (variable).

EXAMPLE:

Solve for t when $a = bt + c$

$a = bt + c$

$a - c = bt + c - c$ (subtract c from each side)

$a - c = bt$ (divide by b)

$\frac{a - c}{b} = \frac{bt}{b}$

$\frac{a - c}{b} = t$

(continues)

(continued)

Check:

$a = bt + c$

$a = b \cdot \frac{a - c}{b} + c$ (substitute $\frac{a - c}{b}$ for t)

$a = a - c + c$

$a = a$ (statement is true)

Variation

Two types of variation will be discussed here—direct and inverse.

Direct Variation. **Direct variation** means that one quantity is a multiple of a second quantity. An example of direct variation is $y = kx$, where k is the constant of proportionality. Here y is a multiple of x, making y directly proportional to x.

Another example is $y = kx^2$, where k is the constant of proportionality, making y directly proportional to the square of x. Another way to think of direct variation is that the quotient of the two quantities is always a constant. It is possible, knowing the values for the quantities, to find the constant.

Inverse Variation. **Inverse variation** means that when two quantities are multiplied their product is a constant.

An example of inverse variation is $y = k/x$, where k is the constant of proportionality. Here the product of x and y is a constant, namely k. This is usually read as y is inversely proportional to x.

Another example is $y = k/x^2$, where k is the constant of proportionality. Here the product of x^2 and y is a constant. This is usually read as y is inversely proportional to the square of x (or x^2).

It is also possible to combine the two variations. As an example, consider $y = kx/z^2$. Here y is directly proportional to x and inversely proportional to the square of z.

UNITS OF MEASUREMENT

In order to quantify scientific phenomena, standard units of measurement have been established. These units allow scientists to describe quantities. In physics, the primary or fundamental units of measurement are **mass, length,** and **time.** These units, although they have the same meaning and have been standardized by international organizations, are measured by the use of two widely different systems. These are the British (foot-pound-second) system, also called the United States customary system, and the metric (MKS [meter-kilogram-second] or CGS [centimeter-gram-second]) system. Although most countries utilize the metric system of measurement, attempts to switch to this system in the United States have not been very successful. In the United States, length is measured in inches and feet rather than meters and kilometers. By combining one or more of the fundamental units, scientists arrive at secondary or derived units. For example, the area of an object is derived from the fundamental unit of length. The area of a rectangle is determined by multiplying the lengths of the two sides of the object.

SI Units

In 1960, at the Eleventh General Conference of Weights and Measures, the Système Internationale d̀ Unites (SI) was defined and officially adopted. This system of units, used to measure various quantities, is now accepted as the metric system. In the SI system, there are seven base units (Table 1-2). All other units are derived from these units, although some derived units are given special names. It is important to become familiar with SI units because they have been internationally adopted.

In addition, although the United States does not use SI/metric units for the public, all scientific inquiries utilize the SI system. As noted earlier, the seven base SI units are mass, length, time, electric current, temperature, amount of substance, and luminous intensity. Radiologically important derived units are the **coulomb per kilogram** (C/kg), formerly the roentgen (R); the **gray** (Gy), formerly the rad (radiation absorbed dose); and the **sievert** (Sv), formerly the rem (radiation equivalent man). These radiologic units are described in greater detail in Chapter 8.

Fundamental Units

Mass. Mass is the amount or quantity of matter. The standard unit of mass is the **kilogram** (kg).

TABLE 1-2. SI Units of Measurement

Base Units

Quantity	Unit Name	Symbol
Mass	kilogram	kg
Length	meter	m
Time	second	s
Electric current	ampere	A
Temperature	kelvin	K
Amount of substance	mole	mol
Luminous intensity	candela	cd

Derived Units

Quantity	Unit Name	Symbol	British Units
Absorbed dose	gray	Gy	rad
Charge	coulomb	C	esu
Electric potential	volt	v	
Dose equivalent	sievert	Sv	rem
Energy	joule	J	ft/lb
Exposure	coulomb/ kilogram	C/kg	roentgen
Frequency	hertz	Hz	cycles per second
Force	newton	N	
Magnetic flux	weber	Wb	
Magnetic flux density	tesla	T	gauss
Power	watt	W	
Radioactivity	bequerel	Bq	curie

It is represented by a cylinder of platinum-iridium, which is kept in a vault at the International Bureau of Weights and Measures in Paris, France.

Length. The unit of length is the **meter** (m). The meter was defined in 1983 as the distance that light travels in a vacuum in 1/299,792,485 second.

Time. The unit of time is the **second** (s). The second was originally defined in terms of the rotation of the earth on its axis (the mean solar day) but, like the meter, the need for greater accuracy resulted in redefining the unit. Time is now measured by the vibrations of cesium-133 atoms. This method is sometimes called the atomic clock.

TABLE 1-3. SI Unit Values

Factors	Prefixes	Symbols
10^{12}	tera	T
10^{9}	giga	G
10^{6}	mega	M
10^{3}	kilo	k
10^{2}	hecto	h
10^{1}	deka	da
10^{-1}	deci	d
10^{-2}	centi	c
10^{-3}	milli	m
10^{-6}	micro	m
10^{-9}	nano	n
10^{-12}	pico	p
10^{-15}	femto	f
10^{-18}	atto	a

Prefixes

The metric system uses prefixes to units to denote different orders of magnitude, as shown in Table 1-3.

To convert from grams to kilograms or micrograms, or to grams with any other prefix, the decimal point is moved. If the prefix moves up the table, the decimal point is moved to the left the number of exponent positions moved. If the prefix moves down the table, the decimal point is moved to the right the number of exponent positions moved. Dimensional analysis can also be used.

EXAMPLES:

23.4 g = 0.0234 kg — Move the decimal point 3 positions left.

23.4 g = 23,400 mg — Move the decimal point 3 positions right.

23.4 mg = 0.0000234 kg — Move the decimal point 6 positions left.

23.4 kg = 2,340,000 cg — Move the decimal point 5 positions right.

Using dimensional analysis:

$$23.4\text{ g} = 23.4\text{ g}\,\frac{\text{kg}}{1000\text{ g}} = 0.0234\text{ kg}$$

Some commonly used prefixes are shown in Table 1-4.

Conversion from one system to another is needed from time to time. For example, 1 inch = 2.54 cm is the conversion fact for changing inches to centimeters. See the section on dimensional analysis under the math review for the procedure to convert from one set of units to another.

TABLE 1-4. Commonly Used SI Prefixes

Unit	Symbol	Meaning
kilovolt	kV	10^3 volts
centimeter	cm	10^{-2} meter
milliampere	mA	10^{-3} amp
milligray	mGy	10^{-3} Gy
nanosecond	ns	10^{-9} second

SUMMARY

A basic review of arithmetic, algebra, and units of measurement has been presented. The arithmetic review includes fractions, decimals, computation with values, powers of 10, scientific notation, and dimensional analysis. The algebra review includes signed numbers, order of operation, algebraic expressions, exponents, evaluating algebraic expressions, equations, and variation. Both SI and British (U.S. customary) units of measurement are introduced.

In order to quantify science, standard units of measurement were established. The fundamental units of measurement are mass, length, and time. Units of measurement were officially defined on an international level through the adoption of the SI units. The seven base SI units are mass, length, time, electric current, temperature, amount of substance, and luminous intensity. Radiologically important derived units are the coulomb per kilogram (C/kg), formerly the roentgen (R); the gray (Gy), formerly the rad (radiation absorbed dose); and the sievert (Sv), formerly the rem (radiation equivalent man).

REVIEW QUESTIONS

1. $\frac{4}{7} + \frac{1}{2} =$
2. $\frac{2}{9} \cdot \frac{3}{8} =$
3. $571.1 - 182.572 =$
4. $725 \div 0.25 =$
5. Change .325 to a percent.
6. What are the significant digits of each of the following:
   a. 20.10
   b. 192
   c. 38.04
   d. 2,700
   e. 1,800.004
7. Add the following numbers, leaving the results with the correct number of significant digits if each number is assumed to be approximate.
   a. 2.1 + 2.824
   b. 3.2 + 4.19
8. Change the following numbers to scientific notation:
   a. .0081
   b. 7,811.2
   c. .00024
   d. 78,432

9. Change the following numbers to ordinary notation:

a. 3.614×10^2

b. 1.876×10^{-4}

c. 1.823×10^3

d. 5.67×10^6

10. Convert 1,500 seconds to hours.

11. Convert 10 meters^2 to centimeters^2.

12. Simplify the following algebraic expressions:

a. $-3(x + y) + 7(2x + 1)$

b. $-4(x + 2y) - 8(2x - y)$

13. Simplify the following expressions, leaving the answer with only positive exponents:

a. $a^2 \cdot b^3 \cdot a^4 \cdot b^2$

b. $(a^4)^3 \cdot (a^2)^{-3}$

14. Evaluate the expression for a = 5 and b = 3.

$\frac{3}{8}(a^2 - b^2)$

15. Evaluate the expression for a = 2, b = −4, and c = 6.

$3(a + b) - c$

16. Solve for x: $2x - 8 = 4$

17. Solve for x: $2(3x - 8) = 3(4 - x) + 6x$

18. Solve for a: $\frac{2}{3} = \frac{a}{15}$

REFERENCES AND RECOMMENDED READING

Aufmann, R. N. (2007). *Basic college mathematics: An applied approach* (8th ed.). Boston: Houghton Mifflin.

Burns, J. E. (1979). The new SI units: Problems with conversion. *The Canadian Journal of Radiography, Radiotherapy, and Nuclear Medicine, 10*(2), 60–70.

Dunworth, J. V. (1976). SI units for ionizing radiations. The use of the "gray." *Radiography, 42*(496), 84.

Martin-Gay, K. E. (2010). *Pre- algebra* (6nd ed.). Upper Saddle River, NJ: PrenticeHall.

The SI for the health profession. (1979). *The Canadian Journal of Medical Radiation Technology, 10*(4), 138.

Washington, A. J. (2004). *Basic technical mathematics with calculus* (8th ed.). Upper Saddle River, NJ: Pearson Addison Wesley.

Wyckoff, H. O. (1978). The international system of units (SI). *Radiology, 128*, 833–835.

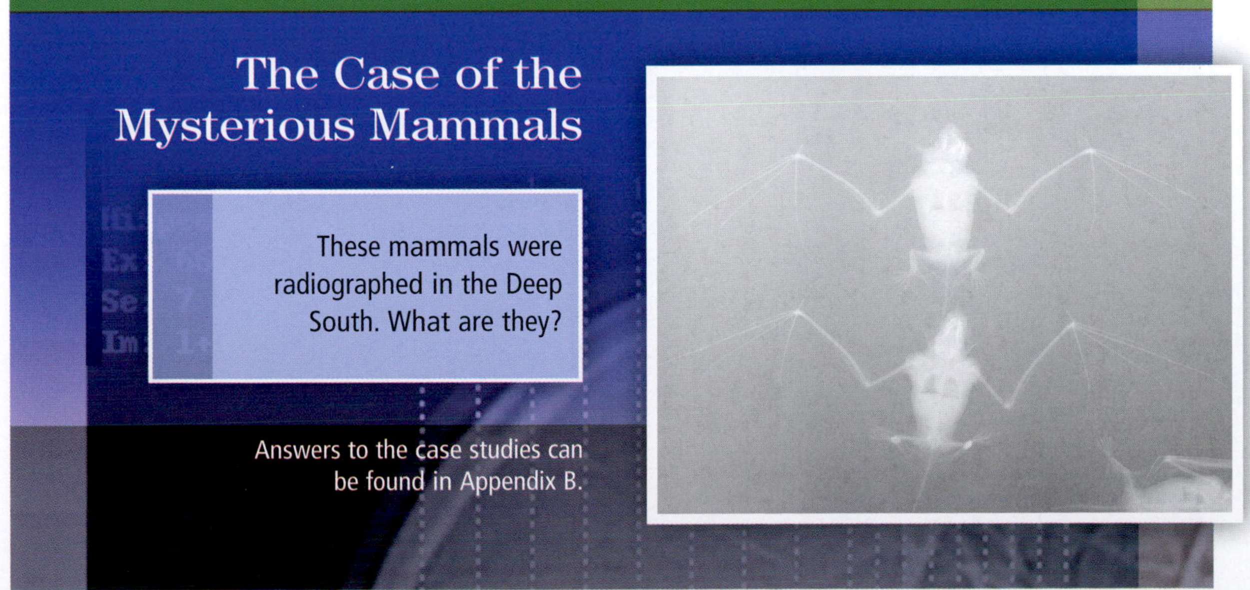

CHAPTER 2

Radiation Concepts

KEY TERMS

amplitude
atom
atomic mass number (A)
atomic mass unit (amu)
atomic number
chemical energy
compound
electrical energy
electricity
electromagnetic energy
electromagnetic radiation (EM)
electromagnetic spectrum
electron (e^-)
electron binding energy E_b
electron volt (eV)
element
excitation
frequency
heat
ion
ionization
isotope
kinetic energy
K-shell
lambda
M theory
mass
mechanical energy

> I have discovered something interesting, but I do not know whether or not my observations are correct.
>
> *W. C. Röntgen to his friend Theodor Boveri in early December 1895.*

OBJECTIVES

Upon completion of this chapter, the student should be able to:

- Describe the branches of science.
- Differentiate between matter and energy.
- Describe the basic structure of matter.
- Identify the various types of energy.
- Explain the basic concepts of atomic theory.
- Differentiate between the radiations along the electromagnetic spectrum.
- Describe the wave and particle theories for electromagnetic radiation.
- Identify the properties of x-rays.
- Explain the standard units of measurement.

KEY TERMS (continued)

mixture
molecule
neutron (n^o)
nu
nuclear energy
nucleon
nucleus
octet rule
period
photon
potential energy
proton (p^+)
quantum
quark
radiation
shell
string theory
substance
temperature
thermal energy
valence
wavelength
weight
Z number

MATTER AND ENERGY

Radiography is the recording of images created by the use of x-ray energy. It is both an art and a science. In order to perform the duties of a radiographer, it is necessary to understand the art of the profession as well as the science.

Science is the use of knowledge in an organized and classified manner. The scientific method has been used by men and women to understand the world in which we live. This method systematically involves collecting facts, studying their relationships, and arriving at conclusions based on analysis. Natural science is the study of the universe and its contents. It can be divided into two categories: (1) the study of nonliving matter, known as physical science; and (2) the study of living matter, known as biological science. Radiographers learn about biological science through a study of human anatomy and physiology and about physical science through a study of x-ray production and imaging processes.

Physics is a branch of physical science that studies matter and energy and their interrelationships. Matter is defined as anything that has mass and occupies space. Energy is the ability to do work.

Matter

Matter is a very general term used to describe the substance that comprises all physical objects. It has shape, form, and it occupies space. A principal characteristic of matter is **mass**. Mass is the quantity of matter contained in an object. It is best described by its energy equivalence, although the term *weight* is generally used to mean the same thing. **Weight** is the force that an object exerts under the influence of gravity. An object may be weightless in a zero-gravity environment, such as in space, but the mass of that object would remain unchanged.

The unit of mass is the kilogram, which equals 1,000 grams. The kilogram represents the weight of a standard piece of platinum-iridium kept at the International Bureau of Weights and Measures in Paris, France. It is equal to the mass of 1,000 cm^3 of water at 0° Celsius (C) or Centigrade.

The structure of matter has been studied throughout history. In nature, matter is most commonly found as a mixture of substances (Figure 2-1). A **substance** is defined as a material that has a definite and constant composition. When two or more substances are combined, they form a **mixture**. For example, air is a mixture of oxygen, hydrogen, nitrogen, and a variety of other substances.

Substances may be either simple or complex. Simple substances are known as **elements** and complex substances are known as **compounds**. An element is a substance that cannot be broken down into any simpler substances by ordinary means.

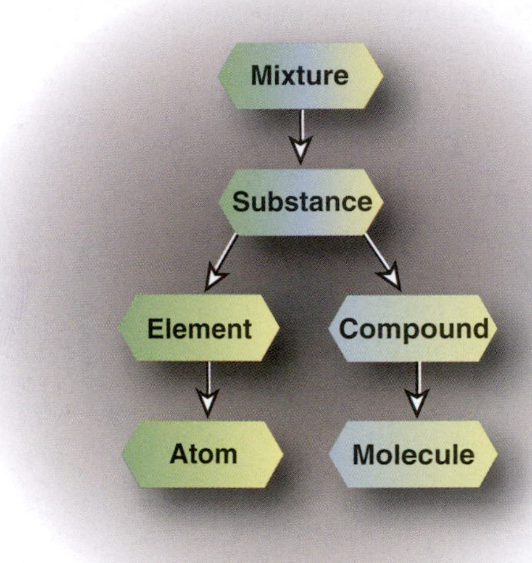

FIGURE 2-1. Structure of matter.

There are 92 naturally occurring elements identified on the periodic table of elements (Figure 2-2). Elements include such substances as hydrogen, oxygen, carbon, calcium, copper, silver, gold, lead, and barium. When two or more elements are chemically united in definite proportion, compounds are formed. Water and salt are both examples of compounds. Water is formed by the chemical union of two hydrogen atoms and one oxygen atom and is referred to as H_2O (Figure 2-3). Each element has an abbreviated letter or letters to identify it. These abbreviations for the elements are outlined on the periodic table. For example, in the compound salt, the element sodium (Na) is chemically combined with the element chlorine (Cl), in equal proportions, to form sodium chloride (NaCl).

When broken down and examined in its purest form, matter is actually comprised of very small invisible particles known as atoms. An **atom** is the smallest particle of an element that still possesses the chemical properties of that element. When two or more atoms are chemically united, they form a **molecule**, which is the smallest particle of a compound that still possesses the characteristics of the compound. For example, in the compound water, two hydrogen (H) atoms combine with one oxygen (O) atom to form one water (H_2O) molecule. With salt, one sodium (Na) atom combines with one chlorine (Cl) atom to form one sodium chloride (NaCl) molecule.

Atoms are tightly bonded to one another when a molecule is formed. These bonds cannot be broken by ordinary physical means, such as crushing. Atoms and molecules are, however, bound to one another by varying degrees of attraction. The degree of attraction between atoms or molecules will determine if the substance is a solid, a liquid, or a gas. The attraction is weakest with a gas and strongest with a solid. For example, depending on the degree of molecular attraction, water can exist in its usual state as a liquid, or it can exist as a gas (steam) or a solid (ice). The state is determined by the heat or thermal energy that the substance possesses.

Energy

Energy is defined as the ability to do work. The unit of energy is the joule (J), named after the English physicist who developed the standard. When energy is emitted and transferred through matter, it is called **radiation**. Radiation is a term applied to many forms of energy, such as heat and light. When the burner on a stove is lit, it can be described as radiating heat. A light bulb is capable of radiating light. When any form of matter is struck by a form of radiant energy, it is described as being exposed or radiated.

There is a unique relationship between matter and energy. They are interchangeable. This relationship was described in 1905 by the German-American physicist Albert Einstein (1879–1955) in his well-known theory of relativity. Einstein mathematically described the relationship between matter and energy in the equation:

$$E = mc^2$$

where: E = energy
m = mass
c = constant (the speed of light in a vacuum)

At the basis of Einstein's work is the Law of Conservation. This law states that the sum total of all matter and energy in the universe is

IUPAC
Periodic Table of the Elements

Key:

atomic number symbol name standard atomic weight

	1	2	3	4	5	6	7	8	9	10	11	12	13	14	15	16	17	18
K or 1	1 **H** hydrogen 1.007 94(7)																	2 **He** helium 4.002 602(2)
L or 2	3 **Li** lithium 6.941(2)	4 **Be** beryllium 9.012 182(3)											5 **B** boron 10.811(7)	6 **C** carbon 12.0107(8)	7 **N** nitrogen 14.0067(2)	8 **O** oxygen 15.9994(3)	9 **F** fluorine 18.998 4032(5)	10 **Ne** neon 20.1797(6)
M or 3	11 **Na** sodium 22.989 770(2)	12 **Mg** magnesium 24.3050(6)											13 **Al** aluminium 26.981 538(2)	14 **Si** silicon 28.0855(3)	15 **P** phosphorus 30.973 761(2)	16 **S** sulfur 32.065(5)	17 **Cl** chlorine 35.453(2)	18 **Ar** argon 39.948(1)
N or 4	19 **K** potassium 39.0983(1)	20 **Ca** calcium 40.078(4)	21 **Sc** scandium 44.955 910(8)	22 **Ti** titanium 47.867(1)	23 **V** vanadium 50.9415(1)	24 **Cr** chromium 51.9961(6)	25 **Mn** manganese 54.938 049(9)	26 **Fe** iron 55.845(2)	27 **Co** cobalt 58.933 200(9)	28 **Ni** nickel 58.6934(2)	29 **Cu** copper 63.546(3)	30 **Zn** zinc 65.409(4)	31 **Ga** gallium 69.723(1)	32 **Ge** germanium 72.64(1)	33 **As** arsenic 74.921 60(2)	34 **Se** selenium 78.96(3)	35 **Br** bromine 79.904(1)	36 **Kr** krypton 83.798(2)
O or 5	37 **Rb** rubidium 85.4678(3)	38 **Sr** strontium 87.62(1)	39 **Y** yttrium 88.905 85(2)	40 **Zr** zirconium 91.224(2)	41 **Nb** niobium 92.906 38(2)	42 **Mo** molybdenum 95.94(2)	43 **Tc** technetium [97.9072]	44 **Ru** ruthenium 101.07(2)	45 **Rh** rhodium 102.905 50(2)	46 **Pd** palladium 106.42(1)	47 **Ag** silver 107.8682(2)	48 **Cd** cadmium 112.411(8)	49 **In** indium 114.818(3)	50 **Sn** tin 118.710(7)	51 **Sb** antimony 121.760(1)	52 **Te** tellurium 127.60(3)	53 **I** iodine 126.904 47(3)	54 **Xe** xenon 131.293(6)
P or 6	55 **Cs** caesium 132.905 45(2)	56 **Ba** barium 137.327(7)	57-71 lanthanoids	72 **Hf** hafnium 178.49(2)	73 **Ta** tantalum 180.9479(1)	74 **W** tungsten 183.84(1)	75 **Re** rhenium 186.207(1)	76 **Os** osmium 190.23(3)	77 **Ir** iridium 192.217(3)	78 **Pt** platinum 195.078(2)	79 **Au** gold 196.966 55(2)	80 **Hg** mercury 200.59(2)	81 **Tl** thallium 204.3833(2)	82 **Pb** lead 207.2(1)	83 **Bi** bismuth 208.980 38(2)	84 **Po** polonium [208.9824]	85 **At** astatine [209.9871]	86 **Rn** radon [222.0176]
Q or 7	87 **Fr** francium [223.0197]	88 **Ra** radium [226.0254]	89-103 actinoids	104 **Rf** rutherfordium [261.1088]	105 **Db** dubnium [262.1141]	106 **Sg** seaborgium [266.1219]	107 **Bh** bohrium [264.12]	108 **Hs** hassium [277]	109 **Mt** meitnerium [268.1366]	110 **Ds** darmstadtium [271]	111 **Uuu** unununium [272]							

57 **La** lanthanum 138.9055(2)	58 **Ce** cerium 140.116(1)	59 **Pr** praseodymium 140.907 65(2)	60 **Nd** neodymium 144.24(3)	61 **Pm** promethium (144.9127)	62 **Sm** samarium 150.36(3)	63 **Eu** europium 151.964(1)	64 **Gd** gadolinium 157.25(3)	65 **Tb** terbium 158.925 34(2)	66 **Dy** dysprosium 162.500(1)	67 **Ho** holmium 164.930 32(2)	68 **Er** erbium 167.259(3)	69 **Tm** thulium 168.934 21(2)	70 **Yb** ytterbium 173.04(3)	71 **Lu** lutetium 174.967(1)
89 **Ac** actinium (227.0277)	90 **Th** thorium 232.0381(1)	91 **Pa** protactinium 231.035 88(2)	92 **U** uranium 238.028 91(3)	93 **Np** neptunium (237.0482)	94 **Pu** plutonium (244.0642)	95 **Am** americium (243.0614)	96 **Cm** curium (247.0704)	97 **Bk** berkelium (247.0703)	98 **Cf** californium (251.0796)	99 **Es** einsteinium (252.0830)	100 **Fm** fermium (257.0951)	101 **Md** mendelevium (258.0984)	102 **No** nobelium (259.1010)	103 **Lr** lawrencium (262.1097)

FIGURE 2-2. Periodic table of elements. *(Copyright ©2003 IUPAC, the International Union of Pure and Applied Chemistry.)*

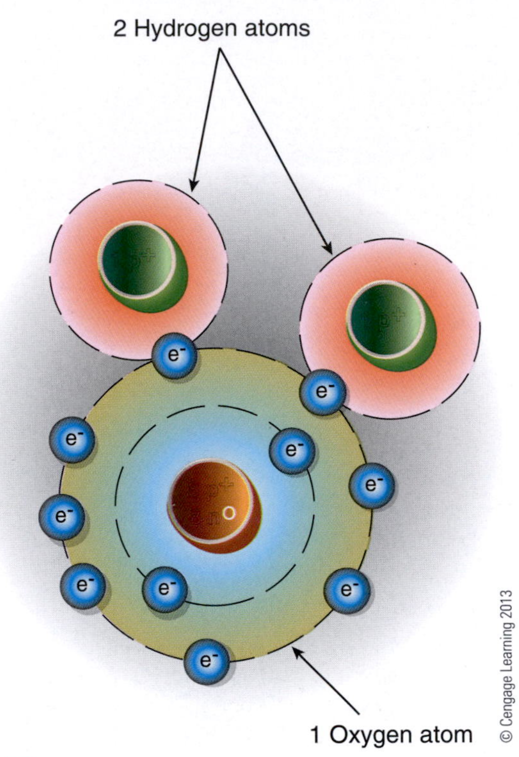

FIGURE 2-3. A water molecule is formed when two atoms of hydrogen combine with one atom of oxygen.

a constant: matter and energy cannot be created or destroyed but can be converted from one form to another. Although recent research has demonstrated certain circumstances when Einstein's theory has been disproved, for practical purposes it is essentially true.

ATOMIC THEORY

Matter is comprised of very small particles known as atoms. To understand how small atoms really are, it has been estimated that one teaspoon of water (about 1 cm^3) contains about three times as many atoms as the Atlantic Ocean contains teaspoons of water.

Atoms can be subdivided into three basic subatomic particles: **protons** (p^+), **neutrons** (n^0), and **electrons** (e^-).

Historical Overview

The composition of the atom has been a topic of scientific investigation for thousands of years. The Greeks theorized that matter has four basic components: air, water, earth, and fire. They named the smallest division of these components the atom. This theory was accepted until the early 1800s, when an English schoolteacher named John Dalton (1766–1844) published his work on atomic theory. Dalton concluded that all elements could be differentiated from one another based on the characteristic of mass. He further concluded that each of the elements was composed of atoms that behaved in an identical fashion during a chemical reaction. During the mid-1800s, a Russian scientist, Dmitri Mendeleev (1834–1907), developed the first periodic table of the elements. This table arranges the elements in order of ascending atomic mass and on the basis of the repetition of similar chemical properties (Figure 2-2). More detailed information on a specific element on the periodic table, including specific characteristics, electron configurations, and electron binding energies, can be found at http://www.webelements.com.

Investigation of the structure of matter continued and, in 1911, English physicist Ernest Rutherford (1871–1937) developed a model for the atom that contained a central, small, dense nucleus, which possessed a positive charge and was surrounded by a negative cloud of randomly placed electrons, which had a negative charge. In 1913, Niels Bohr (1885–1962), a Danish physicist, expanded on Rutherford's work and proposed a model for the atom that is considered the most representative of the structure of matter. Bohr's atom is likened to a miniature solar system where electrons orbit around a central nucleus just as the planets revolve around the sun.

Although the atom is far more complex than Bohr's simple model suggests, this model is still the most widely used in explaining the composition of matter. One key distinction between Bohr's model and an actual atom is that electrons orbit the nucleus in many planes, whereas the planets orbit the sun in essentially the same plane.

Bohr's simple model was difficult to apply to elements with a high atomic number. Both Niels

Bohr and the Austrian physicist Erwin Schrödinger, working with their associates, developed a theoretical approach to understanding atomic behavior. Both Bohr and Schrödinger were successful, but physicists primarily use Schrödinger's concept because it has been found to be more convenient. This approach is the foundation of modern physics and is known as quantum or wave mechanics.

According to the principles of quantum mechanics, orbital electrons are assigned probabilities for occupying any location within the atom. The greatest probabilities are associated with Bohr's original model.

Basic Atomic Particles

The atom is best described as having a small, dense center known as the **nucleus**, which is surrounded by electrons that orbit it at various levels (Figure 2-4). The nucleus contains two of the three basic particles of the atom, protons and neutrons, which are responsible for almost all of the mass of an atom. Protons and neutrons together are referred to as **nucleons**. The third basic particle, the electron, is located outside the nucleus and has a relatively insignificant mass, 1/1,826 that of a proton.

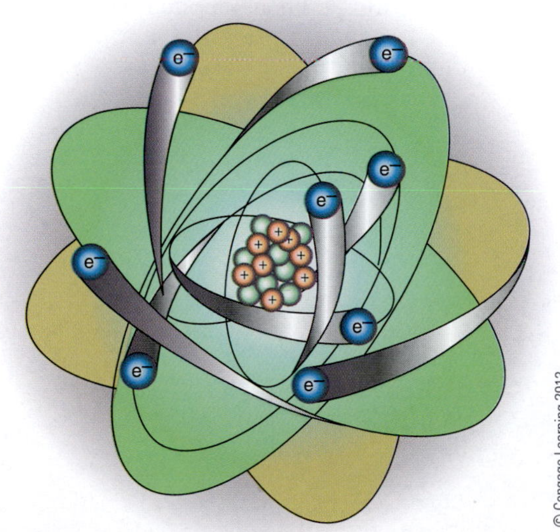

FIGURE 2-4. A three-dimensional diagram of an atom of oxygen, which contains eight protons, eight neutrons located within the center nucleus, and eight electrons within orbital shells moving around the nucleus.

Electrons cannot be divided into smaller parts, but protons and neutrons are both composed of even smaller subnuclear structures called **quarks**. There are new theories that may explain them as well as find a way for quantum physics and relativity theory to work together. The overall concept is being referred to as **M theory**. It postulates that electrons and quarks may not be particles, but instead may be extremely small loops of rapidly vibrating string-like matter. One idea is that matter behaves differently depending on the vibrations of the string (like a guitar string playing many different sounds depending on the position of the fingers on the frets, force applied via finger or pick, and the shape and size of the body of the guitar or the electronics in the pickup). In fact, this concept is now being called **string theory**. There are actually five different string theories and they require the addition of several new dimensions in addition to the four we know (as well as the need to invent new forms of mathematics to figure out how they function). Although this begins to sound like a science fiction story, many physicists are beginning to agree that these new theories may be the next frontier for research and hold hope for better explanations about how matter behaves. It is likely that our knowledge of radiation will expand along with these theories throughout your career in the radiologic sciences.

The subatomic particles possess electrical charges. There are two types of electrical charges: positive and negative. The proton is a positively charged particle and the electron is a negatively charged particle. The neutron contains no charge and is said to be electrically neutral. When the number of positively charged protons equals the number of negatively charged electrons, the atom is neutral or stable. Because of its electrical nature, the atom is dynamic and ever moving. It is in a constant, vibrating motion because of the strong positive nuclear force field, which is surrounded by the negatively charged spinning and orbiting electrons.

Each of the elements has its own specific number of nuclear protons. This is the key characteristic that distinguishes one element from another.

The number of nuclear protons in an atom is known as the **atomic number** or **Z number**. The simplest element, hydrogen, possesses only one proton and therefore has an atomic number of 1. Helium comes next on the periodic table and has two protons, giving it an atomic number of 2. Lead has an atomic number of 82, indicating that within the nucleus of an atom of lead there are 82 protons. The periodic table lists the elements in ascending order according to the element's atomic number (Figure 2-2). In a neutral atom the number of protons is equal to the number of electrons. For example, in a stable, neutral atom of hydrogen there is one proton and one electron. In a stable atom of lead there are 82 protons and 82 electrons.

Although not a common occurrence in nature, when an atom of a given element loses or gains a proton, that atom becomes a different element. For example, if an atom of carbon with atomic number 6 gains a proton, the atom then becomes an atom of nitrogen with atomic number 7. Atoms of one element do change to atoms of another element during the natural process of radioactive decay. Radium, with an atomic number of 88, decays over a very long period of time to form the element radon, which has atomic number 86. Radon is a naturally occurring gas that is also radioactive. Recent studies have found increased radon levels in homes around the country. Radon testing kits are now commercially available to measure radon levels in the home.

Changes in the number of protons change the identity of the element completely, but this is not the case with changes in the number of neutrons or electrons. If an atom gains or loses neutrons, the result is an atom called an **isotope**. Isotopes are atoms that have the same number of protons in the nucleus but differ in the number of neutrons. Deuterium is an isotope of hydrogen. It contains the same number of protons as hydrogen but also contains one neutron.

If an atom gains or loses an electron, it is called an **ion** and the atom is said to be ionized. **Ionization** is the process of adding or removing an electron from an atom. When an electron is removed from an atom, the atom becomes a positive ion; that is, the atom possesses an extra positive charge. When an electron is added to an atom, the atom becomes a negative ion; that is, it possesses an extra negative charge (Figure 2-5). The radiologic technologies use powerful beams of ionizing radiation that have the ability to ionize atoms, thus changing the charges and force fields between atoms. This can cause serious disruption of the metabolic relationships in

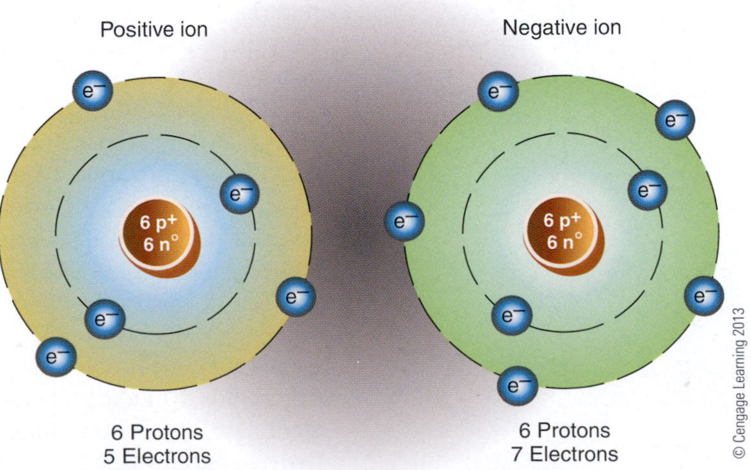

FIGURE 2-5. The ionizations process. When an electron is either added to or removed from an atom, the atom is ionized. A neutral carbon atom contains six protons and six electrons; a positive ion of carbon would contain more protons than electrons, and a negative ion of carbon would contain more electrons than protons.

the body. This is why exposure of patients to ionizing radiation requires an order from someone with a license to practice medicine.

Atomic Mass

The mass of an atom is extremely small; however, it is important to understand the differences in the mass of each of the basic particles of an atom. Each individual particle has its own unique mass. As stated earlier, the mass of an atom is almost entirely concentrated in the nucleus. The mass of a proton is approximately 1.673×10^{-27} kilograms and the mass of a neutron is almost identical, at 1.675×10^{-27} kilograms. Although these numbers seem remarkably small, they are still significantly greater than the mass of an electron, at 9.109×10^{-31} kilograms. Protons have approximately 1,836 times the mass of electrons, and neutrons have approximately 1,838 times more. The mass of the particles of an atom is sometimes described using the **atomic mass unit (amu)**.

In order for science to be as exact as possible, scientists defined an atomic mass unit as equal to one-twelfth of a carbon 12 atom. The amu of a proton is approximately 1.00728, a neutron has an amu of approximately 1.00867, and an electron has an amu of approximately 0.000548. When precision is not necessary, the mass of an atom is described by an **atomic mass number** symbolized by the letter **A.** The atomic mass number is equal to the number of protons and neutrons in the nucleus. For our purposes, each proton and neutron can be considered to have a mass number of one and an electron to have a mass number of zero (Table 2-1).

Orbital Electrons

Each of the electrons around the nucleus is in continuous motion. According to quantum mechanics, each of these electrons resides in an orbit that may be described as a "probability density." The orbital describes the region over which the electron is most likely to be at any given time.

The distance from the nucleus determines the energy level or **shell** the electron occupies. Each energy level has a certain **electron binding energy (E_b)**. The binding energy of an electron is defined as that amount of energy needed to remove the electron from the atom. If a free electron at rest is assumed to have an energy of zero, then the total energy of an orbital electron would be zero minus the binding energy or the negative of the binding energy. The closer an electron is to the nucleus, the more tightly it is bound to its orbit or shell. The charge felt by any electron at various distances from the nucleus is termed the shielded nuclear charge.

Certain forces are responsible for maintaining the electron's position and motion in its orbit. The stability of this orbit is contributed to by two opposing forces: the centrifugal force and the attractive electrostatic force. The centrifugal force tends to cause the electron to fly out in space. The attractive electrostatic force between the positively charged nucleus and the negatively charged electron tends to cause the two to fly together. These forces are exactly equal and opposite in a stable orbital. The end result is an electron that is in motion in a specific orbit around the nucleus. The closer an electron is to the nucleus, the higher the electron binding energy is and the more difficult it is to remove the electron from the atom.

The orbital shell closest to the nucleus is called the **K-shell**; the next shell is called the L-shell, then M-, N-, O-, P-, and, finally, the Q-shell. These letters for the shells are actually no longer used by chemists and physicists. They identify the shells by the principal quantum number (n). The first shell (K) is designated as n = 1. The second shell (L) is n = 2; the third shell (M) is n = 3, and so on. Two additional quantum numbers, the angular momentum quantum number and the magnetic quantum number, are further used by chemists and physicists to describe more precisely the location of an electron within an atom.

In a neutral atom, the number of protons and electrons is equal. This means that each element has a different number of orbital electrons. The element hydrogen has only one proton and one

TABLE 2-1. Atomic Particles

Particle	Mass Number	Mass (Kilograms)	AMU	Charge
Proton	1	1.673×10^{-27}	1.00728	Positive
Neutron	1	1.675×10^{-27}	1.00867	Neutral
Electron	0	9.109×10^{-38}	0.000548	Negative

electron. The electron of a hydrogen atom orbits in the K-shell. There is a maximum number of electrons that can occupy a given shell. The maximum number is determined by the formula $2n^2$, where n equals the shell or principal quantum number, starting with K as the first shell. According to this formula, the maximum number of electrons in each of the shells would be:

$$K = 2(1)^2 = 2$$
$$L = 2(2)^2 = 8$$
$$M = 2(3)^2 = 18$$
$$N = 2(4)^2 = 32$$
$$O = 2(5)^2 = 50$$
$$P = 2(6)^2 = 72$$
$$Q = 2(7)^2 = 98$$

Electrons may begin to appear in the next shell before a shell contains its maximum number of electrons. For example, electrons may appear in the N-shell before the M-shell has 18 electrons in it. This is because the number of electrons in the outermost shell never exceeds eight electrons. This is commonly referred to as the **octet rule**. Atoms that contain exactly eight electrons in their outermost shell are considered inert and chemically stable. The specific electron configuration will determine an element's position within the groups of the periodic table.

As the number of electrons and protons increases, so does the binding energy of a given electron. This is due to the increase in the positive charge in the nucleus. This means that the electrons in atoms of high-atomic-number elements are bound more tightly than the electrons in atoms of lower-atomic-number elements. The binding energy of electrons in the K-shell of lead is much higher than the binding energy of the K-shell electrons in hydrogen or oxygen. In addition, the binding energy of an electron decreases as the distance from the nucleus is increased (Figure 2-6). It takes more energy to remove a K-shell electron from its path than it would to remove an electron from a shell at a greater distance from the nucleus, such as the L-, M-, or N-shell. This will become important to remember when studying the effect of x-rays on atoms.

The binding energy of an electron is measured in a unit called the **electron volt (eV)**. This is the same unit used to describe x-ray energies. The electron volt is the energy one electron will have when it is accelerated by an electrical potential of one volt. Because x-ray and binding energies are great, the usual unit used to express these energies is the kilo-electron volt (keV). One keV equals 1,000 electron volts.

The atomic configuration and the approximate binding energies of certain elements are important because of their significance in radiology. These elements include hydrogen (H), carbon (C), and oxygen (O) because they are the principal elements that comprise the human body; iodine (I) and barium (Ba), because these elements are used as contrast media for a variety of radiologic examinations; tungsten (W) and molybdenum (Mo), because they are x-ray tube target materials; and lead (Pb), because it is the element used for radiation protection devices. A diagram of these elements shows that as the atomic number of an element increases, the K-shell binding energy of the element increases (Figure 2-7). This means that a K-shell electron of lead (Pb) is more tightly bound and more difficult to remove from the atom than a K-shell electron of smaller-atomic-number elements, such as hydrogen (H) or oxygen (O).

To remove the K-shell electron from an atom of tungsten or lead requires much more energy than would be necessary to remove a K-shell electron from an atom of hydrogen, carbon, or oxygen. When an electron is removed from an atom, the atom is said to be ionized. X-rays are capable of ionizing atoms. The x-ray energy must be greater than the binding energy of the electron in order for ionization to occur (Figure 2-8).

The Periodic Table

The present-day periodic table lists the 92 naturally occurring elements and an additional 18 elements that have been created in the laboratory through scientific investigation (Figure 2-2). The elements are listed in ascending order based on the atomic number located above the element's symbol. The relative atomic mass of the element is identified below the symbol. Each of the elements is also arranged into one of seven horizontal periods and one of eight vertical groups. The periods represent elements with the same principal quantum number or

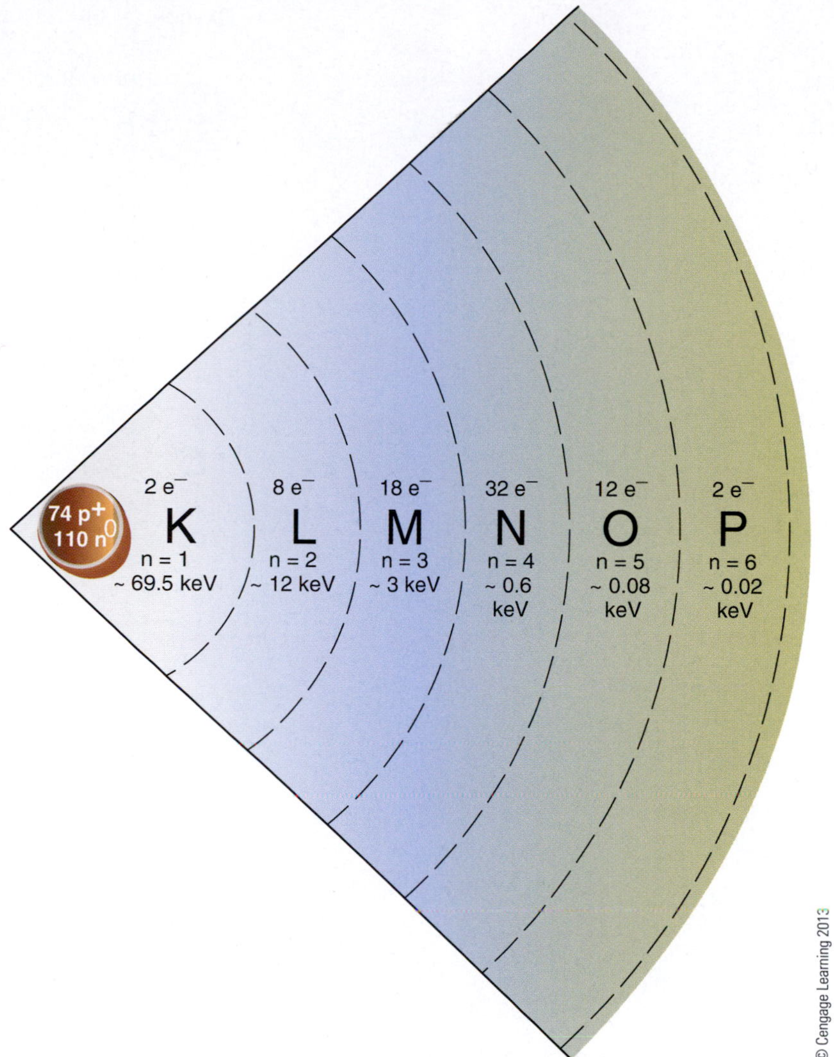

FIGURE 2-6. The closer an electron is to the nucleus, the greater will be the binding energy of the electron.

number of electron shells and the groups represent elements with the same number of electrons in the outermost shell. For example, each element in the last group has eight electrons in its outermost shell. These elements are chemically very stable atoms.

The number of electrons in the outermost shell of an atom determines the chemical combining characteristic or **valence** of the element. An element that has only one electron in the outermost shell is described as having a valence of +1 and would be located in Group 1 on the periodic table. This element will freely give up this electron to bind with another element to form a compound. An element that has seven electrons in its outermost shell has a valence of −1 and would be located in Group 7. This element will freely accept an electron to form a chemical bond because atoms prefer the stable octet configuration. An example of this bond, known as an ionic bond, is the salt molecule. Sodium (Na), having a valence of +1, can easily

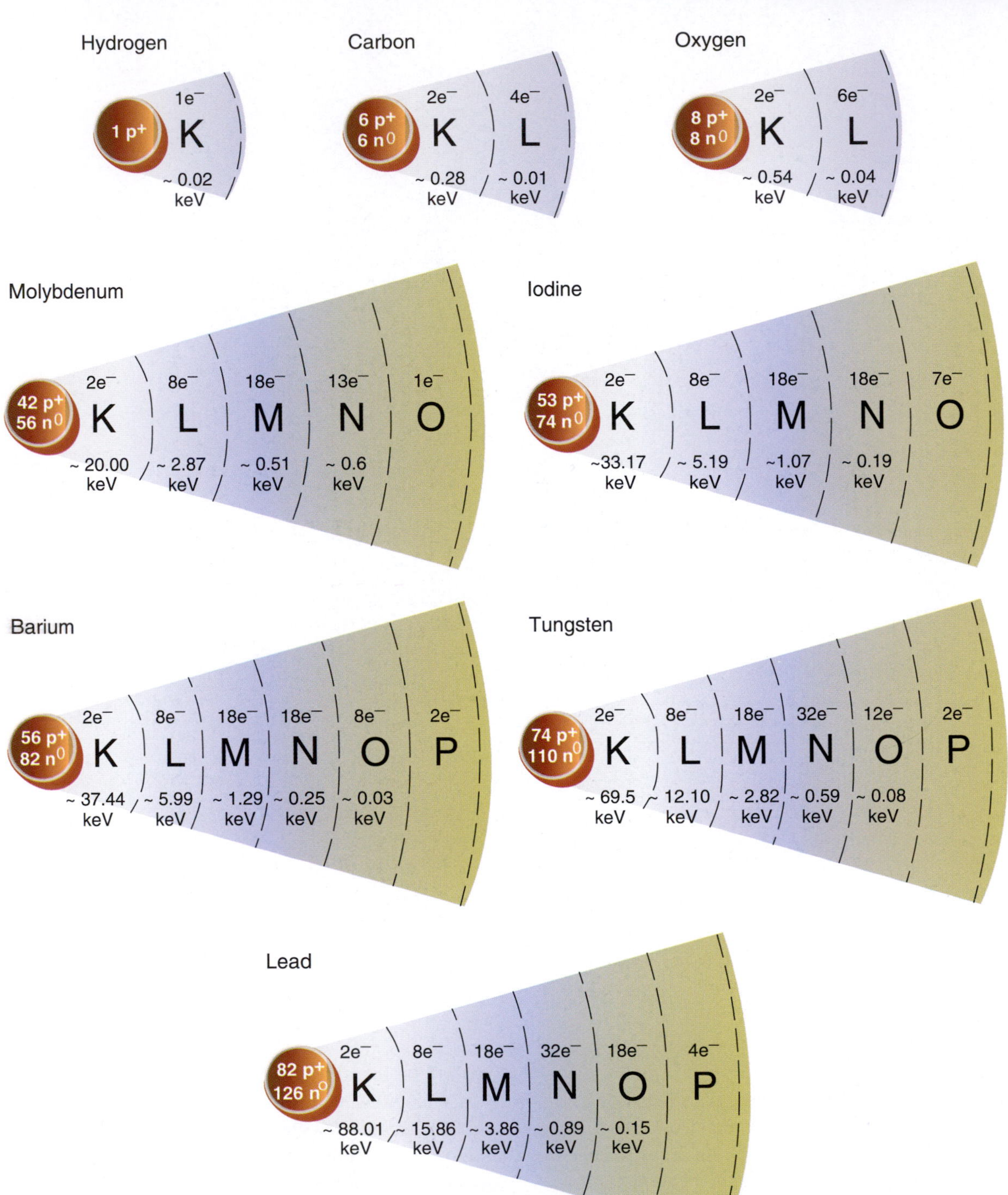

FIGURE 2-7. The atomic configurations and binding energies of elements that have significance in radiology.

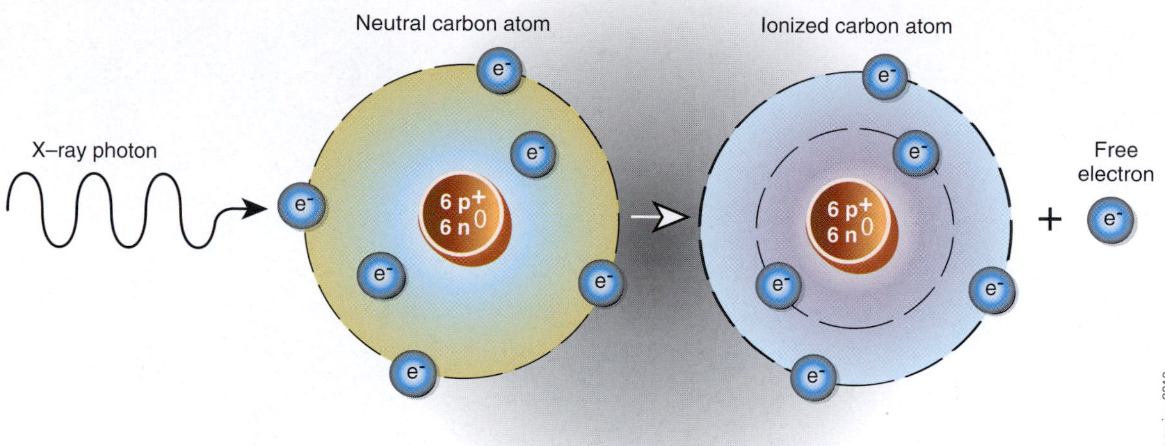

FIGURE 2-8. An x-ray photon can interact with an electron and eject it from an atom. This removal of an electron results in the ionization of the atom.

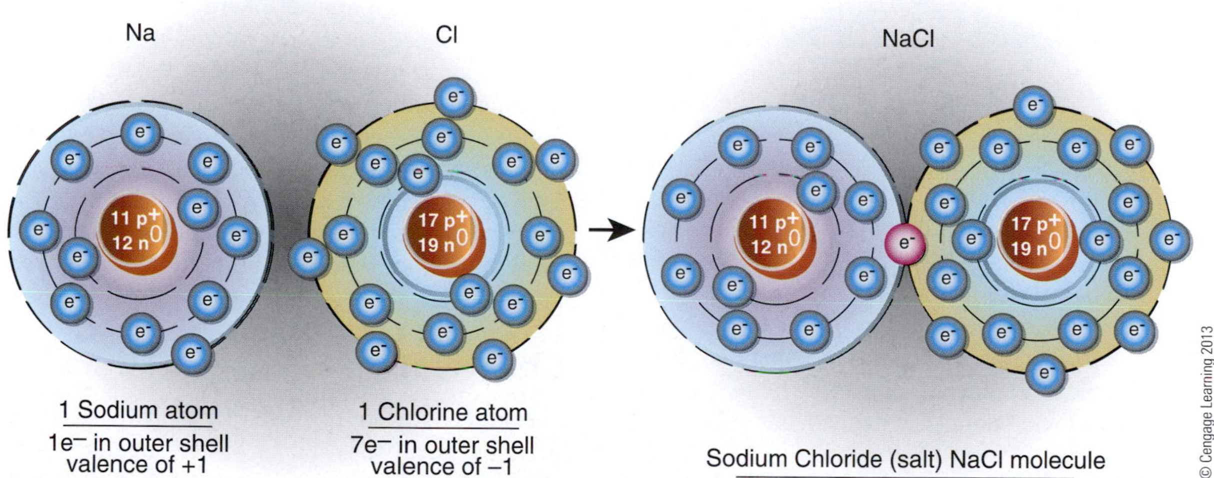

FIGURE 2-9. An ionic bond is formed between sodium (Na) and chlorine (Cl) to form table salt, sodium chloride (NaCl).

combine with chlorine (Cl), with a valence of −1, to form sodium chloride (NaCl), salt (Figure 2-9). The valence of an element determines the way the atoms will combine in definite proportions. Because of the element's valence number, **two** hydrogen atoms combine with **one** oxygen atom to form water. Hydrogen has a valence of +1, while oxygen has a valence of −2. Oxygen has room for two hydrogen atoms and will share electrons, a type of bond known as a covalent bond (Figure 2-10).

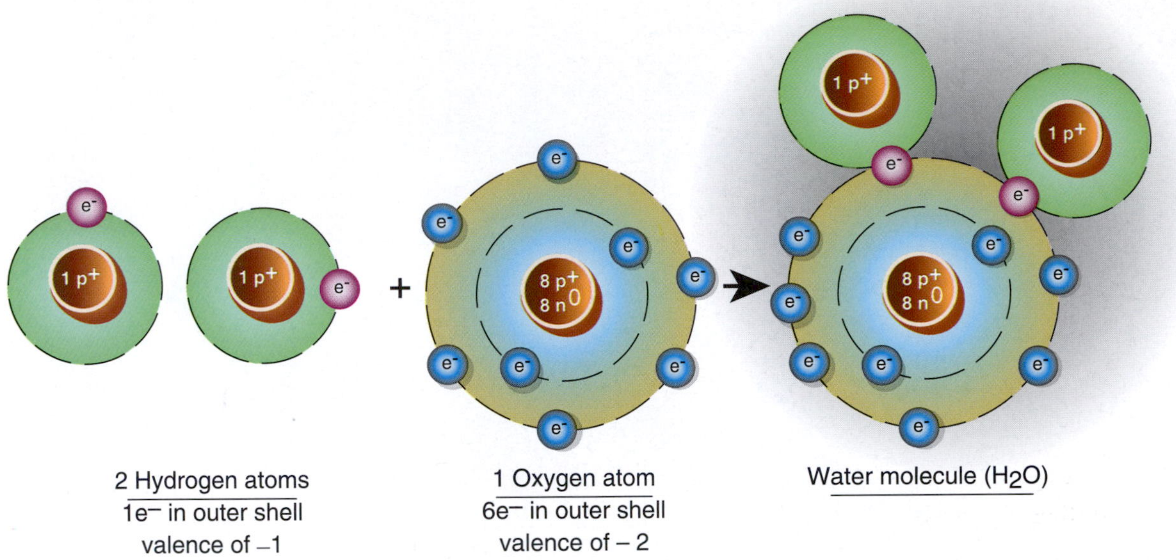

FIGURE 2-10. A covalent bond is formed between two hydrogen atoms and one oxygen atom to form water, H_2O.

TYPES OF ENERGY

Energy is the ability to do work. It exists in many different forms. Regardless of form, all types of energy possess an actual or potential ability to do work. Work is the result of a force acting upon an object over a distance. It is expressed in the equation **work = force × distance**. When a force acts upon an object over a distance, energy is expended. For example, when a book is lifted 1 foot above a table, work is done and energy is expended. If the same book is lifted 2 feet above the table, twice as much work and energy are expended.

Mechanical

Mechanical energy is the result of the action of machines or physical movement. There are two types of mechanical energy: potential and kinetic. **Potential energy** is the energy that an object has because of its position. It is stored, by virtue of its position, in the object until it is converted to another form of energy. A car located at the top of a hill possesses more potential energy than the same car located at the bottom of a hill. If the car's brakes are released, the potential energy is then converted to kinetic energy as the car moves to the bottom of the hill (and a lower energy state). **Kinetic energy** is the energy of motion. An object in motion is able to perform work because it is moving. For example, the energy of water as it moves in a river can be used to perform work. When a dam is built across a river, the kinetic energy of the moving water can be used to produce electric energy. No electricity will be produced if the water is not moving.

Chemical

Chemical energy is the form of energy released during a chemical reaction. A battery operates using chemical energy. The purpose of a battery is to convert chemical energy into electrical energy.

Heat

Heat, also called **thermal energy**, is the result of the motion of atoms and molecules. The faster the atoms and molecules within a substance are moving or vibrating, the greater the thermal energy of the substance. **Temperature** is a measure of thermal energy. As the temperature of a substance increases, the motion of the atoms in the substance increases. When a pan of water is placed on an electric burner, the electrical energy is converted to heat energy, which raises the temperature of the water and increases the motion of its atoms and molecules.

Electrical

Electrical energy, or **electricity**, is the result of the movement of electrons (electrical charges). Electricity is the study of resting or moving electrical charges. Numerous appliances operate by the use of electrical energy. When a lamp is turned on, a flow of electrons passes along a wire in a light bulb. The light bulb is a device that converts electrical energy to light, which is a form of electromagnetic energy. In a toaster, electrical energy is converted to heat, or thermal energy.

Nuclear

Nuclear energy is stored in the nucleus of each atom and holds the nuclear particles in a tight bond. A tremendous amount of energy is stored in the nucleus of an atom. In the 1940s scientists working at the University of Chicago learned how to control the release of this energy and, as a result of this knowledge, developed the atomic bomb. Today, nuclear power plants convert nuclear energy, within a very controlled environment, to electricity.

Electromagnetic

Electromagnetic energy is a form of energy that is the result of electric and magnetic disturbances in space (Figure 2-11). This type of energy travels through space as a combination of electric and magnetic fields and is produced by the acceleration of a charge. There are many familiar forms of electromagnetic energy, including radio waves, microwaves, infrared light, visible light, and cosmic rays. X-rays are a form of man-made electromagnetic energy that is created in an x-ray tube when high-speed electrons are suddenly stopped. Physically they are identical to gamma rays, differing only in origin. Gamma rays originate from the nucleus of radioactive materials, whereas x-rays originate in an x-ray tube.

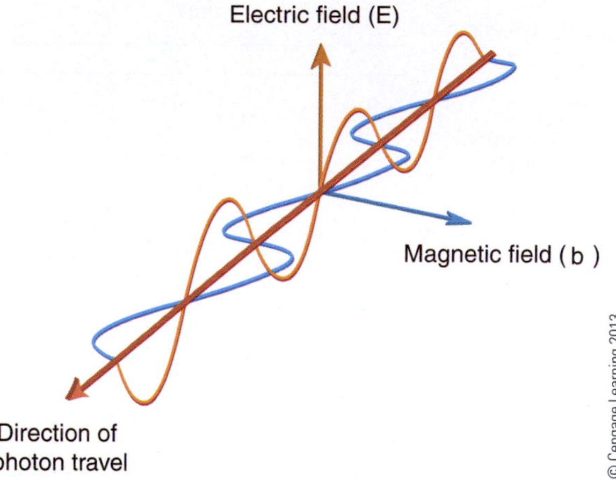

FIGURE 2-11. Overlapping sine waves, one representing an electric field and the other a magnetic field, illustrate electromagnetic radiation.

ELECTROMAGNETIC SPECTRUM

Electromagnetic radiation (EM) is a natural part of the environment in which we live. Although the term may not be a common one, we are all familiar with many forms of this energy. The nature of electromagnetic radiation was discovered in scientific experiments using visible light. Visible light was shown to have both electric and magnetic properties and was therefore described as being electromagnetic. Shortly after these investigations, other forms of electromagnetic radiation, invisible to humans, were studied and a theory to explain this form of energy was proposed.

Electromagnetic radiation spans a continuum of wide ranges of magnitudes of energy. This continuum is termed the **electromagnetic spectrum** (Figure 2-12). The electromagnetic spectrum details all of the various forms of EM radiation. One of the common properties of all forms of EM radiation is velocity. The velocity of EM energy is equal to the speed of light (c), which is 3×10^8 meters/second (186,400 miles per second) in a vacuum.

Electromagnetic radiation with energies of approximately 10 eV and higher is capable of ionizing an atom or molecule. Ultraviolet, x-ray, and gamma radiations are all capable of ionization. When they

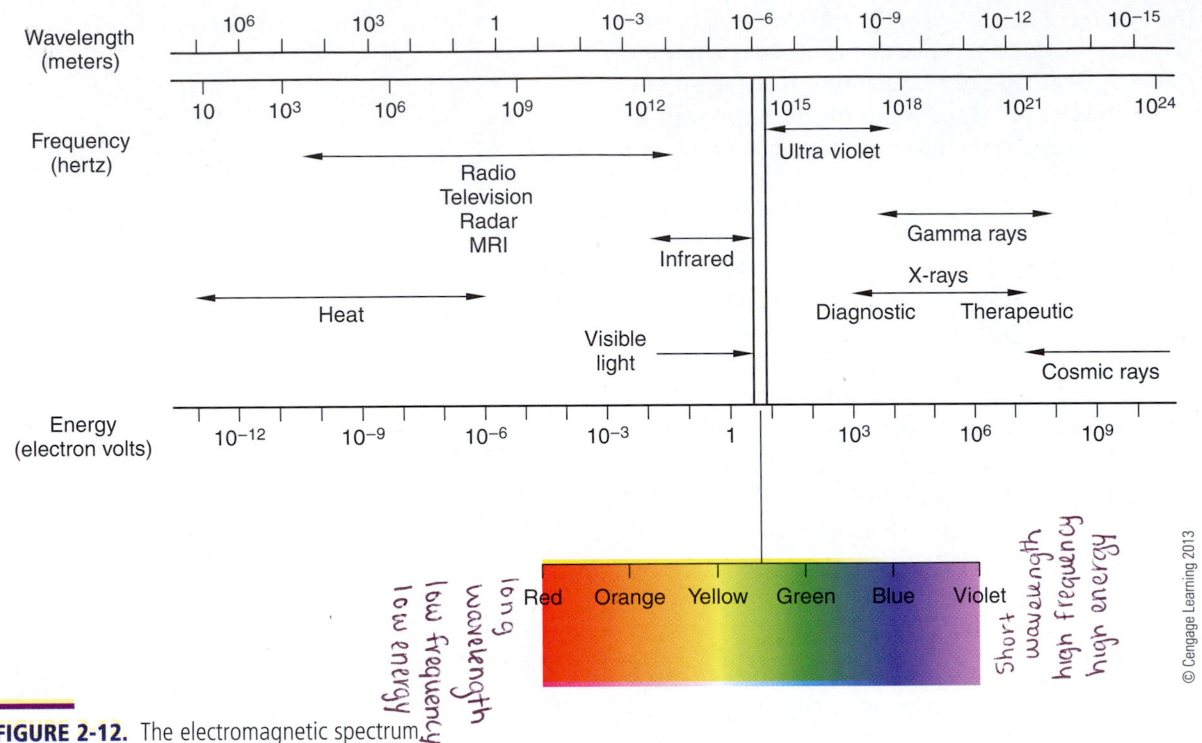

FIGURE 2-12. The electromagnetic spectrum.

interact with matter, they can remove an electron from an orbital shell. Electromagnetic radiation is also capable of transferring energy to an atom by a process known as **excitation**. In the excitation process, electrons in an atom are moved to a higher energy state without actually being removed from the atom.

In studying EM radiation, scientists found that under certain circumstances it behaved as a wave and at other times it behaved as a particle. **This dual nature is known as the wave-particle duality of radiation. To best understand x-rays, it is necessary to consider them as both waves and particles of energy.**

Wave Theory

Electromagnetic energy travels through space in the form of waves. Waves are disturbances in a medium. Ocean waves and sound waves are examples of disturbances of the mediums of water and air. When a rock is dropped into water, waves result. During speech, sound waves are created as disturbances in the air. Electromagnetic waves are unique in that no medium is required. They can travel in a vacuum.

All types of waves have an associated wavelength, frequency, amplitude, and period. To illustrate the wave concept, a sine wave is used because electromagnetic waves travel in the form of a sine wave (Figure 2-13). Sine waves can be mathematically described, but these definitions are beyond the scope of this book. Instead, we will use the primary descriptions of electromagnetic waves: wavelength and frequency. The **wavelength** is the distance between any two successive points on a wave. Wavelength is usually measured from crest to crest or trough to trough. It is represented by the Greek letter **lambda** (λ), the character for length. Wavelengths vary from kilometers to Angstroms. The Angstrom (represented by the symbol Å) is equal to 10^{-10} meters, which is one ten-billionth of a meter. The Angstrom is of special interest because the wavelength of diagnostic x-rays is 0.1–0.5 Å. **Amplitude** is the intensity of the wave defined by its maximal height.

The **frequency** is the number of waves that passes a particular point in a given time frame, or

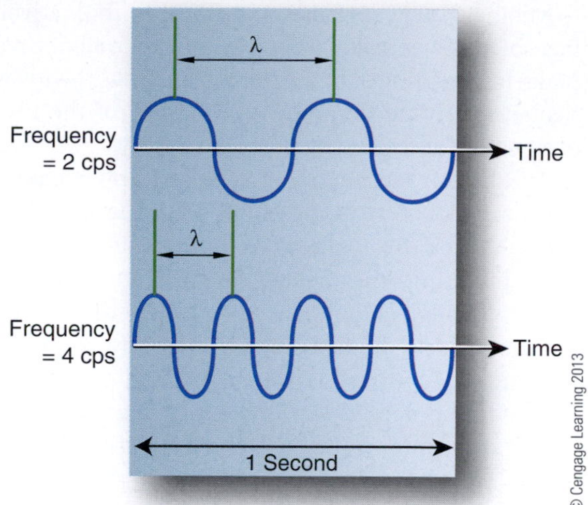

FIGURE 2-13. Two sine waves. With electromagnetic waves, if wavelength decreases, frequency will decrease.

the number of cycles per second. It is represented by the Greek letter **nu** (υ), the initial for number. The unit of frequency is the hertz (Hz) or cycles per second (cps). **Period** is the time required to complete one cycle of the wave.

A relationship exists between the frequency, wavelength, and velocity of a wave. This relationship is expressed by the formula:

velocity = frequency × wavelength,
or $c = \upsilon\lambda$

where: c = constant (the speed of light)

υ = the frequency

λ = the wavelength

This is known as the wave equation. Recall that with electromagnetic waves, velocity was a constant equal to the speed of light. Because velocity is a constant, an increase in frequency would result in an associated decrease in wavelength and vice versa. Therefore, **frequency and wavelength are inversely proportional.**

Radiation along the electromagnetic spectrum will vary according to the associated frequency and wavelength. Low frequencies and long wavelengths are at the bottom end of the spectrum with radio waves and microwaves, visible light is in the center of the spectrum, and at the top of the spectrum are gamma and x-rays, with associated high frequencies and short wavelengths.

Particle Theory

When high-frequency electromagnetic radiation interacts with matter, it behaves more like a particle than a wave. With this model, electromagnetic radiation acts like a small bundle of energy, known as a **photon** or **quantum**. The photon carries a specific amount of energy that is dependent on frequency. **Photon energy and frequency are directly proportional.** If the frequency of an x-ray is doubled, the energy is doubled. This relationship was first described by the German physicist Max Planck (1858–1947). The relationship between photon energy and frequency is mathematically described in the formula:

$$E = h\lambda$$

where: E = photon energy (eV)
h = Planck's constant (4.15×10^{-15} eV-sec)
λ = photon frequency (Hz)

From this formula, it is possible to calculate the frequency of an x-ray when given the x-ray photon's energy.

EXAMPLE: What is the frequency of a 72 keV x-ray photon?

Answer:

$$E = h\upsilon$$

$$v = \frac{E}{h}$$

$$v = \frac{72 \text{ keV}}{4.15 \times 10^{-15} \text{ eV-sec}}$$

$$v = \frac{7.2 \times 10^{4} \text{ eV}}{4.15 \times 10^{-15} \text{ eV-sec}}$$

$$v = 1.73 \times 10^{19} \text{Hz}$$

THE DISCOVERY OF X-RAYS

On November 8, 1895, the German physicist Wilhelm Conrad Röntgen discovered an unusual phenomenon while working in his laboratory at the University of Würzburg. Röntgen had been repeating various experiments with cathode rays, notably those of his colleagues Hertz, Hittorf, Crookes, and Lenard. These investigators had developed equipment for exploring the effects of high-tension discharges in evacuated glass tubes. By late 1895, this small group of physicists was beginning to explore the properties of cathode rays outside the tubes. Early in November of 1895, Röntgen was repeating an experiment with one of Lenard's tubes in which a thin aluminum window had been added to permit the cathode rays to exit the tube. Lenard had supplied the tube with a tightly fitting cardboard covering to protect the aluminum window from damage by the strong electrostatic field necessary to produce the cathode rays. This covering also prevented any visible light from escaping. Röntgen had successfully repeated the experiment and had observed that the invisible cathode rays caused a fluorescent effect on a small cardboard screen painted with barium platinocyanide when it was placed very close to the aluminum window.

It occurred to Röntgen that the Hittorf-Crookes tube, which had a much thicker glass wall than the Lenard tube, might also cause this fluorescent effect. In the late afternoon of November 8, he determined to test his idea. He carefully constructed a black cardboard covering similar to the one he had used on the Lenard tube. He covered the Hittorf-Crookes tube with the covering and attached electrodes to the Ruhmkorff coil to generate an electrostatic charge. Before setting up the barium platinocyanide screen to test his idea, Röntgen darkened the room to test the opacity of his cardboard cover. As he passed the Ruhmkorff coil charge through the tube, he determined that the cover was light-tight and turned to prepare the next step of the experiment. It was at this point that he noticed a faint shimmering from a bench a meter away from the tube. To be sure, he tried several more discharges and saw the same shimmering effect each time. Striking a match, Röntgen discovered the shimmering had come from the location of the barium platinocyanide screen he had been intending to use next.

Röntgen spent the next few hours repeating the experiment again and again. He quickly determined that the screen would fluoresce at a distance from the tube much greater than in his previous tests. He speculated that a new kind of ray might be responsible. November 8 was a Friday, and Röntgen took advantage of the weekend to repeat his experiments and make his first notes. In the following weeks, he investigated nearly all the known properties of the rays, even eating and sleeping in his laboratory.

Röntgen's discovery of x-rays was no accident, and he was not working alone. With the investigations he and his colleagues in various countries were pursuing, the discovery was imminent. The idea that he just happened to notice the barium platinocyanide screen totally misrepresents his investigative powers. He had planned to use the screen in the next step of the experiment.

At one point while he was investigating the ability of various materials to stop the rays, he brought a small piece of lead into position while a discharge was occurring. Imagine Röntgen's astonishment as he saw the first radiographic image, his own flickering ghostly skeleton, on the barium platinocyanide screen. He later reported that it was at this point that he determined to continue his experiments in secrecy, because he feared for his professional reputation if his observations were in error.

Röntgen became the first radiographer when he produced a series of four photographs to accompany the first draft of his paper: the hand of his wife (Figure 2-14), a set of weights, a compass, and a piece of metal. Röntgen's original paper, "On a New Kind of Rays," was published 50 days later on December 28. It is translated in Appendix A. Röntgen assigned the mathematical term for an unknown, X, to the rays he discovered. In later years they were officially given his name to honor his work. Today, either term, x-rays or Röntgen rays, is acceptable. Röntgen published a total of three papers on x-rays between 1895 and 1897. His investigative powers were so phenomenal that none of his conclusions have yet been proven false. Röntgen received many honors for his discovery, including, in 1901, the first Nobel Prize for physics. He died of carcinoma of the bowel in 1923.

X-RAY PROPERTIES

When Röntgen began his study of the invisible x-rays, it was unlikely that he would be able to identify all of the properties of this new discovery. Röntgen's investigation was so thorough, however,

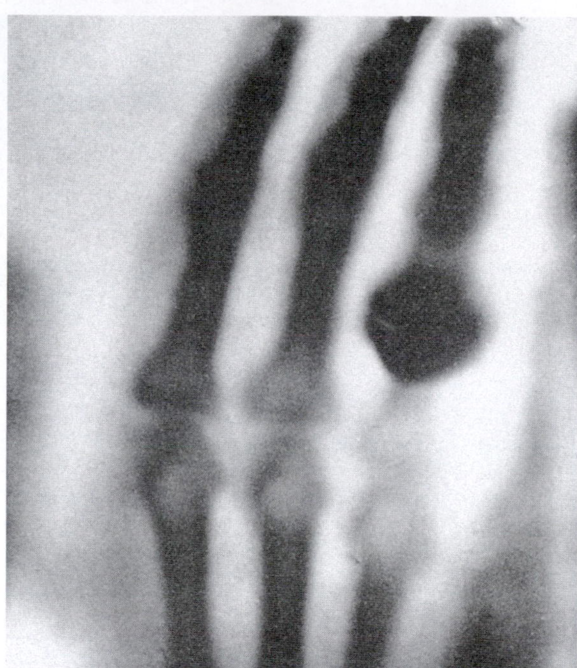

FIGURE 2-14. The first x-ray image of the human hand. The radiograph was taken by Röntgen of his wife's hand. *(Courtesy of American College of Radiology, Chantilly, VA.)*

that no scientist since has been able to add to the list of properties Röntgen identified.

Through his use of the scientific method, Röntgen found that x-rays:

1. Are highly penetrating, invisible rays that are a form of electromagnetic radiation.
2. Are electrically neutral and therefore not affected by either electric or magnetic fields.
3. Can be produced over a wide variety of energies and wavelengths (polyenergetic and heterogeneous).
4. Release very small amounts of heat upon passing through matter.
5. Travel in straight lines.
6. Travel at the speed of light, 3×10^8 meters per second in a vacuum.
7. Can ionize matter.
8. Cause fluorescence (the emission of light) of certain crystals.
9. Cannot be focused by a lens.
10. Affect photographic film.
11. Produce chemical and biological changes in matter through ionization and excitation.
12. Produce secondary and scatter radiation.

SUMMARY

The physical universe can best be understood through physics—the study of matter and energy and their interrelationships. Matter is the substance that comprises all physical objects. The smallest subdivision of matter is the atom, which is comprised of three basic subatomic particles: the proton, the neutron, and the electron. Energy is the ability to do work. There are many forms of energy, including x-rays, which are a form of electromagnetic radiation. Matter and energy cannot be created or destroyed but are interchangeable, as described in Einstein's theory of relativity ($E = mc^2$).

The atom is best described as having a small, dense center, known as the nucleus, that is surrounded by electrons located within orbital shells. Protons and neutrons are located within the nucleus and are responsible for almost all of the mass of an atom. The electron is located outside the nucleus and has a relatively insignificant mass. Protons possess a positive charge, electrons possess a negative charge, and neutrons are electrically neutral.

Each of the elements has its own specific number of nuclear protons. This is the key characteristic that distinguishes one element from another. The number of nuclear protons in an atom is known as the atomic number or Z number. The periodic table lists the elements in ascending order according to the element's atomic number.

Electromagnetic radiation behaves as both a wave and a particle. As a wave, EM radiation has an associated frequency and wavelength. As a particle, it behaves

SUMMARY (continued)

as a bundle of energy, called a photon. X-rays are a man-made form of electromagnetic radiation that is created when high-speed electrons are suddenly stopped. X-rays were discovered by Wilhelm Conrad Röntgen on November 8, 1895, in Germany. From his thorough investigation, 12 properties of x-rays were identified. ■

REVIEW QUESTIONS

1. What are the two major branches of natural science?
2. How do matter and energy differ?
3. Define an atom and a molecule.
4. What are the three basic subatomic particles?
5. What is ionization?
6. What is the formula used to determine the maximum number of electrons that can be contained in a given shell? How many electrons can be contained in the N-shell?
7. The periodic table of elements arranges the elements into periods and groups. How are the elements similar within each period? Within each group?
8. How do radiations differ along the electromagnetic spectrum?
9. List five types of energy.
10. For electromagnetic radiation, what is the relationship between frequency and wavelength? Between frequency and photon energy?
11. List five properties of x-rays.

REFERENCES AND RECOMMENDED READING

Ball, J. L., & Moore, A. D. (2008). *Essential physics for radiographers* (4th ed.). Oxford: Wiley-Blackwell Scientific.

Bushberg, J. T., Seibert, J. A., Leidholdt, E. M., & Boone, J. M. (2003). *The essential physics of medical imaging* (2nd ed.). Philadelphia: Lippincott, Williams & Wilkins.

Bushong, S. C. (2008). *Radiologic science for technologists: Physics, biology, and protection* (9th ed.). St. Louis, MO: Elsevier Mosby.

Curry, T. S., Dowdey, J. E., & Murry, R. C. (1990). *Christensen's introduction to the physics of diagnostic radiology* (4th ed.). Philadelphia: Lea and Febiger.

Eisenberg, R. L. (1992). *Radiology: An illustrated history*. St. Louis, MO: Elsevier C. V. Mosby.

Fuchs, A. W. (1960). Radiography of 1896. *Image*, *9*, 4–17.

Glasser, O. (1958). *Dr. W. C. Röntgen* (2nd ed.). Springfield, IL: Charles C Thomas.

Handbook of chemistry and physics (78th ed.). (1998). Boca Raton, FL: CRC Press.

Hennig, U. (1989). *Deutsches Röntgen-Museum Remscheid-Lennep*. Remscheid, Germany: Westermann.

Meredith, W. J., & Massey, J. B. (1977). *Fundamental physics of radiology* (3rd ed.). Chicago: Yearbook Medical.

Röntgen, W. C. (1896). On a new kind of rays. *Science*, *3*(59), 227–231.

Röntgen, W. C. (1896). On a new kind of rays. *Nature*, *53*(1369), 274–276.

Selman, J. C. (2000). *The fundamentals of imaging physics and radiobiology: For the radiologic technologists* (9th ed.). Springfield, IL: Charles C Thomas.

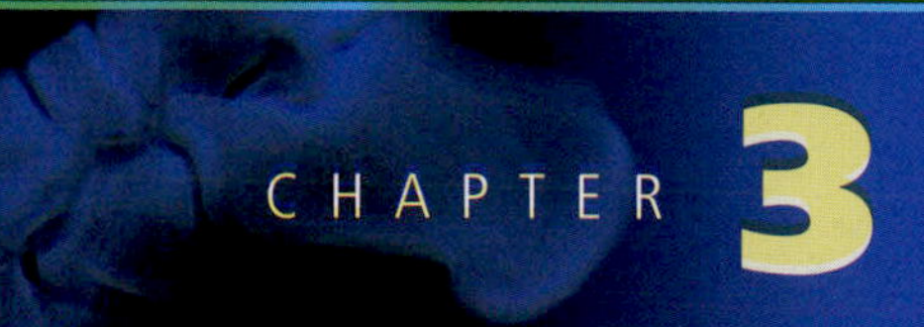

Electricity

KEY TERMS

admittance
alternating current (AC)
amp (A)
ampere (A)
atomic reactor
battery
circuit breaker
concentration
conductance
conduction band
conductor
contact
current
direct current (DC)
distribution
electrical circuit
electric current
electric field
electrification
electromotive force (emf)
electrostatics
friction
fuse
gasses
generator
induction
insulator

> The experience of life itself is the real test … for any … profession.
>
> *W. C. Röntgen*

OBJECTIVES

Upon completion of this chapter, the student should be able to:

- Explain the atomic nature of electricity.
- State the elementary laws of electrostatics.
- Describe the methods of electrification.
- Interpret the results of various electrostatic interactions.
- Differentiate conductors from insulators.
- Describe the basic factors of electrodynamics.
- Calculate the effect of changes in voltage, amperage, and resistance according to Ohm's law.
- Calculate voltage, amperage, and resistance in simple series and parallel circuits.

KEY TERMS (continued)

inverse square law
ionic solution
laws of electrostatics
metallic conductor
milliamperage (mA)
movement
negative charge
ohm (Ω)
parallel circuit
positive charge
potential difference
potentiometer
power loss formula
repulsion-attraction
resistance
rheostat
semiconductor
series circuit
solar converter
static discharge
superconductor
vacuum
valence energy band
volt
voltage (V)
zero or ground potential

To control x-rays it is necessary to understand how they are produced. X-rays are produced when extremely high-energy electricity produces high-speed electrons that interact with matter. Electricity must be understood at the subatomic level for this process to become clear. The distribution and movement of electrons, along with their associated charges, make up electricity. Understanding atomic structure, including how electrons interact both in and outside of atoms, becomes the key to understanding electricity. It is the distribution and movement of atomic charges that can cause forces to interact.

Atoms contain both kinds of electrical charges, the **positive charge** of the proton, which is locked within the nucleus by very strong forces, and the **negative charge** of the electron, which is located outside the nucleus, bound by relatively weak forces. Electrons may not be associated with a nucleus at all, in which case they are called "free" electrons. In either case, **the positive charge of the proton and the negative charge of the electron are equal in strength.** Because electrons, with their negative charges, are free to move between atomic orbital shells and even between atoms, electricity concerns the distribution and movement of electrons and has little to do with the positively charged protons locked within the atomic nucleus.

ELECTROSTATICS

Electrostatics is the study of the distribution of fixed charges, or electrons that are at rest. Just as all atoms are charged (neutral, positive, negative), objects become charged by their composite individual atomic charges. Some atoms include electrons in their outer shells, or beyond the outer shell but within the atom's sphere of influence, that are very easily removed. There are instances, as when walking across a heavy rug in winter, when electrons are easily transferred (literally scooped up) onto another object. It is this type of distribution and redistribution of charged electrons that makes up electrostatics.

The term **electrification** is used to describe the process of electron charges being added to or subtracted from an object. When one object has more electrons than another, it also has more negative charges. Therefore, it can be considered to be negatively electrified, or to have a negative charge. The concept of positive electrification, a positive charge, is more complicated because protons, which carry true positive charges, are not easily distributed. Therefore, a positive charge usually refers to something with a weaker negative charge, or fewer electrons. The so-called positively electrified, or charged, object has a negative charge; it is just a weaker negative charge than the object with which it is being compared. It is less negative, and therefore termed positive, by comparison. It is important to remember that electrification is a relative term and that nearly all objects have negative charges. **When discussing electricity, the terms *negative* and *positive* refer to the relationship between two objects, not to their true atomic charges.**

In conjunction with the idea that negative and positive charges are relative to each other, another concept is required in order to establish a neutral reference point. This is done by defining the earth as **zero or ground potential**. Because the earth contains what is essentially an infinite number of charges, both positive and negative, in equal distribution, it is considered to be neutral and is the reference point for discussing charges. It has zero potential because the equally balanced charges have no potential to perform work and release energy. The symbol for ground is ⏚.

Laws of Electrostatics

Before attempting to understand how objects are electrified, it is helpful to learn five fundamental **laws of electrostatics**. These important laws have many corollaries in physics and will be used again and again throughout this book. The five laws are:

1. **Repulsion-attraction** (Figure 3-1). Like charges repel; unlike charges attract.
2. The **inverse square law** (Figure 3-2). The force between two charges is directly proportional to the product of their magnitudes and inversely proportional to the square of the distance between them. As a charged object gets further away, the influencing charge decreases because of the increased area it affects. The law is expressed as:

$$\frac{I_1}{I_2} = \frac{D_2^{\,2}}{D_1^{\,2}}$$

where: I_1 = old intensity
I_2 = new intensity
$D_1^{\,2}$ = old distance squared
$D_2^{\,2}$ = new distance squared

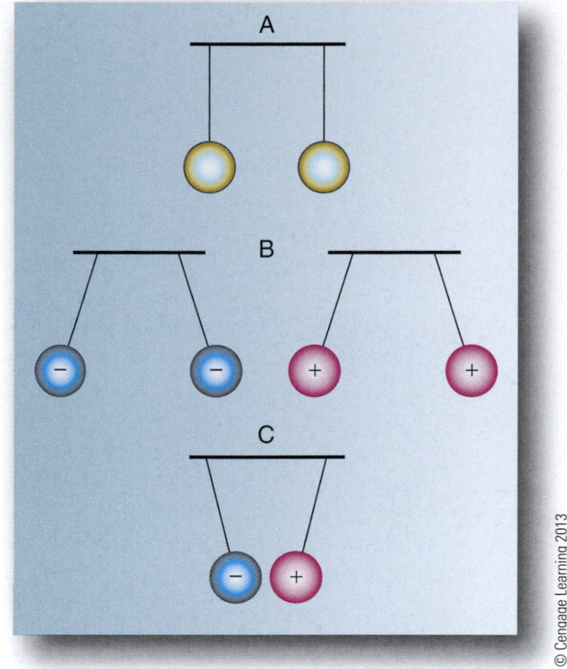

FIGURE 3-1 Repulsion-attraction law: (A) neutral charge; (B) repulsion of like charges; and (C) attraction of unlike charges.

EXAMPLE: If an object has a charge of 4 coulombs at 4 mm, what will the charge be at 8 mm?

Answer:

$$\frac{I_1}{I_2} = \frac{D_2^{\,2}}{D_1^{\,2}}$$

$$\frac{4\text{ coulombs}}{x} = \frac{(8\text{ mm})^2}{(4\text{ mm})^2}$$

$$\frac{4}{x} = \frac{64}{16}$$

$$64x = 64$$

$$x = 1\text{ coulomb}$$

In this example, as the distance doubled, the charge was reduced to 25 percent of its original value. Although this inverse square formula is usually sufficient for radiographic needs, it is

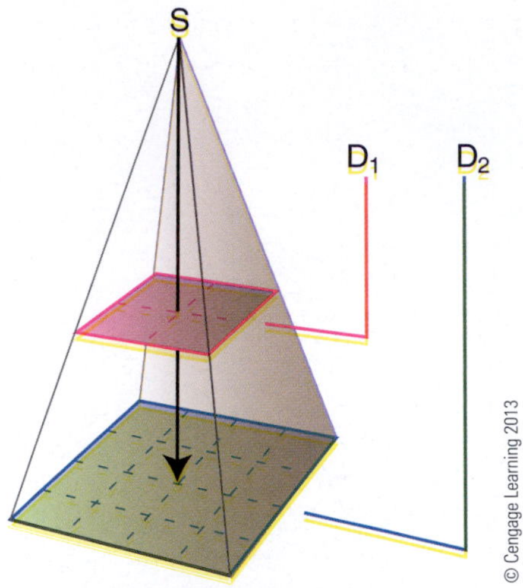

FIGURE 3-2 The inverse square law: If S is the source and D_2 is twice the distance of D_1, the area covered by the diverging field at D_2 is four times the area covered at D_1.

important to understand that the true relationship of the force between two charges is accurately expressed in Coulomb's law:

$$F = \frac{kq_1q_2}{R^2}$$

where: F = electrostatic force in newtons
k = constant of proportionality (9×10^9 for coulombs and meters)
q_1 and q_2 = charges in coulombs
R = distance in meters

This formula takes into account the true definition: the force between two charges (q_1 and q_2) is directly proportional to the product of their magnitudes ($q_1 \times q_2$), and inversely proportional to the square of the distance between them [$(q_1 \times q_2)/R^2$]. Ironically, although the French physicist Coulomb (1736–1806) received the credit for development of this law, the original inquiry was initiated by the American scientist Benjamin Franklin (1706–1790).

3. **Distribution** (Figure 3-3). Charges reside on the external surfaces of conductors and equally throughout nonconductors. This law is a result of the effect of the repulsion-attraction law, as electrons, all with negative charges, attempt to repel each other as much as possible. In a solid conductor this results in equal distribution on the surface, which is the point where electrons can obtain maximum distance from each other. In a nonconductor, such as a cloud, charge movement is not facilitated and equal distribution throughout the object results.

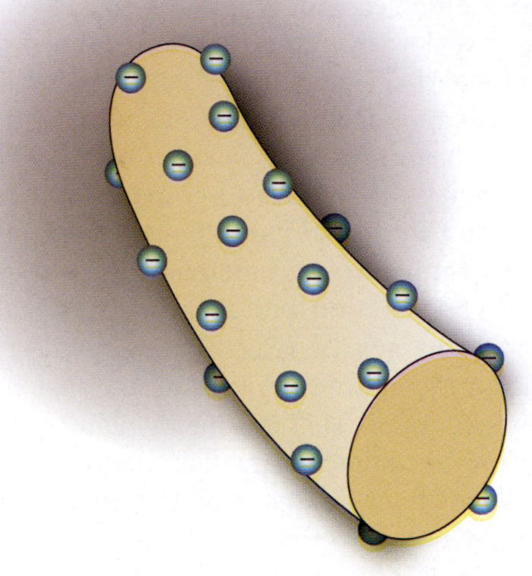

FIGURE 3-3 The law of distribution of charge: As individual electrons are repelled from one another, they distribute at the outer limits of a conductor.

4. **Concentration** (Figure 3-4). The greatest concentration of charge will be on the surface where the curvature is sharpest. If enough electrons congregate they can induce ionization of the surrounding air and even discharge to the nearest point of lower concentration. Therefore, x-ray tubes, which are subjected to extremely high charges, must not have sharp or rough edges where concentrations of electrons could occur and discharge at the wrong moment or in an undesirable direction. Consequently, the interior components of x-ray tubes are rounded and highly polished to eliminate sharply curved surfaces.
5. **Movement**. Only negative charges move along solid conductors. Because the positive charges, the protons, are tightly bound inside

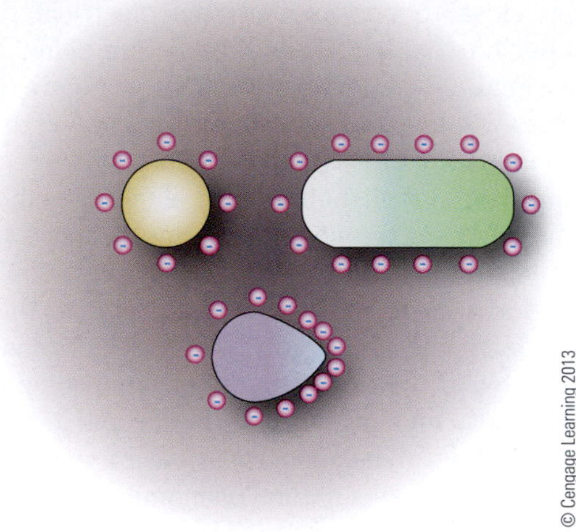

FIGURE 3-4 The law of concentration of charge: Because each negative charge is repelled by all other negative charges, they tend to concentrate at points of greatest curvature.

the atomic nuclear field, only the electrons, which exist outside the nucleus, are easily moved along conductors.

Electrification

Objects can be electrified by three methods: **friction**, **contact**, and **induction**.

Friction. Electrification by friction occurs when one object is rubbed against another and, due to differences in the number of electrons available on each, electrons travel from one to the other. Ideal conditions for electron transfer occur during cold weather when low humidity removes stabilizing electrons from the air, decreasing the resistance to electron movement between objects. An example is a common trick that delights children—rubbing a balloon against a wool sweater will permit the balloon to stick to a wall. In low humidity, electrons will transfer from the wool to the balloon, giving it a negative charge, which can cause it to stick to a smooth wall with a relatively positive charge. This is an example of opposites attracting one another. A common example of like charges repelling one another occurs when hair is electrified by friction during combing in low-humidity conditions. The comb removes electrons from the strands of hair, often accompanied by crackling sounds, leaving each more positively charged. The strands are then repelled by those adjoining, which now also have stronger positive charges. The result is wild strands of hair standing straight out from your head. The solution to the problem is to increase the humidity, or the amount of water in the air, causing a slight condensation on all surfaces. This thin film of moisture becomes a pathway for the distribution of electrons. The use of a humidifier in a radiographic darkroom during cold weather thus helps eliminate electrostatic discharges that can cause artifacts on film.

Contact. Electrification by contact occurs when two objects touch, permitting electrons to move from one to the other. This process is a simple equalization of charges, with both objects having similar charges after the contact. Walking across a woolen carpet in a room with low humidity may cause shoes to scoop electrons from the carpet fibers that are then distributed over the entire body. This is an example of electrification by friction. However, when a positively charged object with fewer electrons is touched, the contact will cause electrons to move to the less negatively charged object in an attempt to equally distribute the charges. A metal doorknob or another person are examples of positively charged objects that would attract electrons from a person who had just walked across a rug. After the contact, both objects would have a more equal distribution of electrons. This is caused by the individual force fields of the electrons satisfying the repulsion-attraction law over the entire surface of the conductors. In many instances, actual physical contact does not occur before the electrons equalize. As soon as the oppositely charged objects are in close proximity, the electrons often jump the gap in the form of a **static discharge**. This occurs as soon as the difference in charges becomes sufficiently great and the intervening distance sufficiently small. In most cases the static discharge releases excess energy in the form of light photons.

An electroscope is a simple device that illustrates the laws of electrostatics. It consists of a rod connected to a pair of thin, easily charged metallic leaves, which are protected from air currents by a glass flask (Figure 3-5A). When a charged object (such as the metallic rod shown in Figure 3-5B) is

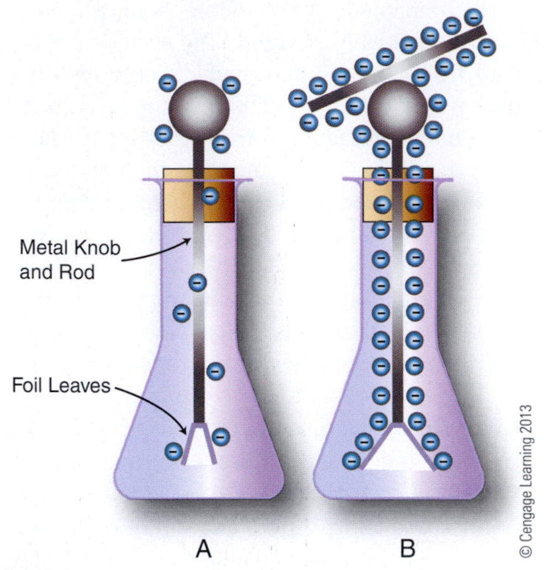

FIGURE 3-5 Charging an electroscope by contact: Electrons distribute equally when they are permitted to move from one object (the road) to another (the electroscope) by contact.

brought into contact with the rod, the excess electrons obey the third law of electrostatics and distribute equally throughout the rod and leaves. The resultant increase in the number of electrons present on both leaves causes the two leaves to obey the first law of electrostatics and, because they possess like charges, repel each other. Consequently, it is possible to see the two leaves move further apart.

If an electroscope is subjected to an intense beam of ionizing x-ray photons, the air becomes ionized. The ionized atoms draw electrons from the leaves, thus causing the charge on the leaves to be reduced. Consequently, the electroscope leaves relax and move closer together.

Induction. Electrification by induction is the most important method because it is the one used in the operation of electronic devices. **Induction is the process of electrical fields acting on one another without contact.** Every charged body is surrounded by a force field, much like the fields that surround individual atoms. Like atoms, force fields are a result of the composite forces of the charges residing within the object. These force fields are called electric fields and they can cause induction. When a strongly and a weakly charged object come close to one another, the electrical fields will begin to act on one another before contact occurs (Figure 3-6A). As can be seen in Figure 3-6B, charges will migrate to one end of an object as the force field interacts with them. However, as seen in Figure 3-6C, when the stronger object is removed before contact, the charges in the weaker object will redistribute themselves as they were before the induction occurred. This temporarily induced movement of charges is useful in many electronic devices, such as motors, transformers, and solenoids.

With an understanding of friction and induction electrification, it becomes possible to understand one of the greatest of natural phenomena—lightning. Lightning discharges occur as the masses of atoms making up the water vapor in clouds move rapidly through the atmosphere. Under conditions where many electrons are available, such as when there are numerous storm clouds, the movement of the water vapor atoms tends to cause electrons to be picked up or lost. As an individual cloud becomes predominantly positively or negatively charged, it becomes a candidate for a huge electrostatic discharge. Clouds often pick up electrons on their upper edges and lose them on their lower edges and vice versa. In these instances the difference in charges makes the cloud a candidate for a cloud-to-cloud discharge as soon as the insulating effect of the vapor between the two surfaces has been overcome. But the most interesting part of lightning is cloud-to-ground discharges. The ground often develops a temporary opposite charge from the underside of the cloud because of the induction effect of the cloud on the ground. This causes the electrons to spread out, which in turn tends to rapidly increase the difference in charges between cloud and ground and can quickly overcome the insulating effect of the air between the cloud and the ground. The result is lightning discharges occurring much more rapidly than if induction had not taken place. Lightning discharges do not occur as a single transfer of electrons from one area to another. Instead, vast numbers of electrons may be transferred from cloud to ground, overloading the ground, which in turn transfers electrons back to the cloud, which again transfers them to the ground, over and over until the charges are somewhat equally distributed. A short lightning discharge

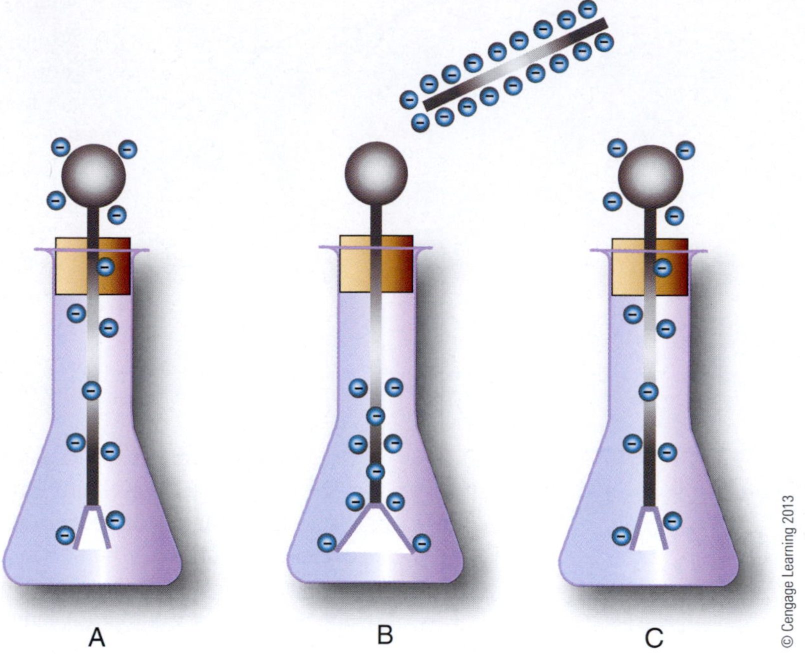

FIGURE 3-6 Charging an electroscope by induction: Electrons are induced to move away from the heavily charged rod (B) but return to their normal distribution when the rod is removed (A and C).

often transfers electrons back and forth between cloud and ground many times within a microsecond.

ELECTRODYNAMICS

Electrons that are moving in predominantly the same direction are often referred to as an **electric current**. Numerous conditions encourage electron movement, thus permitting the flow of electric current. A **vacuum** is a space from which air has been removed. Because it has few atoms to oppose electron flow, it is especially useful in permitting electrons to reach the speed necessary to produce x-rays. Some **gasses** (such as neon) will promote the drift of electrons from a negative electrode (cathode) to a positive electrode (anode). These gasses also promote the drift of positive ions toward the negative cathode while negative ions move toward the positive anode. **Ionic solutions** can cause electrons to migrate to positive or negative poles during electrolysis, when they are subjected to an electric current.

Electrolysis becomes possible when two neutral atoms with complementary valences (e.g., -1 and $+1$) are brought together in a solution. They become ions in the solution when the positive valence atom gives up an outer-shell electron to the negative valence atom. The atom missing an electron becomes a positive ion (because a negative charge has been removed), while the one receiving the electron becomes a negative ion (because a negative charge has been added). When metallic rods are connected to a battery and immersed in the solution, the negative pole will attract the positive ions while the positive pole will attract the negative ions. This migration of electrons during the electrolytic process comprises an electrical current. **Metallic conductors**, such as copper wire, are the most common pathways provided for the movement of electrical current. The atoms of metallic conductors permit valence electrons to drift. In common household wiring the actual physical movement is about 2 mm per second (Figure 3-7). The electrical current, as a whole, is similar to a tube filled with balls, as in Figure 3-8. If the tube is full and

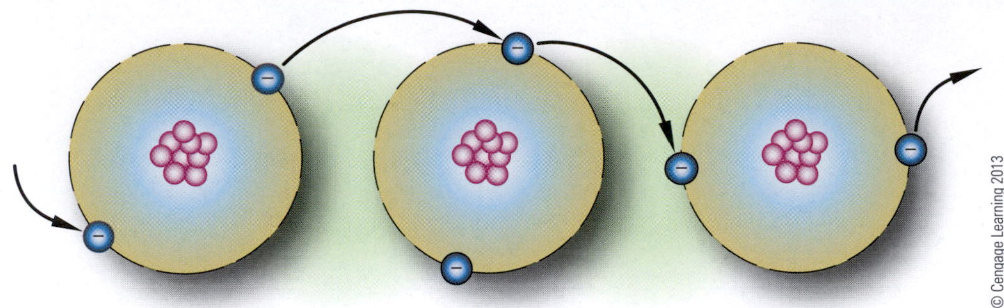

FIGURE 3-7 Electron drift along a conductor.

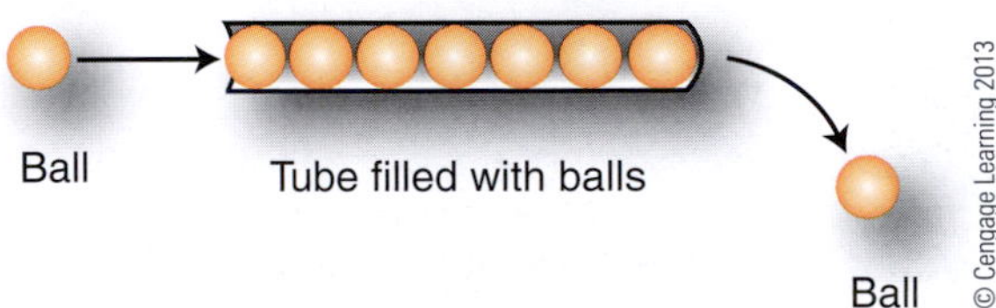

FIGURE 3-8 As when balls are pushed into a tube, each electron needs to move only a short distance for the effect of current movement to be achieved at the other end.

a new ball is pushed into one end, a ball will drop instantly from the far end, although each ball moved or drifted only a short distance. Electrons move along a conductor with a similar domino effect, resulting in movement of electrons at the far end. This movement occurs extremely rapidly, nearly at the speed of light (3×10^8 meters/second).

The movement of electrons is facilitated by materials that easily permit electrons to flow. These materials are called **conductors** and **superconductors**. Examples of conductors are metals such as copper and aluminum. Conversely, electron movement is inhibited by materials that resist the flow of electrons. These nonconducting materials are called **insulators**. Examples of insulators are plastic, rubber, and glass. The third classification of materials is **semiconductors**. They have the ability to conduct under certain conditions and insulate under others. The actual conditions causing these changes in conductivity are complex and are addressed later in this chapter. They result primarily from changes in the energy states of atoms, causing outer-shell electrons to move in a particular direction (Table 3-1).

An **electrical circuit** is a pathway (commonly copper wire) that permits electrons to move in a complete circle from their source, through resisting electrical devices and back to the source. As in electrostatics, an electrical circuit must have an excess charge at one end and a comparative deficiency at the other to allow electrons to flow. There are several sources of the excess electrons necessary to cause current flow. Examples include **batteries**, which convert chemical energy to electrical; **generators**, which convert mechanical energy to electrical; **solar converters**, which convert solar photons to electrical energy; and **atomic reactors**, which convert nuclear energy to electrical. Solar converters remain expensive, and nuclear reactors, although efficient on a large scale, continue to meet significant public opposition. They operate by using the massive energy of the atom to produce steam, which is then used to run turbine generators.

Describing Current Flow

Electrons move from the highest concentration to the lowest. There is much confusion regarding how to describe their movement because early pioneers in electrical phenomena assumed that the moving charges were positive when actually they were negatively charged electrons. The negative pole is the source of electrons that move toward the positive receiving pole. Consequently, **conventional electric current is described as going from positive to negative poles while electron flow is actually from negative to positive poles.**

It is important to specify whether descriptions are of electrical current or electron flow, as they

TABLE 3-1. Properties of Conducting Materials

State	Material	Characteristics
Insulator	Plastic, Rubber, Glass	Large energy difference between conduction and valence bands; resists electron flow.
Semiconductor	Silicon, Germanium	Small energy difference between conduction and valence bands; conducts OR resists, depending on temperature and other conditions.
Conductor	Copper, Aluminum	Overlapping conduction and valence bands; conducts with minor resistance, varying depending on temperature and other conditions.
Superconductor	Titanium	Greatly overlapping conduction and valence bands; conducts with little or no electrical potential; most current systems require extreme cold to function although research indicates room-temperature superconductors may be developed soon.

are exact opposites. It may be useful to think of negative charges moving in one direction as being equivalent to a positive charge effect in the opposite direction. The importance of these definitions will become apparent later in this text, especially when discussing the interactions of both electrical and magnetic forces.

The nature of the flow of electrons that make up an electric current can be described in many different ways. The most common factors used as descriptors are the *quantity* of electrons flowing, the *force* with which they travel, the amount of *opposition* to the current flow in the circuit, and the *direction* of travel.

The direction of travel of the electrons is defined as either **direct current (DC)**, when all electrons move in the same direction, or **alternating current (AC)**, when electrons move first in one direction and then reverse and move in the opposite direction. Through the use of various electrical devices, which we will investigate later, it is possible to change the current from DC to AC and back, as necessary.

Current

The quantity, or number, of electrons flowing is sometimes referred to as the **current**. It is useful to think of the measurement of current as the number of electrons flowing past a given point per unit of time (usually per second). The French scientist André Ampère (1775–1836) did much original work in defining electricity and magnetism. Consequently, the unit of current bears his name. The **ampere** is sometimes called the **amp** for short and is represented by the symbol **A**. It consists of the movement of **6.24×10^{18} electrons per second** past a given point; therefore, the technical definition is **one coulomb of electrical charge flowing per second (1 ampere = 1 coulomb/1 second).** Earlier, the drift of electrons was given as less than 1 mm per second. The fact that 1 ampere flowing in a household wire causes 6,240,000,000,000,000,000 electrons to move less than 1 mm per second should help in understanding the small size of electrons. Diagnostic radiographic equipment utilizes milliamperage units to regulate the number of electrons available to produce x-ray photons. The **milliamperage (mA)** is found on nearly all x-ray machines and adjustment by the radiographer operating the equipment will cause the number of electrons and the number of x-ray photons produced to vary. The adjustment of an x-ray machine to add an additional 100 mA (a common increment) causes 6.24×10^{17} more electrons per second to pass through the x-ray tube.

> ***EXAMPLE:*** If an x-ray machine is operating at 0.01 second and the amperage is 100 mA, how many electrons would move through the tube?
>
> ***Answer:***
>
> $(6.24 \times 10^{17}$ electrons/second$) \times 0.01$ seconds $= 6.24 \times 10^{15}$ (6.24 million billion or 6,240,000,000,000,000

The word *current* is used to describe the presence of electron flow as well as to describe exactly how much current is flowing. It is important to distinguish which use of the word is intended.

Potential Difference

The force with which the electrons travel is a function of the difference between the number of electrons in excess at one end of the circuit and the deficiency at the other end. The attempt of the unequal forces to balance is the cause of the force of electron movement. Because the difference is present while the source is connected into the circuit, **there does not have to be an actual flow of current for the difference to exist.** Therefore, the simple potential for a difference is used to describe the force, or strength of movement, behind electrons.

Potential difference is the best term to describe the force or **strength** of electron flow. It should be remembered that potential difference continues to exist even when a switch is opened in a circuit, breaking the actual flow of electrons (current). Because potential difference is the prime force causing electrical devices to convert electrical energy to mechanical, the term **electromotive force (emf)** has also been used. Electromotive force is actually the total maximum difference of potential between the positive and negative ends of the electron source, but it is not incorrect to use the term in place of potential difference.

The unit of potential difference is the **volt**, represented by the symbol **V** (named for the Italian physicist Alessandro Volta [1745–1827]). The term *voltage* is also used to describe potential difference. The technical definition of a volt is **1 joule (J) of work done on 1 coulomb of charge 1 volt = 1 joule/1 coulomb)**. A joule is the SI unit for both mechanical energy and work.

Thus, for the reasons previously stated, the force with which electrons travel can be described by the terms potential difference, electromotive force (emf), and **voltage (V)**.

As the current flows along the circuit, the potential difference is reduced because the closer the electrons come to the deficient end of the circuit, the farther they are from the excess end (the driving source) and the closer they are to becoming part of the deficiency themselves. With this understanding of potential difference, the concept of grounding electrical circuits for safety should become clear. When equipment is properly grounded and the radiographer, who is also grounded, comes in contact, there is no potential difference. However, when equipment is not properly grounded, the radiographer may become a better path to ground. The passage of electrons (voltage) through the radiographer may be shocking, to say the least.

High voltage is extremely dangerous because there does not have to be an actual flow of current for the potential difference to exist. This means high potential difference or voltage remains a hazard at all times (and explains why warnings must be posted in these areas). All that is required for a high difference in voltage to achieve equalization is for a conductor to present itself. If this happens to be a patient who inadvertently uses a wet hand to grasp a cracked high-voltage cable or a radiographer who touches two connection points inside a control console, the shocking result is the same.

Resistance

The amount of opposition to the current in the circuit is called the **resistance**. Research into the interrelationships of current, potential difference, and resistance was done by the German physicist Georg Ohm (1787–1854). As a result, the unit of resistance is called the **ohm**. It is represented by the symbol Ω (omega). The technical definition of an ohm is the resistance to a flow of current provided by a column of mercury 106.3 cm long with a diameter of 1 mm^2 at 0°C. A practical definition of an ohm will be provided later, based on the interaction of several characteristics of a conductor. Resistance and impedance are the terms used to describe current opposition. There are numerous factors that impede the flow of electrons, thus increasing resistance. The primary factors for electrical circuits are the ability to conduct electrons, the length of the conductor, the cross-sectional diameter, and temperature.

When the expression 1/R is used, the resistance of a DC circuit is measured as **conductance**, whereas that of an AC circuit is measured as

admittance. The SI unit for conductance and admittance is the siemens, which is represented by the symbol S and is named after the English electrical engineer Sir William Siemens (1823–1883), brother of Werner von Siemens, founder of the German electrical and x-ray equipment corporation.

The ability to conduct electrons has already been discussed enough to define a conductor as a material that permits electrons to flow easily, and an insulator as one that inhibits their movement. The tendency of an atom to permit electrons nearby or within one of the orbital shells is the prime factor in determining conductivity, semiconductivity, and insulation properties. The **valence energy band** (the outermost and sometimes next-to-outermost orbital shell) not only determines the chemical properties of the atom, as discussed previously, but has much to do with conductivity as well. Orbital shells lower or closer to the nucleus (and of less energy) than the valence band are normally completely full (Figure 3-9). Valence has much to do with the ability of a material to conduct electrons. Any element with one valence electron is a good conductor (e.g., copper, silver, and gold). In addition, the further the valence electron is from the nucleus, the better a conductor it is. For example, gold is a better conductor than silver because its valence electron is in the sixth shell, while silver's is in the fifth. Silver is a better conductor than copper because copper's valence electron is in the fourth shell. Because copper has a higher melting point and is much cheaper, it is more commonly used than silver or gold.

There is also an area beyond the valence band that is referred to as the **conduction band**. The conduction band is not an orbital shell but is within the force field (area of influence) of the atom (see Figure 3-9). Conductors have conduction bands that are populated by free electrons and, in solid materials, they are able to move freely from one atom's conduction band to another's, as in Figure 3-9C. This is why many of the best conductors are solids. Conversely, insulators have very poor or nonexistent conduction bands. The number of electrons in the conduction band is determined by the energy difference between the valence band and the conduction band. Although the conduction band is always at a higher energy level than the valence band, the energy required of an individual electron to place it in the conduction band will determine how many electrons can possibly exist there. In fact, the difference between the energy levels required of conduction band electrons as compared to valence band electrons is the factor that differentiates conductors from semiconductors from insulators. In Figure 3-9, the differences are shown as (C) a good conductor with overlapping valence

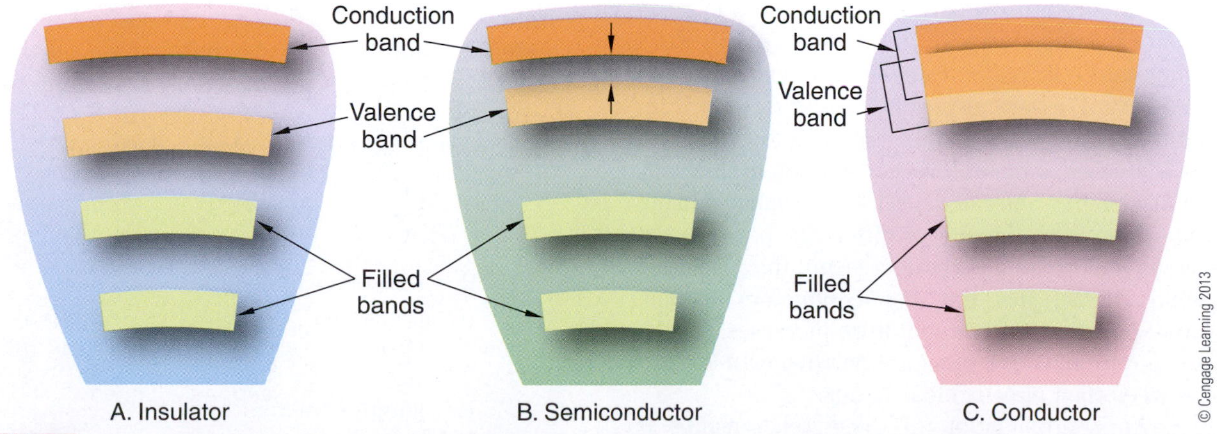

FIGURE 3-9 The arrows demonstrate the difference between the energy levels of conduction and valence bands in an (A) insulator; (B) semiconductor; and (C) conductor. Note that the conduction and valence bands overlap in a good conductor.

and conduction bands; (B) a semiconductor with closely related bands; and (A) a good insulator with a wide gap between the bands. Metals often have overlapping bands with conduction bands, including portions of the valence bands, thus placing large numbers of electrons into the conduction bands. Therefore, metals, especially silver and copper, make the best conductors. The best insulators are materials with complex molecular structures, such as wood, plastic, glass, and rubber.

The length of the conductor has a directly proportional relationship to resistance. In other words, as the length of the conductor doubles, the resistance will also double. Just as a short garden hose will spray water with greater force than a long hose, so a short conductor will permit a greater force of electrons while a longer conductor offers greater resistance.

The cross-sectional diameter of the conductor has an inversely proportional relationship to resistance. In other words, as the cross-sectional diameter doubles, the resistance will be halved. A garden hose with a small diameter will impede water flow more than a large-diameter hose, just as a small-diameter conductor will resist electron flow more than a conductor with a large diameter.

Finally, the temperature of the conductor can also influence the resistance. Heat is simply a measurement of the amount of atomic and molecular energy, often seen as vibration. As temperature increases, atomic collisions provide enough energy to some electrons to permit them to jump into the atom's conduction band. In conductors, increased temperature increases free electron collisions, and this in turn lessens electrical current flow. In insulators the increased number of collisions because of increased temperature causes some electrons to lose energy and fall back into the valence band, thus decreasing the energy difference between the bands and consequently decreasing the insulating ability of the material. Semiconductors become more conductive as temperature increases, for the same reason, with a resultant narrowing of the gap between their already close bands.

An approximation of these relationships is shown in Figure 3-10. A close examination of this figure illustrates that increased resistance from heat is significant. In fact, it becomes a major problem with the large heat-producing transformers used in x-ray equipment, and unique methods have been adopted to overcome its effect. In addition, extrapolation of the conductor curve to the left illustrates that if conductors can be supercooled, as they are in magnetic resonance imaging equipment, a significant increase in conductivity can be achieved.

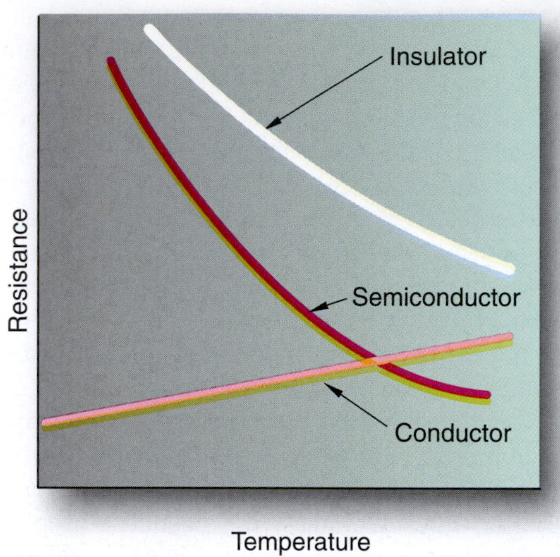

FIGURE 3-10 The effect of temperature on conductors, semiconductors, and insulators.

In recent years, superconductivity has been achieved to reduce resistance to the point where current is apparently flowing without potential difference. Table 3-1 provides information on the conductive properties of materials important in electronics.

The total resistance is calculated as:

$$R = \frac{\rho L}{A}$$

where: R = resistance in ohms
ρ = resistivity (a function of atomic structure and temperature) (ρ is the Greek letter rho)
L = length in meters
A = area in square meters

This total resistance formula is the true technical definition of an ohm as a unit.

Ohm's Law

Georg Ohm discovered a mathematical relationship between the factors of current, potential difference, and resistance that applies to all resistance circuits and is known as Ohm's law. The law describes the relationship between current and potential difference as **the current along a conductor is proportional to the potential difference.** It is easier to remember this relationship as a formula:

$$\frac{V}{I}$$

V = potential difference in volts
I = current in amperes

This expression does not include the resistance factor, which is a critical element. Therefore, Ohm's law is usually expressed as the algebraic derivation with resistance times current equal to potential difference, or:

$$V = IR$$

where: V = potential difference in volts
I = current in amperes
R = resistance in ohms

This version solves for voltage when the current and resistance are known. Of course, Ohm's law can also be stated in its other forms to solve for unknown currents and resistances:

$$I = \frac{V}{R}$$

and

$$R = \frac{V}{I}$$

> ***EXAMPLE:*** What is the amperage in a circuit of 20 volts and 10 ohms?
>
> ***Answer:***
>
> I = V/R
>
> I = 20 volts/10 ohms
>
> I = 2 amperes

> ***EXAMPLE:*** What is the voltage in a circuit of 100 amperes and 5 ohms?
>
> ***Answer:***
>
> V = IR
>
> V = 100 amperes × 5 ohms
>
> V = 500 volts

> ***EXAMPLE:*** What is the resistance in a circuit of 80 kilovolts and 200 milliamperes?
>
> ***Answer:***
>
> R = V/I
>
> R = 80 kV/200 mA
>
> R = 80,000 volts/0.2 ampere
>
> R = 400,000 ohms

A memory device used by many students is known as an Ohm's law triangle (Figure 3-11A). To determine the correct formula for one of the variables in the Ohm's law equation, V = IR, simply write the variables as shown (V over I and R), and then cover the variable to be solved with a finger. For example, Figure 3-11B is to solve for R. The correct relationship is given of V/I equals the covered R. Moving a finger around the triangle produces V/R = I and I • R = V as well.

It is useful to be able to calculate the total amount of power used in an electric circuit. **The unit of power is the watt.** Because the total amount of energy available in a circuit is determined by the current (amperage) and potential difference (voltage), **the watt is defined as 1 ampere flowing through 1 volt.** Power is calculated with the following formula:

$$P = IV$$

where: P = power in watts
I = current in amperes
V = potential difference in volts

Common household appliances tend to operate between 500 and 2,000 watts (most have labels

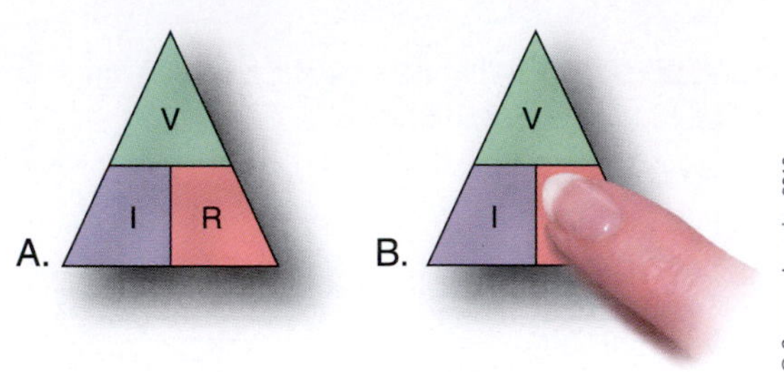

FIGURE 3-11 Ohm's law triangle.

indicating their wattage ratings), and all circuits in buildings have wattage safety limitations. The use of equipment whose total wattage ratings exceed the safety limit of the circuit will cause the circuit to overload and shut down because of excessive heat generation. Radiographic equipment capabilities can be measured by the power rating, usually by calculating the greatest possible energy output.

EXAMPLE: What is the power rating, in kilowatts, of an x-ray generator capable of 800 milliamperes at 100 kilovolts?

Answer:

P = IV

P = 800 mA × 100 kV

P = 0.8 A × 100,000 V

P = 80,000 watts

P = 80 kilowatts

EXAMPLE: If a mobile x-ray machine operates from a 110-V wall receptacle and is rated at a total resistance of 12 Ω, how much current does it draw during exposure?

Answer:

$$I = \frac{V}{R}$$

$$I = \frac{110\,V}{12\,\Omega}$$

$$I = 9.2\,A$$

EXAMPLE: How much power does it use?

Answer:

P = IV

P = 9.2 A × 110 V

P = 1,012 W

With this information it is also possible to calculate the expense of the power for a radiographic examination.

EXAMPLE: If the power company charges 5¢ per kWhr, what is the cost of the power for 10 minutes of fluoroscopy at 5 mA and 100 kV?

Answer:

The power is calculated as:

P = IV

P = 5 mA × 100 kV

P = 0.005 A × 100,000 V

P = 500 W

The total energy consumed is calculated as:

total energy = power × seconds
total energy = 500 W × 10 minutes
total energy = 500 W × 600 seconds
total energy = 300,000 Ws
total energy = 300 kWs

The total cost is calculated as:

total cost = total energy used × \$0.05/kWhr
total cost = 300 kW/second × \$0.05/kWhr
total cost = 0.08 kW/hr × \$0.05/kWhr
total cost = \$0.004, or
total cost = 0.4¢

The heat that is produced during the operation of electrical equipment becomes of great concern as power use increases. The importance of changes in resistance to heat output can best be understood if the power formula, P = IV, is converted to what is sometimes called the **power loss formula, $P = I^2R$**. This is calculated from:

the power formula, $P = IV$
substituting IR for V
(because Ohm's law states that $V = IR$)
resulting in $P = I \times IR$
or $P = I^2R$ (watts).

This equation clarifies that power loss from current heat is proportional to the resistance, and heat power loss increases very rapidly with current increase. As illustrated in the formula, heat power loss is proportional to the square of the amperage. In other words, doubling the amperage increases power loss by a factor of 4, and so forth.

SERIES AND PARALLEL CIRCUITS

An electric circuit can be designed to send electrons through various resistance devices by linking them one after the other in a **series circuit** (Figure 3-12A) or by giving each component an individual branch in a **parallel circuit** (Figure 3-12B). The classic example of the difference is illustrated by comparing strings of Christmas lights in series versus parallel circuits. When a single series-wired light burns out, it breaks the circuit and all the lights go out. When a single parallel-wired light burns out, it breaks the circuit in its parallel branch only and the other lights continue to operate. Electrical devices use a wide variety of both types of circuits, including complicated combinations of both. The effect of each type of circuit on current, potential difference, and resistance is summarized in Table 3-2. The best way to understand the effects of both series and parallel circuitry is to work through a series of problems that demonstrate these differences.

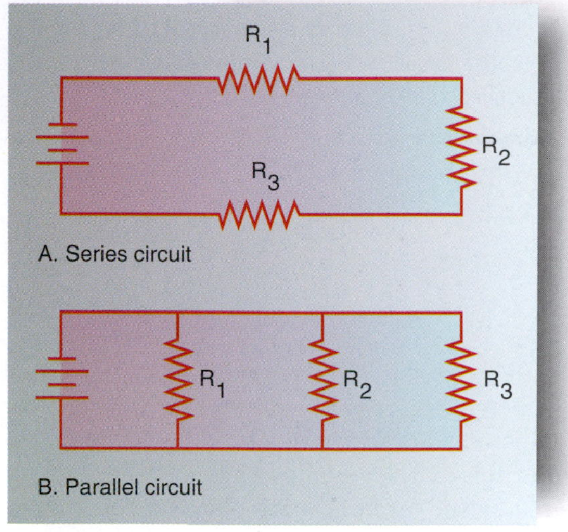

FIGURE 3-12 (A) Series and (B) parallel circuits.

> ***EXAMPLE:*** What is the total current in a series circuit with three resistances, each supplied with 10 amperes?
>
> ***Answer:***
>
> $I_t = I_1 = I_2 = I_3$
>
> $I_t = 10\text{ A} = 10\text{ A} = 10\text{ A}$
>
> $I_t = 10$ amperes

TABLE 3-2. Effect of Circuit Type on Current, Potential Difference, and Resistance (with an example circuit of three resistances)

	Series	Parallel
Current	Same in each element, each element same as total circuit, $I_t = I_1 = I_2 = I_3$	Sum of all elements equals total circuit, $I_t = I_1 + I_2 + I_3$
Voltage	Sum of all elements equals total circuit, $V_t = V_1 + V_2 + I_3$.	Same in each element, each element same as total circuit, $V_t = V_1 = V_2 = V_3$
Resistance	Sum of all elements equals total circuit, $R_t = R_1 + R_2 + R_3$	Sum of reciprocal of each element is inversely proportional to the total, $\frac{1}{R_t} = \frac{1}{R_1} + \frac{1}{R_2} + \frac{1}{R_3}$

NOTE: A reciprocal ohm, as in 1/R, is known as a siemens (S).

EXAMPLE: What is the total current in a parallel circuit with three resistances, each supplied with 10 amperes?

Answer:

$I_t = I_1 + I_2 + I_3$

$I_t = 10\text{ A} + 10\text{ A} + 10\text{ A}$

$I_t = 30\text{ amperes}$

Note that the series circuit supplies a current of 10 amperes, whereas the parallel circuit supplies 30 amperes. Parallel circuits supply a greater total current than series circuits when all other factors are the same. An interesting phenomenon occurs when the effect on voltage is compared, instead of current, using resistances.

EXAMPLE: What is the total voltage in a series circuit with three resistances, each supplied with 10 volts?

Answer:

$V_t = V_1 + V_2 + V_3$

$V_t = 10\text{ V} + 10\text{ V} + 10\text{ V}$

$V_t = 30\text{ volts}$

EXAMPLE: What is the total voltage in a parallel circuit with three resistances, each supplied with 10 volts?

Answer:

$V_t = V_1 = V_2 = V_3$

$V_t = 10\text{ V} = 10\text{ V} = 10\text{ V}$

$V_t = 10\text{ volts}$

Note that the series circuit supplies 30 volts, whereas the parallel circuit supplies 10 volts. Series circuits supply greater total potential difference than parallel circuits when all other factors are the same. The difference between series and parallel circuits when the same resistances are used is also notable.

EXAMPLE: What is the total resistance of a series circuit with resistances of 2.5 Ω, 4.2 Ω, and 6.8 Ω?

Answer:

$R_t = R_1 + R_2 + R_3$

$R_t = 2.5\ \Omega + 4.2\ \Omega + 6.8\ \Omega$

$R_t = 13.5\ \Omega$

EXAMPLE: What is the total resistance of a parallel circuit with resistances of 2.5 Ω, 4.2 Ω, and 6.8 Ω?

Answer:

$$\frac{1}{R_t} = \frac{1}{R_1} + \frac{1}{R_2} + \frac{1}{R_3}$$

$$\frac{1}{R_t} = \frac{1}{2.5\ \Omega} + \frac{1}{4.2\ \Omega} + \frac{1}{6.8\ \Omega}$$

$$\frac{1}{R_t} = 0.4\text{ S} + 0.24\text{ S} + 0.15\text{ S}$$

$$\frac{1}{R_t} = 0.785\text{ S}$$

$$R_t = \frac{1}{0.785\text{ S}}$$

$$R_t = 1.274\ \Omega$$

Note that the series circuit provides 13.5 Ω of resistance, whereas the parallel circuit has only 1.274 Ω. Parallel circuits offer less total resistance to electrical current when all other factors are the same. In addition, parallel circuits are not broken when a single resistance is interrupted (as when a light bulb burns out). Series circuits require all resistances to be operable, otherwise there is no pathway for the current to take. It is also interesting to calculate the effect of both circuit types on amperage by figuring resistance and then applying Ohm's law.

EXAMPLE: What is the total amperage in a series circuit with resistances of 2.5 Ω, 4.2 Ω, and 6.8 Ω with a potential difference of 10 volts?

Answer:

The total resistance is calculated as:

$$R_t = R_1 + R_2 + R_3$$
$$R_t = 2.5\ \Omega + 4.2\ \Omega + 6.8\ \Omega$$
$$R_t = 13.5\ \Omega$$

The total amperage is calculated with Ohm's law:

$$I = \frac{V}{R}$$
$$I = \frac{10\ \text{V}}{13.5\ \Omega}$$
$$I = 0.74\ \text{amperes}$$

Note that the series circuit operates with a current of 0.74 ampere, whereas the parallel circuit operates with a current of 7.1 amperes. Parallel circuits operate with greater current when all other factors are the same. It is also interesting to study the effect of both circuit types on voltage by calculating resistance and then applying Ohm's law.

EXAMPLE: What is the total amperage in a parallel circuit with resistances of 2.5 Ω, 4.2 Ω, and 6.8 Ω and a potential difference of 10 volts?

Answer:

The total resistance is calculated as:

$$\frac{1}{R_t} = \frac{1}{2.5\ \Omega} = \frac{1}{4.2\ \Omega} + \frac{1}{6.8\ \Omega}$$
$$\frac{1}{R_t} = 0.4\ \text{S} + 0.24\ \text{S} + 0.15\ \text{S}$$
$$\frac{1}{R_t} = 0.785\ \text{S}$$
$$R_t = \frac{1}{0.785\ \text{S}}$$
$$R_t = 1.274\ \Omega$$

The total amperage is calculated with Ohm's law:

$$I = \frac{V}{R}$$
$$I = \frac{10\ \text{V}}{1.274\ \Omega}$$
$$I = 7.85\ \text{amperes}$$

EXAMPLE: What is the total voltage of a series circuit with resistances 2.5 Ω, 4.2 Ω, and 6.8 Ω with a current of 50 amperes?

Answer:

The total resistance is calculated as:

$$R_t = R_1 + R_2 + R_3$$
$$R_t = 2.5\ \Omega + 4.2\ \Omega + 6.8\ \Omega$$
$$R_t = 13.5\ \Omega$$

The total voltage is calculated with Ohm's law:

$$V = IR$$
$$V = 50\ \text{A} \times 13.5\ \Omega$$
$$V = 675\ \text{volts}$$

EXAMPLE: What is the total voltage of a parallel circuit with resistances of 2.5 Ω, 4.2 Ω, and 6.8 Ω and a current of 50 amperes?

Answer:

The total resistance is calculated as:

$$\frac{1}{R_t} = \frac{1}{R_1} + \frac{1}{R_2} + \frac{1}{R_3}$$
$$\frac{1}{R_t} = \frac{1}{2.5\ \Omega} + \frac{1}{4.2\ \Omega} + \frac{1}{6.8\ \Omega}$$
$$R_t = 2.5\ \Omega + 4.2\ \Omega + 6.8\ \Omega$$
$$\frac{1}{R_t} = 0.785\ \text{S}$$
$$R_t = \frac{1}{0.785}$$
$$R_t = 1.274\ \Omega$$

The total voltage is calculated with Ohm's law:

$$V = IR$$
$$V = 50\ \text{A} \times 1.274\ \Omega$$
$$V = 63.68\ \text{volts}$$

Note that the series circuit operates at 675 volts, whereas the parallel circuit operates at 64 volts. Parallel circuits operate at lower voltage than series circuits when all other factors are the same.

Parallel circuits are used for the electrical wiring of buildings because the failure of a single device does not break the electrical supply to other devices. As can be seen from these problems, the addition of current-using devices to a series circuit causes the voltage to drop, thus reducing the potential difference to the other devices in the circuit. In a series circuit of lights, for example, the addition of more bulbs will cause all the bulbs to burn dimmer. **As more resistances are added to a parallel circuit, total resistance drops, total amperage increases, and total voltage remains unchanged.** The total resistance of a parallel circuit is always less than the amount of the lowest resistor (usually about half of the lowest resistor).

A disadvantage to parallel circuits is that with the addition of resistances, the increasing amperage can short circuit the entire system. This creates the possibility of wires becoming hot enough to start a fire. To prevent this from occurring, either a **circuit breaker** or a **fuse** is placed in the line. These devices are constructed to permit the breaking of the circuit before a dangerous temperature is reached. Circuit breakers simply pop open and can be reset once the cause of the problem has been located and removed from the circuit. Fuses are constructed with a metal tab that will melt when dangerously heated, thus breaking the circuit. Fuses are not reusable and must be replaced.

A variable resistor called a **potentiometer** or **rheostat** permits a variable contact to slide along a series circuit of resistance coils. When resistors are connected in a series circuit, Ohm's law dictates that an increase in resistance will result in a decrease in voltage and vice versa if the amperage remains unchanged. When a knob is connected to the variable slide contact (as in a radio volume control), a simple twist permits voltage and amperage regulation (with a corresponding increase or decrease in speaker volume). Unfortunately, rheostats cause significant energy waste in heat, and the direct application of Ohm's law results in voltage changing when only an amperage change is desired and vice versa. For these reasons, rheostats are not practical in high-voltage situations. Their prime use is to control current but they have never been adaptable to high-voltage transformers.

SUMMARY

The distribution and movement of electrons, along with their associated charges, make up electricity. Electrostatics is the study of the distribution of fixed charges that are at rest. When one object has more electrons than another, it also has more negative charges and is considered to have an overall negative charge. A positive charge refers to something with a weaker negative charge, or fewer electrons. The terms *negative* and *positive* refer to the relationship between two objects, not to their true atomic charges. Because the earth contains what is essentially an infinite number of charges, it is considered to be neutral, or at zero ground potential. The five laws of electrostatics are: (1) repulsion-attraction, (2) the inverse square law, (3) distribution, (4) concentration, and (5) movement. Objects can be electrified by friction, contact, and induction.

The movement of electrons is facilitated by materials that permit electrons to flow easily. These materials are called conductors or superconductors. Nonconducting materials are called insulators, and materials that conduct under certain conditions and insulate under others are known as semiconductors.

An electrical circuit is a pathway that permits electrons to move in a complete circle from their source,

SUMMARY (continued)

through resisting electrical devices, and back to the source. Electrons move from the highest concentration to the lowest. Conventional electric current is described as going from positive to negative poles, while electron flow is actually from negative to positive poles. It is important to specify whether descriptions are of electrical current or electron flow, as they are exact opposites.

The quantity of electrons flowing is referred to as the current and is measured in amperes. The force with which the electrons travel is referred to as the potential difference, electromotive force, or voltage and is measured in volts. There does not have to be current flow for voltage to exist. The opposition to the current flow is referred to as resistance and is measured in ohms. The relationship between these factors is expressed in Ohm's law: $V = IR$. The resistance of metallic conductors is affected by length, diameter, and temperature. When $1/R$ is used to express resistance in an AC circuit, it is measured in siemens.

The valence energy band of an atom has much to do with the ability of a material to conduct electrons. There is also an area beyond the valence band that is referred to as the conduction band. Conductors have conduction bands that are populated by electrons that are able to move freely from one atom's conduction band to another's. Insulators have widely separated valence and conduction bands, whereas semiconductors have intermediate properties.

Circuits are known by several parameters. These include the direction the electrons travel, which is defined as either direct current (DC) or alternating current (AC). It is possible to change the current from DC to AC and back, as necessary. The total amount of energy in a circuit is described as the power of the circuit and is measured in watts so that $P = IV$. Circuits can be described as series or parallel, depending on how the components are connected. The total resistance of a series circuit is measured in ohms, as $R_t = R_1 R_2 R_3$. The total resistance of a parallel circuit is measured in siemens, as

$$\frac{1}{R_t} = \frac{1}{R_1} + \frac{1}{R_2} + \frac{1}{R_3}$$

Parallel circuits operate with greater current through resistances, and they supply a greater total current from the power supply than series circuits when all other factors are the same. Parallel circuits are often used because the failure of a single device does not break the electrical supply to other devices. Circuit breakers and fuses prevent damage to electrical components by permitting the breaking of an overloaded circuit before a dangerous temperature is reached. A potentiometer or rheostat is a variable resistor. ■

REVIEW QUESTIONS

1. State the five elementary laws of electrostatics.
2. Describe the three methods of electrification.
3. How are conductors different from insulators?
4. Explain the difference between conventional electrical current and actual electron flow.
5. State the four basic factors that are used to describe the nature of the flow of electrons in electrodynamics.
6. What are the units used to describe potential difference, current flow, and opposition to current flow?
7. State Ohm's law.
8. What is the potential difference in a circuit of 20 amperes and 10 ohms? 30 amperes and 6 ohms? 100 mA and 5 ohms?
9. What is the power rating of an x-ray generator capable of 1,000 mA at 110 kV?

10. What is the voltage in a parallel circuit of 20 amperes with resistances of 6, 10, and 15 ohms?

11. What is the amperage in a series circuit of 110 volts with resistances of 5, 10, and 20 ohms?

REFERENCES AND RECOMMENDED READING

Ball, J. L., & Moore, A. D. (2008). *Essential physics for radiographers* (4th ed.). Oxford: Wiley-Blackwell Scientific.

Bushberg, J. T., Seibert, J. A., Leidholdt, E. M., & Boone, J. M. (2003). *The essential physics of medical imaging* (2nd ed.). Philadelphia: Lippincott, Williams & Wilkins.

Bushong, S. C. (2008). *Radiologic science for technologists: Physics, biology, and protection* (9th ed.). St. Louis, MO: Elsevier Mosby.

Carroll, Q. B. (2007). *Practical radiographic imaging (Fuch's radiographic exposure processing & quality control)* (8th ed.). Springfield, IL: Charles C Thomas.

Dendy, P. P., & Heaton, B. (1999). *Physics for diagnostic radiology* (2nd ed.). Bristol, England: Institute of Physics.

Hay, G. A., & Hughes, D. (1997). *First-year physics for radiographers* (3rd ed.) St. Louis, MO: Saunders

Johns, H. E., & Cunningham, J. R. (1983). *The physics of radiology* (4th ed.). Springfield, IL: Charles C Thomas.

Meredith, W. J., & Massey, J. B. (1977). *Fundamental physics of radiology* (3rd ed.). Chicago: Yearbook Medical.

Selman, J. (2000). *The fundamentals of imaging physics and radiobiology for the radiologic technologist* (9th ed.). Springfield, IL: Charles C Thomas.

van der Plaats, G. J. (1980). *Medical x-ray techniques in diagnostic radiology* (4th ed.). The Hague: Martinus Nijhoff.

Wilks, R. J. (2003). *Principles of radiological physics* (4th ed.). Edinburgh: Churchill Livingstone.

Wolbarst, A. B., & Cook, G. (2005). *Physics of radiology* (2nd ed.). Madison: Medical Physics Publishing.

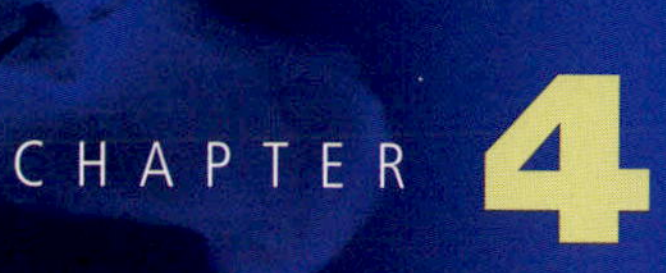

CHAPTER 4

Electromagnetism

KEY TERMS

air-core transformer
ammeter
armature
artificial permanent magnet
autotransformer
brush
capacitor
closed-core transformer
coercivity
commutator ring
diamagnetic
dielectric
diode
dynamometer
eddy current loss
electromagnet
electromagnetic relay
farad (f)
ferromagnetic
Fleming's hand rules
flux density
full-wave rectification
galvanometer
gauss (g)
generator
half-wave rectification
hysteresis loss
I^2R loss
inductive reactance
lines of flux
lines of force

> He expressed his satisfaction and, going back to Joachim, warned him to draw in his breath and hold it until all was over. Joachim's rounded back expanded and so remained; the assistant, at the switch-board, pulled the handle. Now, for the space of two seconds, fearful powers were in play—streams of thousands, of a hundred thousand of volts.
>
> *Thomas Mann, Der Zauberberg (The Magic Mountain)*

OBJECTIVES

Upon completion of this chapter, the student should be able to:

- Explain the atomic nature of magnetism.
- Classify materials according to their magnetic properties.
- State Fleming's hand rules of electromagnetics.
- Explain how a solenoid and an electromagnet function.
- Describe magnetic and electromagnetic induction.
- List the types of movement that will produce electromagnetism.
- State the factors that regulate the strength of electromagnetic induction.
- Explain self-induction.
- Illustrate the generator and motor principles.
- Explain the waveform produced by direct- and alternating-current generators and motors.
- Describe the function of a transformer.

KEY TERMS (continued)

magnet
magnetic dipole
magnetic domain
magnetic field
motor
mutual induction
natural magnet
nonmagnetic
open-core transformer
orbital magnetic moment
paramagnetic
permeability
primary coil
rectification
retentivity
rotor
secondary coil
self-induction
self-rectification
shell-type transformer
silicon-controlled rectifier (SCR)
sine wave
slip ring
solenoid
space charge cloud
spin magnetic moment
stator
step-down transformer
step-up transformer
tesla (T)
thermionic emission
thyristor
transformer
transformer law
voltmeter
Weber (Wb)

- Calculate voltage and amperage according to the transformer law.
- Discuss various factors affecting transformer efficiency and construction.
- Explain the function of an autotransformer and a capacitor.
- Describe the function of a silicon-controlled rectifier at the atomic level.
- Describe the process of thermionic emission.
- Explain the waveforms that are produced by half-wave and full-wave rectification.

MAGNETISM

Magnetism is one of the fundamental forces. Materials that have the ability to attract iron are classified as having a strong magnetic force. To understand magnetism it is important to return to atomic structure for a detailed examination of the effects of particle movement around the nucleus. **When a charged particle is in motion, a magnetic force field perpendicular to the motion will be created** (Figure 4-1). In the case of the

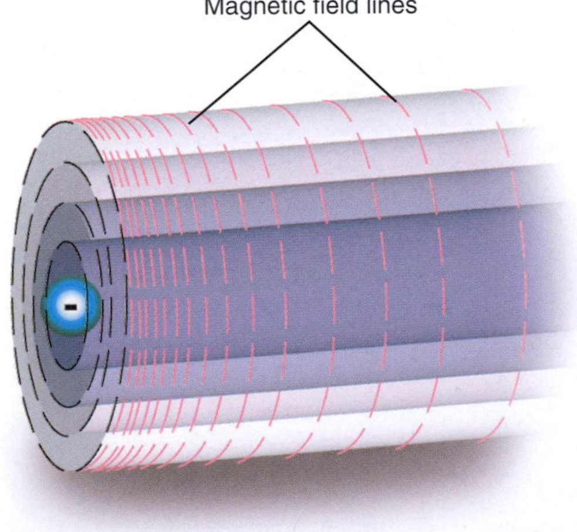

FIGURE 4-1. Magnetic field created by a charged particle in motion. The movement of a charged particle creates a magnetic field perpendicular to the motion of the particle.

negatively charged electrons orbiting the nucleus of an atom, the closed loop of the orbit cancels all but the field that is perpendicular to the plane of the motion (Figure 4-2). This perpendicular magnetic force is called **orbital magnetic moment**.

A magnetic effect is also established by electrons spinning on their axes. The effect created by the movement of these electrons is called **spin magnetic moment**. The disruption of this axial spinning and the energy released as it reorients itself are the physical basis that permits magnetic resonance imaging (see Chapter 42).

Atoms having a significant number of electrons with their magnetic moments in the same direction, especially when the outer shells are involved, will exhibit a net magnetic field in a distinct direction (see Figure 4-2A). Groups of atoms with this net magnetic field are known as **magnetic dipoles** or

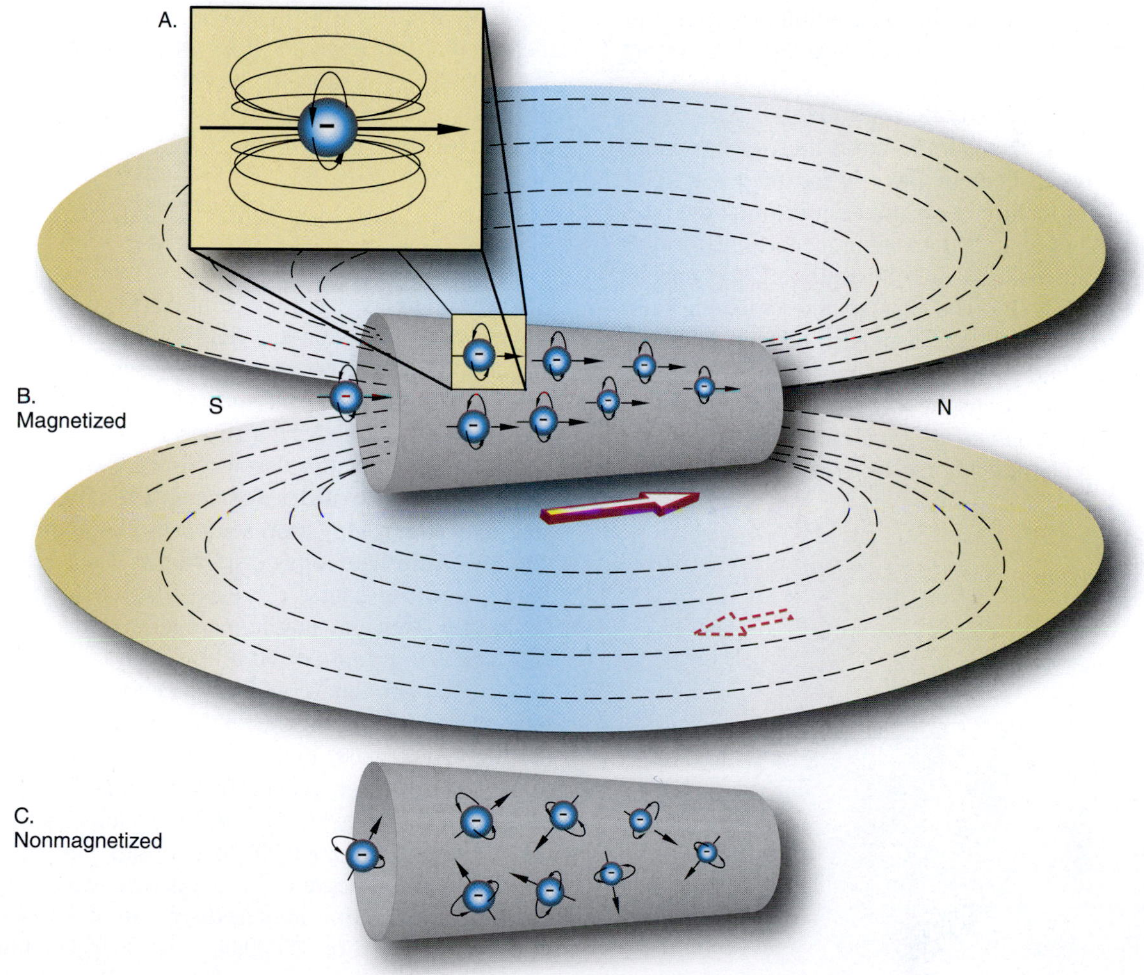

FIGURE 4-2. The concept of magnetism: (A) The spinning of an individual electron is the spin magnetic movement, and the magnetic field created by the spin is the orbital magnetic moment (heavy arrows). Groups of atoms with most of the magnetic moment force in a single direction form a magnetic dipole or domain. (B) When the magnetic dipoles or domains are in a predominant direction, a magnet is formed with an external magnetic field. (C) When the magnetic dipoles or domains are not in predominant direction, the object is not magnetized.

magnetic domains. This is the basis of the domain theory of magnetism. It has been theorized that 10^{15} (1,000,000,000,000,000 or 1 million billion) atoms make up a single dipole. This is not a standard number, as it has been shown that dipoles vary in size and actually grow or shrink, depending on local conditions. In nonmagnetic objects the magnetic dipoles are randomly arranged, essentially cancelling out each other. If an external force field has the time or strength to orient enough of the dipoles in the same direction and/or cause those dipoles to grow in size, the object exhibits a uniformly strong magnetic field and is referred to as a **magnet** (see Figure 4-2B).

The force fields that are created when magnetic dipoles orient to create a magnet are called **lines of force**, **lines of flux**, or the **magnetic field**. These lines of force flow not only through the magnet itself but outside the magnetic material, forming a three-dimensional field surrounding the magnet (see Figure 4-2B). The stronger the magnetic field, the more lines of flux. Placing small iron filings on a surface under which a strong magnet is placed will map out the magnetic lines of flux. Figure 4-3 illustrates the lines of flux emanating from the poles of a bar and a horseshoe magnet. The ends of a magnet are defined as the north and south poles; **lines of force always flow from north to south outside a magnet and from south to north within a magnet** (see Figure 4-2B). It is important to remember that **lines of force never intersect**. In some cases they are described as being parallel. However, many circumstances may cause the magnetic field to contract or expand. Under these conditions the lines of force bend closer or further from one another, making them no longer truly parallel.

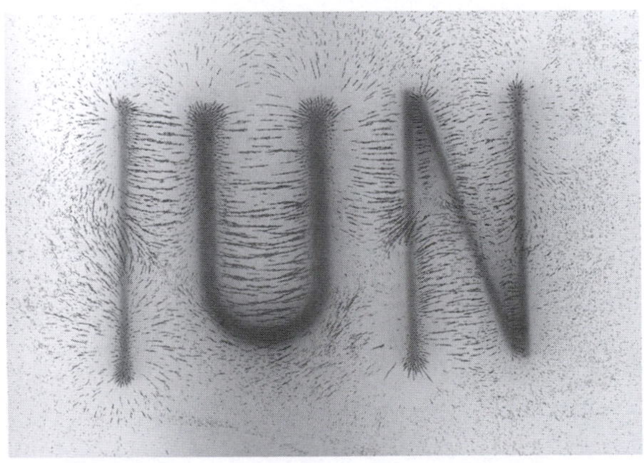

FIGURE 4-3. Strong permanent magnets placed under a surface containing loose iron filings will demonstrate magnetic lines of flux as the filings orient to the magnetic field (forming the initials of Indiana University Northwest). *(Courtesy of Radiologic Sciences Department, Indiana University Northwest.)*

The stronger the magnetic field, the greater the number of lines of flux or the greater the **flux density**. Flux density is determined both by field strength and by the area in which the lines of flux are located.

$$\text{magnetic flux} = \frac{\text{field strength}}{\text{area}}$$

There are two primary units used to measure the strength of magnetic fields. The SI unit for magnetic flux is the **Weber**, represented by the symbol **Wb** (for the German physicist Wilhelm Weber [1804–1891], who proposed the basic theory of magnetism discussed above). 1 Wb = 10^8 lines of flux. **The units for magnetic flux density are the tesla,** represented by the symbol T (for the American physicist Nikola Tesla [1857–1943]), and the **gauss**, represented by the symbol G (for the German mathematician Johann Gauss [1777–1855]). **1 tesla = 10,000 gauss.** 1 T = 1 Wb/m^2, or 1 Wb per square meter. The earth's magnetic field averages about 0.0001 T (1 G or 100,000 lines of flux per square meter), whereas an ordinary household magnet (used, for example, to keep papers on a refrigerator) might have a strength of 0.1 T (1,000 G or 10,000,000 lines of flux per square meter). Modern magnetic resonance imaging (MRI) equipment often operates in the range of 0.3–2.0 T (3,000 to 20,000 G or 30,000,000 to 200,000,000 lines of flux per square meter).

Because the earth itself is a magnet, with a north and a south pole, lines of force, although relatively weak, are present everywhere. This fact is used in the design of a magnetic compass. The pointer is simply a small piece of permanent magnet that will align itself with the earth's magnetic lines of force and indicate direction. Because of this, a compass is a useful tool in detecting magnetic lines of force, including those induced by electrons moving in electrical circuits and devices. Worth noting is the fact that the earth's true magnetic poles are not located in Antarctica and the Arctic Ocean. Instead, the true magnetic north pole is located in Canada's far north, while the true magnetic south pole is near Australia. Both poles tend to drift to new locations as geological conditions beneath the earth's crust change.

Magnets can be classified by type of production as *natural*, *artificial permanent*, and *electromagnets*. **Natural magnets** are created when iron oxide (magnetite) remains in the earth's magnetic field for ages, slowly orienting the magnetic dipoles in the same direction. These natural magnets are called lodestones. They were recognized by primitive man and investigated by Greek academics. In some regions entire mountains of iron ore that have remained undisturbed for eons have magnetic properties. Natives of Thunder Bay, Ontario, delight in watching tourists follow signpost instructions to place their cars in neutral gear at the bottom of a magnetic mountain's gentle grade in hopes that the magnetic field will pull their cars up the hill.

Artificial permanent magnets are manufactured from a steel alloy called alnico, composed of aluminum, nickel, and cobalt. While it is hot, alnico is subjected to the field of a strong commercial magnet to permit easier orientation of the magnetic dipoles. Upon cooling, the magnetic field becomes relatively permanent. Prior to the 20th century, experienced blacksmiths were easy to spot because the tongs they used to handle heated metals had become magnetized. After many years of standing in the same position (in orientation to the earth's magnetic lines of force), heating the tongs in the forge, and then pounding the hot metal into shape on the anvil, the tongs had become well magnetized. A request to see a horseshoe hanging from a rafter would prove a smith's experience when he used the magnetized tongs to easily lift it down.

Electromagnets are temporary magnets produced by moving electric current. Because the electrons comprising the flow of current create magnetic fields in exactly the same manner as do the orbiting and spinning atomic electrons, any flow of current produces a magnetic field. When the current ceases flowing, the magnetic field collapses, making these electrical magnets temporary. It is possible to create a fourth type of magnet by vibration.

The laws governing magnetism are similar to the laws of electrostatics. However, only three are of importance for this text:

1. **Repulsion-attraction.** Like poles repel; unlike poles attract. In addition, like lines of force repel and unlike lines of force attract, when placed within each other's force fields (Figure 4-4).
2. **The inverse square law.** The force between two magnetic fields is directly proportional to the product of their magnitudes and inversely proportional to the square of the distance between them. Exactly as with electrostatics, as an object gets further away, the influencing field decreases because of the increased area it affects.
3. **Magnetic poles.** Every magnet has two poles, a north and a south, as discussed earlier. No matter how much a magnet is divided, even into individual moving electrons, both poles continue to exist.

Because the laws of electrostatics, magnetism, and gravity have so many similarities, physicists

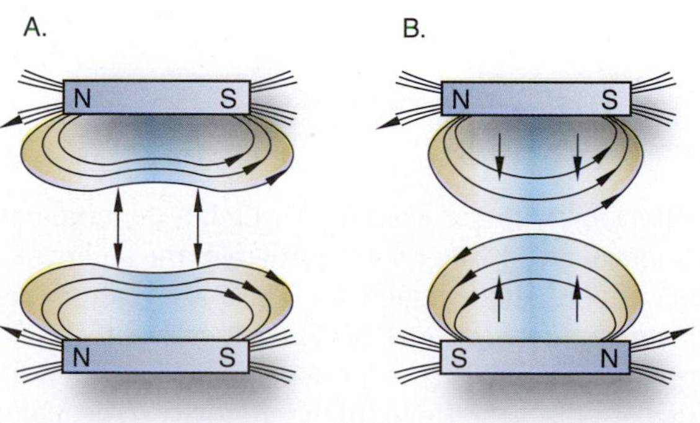

FIGURE 4-4. Repulsion-attraction of magnetic lines of force: (A) Lines of force in the same direction will repel each other. (B) Lines of force in opposite directions will attract each other.

have searched since the 1860s for a mathematical theory to relate the three forces into a unified field theory. Albert Einstein worked unsuccessfully toward this goal until he died, and the search continues to the present time in the work of Stephen Hawking, among other prominent theoretical physicists.

Magnetic Induction

When a nonmagnetized iron bar is brought within the lines of force of a strong magnet, the dipoles will temporarily align themselves with the lines of force passing through the iron bar. If the bar is removed from the field after a short time, the dipoles will return to their random orientation, thus leaving the bar unmagnetized. This process is termed *magnetic induction* and operates like electromagnetic induction. Instead of temporary repulsion of electrons, magnetic poles are induced through the temporary orientation of the dipoles.

The ease with which sensitive devices can be magnetized or demagnetized by stray electrical fields makes magnetic shielding desirable in many situations. Because there is no magnetic insulator, shielding is accomplished by providing a highly permeable ferromagnetic material, such as iron, through which stray magnetic fields can be directed, thus protecting sensitive devices from exposure to the stray field. This technique is used to shield some magnetic resonance imaging (MRI) units, although they require radio frequency (RF) shielding as well.

Magnetic Classification of Materials

Permeability is the ease with which a material can be magnetized, whereas **retentivity** is the ability of a material to stay magnetized. These two factors are inversely proportional because if it is difficult to orient the dipoles (low permeability), it is also difficult to disorient them (high retentivity). The major classifications of the magnetic properties of materials according to their relative permeabilities are:

1. **Ferromagnetic** (or simply magnetic) materials such as iron, cobalt, and nickel are highly permeable and greatly susceptible to induction. These materials have a majority of their dipoles lying in the same direction, thus setting up a natural magnetic field. In addition, the material must permit the atoms to be oriented, thus permitting the growth of magnetic dipoles in predominantly the same direction. Specialized alloys such as alnico, permalloy, or mumetal (some alloys, strangely enough, contain no ferromagnetic elements) are designed to enhance permeability and exhibit dramatically increased magnetic field strength.
2. **Paramagnetic** materials, such as platinum and aluminum, have low permeability and weak attraction to magnetic fields. These materials have only a slight majority of dipoles in the same direction and there is little tendency for the size of the dipoles to grow. MRI contrast media are usually paramagnetic.
3. **Diamagnetic** materials, such as beryllium, bismuth, and lead, are actually weakly repelled by all magnetic fields, including both north and south poles. Strangely, water is slightly diamagnetic. This property is so weak that it is easily obscured by other types of magnetic induction.
4. **Nonmagnetic** materials, such as wood, glass, rubber, and plastic, are not affected by magnetic fields and cannot be magnetized. Nonmagnetic materials are most often composed of atoms locked into crystalline or molecular patterns, thus forming ionic and covalent bonds and eliminating the ability of electrons to freely orient themselves to external magnetic lines of force. This classification includes most materials.

ELECTROMAGNETISM

Electricity and magnetism are actually different aspects of the same force, electromagnetism. Although the study of magnetism dates to ancient times, and the study of electricity to Queen Elizabeth I's physician, William Gilbert (1540–1603), it was not until 1820, when the Danish physicist Hans Oersted (1777–1851) observed the deflection of a compass during a classroom demonstration of electrical phenomena, that the relationships between the two began to be established. Oersted's discovery, and subsequent investigations by many others, permitted the generation, control, and practical use of electricity and initiated the electronic revolution that continues today.

Oersted's experiment proves that when there is no current flowing in the wire, the compass needle aligns itself with the earth's magnetic field (Figure 4-5). However, when current is flowing, the needle is deflected toward the wire and when the current stops, the needle returns to alignment with the earth's field. This led to the conclusion that **any moving charge produces a magnetic field.** As was stated earlier in the section on magnetism, this applies to even a single electron's negative charge in orbit around an atom. A slightly different arrangement of Oersted's experiment (Figure 4-6) permits the mapping of the magnetic field surrounding the flow of current.

The English scientist John Fleming (1849–1945) developed a series of easily remembered aids to help with the relationship between electricity and magnetism. They are known as **Fleming's hand rules**. There are several "hand" rules that are quite useful for remembering various electromagnetic relationships. The rules are divided into four groups: (1) **hand thumb rules along a conductor;** (2) **hand thumb rules for solenoid and electromagnet poles;** (3) **hand generator effect rules;** and (4) **hand motor principle rules.** These are summarized in Table 4-1. Before learning any of the rules, it is critical to remember that **hand rules that are based on current flow (conventional current**

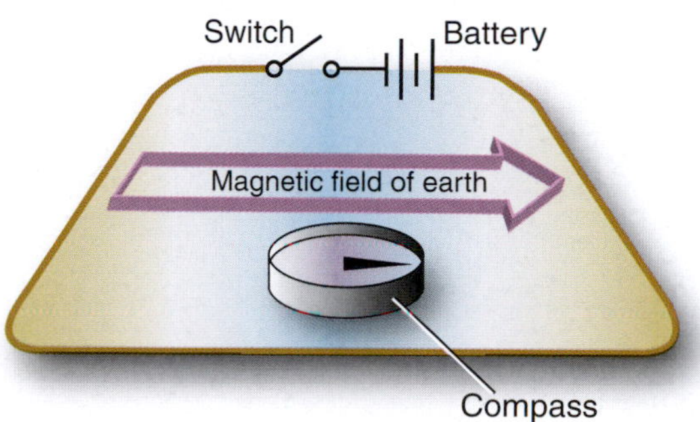

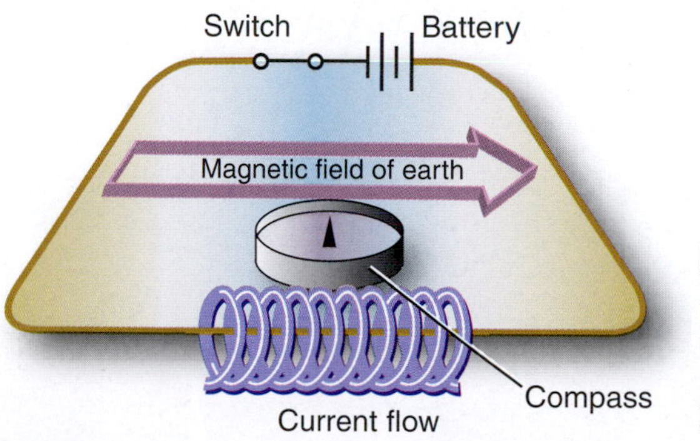

FIGURE 4-5. Oersted's experiment: A compass placed near a wire conductor will indicate the direction of the earth's magnetic field (A) when no current is flowing in the wire. Because flowing current creates a magnetic field around the wire conductor that is stronger than the earth's field, the compass will indicate the direction of the current-induced field while the switch is closed (B).

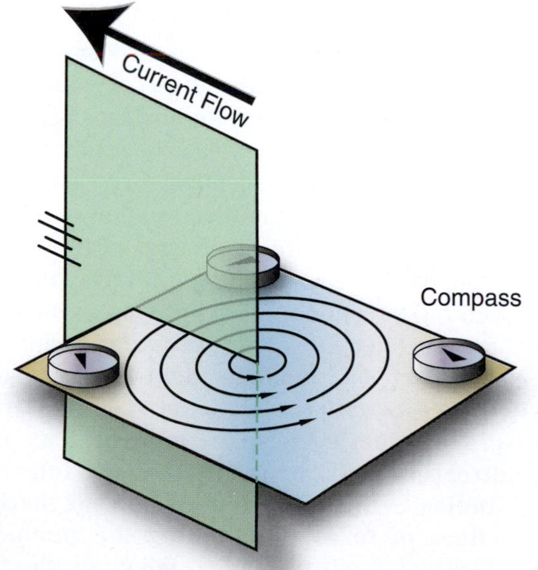

FIGURE 4-6. Relationship of induced magnetic field to direction of current flow: A variation of Oersted's experiment maps out the magnetic field induced by flowing current.

TABLE 4-1. Fleming's Hand Rules for Electromagnetic Relationships

		Conventional Current Flow	Electron Flow
Along a conductor			
thumb	= conventional current or electron flow	right-hand thumb rule (see Figure 4-7)	left-hand thumb rule (left-hand version)
fingers	= magnetic field		
Solenoid and electromagnet poles			
thumb	= direction of north pole	right-hand thumb rule (see Figure 4-9)	left-hand thumb rule (left-hand version)
fingers	= conventional current or electron flow		
Generator effect			
thumb	= movement of conductor on armature	right-hand generator rule (see Figure 4-12)	left-hand generator rule (left-hand version)
index finger	= magnetic lines of force field		
middle finger	= current or electron flow		
Motor principle			
thumb	= movement of conductor on rotor	left-hand motor rule (see Figure 4-18)	right-hand motor rule (right-hand version)
index finger	= magnetic lines of force field		
middle finger	= current or electron flow		

direction) and hand rules that are based on electron flow (actual direction of electron movement) will be exact opposites. For example, the right-hand thumb rule applies to conventional current flow. This is identical to the left-hand thumb rule applied to actual electron flow.

The hand thumb rule, the first of the hand rules, applies to remembering the relationship between the direction of current along a conductor and the direction of the resulting magnetic lines of force field. **Fleming's right-hand thumb rule states that if the right hand is used to grasp a conducting wire with the thumb in the direction of the current flow, the fingers will indicate the direction of the magnetic field lines of force surrounding the conductor** (Figure 4-7). (If the thumb points in the direction of actual electron flow, then a left-hand thumb rule must be used to show the direction of the magnetic field lines of force surrounding the conductor.) Table 4-1 compares this rule with the other "hand" rules.

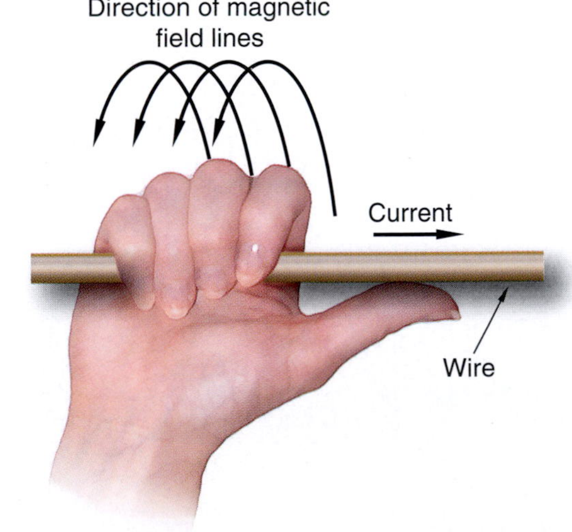

FIGURE 4-7. Fleming's right-hand thumb rule: When the right hand is positioned so the thumb points in the direction of conventional current flow, the fingers indicate the direction of the induced magnetic field. Fleming's left-hand thumb rule does the same for actual electron flow.

SOLENOIDS AND ELECTROMAGNETS

An interesting phenomenon occurs when conducting wire is looped (Figure 4-8A). Using the right-hand thumb rule to determine the direction of the magnetic lines of flux, it is apparent that inside the loop the magnetic fields from both sides join to double the magnetic flux density. If a series of loops is made, creating a coil (Figure 4-8B), the flux density is greatly increased. When current is flowing through this type of coil it is called a **solenoid**. The flux density can be increased further still by adding a ferromagnetic core. This configuration is called an *electromagnet*. **The**

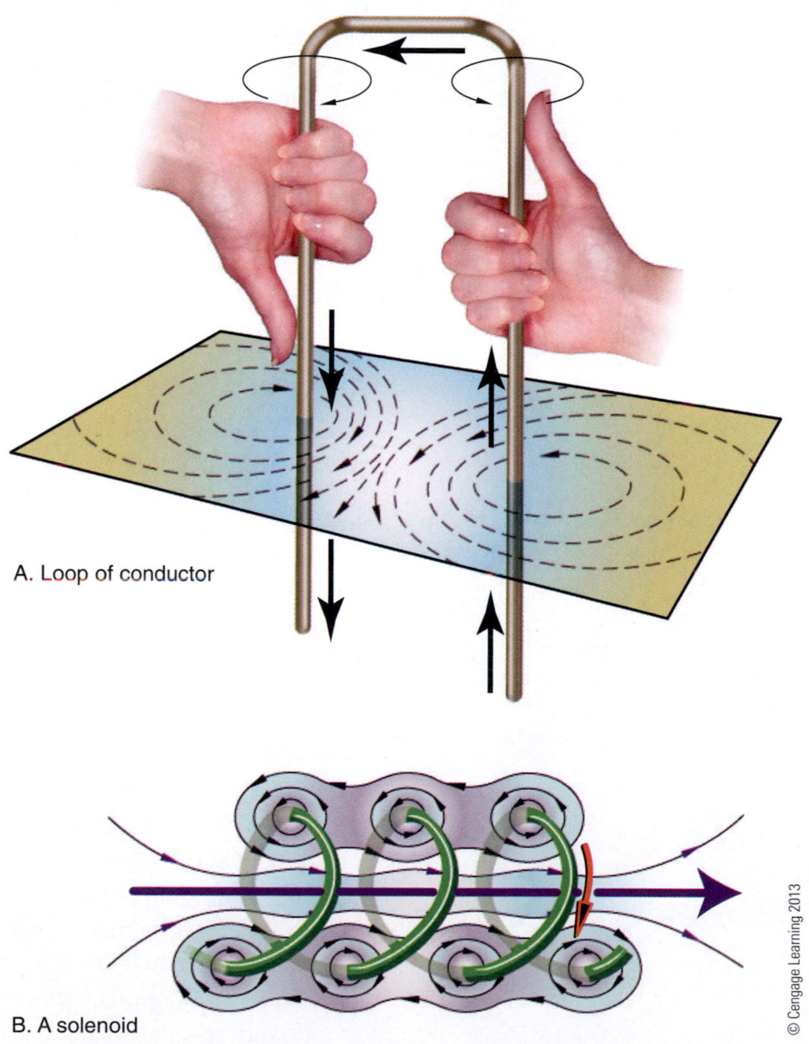

FIGURE 4-8. A solenoid: (A) When a conductor is looped to form a coil, the magnetic fields from both sides join to double the magnetic field strength inside the loop. (B) A solenoid is a helix coil through which current is flowing; it uses the coil loops to produce a greatly strengthened magnetic field.

strength of solenoids and electromagnets is determined by the number of loops (or turns) of wire, the current strength, and the permeability of the core. The right-hand thumb rule can also be applied to a solenoid or an electromagnet to determine the location of the magnetic poles. **If the fingers point in the direction of the current, the thumb will point toward the north pole** (Figure 4-9). (If the fingers point in the direction of actual electron flow, then a left-hand thumb rule must be used for the thumb to point toward the north pole.) Table 4-1 compares this rule with the other "hand" rules.

Both the solenoid and the electromagnet demonstrate magnetic properties only while electric current is flowing. If the current stops flowing, the magnetic properties vanish, and if the current is adjusted up or down, the magnetic strength changes accordingly. The factors that govern the effectiveness of solenoids and electromagnets are the **diameter** of the coil, its **length,** and the **current** passing along the coil. Electromagnets are used as remote control devices in circuit breakers and in the temporary locks, sometimes called detents, on radiographic equipment. In a typical circuit breaker configuration, a wire from the circuit to be protected is incorporated into an electromagnet, which, when the current becomes dangerously high, has been calculated to attract a movable contact, which breaks the circuit.

Solenoids are often used as detent locks on the overhead crane of x-ray tubes. The detent can be activated by a switch at the x-ray tube controls. The switch activates the magnetic properties of the solenoid, which in turn attracts a metal latch or bolt. This temporarily locks the tube to the center of the x-ray table or at the proper distance from a film holder. **Electromagnetic relays** are similar to circuit breakers. They are used to protect radiographers from electrical shock by isolating control buttons on the x-ray console from the actual circuit in which high voltage is flowing.

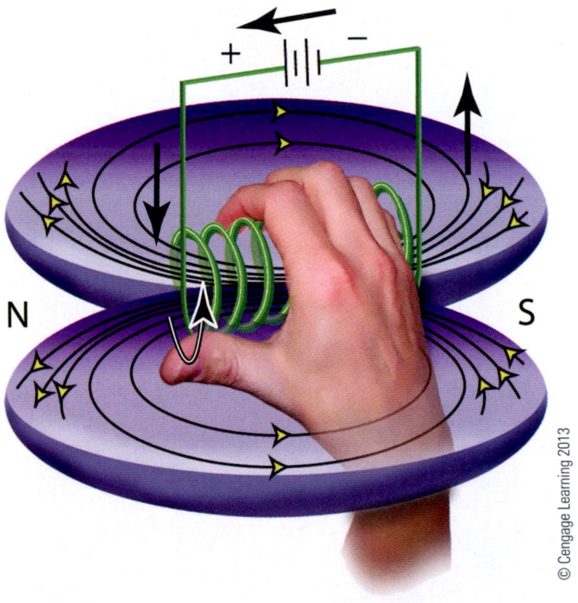

FIGURE 4-9. Fleming's right-hand thumb rule applied to determining the pole of a solenoid or electromagnet. When the fingers point in the direction of the current, the thumb will point toward the north pole.

Electromagnetic Induction

Once it became known that electrical current could generate a magnetic field, the obvious question was whether the reverse was true. In fact it was demonstrated by the English physicist Michael Faraday (1791–1867) the year after Oersted's discovery. The simple presence of a magnetic field is not sufficient to cause electrons to move along a wire. Faraday discovered that the magnetic lines of force and the wire must have a motion relative to each other to induce an electrical current (Figure 4-10). There are three ways to create the motion between lines of force and a conductor:

1. **Move the conductor** through a stationary, unchanging-strength magnetic field.
2. **Move magnetic lines of force** through a stationary conductor with an unchanging-strength magnetic field.
3. **Vary the magnetic flux** strength from a stationary magnet through a stationary conductor. As the flux strength varies, the lines of force will expand and contract, in effect causing the relative motion necessary to induce current.

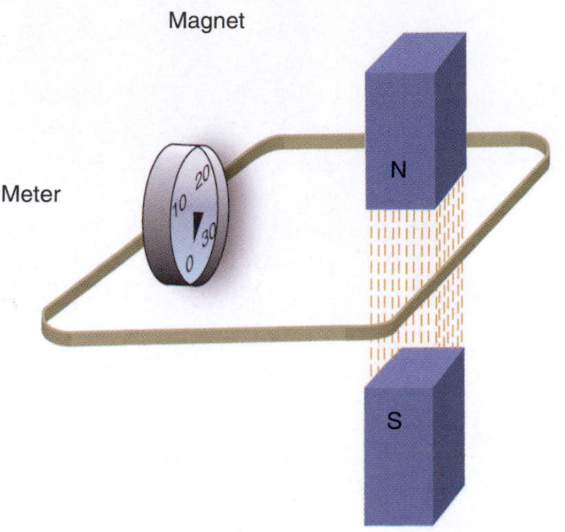

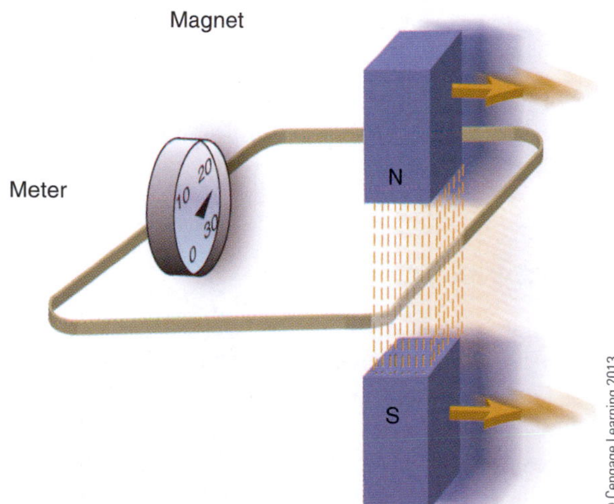

FIGURE 4-10. Faraday's experiment: A meter will not indicate current flow (A) until the magnetic lines of force from the magnet and wire have a motion relative to one another (B).

The exact definitions of "magnetic flux strength" and "lines of force" are critical to understanding these differences.

There are two primary laws that govern the induction of current by magnetic fields. Faraday's law (sometimes called the First Law of Electromagnetics) states that four factors regulate the strength of induced current when magnetic lines of force and a conductor are in motion relative to one another:

1. the **strength** of the magnetic field,
2. the **speed** of the motion between lines of force and the conductor,
3. the **angle** between the magnetic lines of force and the conductor, and
4. the **number of turns** in the conducting coil.

This law makes it possible to determine the direction in which the induced current will flow. This application of the law was established by the Russian scientist Heinrich Lenz (1804–1865). Lenz's law (sometimes called the Second Law of Electromagnetics) states that induced current flow sets up a magnetic field opposing the action that produced the original current, or, simply, that induced current opposes any flux change.

These two laws apply to both forms of induction: mutual induction and self-induction. **Mutual induction** occurs when two coils are placed in proximity and a varying current supplied to the first coil (as an electromagnet) induces a similar flow in the second coil (Figure 4-11). The coil supplied with current is called the **primary coil**, whereas the coil in which the current is inducted is called the **secondary coil**. The flow occurs in the secondary coil because the primary current alternates. This follows the rule that moving lines of force from a varying-intensity current will induce electron flow in the wire through which it passes. In this case the secondary coil is cut by the varying (and therefore moving) lines of force from the current in the primary coil.

Self-induction is much more complicated but is more understandable when comparing a coil supplied with direct current, where there is self-induction only at the turn-on moment, with a coil supplied with alternating current, where self-induction occurs regularly. Alternating current is present when the electrons constantly change direction. A coil supplied with alternating current permits a steady flow of electrons and establishes an electromagnetic effect for half the cycle. However, at the instant the current supply reverses, the previously established electromagnetic north and south

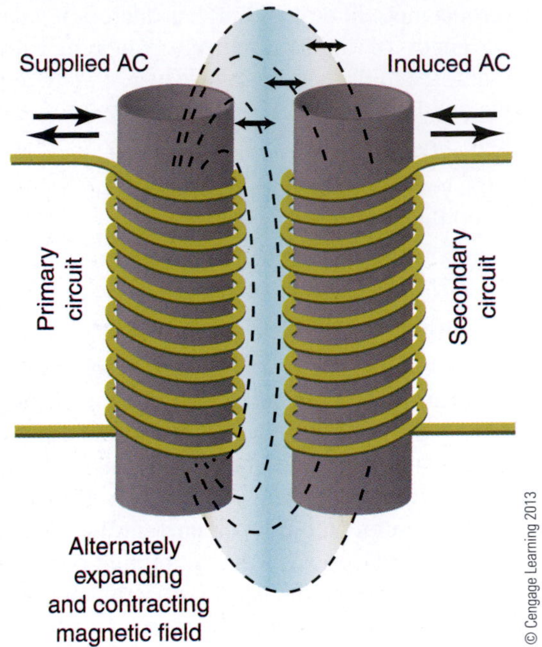

FIGURE 4-11. Mutual induction: A varying current supplied to the primary coil induces a similar flow in the second coil. The constantly expanding and contracting magnetic lines of force induced in the primary coil provide the relative motion, with the secondary coil necessary to induce current flow in the secondary coil.

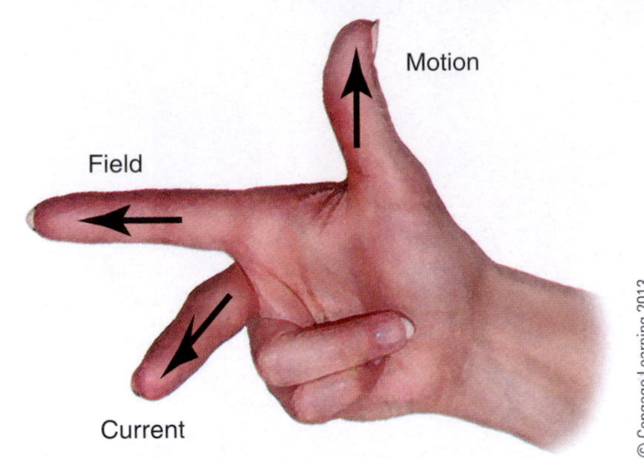

FIGURE 4-12. Fleming's right-hand generator rule: When the thumb points in the direction the conductor (or armature) is moving and the index finger points in the direction of the magnetic lines of force field, the middle finger indicates the direction of conventional current flow. Fleming's left-hand generator rule does the same for actual electron flow.

poles will induce an opposing potential difference, thus attempting to induce against the incoming supply of electrons. This tendency of an alternating current is called **inductive reactance** and is measured in ohms of resistance. Self-induction is useful when it is desirable to permit direct current to flow while at the same time hindering alternating current.

An important relationship exists between the direction of movement of a wire coil (the **armature**), the direction of the magnetic lines of force field, and the direction in which the induced current will flow. This relationship is best remembered by the use of another "hand" rule (Figure 4-12). **Fleming's right-hand generator rule states that if the thumb points in the direction the conductor (or armature) is moving and the index finger points in the direction of the magnetic lines of force field, then the middle finger will indicate the direction of the conventional current.** (If the direction of actual electron flow is desired, then a left-hand generator rule must be used.) Table 4-1 compares this rule with the other "hand" rules.

Generators

A **generator,** or dynamo, is a device that converts mechanical energy to electrical energy using Faraday's discovery of moving lines of flux in relationship to a conductor to induce current. This process converts the mechanical energy of the motion (any of the three ways) to electrical energy. A simple generator is composed of a conductor and magnets arranged as shown in Figure 4-13. The conductor is an armature, set between opposing magnetic poles so that it encounters the strongest lines of force. If the armature is rotated by a strong source of mechanical energy (such as a steam or water turbine), the generator can produce massive amounts of electrical energy. It is important to note the method that is used to convey the electrical current from the armature to the circuit. A set of **slip rings** and **brushes** permits the circuit to remain stationary while the armature rotates without breaking the electrical contact between them. This

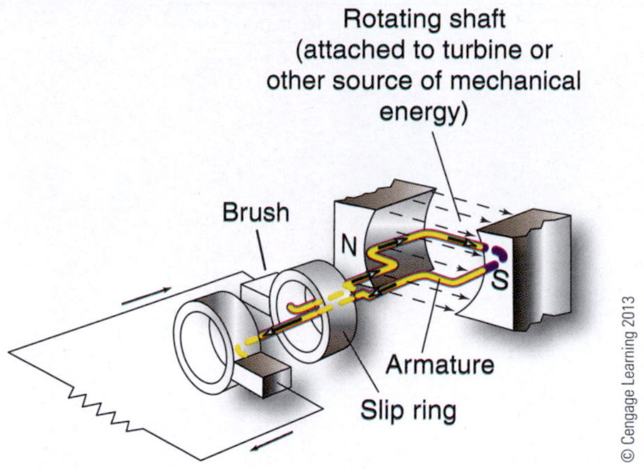

FIGURE 4-13. An AC generator: Mechanical energy rotates the shaft to which the armature is attached. As the wires of the armature rotate, they cut through the magnetic lines of flux from the magnets and produce electrical current. The slip rings and brushes permit the armature to rotate while maintaining contact with the wires of the circuit.

allows the electrons to flow without interruption. **Each slip ring connects to one end of the armature wire** (see Figure 4-13).

To understand exactly how the current is produced, it is necessary to follow the production step by step (Figure 4-14). Notice that the armature coil wire is shown in cross-section at the top, three-dimensionally in the middle, and that the graph at the bottom represents the voltage produced. It is important to understand the relationship of the angle between this wire's motion and the lines of force between the stationary magnets. In Figure 4-14A the wire's motion is parallel to the lines of force. This produces no emf, as shown on the graph. In Figure 4-14B the rotation of the armature has changed the wire's motion until it is at a 45° angle to the lines of force. Fleming's right-hand generator rule demonstrates that the conventional electrical current is moving into the page (electron flow would be out of the page). Because of the 45° angle, the magnitude of the emf, although rising, has not yet reached its peak. In Figure 4-14C, the motion of the wire is 90° to the lines of force (the maximum angle), resulting in the peak emf. As the wire begins to turn back to parallel in Figure 4-14D, the emf begins to drop back toward zero. When the wire reaches a parallel position, as in Figure 4-14E, the emf has returned to zero. As the wire begins to move into a 270° position (which is a 90° position in the opposite direction), notice that the relationship between the wire's motion and the lines of force has changed. Using Fleming's right-hand generator rule again, it is simple to see that the conventional electrical current has now reversed and is moving out of the page (while the electron flow has reversed to move into the page). **It is at this point that alternating current is produced.** This has occurred because **alternating current is produced when the wire's motion relative to the lines of force is reversed.** In Figures 4-14F, G, H, and I, the rise to peak and drop back to zero emf is repeated but in the opposite direction. This explains not only why generator-produced current must be alternating but also accounts for its pulsating nature.

The type of curve produced by an AC generator will always appear as in Figure 4-14. It is called a **sine wave** because it depends on the mathematical sine (a smooth repetitive oscillation) between the plane of the armature and a plane perpendicular to the lines of force. **One complete turn of the generator armature represents one cycle.** The sine wave illustrates one complete turn of the armature as the distance between two corresponding points. Note that this would be represented by the distance between **a** and **i** in Figure 4-14. **The frequency of the sine wave is determined by the number of cycles per second (cps). The unit of frequency is the hertz, represented by the symbol Hz. 1 cps = 1 Hz.** American and Canadian generators operate at 60 Hz. Most of the rest of the world operates at 50 Hz.

EXAMPLE: How many times per second do the electrons in a 60-Hz alternating current change their direction of movement?

Answer:

60 Hz × 2 directions = 120 changes per second

From Figure 4-14, it also becomes apparent that the **peak voltage is not the same as the average voltage** throughout the entire sine

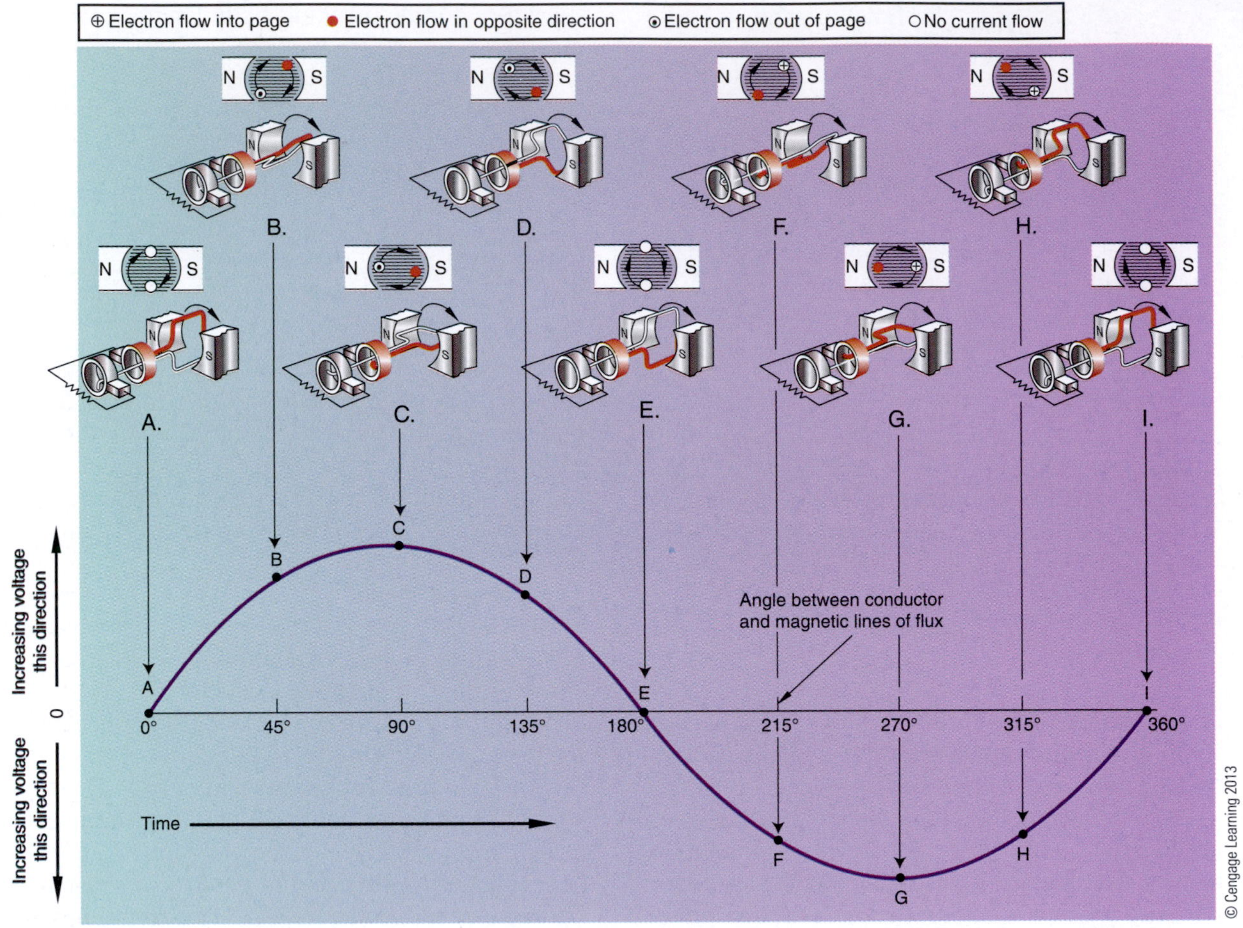

FIGURE 4-14. The production of alternating current: Armature coil wire is shown in cross section (top). Three-dimensional view of generator (middle). Graph of the voltage produced (bottom). See text for step-by-step description.

wave. The same is true of amperage and resistance (Ohm's law). This makes the measurement of all factors very difficult in pulsating alternating current because of the constant fluctuation of the sine wave. This is solved by using the root mean square (rms) values of the amperage and voltage. **Root mean square (rms) values of the total voltage and amperage in an alternating current are equivalent to the effect that would be produced in a direct-current resistance by the same factors.** Resistance in alternating currents is calculated from a complicated series of factors, resulting in measurement of the apparent total resistance. **Apparent total resistance of an alternating current is called impedance, which is represented by the symbol Z.** This permits a revised version of Ohm's law to be applied for alternating current as:

$$I = \frac{V}{Z}$$

where: I = rms amperage
V = rms voltage
Z = impedance

When using an x-ray machine, it is worth remembering that the **kilovoltage settings represent peak kilovoltage, not average or rms values.**

A direct-current generator is made by exchanging the slip rings for a commutator ring, as shown in Figure 4-15. **A commutator is a single ring that is divided in half, with each half connected to one end of the armature wire.** The single commutator's two halves replace the pair of slip rings. Instead of each end of the armature wire being connected to its own slip ring, each end of the armature wire is connected to half of the commutator ring. When a generator has its armature connected to a commutator, the sine wave of the output is dramatically different from that produced by a pair of slip rings. Although the armature turns exactly as in an alternating-current generator, the commutator routes the current very differently. This current produces a sine wave exactly as in an alternating-current generator (Figures 4-15A–C). The use of Fleming's right-hand generator rule demonstrates that the conventional electrical current is moving into the page (electron flow would be out of the page). In Figure 4-15D the wire has begun to move toward the second phase of the cycle. As in the alternating-current generator, the relationship between the wire's motion and the lines of force has changed. Using Fleming's right-hand generator rule again, it is simple to see that the conventional electrical current has now reversed and is moving out of the page (while the electron flow has reversed to move into the page). However, it is extremely important to note that in Figure 4-15D, the commutator ring has also changed the brush with which it was in contact. This has the same effect as switching the exiting connections on the armature wires. **Although Fleming's right-hand generator rule demonstrates the change in direction of current within the armature wire, the**

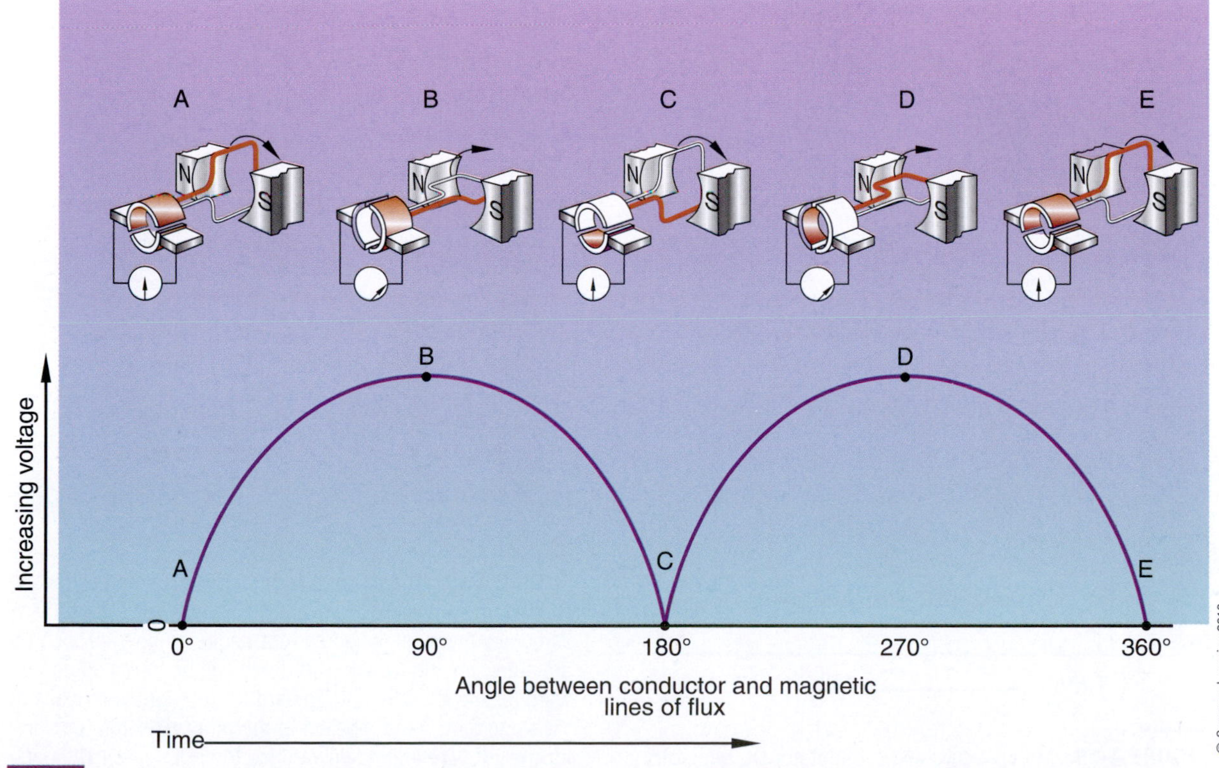

FIGURE 4-15. A DC generator: The slip rings have been exchanged for a commutator ring, with each half connecting to one end of the armature wire. Although the armature turns exactly as in an AC generator, the commutator routes the current as shown on the graph. See text for step-by-step description.

commutator ring has also reversed the exiting connections, thus keeping the current in the circuit flowing in the same direction. It is at this point that direct current is produced. Note that the direct current is not as steady as would be expected with a battery source. Instead a pulsating direct current has been produced.

Multiple-coil direct-current generators are used in place of the simple single-coil generators diagrammed in Figures 4-14 and 4-15. These DC generators utilize numerous coils and a commutator divided into a corresponding number of segments, as shown in Figure 4-16A. This type of generator produces a sine wave, as shown in Figure 4-16B. The combined current generated never drops to zero and has the advantage of a much steadier flow, although the pulsations have not been completely eliminated.

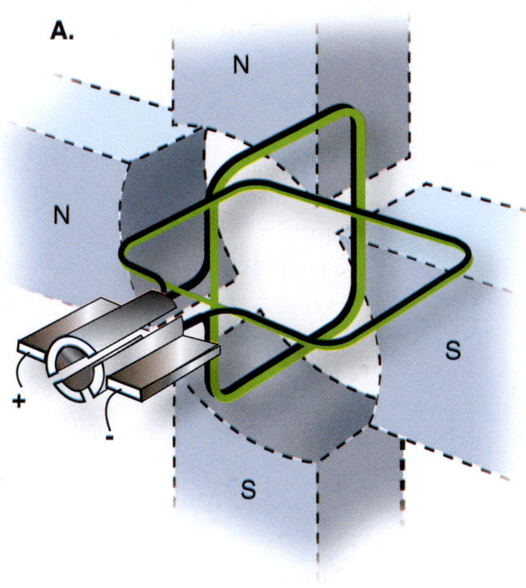

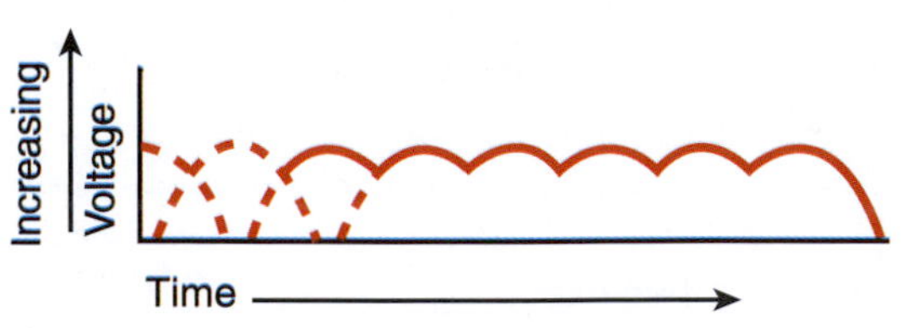

FIGURE 4-16. Multiple coil, split commutator DC generator: More than one coil, or armature, with a split commutator (A) will produce DC current as shown in the graph (B).

Motors

A device that is supplied with electrical current to produce mechanical motion is called a **motor**. Motors have essentially the same parts as generators and operate on the same principles but in reverse. In addition, some of the parts have been slightly redesigned and carry names different from those in a generator.

The motor principle is a result of the interaction of magnetic fields when an electric current is sent along a conductor that is residing in a magnetic field. As current flows through the conducting coil, a magnetic field is established, according to Fleming's right-hand thumb rule (Figure 4-17). Because the conducting coil lies within the lines of force from the stationary magnets, the induced lines of force will be attracted in one direction (downward for the left wire and upward for the right wire) while at the same time

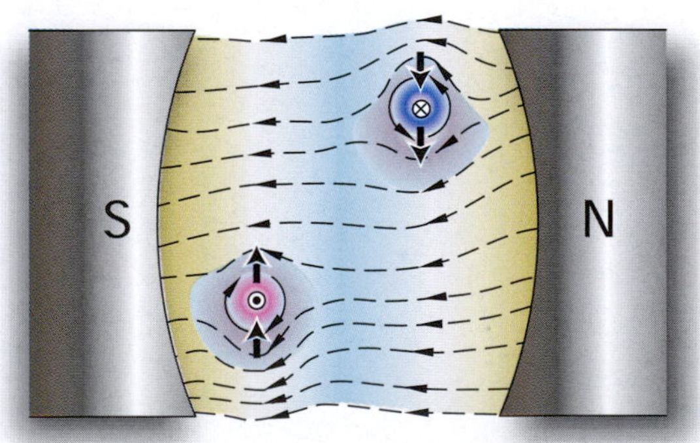

FIGURE 4-17. The motor principle: Because the conducting wires of the armature lie within the lines of force from the stationary magnets, when current begins to flow through the armature, the induced lines of force will be attracted downward for the left wire and upward for the right wire while at the same time being repelled in the other direction (upward for the left wire and downward for the right wire). The net result is that the conductor begins to move in the direction of the arrows.

being repelled in the other direction (upward for the left wire and downward for the right wire). The net result is that the conductor begins to move in the direction of the arrows.

Fleming's left-hand motor rule states that if the index finger points in the direction of the magnetic lines of force field and the middle finger points in the direction of the conventional current, the thumb will indicate the direction the conductor will move (Figure 4-18). (This would be a right-hand motor rule if the direction of electron flow is being considered.) Table 4-1 compares this rule with the other "hand" rules.

Different motor configurations are required depending on whether alternating or direct current is supplied. **Direct-current motors use commutator rings.** As with a DC generator, the commutator is required in order to switch the flow of current when the conducting coil begins to reach a 180° position, where the induced and stationary lines of force no longer attract or repel one another. When the current flow is switched by the commutator ring, the magnetic lines of force also reverse. Continuing this switching of current flow results in the conductor continually being simultaneously repelled and attracted in a circle, thus turning a shaft and supplying the mechanical motion as a conversion of the applied electrical energy.

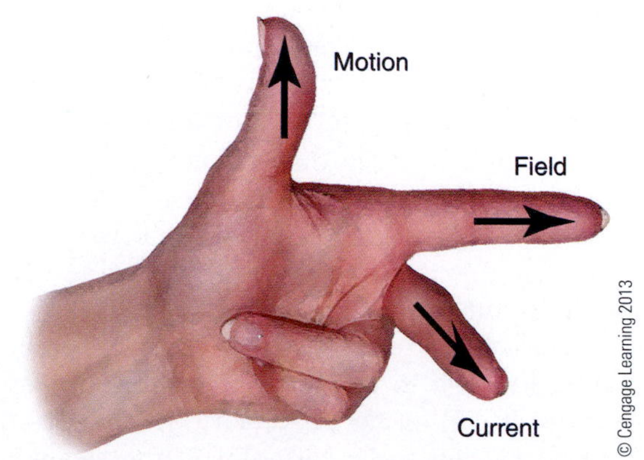

FIGURE 4-18. Fleming's left-hand motor rule: If the index finger points in the direction of the magnetic lines of force and the middle finger points in the direction of the conventional current flow, the thumb will indicate the direction the conductor will move. (This would be a right-hand motor rule if the direction of actual electron flow is being considered.)

These direct-current motors use many turns of wire in the conductor coil to increase the strength of the field. This requires numerous pairs of stationary magnets to force the conductor coil to cut the stationary lines of force as near to 90° (the maximum inducing angle) as often as possible.

Alternating-current motors use slip rings. Unlike direct-current motors, the incoming current switches direction, making the commutator unnecessary. There are two major types of alternating-current motors.

Synchronous alternating-current motors have conducting coils that turn at the same speed as the generator armature supplying the current (or a multiple of the armature's speed). Synchronous motors are useful when a steady speed is necessary, as in a timing device. They tend to be relatively weak because insufficient motor principle force is established at the conducting coil.

Alternating-current induction motors utilize a rotor coil with the exterior magnetic field supplied by several pairs of electromagnets, thus producing a strong magnetic field, increasing the power of the motor and permitting it to run at any desired speed. Instead of supplying current to the coil in the magnetic field, an induction motor uses a device called a **rotor**. **A rotor consists of bars of copper around an iron core** (Figure 4-19). No commutator or slip rings are required. Instead, a device called a **stator** is used. **A stator consists of pairs of stationary magnets (or, more commonly, electromagnets) arranged around the rotor. The stator must be supplied with multiphase current.** The stator electromagnets are energized in sequence. As the copper bars of the rotor reach a point where the motor principle forces are equalized, the multiphase current activates the next pair of electromagnets and the motor principle forces pull the rotor around to the next position. This continuing sequential energization causes the motor principle forces to continually turn the rotor. Extremely powerful induction motors are made by increasing

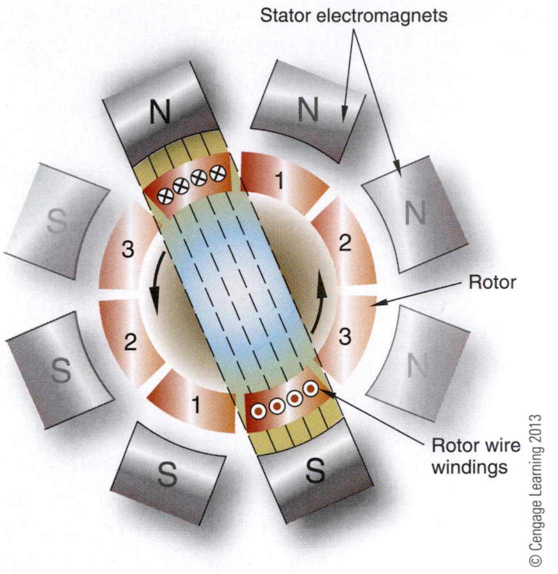

FIGURE 4-19. Alternating-current induction motor: The rotor windings obey the motor principle as they move perpendicular to the magnetic lines of flux, in the direction of the arrows. The stator electromagnets are supplied with multiphase current to activate them in sequential pairs to maintain maximum perpendicular motor principle force.

the strength and number of pairs of electromagnets; these motors are popular for industrial and consumer uses.

Induction motors are used in rotating anode x-ray tubes where the target anode is attached to the induction motor rotor inside the glass vacuum tube. Because magnetic lines of force will pass through glass and a vacuum, the electromagnets can be positioned outside the vacuum tube, thus avoiding interference with the high voltages required to produce x-rays.

The motor principle is also used in meters: **galvanometers** for direct current, when permanent magnets are used, to indicate current, and **dynamometers** for alternating current, when electromagnets are used (Figure 4-20A). To a great extent they are being replaced by digital meters that provide numerical indications of current. When a meter is connected in series, it measures current in amperes and is called an **ammeter** (see Figure 4-20B). When connected in parallel, it measures potential difference in volts and is called a **voltmeter** (see Figure 4-20C).

CONTROLLING ELECTRICAL CURRENT

Although nearly all electrical components in x-ray units are now embedded in silicon chips on printed circuit (PC) boards, transformers continue to operate as discussed below, although they are much smaller than they were 20 to 30 years ago.

Although the concepts behind the operation of most of these components are more easily understood when presented from a hard-wired perspective, readers should remember that these devices and circuits are now miniaturized within chip technology.

Transformers

Alternating current, because of its changing direction, constantly establishes, collapses, reestablishes, and re-collapses its surrounding magnetic field. This aspect can be used to change electricity by combining electromagnetic mutual induction with an application of Ohm's law to form a device called a **transformer**. Transformers are composed of two coils placed near one another (but without electrical connection). If current is supplied to one coil, the lines of force that are induced will pass through the other coil and induce a flow of electrons (see Figure 4-11). The coil that is supplied with current is the **primary,** and the coil in which current is induced is the **secondary.**

The number of turns of wire in the primary coil is designed to be different from the number of turns of wire in the secondary. This causes the induced current to be different in the secondary coil. For example, the lines of force induced by a single primary coil loop may cut two loops of the secondary. In this case the voltage in the primary would be induced in **both** secondary loops, thus doubling the secondary voltage. When the voltage is increased from primary to secondary it is called a **step-up transformer.** When the voltage is decreased from primary to secondary it is called

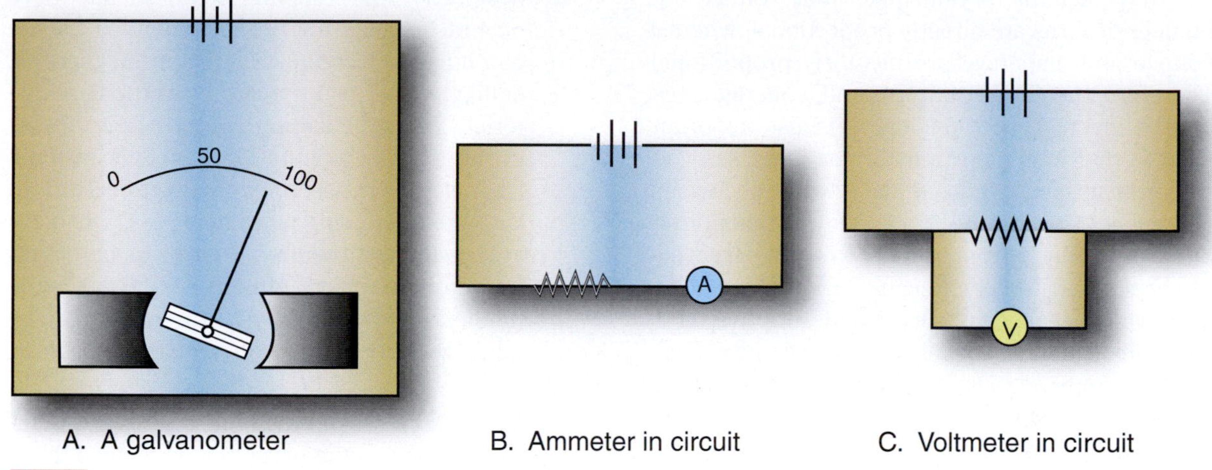

FIGURE 4-20. (A) A simple galvanometer uses an electromagnet to attract a coil of wire to which a needle is attached. When a scale is calibrated, amperage or voltage can be measured. (B) Ammeter connection. (C) Voltmeter connection.

a **step-down transformer.** The **transformer law** expresses this phenomenon:

$$\frac{V_s}{V_p} = \frac{N_s}{N_p}$$

where: V = potential difference in volts
N = number of turns of wire in the coil
p = primary coil
s = secondary coil

EXAMPLE: If a transformer is supplied with 400 volts to the primary coil, has 100 turns of wire on the primary coil and 20,000 turns of wire on the secondary coil, what will the voltage be in the secondary coil?

Answer:

$$\frac{V_s}{V_p} = \frac{N_s}{N_p}$$

$$\frac{V_s}{400\text{V}} = \frac{20{,}000 \text{ turns}}{100 \text{ turns}}$$

$$100\ V_s = 400\text{ V} \times 20{,}000 \text{ turns}$$

$$V_s = \frac{8{,}000{,}000}{100}$$

$$V_s = 80{,}000 \text{ volts or } 80 \text{ kilovolts.}$$

EXAMPLE: If a transformer has 120 turns of wire on the primary coil, 80 volts in the primary coil, and 20 volts in the secondary coil, how many turns of wire must there be in the secondary coil?

Answer:

$$\frac{V_s}{V_p} = \frac{N_s}{N_p}$$

$$\frac{20\text{V}}{80\text{V}} = \frac{N_s}{120 \text{ turns}}$$

$$\frac{2{,}400 \text{ turns}}{80} = N_s$$

$$N_s = 30 \text{ turns}$$

Transformers are used to change voltage. However, Ohm's law is in effect and the effect of the transformer on amperage, voltage, and number of turns in the coils can be calculated by combining the transformer law with Ohm's law:

$$\frac{I_s}{I_p} = \frac{V_p}{V_s}$$

and:

$$\frac{I_s}{I_p} = \frac{N_p}{N_s}$$

It is helpful to remember that voltage and number of turns are directly proportional, whereas voltage and amperage are inversely proportional. Therefore, the number of turns and amperage must also be inversely proportional. It is also important to note that a step-up transformer increases voltage from primary to secondary while decreasing amperage. Conversely, a step-down transformer decreases voltage from primary to secondary while increasing amperage. Because transformers are designed to change voltages, the descriptive terms *step-up* and *step-down* refer to the voltage change, not the amperage change. You should remember that Ohm's law requires the consideration of resistance, and this is indeed an important factor. However, this book will not address that aspect. **All transformers must operate on alternating current to provide the establishing and collapsing magnetic fields that induce the voltage changes in the secondary coil.**

Although transformer efficiency, the ability of a transformer to avoid power loss, is usually above 95 percent, a number of factors influence how much energy is lost. Because the high-voltage transformer used in x-ray equipment must step up voltage into the kilovolt range, it uses large amounts of secondary coil windings. This massive amount of wire and the high induced voltage cause several problems that greatly affect the efficiency of the transformer.

1. **I^2R loss**, sometimes called copper loss, is caused by the inherent resistance to current flow that is found in all conductors. The power lost due to this resistance is proportional to the square of the current. It is minimized by using low-resistance wire, such as large-diameter copper, and by using high voltage and low amperage. Lost power is given off as heat. This is the reason why power transmitted long distances between cities is carried on high-voltage power lines. The high voltage permits low amperage and greatly reduced I^2R loss. Because high voltages are extremely dangerous, they are carried on high towers. Step-down transformers are used at receiving stations to lower the voltage (and increase the amperage) to make the power safe for use in buildings.
2. **Hysteresis loss** (lagging loss) in the core occurs because energy is expended as the continually changing AC current magnetizes, demagnetizes, and remagnetizes the core material. Demagnetization leaves some dipoles in the original orientation, and this residual magnetism causes the remagnetic effort to lag, thus producing more heat loss. The characteristic that requires energy to carry out this constant reorientation of the magnetic dipoles is called **coercivity**. Coercivity can be minimized by using a core material such as silicon iron.
3. **Eddy current loss** in the core is a result of currents opposing the cause that produced them, according to Lenz's law, as discussed earlier. They are produced in any conducting material subjected to changing magnetic fields. Laminating the transformer core reduces the eddy current loss by dividing the core into thin layers. This reduces the strength of the eddy currents (Figure 4-21).

These factors result in a great amount of heat build-up, which can be felt by placing your hand on the exterior of the transformer cabinet in a diagnostic x-ray room. Although the transformer is highly insulated and immersed in insulating dielectric oil, there is a definite warmth to the cabinet after the machine has been in use for a few hours. The size of the x-ray transformer makes its efficiency an important factor.

There are numerous types of transformer configurations. The simple arrangement of two coils of wire in proximity to facilitate induction, which has been used so far to explain transformer function, is called an **air-core transformer**. If the primary and secondary coils are filled with an iron core, the strength of the magnetic field is greatly increased, forming an **open-core transformer**. Various types of cores have been designed to enhance the lines of force and thereby increase the magnetic field strength (Figure 4-22). The field from an open core tends to diverge as it forms the external lines of force. Closing the core to form a **closed-core transformer** (by placing a top and bottom to the cores) will direct the lines of force from primary and secondary cores toward each

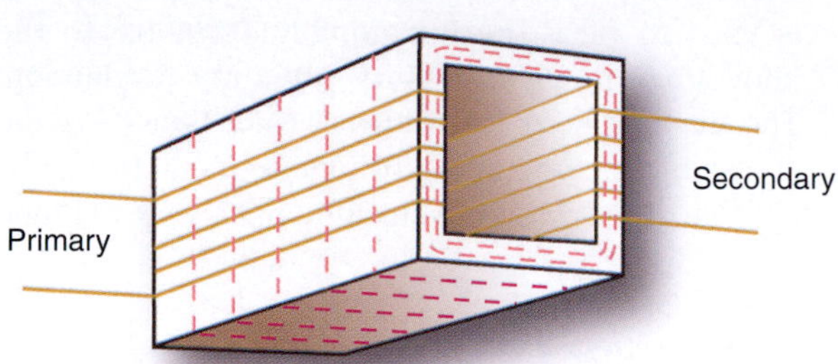

A. Closed core transformer

B. Nonlaminated core

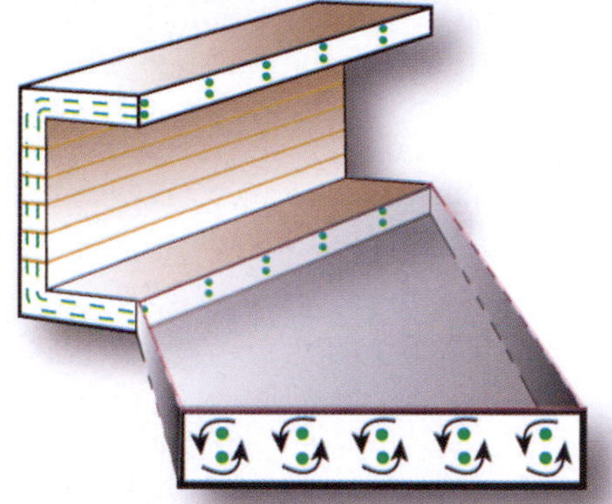

C. Eddy currents

D. Laminated core

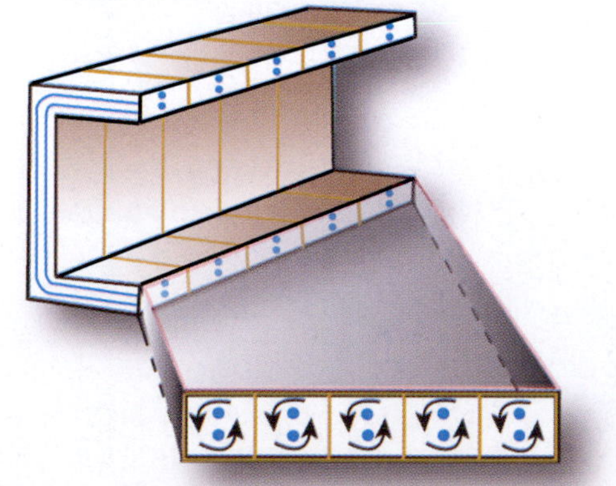

E. Eddy currents

FIGURE 4-21. (A) Closed-core transformer; (B) nonlaminated core; (C) nonlaminated core eddy currents; (D) laminated core; and (E) laminated core eddy currents.

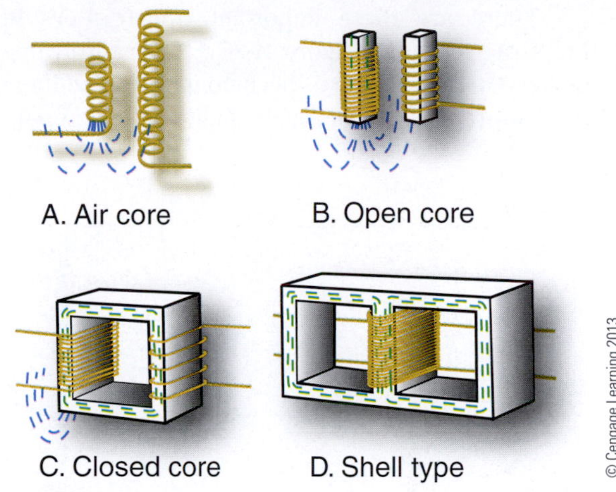

FIGURE 4-22. Various types of transformer core configurations; (A) air core; (B) open core; (C) closed core; and (D) shell type.

other and result in a significant system net increase in field strength. The **shell-type transformer** goes one step further by converging both the inside and outside lines of force through an iron core. In addition, a great efficiency is obtained by insulating the wiring and wrapping the primary and secondary coils atop one another, thus minimizing the distance between coils and maximizing the coupling effectiveness of the induction. X-ray generators use laminated core, shell-type transformers, which are the most common type in use today.

Autotransformers

It is possible to construct a variable transformer, called an **autotransformer**, by connecting both primary and secondary coils in series instead of insulating them. This also permits a single coil on a central core. Connections are made along a single coil at different points for primary and secondary. The primary side has a selection of taps available to permit a variable number of turns in the primary coil (Figure 4-23). When the connections to the taps are attached to control buttons, an effective means of changing voltage is available.

There are three important transformers in the x-ray circuit (Figure 4-24). The autotransformer is used to vary the incoming-line voltage to an appropriate level for the high-voltage step-up transformer. The high-voltage step-up transformer is used to raise the incoming-line voltage to the kilovoltage range necessary for x-ray production. The filament step-down transformer is used to decrease the incoming-line voltage to the 5- to 15-volt and 3- to 5-ampere range used to heat the x-ray tube filament.

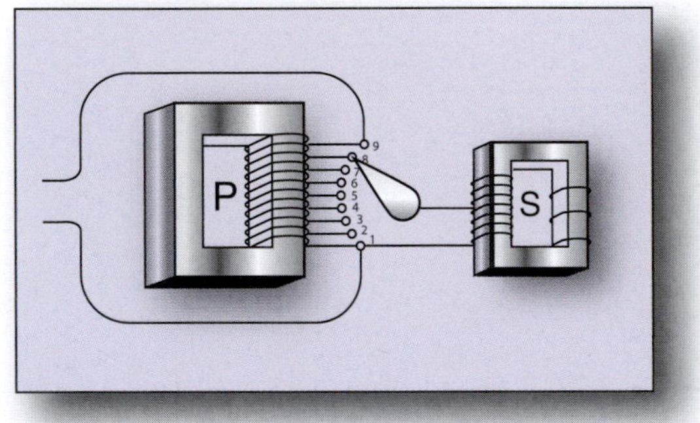

FIGURE 4-23. An autotransformer.

Capacitors

A **capacitor** is a device capable of accumulating and storing an electrical charge. A simple capacitor consists of two insulated metal plates with opposite charges (Figure 4-25). The repulsion between the charges on the two plates permits a greater number of electrons to be stored on each. The insulation between the plates is called the **dielectric**, and its value is determined by the insulating ability as well as the plate size, distance between the plates, and charge. The unit of capacitance is named for

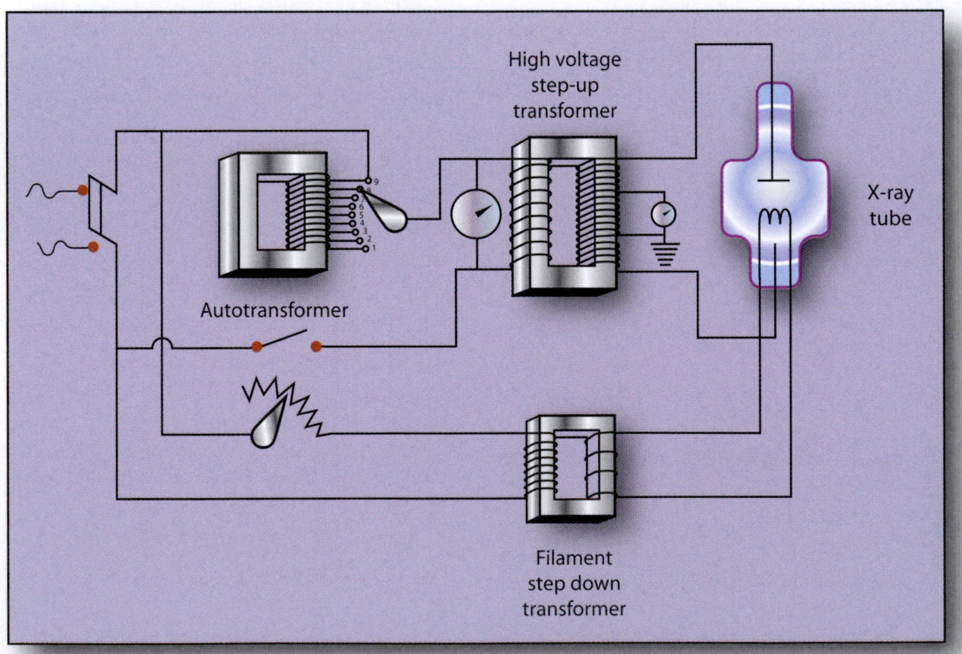

FIGURE 4-24. Three critical transformer locations in the diagnostic x-ray circuit. The autotransformer permits selection of the voltage (by controls labeled kV on the console). The high-voltage transformer steps the incoming-line voltage up to the kV range before sending it to the x-ray tube. The filament transformer steps the incoming-line voltage down to heat the x-ray tube filament.

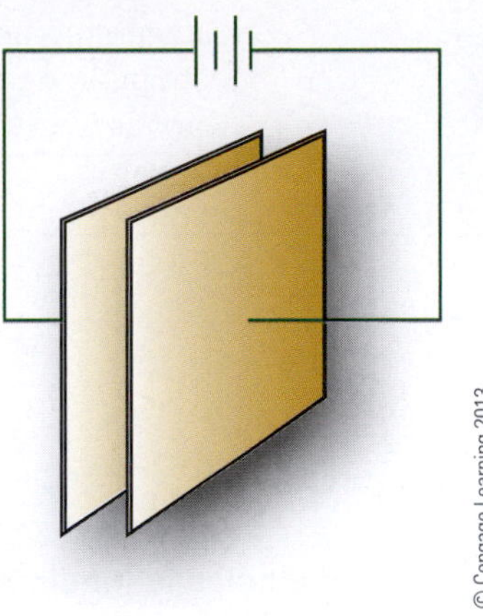

FIGURE 4-25. A simple parallel plate capacitor.

Faraday but has been shortened to **farad**. It is represented by the symbol **f** and is expressed as:

$$C = \frac{q}{V}$$

where: C = capacitance in farads
q = charge on either plate in coulombs
V = potential difference between plates in volts

Because of the immense size of the coulomb, the farad is very large, making the microfarad (μf) the more common unit.

Capacitors must be charged to be operable; this is done by applying a direct-current voltage. The capacitor will accept a charge until it equals the DC voltage. When discharged, the capacitor has the ability to deliver the stored charge in short and easily controlled intervals. This uniform direct current is especially useful in mobile x-ray units where it is convenient to have a battery charge a capacitor and then initiate a burst of high voltage for the x-ray exposure. Capacitors are also used to supply a more constant voltage to the x-ray tube in some stationary units.

RECTIFICATION

X-ray tubes operate best when receiving direct current. In fact, there is a danger in supplying alternating current because if a flow of electrons occurs in the wrong direction the tube may be damaged beyond repair. **Rectification** is the process by which alternating current is changed to pulsating direct current, and requires the use of one-way electrical devices called rectifiers. Although solid-state semiconductor diodes are most commonly used, it is easier to understand the operation of a vacuum-tube rectifier. Both of these devices create electrical "one-way streets" by permitting electrons to flow easily in one direction while offering a high resistance to movement in the other direction.

The operation of semiconductors was mentioned earlier, in Chapter 3, during the discussion of conductor valence bands. There are numerous types of semiconductors but they all operate in the same manner. The simplest to explain is the p-n junction semiconductor, which is composed of solid materials of two predominant categories, n-type and p-type. The n-type materials have loosely bound electrons that move freely between an atom's conduction bands. The p-type materials have electron traps made up of positively charged holes that tend to attract and hold electrons instead of permitting them to move freely to another atom. Both types of materials are affected by slight amounts of impurities that are intentionally added to change the conduction properties. For example, arsenic has a valence that permits it to form covalent bonds with silicon crystals, but it makes an extra electron available for conduction, thus forming an n-type material. Conversely, gallium also has a valence permitting covalent bonding with silicon, but it leaves a need for an additional electron, thus forming an electron "hole" and a p-type material.

A rectifying semiconductor called a **diode** is made by sandwiching a p-type crystal with an n-type to form a p-n junction (Figure 4-26). When a potential difference is established with the positive charge at the p side of the junction and the negative charge at the n side, the positive holes from the p side are attracted to the junction, as are the available electrons from the n side. This permits easy movement of electrons into the p holes. **In a diode, electrons flow from the n to the p side of the p-n junction and conventional electrical current moves from the p to the n side.** When alternating current reverses and the positive charge is

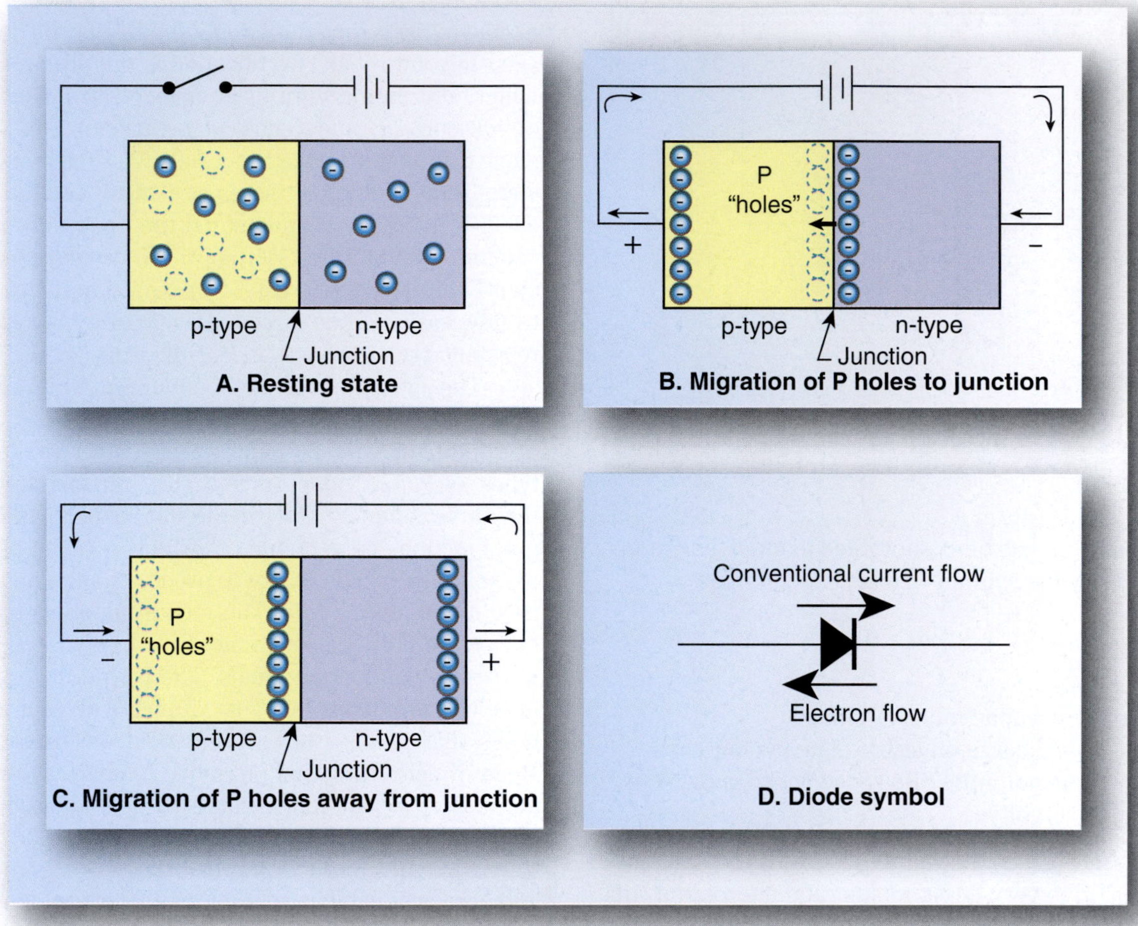

FIGURE 4-26. The functioning of a p-n junction of a solid-state semiconductor diode.

at the n side of the junction and the negative charge is at the p side, the positive holes from the p side are repelled from the junction, as are the available electrons from the n side. This makes movement of electrons from the n side of the junction to the p side very unlikely, as both the repulsion-attraction of the charges and the distance between p holes and electrons are working against the electron movement. The result is that no electrons move across the junction, thus creating a one-way street for electrons. The electronic symbol for a diode reflects this movement for conventional electrical current (see Figure 4-26D). Remember that electron flow will be opposite the direction of the arrow.

A **thyristor**, or **silicon-controlled rectifier (SCR)**, is a more complex semiconductor that has proven useful for high-speed switching of the primary high-voltage x-ray circuit. The term SCR is actually a General Electric trade name for a specific type of thyristor. SCRs are composed of two p-type and two n-type layers, making three p-n junctions (Figure 4-27). Both n-p-n-p and p-n-p-n sequences are possible. In either case, the third section serves as a gate. This gate can change the polarity of the entire SCR by receiving a given charge. Rapid pulses of current to the gate permit it to hold or release large amounts of current. The SCR functions extremely rapidly in high-kilowattage x-ray generators.

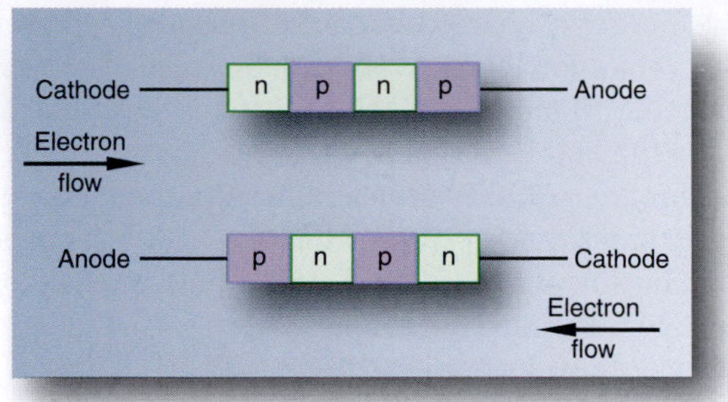

FIGURE 4-27. Silicon-controlled rectifier (SCR) n-p-n-p and p-n-p-n junctions.

A valve tube was a vacuum tube that operated in the same manner as a diode but was constructed like an x-ray tube. Although they are no longer used in x-ray circuitry, they are a useful example in learning how a modern diode circuit functions. The difference between a valve tube and an x-ray tube is that a valve tube operated at energies below the range necessary to produce x-ray photons. The cathode and anode were arranged to permit electrons to jump without requiring the energy necessary to produce x-rays (Figure 4-28). Current could flow from cathode to anode because the jump to the massive anode was easy. However, as electrons repelled one another, they spread out over the entire surface of the anode and could not develop sufficient repulsive force to jump to the cathode. This made the tube a one-way street for electrons to move from cathode to anode.

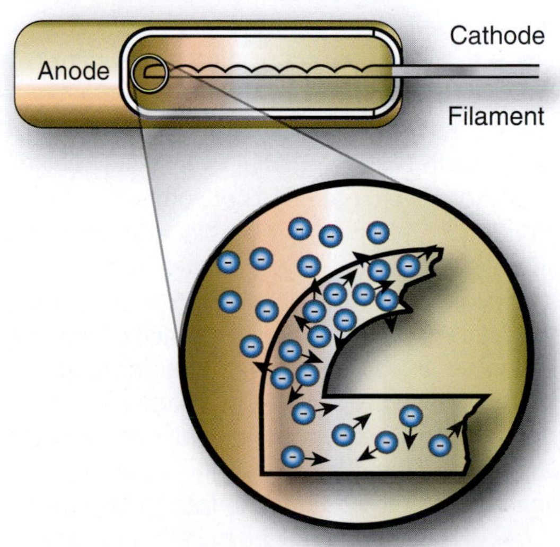

FIGURE 4-28. Anode and cathode of a valve tube.

The cathode included a coil of small-diameter tungsten wire, called the filament, through which current was passed. Of course the small diameter of the wire caused a greatly increased resistance to the flow of electrons. This resulted in heat increase to the extent that electron movement actually ejected individual electrons from the surface of the wire. Sometimes this phenomenon is described as a boiling of electrons from the surface. The result was the formation of an electron cloud (see Figure 4-28B). This process is called **thermionic emission** because the heat (therm) has caused ionization (ionic), resulting in electrons being expelled (emission) from the surface of the wire. This effect is sometimes called a **space charge cloud.** It is important to note that the small diameter of the cathode's thin filament wire makes it extremely fragile. At the high kilovoltages supplied to x-ray tubes, a single electron striking the heated filament would cause it to break, thus rendering the tube useless. All modern x-ray machines use safety devices to prevent the anode side of the tube from receiving electrons, even during the opposing flow of alternating current.

The anode is a relatively large metallic surface, usually a cup, disk, or flat plate, depending on the desired function of the tube. The shape of the anode varies between a valve tube and an x-ray tube and this accounts for the fact that x-ray tubes emit primarily x-ray-range photons whereas valve tubes do not. Diagnostic x-ray tubes utilize angled disks, whereas dental x-ray tubes and other types of relatively low-voltage tubes use flat-plate anodes. A valve-tube anode consists of a cold metallic cup that surrounds the coiled filament (see Figure 4-28).

Valve tubes permit electrons to flow from cathode to anode when a large enough potential difference exists to cause the electrons of the thermionically emitted cloud to be simultaneously repelled from the cathode and attracted to the anode. This is done by creating a **negative charge at the cathode and a positive charge at the anode (Figure 4-29). Remember that electron flow will always be from cathode to anode and this means conventional electrical current will always be from anode to cathode.** It is important to note that electrons cannot move from anode to cathode due to the charges and to the shapes of the anode and cathode. The anode is shaped much larger than the cathode filament, and this causes the electrons to distribute themselves over the entire surface as they follow the law of repulsion in regard to one another (see Figure 4-29). With such a large distribution surface, the electrons should not build up enough repulsion or heat to make movement from anode to cathode possible. When direct current causes the anode to remain positive at all times, there is a force of attraction working to keep the electrons on the anode. On the other hand, the cathode is relatively small and carries a negative charge at all times. The small size not only causes heating, it also restricts the flow of electrons so much that thermionic emission is enhanced.

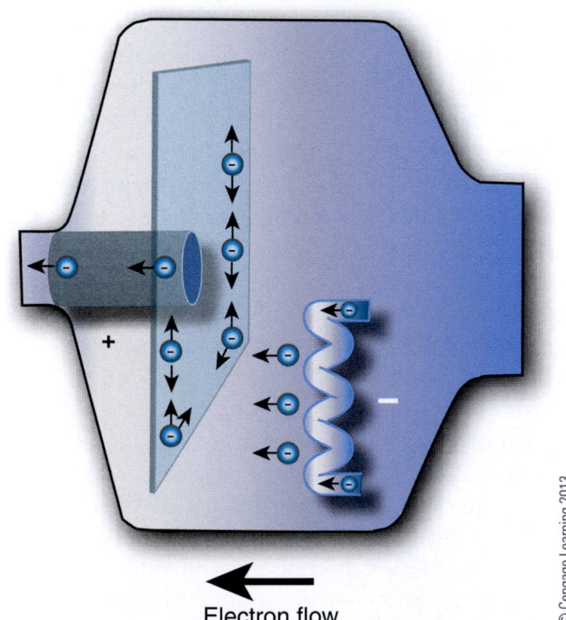

FIGURE 4-29. Electron flow through an x-ray tube.

The negative charge works to encourage thermionic emission by actively repelling the electrons from the filament surface. Together these forces make the anode very attractive to electrons, while making the cathode undesirable. Consequently, as electron movement from cathode to anode is made easy, movement from anode to cathode is made extremely difficult. This creates a one-way street for electron flow, just as in a diode.

Half-Wave Rectification

In both solid-state diodes and valve tubes the forces create an electronic one-way street and effectively suppress the opposing half of the incoming current flow. This effect can be used to protect an expensive and sensitive device, such as an x-ray tube, from current that could potentially damage it. A supply of alternating current to either type of rectifier will result in a pulsating direct current due to the suppression of half of the incoming wave (Figure 4-30). This type of suppression rectification is called **half-wave rectification** because only half of the incoming alternating current is being converted to pulsating direct current. The opposing half of the flow is simply ignored and not utilized. The electrons simply cease moving and stop transferring energy. In early radiography this type of circuit was called **self-rectification** (Figure 4-31). The danger was that overheating of the anode might cause thermionic emission. This condition could result in electrons moving to the cathode filament during the half of the alternating-current cycle when the anode was negatively charged. This of course would break the filament and destroy the x-ray tube. In even the simplest of modern x-ray equipment the x-ray tube is protected from this occurrence by the addition of a single rectifier on the anode side of the circuit (see Figure 4-30). This protects the x-ray tube anode from receiving a negative charge. In addition, if overheating should occur, the protecting rectifier would be destroyed and could be replaced, costing much less than it would to replace the x-ray tube.

Full-Wave Rectification

It is possible to convert the opposing half of the incoming electron flow so that electrons

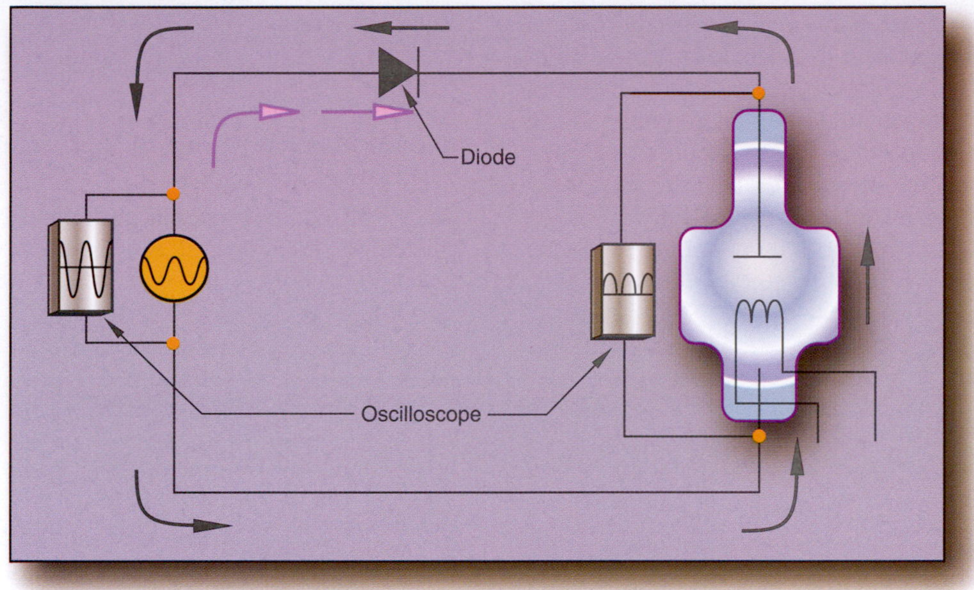

FIGURE 4-30. Half-wave rectification with one diode rectifier on the anode side of the x-ray tube circuit. Note the waveforms that would result if an oscilloscope was connected to the circuit.

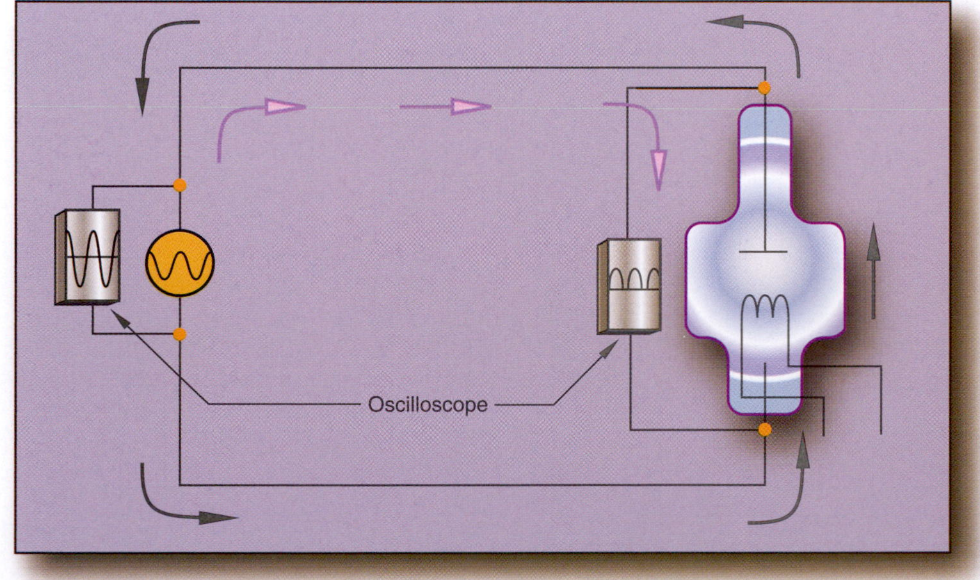

FIGURE 4-31. Half-wave rectification without a diode rectifier (self-rectification).

are always moving in the same direction, instead of discarding half the cycle by suppression. This is done through an ingenious arrangement of four rectifiers in a bridge circuit called a **full-wave rectification** circuit (Figure 4-32). A full understanding of the circuit requires following the electron flow completely from the secondary coil of the high-voltage step-up transformer to the x-ray tube during both halves of the AC cycle. Figure 4-32A illustrates the electron flow by the sequence of numbered arrows.

1. Electron flow is induced from the secondary coil of the high-voltage step-up transformer.
2. Electron flow reaches the first circuit junction and flows both ways.
3. Electron flow on this path reaches the anode of valve tube II and distributes over the

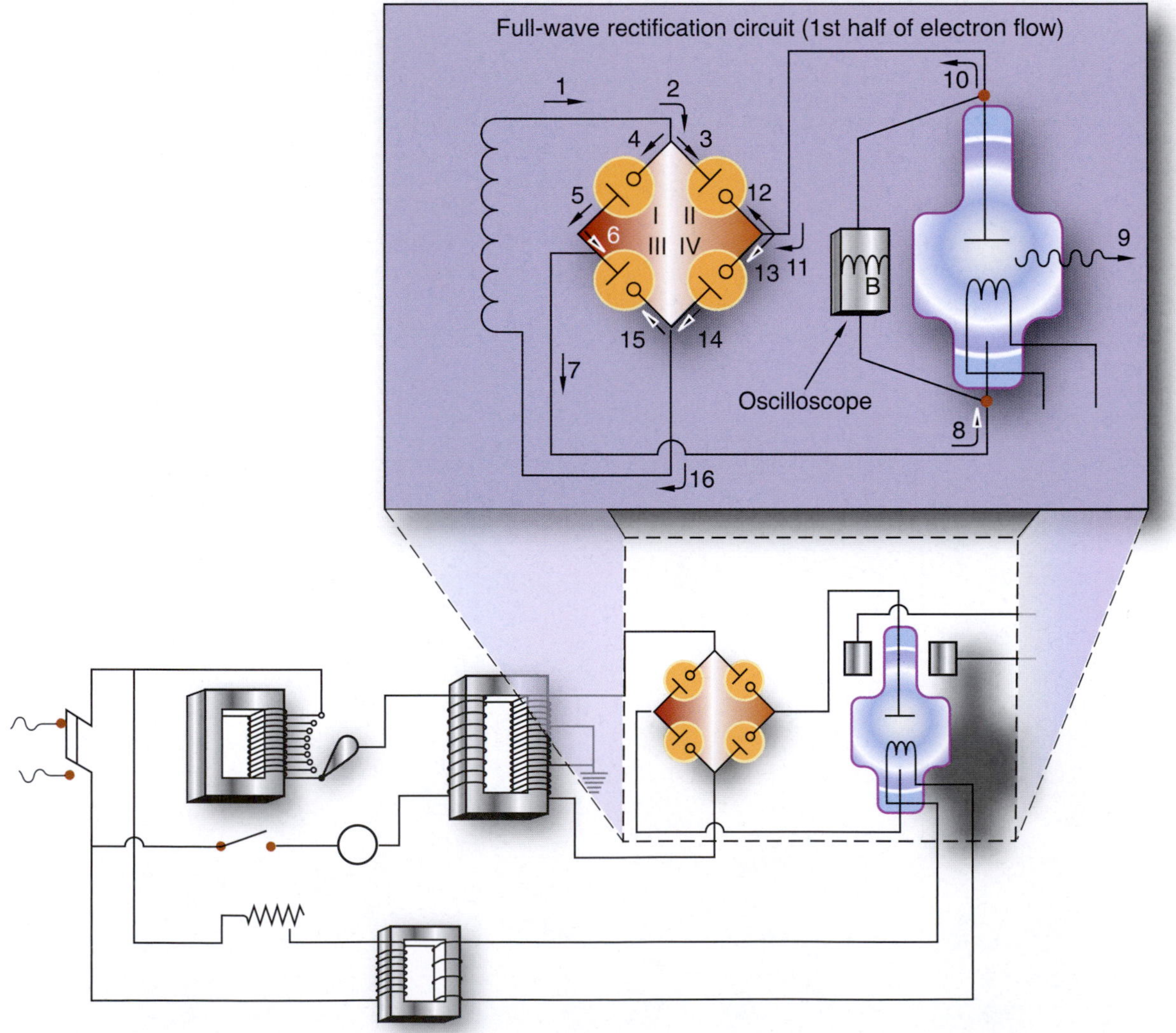

FIGURE 4-32. Full-wave rectification circuit from within a basic diagnostic x-ray circuit. (See text for description of electron flow.)

large, unheated surface, attempting to build up enough charge to jump to the cathode.

4. Electron flow on this path reaches the heated cathode of valve tube I and easily jumps to the anode (thus never permitting enough charge to accumulate for the electron flow at arrow 3 to jump across valve tube II).
5. Electron flow reaches the second junction and flows both ways.
6. Electron flow on this path reaches the an ode of valve tube III and distributes over the large, unheated surface, attempting to build up enough charge to jump to the cathode.
7. Electron flow on this path moves without resistance toward the x-ray tube.
8. Electron flow reaches the x-ray tube's heated cathode and jumps to the anode.
9. X-rays are produced as a result of the electrons striking the anode.
10. Electron flow from the anode moves without resistance back toward the rectification circuit.
11. Electron flow reaches the third junction and flows both ways.
12. Electron flow on this path reaches the heated cathode of valve tube II but cannot jump to the anode because the anode is still loaded with the charge moving at arrow 3. Because these are like charges, they repel one another.
13. Electron flow on this path reaches the heated cathode of valve tube IV and easily jumps to the anode.
14. Electron flow reaches the fourth junction and flows both ways.
15. Electron flow on this path reaches the heated cathode of valve tube III but cannot jump to the anode because the anode is still loaded with the charge moving at arrow 6. Because these are like charges, they repel one another.
16. From this point on, electron flow on this path moves without resistance toward the secondary coil of the high-voltage step-up transformer. This completes the circuit.

Following the same logic, to trace the current path for the opposite half of the alternating-current cycle in Figure 4-32 results in reorientation of the direction of electron flow. This is full-wave rectification and it produces the sine wave shown in Figure 4-14.

Note that **the x-ray tube will emit x-ray photons during both halves of the full-wave rectified AC cycle.** The double efficiency of full-wave rectification permits a significant increase in the power output capability of radiographic equipment. This results in an ability to use higher mA and kVp settings. Consequently, all modern x-ray equipment is full-wave rectified.

SUMMARY

A magnetic force field surrounds all charged particles when they are in motion. These force fields are magnetic lines of force. Electromagnets are temporary magnets produced by moving electric current. The laws governing magnetism are similar to the laws of electrostatics. Electromagnetic induction is an important phenomenon basic to nearly all electrical devices. It is produced by movement between magnetic lines of force and a conductor.

A generator is a device that converts mechanical energy to electrical energy. Either AC or DC current can be produced through the use of either slip rings or a commutator ring. One complete turn of the generator armature represents one cycle (1 Hz). A device that is

SUMMARY (continued)

supplied with electrical current to produce mechanical motion is called a motor. Motors have essentially the same parts as generators and operate on the same principles, but in reverse. A meter may be connected in parallel to measure current or in series to measure voltage.

A transformer is used to change voltage through the use of Ohm's law. A capacitor is a device capable of accumulating and storing electrical charge. Rectification is the process by which alternating current is changed to pulsating direct current. Silicon-controlled rectifiers are solid-state semiconductors that are used for high-speed switching of the primary high-voltage x-ray circuit. Both self-wave and half-wave rectification are infrequently used in modern x-ray equipment. Diodes replaced valve tubes as one-way circuits that permit full-wave rectification. ■

REVIEW QUESTIONS

1. What is magnetism?
2. What is an electromagnet?
3. Explain the difference between electron flow and conventional current flow.
4. What is indicated by the direction of the thumb, index, and middle finger in one of Fleming's hand rules?
5. What are the three ways to induce electromagnetic current flow in a conductor?
6. Name the four factors controlling the strength of electromagnetically induced current.
7. What is the difference between a generator and a motor?
8. Describe the functions of slip rings and of a commutator ring.
9. How is an ammeter different from a voltmeter?
10. What is the function of a transformer?
11. State the transformer law.
12. What is the function of an autotransformer?
13. What is a diode?
14. What is rectification?
15. What components are necessary to produce a full-wave rectified circuit?

REFERENCES AND RECOMMENDED READING

Ball, J. L., & Moore, A. D. (2008). *Essential physics for radiographers* (4th ed.). Oxford: Wiley-Blackwell Scientific.

Brumbach, M. (2010) *Industrial electricity* (10th ed.) Clifton Park, NY: Delmar Cengage Learning.

Bushberg, J. T., Seibert, J. A., Leidholdt, E. M., & Boone, J. M. (2003). *The essential physics of medical imaging* (2nd ed.). Philadelphia: Lippincott, Williams & Wilkins.

Bushong, S. C. (2008). *Radiologic science for technologists: Physics, biology, and protection* (9th ed.). St. Louis, MO: Elsevier Mosby.

Carroll, Q. B. (2007). *Practical radiographic imaging (Fuch's radiographic exposure processing & quality control)* (8th ed.). Springfield, IL: Charles C Thomas.

Dendy, P. P., & Heaton, B. (1999). *Physics for diagnostic radiology* (2nd ed.) Bristol, England: Institute for Physics.

Gates, E. D. (2006). *Introduction to electronics* (5th ed.). Clifton Park, NY: Delmar Cengage Learning.

Glasser, O., Quimby, E. H., Taylor, L. S., Weatherwax, J. L., & Morgan, R. H. (1961). *Physical foundations of radiology* (3rd ed.). New York: Paul B. Hoeber Division of Harper & Brothers.

Hay, G. A., & Hughes, D. (1997). *First-year physics for radiographers* (3rd ed.) St. Louis, MO: Saunders

Hendee, W. R., & Ritenour, R. (2002). *Medical imaging physics* (4th ed.) New York: Wiley-Liss.

Johns, H. E., & Cunningham, J. R. (1983). *The physics of radiology* (4th ed.). Springfield, IL: Charles C Thomas.

Roller, D., & Roller, H. D. (1967). The development of the concept of electric charge: Electricity from the Greeks to Coulomb, case 8. *Harvard Case Histories in Experimental Science.* Cambridge, MA: Harvard University Press.

Wayne, D. F. (2005). *Newnes electrical power engineer's handbook* (2nd ed.). St. Louis, MO: Elsevier Newnes.

Wilks, R. J. (2003). *Principles of radiological physics* (4th ed.). Edinburgh: Churchill Livingstone.

Wolbarst, A. B., & Cook, G. (2005). *Physics of radiology* (2nd ed.). Madison: Medical Physics Publishing.

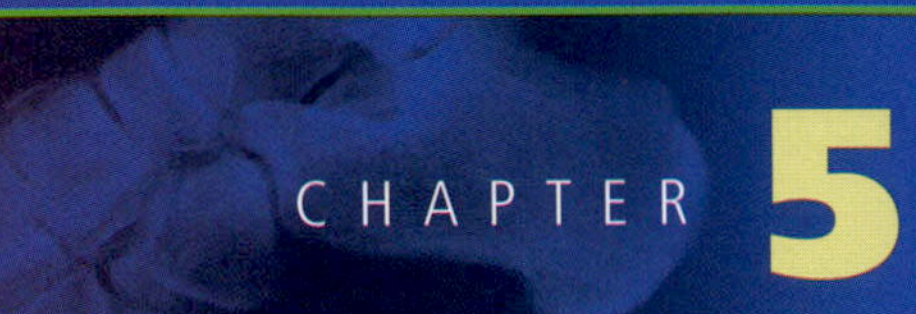

CHAPTER 5 X-Ray Equipment

KEY TERMS

automatic exposure control
automatic exposure device
C-arm tube suspension system
compression band
computed tomography unit
diagnostic
exposure switch
filament circuit
fixed
floor suspension system
floor-to-ceiling suspension system
footboard
handgrip
head unit
incoming-line current
ionization chamber
main circuit
main switch
mains
mammography unit
milliampere-second timer
minimum reaction (or response) time
mobile system
multiphase power
overhead suspension system
panoramic dental and facial unit
phototimers

Suspended in icy silence
I look at myself from far off
Calmly, I feel free

Even though I'm not, now
Or ever:

The metal teeth of death bite
But spit me out
One more time:

When the technologist says
Breathe
I breathe.

OBJECTIVES

Upon completion of this chapter, the student should be able to:

- Describe various diagnostic equipment, table, tube-support, and ancillary equipment configurations.
- State incoming-line current characteristics.
- Describe the differences between single-phase and three-phase power.
- Explain the functions of the basic components of the main and filament x-ray circuits.
- Discuss the differences between single-phase, three-phase, six- and twelve-pulse, and high-frequency waveforms on generator output.

KEY TERMS (continued)

shoulder supports
simulator unit
single-phase power
therapeutic
tilting
timer
tomography unit
urologic unit
voltage ripple

- Describe the function of capacitor discharge and battery-operated mobile units.
- Explain the function of a falling-load generator.
- Differentiate phototimers from ionization chamber automatic exposure controls.
- Describe the placement and function of a phototimer and an ionization chamber automatic exposure control.
- Describe potential problems that could be caused by minimum reaction times.
- Justify the use of backup time when using automatic exposure controls.

TYPES OF X-RAY EQUIPMENT

A vast number of uses for x-rays have been found in medicine and this has led to the development of a wide variety of categories and types of equipment (Figure 5-1). Medical x-ray units can be classified as **diagnostic** or **therapeutic**. Most diagnostic units are designed for specific procedures, such as general radiographic procedures, cardiac catheterization, head procedures, fluoroscopy, and so forth. All of these units operate within the diagnostic x-ray range. This range is approximately 10–1,200 milliamperes (mA), 0.001–10 seconds, at a peak kilovoltage (kVp) of approximately 25–150.

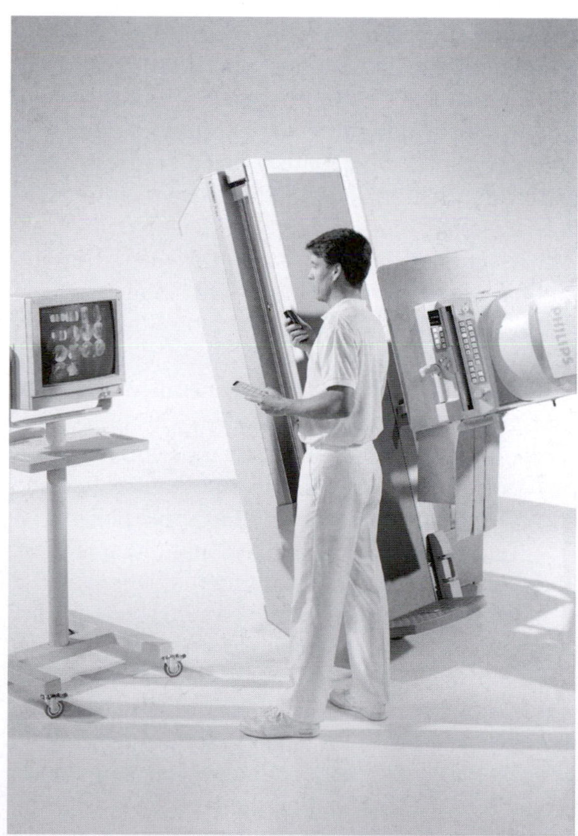

FIGURE 5-1. A typical diagnostic radiographic and fluoroscope room. *(Courtesy of Philips Medical Systems.)*

Tables

The radiographic table is designed to support the patient in a position that will enhance radiographic examination. As any patient can attest, comfort is not the primary purpose of the table, although some institutions permit foam pads for lengthy examinations.

The tabletop must be uniformly radiolucent to easily permit x-rays to pass through. Most tabletops use carbon graphite fiber to reduce absorption of photons. Although flat tops are most common, curved tops are available. Curved (or dished) tops are usually used for fluoroscopic examinations.

They are usually more comfortable for the patient and permit the body part to be placed slightly closer to the image receptor for a more accurate image. Curved tops have two serious disadvantages. It is difficult for the radiographer to maintain a patient accurately in an oblique or lateral position on a curved top, and the top is entirely useless as a level support surface for a film cassette during tabletop radiography.

The tabletop must be **easily cleaned, hard to scratch, and without crevices where radiographic contrast media can accumulate.** It is sometimes necessary to remove body fluids after an examination, and this must be possible to achieve in a quick and sanitary manner.

The table must **include space for a tray to hold cassettes and a radiographic grid.** The tray is often called a "Bucky tray" in honor of Dr. Gustav Bucky (1880–1963), the inventor of the radiographic grid that is installed over the cassette tray. The grid installation usually consists of a mechanism that will automatically move the grid during exposure. Many units include automatic exposure control sensors in the tray. Some tables use a stationary tray with a movable tabletop. Others use a tray that is movable along rails extending the length of the table with a stationary tabletop. Still others use a tray and top that are both partially movable. Some tabletops are motor driven and movable along their length. Others are floating tops that can be moved along their length and width simultaneously when an electromagnetic brake is released. The brake may be controlled by hand, knee, or foot. Floating tops save radiographers significant amounts of time and effort, especially when positioning large patients.

Tables are available in **fixed** and **tilting** models. Fixed tables do not permit tilting the patient's head or feet down. They are designed for diagnostic radiographic work only. Tilting tables are sometimes described by their tilting capability (for example, 90–15 would indicate a table capable of tilting 90° in one direction and 15° in the other). Rooms designed to perform both diagnostic radiographic and fluoroscopic (R & F) examinations are equipped with tilting tables, although some rooms designed only for radiographic examinations may also use them.

The table is usually at a height that reduces physical strain on the radiographer, who must stretch and bend over and around the table as the patient, ancillary equipment, cassette, and x-ray tube are positioned. This is usually 30–40 inches or 75–100 cm from the floor. This is not a safe or convenient height for patients and it causes problems for ambulatory patients who are not in good physical condition. A primary concern for all radiographers must be proper assistance to these patients when they are getting onto and down from the table. Fixed tables are available in adjustable models that can be lowered while a patient is assisted onto the table and then raised to a working height.

Ancillary equipment for tilting tables includes a **footboard** for patients to stand on when the table is upright. The footboard is often used for gastrointestinal studies when the patient begins the examination in an erect position and is then brought horizontal during the procedure, or vice versa. In these instances it is critical to ascertain that the footboard is securely in place and will support the full weight of the patient. This is best done when the table is horizontal by pulling hard on the footboard. Procedures requiring tilting the patient's head down, such as myelography, may require the use of **shoulder supports** to keep patients from sliding off the table. In these instances, **handgrips** give the patient an added feeling of security.

Compression bands serve three functions: they restrain patients who are unable to cooperate, they compress abdominal tissue for a more uniform subject density, and they can be used to compress the renal ureters to restrict the flow of urine to the bladder until they are released (which allows production of an image with both ureters full of contrast media). A compression band should never be used as the sole restraint device.

Tube Supports

The tube-support system is designed to permit the x-ray tube to be manipulated to the various locations necessary to obtain examination procedure projections and to hold the tube immobile during the exposure. Tube suspension systems are available in numerous configurations, such as: overhead, floor-to-ceiling, floor, mobile, and C-arm. Overhead supports are the most flexible and the most costly.

The **overhead suspension system**, sometimes called ceiling suspension, allows controls of longitudinal and transverse positioning as well as vertical distance.

Each of these complex motions is locked into place by a solenoid with a control placed where it can be easily reached by the radiographer. Also included in the control mechanisms are "detents," or centering locks, to verify common tube positions (for example, centered to the cassette in the Bucky tray or at a routine distance from the table or upright Bucky unit). Unfortunately, each manufacturer uses a different placement and labeling for these controls. For this reason, it is helpful to practice manipulating the controls prior to using the equipment to perform radiographic procedures.

The **floor-to-ceiling suspension system** uses a pair of rails, one on the ceiling and one on the floor, for longitudinal positioning. Rooms with extremely high ceilings may use an overhead rail suspended from a wall.

A **floor suspension system** uses a tube-support column mounted on the floor. The system must be carefully counterbalanced to avoid tipping. This is usually accomplished by adding a counterweight to the back of the telescoping tube arm and requires that both tube system and table be installed further from the back wall than other systems.

There are many types of **mobile systems** as well. The tube suspension systems for mobile units vary tremendously but most are based on the floor suspension system.

A **C-arm tube suspension system** utilizes a C-shaped arm to support the tube and image receptor (Figure 5-2). The tube and image receptor are fixed to opposite ends of the C-arm. When the clamp or lock holding the C-arm in position is released, it permits both tube and image receptor to be rotated to a new position. C-arms (or U-arms) are used in **head units**, mobile fluoroscopy units, and ceiling-suspended angiography and surgical units.

Upright Units

An upright cassette holder or Bucky unit is a common and useful ancillary piece of equipment in any radiographic room (Figure 5-3). Chest radiography

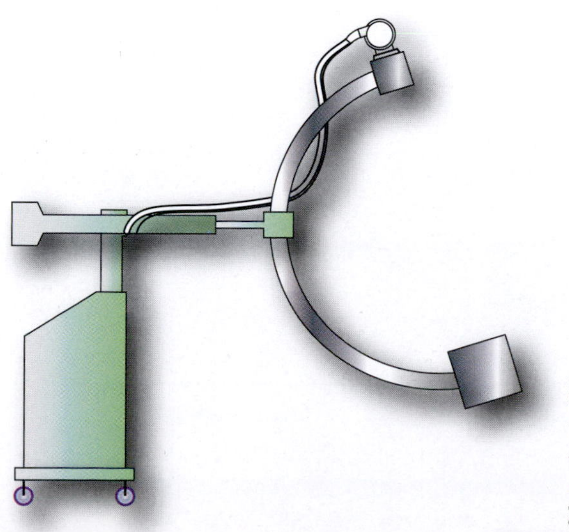

FIGURE 5-2. A C-arm tube suspension system.

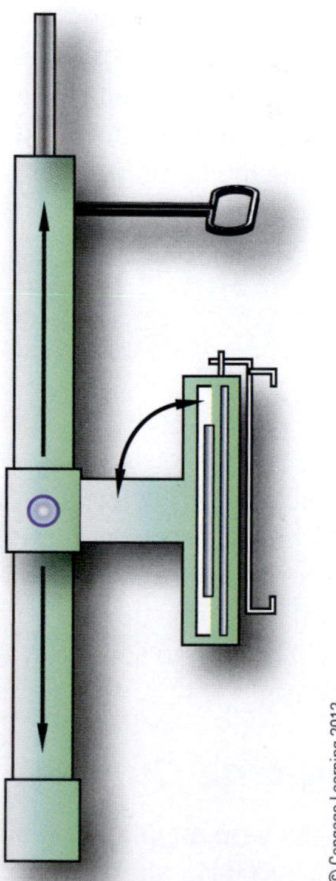

FIGURE 5-3. An upright Bucky unit.

should routinely be done in an upright position and there are numerous other procedures that are best done upright (for example, acromioclavicular joints, abdominal obstructive procedures, cervical spine, etc.). Upright cassette holders may or may not include a radiographic grid. Upright Bucky units may include the same equipment as the Bucky tray located in a table (movable radiographic grid, cassette tray, and automatic exposure control sensors).

Other Specialized Diagnostic Equipment

Other types of equipment have been developed to meet specialized needs. They include chest units designed to automate chest radiography by combining an upright Bucky unit with an automatic film-handling mechanism, **mammography units** for breast studies, **tomography units** with tubes that move in an arc during exposure, **panoramic dental units** for combined tomography of facial structures, **computed tomography units** for computerized sectional images, radiation therapy **simulator units** to verify radiation therapy treatment set-ups prior to actual treatment, **urologic units** to facilitate urological and genital studies, and units custom built to nearly any specifications.

POWER FOR X-RAY GENERATION

A diagnostic x-ray generator is composed of numerous basic electrical devices. An x-ray circuit is established when these devices are connected in a sequence capable of accelerating electrons to the speed necessary to cause the production of x-ray photons within an x-ray tube. The incoming line power may be modified in several ways to establish these conditions.

Incoming-Line Current

Electricity is usually supplied to buildings in the United States by 60-Hz alternating current with a nominal root mean square (rms) voltage of 200–240. These are termed nominal because, as users operate various resistances, the voltages constantly fluctuate, as illustrated by Ohm's law. This power is called the **incoming-line current** (sometimes called the **mains**) and is supplied in the form of a three-phase power cycle (Figure 5-4). One of the "hot" wires is always half the incoming voltage above-ground potential, while the other is always the same voltage below-ground potential. In the United States each carries 110–120 volts. With 60-Hz alternating current, the two hot wires reverse their polarity 120 times per second. Bringing incoming-line current from the neutral (or ground) wire and one of the hot wires produces

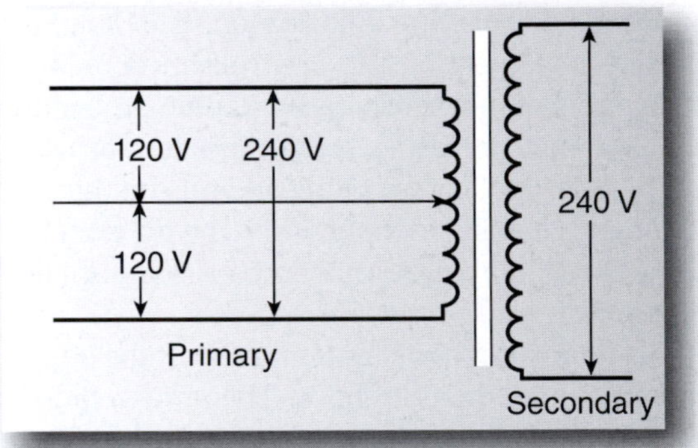

FIGURE 5-4. Three-phase, 60-Hz, 240-V incoming-line current.

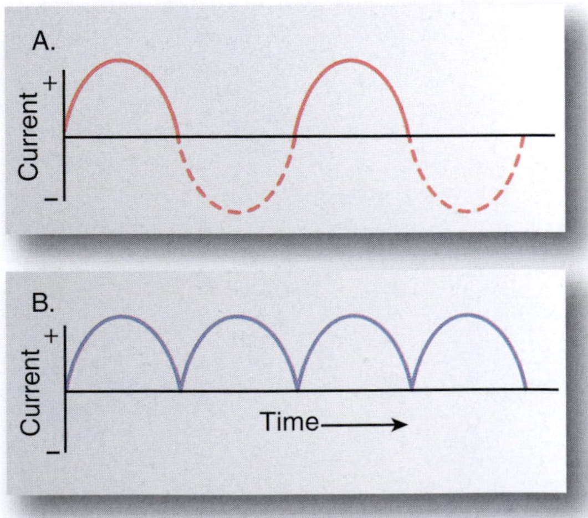

FIGURE 5-5. Single-phase power: (A) incoming line; (B) full-wave rectified.

a potential difference of 110–120 volts. Because the two lines are not in phase with one another, using incoming current from both hot wires produces a potential difference that is less than the sum of the two single phases. The usual result is about 210 volts. Nearly all x-ray equipment operates from an incoming line of 210–220 volts.

Single-Phase Power

Single-phase power permits the potential difference to drop to zero with every change in the direction of current flow (Figure 5-5A) and is represented by the symbol 1φ. In a full-wave rectified circuit (direct pulsating current), this means the x-ray tube is experiencing no potential difference and is producing no x-ray photons 120 times each second on a 60-Hz line (see Figure 5-5B). With the 60-Hz line, an exposure of 0.1 second with a single-phase full-wave rectified unit results in twelve intervals of no photon production (Figure 5-6). In addition, the photons produced during the low-voltage periods are of such low energy that they may not exit the tube, or they do not contribute to the radiographic image because they are absorbed before reaching the image receptor. The rms voltage of

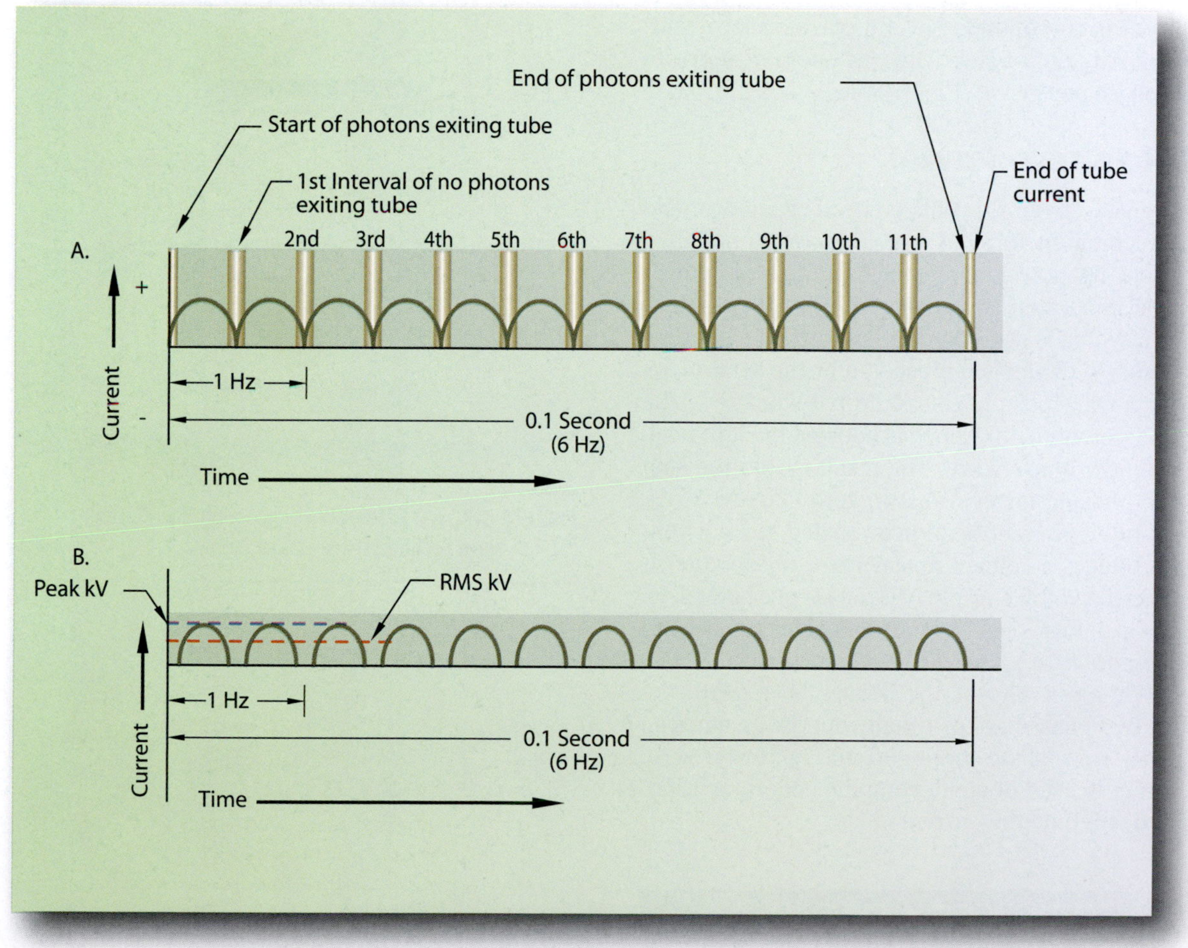

FIGURE 5-6. The difference between the photons produced inside the x-ray tube during an exposure and the photons emitted from the tube during the same exposure. (A) X-ray production during an exposure of 0.1 second with a 1φ full-wave rectified circuit.

a single-phase sinusoidal wave is usually given as 70.7 percent of the peak voltage.

EXAMPLE: What is the approximate rms voltage of a single-phase sine wave with a peak of 80 kVp?

Answer:

rms voltage = 70.7% peak kVp

rms voltage = 70.7% × 80 kVp

rms voltage = 56.6 kVp

Obviously this is not as efficient as desired. A solution is to combine several waveforms of current slightly out of step with one another to create **multiphase power**.

Multiphase Power

Multiphase power is produced by the generator and is the common form in which power is supplied to users by power companies. Multiphase power will be illustrated by a description of three-phase power, which is generated as is shown in Chapter 4 by Figure 4-16 and is represented by the symbol 3φ. As each wave peak begins to drop toward zero, the overall potential difference is boosted back to peak by the next phase wave. The result is that the sum of the phasing never drops to zero (Figure 5-7A). When full-wave rectification is applied, the net voltage produces a **voltage ripple**. Three-phase current produces a voltage ripple of 3 pulses per half cycle, which is 6 pulses per Hz and 360 pulses per second (see Figure 5-10.)

Whenever any of the phases is at zero, the other two phases are of equally opposite values so that the sum of the three currents is always zero. This fact is used in connecting the generator windings to combine the current.

A BASIC X-RAY CIRCUIT

The basic x-ray circuit can be divided into the **main** and **filament circuits**. **The main circuit supplies the x-ray tube with properly modified power.** Its purpose is to produce x- rays. **The filament circuit supplies the filament of the x-ray tube with properly modified power.** Its purpose is to create the appropriate thermionically emitted electron cloud at the filament. These two circuits are distinct from each other although they are interconnected (Figure 5-8).

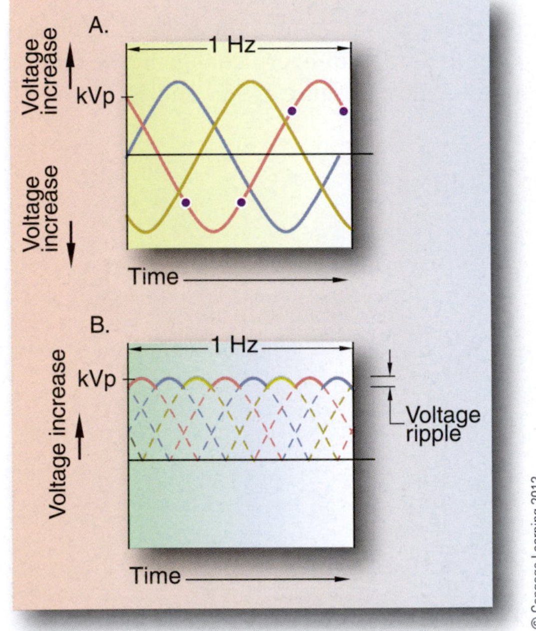

FIGURE 5-7. (A) Three-phase incoming-line current. (B) Full-wave rectified three-phase current.

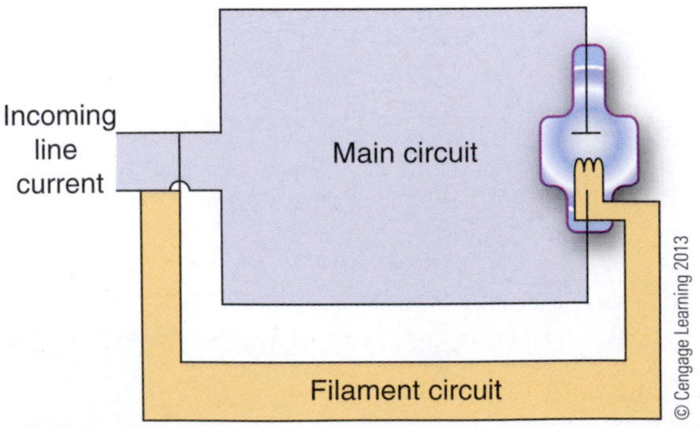

FIGURE 5-8. Main and filament circuits.

The Main X-Ray Circuit

The main x-ray circuit modifies the incoming-line power to produce x-rays by a sequence of devices, as shown in Figure 5-9. The circuit must boost the voltage to the range necessary to produce x-rays and to permit the radiographer to adjust the amperage, voltage, and length of exposure, as well as incorporate appropriate circuitry to increase the efficiency of x-ray production.

The **main switch** and circuit breakers are usually enclosed in an electrical power box. The **exposure switch** is simply a connection that permits current to flow through the circuit. The **timer** circuit is intended to end the exposure at an accurately measured, preset time. For this reason, whenever the exposure switch is depressed it must be held until both the audible and visible indicators (usually a buzzer and a light) have ceased. For example, if a radiographer is accustomed to making short exposures of less than 0.5 second, failure to hold the exposure switch for a 2.5-second exposure of a large abdomen would prematurely terminate the exposure.

The Exposure Switch

The exposure switch also activates the rotating anode of the x-ray tube. The anode must be turning at a sufficiently high speed to avoid melting of the target area by the high-kilovoltage exposure. To avoid the possibility of error, all x-ray units that utilize rotating anodes have circuitry that prevents an exposure until the anode is turning at the correct speed. It is usually convenient to combine the anode rotor and the exposure switch in a two-step

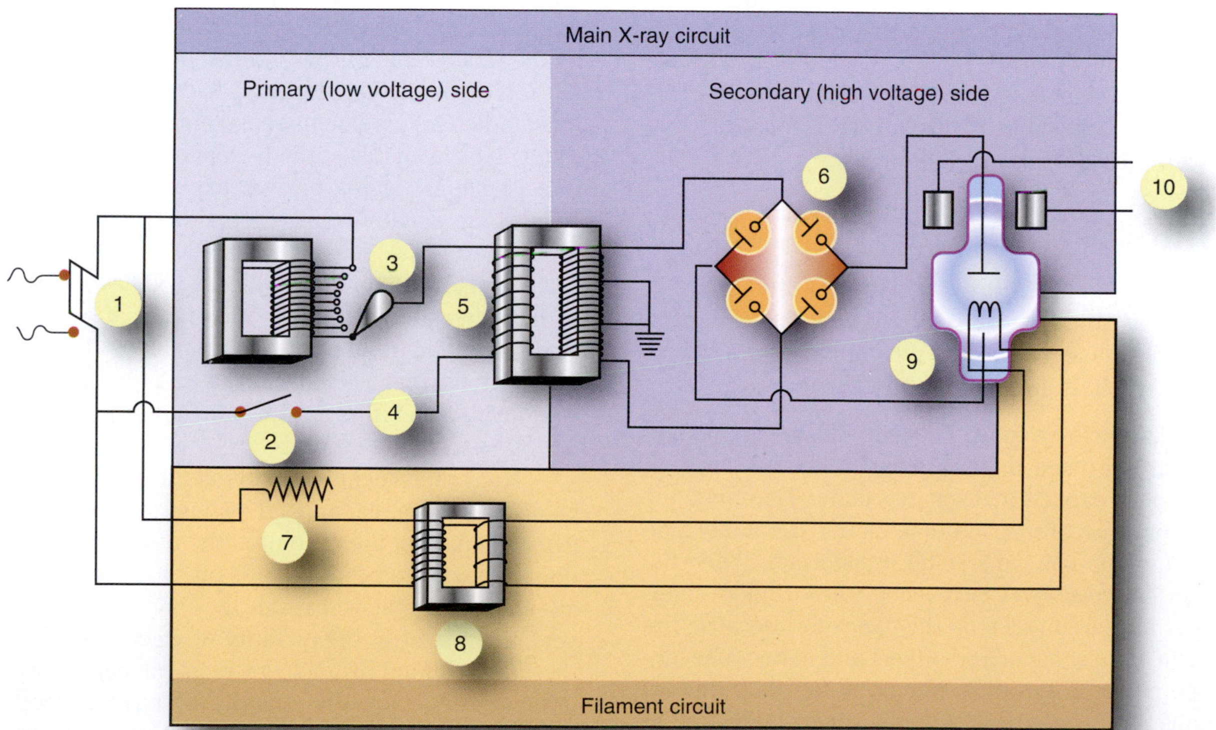

FIGURE 5-9. The complete basic x-ray circuit: (1) main breaker; (2) exposure switch; (3) autotransformer; (4) timer circuit; (5) high-voltage step-up transformer; (6) four-diode rectification circuit; (7) filament circuit variable resistance; (8) filament step-down transformer; (9) x-ray tube; and (10) rotor stator.

button, although separate anode and exposure switches can also be used. Therefore, most exposure switches are depressed halfway to activate the anode rotation and then depressed completely to initiate the x-ray exposure. Tube manufacturers recommend that these buttons be depressed completely in one motion. This helps to extend the life of the x-ray tube. If separate switches are used, the rotor (or "prep") switch should be activated first, followed by the exposure switch.

The exposure switch must be attached to the control console in such a manner that it is impossible for the operator to be exposed. In addition, the equipment must be designed to prohibit the x-ray tube from being manipulated into a position where it could expose the user. On mobile equipment the switch must be on a cord with a minimum length of 6 feet. This is to permit the radiographer to move as far as possible from the x-ray tube during an exposure. All exposure switches must be of the "dead-man" type, in which x-ray exposure may occur only while the switch is depressed. Release of the switch must terminate the exposure. This prevents the exposure from continuing when the operator enters the radiation area.

The Timer Circuit

Electronic timers are capable of accurate exposures as short as 0.001 second with only a 1-msec delay. This level is set by the variation of the timer controls on the console unit by the radiographer.

Milliampere-Second Timers. **Milliampere-second timers** are used in falling-load generators as well as some capacitor discharge units. They monitor the product of mA and time on the secondary side of the high-voltage step-up transformer. When the desired mAs level is reached, these timers interrupt the circuit to stop the exposure. Because the high-voltage capacitor, timer, and x-ray tube are operating on the same circuit, mAs value remains constant even when there is a slight fluctuation in the capacitor charging current.

Automatic Exposure Control Timers. **Automatic exposure controls** or **automatic exposure devices** are also used, as described later in this chapter. The autotransformer, which is controlled by the kVp selectors on the control console, modifies the incoming-line voltage in anticipation of the kilovoltage that will be produced by the step-up transformer. Some units divide the kVp adjustments into major and minor regions. Usually a major adjustment will change in units of 10 kVp, while minor adjustments will change in units of 1 or 2 kVp.

The Filament Circuit

The filament circuit modifies the incoming-line power to produce the thermionic emission from the filament wire of the x-ray tube by a sequence of devices (see Figure 5-9). The incoming line must be modified to about 3–5 amperes and 6–12 volts. The filament circuit's supply is drawn directly from the main circuit's supply. Current control devices regulate the amperage supplied to the filament in the x-ray tube. This control device can be adjusted by the radiographer at the control console. It is not labeled by the actual amperage it controls. Instead it is marked in increments representative of the mA that will be available at the filament when the high-voltage supply is released at exposure. Filament circuits are usually adjustable to the equivalent of mA ratings of 50, 100, 200, 300, 400, 500, 600, 800, 1,000, and 1,200. Not all equipment will have all mA settings and some may have other unusual settings, as discussed in the section on timers. Most 1φ units do not go beyond 500 mA. Specialized tomographic equipment generators may also include 10-, 15-, 20-, 25-, 30-, and 40-mA stations.

Many units include a meter at this point to provide an accurate reading of the amperage delivered. After regulation, the current is then sent to a step-down transformer that modifies it to the appropriate amperage that will reach the filament itself. A very slight shift in the quantity of electrons in the thermionic cloud around the filament can have a dramatic effect on the quantity of x-ray photons produced when the kilovoltage exposure occurs. Therefore, filament circuits also incorporate several types of current stabilization devices, including frequency compensators, voltage stabilizers, and space charge compensators.

TABLE 5-1.

Control	Factor	Electrical Device and Location in Circuit
kVp selection	kVp level	Autotransformer (between incoming line and exposure switch)
mA selection	Filament current	Variable resistor (in filament circuit between incoming line and step-down transformer)
Time selection	Length of exposure	Timer circuit (between exposure switch and step-up transformer)
Rotor switch	Speed of rotating anode	Stator (separate circuit from stator of anode motor)
Exposure switch	Moment of exposure	Switch (between autotransformer and timer circuit)

The main and filament circuits are combined to form the complete basic x-ray circuit (see Figure 5-9). The radiographer adjusts the various factors from a control console, which must be located in a radiation-shielded location outside the radiographic exposure room. **All of the radiographer-operated controls are located on the low-voltage side of the circuit to protect operators from high-voltage shock hazards.** The controls that are likely to be located on this console are included in Table 5-1.

GENERATORS

Single-Phase Generators

Single-phase generators with full-wave rectification produce a voltage ripple of 2 pulses per hertz or 120 pulses per second. This produces two usable pulses per cycle (1φ 2P waveform) with a ripple of 100 percent. This means the voltage in the tube drops to 0 twice per period or cycle. These relationships are shown in Figure 5-10.

Multiphase Generators

When full-wave rectification is applied to 3φ current, it produces a voltage ripple of 6 pulses per hertz or 360 pulses per second. This produces six usable pulses per cycle, which is known as a three-phase, six-pulse (3φ 6P) waveform. Three-phase, six-pulse power produces a ripple of 13–25 percent. This means the voltage in the x-ray tube never falls below 75–87 percent of the peak kilovoltage setting on the console. These relationships are shown in Figure 5-10. **A full-wave rectified, three-phase, six-pulse waveform produces approximately 35 percent more average photon energy than a full-wave rectified, single phase.** Similar changes occur with high-frequency equipment, which can operate as high as 10,000–12,000 Hz. This will become an important point to remember when setting technical factors.

Generator power ratings are determined by the greatest load the generator is capable of sending to the x-ray tube. Power is calculated as voltage times amperage. The unit of power is the watt, so $V \times A = W$. This formula applies to a 3φ generators. Because 1φ generators have a lower average photon emission energy, the formula must be corrected by using a constant. For a 1φ generator the power rating formula $V \times A \times 0.7 = W$. Because x-ray generators operate in the kilovoltage and milliamperage range, their power ratings are stated in kilowatts.

> ***EXAMPLE:*** What is the power rating for a 3φ generator capable of delivering 150 kVp at 1,000 mA to the tube?
>
> ***Answer:***
>
> $V \times A = W$
>
> $150\ kV \times 1{,}000\ mA = W$
>
> $150{,}000\ V \times 1.0\ A = 150{,}000\ W$
>
> $= 150\ kW$

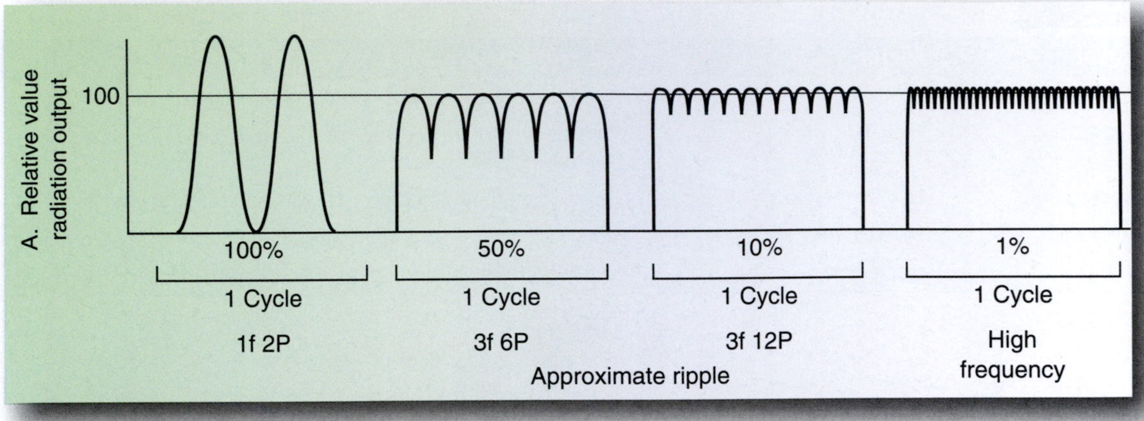

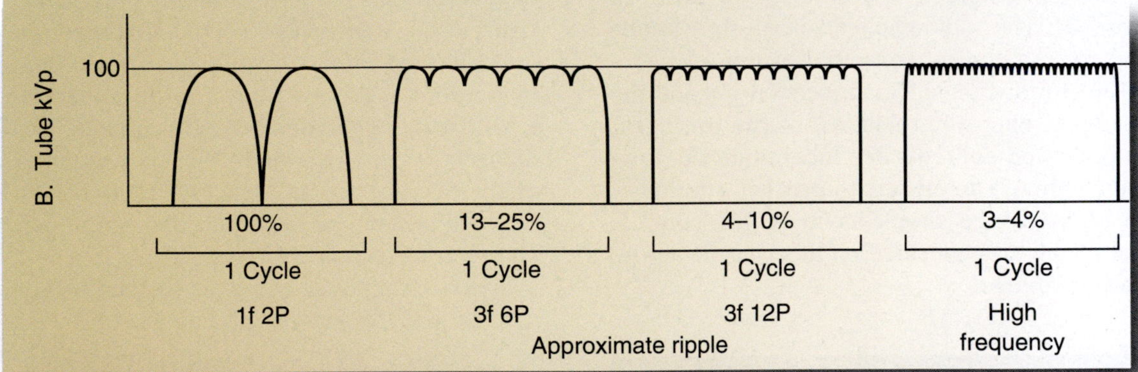

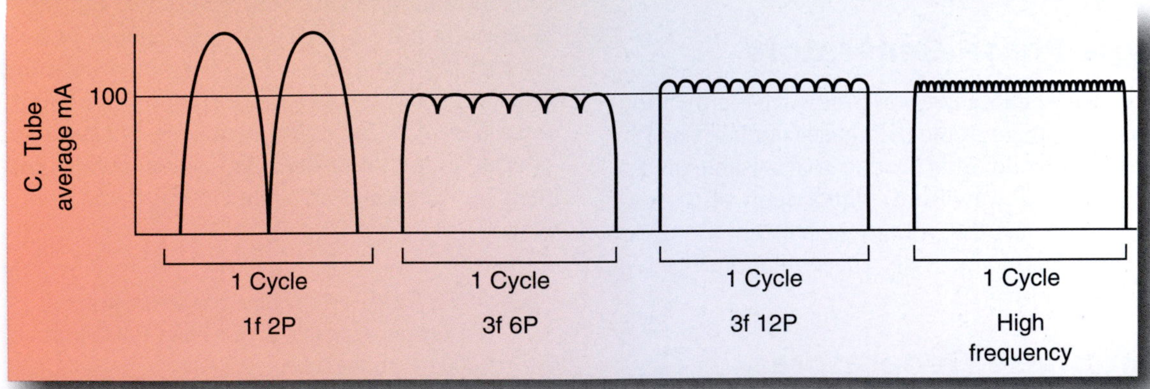

FIGURE 5-10. The relationships between (A) relative value radiation output and approximate ripple; (B) tube kVp and approximate ripple; and (C) tube average mA. Each relationship is shown for one cycle of 1 2P, 3 6P, 3 12P, and high-frequency generator configurations.

> ***EXAMPLE:*** What is the power rating for a 1φ generator capable of delivering 120 kVp at 300 mA to the tube?
>
> ***Answer:***
>
> $V \times A \times 0.7 = W$
>
> $120\ kV \times 300\ mA \times 0.7 = W$
>
> $120{,}000\ V \times 0.3A \times 0.7 = 25{,}200\ W$
>
> $= 25.2\ kW$

These ratings serve as a guideline for comparing the capability of various generators. Generator power often varies as kilovoltage changes, so a high-power generator at 150 kVp may not be as powerful when the kVp is lowered into the middle diagnostic range.

High Frequency

High-frequency generators use AC and DC power converters to change the incoming-line voltage frequency from 60 Hz to the 6,000 Hz range (Figure 5-11A).

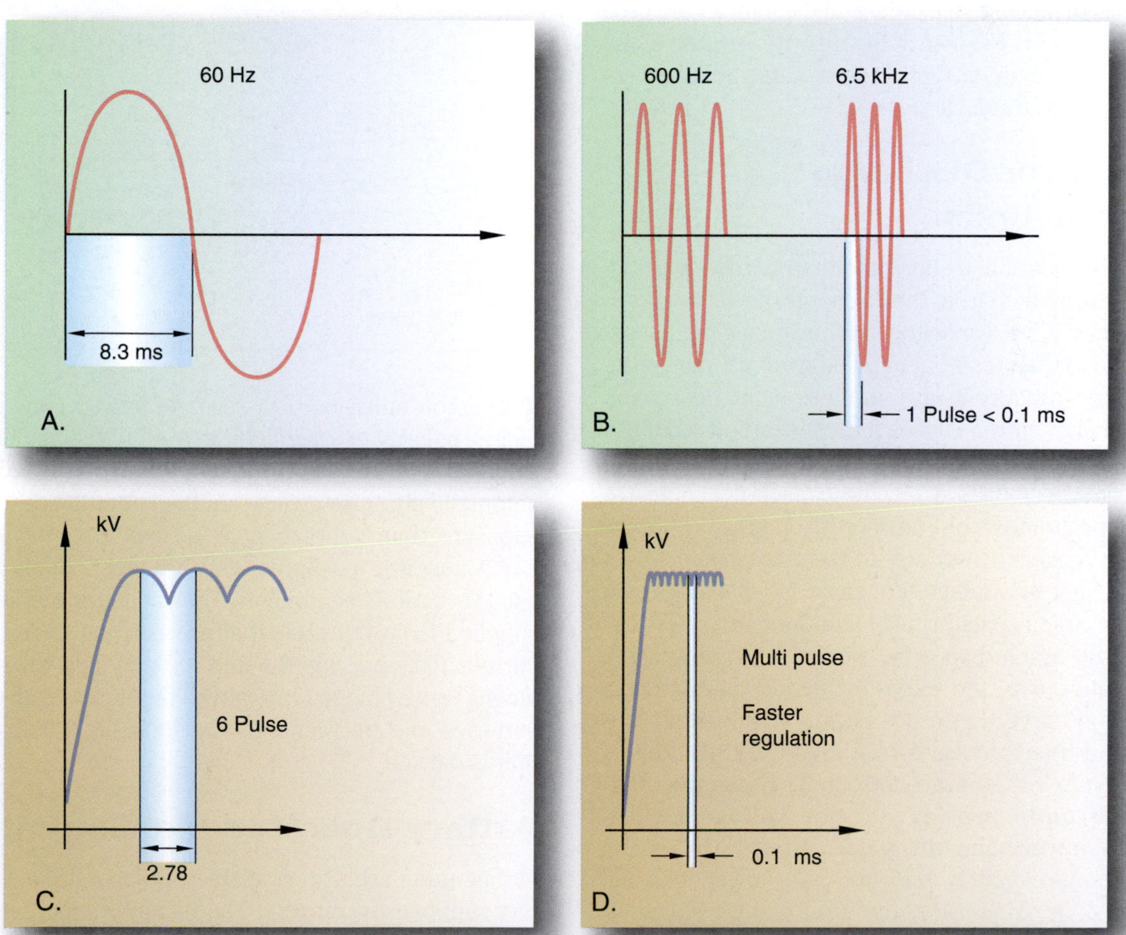

FIGURE 5-11. High-frequency waveforms; (A and B) Conversion of 1φ 2P to 3φ 6P to high frequency; (C and D) comparison of time interval necessary to reach peak kV on 3φ 6P and high-frequency generators. *(Courtesy of Siemens Medical Solutions USA, Inc.)*

When a high-frequency current is supplied with full-wave rectified power, a 12- to 13-kHz waveform can be produced. An oscillator or inverter unit controls the pulses sent through the circuit, sending them at a much higher frequency (closer together), as shown in Figure 5-11B. When this wave is applied to the x-ray tube, the peak kilovoltage is achieved in about 10 percent of the time necessary for 3φ generators and with only 3–4 percent voltage ripple. Figure 5-10 illustrates the complex conversions used in a high-frequency generator to create the various waveforms prior to achieving the final multipulsed radiation beam. Full-wave rectified high-frequency generator ripple ranges from 4–15 percent, depending on the total load. These relationships are shown in Figure 5-10. Because of the higher-frequency current, transformers for these units are significantly smaller.

Capacitor Discharge Mobile Units

It is also possible to operate an x-ray tube with the power generated from the discharge of a high-voltage capacitor. The capacitor operates exactly as explained in Chapter 4 but in the kilovoltage range necessary to produce x-rays. In these units, depression of a charge button causes the rectification circuit to charge a capacitor instead of the x-ray tube. A signal indicates readiness when the capacitor charges to the appropriate level, and depression of the exposure switch triggers a discharge to the x-ray tube.

The disadvantage of a capacitor discharge unit is that the capacitor may continue to discharge after the usable exposure. Figure 5-12A shows the charging curve, the exposure period, and the discharging curve. Exposure begins at the peak voltage and then decreases (see Figure 5-12B). This is sometimes called wavetail cutoff. **Capacitor discharge units provide an rms voltage significantly lower than the peak voltage.** The ending kV is approximately 1 kV per mAs lower than the initial kVp. Therefore, the rms voltage is about 0.5 kV/mAs lower than the initial kVp. Because capacitors discharge more slowly as potential difference decreases, considerable residual kV may exist after the desired exposure time. This can create a leakage of radiation, although several devices help avoid the problem. Grid-biased x-ray tubes can be used to cut the photon emission at a set time by reversing the charge polarity of a wire grid in front of the filament. Additionally, the tube collimator can be designed to automatically close its lead shutters after the desired exposure, thus stopping radiation leakage.

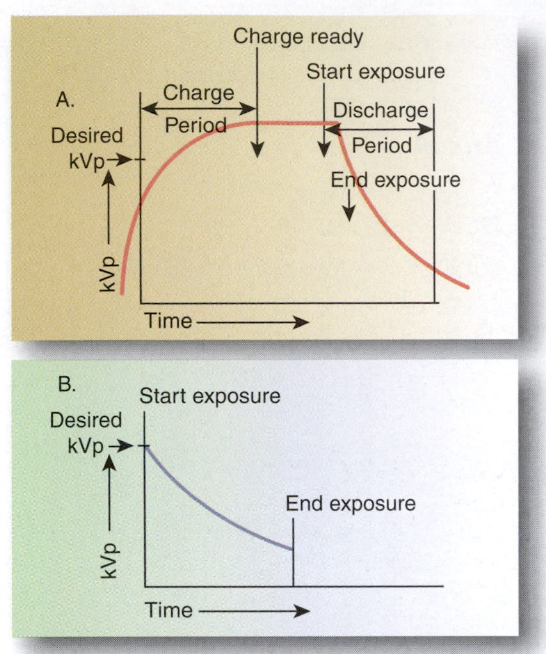

FIGURE 5-12. (A) Capacitor discharge unit waveform; (B) wavetail cutoff.

Capacitor discharge units are most commonly used for mobile equipment. The capacitor circuit is supplied from batteries that are charged from line current. This permits the unit to be mobile without having to be plugged into a wall outlet. Instead, the batteries can be recharged periodically when the unit is parked.

Battery-Operated Mobile Units

Mobile units are also available that operate on battery-supplied AC current. The batteries supply nonpulsating direct current to a rotary converter, which provides current similar to 3φ 12P or even greater frequencies. Compared to capacitor discharge machines, these units have the obvious advantage of 3φ exposure consistency, higher rms voltage, and no leakage possibility. They also have all the advantages of mobility, with recharging capabilities, and for these reasons they have become extremely popular.

Falling-Load Generators

Falling-load generators usually are specially designed high-frequency generators. They take full advantage of the current-loading capability of the x-ray tube by beginning the exposure with a high amperage and then allowing it to fall during the exposure. This can be accomplished with a constant-potential generator. It requires that both the mA and the kV be regulated independently.

Falling-load generators are a solution to this problem as they permit greater use of the acceptable tube limits. They do so without requiring a higher-power (and more expensive) generator that would permit higher mA loading. For example, in Figure 5-13, a constant-potential generator exposure of 240 mAs is compared to the same falling-load exposure. A falling-load generator permits the same tube to achieve 240 mAs in 0.5 second. This is accomplished by beginning the exposure at 600 mA for the first 0.1 second. At this time the 600-mA tube limit is reached and the generator is programmed to automatically reduce the mA to 500 until the tube limit is again reached (0.2 second later, or 0.3 second from exposure start). Once again the generator reduces the mA to 400 until the limit is reached (0.2 second later, or 0.5 second from exposure start). This produces 240 total mAs.

A falling-load generator utilizes the tube's loading potential to a much greater extent than the constant-potential generator. This is made evident by comparing the falling load of the 240-mAs example with a constant-potential load for the same mAs. In actual practice a margin of error is allowed for the tube loading. Most falling-load generators will step down the mA at 70–80 percent of the tube loading capacity. This feature has a disadvantage in that constant-potential generators may actually make better use of tube loading capacity on very

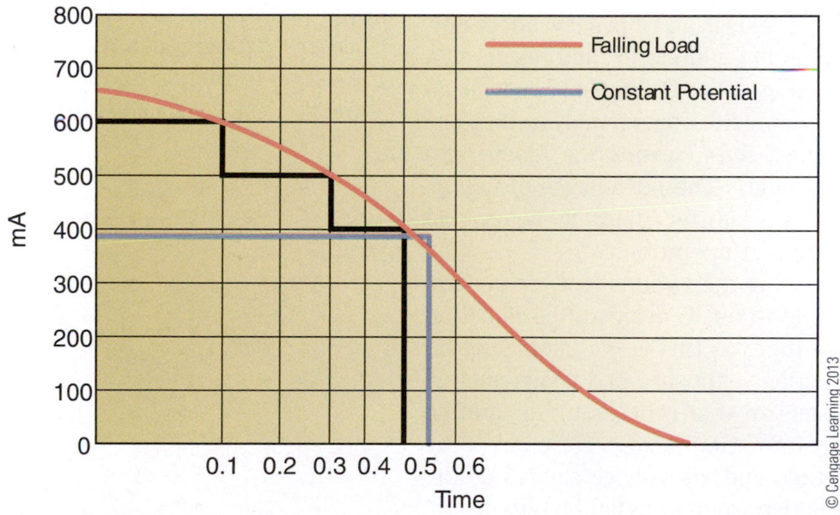

FIGURE 5-13. Falling-load generator versus constant-potential tube limit curve. In the example shown, the mAs is calculated as follows:

mA	Time in sec	mAs achieved
600	0.1	60
500	0.2	100
4000	0.2	80
Total	0.5	240

short exposures, where they may use 80–90 percent of the tube loading capacity.

Falling-load generators begin exposures at the highest possible mA. This removes control of the mA from the radiographer, and there are instances when this is undesirable. For example, some examinations, such as those for the lateral thoracic vertebra (spine) and sternum, require a "breathing technique" in which low mA and long-time exposures are used to blur superimposing structures from the image. Unless falling-load consoles are equipped with special controls (often as tomographic options) to permit starting exposures at low mA, these examinations cannot be performed correctly.

There are several factors that should be understood before using falling-load generators. Because they function with an mA that is unknown to the operator, it is impossible for the operator to set the correct time to achieve the desired mAs. Therefore, falling-load generators must be used with automatic exposure controls, or rely on an mAs timer, instead of independent mA and time controls. The kVp across the tube varies for a brief moment as the mA is adjusted. This is an Ohm's law effect during the continuous mA reductions and results in a slightly lower average kVp. Falling-load generators can shorten x-ray tube life considerably as they use higher mA settings, thus causing the filament to wear out more quickly. The advantages of falling-load generators are shorter times in heavy-load situations, and simpler operation.

When comparing the various types of generators it is most important to evaluate the radiation output from the tube, as this is the factor that influences both patient exposure and image quality. Figure 5-10 assists in this process by illustrating the various transformations that occur in the x-ray tube milliamperage and kilovoltage as well as the all-important relative value of radiation output.

AUTOMATIC EXPOSURE CONTROLS

All automatic exposure controls do exactly what their name indicates; they are programmed to terminate the radiographic exposure time. It is important to remember that automatic exposure controls do not control any factor except time. Milliampere-seconds and kVp remain under the control of the radiographer in all but falling-load generators. Even falling-load units leave the kVp under the radiographer's control.

Although antiquated, the term **phototimer** is often used to refer to all automatic exposure controls. They are also referred to as automatic exposure devices, and the acronyms AEC and AED occasionally appear in professional literature.

All automatic exposure controls function by measuring a preset quantity of radiation and breaking the timer circuit when a dose sufficient to produce the desired exposure has been reached.

Ionization Chambers

Ionization chamber automatic exposure controls (Figure 5-14) use a thin, parallel-plate ionization chamber, which is positioned immediately above the image receptor. Because thin, parallel-plate chambers are only about 5 mm in thickness, they do not cause an appreciable shadow on the image (Figure 5-15). It is critical that the exact size, shape, and position of the ionization chamber be known to the radiographer. It is possible to image the location of the ionization chambers by using an automated AEC exposure at the lowest kVp possible.

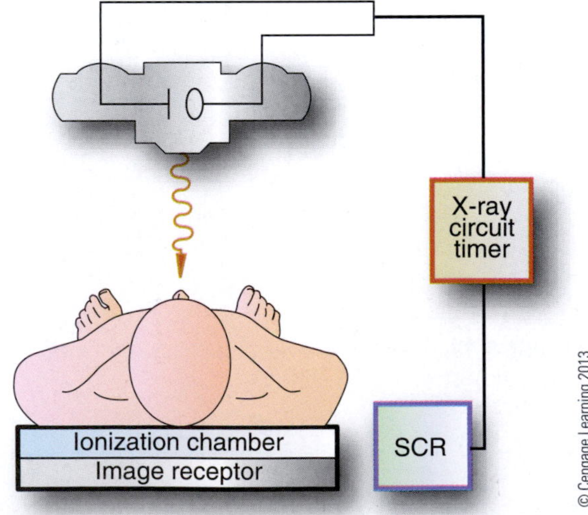

FIGURE 5-14. Ionization chamber AEC circuit.

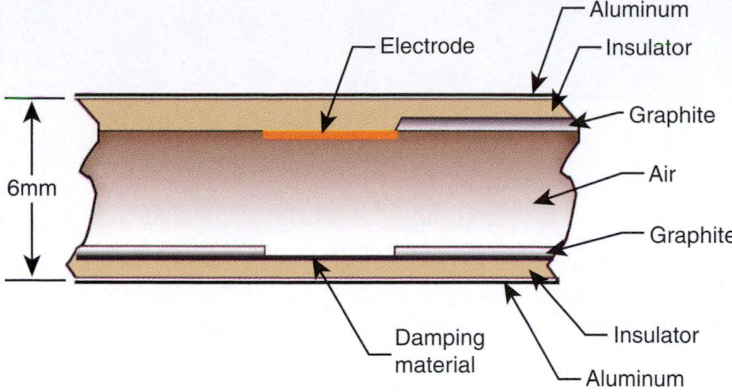

FIGURE 5-15. Parallel-plate ionization chamber AEC. *(Courtesy of Siemens Medical Solutions USA.)*

Minimum Reaction Time

All automatic exposure controls have a **minimum reaction (or response) time**, which is determined by the length of time necessary for the AEC to respond to the radiation and for the generator to terminate the exposure. This delay is caused primarily by the turn-off delay in the high-voltage circuits. Old phototimers had a minimum reaction time of 0.05 second or less. Modern ionization chambers with SCRs may have a minimum reaction time of less than 0.001 second. Automatic exposure controls are sometimes incapable of terminating exposures quickly enough, especially with extremely high-speed image receptors during high-kVp chest radiography. In this instance, radiographic technology has outstripped itself and either a manual time or a slower image receptor must be used, although some manufacturers use an exposure-monitoring circuit to terminate low-dose-rate exposures quickly.

Imaging small body parts with an AEC may not be possible. If such an image is overexposed, the AEC should be turned off and a manual exposure should be used.

Backup Time

Nearly all units equipped with automatic exposure permit (and may have electronic interlocks that require) a manual backup time to be set. There are numerous reasons why an automatic exposure control may be improperly set. For example, if one forgets to activate the AEC in a wall unit, this may leave an AEC in a table unit waiting for exposure by a tube that is directed toward the wall (and through a patient). Because the wall AEC is not receiving any radiation dose, the exposure would not cease until the tube overload protector activated. Not only is this an expensive waste of tube life, but the radiographer error causing excessive radiation dose to the patient is completely unwarranted. The fact that the image would be overexposed, requiring it to be repeated, adding to the patient's dose again, simply makes matters worse. **Backup times cannot exceed the tube limit and should be set at 150 percent of the anticipated manual exposure mAs.** According to U.S. Public Law 90–602, generators must terminate the exposure at 600 mAs for exposures above 50 kVp and 2,000 mAs for exposures below 50 kVp (primarily during mammography).

SUMMARY

Medical x-ray units can be classified as diagnostic or therapeutic. Diagnostic units operate within a range of 10–1,200 milliamperes (mA), 0.001–10 seconds, and at a peak kilovoltage (kVp) of approximately 25–150.

Radiographic equipment includes a wide variety of units with different tube stand configurations, including ceiling suspension, floor-to-ceiling, floor mounted, and C-arms. Nearly all x-ray equipment operates from an incoming line of 210–220 volts, which is then used for single-phase or three-phase power.

The basic x-ray circuit can be divided into the main and filament circuits. The main circuit supplies the x-ray tube with properly modified power, and the filament circuit supplies the filament of the x-ray tube with properly modified power. The basic circuit includes the exposure switch, timer, high-voltage step-up transformer, and rectifier circuit.

Although waveforms differ depending on incoming line and rectification, differences occur in both voltage ripple and the interval between initiation of the exposure and the peak kilovoltage.

Generator power ratings are determined by the greatest load the generator is capable of sending to the x-ray tube. Power is expressed in watts and varies by incoming-line current and rectification. Falling-load generators permit more effective use of the tube loading capacity but eliminate mA and time settings from consideration.

Although often called phototimers, automatic exposure controls (AECs) today are almost always ionization chambers. When using an AEC, problems may be avoided by considering the minimum reaction time and the backup time. ■

REVIEW QUESTIONS

1. Name three types of diagnostic radiographic tube-support systems.
2. What are the two types of incoming-line current?
3. How many pulses are there per Hz for 1φ and 3φ power?
4. What device in the x-ray circuit controls kVp? mA? time? rectification?
5. What is the approximate voltage ripple for 1φ 2P equipment? 3φ 6P? 3φ 12P?
6. What happens to the tube mA during an exposure using a falling-load generator?
7. What is the difference between an ionization chamber and a phototimer?
8. What factor determines the minimum reaction time?

REFERENCES AND RECOMMENDED READING

Braun, M. (1976). Considerations on the falling load principle. *Optical Engineering, 15*(4), 338–343.

Brumbach, M., & Nadon, J. (2004). *Industrial electricity* (7th ed.). Clifton Park, NY: Delmar Cengage Learning.

Bushberg, J. T., Seibert, J. A., Leidholdt, E. M., & Boone, J. M. (2003). *The essential physics of medical imaging* (2nd ed.). Philadelphia: Lippincott, Williams & Wilkins.

Bushong, S. C. (2008). *Radiologic science for technologists: Physics, biology, and protection* (9th ed.). St. Louis, MO: Elsevier Mosby.

Curry, T. S., Dowdey, J. E., & Murry, R. C. (1990). *Christensen's introduction to the physics of diagnostic radiology* (4th ed.). Philadelphia: Lea and Febiger.

Evans, S. A., Harris, L., Lawinski, C. P., & Hendra, I. R. F. (1985). Mobile x-ray generators: A review. *Radiography, 51*(595), 89.

McClelland, I. (2004). *X-ray equipment maintenance and repairs workbook for radiographers and radiological technologists.* Geneva, Switzerland: World Health Organization.

Morgan, J. A. (1968). The development and application of multi-phase x-rays in medical radiography. *Radiologic Technology, 40*(2), 57.

Panichello J. (2004). *X-ray repair: A comprehensive guide to the installation and servicing of radiographic equipment.* Springfield, IL: Charles C Thomas.

Seeram, E. (1985). *X-ray imaging equipment.* Springfield, IL: Charles C Thomas.

Selman, J. (2000). *The fundamentals of imaging physics and radiobiology for the radiologic technologist* (9th ed.). Springfield, IL: Charles C Thomas.

Sobol, W. T. (2002). High frequency x-ray generator basics. *Medical Physics, 29*(2), 132–144.

Stears, J. G., Gray, J. E., Webbles, W. E., & Frank, E. D. (1988). Radiologic exchange (automatic exposure control function). *Radiologic Technology, 59*(6), 521–522.

Sterling, S. (1988). Automatic exposure control: A primer. *Radiologic Technology, 59*(5), 421–427.

Thornburn, D. S. *Physical characteristics of falling load generators.* Shelton, CT: Philips Medical Systems, Inc.

Weigl, W. (1988). Design of falling load generators. Unpublished paper presented at American Association of Physicists in Medicine seminar.

Weigl, W. (1989). A new high-frequency controlled x-ray generator system with multi-pulse wave shape. *Journal for Radiological Engineering, 1*(1), 7–19.

Wilks, R. J. (2003). *Principles of radiological physics* (4th ed.). Edinburgh: Churchill Livingstone.

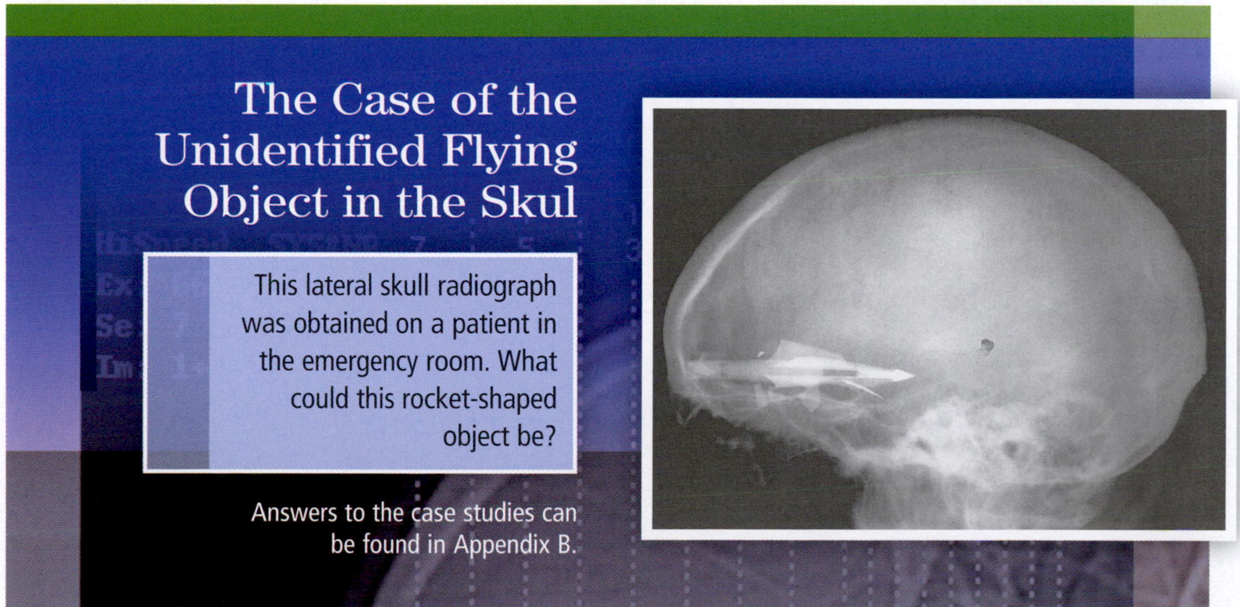

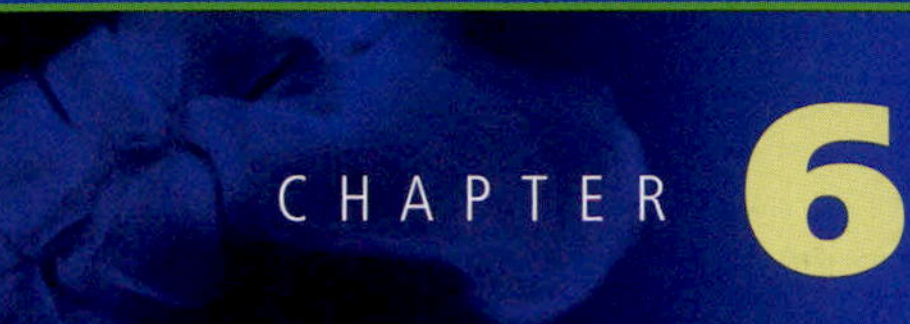

The X-Ray Tube

KEY TERMS

actual focal spot
anode
anode assembly
anode cooling chart
anode heel effect
cathode
cathode assembly
dual focus
effective focal spot
envelope
extrafocal radiation
filament
focal point
focal spot
focal track
focus
focusing cup
fractional focal spot
grid-biased
grid-controlled
grid-pulsed
housing cooling chart
leakage radiation
line-focus principle
off-focus radiation
protective housing
radiographic tube rating chart
rotating anode
rotor

> . . . circumstances led me to the construction of experimental high vacuum tubes with a heated tungsten filament as cathode and a tungsten disc as anode. . . . The tube was then stable and controllable. . . .
>
> *W. D. Coolidge, "Experiences with the Röentgen-ray tube"*

OBJECTIVES

Upon completion of this chapter, the student should be able to:

- Draw a complete dual-focus cathode assembly.
- Discuss the necessary characteristics of filament metals and construction.
- Describe the control of thermionic emission from the filament.
- Select exposure factors and techniques that will extend tube life.
- Explain the function and design of a grid-biased focusing cup.
- Draw a complete rotating anode assembly.
- Discuss the characteristics of anode targets.

KEY TERMS (continued)

saturation current
space charge effect
stationary anode
stator
target
tube rating chart
window
wiring

- Explain the line-focus principle and its effect on anode target design.
- Explain the anode heel effect and its effect on primary beam intensity.
- Explain the production of off-focus radiation.
- Describe the function of a rotating anode induction motor, stator, and rotor.
- Discuss the construction of the envelope and protective housing.
- Calculate safe exposures when provided with a tube rating chart, anode cooling curve, and housing cooling curve.

The electrical production of x-rays is only possible under very special conditions, including a source of electrons, an appropriate target material, a high voltage, and a vacuum. The x-ray tube is the device that permits these conditions to exist, and it is within the tube that x-ray photons come into existence. The tube consists of a **cathode** and an **anode** enclosed within an **envelope** and then encased in a **protective housing** (Figure 6-1). X-ray tubes, whose useful life can be significantly extended by proper care and handling by professional radiographers, can cost over $10,000.

THE CATHODE ASSEMBLY

The cathode is the negative side of the x-ray tube. The function of the cathode is to produce a thermionic cloud, conduct the high voltage to the gap between cathode and anode, and focus the electron stream as it heads for the anode. The cathode is a complex device and is referred to as the **cathode assembly.** This assembly consists of the **filament** or filaments, **focusing cup,** and associated **wiring** (Figure 6-2).

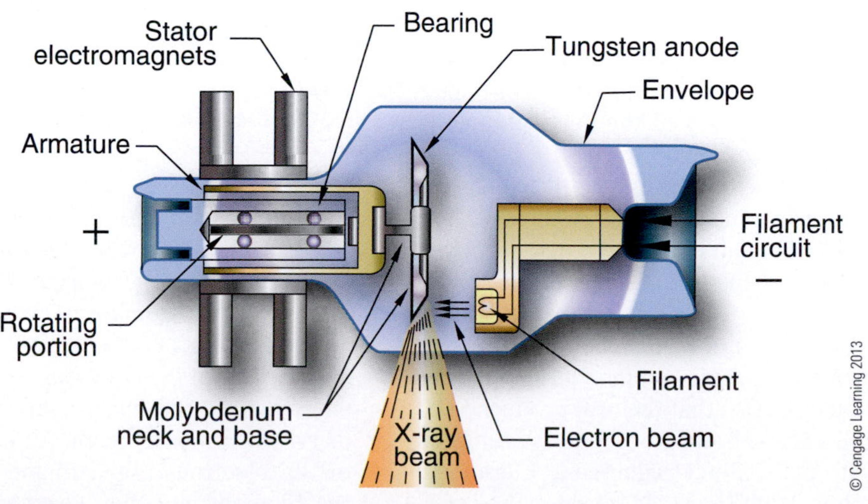

FIGURE 6-1. A rotating anode x-ray tube.

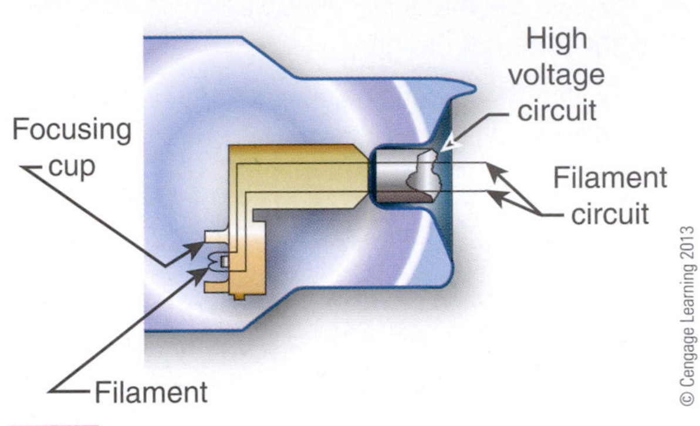

FIGURE 6-2. A cathode assembly.

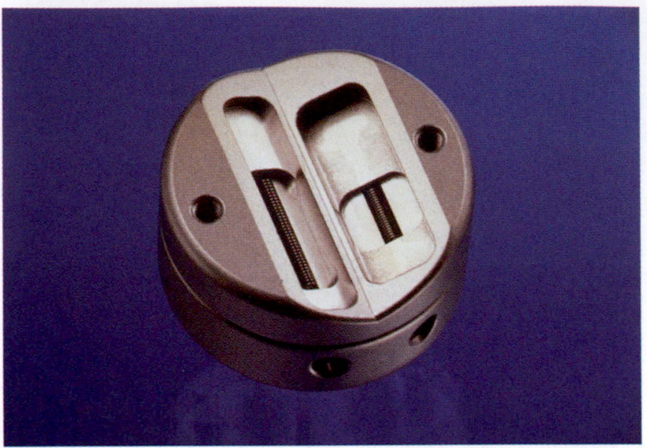

FIGURE 6-3. Dual filaments in a focusing cup. *(Photography courtesy of Dunlee, Division of Philips Medical Systems.)*

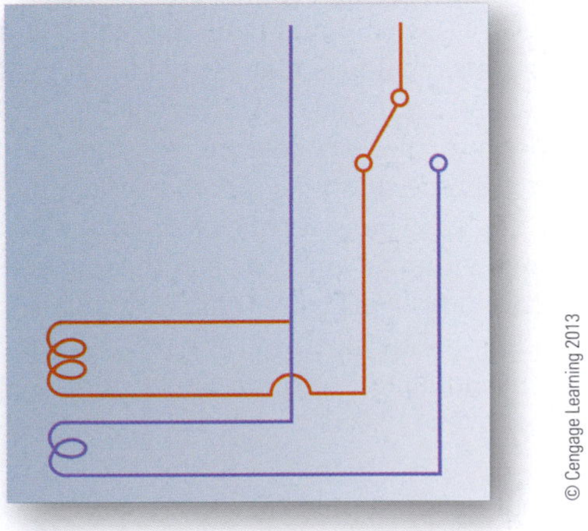

FIGURE 6-4. Dual-filament wiring.

The Filament

The filament is a small coil of thin thoriated tungsten wire. The wire is about 0.1–0.2 mm thick and the coil 1–2 mm wide by 7–15 mm long. It is set in the cathode assembly within the focusing cup (Figure 6-3). Tungsten is the material of choice because of its high melting point (3,370°C) and because it is difficult to vaporize (turn into a gas). Rhenium (melting point of (3,170°C) and molybdenum (melting point of (2,620°C) are also desirable materials. The high melting point permits the filament to operate at the high temperatures required of an x-ray tube. In addition, tungsten is not easily vaporized. Vaporization produces particles that deposit on other surfaces and reduce the vacuum within the tube. The length and width of the filament have a great effect on the ability of the particular x-ray tube to image fine details.

Most diagnostic x-ray tubes have dual filaments called a **dual focus** arrangement (see Figure 6-3). The wiring for dual filaments does not require separate ground conductors. Instead a common ground is used (Figure 6-4).

As we have discussed previously, the function of the filament is to provide sufficient resistance to the flow of electrons so that the heat produced will cause thermionic emission to occur. (A tungsten filament will not exhibit significant thermionic emission below 2,200°C). This process causes electrons to leave the surface of the filament wire and form a thermionic cloud. When the high voltage is released at exposure, the entire cloud is available to be driven toward the anode target where x-ray photons will be produced. This provides many more times the number of electrons than would be available from a cold cathode.

Not all of the electrons that are thermionically emitted from the filament are driven to the anode or return to the filament. A very small percentage of the electrons are permanently vaporized from the filament and they contribute to reducing the vacuum, thus making the tube gassy. Vaporized tungsten (from both filament and anode) is also gradually deposited on the inner surface of a glass envelope. This deposit causes old tubes to have a mirrored appearance and can eventually cause high-voltage arcing when sufficient current is attracted to a deposit during an exposure. Arcing of this type immediately destroys the tube. Evaporization deposits on the glass envelope also cause increased filtration of the primary beam, and this decreases tube efficiency. Tubes with a metal envelope can be grounded to significantly reduce this problem.

Another major cause of tube failure is the breaking of the filament itself. Filaments become increasingly thin as vaporization continues. When about 10 percent of the diameter has vaporized, a filament becomes subject to breaking, exactly the way a tungsten light bulb filament will burn out. However, older tubes are much more sensitive to rough handling and a thin filament that is jarred can break prematurely. For this reason, radiographers must move tube units gently, never allowing them to be heavily jarred by jamming against overhead stops and detents.

When the x-ray machine is first turned on, a mild current is sent to the filament. The filament remains in this preheated mode until immediately prior to an exposure. When the switch labeled "rotor" is activated prior to an exposure, not only does the rotor begin to turn but a higher current is sent to the filament to bring the thermionic cloud to the proper size for the mA selected. This increase in filament heating is what causes most of the vaporization of the filament. An average diagnostic x-ray tube filament life is only about 6–9 hours (10,000–20,000 exposures) at this heating level. One of the primary causes of premature tube failure is the radiographer's habit of holding the rotor switch prior to making exposures. Every second the rotor switch is depressed, life is removed from the filament. Routinely delayed exposures while the filament is enduring maximum current can shorten tube life by 50–60 percent (to 5,000–12,000 exposures).

Most tube manufacturers recommend that two-step exposure switches be **fully depressed in one motion.** All units have electronic interlocks that will not permit the exposure to occur until the rotor has brought the anode up to the proper speed. Holding the rotor switch (and filament heat) can be justified in cases where the patient is unable to cooperate. In these instances (such as with pediatric patients) the rotor and filament must be readied to permit an instant exposure to avoid patient breathing and motion. Single-phase generators are usually capable of initiating exposure within 10 milliseconds (0.01 second), whereas high-frequency generators may be a quick 1 millisecond (0.001 second). Routine clinical examinations seldom need to be timed closer than these limitations.

Historical Notes. In the earliest days of radiography a cold cathode with an unheated filament was used. It was not until the American physicist William D. Coolidge (1873–1975) developed the Coolidge tube for the General Electric Corporation in 1915 that the hot filament became available. Prior to the development of the Coolidge tube, the radiographer kept a selection of tubes of various mA values on a rack, usually in the darkroom (Figure 6-5). When a change of mA was required, the radiographer disconnected the tube and replaced it with a different one from the rack. Coolidge's contributions to radiography included not only the hot filament, but also the focusing cup, the imbedded anode target, and various anode cooling devices (including the unique water-cooled tube).

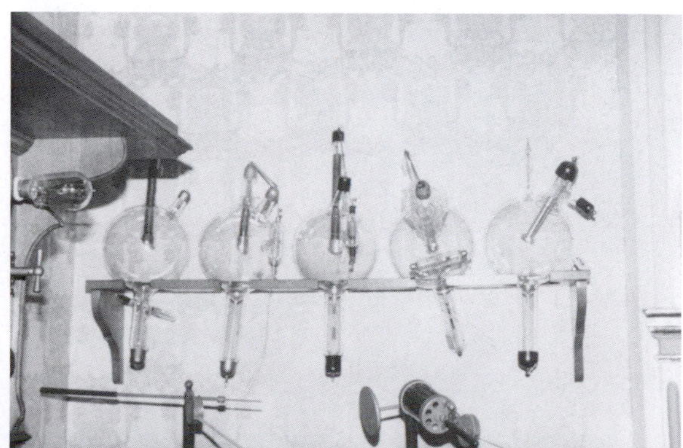

FIGURE 6-5. A selection of cold filament tubes as displayed at the Deutsches Röntgen Museum, Remscheid-Lennep, Germany. *(Photography courtesy of Phillip W. Ballinger.)*

The Focusing Cup

The focusing cup is a shallow depression in the cathode assembly designed to house the filament (see Figure 6-2). It is made of nickel and its purpose is to narrow the thermionic cloud as it is driven toward the anode. Because electrons all possess negative charges, their tendency is to diverge rather than to travel in straight lines. The focusing cup is provided with a low negative potential, which, because of its geometry, focuses the electrons toward one another in a convergence pattern (Figure 6-6). Most x-ray tubes have the focusing cup at the same potential as the filament. It is possible to decrease the size of the focal spot by using a biased focusing cup. A biased focusing cup maintains the cup at a more negative voltage than the filament. This causes the exiting electron beam to be focused into a narrower stream as it heads toward the anode. In mammographic x-ray tubes focusing cup biasing is used when the small focal spot is selected.

As more and more electrons build up in the area of the filament, their negative charges begin to oppose the emission of additional electrons. This phenomenon is called the **space charge effect** and it limits x-ray tubes to maximum mA ranges of 1,000–1,200.

Saturation current is another filament phenomenon that affects the efficiency of the x-ray tube. As kVp increases, a greater percentage of the thermionically emitted electrons are driven toward the anode. This relationship is shown by a filament emission chart (Figure 6-7). The filament amperage curve flattens out when the kVp is driving the entire thermionic cloud toward the anode. The filament saturation current has been achieved when there are no further thermionic electrons to be driven toward the anode. At this point an increase in kVp will not increase the tube mA. Further mA increases must be achieved by increasing the filament amperage. Close examination of a filament emission chart demonstrates that something must be done to compensate for the tube mA increase when kVp is changed. For example, an exposure at 100 kVp will produce a significantly greater tube mA than the same exposure at 60 kVp. The filament amperage must be adjusted to compensate for these changes, and the x-ray circuitry is programmed to do this automatically whenever factors are changed by the operator.

Grid-Biased Tubes. In some applications, such as angiography or capacitor discharge generators, it is desirable to quickly regulate the flow of

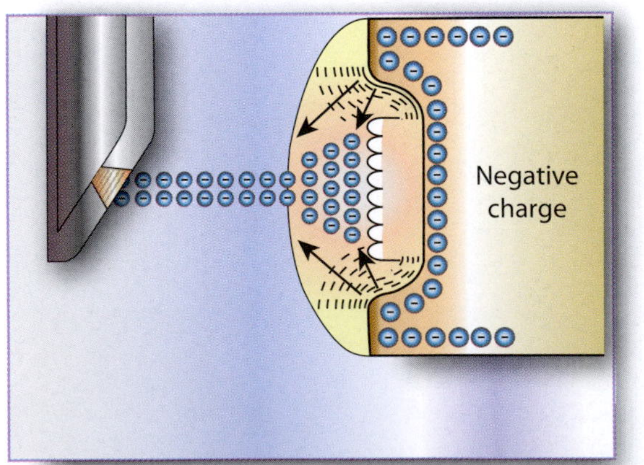

FIGURE 6-6. The geometry of the negative charge on the cathode focusing cup.

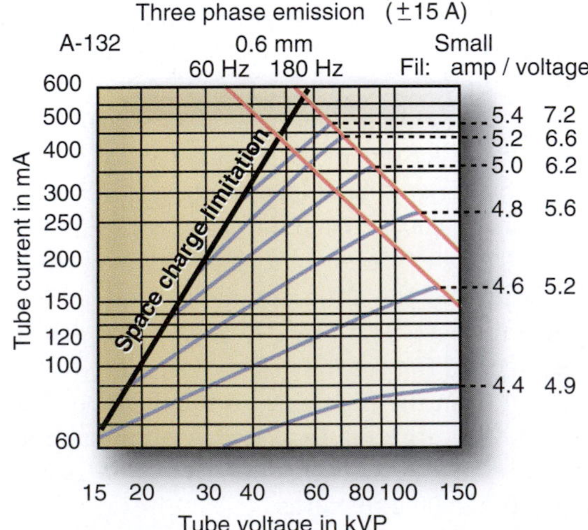

FIGURE 6-7. A filament emission chart showing saturation as a function of filament amperage, tube voltage, and tube current. *(Courtesy of Varian EIMAC.)*

electrons producing x-ray photons. The addition of a positive or negative potential difference (approximately 2,000 volts) at the focusing cup causes the cup to attract or repel the thermionic cloud. This very cleanly removes electrons from use for x-ray production when the focusing cup charge is pulsed from negative to positive in synchrony with another device, and it becomes possible to regulate, pulse, and synchronize x-ray production very precisely. These types of tubes are sometimes called **grid-pulsed, grid-biased,** or **grid-controlled,** and are also used in pulsed fluoroscopy.

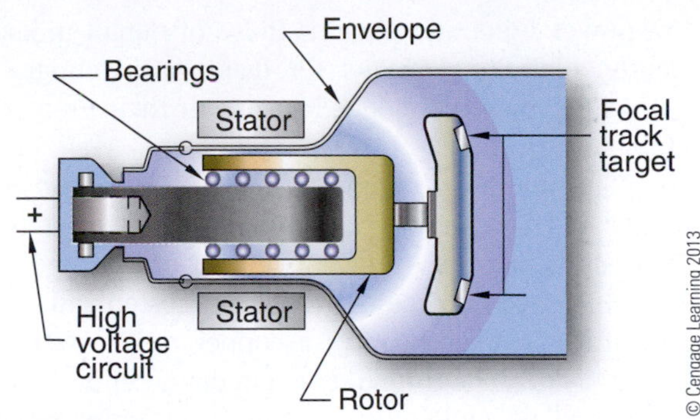

FIGURE 6-8. The anode assembly with anode, target, rotor, bearings, and stator.

THE ANODE ASSEMBLY

The anode is the positive side of the x-ray tube and has three functions: it serves as a target surface for the high-voltage electrons from the filament, thereby becoming the source of the x-ray photons; it conducts the high voltage from the cathode back into the x-ray generator circuitry; and it serves as the primary thermal conductor. The anode target surface is where the high-speed electrons from the filament are suddenly stopped, resulting in the production of x-ray photons. The entire anode is a complex device referred to as the **anode assembly.** This assembly consists of the anode, **stator,** and **rotor** (Figure 6-8) and serves as the path for the high-voltage flow during exposure.

The Anode

Anodes are divided into two types: **stationary** and **rotating** (Figure 6-9). Rotating anodes, developed in 1936, turn during the exposure, thus presenting a much larger target area. Modern rotating anodes permit bombardment of a given area of the target for only 7–50 microseconds. The faster the anode rotates, the better the heat dissipation. The use of stationary anode x-ray tubes has become limited to

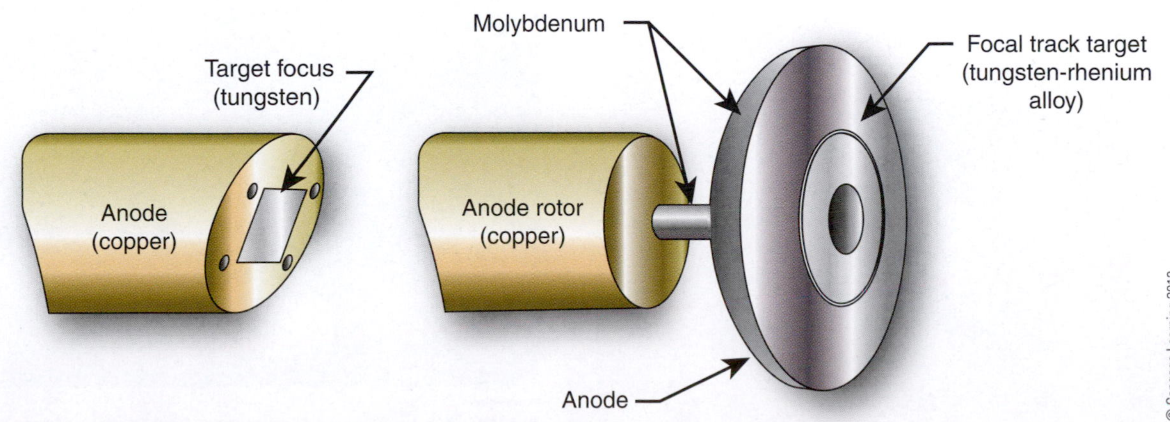

FIGURE 6-9. A stationary and a rotating anode.

low-power functions, such as those of dental units. Nearly all units designed for diagnostic radiography utilize rotating anodes because of their greater efficiency.

The anode is composed of several different metals, each designed to contribute the maximum to the overall function of the anode. Stationary anodes are composed of rhenium-alloyed tungsten imbedded in a 45° angled end of a copper rod. Rotating anode disks range from 5–13 cm in diameter and are composed of molybdenum. The anode's function as the source of x-ray photons and as the primary thermal conducting device is enhanced by the use of rhenium-alloyed tungsten as the target focal track material (Figure 6-10). Tungsten is the metal of choice for the source of x-ray photons for three primary reasons:

1. High atomic number
2. High melting point
3. Heat-conducting ability

Tungsten's atomic number (74) enhances the production of diagnostic-range photons. During normal use, the focal track reaches a temperature between 1,000°C and 2,000°C but the temperature can go higher if the tube load increases. Because of tungsten's high melting point, it can withstand normal operating temperatures. Tungsten also conducts heat very well. The rhenium provides greater elasticity when the focal track expands rapidly due to the intense heat. To assist in the dissipation of heat in heavy-load situations, specialized anodes may have the anode disk backed by a thicker layer of molybdenum or graphite. Graphite-backed anodes can double heat-loading capabilities without increasing bearing wear.

Specialized x-ray tubes for mammography utilize molybdenum (atomic number 42) as the primary target material due to its ability to emit a more uniform range of lower-energy photons. The lower characteristic energy photons permit a better soft tissue image. Molybdenum also has a high melting point, as discussed earlier. These tubes also utilize a specialized glass envelope window made of beryllium because the glass used in most x-ray tubes absorbs too much of the low-energy beam.

Normal use of a rotating anode will eventually vaporize sufficient target focal track material to roughen or pit the target area (Figure 6-11). Pitting reduces the efficiency of the tube; the term *pitted*, or *pitting*, is often used to describe an older tube's focal track.

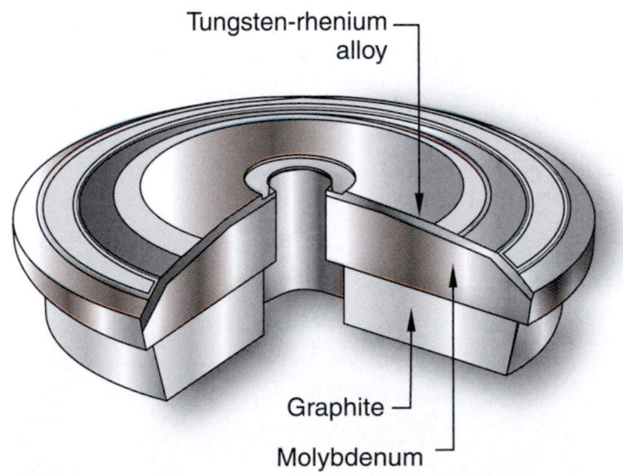

FIGURE 6-10. Rotating anode construction.

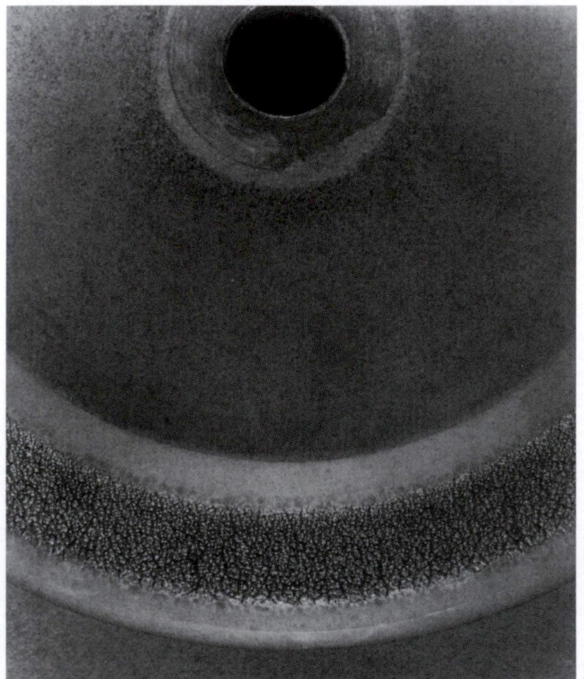

FIGURE 6-11. Pitting of a rotating anode focal track from extended use.

When first activating an x-ray unit, it is important to use an **anode warm-up procedure.** These procedures are specified by the tube manufacturers and are designed to bring the anode heat from room temperature to near the range of operation. The procedure also permits the heat from the hot anode to serve as a "vacuum pump" to maintain a strong vacuum inside the envelope. This is why x-ray tubes should be warmed up regularly, even when the unit is not being used for patients. A normal procedure might require an average kVp and mA station for a 1-second exposure to be followed by two more 2-second exposures. Failure to follow the warm-up procedure can cause the entire anode to crack if the molybdenum absorbs the heat too rapidly and exceeds its expansion capability. Many anodes are stress relieved (Figure 6-12). A stress-relieved anode dissipates heat much more efficiently and does not require an elaborate tube warm-up procedure.

The Target Area. The portion of the anode where the high-voltage electron stream will impact is called by various names: the **target,** the **focus,** the **focal point,** the **focal spot,** or the **focal track** (although this last term has a more specific definition, it is the target area). This is the precise point at which the x-ray photons are created. The target is considered to be a point source of x-ray photons and it is from this point that all tube-to-object and image-receptor distances are measured. Some x-ray tube housings have a line drawn on them to indicate the exact level of the target within. All measuring devices have their zero point at this level. This is why a tape measure attached to the side or bottom of a tube collimator may begin at 12 cm. It is attached 12 cm from the target but is calculated to measure target-to-image-receptor distances.

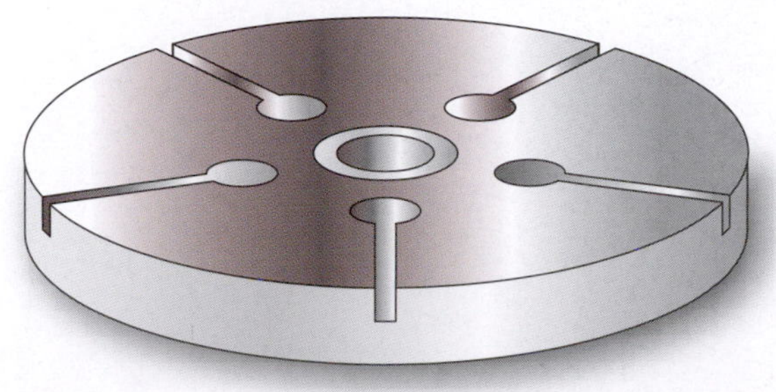

FIGURE 6-12. The back of a stress-relieved anode.

Stationary anodes have a static target area. Rotating anodes have a dynamic target area and are designed to greatly increase the target area (see Figure 6-9). A rotating anode can increase the target area up to 300 times, depending on the diameter of the anode disk. Rotating anodes have much greater heat loading capacities than stationary anodes. High-speed anodes have higher heating capacities than regular-speed anodes (often 50 percent greater).

When discussing a rotating anode target area, the term *focal track* is used to represent the circular path that will be impacted by the electron beam. The terms *target*, *focus*, *focal points*, and *focal spot* refer to the area of the focal track that is impacted by the electron beam at one time. In addition, the term **actual focal spot** is used to describe the physical area of the focal track that is impacted. The term **effective focal spot** is used to describe the area of the focal spot that is projected out of the tube toward the object being radiographed (Figure 6-13).

Line-Focus Principle. The **line-focus principle** is used to reduce the effective area of the focal spot. This permits the best resolution of detail while permitting as large an actual area as possible (to increase thermal conductivity). **The effective focal-spot size is controlled by the size of the actual focal spot (which is controlled by the length of the filament) and the anode target angle.** As the actual focal-spot size increases, the effective focal-spot size also increases (see Figure 6-13).

When the target angle is less than 45°, the effective focal spot is smaller than the actual focal spot (Figure 6-14). This is accomplished by the line-focus principle. This principle can best be understood by holding a pencil straight up and then sloping it toward oneself so that the pencil is seen end on. The perceived dimensions of the pencil change as the angle changes. In the x-ray tube, changing the angle of the target changes the effective focal spot.

The most common diagnostic radiography target angle is 12°. However, tubes are available with angles ranging from 7° to 17°. When the angle

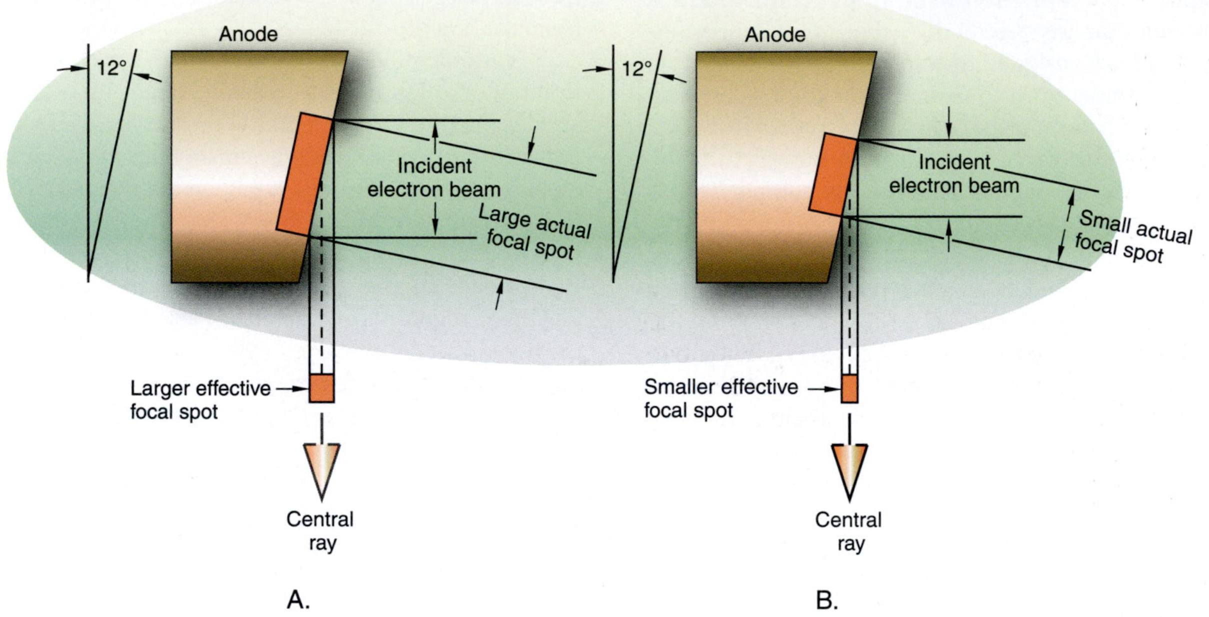

FIGURE 6-13. Effect of actual focal-spot size on effective focal-spot size.

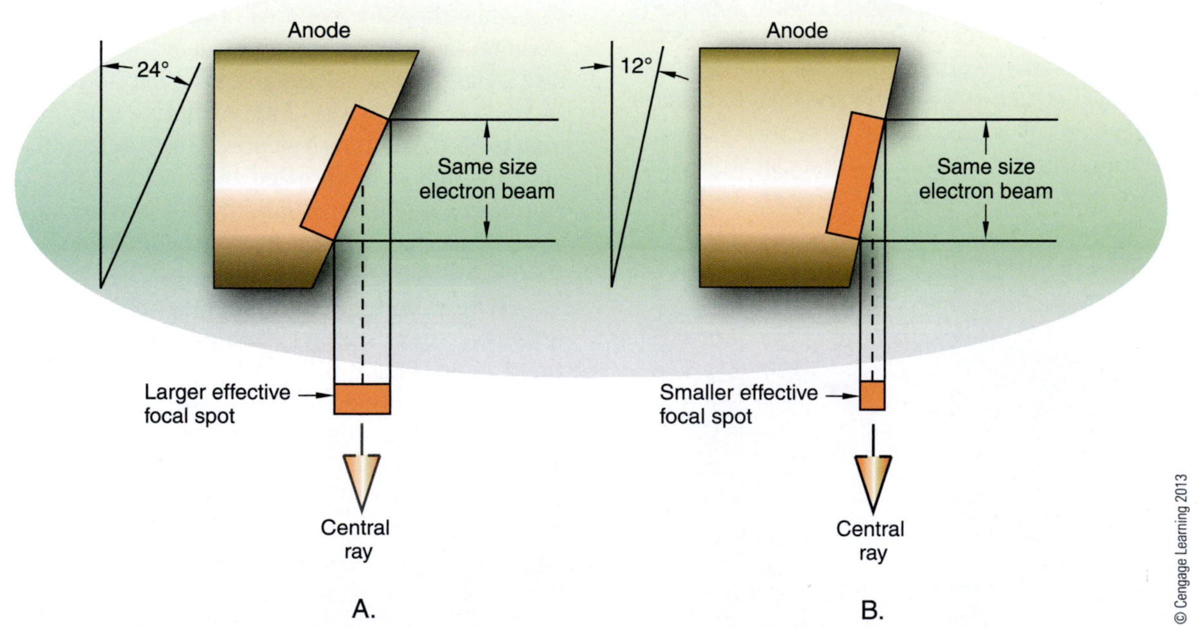

FIGURE 6-14. Use of the line-focus principle to obtain an effective focal spot smaller than the actual focal spot.

is decreased, smaller focal spots can be achieved. A disadvantage of extremely small target angles is that the geometry of the angle can limit the size of the primary beam field at short source-to-image receptor distances (Figure 6-15). To cover a 14" × 17" field at 40", a minimum of a 12° target angle is required. It has been shown that at large heat loads, target angles can decrease due to "warping" of the anode. In these instances, the anode end of the primary beam field can be reduced enough to cut off structures near the collimated edge. A slight angle of the tube will compensate for this effect. Target angles of less than 14° have been shown to produce some degree of cutoff as they age. Some tubes have offset filaments with two different focal tracks, which can be set at different target angles.

X-ray tube focal spots are rectangular because the line-focus principle applies only in the direction of the angle. It does not apply horizontally across the anode focal track because there is no angle in this direction. X-ray tube targets must be narrow to maintain the small effective focal-spot size in the horizontal direction, usually not over 2 mm. The line-focus principle permits the actual focal spot's vertical dimension to be as much as 6 mm to gain the maximum thermal conductivity. **The effective focal spot's vertical dimension is the one that is stated as the focal-spot size.**

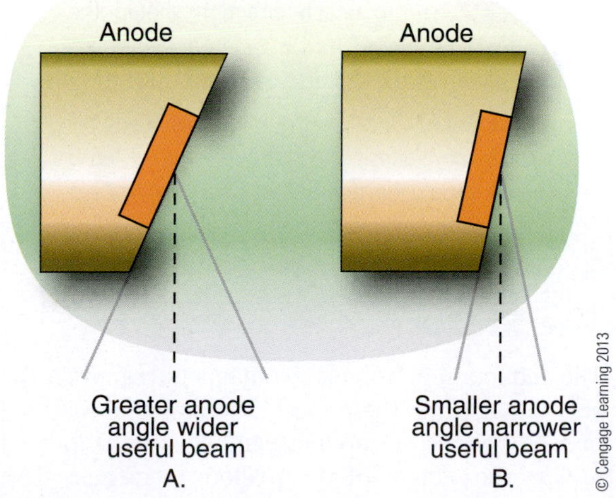

FIGURE 6-15. Anode target angle as a function of maximum primary beam field size.

The National Electrical Manufacturers Association (NEMA) establishes standards for focal-spot size. These standards provide tolerance ranges for 23 focal-spot sizes. For example, a 1.0-mm focal spot is within tolerance if it measures up to 1.4 mm in width and 2.0 mm in length. It is important to remember that, in some instances, focal spots may be considerably larger than their stated size. Diagnostic tubes are available with focal spots of 0.1 mm to 3.0 mm. Occasionally, the term **fractional focal spot** is used to refer to a very small focal spot, one that is a fraction of a millimeter in size.

In normal usage, the term *focal-spot size* refers to the effective focal-spot size. Most diagnostic x-ray tubes have dual focal spots to include one for fine detail studies and the other for heavy tube loads. The small focal spot will not permit the use of higher-mA stations. If the x-ray unit allows the radiographer to choose the focal-spot size, an exposure cannot be made with a high-mA station and the small focal spot. Automatic systems link the focal-spot size selection with the appropriate mA station. Therefore, the radiographer should realize that the focal-spot size may be mandated by the mA station. When a small focal spot is desired, it is important to use only low-mA stations, even though this may require a longer exposure time.

Focal-spot size increases, or blooms, as milliamperage is increased. For example, the focal spot is slightly larger during an exposure of 80 kVp, 800 mA, and 0.1 second than it is during an exposure of 80 kVp, 100 mA, and 0.8 second. Although originally considered to be a significant factor, research has indicated that focal-spot blooming does not have a resounding effect on recorded detail.

Anode Heel Effect. The use of the line-focus principle causes a problem that is known as the **anode heel effect** (Figure 6-16). Because of the geometry of an angled anode target, the **radiation intensity is greater on the cathode side.** As electrons bombard the target, x-rays are produced and most are emitted at angles between 45° and 90° in the direction of the electron travel. These are absorbed by the anode itself or by the tube housing. Those photons that are emitted from the surface of

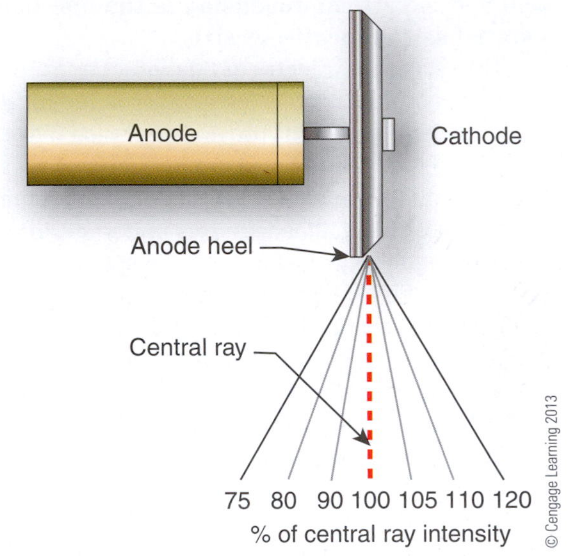

FIGURE 6-16. The anode heel effect.

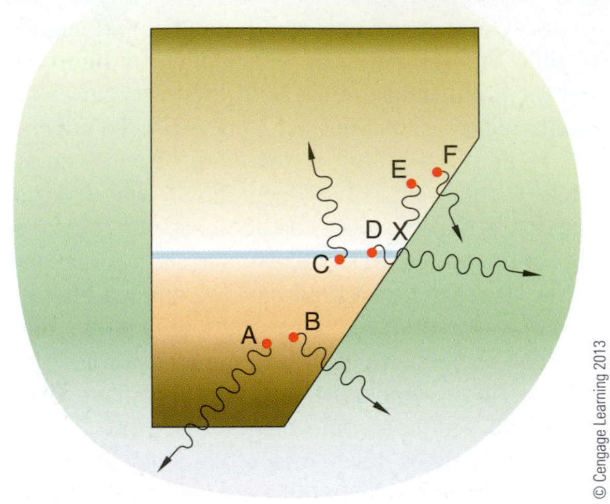

FIGURE 6-17. A–F represent photons created in the target. A exits at the anode end of the tube, whereas B exits at the cathode end of the tube. Notice the greater distance that photon A must travel through the target material itself as compared to photon B. Most photons are absorbed as in C. C is absorbed in anode D, which exits the anode but is absorbed in the housing, and E, which is heading toward the anode end but does not exit the anode. F exits at the cathode end because it has a shorter distance to travel through the anode.

the target are emitted in all directions. The intensity of the radiation that is emitted will vary between the cathode end of the tube and the anode end of the tube. This is because photons that are emitted toward the anode end are more likely to be absorbed by the target material itself than those that are emitted toward the cathode end (Figure 6-17). This can cause as many as 20 percent more photons at the cathode end of the tube and 25 percent fewer photons at the anode end (Figure 6-18). A total variation of approximately 45 percent exists parallel to the anode-cathode axis. No significant variation occurs perpendicular to the anode-cathode axis.

The 45 percent variation is significant enough to cause a visible difference in exposure during radiographic examinations **when large film sizes are used at short distances.** The anode heel effect is the reason why each radiographic table has a standard or natural "head" end. The tube anode is established at the head of the table to utilize the anode heel effect to best advantage. No significant variations will be seen in exposure from side to side.

Because the cathode end of the x-ray tube has a more intense beam, it should be positioned toward the denser (thicker) part of the body.

> ***EXAMPLE:*** In which direction should the cathode be placed for an anteroposterior examination of the thoracic vertebral column?
>
> ***Answer:*** Because the inferior thoracic region is more dense, the cathode's more intense beam should be positioned inferiorly to help increase the exposure in that region.

The Stator

The induction-motor electromagnets comprise the stator that turns the anode. The stator is the only part of cathode or anode assemblies that is located *outside* the vacuum of the envelope (see Figure 6-8). The electromagnetic effect that causes the rotor to turn can function through the envelope, permitting electrical isolation of the stator coils from the high voltage of the exposure. The kilovoltage range of

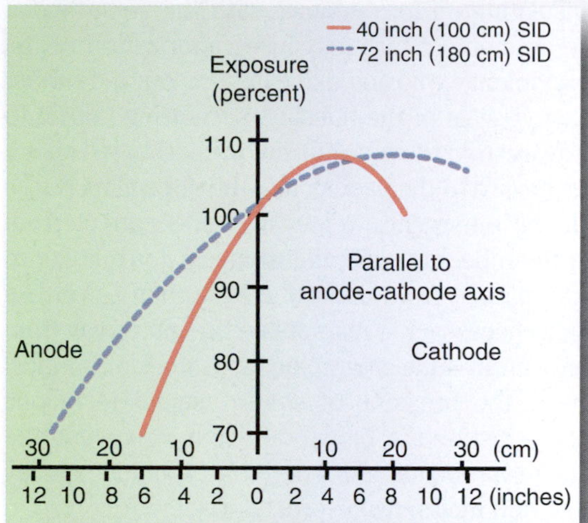

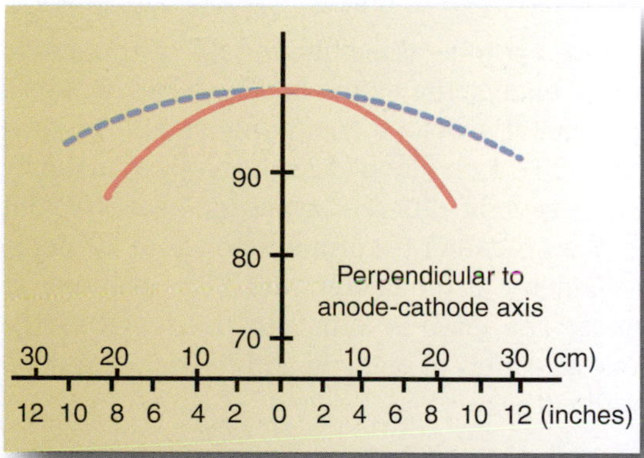

FIGURE 6-18. Variation in intensity of x-ray emissions parallel and perpendicular to anode-cathode axis. *(Note: From Quality Control in Diagnostic Imaging, by the Mayo Foundation, 1983, Rockville, MD: Aspen. Reprinted by permission of the Mayo Foundation for Medical Education and Research. All rights reserved.)*

the exposure would destroy the stator's electromagnets. The switch labeled "rotor" that must be activated prior to an exposure actually sends current to the stator, which then causes the rotor to turn the anode. If the stator fails, the rotor will cease to turn the anode, resulting in the immediate melting of a spot on the target because rotating anode targets

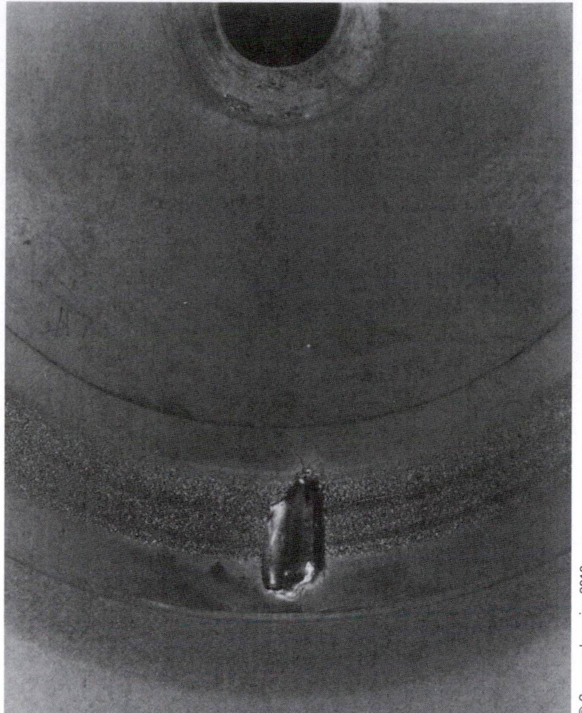

FIGURE 6-19. Anode melt due to rotor-bearing failure.

are not designed to absorb the heat of a high-voltage exposure while stationary (Figure 6-19).

The Rotor

The rotor is located inside the stator and inside the envelope. It is composed of a hollow copper cylinder or cuff that is attached to the anode disk by a molybdenum shaft. The cuff is the true rotor that is affected by the electromagnetic field of the stator, causing it to turn. Common rotating anodes revolve at 3,200–3,600 revolutions per minute (rpm). High-speed rotating anodes that operate at 10,000–12,000 rpm are also available to assist in dissipating heat.

The inside of the rotor contains silver-plated steel ball bearings around a shaft that is anchored to the envelope (see Figure 6-8). The ball bearings use silver plating as a high-temperature lubricant between the cuff and the anode shaft. Liquids tend to produce gas at high temperatures, and this would reduce the vacuum in the tube. When the rotor switch is depressed prior to an exposure, the sound that is heard from the tube is actually the sound of the ball bearings turning at high speed. A new tube rotor with fresh bearings should coast for about 60 seconds after a 3,000-rpm exposure before stopping. When the coasting time slows to less than 20 seconds, the bearings are usually near binding.

High-speed anodes have a particular problem that is caused by the tone produced by their rotating. At between 5,000 and 7,000 rpm, the harmonics produced by the rotating cuff are at a frequency capable of shattering the glass envelope. Consequently, at the end of an exposure, direct current is run through the stator to quickly slow (or brake) the rotor safely through the dangerous harmonic range. Another problem associated with high-speed anodes is the gyroscopic effect produced by the centrifugal force of the rotation. This force is great enough that if a high-speed anode tube housing is quickly rotated from one position to another (for example, from horizontal to vertical), the gyroscopic effect can cause trauma to the anode disk and bearing, causing the destruction of the tube. Usually the reversal of the stator prevents this problem, but constant rough handling of this sort can cause undue wear on the rotor bearings. Any rough or extremely fast movement of the housing is not healthy for an x-ray tube and should be avoided.

A common cause of tube failure is bad bearings caused by long use at high temperatures. Although the molybdenum shaft that attaches the anode disk is designed to conduct a minimal amount of heat, the ball bearings eventually become imperfectly round. This leads to a grinding noise and wobbling of the rotor. Rotor wobble throws the focal track off center and tube efficiency drops dramatically.

Another effect of stator or rotor failure is that the electron stream overheats the target area of the anode focal track. When the temperature exceeds the melting point of tungsten, melting will occur. Superheated melted tungsten that drips onto the envelope will destroy the tube.

Any tube is dangerous to use when these events occur. A wobbling or melting anode disk can crack from the heat of exposure. A cracked anode can divert the electron and/or photon stream toward the envelope. Either instance will crack the envelope, permitting implosion of the vacuum, which can suck the insulating oil into contact with the superheated anode assembly. This can cause vaporization of the oil in a violent explosion that can blow out the rubber expansion seals of the housing, permitting hot oil to blow away from the tube housing. Superheated oil is a severe hazard to the patient, and the normal response should be emergency removal of the patient from under the tube. In nearly all instances, it is quicker to pull the patient from under the tube than to release the locks necessary to manipulate the tube away from the patient. In an angiographic laboratory or surgical situation, the breaking of sterile aseptic technique would be justified. A blown tube is a rare event and should never occur if proper tube loading, quality control, and maintenance procedures are followed.

THE ENVELOPE

The entire cathode assembly and all of the anode assembly except the stator are enclosed within a glass or metal envelope commonly called the tube (Figure 6-20). A common glass envelope is made by sculpting several different types of heat-resistant Pyrex glass together to form a tube about 10" long, 6" in diameter at the center, and 2" in diameter at the ends. The glass is joined to the metal of the cathode assembly at one end and the anode assembly at the other.

The Envelope

Metal envelopes are increasingly becoming more common. They prolong tube life because they eliminate the problem of tungsten vaporization, as discussed earlier. The vast majority of high-output x-ray tubes are now made with metal envelopes.

The envelope is constructed around both the cathode and anode assemblies and must be sealed tight to maintain a high vacuum. At the point where the primary x-ray beam exits the envelope, a **window** segment is constructed. In some tubes this is simply a thinner section of the envelope to allow less absorption or scatter of the photons. Some special application tubes have other types of windows. For example, a molybdenum target tube for mammography uses a special metallic beryllium window to avoid attenuating the lower-energy photons, as discussed earlier.

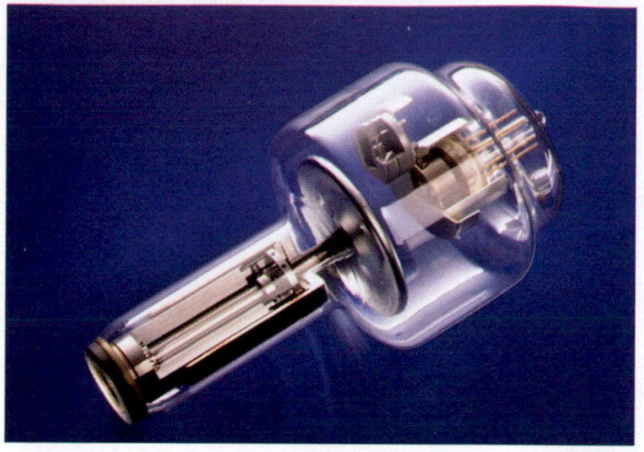

(A)

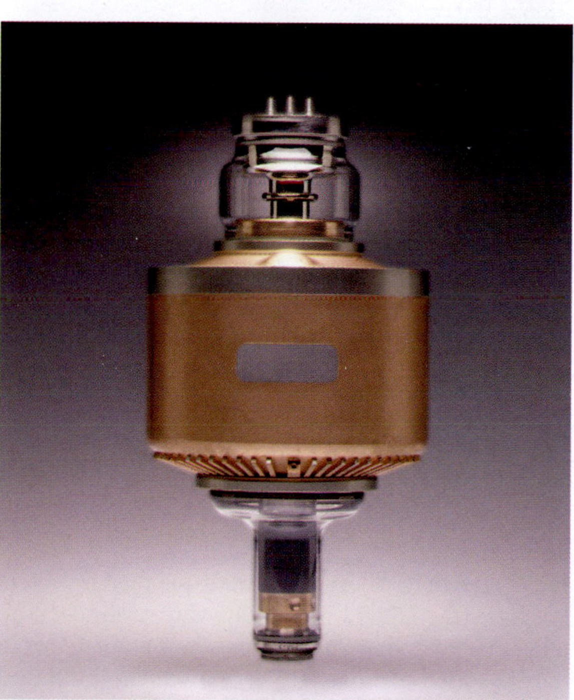

(B)

FIGURE 6-20. A complete diagnostic x-ray tube with envelope, cathode assembly, anode disk, and rotor. (A) Glass envelope. (B) Metal envelope. *(Photo courtesy of Dunlee, Division of Philips Medical Systems.)*

The Vacuum

The primary function of the envelope is to maintain the vacuum between the cathode and anode. After construction, the air is removed from the tube until a pressure of less than 10^{-5} mm mercury (Hg) is achieved. This is done by use of a vacuum pump through a special vent, which is then permanently sealed. **The removal of the air permits electrons to flow from cathode to anode without encountering the gas atoms of air** and greatly increases the efficiency of the tube's operation.

Historical Notes. Röntgen discovered x-rays with a Crookes or Hittorf tube, which did not enclose a vacuum but instead contained known volumes of various gasses. Specialized tubes were quickly developed to meet the increasing need for x-ray production, and the vacuum tube was an early improvement. The x-ray pioneers simply placed the glass envelope within a leaded glass bowl. This was convenient when tubes had to be changed manually during the era of cold cathodes. Rapidly increasing awareness of the biological effects of ionizing radiation led to the development of metallic housings for x-ray tubes.

PROTECTIVE HOUSING

Modern x-ray tubes must be mounted inside a protective housing (Figure 6-21). **The housing controls leakage and scatter radiation, isolates the high voltages, and provides a means to cool the tube.**

Control of Leakage Radiation and Scatter Radiation

When x-ray photons are produced at the anode, they are emitted isotropically (in all directions). The primary beam consists of photons emitted through the window. The remaining photons are unwanted and the tube housing is designed to absorb them. The protective housing is composed of cast steel and is capable of absorbing most of the unwanted photons. The housing is usually lined with lead for additional absorption only at the cathode end because of the direction of the photons being emitted from the anode. The housing is equipped with a window to permit unrestricted exit for the useful photons from the envelope window. Any photons that escape from the housing except at the port are **leakage radiation.** **Leakage radiation must not**

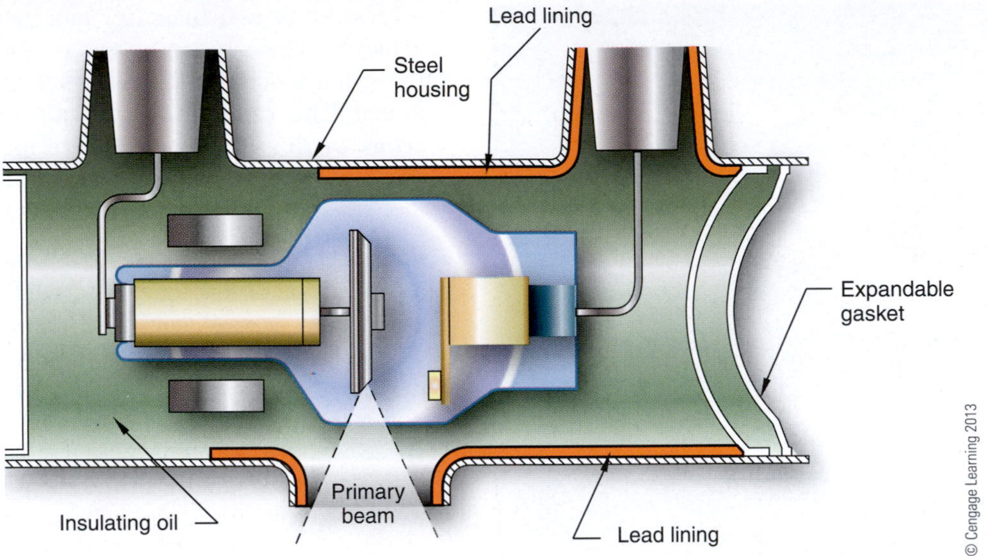

FIGURE 6-21. A diagnostic x-ray tube housing.

exceed 100 mR/hr at 1 meter. The housing also serves to cushion the x-ray tube from rough handling by operators.

High-Voltage Isolation and Tube Cooling

A special dielectric oil is used to fill the space between the envelope and the tube housing. The dielectric property of the oil insulates the high-voltage components from the tube housing, which is handled by the radiographer. In addition, the oil absorbs much of the heat that is produced by x-ray production. One end of the tube housing is sealed with an expandable gasket to permit the oil to expand as it is heated (see Figure 6-21). This gasket can be blown out by an imploded tube that has vaporized some of the insulating oil, thereby presenting a hazard to the patient. Many tube housings include a small air fan to remove heat from the housing itself. In tubes that are subjected to extremely high loads, such as computed tomography tubes, the oil may be routed through a recirculation system (heat exchanger) to further cool it. Under no circumstances should anyone be in contact with a tube housing during an exposure.

Off-Focus Radiation

An often overlooked factor that can cause serious degradation of radiographic image quality is **off-focus,** or **extrafocal, radiation. Off-focus radiation is composed of photons that were not produced at the focal spot.** It occurs when the high-voltage electrons striking the focal spot produce scattered electrons or photons. In some cases these scattered electrons or photons have sufficient energy remaining that when they strike another object in the tube (the cathode assembly, vaporized metal on a glass envelope, off-target sites on the anode, etc.), they produce photons. These photons are produced away from the focal spot and are therefore considered off-focus. The tube housing will absorb the majority of off-focus radiation but enough will be produced at a proper angle that it will exit through the tube window, housing port, and collimator (Figure 6-22). These photons can cause "ghosting" of structures adjacent to the edge of the primary beam (Figure 6-23). This is not the result of scatter from the patient. Patient scatter is not capable of creating a diagnostic image of anatomical structures. Off-focus radiation may contribute as much as 25–30 percent of the total primary beam and is a special problem

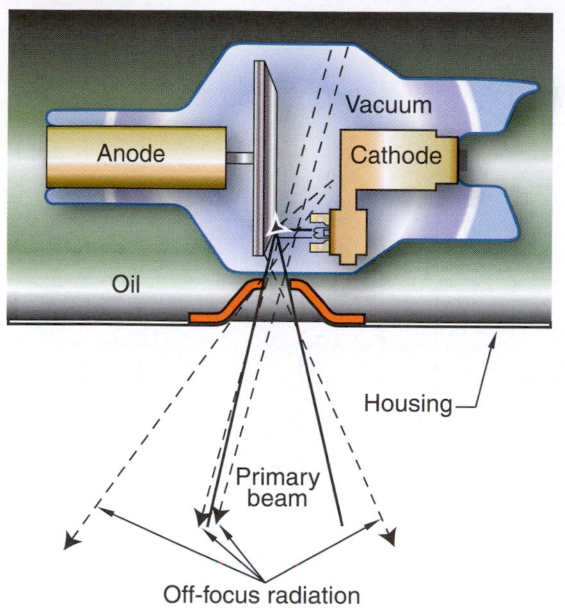

FIGURE 6-22. The production of off-focus radiation.

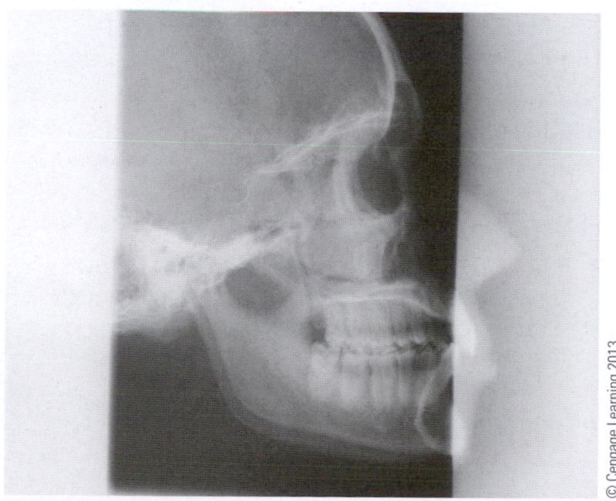

FIGURE 6-23. Off-focus radiation producing an image of the nose on a collimated sinus radiograph.

in digital radiographic units, as it may be perceived as primary beam, thus dramatically changing the histogram during post-processing. All off-focus radiation is of significantly lower energy than the primary beam itself. X-ray tubes are available with a grounded metal and ceramic envelope to absorb off-focus radiation. These tubes may also use two sets of bearings to increase the heat-loading capacity. They have received limited acceptance because of their cost and the fact that they will not fit most existing tube housings. However, they can increase the total tube life by up to three times.

RATING CHARTS AND COOLING CURVES

Three types of rating charts are available to help radiographers avoid thermal damage to x-ray tubes: **radiographic tube rating charts, anode cooling charts,** and **housing cooling charts.** Radiographic rating charts, sometimes called **tube rating charts,** are the most valuable because they provide a guide regarding the maximum technical factor combinations that can be used without overloading the tube. All radiographic tube rating charts plot milliamperage, kilovoltage, and time (the three most important factors set by the radiographer). Various manufacturers plot these factors in different ways (Figure 6-24). In most instances, any combination of factors at or under the curve is safe. However, the radiographer should verify this fact by establishing that

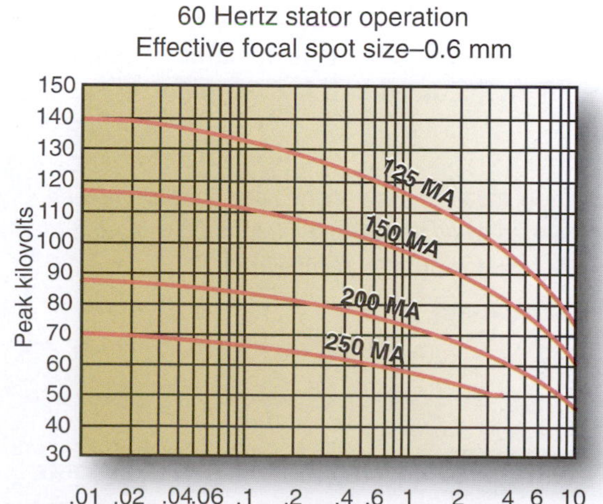

FIGURE 6-24. Example tube rating chart for 1ϕ full-wave rectification. *(Courtesy of Varian EIMAC.)*

lower technical combinations lie under the curve. (If both the x and the y axes have lower values at the lower left corner of the chart, safe factors are under the curves.) **Each filament of each tube has a unique radiographic tube rating chart.** The radiographer must ascertain that the correct chart for the **tube and filament** is being used.

> ***EXAMPLE:*** Is an exposure of 80 kVp, 0.1 second, and 200 mA within the limits of the 1φ, 0.6-mm focal-spot tube rating chart shown in Figure 6-24?
>
> ***Answer:*** When the intersection of the 80-kVp and 0.1-second lines is located on the tube rating chart, it is below the 200-mA line. Because the lower technical combinations lie below the mA lines, this is within limits.

Anode cooling charts permit the calculation of the time necessary for the anode to cool enough for additional exposures to be made (Figure 6-25). All cooling charts are calculated in terms of radiographic heat units. **A heat unit is calculated as kVp × mA × time × rectification constant.** The heat unit (HU) constants are given in Table 6-1. (Radiographic heat units are based on 1 kVp × 1 mA = 1 watt × 1 sec = 1 watt/sec × 0.71 rms voltage = 1 head unit. Technically, 1 radiographic head unit = 0.78 joule.

> ***EXAMPLE:*** How many heat units are generated by an exposure of 80 kVp, 200 mA, and 0.2 second on a 1φ rectified unit?
>
> ***Answer:***
>
> 80 kVp × 200 mA × 0.2 sec × 1.00 = 3,200 HU

TABLE 6-1. Heat Unit Rectification Constants

Rectification	Constant
1φ	1.00
High frequency	1.40

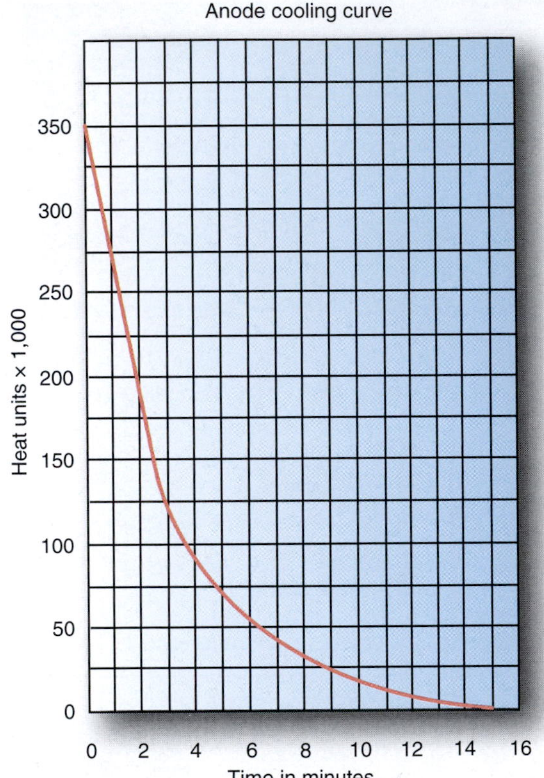

FIGURE 6-25. Example anode cooling chart.

> ***EXAMPLE:*** How many heat units are generated by an exposure of 70 kVp, 300 mA, and 0.15 second on a high-frequency rectified unit?
>
> ***Answer:***
>
> 70 kVp × 300 mA × 0.15 sec × 1.40 = 4,410 HU

> ***EXAMPLE:*** How many heat units are generated by two exposures of 65 kVp, 400 mA, and 0.05 second on a high-frequency unit?
>
> ***Answer:***
>
> 65 kVp × 400 mA × 0.05 sec
> × 1.40 × 2 exposures
> = 3,640 HU

To use the chart, the exposure factors must first be calculated in heat units. The length of time for the anode to cool can then be calculated by the following steps:

1. Find the total heat units applied on the vertical scale.
2. Read from the heat units over to the cooling curve and then down to read the corresponding time.
3. Calculate the time necessary for the anode to cool to any desired level and subtract the corresponding time of the initial exposure. (Or make the corresponding time of the initial exposure zero and calculate the time necessary for the anode to cool to any desired level from this point.)

For example, with the anode cooling chart in Figure 6-25, if a series of exposures produces 200,000 HU, the corresponding time is 2 minutes. The anode will cool to 150,000 HU in 2.5 minutes, so it will take 0.5 minute for the anode to cool from 200,000 HU to 150,000 HU. Similarly, the anode will cool to 100,000 HU in 1.5 minutes, to 50,000 HU in 4 minutes, and to room temperature (0) in 13 minutes.

EXAMPLE: Use the anode cooling curve in Figure 6-25 to calculate the length of time necessary for the anode to cool to 50,000 HU after five exposures of 80 kVp, 500 mA, and 0.5 second on a 1φ unit.

Answer:

80 kVp × 500 mA × 0.5 sec × 1.00 × 5 = 100,000 HU

50,000 HU = 6 minutes on cooling curve
100,000 HU = 3.5 minutes on cooling curve, so 6 min − 3.5 min = 2.5 min to cool from 100,000 to 50,000 HU

A more practical application of an anode cooling curve is to solve a problem regarding whether a desired exposure will overload the anode. For example, again using Figure 6-25, how long would it be after a load of 250,000 HU before a series of exposures equal to 150,000 HU could be made? Because the total HU capacity of the anode is 350,000 HU, it must cool to 200,000 HU in order to take the additional 150,000 HU. The question becomes "How long will it take the anode to cool from 250,000 to 200,000 HU?" It will take 0.75 minute (2–1.25 min), or 45 seconds, before the new series of exposures can be made because 250,000 HU corresponds to 1.25 minutes and 200,000 HU corresponds to 2 minutes.

EXAMPLE: Use the anode cooling curve in Figure 6-25 to calculate the length of time necessary for the anode to cool sufficiently from 350,000 HU to accept a series of exposures totaling 150,000 HU on a 1φ unit.

Answer:

350,000 HU − 150,000 HU = 200,000 HU as level to which anode must cool

350,000 HU = 0 minute

200,000 HU = 2 minutes

It will be 2 minutes (2−0 min) before the series of exposures can be made.

After working through several of these problems for most tube anodes, it becomes apparent that modern x-ray tubes are designed to withstand most exposures within the diagnostic range for average patients. It is when a series of exposures must be made (as occurs routinely in angiographic procedures) that most radiographic tube rating and anode cooling charts must be consulted.

Housing cooling charts permit the calculation of the time necessary for the housing to cool enough for additional exposures to be made (Figure 6-26). As with anode cooling charts, they are calculated in terms of radiographic heat units. They are used in exactly the same manner as an anode cooling chart. In actual practice the anode will usually reach its limits long before the housing. However, there are instances, as when the forced-air fan for the housing is not functioning, when these charts can be useful.

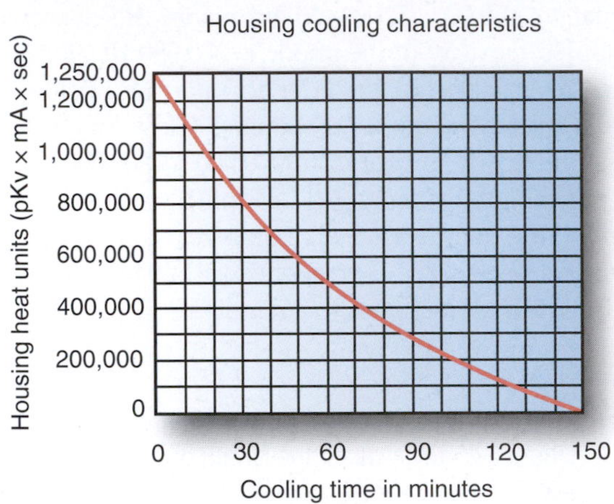

FIGURE 6-26. Example housing cooling chart. *(Courtesy of Varian EIMAC.)*

RECOMMENDATIONS FOR EXTENDING TUBE LIFE

There are many things that the professional radiographer can do to extend the life of an x-ray tube. Warming up the anode according to the manufacturer's recommendations prevents thermal shock (cracking of a cold anode). Cracking can occur when a nonstress-relieved anode is unable to expand rapidly enough to absorb a room temperature-to-operating heat level exposure. Holding the rotor switch unnecessarily should be avoided. The rotor switch increases the filament's thermionic emission to exposure levels. Thermionic emission removes the electrons from the filament, deposits vaporized electrons on tube surfaces, and decreases the tube vacuum, all of which can cause tube failure. In addition, the rotor switch causes stress to the rotor bearings, which can also decrease tube life. To avoid these problems, double-press switches should be completely depressed in one motion and dual switches should have the exposure switch depressed first, followed by the rotor switch. Lower-mA stations should be used when possible because high mA increases filament thermionic emission. The lower-speed rotor should be used when possible because the high-speed rotor increases rotor bearing wear. Repeated exposures near tube loading limits should not be made, as total heat units may approach anode or housing loading limits. Rotating the tube housing rapidly from one position to another should be avoided because the gyroscopic effect may crack or otherwise damage the rotor. A tube should not be used when loud rotor bearings can be heard (unless it has been checked by a qualified service person) because a wobbling anode disk can cause tube failure. These recommendations are summarized in Table 6-2.

TABLE 6-2. Recommendations for Extending Tube Life

1. Warm up the anode following the manufacturer's recommendations.
2. Do not hold the rotor switch unnecessarily. Double-press switches should be completely depressed in one motion. Dual switches should have the exposure switch depressed first, followed by the rotor switch.
3. Use lower-mA stations when possible.
4. Use a lower-speed rotor when possible.
5. Do not make repeated exposures near tube loading limits.
6. Do not rotate the tube housing rapidly from one position to another.
7. Do not use a tube when you can hear loud rotor bearings (unless it has been checked by a qualified service person).

SUMMARY

X-ray production requires a source of electrons, an appropriate target material, a high voltage, and a vacuum. The x-ray tube is the device that permits these conditions to exist. It consists of a cathode and an anode enclosed within an envelope and then encased in a protective housing.

The cathode is the negative side of the x-ray tube. The function of the cathode is to produce a thermionic cloud, conduct the high voltage to the gap between cathode and anode, and focus the electron stream as it heads for the anode. The cathode assembly consists of the filament or filaments, focusing cup, and associated wiring. The filament is a small coil of thin, thoriated tungsten wire. The focusing cup serves to narrow the thermionic cloud as it is driven to the anode.

The anode is the positive side of the x-ray tube. Anodes are divided into two types: stationary and rotating. Anodes are made using tungsten because of its high atomic number, high melting point, and good heat-conducting ability. The anode assembly consists of the anode, the stator, and the rotor. The portion of the anode where the high-voltage electron stream impacts is called the target, focus, focal point, focal spot, or focal track. The term *actual focal spot* is used to describe the physical area of the focal track that is impacted. The term *effective focal spot* is used to describe the area of the focal spot that is projected out of the tube toward the object being radiographed.

The line-focus principle is used to reduce the effective area of the focal spot. This permits the best resolution of detail in as large an actual area as possible. The effective focal-spot size is controlled by the filament size and the anode target angle. When the target angle is less than 45°, the effective focal spot is smaller than the actual focal spot.

The anode heel effect states that radiation intensity is greater on the cathode side than on the anode side.

An often overlooked factor that can cause serious degradation of radiographic image quality is off-focus or extrafocal radiation. Off-focus radiation is composed of photons that were not produced at the focal spot.

Three types of heating charts are available to help radiographers avoid thermal damage to x-ray tubes: radiographic tube rating charts, anode cooling charts, and housing cooling charts. Radiographic rating charts, sometimes called tube rating charts, are the most valuable because they provide a guide regarding the maximum technical factor combinations that can be used without overloading the tube. There are many things a radiographer can do to extend the life of an x-ray tube. ■

REVIEW QUESTIONS

1. What conditions must exist for x-rays to be produced?
2. What are the basic parts of a cathode assembly?
3. What is the purpose of the focusing cup?
4. Explain the space charge effect.
5. Why is tungsten the best metal for the x-ray source?
6. Explain the line-focus principle.
7. How does the anode heel effect affect radiation intensity?
8. What is the advantage of a high-speed rotor?
9. Why is it necessary for a vacuum to exist within the envelope?
10. Define leakage radiation.
11. How is off-focus radiation produced?

12. What is the function of rating charts and cooling curves?
13. Define a heat unit.
14. Name five things a radiographer can do to extend the life of an x-ray tube.

REFERENCES AND RECOMMENDED READING

Bushberg, J. T., Seibert, J. A., Leidholdt, E. M., & Boone, J. M. (2003). *The essential physics of medical imaging* (2nd ed.). Philadelphia: Lippincott, Williams & Wilkins.

Coolidge, W. D. (1913). A powerful Röntgen ray tube with a pure electron discharge. *The Physical Review, 2*(6).

Coolidge, W. D. (1945). Experiences with the Röentgen-ray tube. *American Journal of Roentgenology, 54*, 583–589.

Curry, T. S., Dowdey, J. E., & Murry, R. C. (1990). *Christensen's introduction to the physics of diagnostic radiology* (4th ed.). Philadelphia: Lea and Febiger.

Dendy, P. P., & Heaton, B. (1999). *Physics for diagnostic radiology* (2nd ed.). Bristol, England: Institute of Physics.

Eisenberg, R. L. (1992). *Radiology: An illustrated history*. St. Louis, MO: Elsevier/C. V. Mosby.

Engel, T. L. (1979). Effect of kilovoltage and milliamperage on focal spot size. *Radiologic Technology, 50*(5), 559–561.

Everson, J. D., & Gray, J. E. (1987). Focal-spot measurement: Comparison of slit, pinhole, and star resolution pattern techniques. *Radiology, 165*(1), 261–264.

Fairbanks, R., & Doust, C. (1979). Methods for studying the focal spot size and resolution of diagnostic x-ray tubes. *Radiography, 45*(533), 89.

Fuchs, A. W. (1947). The anode "heel" effect in radiography. *The X-Ray Technician, 18*, 158–163.

Glasser, O. (1936). What kind of tube did Röntgen use when he discovered x-ray? *Radiology, 27*, 138–140.

Glasser, O. (1958). *Dr. W. C. Röentgen* (2nd ed.). Springfield, IL: Charles C Thomas.

Grigg, E. R. N. (1965). *The trail of the invisible light: From x-Strahlen to radio(bio)logy*. Springfield, IL: Charles C Thomas.

National Electrical Manufacturers Association. (1985). *Measurements of dimensions and properties of focal spots of diagnostic x-ray tubes* (NEMA Standards Publication No. XR-5-1984). Rosslyn, VA: Author.

Selman, J. (2000). *The fundamentals of imaging physics and radiobiology: For the radiologic technologist* (9th ed.). Springfield, IL: Charles C Thomas.

Stears, J. G., Gray, J. E., & Frank, E. D. (1986). Half-value layer increase owing to tungsten buildup in the x-ray tube: Fact or fiction? *Radiology*, 837.

Stears, J. G., Gray, J. E., Webbles, W. E., & Frank, E. D. (1988). Radiologic exchange (tube warm-up and leaving x-ray units on). *Radiologic Technology, 59*(4), 325–326.

Stears, J. G., Gray, J. E., Webbles, W. E., & Frank, E. D. (1989). Radiologic exchange (resolution according to focal spot size). *Radiologic Technology, 60*(5), 429–430.

Trigg, C. N. (1979). X-ray tube failures and prevention: A preliminary report. *Radiologic Technology, 50*(4), 430.

Wilks, R. J. (2003). *Principles of radiological physics* (4th ed.). Edinburgh: Churchill Livingstone.

Wolbarst, A. B. (1993). *Physics of radiology*. Norwalk, CT: Appleton & Lange.

CHAPTER 7

X-Ray Production

KEY TERMS

bremsstrahlung interaction
characteristic cascade
characteristic interaction
characteristic peak
incident electron
target interaction

I did not think, I investigated.

Professor Wilhelm Röntgen to Sir James Mackenzie-Davidson during his only recorded interview, when asked what he thought when he discovered x-rays

OBJECTIVES

Upon completion of this chapter, the student should be able to:

- State the percentage of electron energy that is converted to x-ray photon energy in the x-ray tube.
- Describe a bremsstrahlung target interaction.
- Describe a characteristic target interaction.
- Identify factors affecting characteristic K-shell photon production.
- Explain the shape of the x-ray photon emission spectrum curve.

CONDITIONS

X-ray photons are produced when the high-speed electrons from the cathode strike an anode target. The fact that they are man-made is the primary difference between x-rays and gamma rays (which are products of nuclear radioactive decay). An understanding of how x-ray photons are created from the atoms of the target material permits the radiographer to assert full control over the production of the primary beam.

The electrons that form the thermionic cloud around the filament arrive at the anode target (~2 cm distant) traveling at nearly half the speed of light. A true understanding of the force contained in a kilovoltage-level exposure can be obtained by realizing that these electrons were accelerated from zero to half the speed of light in about 2 cm. These incoming electrons are called **incident electrons** and are represented in drawings by a solid arrow. In contrast, photons are represented by a wave arrow.

When incident electrons strike the target, they transfer their tremendous kinetic energy to the atoms of the target material and this interaction produces x-ray photons. The greater the mass or speed of the incident electrons, the greater the quality (energy) and quantity (number) of photons produced. This process occurs through two very different **target interactions**. All target interactions occur within 0.25 to 0.5 mm of the surface of the target. After giving up their energy to the target atoms, the electrons slow down enough to be conducted through the anode and the remainder of the high-voltage circuit. However, the incident electrons often experience 1,000 or more interactions before reaching this state.

TARGET INTERACTIONS

Heat Production

The target interactions that produce the x-ray photons consist of **less than 1 percent** of the total kinetic energy of the incident electrons. **Over 99.8 percent** of the kinetic energy of the incident electrons is converted to heat. This is the reason why so much technical research has gone into the development of the thermal aspects of x-ray tubes. In spite of the cost and performance capabilities of modern x-ray tubes, they are tremendously inefficient because they waste over 99 percent of the energy they use. This is true only in the range of diagnostic x-rays. As the kinetic energy of the incident electrons increases, so does the efficiency of photon production. By the time the therapeutic MeV range is reached, the majority of the energy is producing photons of heat.

Because they have such high kinetic energy, incident electrons seldom transfer enough energy to the outer shells of target atoms to cause ionization. Instead, they transfer enough energy to excite the outer-shell electrons to the point where they will emit infrared radiation as heat. These electrons then return to their normal state—where they will be re-excited again and again, each time emitting infrared radiation as heat.

There are two types of target interactions that can produce diagnostic-range x-ray photons: **bremsstrahlung interactions** and **characteristic interactions**. The interaction that will occur depends on the **electron kinetic energy** and the **binding energy of the electron shells** of the atom. Tungsten and rhenium are used as target materials in an effort to provide appropriate-atomic-number atoms and a maximum number of similar electron-shell binding energies.

Bremsstrahlung Interactions

Bremsstrahlung interactions are named by the German word for braking or slowing. The abbreviation "brems" is also used. **Brems interactions may occur only when the incident electron interacts with the force field of the nucleus.** The incident electron must have enough energy to pass through the orbital shells and approach the nucleus of the atom. Because atomic nuclei have a positive charge and the incident electron has a negative charge, there is a mutual attraction between them. When the incident electron gets close to the nucleus, the powerful nuclear force field is much too great for the electron to penetrate. Instead, the force field causes the incident electron to slow down (or brake) and then it diverts the electron's course. As a result, the electron loses energy and changes direction. The energy that is lost during the braking (or bremsstrahlung) is emitted as an x-ray photon. **These emissions are called bremsstrahlung photons and their energy is exactly the difference between the entering and exiting kinetic energy of the electron** (Figure 7-1). The amount of kinetic energy lost by the incident electron in a brems interaction is determined by the distance the electron is from the nucleus. At larger distances very little kinetic energy is lost, resulting in low-energy brems radiation. At closer distances more energy is lost, resulting in higher-energy brems radiation. The incident electron can also have a direct impact with the nucleus, resulting in the loss of all of the electron's kinetic energy. Because of the relatively small size of the nucleus, the chance of a direct impact is very low.

These energies are individually unpredictable and can range from the total value of the incident electron (which could be as high as the peak kilovoltage) to such a minimal amount of energy that it is nearly immeasurable. Statistically, it is possible to predict the energies quite accurately by a study of the x-ray emission spectrum, as will be discussed later in this chapter. Only when the incident electron loses all of its excess kinetic energy would the electron drift away to join the current flow. A single incident electron can cause numerous brems interactions in many different atoms before losing enough energy to become included in the current flow.

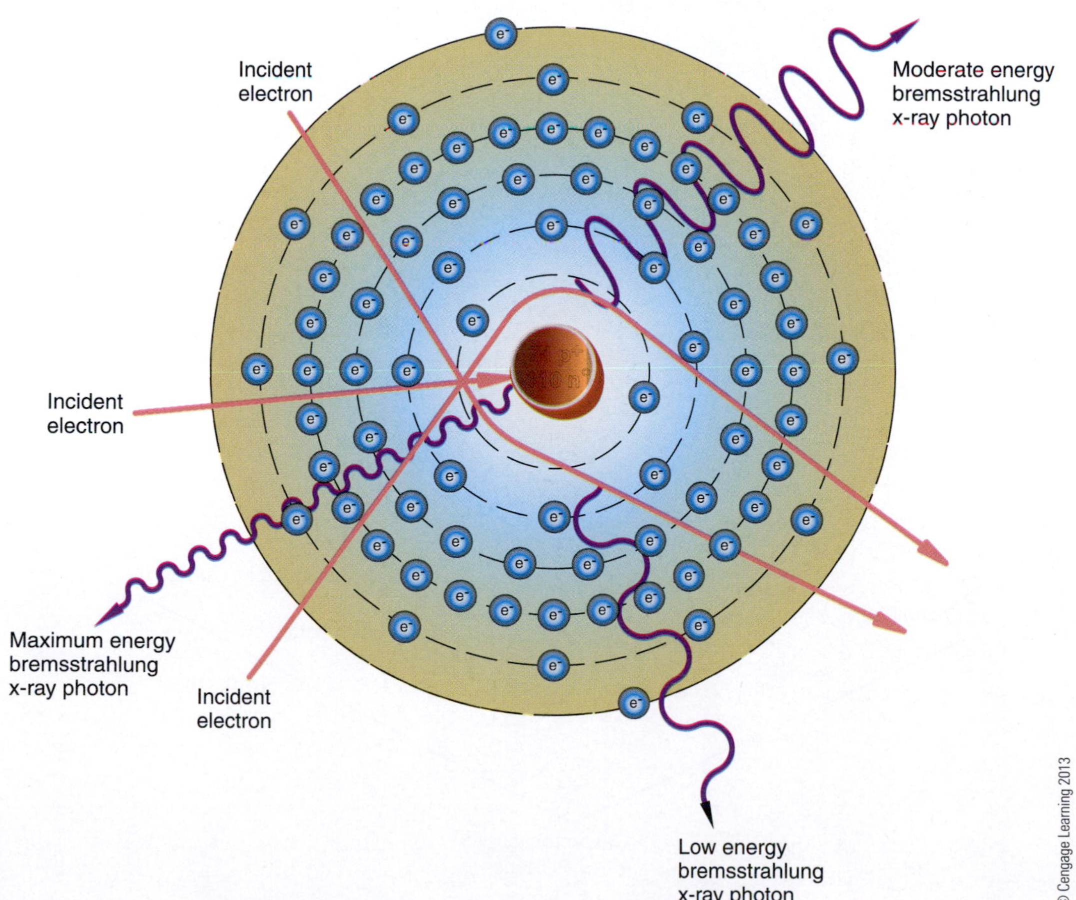

FIGURE 7-1. The bremsstrahlung interaction in a tungsten atom.

Characteristic Interactions

Characteristic interactions may occur only when the incident electron interacts with an inner-shell electron (Figure 7-2). The incident electron must have enough energy to knock an inner-shell electron from orbit, thereby ionizing the atom. The incident electron will usually continue but in a slightly different direction. More important is the fact that the electron "hole" that has been created in the inner shell makes the atom unstable. An electron from another shell will immediately drop into the "hole." This dropping of an electron from an outer, higher-energy state into an inner, lower-energy state results in the energy difference between the two shells being emitted as an x-ray photon. **These emissions are called characteristic photons because their energy is exactly the difference between the binding energy of the outer and inner shells between which the**

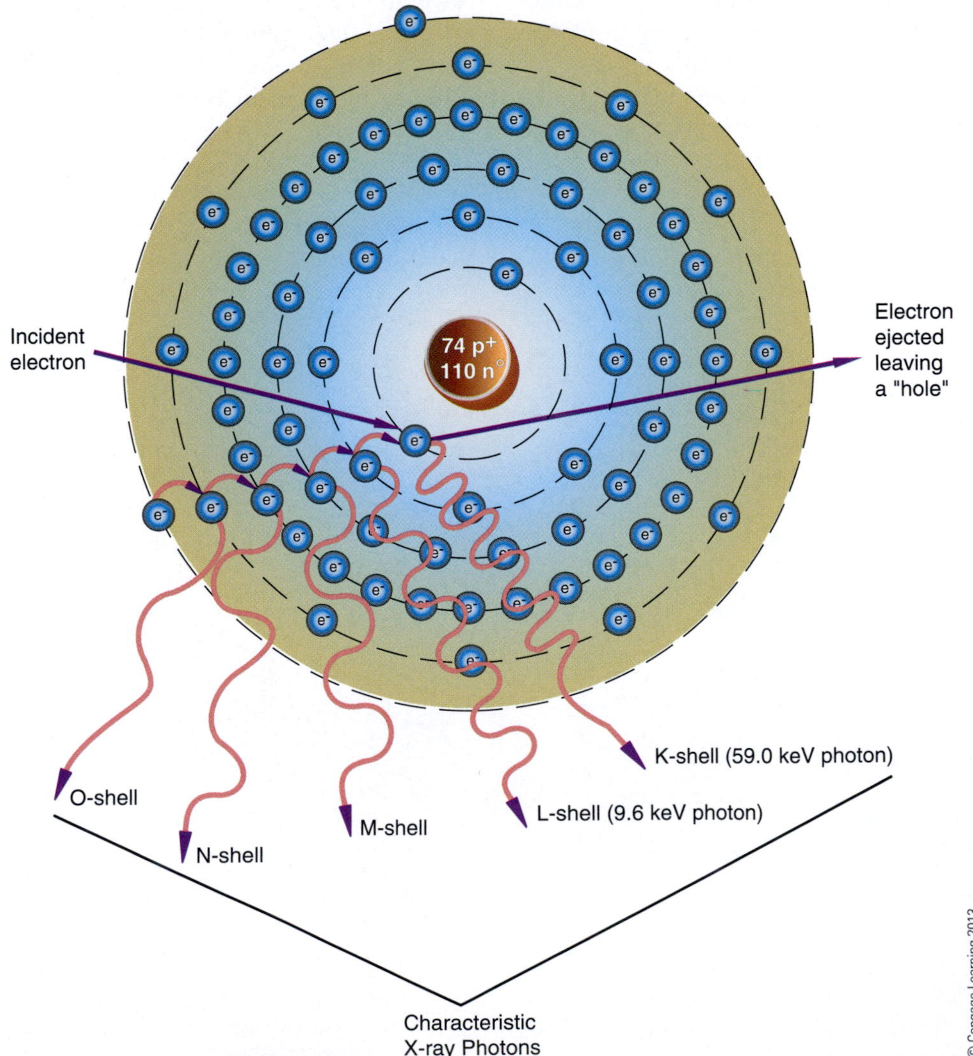

FIGURE 7-2. The characteristic interaction in a tungsten atom. Only the K-shell characteristic photon has sufficient energy to be a part of the useful beam.

electron dropped. After an outer-shell electron has dropped to fill the "hole," another electron will drop to fill the "hole" it left and so on until only the outermost shell is missing an electron. This process is called a characteristic cascade and it can produce numerous x-ray photons for each electron that leaves the atom.

The first electron that was knocked from position in an inner orbital shell often has sufficient energy that it, too, may cause further interactions before it loses enough energy to become part of the current flow. Of course, this will also contribute to the total number of photons created.

Unlike brems photons, characteristic photon energies are so predictable that the science of x-ray spectroscopy uses measurements of these photon energies to determine what types of atoms make up the sun, stars, and other celestial bodies.

A tungsten atom, with its high atomic number of 74, has sufficient electron shells to produce relatively high-energy characteristic photons. Tungsten has a total of 74 electrons, with 2 electrons in the K-shell, 8 in L, 18 in M, 32 in N, 12 in O, and 2 in the P-shell (see Figure 2-6). The binding energies of the electrons in these shells are 69.5 keV for the K-shell electrons, 12.1 keV for L-shell electrons, 2.8 keV for M, 0.6 keV for N, and 0.08 keV for the O-shell electrons. The electron that drops into the "hole" may be from any shell further away from the nucleus. Of course, the further out the dropping electron's original position, the greater the energy imparted to the characteristic photon.

Characteristic photons can be created from incident electron ionization of any shell and "hole" filling from any shell. For example, K-shell ionizations can result in characteristic photons from electron drops between shells L and K, M and K, N and K, etc. Characteristic photons can also result from L-shell ionizations with electron drops between shells M and L, N and L, and so on. A wide variety of characteristic photon energy levels are thus produced (Table 7-1). The filling of a "hole" from an adjacent shell results in a lesser-energy photon than nonadjacent shell transitions. For example, a K-shell vacancy filled by an L-shell electron will result in a weaker characteristic photon than the same vacancy filled by an M-shell electron. That is the result of the lower binding energy for the M-shell electrons. In addition, within each shell there are discrete energy states for individual electrons. As a result, slightly different energies can result from an L-to-K transition depending on the specific energy state of the electron involved in the transition. Note that only electron drops into the K-shell will produce characteristic photons within the diagnostic x-ray range. Characteristic photons from the other shells (L, M, N, etc.) have energies that are too low to be significant in diagnostic radiology.

TABLE 7-1. Characteristic Photon Emissions from X-Ray Target Materials

Tungsten			
K-Shell Characteristic Photons		**L-Shell Characteristic Photons**	
L to K	59.0 keV		
M to K	67.2 keV	M to L	9.6 keV
N to K	69.1 keV	N to L	11.0 keV
Effective energy	69.5 keV	Effective energy	12.1 keV
Molybdenum			
K-Shell Characteristic Photons			
L to K	17 keV		
M to K	20 keV		
Effective energy	18 keV		

A single incident electron can cause a variety of interactions in many different atoms before losing enough energy to become included in the current flow (Figure 7-3). Remember, most of these interactions will result in the production of heat.

EMISSION SPECTRUM

Within the diagnostic x-ray range most photons are produced by bremsstrahlung target interactions. Characteristic photons will not comprise any of the useful beam until the kVp is above 70 because removal of a K-shell electron from tungsten requires 69.5 keV. Between 80 and 100 kVp, about 80–90 percent of the primary beam is

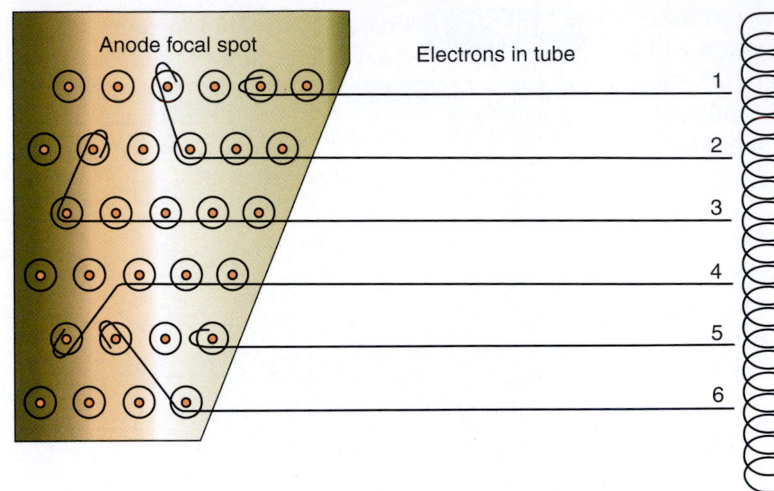

FIGURE 7-3. Sample paths of interactions for incident electrons striking the tube target.

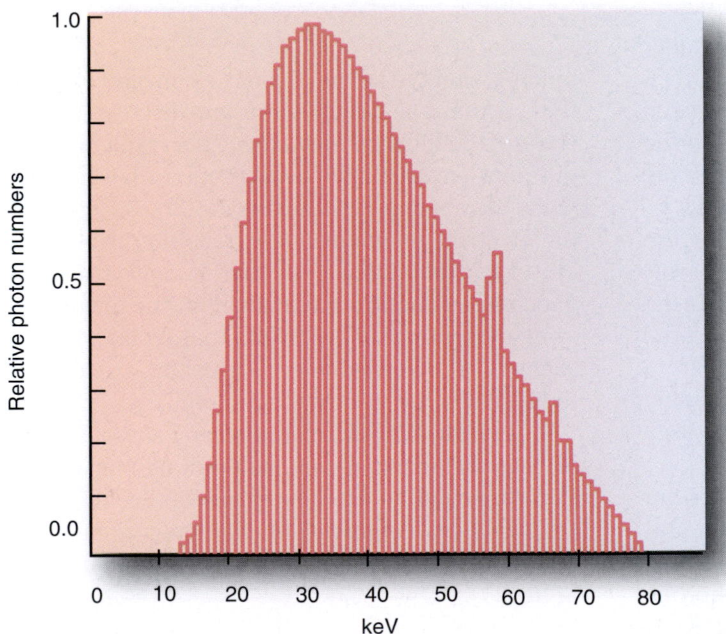

FIGURE 7-4. The x-ray emission spectrum with a tungsten target. This graph is the result of an exposure made with 2.8-mm Al/Eq filtration at constant potential, producing 17.8 mP/mAs at 30 in. (75 cm). The effective photon energy was 31 keV. *(Courtesy of Raymond P. Rossi, University of Colorado Health Science Center.)*

produced by brems interactions and 10–20 percent by characteristic interactions.

As mentioned previously, the K-shell emissions are the only ones within the diagnostic x-ray range, although the L-shell emissions form a similar group and the M- to P-shell emissions form a third group. Both brems and characteristic emissions combine to form the complete primary beam spectrum (Figure 7-4). The L-shell characteristic emissions are included within the total spectrum, but when filtration is added to the tube these photons do not have sufficient energy and are absorbed by the filter. The K-shell emissions form a **characteristic peak** at their effective energy range of 69 keV. This characteristic peak is worthy of special note as it can cause strange results for the radiographer who is operating the x-ray tube slightly above the K-shell peak and needs a slight decrease in radiation output. A slight decrease that sets the tube potential directly on the 69-keV K-shell peak would greatly increase the tube output instead of decrease it, as anticipated. Modern x-ray equipment is capable of somewhat overcoming these fluctuations by programmed switching and the use of tungsten alloys (such as molybdenum) in the target to smooth out characteristic peaking. However, characteristic peaks are a point of consideration, not only in the target material but in the construction of x-ray tabletops, grids, cassettes, intensifying screens, and any other object through which the primary beam must pass. **The kilovoltage peak of the exposure is the maximum possible energy for any photon that exits the x-ray tube.**

> ***EXAMPLE:*** At what kVp was the exposure made that produced the graph in Figure 7-4?
>
> ***Answer:***
>
> As the maximum brems photons were at 80 keV, the kVp was set at that level.

What is interesting about Figure 7-4 is that it clearly demonstrates an often overlooked fact about radiographic exposures. **The average primary beam photon has a keV energy of only about 30–40 percent of the kVp.**

The emission spectrum for a mammographic molybdenum target is quite different from that of a tungsten target. The K-shell characteristic peak is about 18 keV and the average photon energy range is between 20 and 40 keV, which is perfect for soft tissue visualization.

It is very useful to examine the effect on the primary beam emission spectrum of various factors under the control of the radiographer. When **mA, time,** or **mAs** is changed, all of which control the quantity (number) of electrons striking the target, the result is a change in the **amplitude** of the emission graph (Figure 7-5). Note that each point on the higher curve represents exactly twice the number of photons on the lower curve. When **kVp,** which controls the quality (energy) of electrons striking the target, is changed, the result is a change in the **number of higher-energy photons as well as in the amplitude** of the emission graph (Figure 7-6). Note that there are more higher-energy photons on the higher curve, as well as an increase in the number of photons (seen in the increased amplitude). There was no increase in the total number of electrons striking the target. The increase in amplitude represents more emitted photons due to the higher energy of each incident electron striking the target.

The x-ray emission spectrum is affected by the quantity and composition of the materials through which it must pass to exit the x-ray tube and housing. This is the filtration, which is the subject of Chapter 10. As the x-ray beam passes

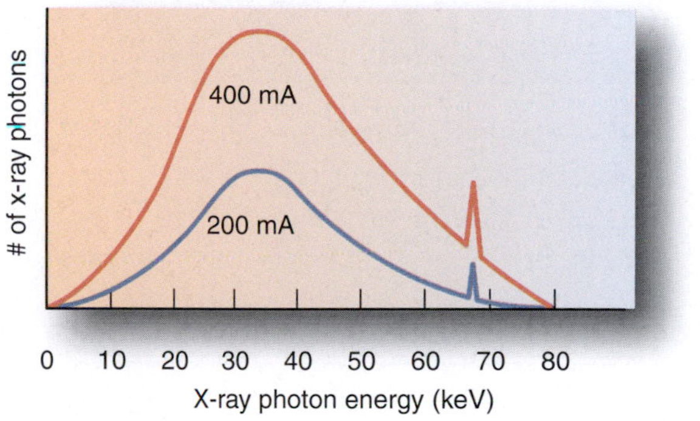

FIGURE 7-5. The effect of mA changes on the x-ray emission spectrum.

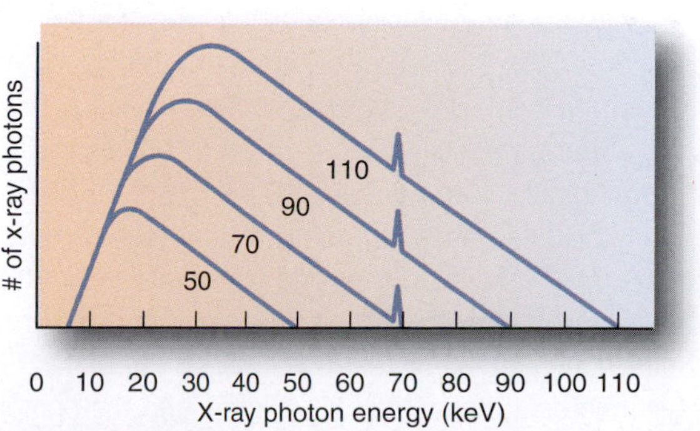

FIGURE 7-6. The effect of kVp on the x-ray emission spectrum.

through the filtering materials, some of the lower-energy photons are absorbed. This **decreases** the intensity of the beam but at the same time **increases** the average photon energy. Increased filtration decreases image receptor exposure, and vice versa.

The generator phasing also has an effect on the emission spectrum. As the efficiency of x-ray production increases, the emission spectrum changes (Figure 7-7). As generator phasing efficiency increases, the x-ray beam increases in intensity, and there is also an increase in the average photon energy. Decreased phasing efficiency decreases both intensity and average photon energy.

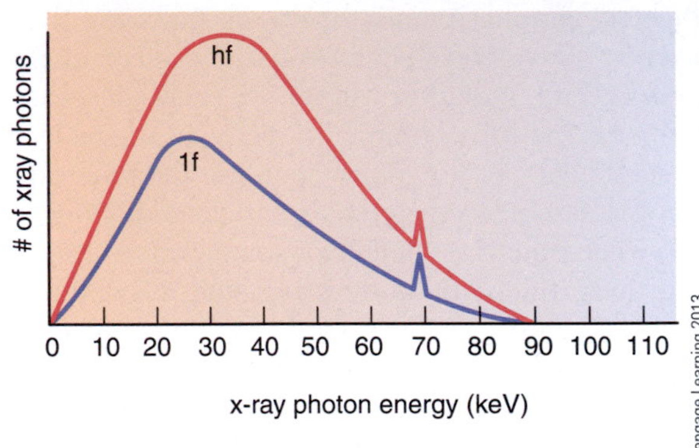

FIGURE 7-7. The effect of generator phase on the x-ray emission spectrum. 1φ = single phase, hf = high frequency.

SUMMARY

X-ray photons are produced when the high-speed electrons from the cathode strike an anode target. When incident electrons strike the target, they convert their tremendous kinetic energy to the atoms of the target material and this interaction produces x-ray photons. The greater the mass or speed of the incident electrons, the greater the quality (energy) and quantity (number) of photons produced.

The two target interactions that produce x-ray photons are bremsstrahlung (brems) and characteristic interactions. Less than 1 percent of the total kinetic energy of the incident electrons produces these interactions. Over 99 percent of the kinetic energy of the incident electrons is converted to heat.

Brems interactions occur when the incident electron interacts with the force field of the nucleus. This force field causes the incident electron to slow down (or brake), and then it diverts the electron's course. As a result, the electron loses energy and changes direction. The energy that is lost during the braking is emitted as a bremsstrahlung photon, and the photon energy is exactly the difference between the entering and exiting kinetic energy of the electron.

Characteristic interactions occur when the incident electron interacts with an inner-shell electron. The incident electron knocks out an inner-shell electron and continues in a slightly different direction. An electron "hole" is created in the inner shell, making the atom unstable. An electron from another shell will immediately drop into the "hole," which results in the emission of an x-ray photon. This emission is called a characteristic photon because the energy is exactly the difference between the binding energy of the outer and inner shells between which the electron dropped.

Within the diagnostic x-ray range, most photons are produced by bremsstrahlung target interactions. An x-ray emission spectrum graph illustrates the relationship between the two target interactions within the primary beam. The average primary beam photon has a keV energy of only about 30–40 percent of the kVp.

When mA, time, or mAs is changed, all of which control the quantity (number) of electrons striking the target, the result is a change in the amplitude of the emission spectrum graph. When kVp is changed, which controls the quality (energy) of electrons striking the target, the result is a change in the number of higher-energy photons, as well as in the amplitude of the emission spectrum graph. ■

REVIEW QUESTIONS

1. What is the approximate percentage of electron energy that is converted to x-ray photon energy in the x-ray tube?
2. The majority of the electron energy in the x-ray tube is converted to what form of energy?
3. Describe a bremsstrahlung target interaction.
4. Describe a characteristic target interaction.
5. What is a characteristic cascade?
6. What is the average keV of the primary beam as compared to the kilovoltage peak?
7. What effect does increasing mAs and kVp have on the total x-ray emission spectrum?

REFERENCES AND RECOMMENDED READING

Ball, J. L., & Moore, A. D. (2008). *Essential physics for radiographers* (4th ed.). Oxford: Wiley-Blackwell Scientific.

Bushberg, J. T., Seibert, J. A., Leidholdt, E. M., & Boone, J. M. (2003). *The essential physics of medical imaging* (2nd ed.). Philadelphia: Lippincott, Williams & Wilkins.

Bushong, S. C. (2008). *Radiologic science for technologists: Physics, biology, and protection* (9th ed.). St. Louis, MO: Elsevier Mosby.

Carroll, Q. B. (2007). *Practical radiographic imaging (Fuch's radiographic exposure processing & quality control)* (8th ed.). Springfield, IL: Charles C Thomas.

Coolidge, W. (1945). Experiences with the Roentgen ray tube. *American Journal of Roentgenology, 54*, 583–589.

Dendy, P. P., & Heaton, B. (1999). *Physics for diagnostic radiology* (2nd ed.). Bristol, England: Institute of Physics.

Hendee, W. R., & Ritenour, R. (2002). *Medical imaging physics* (4th ed.). New York: Wiley-Liss.

Irfan, A. Y., Pugh, V. I., & Jeffery, C. D. (1985). Some practical aspects of peak kilovoltage measurements. *Radiography, 51*(599), 251–254.

Johns, H. E., & Cunningham, J. R. (1983). *The physics of radiology* (4th ed.). Springfield, IL: Charles C Thomas.

Stears, J. G., Gray, J. E., Webbles, W. E., & Frank, E. D. (1989). Radiologic exchange (kVp measurements). *Radiologic Technology, 60*(3), 233–236.

Storm, E., & Israel, H. I. (1970). *Photon cross sections from 1 keV to 100 MeV. Nuclear data tables.* Boca Raton, FL: CRC Press.

Wilks, R. J. (2003). *Principles of radiological physics* (4th ed.). Edinburgh: Churchill Livingstone.

Wolbarst, A. B., & Cook, G. (2005). *Physics of radiology* (2nd ed.). Madison: Medical Physics Publishing.

Unit II

Protecting Patients and Personnel

8 Radiation Protection Concepts and Equipment / 140

9 Radiation Protection Procedures for Patients and Personnel / 155

10 Filtration / 170

11 The Prime Factors / 178

12 X-Ray Interactions / 191

13 Minimizing Patient Dose / 204

A critical skill of the radiographer is the ability to protect both patients and other personnel from excessive exposure to ionizing radiation. This includes the radiographer as well. A thorough knowledge of basic radiation physics, personnel monitoring procedures, and advanced procedures for reducing exposure are expected of all radiographers.

Prior to beginning to function in a clinical setting, the radiographer must learn the **basics of radiation protection concepts and equipment**. The critical skill is the ability to apply this information to the **radiation protection procedures for patients and personnel**.

The chapters on **filtration** and the **prime factors** explain how to shape and mold the beam to minimize radiation exposure while obtaining maximum diagnostic information. **X-ray interactions** open the door to exactly what occurs to the biological systems that are being imaged as well as laying groundwork for future understanding of problems in image production.

Finally, advanced procedures for **minimizing patient dose** are covered to provide the practicing radiographer with real clinical skills that will achieve the theory presented in this unit.

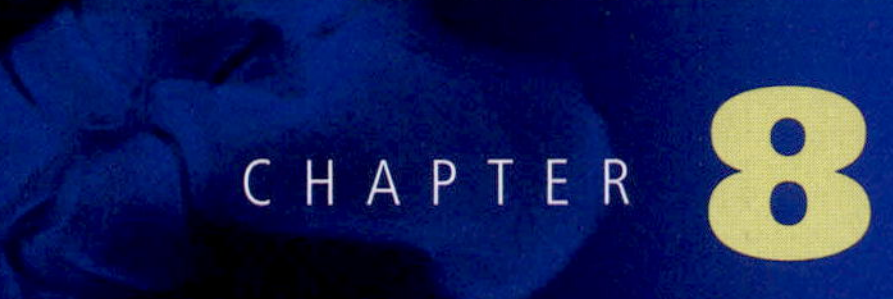

CHAPTER 8 Radiation Protection Concepts and Equipment

KEY TERMS

activity
air kerma
alpha particle
becquerel
beta particle
Compton scattering
curie (ci)
dosimeter
effective dose
electromagnetic radiation
field survey instrument
film badge dosimeter
genetic
gray (Gy)
integral dose
kerma
optically stimulated luminescence (OSL) dosimeter
particulate radiation
personnel monitoring device
photoelectric absorption
pocket dosimeter
quality factor
rad
rem
roentgen (R)
sievert (Sv)

> One aspect of the wide use of the x-rays perturbed Röntgen greatly. From laboratories in the United States, England, Germany, and France came more and more reports of a peculiar skin reaction similar to a sunburn in persons working with the rays, some of these reactions being particularly serious. . . . It distressed Röntgen to believe that these effects were due to x-rays . . .
>
> *Otto Glasser from the biography Dr. W. C. Röntgen.*

OBJECTIVES

Upon completion of this chapter, the student should be able to:

- Describe the nature of ionizing radiation.
- Identify the types of biological effects of ionizing radiation.
- Identify the principal sources of ionizing radiation.
- Define the quantities and units used for measurement of radiation.
- Describe devices used to detect and measure radiation, including field survey instruments and personnel monitoring devices.

KEY TERMS (continued)

somatic
Système Internationale d'Unites (SI units)
thermoluminescent dosimeter (TLD)

THE BASICS OF RADIATION PROTECTION PRINCIPLES AND PRACTICE

In medical applications, exposure to ionizing radiation carries with it both a benefit and a risk. The benefit of information from an x-ray examination regarding the clinical management of the patient examination is weighed against the small, but nonetheless finite, risk when a physician requests the examination. The diagnostic benefit of a radiologic procedure often far outweighs the risk resulting from the associated x-ray exposure. The information about the clinical condition of a patient received by the physician from a radiologic examination is an essential part of the practice of modern medicine.

It is the responsibility of the radiographer to ensure that each patient receives the minimal dose of radiation that will produce a diagnostic image consistent with the requirements of the examination. Radiographers must also ensure that all individuals are properly protected from unnecessary radiation exposure.

The Nature of Ionizing Radiation

Ionizing radiation is capable of creating positively and negatively charged particles when it interacts with matter. It arises from both natural and man-made sources and has the ability, as a consequence of its interactions with matter, to affect the various organs and tissues within the body. The energy possessed by ionizing radiation is capable of displacing atomic electron bonds and breaking the electron bonds that hold the molecules of matter together, resulting in chemical changes that can lead to metabolic changes in the body with resulting harmful effects.

Ionizing radiations are grouped as either **particulate** or **electromagnetic radiations**. Particulate radiations include high-energy electrons, neutrons, and protons that produce ionization in matter by direct atomic collisions. Two principal types of particulate radiation are associated with radioactive decay, **alpha particles** and **beta particles**. An alpha particle contains two protons and two neutrons and, as a result, is equivalent to a helium nucleus. Alpha particles are emitted from the nuclei of very heavy elements as they undergo radioactive decay. Compared to other types of particulate radiation, alpha particles have great mass and a positive charge. The energy of an alpha particle is transferred over a very short range in matter. In air, alpha particles can travel about 5 cm. As a result, alpha particles from external sources are essentially harmless. Beta particles are identical to electrons, with the exception of their origin. Beta particles are emitted from the nuclei of radioactive material, whereas electrons exist in shells around the nucleus. Beta particles are negatively charged and very light. As a result, they travel farther in matter than alpha particles. Beta particles are capable of traveling approximately 10–100 cm in air.

Electromagnetic radiations include x-rays and gamma rays, which produce ionization in matter by other types of interactions. X-ray and gamma rays are essentially the same with the exception of their origin. Gamma rays are emitted by the nuclei of radioactive materials, whereas x-rays are man-made in an x-ray tube. For electromagnetic radiation in the medically useful x-ray energy range (<200 keV), the transfer of energy from the photon to matter, resulting in ionization, occurs by processes known as **photoelectric absorption** and **Compton scattering**.

During such interactions with matter, photon energy is transferred by a two-step process. First, the incident photon interacts with an atom, causing an electron to be set in motion, which results in kinetic energy being released in the material. Second, the absorption of the released kinetic energy from the electron occurs via excitation and ionization. The excitations and ionizations that occur along the tracks of the charged particles set in motion give rise to biological damage in tissue. The biological damage may be a result of a direct interaction between the charged particle set in motion by the photons, in which cellular macromolecules are directly excited or ionized, or may be a result of an indirect interaction in which the absorption of radiation occurs in a water molecule, producing highly reactive species such as free radicals, which diffuse from the site of origin and subsequently cause biological damage. For x-rays and gamma rays approximately two-thirds of the biological effects on tissue are the result of indirect actions.

Biological Effects of Ionizing Radiation

Exposure to ionizing radiation affects various organs and tissues in the body and may result in a finite probability for radiation-induced disease in persons exposed to the radiation, and in their descendants. Health effects are known to be influenced by radiation characteristics and biological factors and include cancer induction, genetically determined ill health, nonspecific life shortening, developmental abnormalities, and degenerative diseases. The effects from the exposure to ionizing radiation may be classified as either **somatic** or **genetic**.

Somatic effects may become evident in the irradiated individual. Such effects are not usually to be expected in individuals exposed in the course of their work in the medical environment. To demonstrate a radiation response in humans within a few days to weeks, the dose must be quite high. Among the somatic effects of radiation are skin erythema, cataracts, and radiation-induced malignancies.

Genetic effects do not produce any significantly observable effect in the exposed individual but may appear in descendants of the exposed individual. They may not be manifest in the children of the exposed individual but may lie dormant for several generations and, eventually, may be eliminated completely from the genetic pool. Such effects result from alterations in the reproductive cells that can lead to defects in the offspring. Detectable radiation-induced mutations can result if the individual's reproductive cells have been exposed to an appreciable amount of radiation. It is unlikely that any worker in the medical environment would be exposed to ionizing radiation at a level high enough to cause the transmission of appreciable genetic effects.

Among the many factors that will influence the effect of exposure to ionizing radiation are the total dose received, the rate at which the dose was received, the age at exposure, the type of radiation, the sensitivity of the irradiated cells, and the portion of the body that was irradiated.

When x-rays were initially investigated, scientists were unaware of any harmful effects of their use and a number of the early radiation workers suffered injuries that are easily prevented today. Injuries from exposure were reported in Europe within the first year of investigation of x-radiation. In 1904 the first radiation fatality, a radiation-induced cancer, was reported in the United States. Over the next decade blood disorders such as leukemia and anemia, cancerous skin lesions, and cancer deaths were reported among radiation workers and linked to x-ray exposure. As a result of the high rate of documented radiation-related injuries, the British X-Ray and Radium Protection Committee was formed in 1921 to study ways to reduce radiation exposure to patients and medical personnel. The International Commission on Radiological Protection was established in 1928, and in 1929, "The Advisory Committee on X-Ray and Radium Protection" evolved into the National Council on Radiation Protection and Measurements (NCRP) in the United States.

The goal of radiation protection is to limit human exposure to ionizing radiation to a degree that is reasonable and acceptable in relation to the benefit gained from the activities that involve the exposure, thereby reducing the likelihood of occurrence of somatic and genetic effects.

Sources and Magnitude of Ionizing Radiation Exposure

Everyone is exposed to sources of ionizing radiation. Some individuals will be exposed to a wide variety of such sources, whereas others will be exposed to only a few. The sources include those of natural origin either undisturbed by human activities or that have somehow been affected by human activities and man-made sources. The NCRP regularly collects data to assess the ionizing radiation exposure to the U.S. population. NCRP Report No. 160, *Ionizing Radiation Exposure of the Population of the United States* (2009), has recently replaced the data presented in the previous NCRP Report No. 93, *Ionizing Radiation Exposure of the Population of the United States* (1987). The data presented in NCRP Report No. 93 detailed radiation exposure in the early 1980s and NCRP Report No. 160 details radiation exposure from 2006. The new report categorizes radiation exposure into the following five major areas:

1. exposure from ubiquitous background radiation, including radon in the home;
2. exposure to patients from medical procedures;
3. exposure from consumer products or activities involving radiation sources;
4. exposure from industrial, security, medical, and educational and research radiation sources; and
5. exposure to workers resulting from their occupations.

Ubiquitous background radiation includes external exposure from space such as solar particles and cosmic radiation, external exposure from terrestrial radiation from naturally occurring radioactive sources in the ground, radionuclides naturally present in the body, and inhaled radionuclides of natural origin, such as radon, the common name for the radionuclide ^{222}Rn, and thoron, the common name for the radionuclide ^{220}Rn. Human exposure to these natural sources varies depending on locality and other circumstances. When human exposure to natural sources increases as a result of a human's actions, deliberate or otherwise, the natural sources are enhanced.

Man-made sources of radiation result from various man-made materials and devices and include such sources as x-rays and radiopharmaceuticals used for medical procedures; consumer products and activities, such as building materials, commercial air travel, cigarette smoking, and combustion of fossil fuels; industrial, security, medical, and educational and research activities; and occupational exposures.

Exposure from medical procedures to the U.S. population in Report No. 160 separates out five different sources to further detail the extent of the exposures. These five categories are computed tomography, conventional radiography and fluoroscopy, interventional fluoroscopy, nuclear medicine, and external-beam radiotherapy.

Figure 8-1 shows the distribution of the collective effective dose (S) (person-Sv) and the effective dose per individual in the U.S. population (E_{US}) (mSv) as reported in the 2006 data. The collective

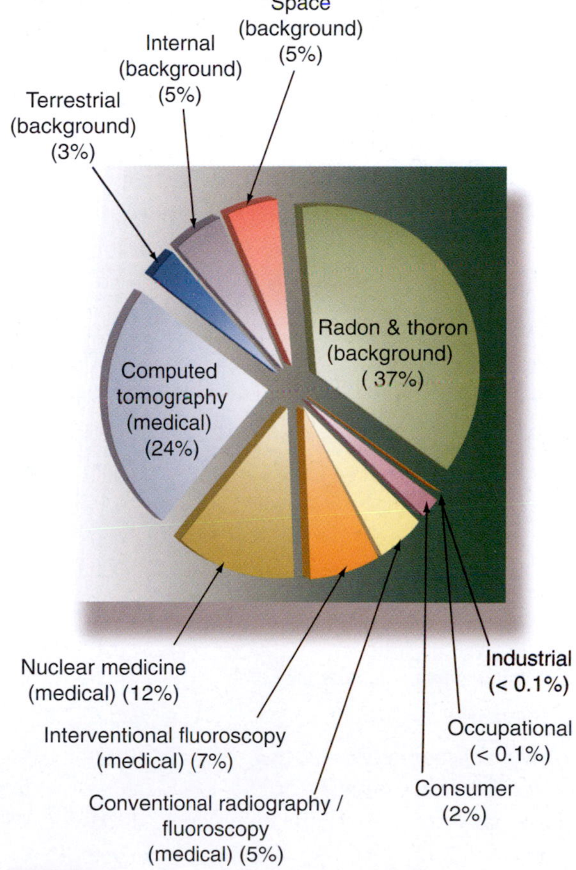

FIGURE 8-1. Percent contribution of various sources of exposure to the total collective effective dose (1,870,000 person-Sv) and the total effective dose per individual in the U.S. population (6.2 mSv) for 2006. Percent values have been rounded to the nearest 1%, except for those <1%. NCRP Report 160, *(courtesy NCRP.)*

effective dose (S) is the product of the mean effective dose for a population and the number of persons in the population. The population of the United States in 2006 was 300 million.

Table 8-1 details the comparison of the exposures collected in 2006 to the exposures collected in the early 1980s. The total effective dose per individual has significantly increased from the early 1980s to 2006 as the result of the increased use of ionizing radiation for medical procedures. In the early 1980s the total E_{US} was 3.6 mSv, and the 2006 data shows a total E_{US} of 6.2 mSv. This increase can be attributed almost exclusively to the change in medical procedure exposures, which rose from 0.53 mSv in the early 1980s to 3.00 mSv in 2006. This reflects a percentage change from 15 percent of the total in the early 1980s to 48 percent of the total in 2006. Although the increased use of ionizing radiation for medical procedures has had tremendous benefits to the population and has resulted in saved lives, there is an increased awareness for searching for ways to reduce this dose, particularly in computed tomography.

QUANTITIES AND UNITS RELEVANT TO RADIATION PROTECTION

Various quantities, units, and radiation dosimetry concepts have been developed and defined to quantify the amount of radiation received by individuals. Historically the quantities and units associated with

TABLE 8-1. Comparison of collective effective dose(S) and effective dose per individual in the U.S. population(E_{US} as reported in NCRP (1987a) and in this Report (annual values for percent are rounded to the nearest 1 %)

Exposure Category	This Report [for 2006]			NCRP (1987a)[a] [for the early 1980s]		
	S (person-Sv)	E_{US} (mSv)	Percent of Total *S* or E_{US}	*S* (person-Sv)[a]	E_{US} (mSv)[a]	Percent of Total *S* or E_{US}
Ubiquitous background	933,000	3.11	50	690,000	3.0	83
Radon and thoron[b]	684,000	2.28	37	460,000	2.0	55
Other	249,000	0.83	13	230,000	1.0	28
Medical	*899,000*	*3.00*	*48*	*123,000*	*0.53*	*15*
CT (2006)	440,000	1.47	24			
Conventional radiography and fluoroscopy (2006)	100,000	0.33	5			
All diagnostic (1980)				91,000[c,d]	0.39	11
Nuclear medicine	231,000	0.77	12	32,000[d]	0.14	4
Interventional fluoroscopy (2006)	129,000	0.43	7			
Consumer	*39,000*	*0.13*	*2*	*12,000–29,000*	*0.05–0.13*	*<2*
Industrial, security, medical, educational, and research	*1000*	*0.003*	*0.05*	*200*[e]	*0.001*	*0.03*
Occupational	*1,400*	*0.005*[f]	*0.08*	*2,000*	*0.009*[f]	*0.3*
Total	*1,870,000*[g]	*6.2*[g]		*835,000*	*3.6*	

[a]The quantities used in NCRP (1987a) were expressed in H_g.
[b]Radon plus thoron for 2006; radon only for the early 1980s.
[c]Included 3,700 person-S_v from CT and 4,200 person-S_v from interventional fluoroscopy [listed as "other" in NCRP (1987a)].
[d]Values differ slightly from those reported in NCRP (1989a) and Table 4.19.
[e]Consisted ot the nuclear fuel cycle and miscellaneous environmental sources.
[f]The values of E_{Exp} are 1.1 mSv for 2006 and 2.3 mSv for the early 1980s.
[g]Rounded values.
NCRP Report 160, *courtesy NCRP.*

radiation dosimetry have included the **roentgen (R)**, used for specifying exposure; the **rad** (radiation absorbed dose), used for specifying energy absorbed; and the **rem** (radiation equivalent in man), used for specifying biologically equivalent dose.

Other radiation quantities of importance are the **kerma**, used to describe the kinetic energy released per unit mass; the **air kerma**, used to describe the kinetic energy released per unit mass of air; **integral dose**, used to describe the total radiation energy imparted to matter; **effective dose**, used to measure the radiation and organ-system-specific damage in man; and **activity**, used to measure the amount of a radioactive material as it undergoes decay.

In 1948, the International Committee for Weights and Measures was charged with developing an international system of units based on the metric system. The committee developed the **Système Internationale d'Unites**, or **SI units**. In recent years the international system of units has been adopted for radiation protection, and within this system of units the older units are no longer applicable. Although the National Council on Radiation Protection and Measurement (NCRP) adopted the SI units for use with ionizing radiation in 1985, traditional units are still very much in use. The following discussion will serve to review the conventional and more familiar units and SI units. Table 8-2 provides conversions between conventional units and SI units.

TABLE 8-2. Conversions between Conventional and SI Units

Conventional Unit (Column A)	Conversion Factor (Column B)	SI Unit (Column C)
roentgen	2.58×10^{-4}	coulomb/kilogram
rad	0.01	gray
rem	0.01	sievert
curie	3.7×10^{10}	becquerel

Column A amount multiplied by Column B equals Column C amount.

Column C amount divided by Column B equals Column A amount.

Exposure

The roentgen (R) represents a unit of exposure in air and was defined as that quantity of x-rays or gamma rays required to produce a given amount of ionization (charge) in a unit mass of air. One roentgen creates 2.08×10^9 ion pairs per cubic centimeter of air to produce a total ion charge of 2.58×10^{-4} coulomb (C) per kilogram (kg). The roentgen is limited to the measurement of exposure in air only and is not applicable to photons of energy above 3 Mev or to particulate radiations. The roentgen has no direct equivalent or special unit in the SI system of units and is no longer used. Exposure may be expressed directly in C/kg or its equivalent Ckg^{-1}.

Absorbed Dose

The rad was developed as a unit of absorbed energy or dose and is applicable to any material. The rad was defined as 100 ergs of energy absorbed in 1 gram of absorbing material. In the SI system of units the rad has been replaced by the **gray (Gy)**, which is defined as 1 joule (J) of energy absorbed in each kilogram (kg) of absorbing material. One gray is equivalent to 100 rads; therefore, 1 rad equals 10 mGy. This unit is not restricted to air and can be measured in other absorbing materials.

Kerma/Air Kerma

The rad is also a unit of kerma, an acronym for kinetic energy released in matter. As radiation passes through matter it interacts and the energy carried by the photons is transformed to kinetic energy of charged particles such as the electrons in the photoelectric and Compton interactions. The energy imparted directly to the electrons, per unit mass, is the kerma. Some of the kerma may be radiated away as bremsstrahlung if any of these electrons interact with the nuclei of the atoms in the matter. In these instances, kerma and absorbed dose would not be identical. At diagnostic energies, however, practically no brems is produced in the tissues and, as a result, kerma will equal dose. The SI unit for the kerma is the gray.

Air kerma is the kinetic energy released per unit mass of air. X-ray tube outputs and inputs to image receptors are sometimes described in air kerma. An air kerma of 1 cGy (1 rad) corresponds to an exposure of about 1 R.

Integral Dose

The integral dose describes the total amount of energy imparted to matter. It is a product of the dose and the mass over which the energy is imparted. For example, when a patient has a CT scan of the abdomen, the dose per section (irradiated volume) might be 1 rad (10 mGy). Regardless of the number of scan sections, the dose to the irradiated volume would be defined as 1 rad (10 mGy). If the patient has 20 scan sections, the integral dose would be approximately 20 rad (200 mGy).

Equivalent Dose

Different types of radiation, such as alpha and beta particles and neutrons, produce different degrees of biological damage as compared to gamma or x-radiation. To account for the fact that the same absorbed dose of radiation may result in different biological responses for different types of radiation, a unit known as the rem (radiation equivalent man) was developed. The rem is the conventional unit for equivalent dose (H_T). **In NCRP Report No. 116, *Limitations of Exposure to Ionizing Radiation* (which replaces NCRP Report No. 91), the term *equivalent dose* replaces the previously used term, *dose equivalent* (H), in defining dose limits.** These two terms are conceptually different. Dose equivalent (H) is based on the absorbed dose at a "point" in tissue and equivalent dose (H_T) is based on the average absorbed dose in the tissue or organ.

Equivalent dose (H_T,R) is the product of the average-absorbed dose (D_T,R) in a tissue (T) due to radiation (R) and a radiation weighting factor (W_R), previously known as the **quality factor** (Q), which is specific to specific types of radiation and accounts for the biological effectiveness of the specific radiation. The radiation weighting factor for gamma or x-radiation equals 1. This means that 1 rad equals 1 rem for gamma or x-radiation. For alpha particles, however, the radiation weighting factor is 20. This means that 1 rad equals 20 rem for alpha particle absorption. In the SI system of units the rem has been replaced by the **sievert (Sv)**, which is defined as the product of the absorbed dose in gray and the radiation weighting factor. One sievert is equal to 100 rem, and 1 rem is equal to 10 mSv.

Effective Dose

Effective dose (E) is the sum of the weighted equivalent doses for all irradiated tissues and organs. It takes into account the fact that not all tissues are equally sensitive to the effects of ionizing radiation. As was seen with equivalent dose and dose equivalent, in NCRP Report No. 116, *Limitations of Exposure to Ionizing Radiation*, the term *effective dose* (E) replaces the previously used term, *effective dose equivalent* (H_E), in defining dose limits.

Because exposure received from ionizing radiation is rarely uniform over the whole body, the concept of effective dose is used to compare the detriment from irradiation of a limited portion of the body with the detriment from irradiation of the entire body and employs weighting factors for the relative risks associated with irradiation of various body tissues. The effective dose is defined as the sum over specified tissues of the products of the equivalent dose in a tissue (T) and the weighting factor for that tissue.

Activity

Activity (A) describes the quantity of radioactive material. It is expressed as the number of radioactive atoms that undergo decay per unit time. The unit of activity has traditionally been the **curie (Ci)**. The curie is defined as 3.7×10^{10} disintegrations per second (dps). One curie is a very large amount of radioactive material. In a typical nuclear medicine procedure, activities from 0.1–30 millicuries (mCi) are used. The SI unit for activity is the **becquerel**. The becquerel is defined as 1 dps.

Further information regarding the international system of units and its application in radiation protection and measurements may be found in NCRP Report No. 82, *SI Units in Radiation Protection and Measurements*. A comparison between SI units and conventional ones is displayed in Table 8-3.

TABLE 8-3. Comparison between SI and Conventional Units

Quantity	Symbol for Quantity	Expression in SI Units	Expression in Symbols for SI Units	Special Name for SI Units	Symbol Using Special Name	Conventional Unit	Symbol for Conventional Unit	Value of Conventional Unit in SI Units
Activity	A	1 per second	s^{-1}	becquerel	Bq	curie	Ci	3.7×10^{10} Bq
Absorbed Dose	D	joule per kilogram	J/kg	gray	Gy	rad	rad	0.01 Gy
Dose Equivalent	H	joule per kilogram	J/kg	sievert	Sv	rem	rem	0.01 Sv
Exposure	X	coulomb per kilogram	C/kg			roentgen	R	2.58×10^{-4} C/kg

DETECTION AND MEASUREMENT OF IONIZING RADIATION

Numerous different dose-measuring devices, known as dosimeters, are employed for detection and measurement of radiation exposure from x-rays. These **dosimeters** may be classified as either **field survey instruments** or **personnel monitoring devices**.

Field Survey Instruments

Numerous portable field survey instruments are available for use in radiation detection and measurement. They include the Geiger-Mueller (GM) survey instruments, scintillation detection devices, and ionization chamber instruments. Regardless of the type, field survey instruments should be calibrated at least annually.

Geiger-Mueller Survey Instruments. Geiger-Mueller survey instruments or counters are primarily used to detect the presence of radiation rather than provide exact measurements. A GM counter is a gas-filled detector. It consists of a volume of gas between two electrodes. Ionizing radiation produces ion pairs in the gas that can be collected and measured. GM counters are very efficient at detecting charged particles, such as beta particles, but are relatively inefficient at detecting x- and gamma radiation. GM counters are most commonly used in nuclear medicine as radioactive contamination survey instruments.

Scintillation Detection Devices. Scintillation detectors combine the use of a scintillator with a device that can convert light to an electric signal. Scintillators are materials that emit visible or ultraviolet light when exposed to ionizing radiation. In a scintillation detector, this light is converted to an electric signal and is measured. The most common applications for scintillation detectors are in gamma cameras in nuclear medicine.

Ionization Chamber Instruments. Ionization chamber instruments are commonly employed for the measurement of the primary and secondary radiation beam for purposes of evaluation of equipment performance, environmental exposure assessment of scatter and leakage radiation, and for measurement of patient exposure. An ionization chamber works on the principle that when radiation interacts with air electrons, positive ions are produced, giving rise to an electrical charge that can be measured.

A typical ionization chamber dosimeter consists of a chamber with a known volume of air and an electrode (Figure 8-2). A small voltage is applied between the electrode and the wall of the chamber, so the electrode is positive and the chamber wall is negative. As x-ray photons pass through the chamber they ionize the air. The free electrons from these ionizations are attracted to the positive electrode, where they can be measured with

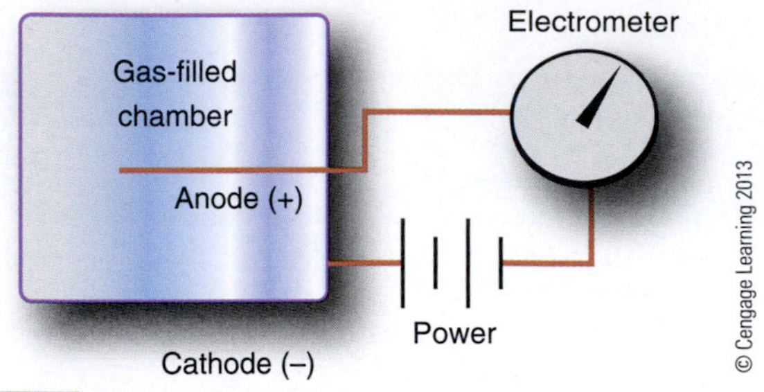

FIGURE 8-2. An ionization chamber dosimeter. The chamber encloses a known volume of air, inside of which a chargeable electrode is positioned to attract electrons freed by the ionization of the gas by the radiation. The difference in the electrode's charge before and after exposure is measured by an electrometer and displayed in radiation units.

an electrometer. The intensity of the signal that is produced on the electrode is proportional to the radiation exposure that occurred in the air volume of the chamber. This relationship can be displayed on a digital readout in R or C/Kg units. Ionization dosimeters can be designed to measure specific ranges of radiation intensity.

Personnel Monitoring Devices

Individuals who are regularly exposed to ionizing radiation should be supplied with personnel monitoring devices that will provide an estimate of the exposure they received. Personnel monitoring is recommended whenever a possibility exists that an individual will receive more than 1/10 of the recommended dose limit as a result of his or her occupational activities. A personnel monitoring device measures the quantity of exposure it has received. It is not a radiation protection device.

When only one personnel monitoring device is issued, it should be worn on the anterior surface of the body between the chest and waist level. When a lead apron is worn and only one personnel monitoring device is issued, it is recommended that it be worn outside the apron at the collar level. Because of the considerable controversy regarding the proper location of the dosimeter when a lead apron is worn, the local radiation safety officer should be contacted for specific guidance. It is important that all persons wear their dosimeters at the same locations.

An additional dosimeter, usually designated as a whole-body dosimeter, may be worn in addition to the collar dosimeter when the potential for significant exposure to the thyroid or eyes exists. This dosimeter is usually positioned near the waist under the lead apron and may be used in conjunction with the collar dosimeter to determine the effective dose. The whole-body dosimeter and collar dosimeter must never be interchanged.

The most common types of personnel monitoring devices are the **optically stimulated luminescence (OSL) dosimeter**, **film badge dosimeter**, **thermoluminescent dosimeter (TLD)**. and **pocket dosimeter**.

Optically Stimulated Luminescence (OSL) Dosimeter. The most common type of radiation monitoring device is the optically stimulated luminescence (OSL) dosimeter. The OSL dosimeter measures radiation that passes through a thin strip of aluminum oxide (Al_2O_3). A laser light is used to stimulate the aluminum oxide, which becomes luminescent in proportion to the amount of radiation exposure it has received.

The OSL dosimeter has distinct advantages over both the film badge and the TLD. It can report doses along a wide range from as low as 1 mrem with a precision of ±1 mrem. In addition, it can undergo complete reanalysis to confirm the radiation exposure received with no loss of information. It also has excellent long-term and environmental (temperature and humidity) stability.

Laudauer, Inc. offers the Luxel® OSL Dosimeter with a variety of color-coding options for both department/series and exchange frequencies. The Luxel® dosimeter is a self-contained packet that contains an aluminum oxide strip located between three filters and an open window (Figure 8-3). The open window and the copper and tin filters are used to determine the energy levels of the exposure to the dosimeter. The imaging filter is used to determine whether the exposure was a static or dynamic exposure. A static image indicates that the dosimeter was not moving at the time of exposure. This may imply that the dosimeter was not worn during the time of exposure and an accidental exposure may have occurred. A dynamic exposure image will have a blurred appearance and indicates that

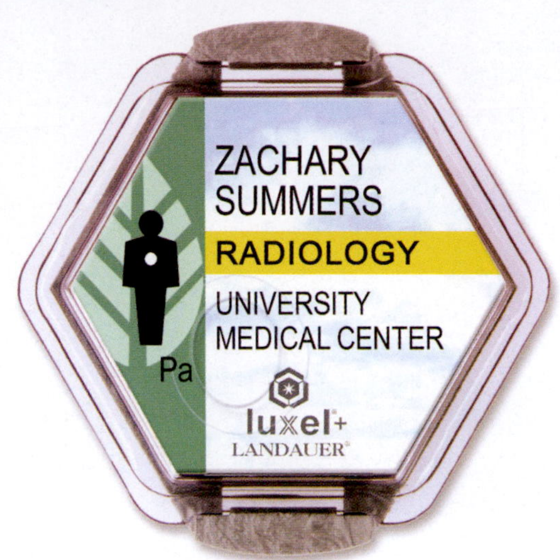

FIGURE 8-3A. The Luxel Dosimeter. *(Courtesy of Landauer Inc.)*

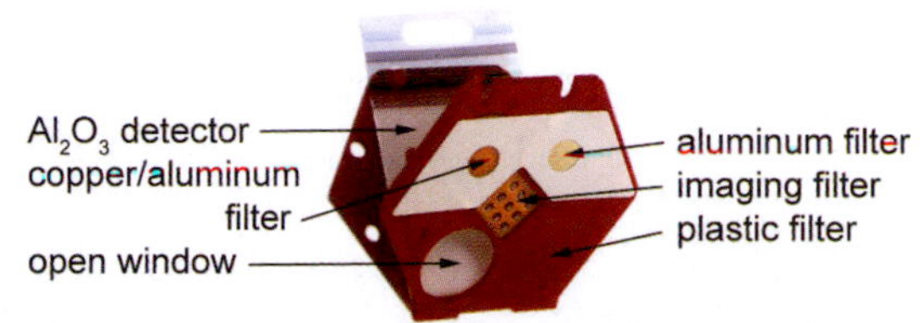

FIGURE 8-3B. The Luxel Filter Pack. *(Courtesy of Landauer Inc.)*

the dosimeter was being worn during the time of exposure and the dose is valid.

Film Badge Dosimeter. Film badge dosimeters are usually issued on a monthly basis and consist of two pieces of film having different sensitivities to x-rays and contained within a light, tight envelope. This film packet is placed within a holder, which contains a number of different filter elements held in a fixed position with respect to the film. Printed on the front of the film packet is the name of the individual, the beginning date for which the film badge is issued, and other coded information.

When the badge is exposed to ionizing radiation, the film emulsion darkens in proportion to the degree of radiation exposure received. The resultant optical density can be measured with a densitometer and calibrated to the degree of radiation exposure received.

The filters in the film badge holder provide a means of determining the energy of the incident radiation. Because the absorption of radiation by a specific thickness of given material will depend on the energy of the radiation, the measurement of the relative film densities under the different filters provides a means of estimating the energy of the exposing x-ray beam. Typically copper, cadmium, and aluminum are used as filtering metals.

Film badges are capable of measuring exposures over the range of approximately 10 mrem (0.1 mSv) to 2,000 rem (20 Sv) and are most commonly used to measure the total body exposure of the individual. Readings of less than 10 mrem (0.1 mSv) are generally not detectable and may be reported as minimal (M).

Thermoluminescent Dosimeter (TLD). Personnel monitoring devices using thermoluminescent dosimeters contain small chips of a thermoluminescent material, usually lithium fluoride (LiF). When exposed to radiation, a portion of the absorbed energy is stored in the crystal structure of the LiF chips in metastable states. This absorbed energy will remain in these states for long periods of time. If the LiF chips are heated, the absorbed energy is released as visible light. The heating and measurement of the LiF chips are carried out in a device called a reader, and the amount of measured light is proportional to the absorbed radiation dose. TLDs provide approximately the same measurement range as film badges and can be used as whole-body badges or collar badges. Because of their small size, TLDs are commonly used for monitoring exposure to the extremities in the form of ring badges.

Pocket Dosimeter. Although technically known as direct reading conductive fiber electroscopes, there are now electronic personal dosimeters available. Both types of devices look like large pens or flash drives. These devices provide immediate personal dosimetry, which is useful especially in interventional radiology laboratories where waiting several months for readings is not reasonable. Figure 8-4 shows the older direct reading conductive fiber electroscope type. When irradiated, ionization of the air in a small chamber occurs, which partially neutralizes a previously positively charged electrode (quartz fiber on a wire frame), causing a

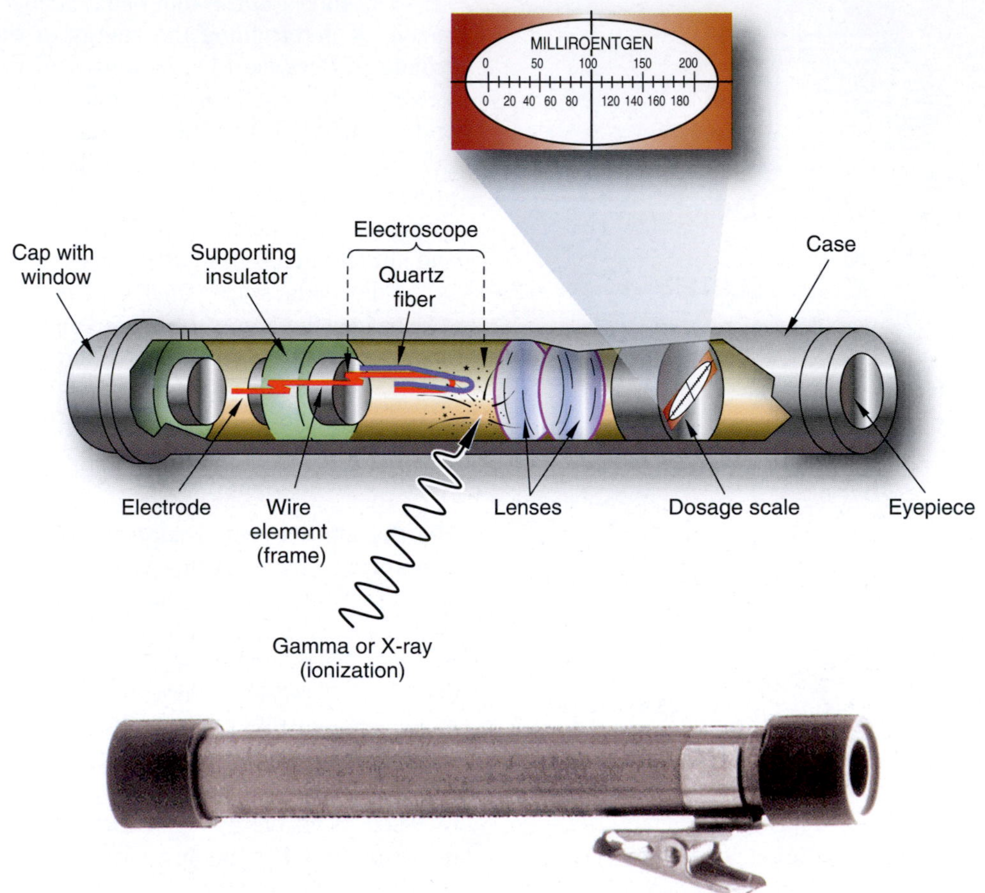

FIGURE 8-4. Cross section of a pocket ion chamber (dosimeter). *(Courtesy of Bushberg, J. T., Seibert, J. A., Leidholdt, E. M., Boone, J. M. [1994].)* The essential physics of medical imaging. *Baltimore: Lippincott Williams & Wilkins.*

hairline fiber to move on an exposure scale. The amount of ionization and the movement of the fiber are proportional to the radiation exposure to the chamber. Older devices required a charging unit and the pocket dosimeter had to be returned to this unit for a reading. The newer electronic personal dosimeters utilize a similar system of ionization of air in a small chamber, but the readout occurs digitally and can be read from a display on the side of the dosimeter.

Care of Personnel Monitoring Devices. The proper care and handling of personnel monitoring devices is essential to obtaining accurate results. The personnel monitoring device must be worn only by the individual to whom it is assigned, must be worn in the proper location for the prescribed time period, and must be turned in for processing when due.

The OSL dosimeter has distinct advantages because it can report a wide range of doses from as low as 1 mrem with precision, and it has excellent long-term environmental stability.

Both film badge dosimeters and TLD dosimeters may be adversely affected by heat, humidity, mechanical pressure, inadvertent exposure to light, and prolonged delay between exposure and processing. Exposure from the rear or from oblique angles may also result in inaccurate results.

SAMPLE ORGANIZATION
RADIATION SAFETY OFFICER
1000 HIGH TECH AVENUE
GLENWOOD, IL 60425

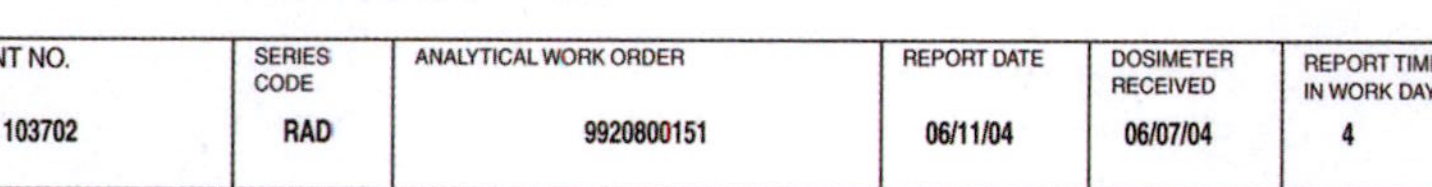

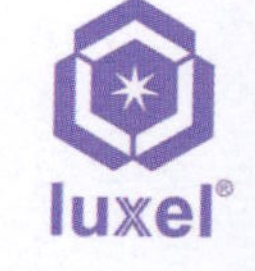

RADIATION DOSIMETRY REPORT

ACCOUNT NO.	SERIES CODE	ANALYTICAL WORK ORDER	REPORT DATE	DOSIMETER RECEIVED	REPORT TIME IN WORK DAYS	PAGE NO.
103702	RAD	9920800151	06/11/04	06/07/04	4	1

PARTICIPANT NUMBER	NAME / ID NUMBER	BIRTH DATE	SEX	DOSIMETER	USE	RADIATION QUALITY	DOSE EQUIVALENT (MREM) FOR PERIODS SHOWN BELOW			QUARTERLY ACCUMULATED DOSE EQUIVALENT (MREM)			YEAR TO DATE DOSE EQUIVALENT (MREM)			LIFETIME DOSE EQUIVALENT (MREM)			RECORDS FOR YEAR	INCEPTION DATE (MM/YY)
							DEEP DDE	EYE LDE	SHALLOW SDE	DEEP DDE	EYE LDE	SHALLOW SDE	DEEP DDE	EYE LDE	SHALLOW SDE	DEEP DDE	EYE LDE	SHALLOW SDE		
FOR MONITORING PERIOD:							05/01/04 - 05/31/04			QTR 2			2004							
0000H	CONTROL CONTROL CONTROL			Ja Pa U	CNTRL CNTRL CNTRL		M M	M M	M M M										5	07/97 07/97 07/97
00191	ADDISON, JOHN 336235619	08/31/1968	M	Ja	WHBODY	PN P NF	90 60 30	90 60 30	90 60 30	90 60 30	90 60 30	90 60 30	100 70 30	100 70 30	100 70 30	200 170 30	200 170 30	200 170 30	5	07/97
00192	JORGENSON, MIKE 471740095	10/04/1968	M	Pa U	WHBODY RFINGR		M	M	M M	M	M	M M	M	M	M 70	M	M	M 100	5	07/97 07/97
00193	THOMAS, LEE 384846378	11/22/1964	M	Pa U	WHBODY RFINGR		ABSENT ABSENT			M	M	M M	M	M	M M	M	M	M M	5	07/97 07/97
00196	WALKER, JANE 587336640	06/09/1960	F	Pa	WHBODY		3	3	3	12	11	11	12	11	11	22	21	21	5	11/97
00197	EDWARD, CHRIS 489635774	02/14/1966	M	Pa	WHBODY		M	M	M	M	M	M	M	M	M	M	M	M	5	01/98
00198	ZERR, ROBERT 982446591	07/15/1945	M	Pa	WHBODY NOTE		40 CALCULATED	40	40	160	160	160	200	200	200	240	240	240	5	07/98
00199	ADAMS, JANE 335148621	08/25/1951	F	Pa	WHBODY		M	M	M	M	M	M	9	10	12	9	10	12	5	07/98
00200	MEYER, STEVE 416395887	03/21/1947	M	Pa Pa U	COLLAR WAIST ASSIGN NOTE RFINGR	PL	105 M 4 ASSIGNED DOSE BASED ON EDE 1 CALCULATION	105 M 105	105 M 105 140	6	162	165 400	11	327	334 690	51	1247	1284 2180	5	08/98 08/98 08/98
00202	HARRIS, KATHY 352235619	06/15/1972	F	Pa U	WHBODY RFINGR		M	M	M M	M	M	M M	M	M	M 30	M	M	M 30	4	02/99 02/99

M: MINIMAL REPORTING SERVICE OF 1 MREM
ELECTRONIC MEDIA TO FOLLOW THIS REPORT

QUALITY CONTROL RELEASE: VS

20 - PR 6774 - RPT130 - N1 - 02013

NVLAP®
NVLAP LAB CODE 100518-0**

FIGURE 8-5. A sample radiation dosimetry report. *(Courtesy Landauer, Inc.)*

Generally, groups of personnel dosimeters are provided with a control that must be stored in an unexposed area at the facility and returned with the group for processing. This control provides an unexposed level against which the personnel dosimeters are evaluated.

Personnel monitoring devices should not be worn during medical or dental exams and should never be intentionally exposed to the primary radiation beam. Individuals should be aware of the exposure they receive by reviewing their exposure readings on the reports posted in the facility on a routine basis. Should any aspect of the reported exposure be unclear or cause concern, the individual should seek the counsel of the facility radiation safety officer.

Dosimetry Reporting

After each wear date period, the dosimeters are returned to the company's laboratory for analysis. Wear date periods can range from weekly to biweekly to monthly to bimonthly to quarterly. A report is generated for the facility and includes a wide variety of information (Figure 8-5). For the Luxel® OSL dosimeters, Landauer, Inc. provides participant identification information, the type of dosimeter used, the radiation quality that exposed the dosimeter (e.g., x or gamma photons, beta, neutrons), and the radiation exposures that were received. The radiation exposure is expressed as the dose equivalent in millirem for the wear period, a quarterly accumulated dose equivalent, a year-to-date dose equivalent, and a lifetime dose equivalent for each participant. In addition, for each column, exposures are provided for deep dose, lens of the eye dose, and shallow dose equivalents. The deep dose equivalent applies to the external whole-body exposure at a tissue depth of 1 cm, the eye dose equivalent applies to the external lens of the eye at a tissue depth of 0.3 cm, and the shallow dose equivalent applies to the external exposure of the skin at a tissue depth of 0.007 cm. Participants should check their dosimetry report for each wear period.

SUMMARY

Exposure to ionizing radiation carries with it both a benefit and a risk. With few exceptions, the diagnostic benefit of a radiologic procedure far outweighs the minimal risk resulting from the x-ray exposure. The information received by the physician from a radiologic examination about the clinical condition of the patient is an essential part of the practice of modern medicine.

Ionizing radiation is any form of radiation that possesses energy capable of displacing atomic electron bonds and breaking the electron bonds that hold the molecules of matter together. The potential biological damage from the ionization process is the reason for the need to understand proper radiation protection practices. Ionizing radiation comes from two major sources: natural background radiation and man-made radiation.

The biological effects of radiation exposure are either somatic, occurring in the individual exposed, or genetic, occurring in the descendants of the individual exposed. It is the responsibility of the radiographer to ensure each patient receives the minimal dose of radiation necessary to produce a diagnostic image. Radiographers must also be properly shielded from unnecessary radiation exposure.

Radiation quantities and units that are important in radiation protection are exposure, absorbed dose, and equivalent dose. The SI units that correspond to these quantities are the coulomb per kilogram (C/kg),

SUMMARY (continued)

the gray (Gy), and the sievert (Sv). The corresponding traditional units are the roentgen (R), the rad, and the rem. Other radiation quantities of importance are the kerma, the air kerma, integral dose, effective dose, and activity.

Various devices are available to detect and measure exposure to ionizing radiation. Portable field survey instruments include the Geiger-Mueller (GM) survey instruments, scintillation detection devices, and ionization chamber instruments. Personnel monitoring devices include the optically stimulated luminescence dosimeter, film badge dosimeter, thermoluminescent dosimeters, and pocket dosimeters. ■

REVIEW QUESTIONS

1. Explain the differences between alpha and beta particles.
2. Differentiate between somatic and genetic effects.
3. What are the primary sources of ionizing radiation? Give examples of each.
4. What are the three basic quantities of radiation measurement and their associated conventional and SI units?
5. What is the kerma?
6. Describe the function of a GM survey instrument.
7. List three types of personnel monitoring devices.
8. Explain the function of the filters in a dosimeter.

REFERENCES AND RECOMMENDED READING

Birnbaum, S. (2010). Radiation protection in the era of helical CT: Practical patient based programs for decreasing patient exposure. *Semin Ultrasound CT MR, 31*(1), 46–52.

Bushberg, J. T., Seibert, J. A., Leidholdt, E. M., & Boone, J. M. (2003). *The essential physics of medical imaging* (2nd ed.). Philadelphia: Lippincott, Williams & Wilkins.

Bushong, S. C. (2008). *Radiologic science for technologists: Physics, biology, and protection* (9th ed.). St. Louis, MO: Elsevier Mosby.

Chaffins, J. A. (2008). Radiation protection and procedures in the OR. *Radiologic Technology, 79*(5), 415–431.

Colangelo, J. E., Johnston, J., Killion, J. B., Wright, D. L. (2009). Radiation biology and protection. *Radiologic Technology, 80*(5), 421–441.

Dowd, S. B. (1994). *Practical radiation protection and applied radiobiology.* Philadelphia: W. B. Saunders.

Elsberry, J. S. (1979). A technique for scatter dose calculations. *Radiologic Technology, 51*(1), 51.

Engle-Hills, P. (2006). Radiation protection in medical imaging. *Radiography, 12*(2), 153–160.

Forshier, S. (2008). *Essentials of radiation, biology and protection* (2nd ed.). Clifton Park, NY: Delmar Cengage Learning.

Hall, E. J., & Giaccia, J. (2005). *Radiobiology for the radiologist* (6th ed.). Philadelphia: J. B. Lippincott.

Hendee, W. R. (Ed.). (1984). *Health effects of low-level radiation.* Norwalk, CT: Appleton-Century-Crofts.

Hendee, W. R., & Ritenour, R. (2002). *Medical imaging physics* (4th ed.) New York: Wiley-Liss.

International Commission on Radiation Protection. (1970). *Protection of the patient in x-ray diagnosis publication number 16.* Oxford: Pergamon Press.

Mettler, F. A., & Moseley, R. D. (1985). *Medical effects of ionizing radiation.* Orlando, FL: Grune & Stratton.

National Council on Radiation Protection and Measurements (NCRP). (1976). *Structural shielding design and evaluation for medical use of x-rays and gamma rays of energies up to 10 mev* (NCRP Report No. 49). Bethesda, MD.

National Council on Radiation Protection and Measurements (NCRP). (1977). *Medical exposure of pregnant and potentially pregnant women* (NCRP Report No. 54). Bethesda, MD.

National Council on Radiation Protection and Measurements (NCRP). (1985). *SI units in radiation protection and measurements* (NCRP Report No. 82). Bethesda, MD.

National Council on Radiation Protection and Measurements (NCRP). (1987). *Ionizing radiation exposure of the population of the United States* (NCRP Report No. 93). Bethesda, MD.

National Council on Radiation Protection and Measurements (NCRP). (1989). *Medical x-ray, electron beam and gamma-ray protection for energies up to 50 mev (equipment design, performance and use)* (NCRP Report No. 102). Bethesda, MD.

National Council on Radiation Protection and Measurements (NCRP). (1989). *Radiation protection for medical and allied health personnel* (NCRP Report No. 105). Bethesda, MD.

National Council on Radiation Protection and Measurements (NCRP). (1990). *Implementation of the principle of ALARA for medical and dental personnel* (NCRP Report No. 107). Bethesda, MD.

National Council on Radiation Protection and Measurements (NCRP). (1993). *Limitations of exposure to ionizing radiation* (NCRP Report No. 116). Bethesda, MD.

National Council on Radiation Protection and Measurements (NCRP). (2000). *Radiation protection for procedures performed outside the radiology department* (NCRP Report No. 133). Bethesda, MD.

National Council on Radiation Protection and Measurements (NCRP). (2001). *Evaluation of the linear-nonthreshold dose-response model for ionizing radiation* (NCRP Report No. 136). Bethesda, MD.

National Council on Radiation Protection and Measurements (NCRP). (2004). *Structural shielding design for medical x-ray imaging facilities* (NCRP Report No. 147). Bethesda, MD.

National Council on Radiation Protection and Measurements (NCRP). (2007). *Radiation protection in educational institutions* (NCRP Report No. 157). Bethesda, MD.

National Council on Radiation Protection and Measurements (NCRP). (2009). Ionizing Radiation Exposure of the Population of the United States. (NCRP Report No. 160). Bethesda, MD.

Noz, M. E., & Maguire, G. Q. (1985). *Radiation protection in the radiologic and health sciences* (2nd ed.). Philadelphia: Lea & Febiger.

Stabin, M. (2007). *Radiation protection and dosimetry: An introduction to health physics.* New York: Springer.

Watkins, G. L. (1988). Public health risks from low dose medical radiation. *Radiologic Technology, 59*(2), 160.

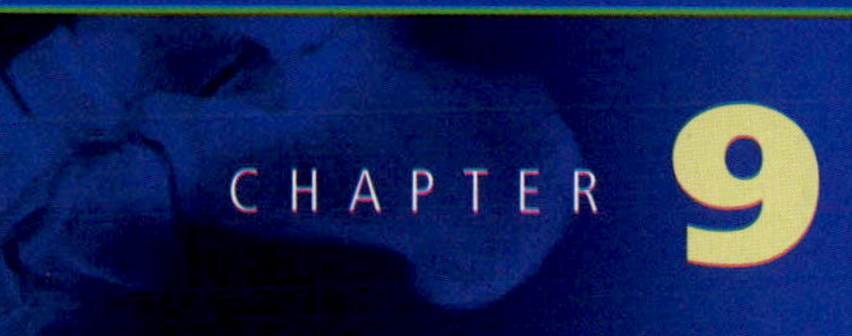

Chapter 9 Radiation Protection Procedures for Patients and Personnel

KEY TERMS

10-day rule
ALARA
deterministic effect
dose limit
occasionally exposed worker
occupationally exposed worker
primary barrier
protective device
radiation worker
secondary barrier
stochastic effect
structural protective barrier

> Röntgen almost from the beginning had conducted all his experiments in his big zinc box.... Then he had added a lead plate to the zinc between the tube and himself, and in doing so he had unknowingly protected himself completely. With an accurate appreciation of the import of these unexplained effects, Röntgen foresaw the suffering consequent to the careless handling of the rays.
>
> *Otto Glasser from the biography Dr. W. C. Röntgen*

OBJECTIVES

Upon completion of this chapter, the student should be able to:

- Differentiate between the various advisory groups and regulatory agencies involved in developing radiation protection standards.
- Explain the concept of dose limits related to the use of radiation.
- Describe the ALARA concept.
- Explain the basic principles of reducing exposure to radiation.
- Describe techniques used to minimize radiation exposure to patients and personnel.
- Discuss the precautions that should be taken to minimize potential fetal exposures.

ADVISORY GROUPS AND REGULATORY AGENCIES

A number of different organizations and agencies are involved in the development of standards for radiation protection and the establishment of regulations for the protection against the hazards that can result from the use of ionizing radiation.

The advisory groups that have shared in the establishment of radiation protection standards include: the **International Commission on Radiological Protection (ICRP)**, the **National Council on Radiation Protection and Measurements (NCRP)**, the **National Academy of Sciences Advisory Committee on the Biological Effects of Ionizing Radiation (NAS-BEIR)**, and the **United Nations Scientific Committee on the Effects of Atomic Radiation (UNSCEAR).**

The ICRP was formed in 1928 and has an international membership. It provides a variety of perspectives on radiologic health issues. In 1929 the ICRP established the National Committee on Radiation Protection and Measurements, which was later chartered by Congress in 1964 as the National Council on Radiation Protection and Measurements (NCRP). The NCRP is a nonprofit organization that is charged with collecting, analyzing, developing, and disseminating information in the public interest, and recommendations about radiation protection and radiation measurements, quantities, and units. It works cooperatively with the ICRP and other agencies to accomplish its mission.

The NAS-BEIR and UNSCEAR are two additional advisory groups that study and report on the risks from exposure to ionizing radiation.

In addition to the advisory groups, there are a number of regulatory agencies responsible for protecting the public and occupationally exposed individuals from the effects of ionizing radiation. Regulatory agencies carry the force of law and can inspect facilities, issue fines, and revoke radiation use authorizations. Two such agencies are the **U.S. Nuclear Regulatory Commission (NRC)** and the **U.S. Food and Drug Administration (FDA).** The NRC has been given the regulatory authority for special nuclear materials and by-products. In a number of instances, the NRC has entered into agreements with the states to oversee and enforce the regulations. In these "agreement states," it becomes the state's responsibility to enforce NRC regulations. The FDA regulates radiopharmaceuticals as well as the performance and radiation safety requirements of commercial x-ray equipment.

The two primary sources of radiation protection standards in the United States are the NRC, which is a U.S. federal agency charged with licensing facilities and controlling the use of radioactive materials, and the NCRP, an advisory group that makes recommendations for radiation protection. Both sources are used when setting radiation protection policies and procedures. The NRC regulations are available on the Internet at *www.nrc.gov*, and the NCRP reports are available at *www.ncrp.com.*

LIMITING EXPOSURE TO IONIZING RADIATION

It is important to set limits for the protection of the radiation worker and the general public because of the known biological effects of exposure to ionizing radiation. The primary purposes for establishing dose limits are to limit the risks of **stochastic effects** and to prevent **deterministic effects** (also known as nonstochastic effects). Stochastic effects are those for which no threshold dose of radiation exists, such as cancer and genetic effects. They are random in nature. Regardless of dose, some will experience an effect. As dose goes up, the chance of experiencing an effect also goes up. Deterministic effects, such as cataracts, skin erythema, and sterility, are those for which a threshold dose is assumed. As dose increases, the severity of the effect increases. Although the dose has to be high to demonstrate the effect, once that dose is reached, the probability of demonstrating the effect is very high.

For radiation protection purposes, individuals may be divided into two groups. First are those classified as **radiation workers**, who incur, as an occupational risk, a certain likelihood of exposure to ionizing radiation in the course of their normal duties. The second group includes members of the general public.

Radiation workers may be further classified as **occupationally exposed workers** and **occasionally exposed workers**. Occupationally exposed workers are individuals who have a significant potential for exposure to radiation in the course of their employment. Occasionally exposed workers are individuals whose duties may occasionally bring them into areas where radiation exposure may occur. Both occupationally exposed workers and occasionally exposed workers should receive instruction and training regarding hazards of radiation exposure and radiation protection practices.

Dose Limits

Radiation exposure limits pertinent to the protection of radiation workers are known as **dose limits** and are specified for both **whole-body** exposure and for exposure to **certain tissues and organs.** Several terms have been used to describe dose limits, including maximum permissible dose, dose equivalent limits, and equivalent dose limits. Prior to 1987, the term *maximum permissible dose* (MPD) was used to describe dose limits; this is no longer acceptable terminology because no dose is considered permissible.

Dose equivalent limits and *cumulative effective dose equivalent* replaced MPD, and this philosophy was described in NCRP Report No. 91, *Recommendations on Limits for Exposure to Ionizing Radiation.* In 1993, **NCRP Report No. 116, *Limitation of Exposure to Ionizing Radiation***, replaced NCRP Report No. 91. This report follows the same basic framework to dose limits as the previous report but incorporated some changes as provided in ICRP Publication 60. Of particular note is the change in terminology, from effective dose equivalent limits (Report No. 91) to effective dose limits (Report No. 116) and dose equivalent limits for tissues and organs (Report No. 91) to equivalent dose limits for tissues and organs (Report No. 116). Equivalent dose (H_T) replaces the previously used term, *dose equivalent* (H), in defining dose limits. These two terms are conceptually different. Dose equivalent (H) is based on the absorbed dose at a "point" in tissue and equivalent dose (H_T) is based on the average absorbed dose in the tissue or organ.

TABLE 9-1. Effective Dose Limit Recommendations

Occupational Exposures		
Effective dose limits		
Annual	50 mSv	(5 rem)
Cumulative	10 mSv × age	(1 rem × age)
Dose equivalent annual limits for tissues and organs		
Lens of eye	150 mSv	(15 rem)
Skin, hands, and feet	500 mSv	(50 rem)
Public Exposures (Annual)		
Effective dose limit		
Continuous or frequent exposure	1 mSv	(0.1 rem)
Infrequent exposure	5 mSv	(0.5 rem)
Equivalent dose limits for tissues and organs		
Lens of eye	15 mSv	(1.5 rem)
Skin, hands, and feet	50 mSv	(5 rem)
Embryo-Fetus Exposures (Monthly)		
Equivalent dose limit	0.5 mSv	(0.05 rem)
Education and Training Exposures (Annual)		
Effective dose limit	1 mSv	(0.1 rem)
Dose equivalent limit for tissues and organs		
Lens of eye	15 mSv	(1.5 rem)
Skin, hands, and feet	50 mSv	(5 rem)

Adapted from NCRP Report No. 116, *Limitations of Exposure to Ionizing Radiation,* Table 19.1.

Currently recommended values for occupational and public dose limits are given in Table 9-1 and reflect the recommendations of the NCRP as put forth in Report No. 116. The effective dose limit for whole-body exposure of a radiation worker is 5 rem (50 mSv) per year.

The cumulative effective dose (E) limit is age in rem, which is determined in SI units by the formula:

$$E = 10 \text{ mSv} \times N$$

where: E = effective dose limit

N = age in years

EXAMPLE: What is the dose limit for a 19-year-old radiation worker?

Answer:

E = 10 mSv × N

E = 10 mSv × 19

E = 190 mSv (19 rem)

EXAMPLE: What is the dose limit for a 35-year-old radiation worker?

Answer:

E = 10 mSv × N

E = 10 mSv × 35

E = 350 mSv (35 rem)

Irradiation at the upper level of the dose limits is not to be considered as desirable, and in every case efforts to reduce exposures to the lowest possible level should be taken.

Individuals not classified as radiation workers are considered members of the **general public.** For purposes of protection of these individuals, the level of recommended dose limits, exclusive of any exposure received as the result of a medical procedure, has been established as one-tenth of the effective dose limit for radiation workers—that is, 0.5 rem (5 mSv) per year for infrequent exposure and one-fiftieth of the effective dose limit for radiation workers, which is 0.1 rem (1 mSv) per year for continuous exposure. Individuals in education and training have the same effective dose limit (for continuous or frequent exposure) as the general public, that is, 0.1 rem (1 mSv).

Nuclear Regulatory Commission (NRC)

The NRC regulations for radiation protection are known by their Code of Federal Regulations (CFR) No. 10CFR20. Unlike the NCRP, which is an advisory body, the NRC is a U.S. federal government agency and its regulations are law in the United States. NRC licensees are required to implement these standards. The standards for occupational dose limits for adults are shown in Table 9-2.

The most critical of the NRC regulations is the whole-body exposure regulation that limits exposure to 500 mSv (50 rem)/year to any organ or 50 mSv (5 rem)/year whole body. Also worthy of note are the regulations for exposure to the extremities, lens of the eye, and pregnancy (which is discussed in detail later in this chapter).

Maintaining Exposure as Low as Reasonably Achievable (ALARA)

A basic philosophical principle of radiation protection concerning the use of ionizing radiation emphasizes the need to maintain exposure to ionizing radiation at a level **A**s **L**ow **A**s **R**easonably **A**chievable (ALARA), with economic and societal factors being taken into consideration. This premise has been accepted by advisory and regulatory agencies and requires that radiologic personnel take on the responsibility of minimizing the exposure to their patients and any other individuals involved in a radiologic procedure. Implementation of the ALARA principle is achieved by application of the basic principles of

TABLE 9-2. Occupational Dose Limits for Adults—NRC Regulation IOCFR20

Whole-body definition	Head, trunk, gonads, arms above elbow, legs above knee
Extremities definition	Arms, elbows, and below; legs, knees and below
Whole-body exposure limits	Most limiting of: 500 mSv (50 rem)/yr to any organ or 50 mSv (5 rem)/yr whole body
Lens of the eye	150 mSv (15 rem)/yr
Skin of the whole body	500 mSv (50 rem)/yr
Extremities	500 mSv (50 rem)/yr applied to each extremity
Embryo/fetus/pregnancy	5 mSv/term (0.5 rem or 500 mrem)

radiation protection and a thoughtful approach to all work involving exposure to ionizing radiation.

PROTECTION OF PERSONNEL

When radiological procedures are performed, there is a possibility that individuals other than the patient will receive some radiation exposure. Although the patient should be the only person exposed to the primary beam, others involved in the procedure may be exposed to radiation scattered from the primary beam or to leakage radiation from the x-ray tube. This occurs particularly during fluoroscopy, mobile examinations, interventional special procedures, and cardiac catheterization. For most radiographic exposures, personnel should be behind protective barriers. Radiologic personnel should not be involved in holding patients who are unable to cooperate during an x-ray exposure. Immobilization devices should be used or, if absolutely necessary, assistance should be requested from the patient's family or friends.

Figure 9-1A and B represent diagrams of two iso-exposure curves that illustrate the percentage of scattered radiation that personnel are exposed to during a single exposure of 20 mAs to a chest phantom. The curves represent the percentage of the exposure to the skin at various distances from the patient using two different kilovoltages (60 kVp and 80 kVp) and two different field sizes (20 × 20 cm and 28 × 32 cm). The effect of kVp is illustrated in Figure 9-1A for the transverse plane. The effect of beam restriction (collimation) is shown in Figure 9-1B for the coronal plane. In both instances, an obvious reduction in exposure to scattered radiation occurs as the distance away from a patient increases. In addition, the amount of scatter around a patient is affected to a greater extent by changes in collimation rather than changes in kVp.

Principles of Personnel Exposure Reduction

Reduction of an individual's exposure to ionizing radiation may be accomplished by application of three basic principles: (1) reduce the amount of **time** spent in the vicinity of the radiation source while it is operating; (2) increase the **distance** between the radiation source and the individual to be protected; and (3) interpose a **shielding** material, which will attenuate the radiation from the source. These three basic principles are sometimes referred to as the three cardinal rules of radiation protection.

Time. X-ray imaging equipment produces radiation only during the actual exposure used to form the image during a procedure. The time of exposure on a per-image basis is very short (typically much less than 1 second) during radiographic procedures. During fluoroscopic procedures, which are used when dynamic information is required, the x-ray source may be on (usually intermittently) for several minutes to as long as an hour or more. To minimize exposure to radiation, individuals should reduce the amount of time they spend in the vicinity of an operable radiation source. The simplest way to do this is to ascertain whether their presence is needed during the procedure. Whenever possible, individuals should remain behind protective barriers.

Distance. Increasing the distance between the individual and the source of radiation is an effective method to reduce exposure to radiation. As distance from the source of radiation is increased, the radiation level will decrease significantly. Maximizing the distance from an operable source of radiation is a particularly effective method of exposure reduction during mobile radiographic and fluoroscopic procedures.

The amount of exposure reduction can be calculated using the inverse square law, which describes the relationship between distance and radiation intensity. The inverse square law states that the intensity of radiation at a given distance from a point source is inversely proportional to the square of the distance. For example, if the distance between the individual and the source of radiation is doubled, the exposure to the individual will be reduced by a factor of 4 (2^2); if the distance between the individual and the source of radiation is tripled, the exposure to the individual will be reduced by a factor of 9 (3^2). The relationship between distance

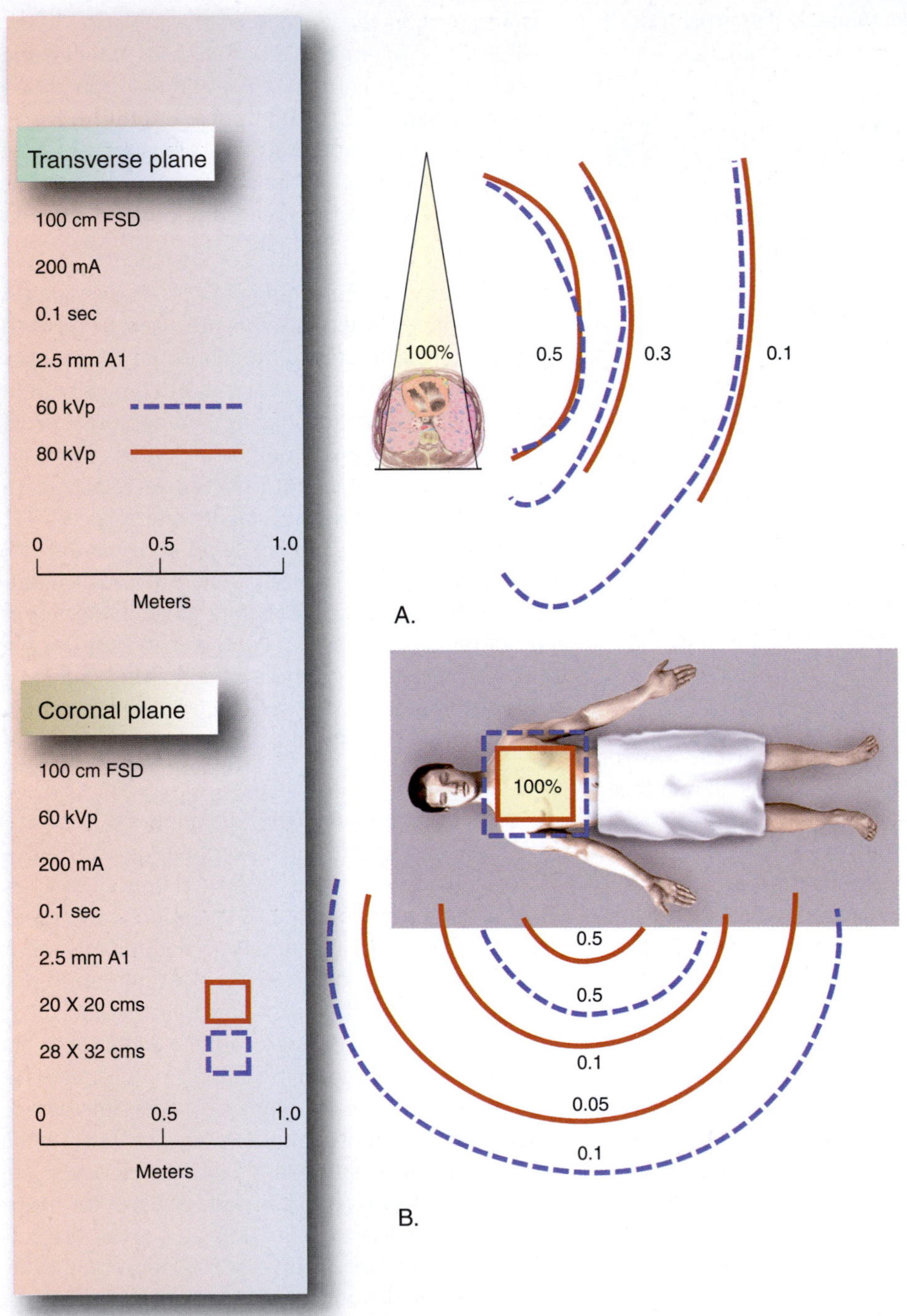

FIGURE 9-1. The iso-exposure curves represent the percentage of the exposure to the skin at various distances from the patient using two different kilovoltages (60 kVp and 80 kVp) and two different field sizes (20 × 20 cm and 28 × 32 cm). The effect of kVp is illustrated in (A) for the transverse plane. The effect of beam restriction (collimation) is shown in (B) for the coronal plane. *(Reprinted with permission from P. Cartwright 1992, "Distribution and Relative Intensity of Scattered Radiation,"* Radiography Today, *58[664], 12–13.)*

and radiation exposure is explained in further detail in Chapter 11.

Shielding. Shielding is used when neither time nor distance is effective in achieving the desired degree of reduction in exposure. By interposing any material between the source of radiation and the point at which it is desired to reduce the exposure, a certain reduction in exposure will be achieved. The degree of exposure reduction will depend on the physical characteristics of the material (atomic number, density, and thickness). For fixed x-ray imaging facilities, the most common materials are lead and concrete. Such facilities are designed in accordance with specific recommendations (NCRP Report No. 49) depending on the configuration of the equipment, its intended use, and the surrounding area. Additional devices, such as mobile shields, lead-equivalent aprons, and lead-equivalent gloves should be used when it is not possible to take advantage of fixed structural barriers.

Protective Barriers

During the design of fixed x-ray imaging facilities it is necessary to ensure that the layout of the equipment and shielding of the room are such that the exposure to personnel and members of the public within adjacent areas is within the recommended equivalent dose limits. This is accomplished through the use of **structural protective barriers** made of materials having effective x-ray attenuating properties and of thicknesses sufficient to reduce exposures to the desired levels. Commonly used materials include lead sheet, concrete, lead glass, steel, and leaded acrylic.

Protective barriers are classified as either **primary barriers** or **secondary barriers**. Primary barriers can be struck by the primary or useful beam exiting the x-ray tube. Secondary barriers can only be struck by scattered and leakage radiation. The primary beam cannot be directed at secondary barriers. Secondary barriers are always thinner than primary barriers.

The design of structural shielding for x-ray imaging facilities is treated in detail in **NCRP Report No. 49, *Structural Shielding Design and Evaluation for Medical Use of X Rays and Gamma Rays of Energies Up to 10 MeV.*** Barrier requirements are dependent on the type of equipment, its layout within the room, the occupancy of adjacent areas, and other factors. Such shielding should always be designed by a qualified diagnostic radiological physicist.

Protective Devices

When it is not possible for personnel to remain behind a protective barrier, it is the radiographer's responsibility to ensure that **protective devices** are worn by all personnel, including physicians, nurses, aides, and so forth. These situations arise frequently during fluoroscopy and some mobile procedures. The most common protective devices are lead aprons and lead gloves. Special devices include leaded glasses and thyroid shields.

During fluoroscopy and mobile radiography, personnel should always wear a protective apron. Lead gloves should also be worn if the hands will be in close proximity to the primary beam. Protective aprons and gloves are usually made of lead-impregnated vinyl within the range of 0.25–1.0 mm of lead equivalency. The greater the lead equivalence, the greater the protective ability and the weight of the item. Aprons vary in weight from a few pounds to over 20 pounds depending on design and lead content. For example, a lead apron that wraps completely around the body, extending from shoulders to knees with a 1-mm lead equivalent, will possess a significant weight. This weight can be a serious consideration if personnel are expected to wear the apron for long periods of time. The protective aprons must possess a minimum of 0.5-mm lead equivalent if the peak energy of the x-ray beam is 100 kVp. Most departments use aprons with 0.5-mm lead equivalent to provide personnel with a balance between protection and weight. Lead gloves usually possess 0.25 mm of lead equivalency.

PROTECTION OF THE PATIENT

Proper radiation protection of the patient is achieved through both medical and technical decisions. Medical decisions lie with the patient and are based on the professional judgment of physicians and other practitioners of the healing arts in consultation with the patient.

Technical decisions include a number of factors that affect the amount of radiation a patient receives during a diagnostic x-ray examination. Many of these factors are under the direct control of the radiographer. It is a radiographer's responsibility to understand these factors and to minimize patient exposure while producing a satisfactory diagnostic image.

Although it is desirable to minimize the exposure to a patient undergoing a radiologic procedure, it must be kept in mind that the goal of any radiologic imaging procedure is to provide information about the medical condition of the patient to aid in clinical management. Overzealous attempts to reduce patient exposure may significantly compromise the information to be obtained from the examination. Keeping these concepts in mind, the following principles should be applied to minimize exposure to the patient.

Beam Limitation

The size of the x-ray beam should always be restricted to the area of clinical interest and should never exceed the size of the image receptor. Proper collimation not only reduces patient dose but also improves the overall quality of the radiographic image because less scatter radiation is created with smaller field sizes. Ideally, evidence of proper collimation, as demonstrated by an unexposed border on all sides of the radiographic image, should be present.

Technique Selection

Technique factors for a given examination should be selected to minimize dose to the patient. High-kVp/low-mAs techniques are preferred to decrease patient dose. However, the selected kVp should be chosen so the required contrast in the radiographic image is not compromised as a result of a more penetrating x-ray beam or because of an increase in the amount of scatter radiation reaching the image receptor, which can impair image quality. Tube current and exposure time should be chosen to minimize the degrading effects of anatomical motion. Proper technical factor selection is the responsibility of the radiographer. This decision must take into account the information needed to make a proper diagnosis. It is important to remember that increasing kVp alone does not decrease patient dose but instead will increase patient dose. To reduce patient dose, the increase in kVp must be accompanied by a reduction in mAs to maintain an acceptable exposure.

Distance also has an impact on patient dose. Exposure decreases as distance increases. For this reason routine procedures traditionally done at 40″ are now recommended to be done at 44–48″.

Filtration

Filters are placed at the x-ray port to selectively absorb low-energy photons that would be absorbed by the patient and not contribute to the image. These low-energy photons would be absorbed by the patient, resulting in an increase in the patient dose. Specialized filtration is also available. It allows for additional exposure reduction by the selective removal of photons from the beam.

Aluminum is the most common filtering material used and filtration is expressed in terms of the thickness of aluminum equivalency (Al/Eq). The NCRP recommends a minimum total filtration of 2.5 mm Al/Eq for x-ray equipment operating above 70 kVp. When filtration is increased, technical factors need to be increased to compensate for the reduction in exposure associated with the filtration. Despite the need to increase exposure to maintain exposure, the overall dose to the patient decreases with the use of filtration.

Grids

Radiographic grids are placed between the patient and the image receptor to preferentially absorb scatter radiation. Because grids absorb primary as well as scatter radiation, technical factors must be increased to produce an image of acceptable exposure. This increase in technical factors results in an increase in patient dose but image quality is significantly improved. The lowest possible grid ratio consistent with effective scatter removal should be utilized to keep patient dose as low as reasonably achievable.

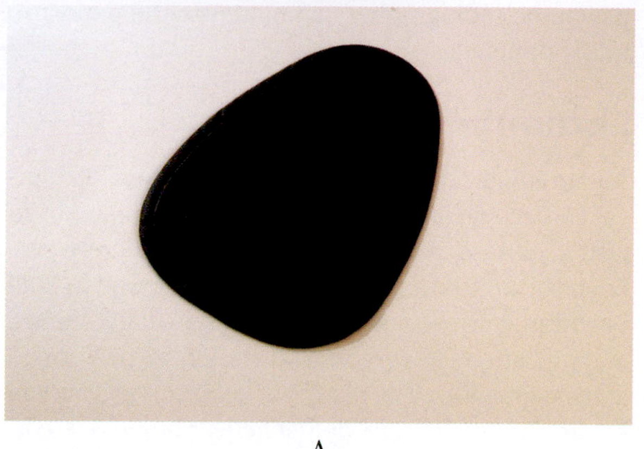

A

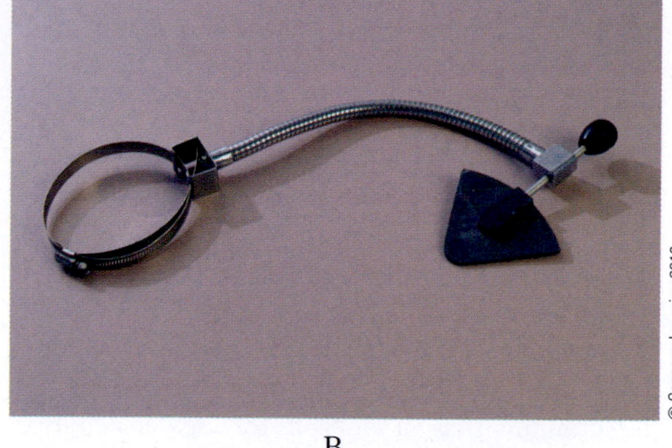

B

FIGURE 9-2. Gonadal shields: A. flat shield, B. shadow shield.

Gonadal Shielding

Shielding the gonads (ovaries or testes) is especially important to minimize the possibility of any genetic effect on the future children of an exposed individual. Special attention should be paid to shielding the gonads of children and adults of child-bearing age.

Proper collimation is important when decreasing gonadal dose, but special gonadal shields should be used any time the gonads are within 4 to 5 cm of the primary beam. The three basic types of gonadal shields are **flat contact shields, shaped contact shields,** and **shadow shields** (Figure 9-2).

Flat contact shields are usually made of various sizes of lead-impregnated vinyl and are placed between the patient's gonads and the source of radiation. During fluoroscopy, the shield usually needs to be placed underneath the patient because that is where the source of radiation is most often located. Flat contact shields may need to be secured in place to ensure correct placement for a variety of patient positions.

Shaped contact shields are cup-shaped and designed to enclose the male gonads. These shields provide maximum protection in a number of patient positions.

Shadow shields are mounted to the tube and are placed in the x-ray beam near the collimator. The collimator's light field must be precise for accurate shield placement. The device is adjusted to cast a shadow over the patient's gonads.

Image Receptors

The response (speed) of the image receptor should be as high as possible, consistent with the required information of the radiologic procedure. Both digital image and conventional film/screen image receptor systems reduce patient dose by reducing the quantity of x-ray photons needed to create an image. Digital systems convert x-ray photons either directly to electronic image signals or to light, while intensifying screens convert x-ray photons to light photons, which expose film within a cassette. The response or speed of the image receptor is influenced by the sensitivity of the materials that make up the receptor.

With digital image receptor systems, the speed of the system is selected based on the specific exam being performed and is not as closely linked to patient dose as film/screen image receptor systems are. With digital systems, it becomes the responsibility of the department to establish exposure ranges based on the image quality desired for a particular examination. A wide range of patient exposures can produce acceptable images, and it is the technologist's responsibility to keep the patient dose for a given exam as low as possible without compromising image quality. Gross over- or under-exposure errors are not as obvious to the eye but do significantly affect image quality and require repeating the procedure. All digital radiography systems have a method for evaluating the image receptor exposure although this varies from vendor to vendor.

Projection

The projection used for a particular exam will have an impact on patient dose to specific body tissues. For example, the lens of the eye receives a greater dose during anteroposterior (AP) projections of the cranium than it does if the posteroanterior (PA) projection is used. Or, a contrast-filled bladder will serve as a gonadal shield for females if the exposure is made with the patient in the AP projection but will not shield the ovaries in the PA projection.

Repeat Images

Any time an image must be repeated, patient dose increases as a direct result of the exposure from the poor image. Radiographers must possess a complete understanding of the entire radiographic process to minimize repeat exposures. Images generally need to be repeated for such reasons as improper exposure factor selection, poor positioning (tube/part/image receptor alignment), poor patient instruction, or improper film or post-processing. Images should only be repeated when the quality compromises the diagnostic information of the procedure. It is important for the radiographer to communicate effectively with the patient and provide the patient with clear instructions during the procedure to minimize the possibility of needing to repeat the exposure.

Patient Exposure Estimates

Estimates of the exposure received by patients undergoing radiographic procedures should be available. These estimates should be developed for the average patient based on standard technique charts and measured exposure characteristics of the radiological imaging equipment. Chapter 13 provides information on calculating the patient exposure for a given procedure and describes ways in which the radiographer can minimize the exposure to the patient.

Equipment

All radiologic imaging equipment should be surveyed periodically by a diagnostic radiologic physicist to assess its radiation safety characteristics. Such surveys should normally be conducted in conjunction with scheduled preventive maintenance and performance surveys and should be performed at least annually. The results of such surveys should be documented. Any deficiencies should be corrected prior to returning the equipment to clinical service.

RADIATION EXPOSURE AND PREGNANCY

A situation deserving special consideration is the possibility of radiation exposure during the early weeks of pregnancy, generally before the woman is aware of her condition. The dose to the fetus is of concern, particularly in the early stages of development when certain tissues and organs are especially sensitive to radiation. Recent studies, as summarized in the report BEIR V, suggest the fetus may be particularly radiosensitive during the period of 8 to 15 weeks postconception. As a result, care must be taken to reduce radiation exposure to any pregnant individual, including pregnant (or potentially pregnant) patients and pregnant personnel. It is currently recommended by the NCRP that the monthly equivalent dose limit (excluding medical exposure) for the embryo not exceed 0.05 rem (50 mrem, 0.5 mSv) once the pregnancy becomes known.

NCRP Report No. 54, *Medical Exposure of Pregnant and Potentially Pregnant Women*, discusses the risks associated with fetal exposure: This risk is considered to be negligible at 5 rad or less when compared to other risks of pregnancy, and the risk of malformations is significantly increased above control levels only at doses above 15 rad. Therefore, the exposure of the fetus to radiation arising from diagnostic procedures would very rarely be cause, by itself, for terminating a pregnancy. If there are reasons, other than the possible radiation effects, to consider a therapeutic abortion, such reasons should be discussed with the patient by the attending physician, so that it is clear that the radiation exposure is not being used as an excuse for terminating the pregnancy (NCRP, 1977).

Pregnant Radiation Worker Exposure Standards

There are two sets of standards that are applied to pregnant radiation workers. These standards include students under the definition of those who are "occupationally" exposed to ionizing radiation because students in radiologic sciences programs are classified as students by occupation, and the exposure occurs during duties in their occupation.

The two standards complement one another. The NRC is a U.S. federal agency charged with licensing facilities and controlling the use of radioactive materials. The NCRP is an advisory group that makes recommendations for radiation protection.

NRC regulations state that the dose equivalent to the embryo/fetus during the entire pregnancy, due to the occupational exposure of a declared pregnant woman, cannot exceed 5 mSv (0.5 rem or 500 mrem). The NCRP recommends that fetal exposure be restricted to an equivalent dose limit of 0.5 mSv (0.05 rem or 50 mrem) per month. These two limits are complementary as a normal human gestation spans a 10-month period. Therefore, 0.5 mSv (0.05 rem) for 10 months equals 5 mSv (0.5 rem) for the entire gestational period. The specific citations (which are often referred to in pregnancy policies and state regulations) are NRC regulation 10CFR20.1208 and NCRP Reports No. 54, No. 116, and No. 128, with the primary recommendation issued in Report No. 116.

Declaring Pregnancy. Pregnant radiation workers are referred to in U.S. federal regulations as "declared pregnant" because a woman has the right to choose whether or not to declare her pregnancy (this was established in a U.S. Supreme Court decision in the case of *United Auto Workers vs. Johnson Controls*). The government currently interprets this as including the right to revoke her declaration at any time. In addition, a female worker can legally declare pregnancy without documented medical proof and there is no limit on how frequently or for how long a duration a person can declare she is pregnant.

Although the idea of declaring and undeclaring a pregnancy may sound bizarre, it is legitimate in the light of recent legal decisions that give women the right to choose for their embryo/fetus. This concept requires women to make a decision as to what radiation regulations will be applied to a pregnancy. Therefore, the NRC requires a voluntary declaration of pregnancy to be in writing, dated, and include the estimated month of conception. In addition, **NRC regulation 10CFR19.12 requires that instructions to women assigned to radiation exposure areas must include explanation of the right to declare or not declare pregnancy status as well as requiring that all information in NRC Regulatory Guide 8.13 be discussed.** This mandatory guide has details about the risk of radiation exposure in order to permit women to make an informed decision about declaring a pregnancy. The guide is downloadable at *www.nrc.gov.*

ALARA and Pregnancies

It has become common practice to assign declared pregnant women to areas where exposure is likely to be lower. This approach is now being discouraged in compliance with ALARA concepts of keeping all occupational exposure as low as reasonably achievable. The rationale is that any displacement of normal duties places additional radiation exposure burden on fellow workers, both male and female, which they may find unacceptable. Therefore, reassigning declared pregnant women to lower-exposure areas causes increased risk to others.

In addition, because most women are not aware of pregnancy until after the most sensitive first trimester has passed, it is very possible that another as-yet-undeclared pregnant woman could be assigned additional time in a high-exposure area, thus increasing risk to her embryo/fetus at the worst possible time.

Some authors are recommending that if institutions choose to reassign declared pregnant women in opposition to recommended ALARA guidelines, all workers (or students) must clearly understand the ramifications of such a policy. To avoid legal complications, it is recommended that all occupationally exposed persons in the institution agree to the policy in writing and that this documentation include specific statements indicating agreement to be placed in higher-exposure areas from time to time as necessary to accommodate those women who have declared pregnancy.

The authors of this book recognize the controversial nature of these recommendations and acknowledge that administrative ethical beliefs about abortion are often linked to pregnancy policies in institutions. However, we believe that radiologic sciences professionals should have a part in the determination of these policies as it is their bodies and future children that are at risk. Informed decisions cannot be made without the information we have supplied here.

The Pregnant Patient

To minimize the possible exposure to an embryo in the earliest days of a pregnancy, a guideline known as the **10-day rule** was recommended by a number of advisory agencies. This guideline stated that elective abdominal x-ray examinations of fertile women should be postponed until the 10-day period following the onset of menstruation, as it would be improbable that a woman would be pregnant during these 10 days. Based on the current understanding of radiobiology, this rule is now considered obsolete, primarily because the egg for the next cycle reaches maximum sensitivity during the 10-day period. The application of this guideline within the radiology department has always proven difficult.

It is now the general belief that postponement of abdominal x-ray examinations is not necessary when the physician requesting the examination has considered the entire clinical state of the patient, including the possibility of pregnancy. The potential pregnancy status of all female patients of childbearing age should always be determined; in the event of known pregnancy, steps should be taken to minimize exposure to the fetus. One way to ensure against irradiating a woman in the early stages of pregnancy is to institute elective scheduling for nonemergency procedures. In many departments, female patients of childbearing ages are asked to provide the date of their last menstrual period (LMP). If there is a concern about a possible pregnancy, the patient's exam may be rescheduled. If a radiologic exam on a pregnant patient is deemed necessary, a diagnostic radiological physicist should perform calculations to estimate the actual fetal dose.

SUMMARY

It is important to set limits for the protection of the radiation worker and the general public because of the known biological effects of exposure to ionizing radiation. Occupational radiation exposure limits pertinent to the protection of radiation workers are known as dose equivalent limits and are specified for both total body exposure and for exposure to certain tissues and organs.

To minimize dose to personnel the basic principles of time, distance, and shielding should be applied. There are two types of fixed x-ray installation protective barriers. Primary protective barriers are designed to protect against the direct exposure of the primary x-ray beam. Secondary protective barriers are designed to protect against exposure from scatter and leakage radiation. When it is not possible for personnel to

SUMMARY (continued)

remain behind a protective barrier, protective devices, such as lead aprons and lead gloves, should be worn.

To minimize patient dose while creating a diagnostic image, the radiographer must understand the factors that have a significant relationship to patient dose, such as beam limitation, technique selection, filtration, grids, gonadal shielding, image receptors, and repeat images.

Care must be taken to reduce radiation exposure to any pregnant individual, including pregnant (or potentially pregnant) patients and pregnant personnel. It is currently recommended by the NCRP that the equivalent dose limit (excluding medical exposure) for the embryo-fetus not exceed 0.05 rem (0.5 mSv) in any month once the pregnancy becomes known. ■

REVIEW QUESTIONS

1. What is the annual effective dose limit for whole-body exposure of a radiation worker?
2. What is the cumulative effective dose limit for a 28-year-old radiation worker (in rem and mSv)?
3. Explain the ALARA concept.
4. What are the three basic principles used for minimizing an individual's exposure to ionizing radiation?
5. What is the difference between a primary and secondary protective barrier?
6. How can a radiographer minimize radiation exposure to the patient?
7. What is the equivalent dose limit for the embryo-fetus per month?
8. According to NRC regulations, how does a woman declare herself pregnant?

REFERENCES AND RECOMMENDED READING

Barrett, J. (1993). An investigation of radiation dose levels to patients during lumbar spine examinations. *Radiography Today, 59*(675), 19–22.

BEIR V health effects of exposure to low levels of ionizing radiation. (1990). Washington, DC: National Academy Press.

Boice, J. D., Mandel, J. S., & Doody, M. M. (1992). A health study of radiologic technologists. *Cancer, 69*, 586–597.

Boone, J. M., & Levin, D. C. (1991). Radiation exposure to angiographers under different fluoroscopic imaging conditions. *Radiology, 180*, 861–865.

Bushberg, J. T., Seibert, J. A., Leidholdt, E. M., & Boone, J. M. (2003). *The essential physics of medical imaging* (2nd ed.). Philadelphia: Lippincott, Williams & Wilkins.

Bushong, S. C. (2008). *Radiologic science for technologists: Physics, biology, and protection* (9th ed.). St. Louis, MO: Elsevier Mosby.

Butler, P., Thomas, A. W., Thompson, W. E., Wollerton, M. A., & Rachlin, J. A. (1986). Simple methods to reduce patient exposure during scoliosis radiography. *Radiologic Technology, 57*(5), 411.

Caprio, M. L. (1980). The pregnant x-ray tech—providing adequate radiation safety for the fetus. *Radiologic Technology, 52*(2), 161.

Chaffins, J. A. (2008). Radiation protection and procedures in the OR. *Radiologic Technology, 79*(5), 415–431.

Curry, T. S., Dowdey, J. E., & Murry, R. C. (1990). *Christensen's introduction to the physics of diagnostic radiology* (4th ed.). Philadelphia: Lea and Febiger.

Detain, J. (1984). Is it time to question the 10-day rule? *Radiography, 50*(592), 149–150.

Dowd, S. B. (1994). *Practical radiation protection and applied radiobiology.* Philadelphia: W. B. Saunders.

Dowd, S. B., & Archer, J. (1994). Radiation safety regulations: The evolution and development of standards. *Radiology Management*, *16*(1), 39–45.

Engle-Hills, P. (2006). Radiation protection in medical imaging. *Radiography*, *12*(2), 153–160.

Floyd, C., Baker, A., Lo, J., & Ravin, C. (1992). Measurement of scatter fractions in clinical bedside radiography. *Radiology*, *183*(3), 857–861.

Forshier, S. (2008). *Essentials of radiation, biology and protection* (2nd ed.). Clifton Park, NY: Delmar Cengage Learning.

Frank, E., Stears, J., Gray, J., Winkler, N. T., & Hoffman, A. D. (1984). Use of the P. A. projection: A method of reducing x-ray exposure to specific radiosensitive organs. *The Canadian Journal of Medical Radiation Technology*, *15*(2), 63.

Glaze, S., LeBlanc, A. D., & Bushong, S. C. (1984). Defects in new protective aprons. *Radiology*, 217.

Gray, J. E., Stears, J. G., & Frank, E. D. (1983). Shaped, lead-loaded acrylic filters for patient exposure reduction and image-quality improvement. *Radiology*, 825.

Gur, D., & Wald, N. (1986). Probability of causation tables and their possible implications for the practice of diagnostic radiology. *Radiology*, *158*, 853–854.

Hall, E. J., & Griacci, J. (2005). *Radiobiology for the radiologist* (6th ed.). Philadelphia: J. B. Lippincott.

Hendee, W. R. (1992). Estimation of radiation risks: BEIR V and its significance for medicine. *Journal of the American Medical Association*, *268*, 620–624.

Hendee, W. R. (Ed.). (1984). *Health effects of low-level radiation*. Norwalk, CT: Appleton-Century-Crofts.

Hilger, M. T. J. (1983). Radiation exposure to nursing personnel from portable radiographic procedures. *Radiology Management*, *6*(2), 16.

Huda, W., & Gordon, K. (1986). Radiation risks to medical radiation technologists during pregnancy. *The Canadian Journal of Medical Radiation Technology*, *17*(3), 121.

International Commission on Radiation Protection. (1970). *Protection of the patient in x-ray diagnosis publication number 16*. Oxford: Pergamon Press.

Jeans, S. P., Faulkner, K., Love, H. G., & Bardsley, R. A. (1985). An investigation of the radiation dose to staff during cardiac radiological studies. *British Journal of Radiology*, *58*, 419–428.

Mahesh, M. (2009). NCRP Report Number 160: Its significance to medical imaging. *J. Am. Coll. Radiol*, *6(12)*, 890–892.

Miller, D. L., Vano, E., & Bartal, G. (2010). Occupational radiation protection in interventional radiology: A joint guideline of the Cardiovascular and Interventional Radiology Society of Europe and the Society of Interventional Radiology. *J. Vasc. Interv. Radiol.*, *21*, 607–615.

Minigh, J. (2005). Pediatric radiation protection. *Radiologic Technology*, *76(5)*, 365–378.

Mole, R. H. (1979). Radiation effects on pre-natal development and their radiological significance. *The British Journal of Radiology*, *52*(614), 89–101.

Mole, R. H. (1982). Consequences of pre-natal radiation exposure for post-natal development: A review. *International Journal of Radiation Biology*, *42*(1), 1–12.

Mole, R. H. (1984). The 10-day rule: A misnomer. *Radiography*, *50*(593), 229–230.

National Council on Radiation Protection and Measurements (NCRP). (1976). *Structural shielding design and evaluation for medical use of x rays and gamma rays of energies up to 10 mev* (NCRP Report No. 49). Bethesda, MD.

National Council on Radiation Protection and Measurements (NCRP). (1977). *Medical exposure of pregnant and potentially pregnant women* (NCRP Report No. 54). Bethesda, MD.

National Council on Radiation Protection and Measurements (NCRP). (1985). *SI units in radiation protection and measurements* (NCRP Report No. 82). Bethesda, MD.

National Council on Radiation Protection and Measurements (NCRP). (1987). *Ionizing radiation exposure of the population of the United States* (NCRP Report No. 93). Bethesda, MD.

National Council on Radiation Protection and Measurements (NCRP). (1989). *Medical x-ray, electron beam and gamma-ray protection for energies up to 50 mev (Equipment design, performance and use)* (NCRP Report No. 102). Bethesda, MD.

National Council on Radiation Protection and Measurements (NCRP). (1989). *Radiation protection for medical and allied health personnel* (NCRP Report No. 105). Bethesda, MD.

National Council on Radiation Protection and Measurements (NCRP). (1990). *Implementation of the principle of ALARA for medical and dental personnel* (NCRP Report No. 107). Bethesda, MD.

National Council on Radiation Protection and Measurements (NCRP). (1993). *Limitation of exposure to ionizing radiation* (NCRP Report No. 116). Bethesda, MD.

National Council on Radiation Protection and Measurements (NCRP). (1994). *Considerations regarding the unintended radiation exposure of the embryo, fetus or nursing child* (NCRP Commentary No. 9). Bethesda, MD.

National Council on Radiation Protection and Measurements (NCRP). (1998). *Radionuclide exposure of the embryo/fetus* (NCRP Report No. 128). Bethesda, MD.

National Council on Radiation Protection and Measurements (NCRP). (2000). *Radiation protection for procedures performed outside the radiology department* (NCRP Report No. 133). Bethesda, MD.

National Council on Radiation Protection and Measurements (NCRP). (2001). *Evaluation of the linear-nonthreshold dose-response model for ionizing radiation* (NCRP Report No. 136). Bethesda, MD.

National Council on Radiation Protection and Measurements (NCRP). (2009). *Ionizing Radiation Exposure of the Population of the United States* (NCRP Report No. 160). Bethesda, MD.

Noz, M. E., & Maguire, G. Q. (1985). *Radiation protection in the radiologic and health sciences* (2nd ed.). Philadelphia: Lea & Febiger.

Osborn, S. B. (1955). Radiation doses received by diagnostic x-ray workers. *British Journal of Radiology, 28*, 650–654.

Parkinson, L. (1991). Assessment of dose in computerised tomography. *Radiography Today, 57*(650), 23–28.

Ragozzino, M. W. (1986). Average fetal depth in utero: Data for estimation of fetal absorbed radiation dose. *Radiology, 158*(28), 513–515.

Seeram, E., & Travis, E. L. (1997). *Radiation protection.* Baltimore: Lippincott, Williams & Wilkins.

Shrimpton, P. (1994). Patient dose in CT and recommendations for reduction. *Radiography Today, 60*(683), 9–11.

Shrimpton, P. C. (1989). Monitoring the dose to patients undergoing common x-ray examinations. *Radiography Today, 54*(619), 38.

Stabin M. (2007). *Radiation protection and dosimetry: An introduction to health physics*. New York: Springer.

Statement from the 1985 Paris meeting of the International Commission on Radiological Protection. (1985, September). *Radiology.*

Stewart, A., & Kneale, G. W. (1970). Radiation dose effects in relation to obstetric x-rays and childhood leukemias. *Lancet, 1*, 1185–1188.

Wade, P. (1994). Science and practicalities of patient dose measurement procedures. *Radiography Today, 60*(681), 13–16.

Waldron, L., & Wade, J. (1992). Skin dose reduction as part of a regional x-ray dose assessment programme. *Radiography Today, 58*(659), 9–10.

Warner, R. (1993). Using technique factors to predict patient ESE. *Radiologic Technology, 65*(1), 21–26.

Young, A. T. (1986). Surface shield: Device to reduce personnel radiation exposure. *Radiology*, 801.

CHAPTER 10

Filtration

KEY TERMS

added filtration
compensating filter
compound filter
filter
half-value layer (HVL)
inherent filtration
K-edge filter
Thoreaus filter
total filtration
trough filter
wedge filter

the bones gleam out of the dark. like the ghost of a fern in stone here are spine and ribs.

Celia Gilbert, "X-Ray."

OBJECTIVES

Upon completion of this chapter, the student should be able to:

- Define filtration, inherent filtration, added filtration, compound filtration, compensating filtration, and total filtration.
- Explain the concept of half-value layer equivalency measurements of filtration.
- Appraise various types of filters for specific clinical situations.
- Describe the effect of filtration on the entire x-ray beam.

Filtration is the process of eliminating undesirable low-energy x-ray photons by the insertion of absorbing materials into the primary beam. When inserted properly, filtration permits the radiographer to shape the photon emission spectrum into a more useful beam. Filtration is sometimes called hardening the beam because it removes the low-energy (soft) photons (Figure 10-1). The primary reason for filtration is the elimination of photons that would cause increased radiation dose to the patient but would not enhance the radiographic image.

At 20 keV, about 45 percent of the incident photons will penetrate 1 cm of soft tissue but only about 0.0006 percent will penetrate 15 cm. At 50 keV, 3.5 percent of the incident photons (a significant percentage) will penetrate 15 cm. Significant soft tissue penetration occurs between 30 and 40 keV. Although they contribute to the patient dose, low-energy photons have insufficient energy to exit the patient and make any contribution to the image. Therefore, their elimination is desirable.

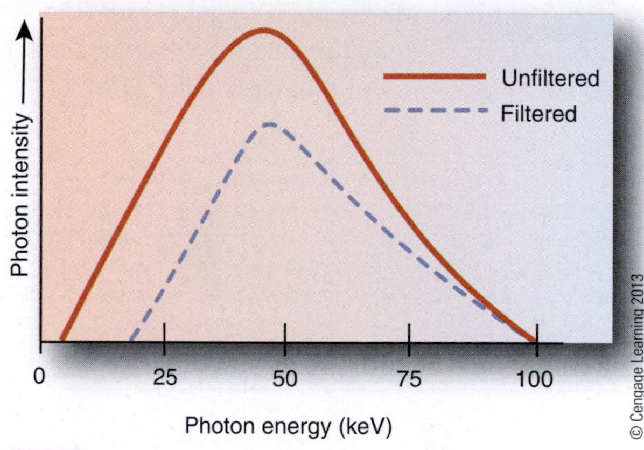

FIGURE 10-1. Effect of filtration on the x-ray beam.

MEASUREMENT

Any material designed to selectively absorb photons from the x-ray beam is called a **filter**. In diagnostic radiology, filtration is typically added between the source and the patient. Aluminum is the most common filter material used, although other materials, such as glass, oil, copper, and tin, are used as or become filters in various instances. **Aluminum is considered the standard filtering material and all filtration can be expressed in terms of the thickness of aluminum equivalency (Al/Eq).** For example, the attachments, mirror, and plastic of a collimator might be the equivalent of 0.5 mm of aluminum (Figure 10-2). This would be expressed as 0.5 mm Al/Eq.

Filtration is also expressed in terms of half-value layer. The **half-value layer (HVL)** is that amount of absorbing material that will reduce the intensity of the primary beam to one-half its original value. It is an indirect measure of the total filtration in the path of the x-ray beam. Half-value layers are usually expressed in terms of aluminum filtration equivalency; for example, HVL = 2.0 mm Al/Eq.

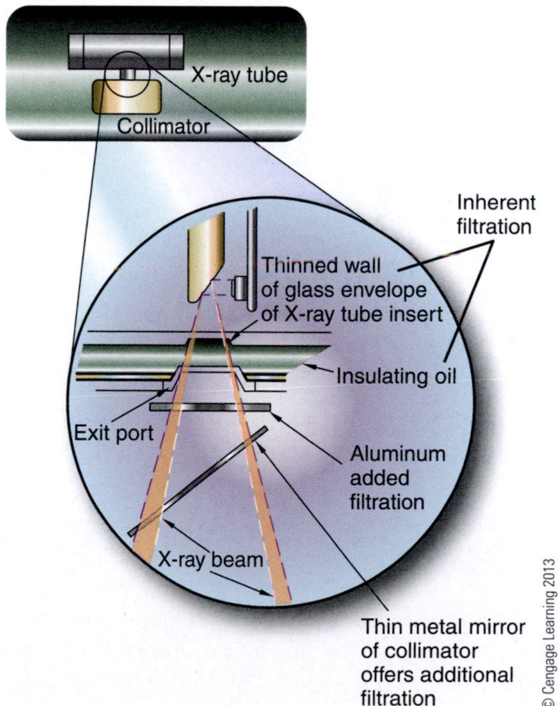

FIGURE 10-2. Total filtration of the x-ray beam.

The federal government specifies the minimum HVLs for all diagnostic x-ray tubes. Table 10-1 outlines this requirement as specified in Title 21 of the Code of Federal Regulations (21 CFR 1020.30).

TABLE 10-1. Minimum Half-Value Layer (HVL) Requirements for X-Ray Systems in United States (Title 21 of 21 CFR 1020.30)

X-Ray Tube Voltage (Kilovolt Peak)		
Designed operating range	Measured operating potential	Minimum HVL (mm of aluminum)
Below 51	30	0.3
	40	0.4
	50	0.5
51 to 70	51	1.2
	60	1.3
	70	1.5
Above 70	71	2.1
	80	2.3
	90	2.5
	100	2.7
	110	3.0
	120	3.2
	130	3.5
	140	3.8
	150	4.1

If the HVL is at the appropriate level, the total filtration in the x-ray tube is adequate to protect the patient from unnecessary radiation.

TYPES OF FILTRATION

Filtration occurs at various points between the x-ray tube and the image receptor. It is either *inherent* in the design of the tube or *added* between the tube and the image receptor.

Inherent Filtration

Filtration that is a result of the composition of the tube and housing is often called **inherent filtration** because it is a part of these structures. The thickness of the glass envelope of the tube, the dielectric oil that surrounds the tube, and the glass window of the housing all contribute to the inherent filtration. A typical x-ray tube might have a total inherent filtration of 0.5–1.0 mm Al/Eq. Most of the inherent filtration comes from the window of the glass envelope.

Because of this, mammographic tubes with special molybdenum targets that are designed to produce lower-energy photons for soft tissue imaging often have special beryllium (atomic number 4) windows in the glass envelope to eliminate the majority of the inherent filtration. Beryllium windows can reduce the inherent filtration to 0.1 mm Al/Eq (see Chapter 38).

As tubes age they become gassy, the anode begins to pit, and the glass envelope may gain a mild coating of vaporized metal. All of these factors will cause an increase in the inherent filtration, thus reducing the tube efficiency. This is the reason why HVL testing of tubes is a recommended quality control procedure for evaluation of tube efficiency and age.

Added Filtration

Any filtration that occurs outside the tube and housing and before the image receptor is considered **added filtration**. Filtration materials are selected to absorb as many low-energy photons as possible while transmitting a maximum number of high-energy photons. Aluminum, with an atomic number of 13, functions very well as a low-energy absorber.

The collimator device also adds filtration to the beam and is considered to be added filtration. Collimators average 1.0 mm Al/Eq, most of which comes from the silver on the mirror situated in the beam. The mirror is designed to reflect the collimator light to simulate the primary beam field size for positioning purposes. This addition to the inherent filtration is why mammographic units often do not use collimators. The filtering effect would cause absorption of the low-energy photons that are desirable for soft tissue imaging.

Compound Filtration

A **compound filter** uses two or more materials that complement one another in their absorbing abilities. Most compound filters are constructed so that each layer absorbs the characteristic photons created by the previous layer. For this reason, compound filters are also referred to as **K-edge filters**. Compound filters place the highest-atomic-number material closest to the tube and the lowest-atomic-number material closest to the patient. The final layer is usually aluminum, which has an atomic number of 13.

Although aluminum is the most common filtering material, copper, with an atomic number of 29, functions well for slightly higher energies. When a copper filter is used, it must be backed by an aluminum filter to absorb the 8-keV K-shell characteristic radiation produced by the copper. Copper filters should be at least 0.25 mm thick and backed with a minimum of 1 mm of aluminum.

A good example of a compound filter is the **Thoreaus filter** used in radiation therapy. This filter combines tin, copper, and aluminum, in that order. Tin has the highest atomic number (50) and is placed first in the beam. Next, a copper filter is added to absorb the 29.3-keV characteristic photons created by the tin. Finally, aluminum is added to the copper to absorb copper's characteristic photons, which would only contribute to increasing patient dose. The 1.5 keV K-shell characteristic radiation produced by the aluminum filter is absorbed in the air between the filter and the patient.

Compensation Filtration

A **compensating filter** is usually designed to solve a problem involving unequal subject densities. The goal is to add an absorber to compensate for unequal absorption within the subject, thus making the overall absorption of the primary beam more equal. This helps in producing a more uniform image receptor exposure. Compensating filters can be made of aluminum, leaded plastic trademarked under the name ClearPb™, or plastic. Even an ordinary saline solution bag can be a useful compensating filter.

The two most popular compensating filters are the **wedge filter** and the **trough filter** (sometimes called a double wedge). The thicker portions of the filter are matched to the less dense patient body parts (Figure 10-3). A wedge filter can be

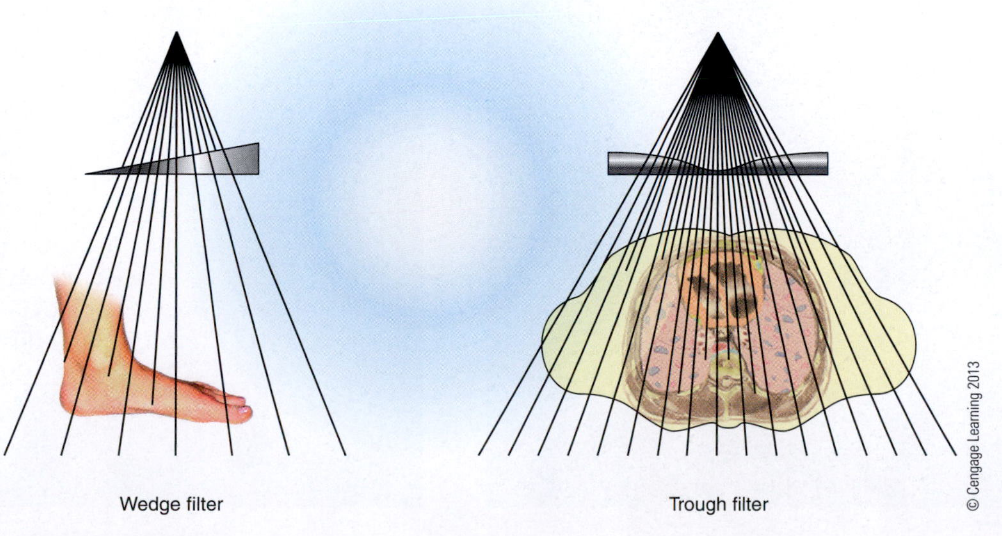

FIGURE 10-3. Compensating filters.

useful for procedures on the thoracic spine, the feet (Figure 10-4), and the lower extremities, particularly during venography and femoral angiography. A trough filter is useful to even the density differences between the mediastinum and the lungs on a chest radiograph.

It is also possible to custom design filters by several methods. Aluminum, ClearPb™, or plastic pieces may be attached by magnets or rods underneath the collimator to permit movement into or out of the primary beam. The advantage of the ClearPb™ is its ability to use the collimator light to project the filter position onto the patient's body. Some plastic filters, such as the boomerang filter, are designed to be placed under the patient. Radiologists may object to the use of compensating filters on the justifiable grounds that they cast artifacts onto the radiographic image.

Explorations have been made into the use of various heavy elements, including some of the rare earths, to utilize K-shell characteristic production to enhance energy ranges that are especially useful. For example, studies have been done using rare earths to increase photon emissions at the energies needed by iodine contrast agents. Difficulties in making these filtration techniques practical have kept them from becoming popular. However, very good results have been obtained for mammography by using a 0.05-mm molybdenum filter and operating the tube at a constant 35 kVp.

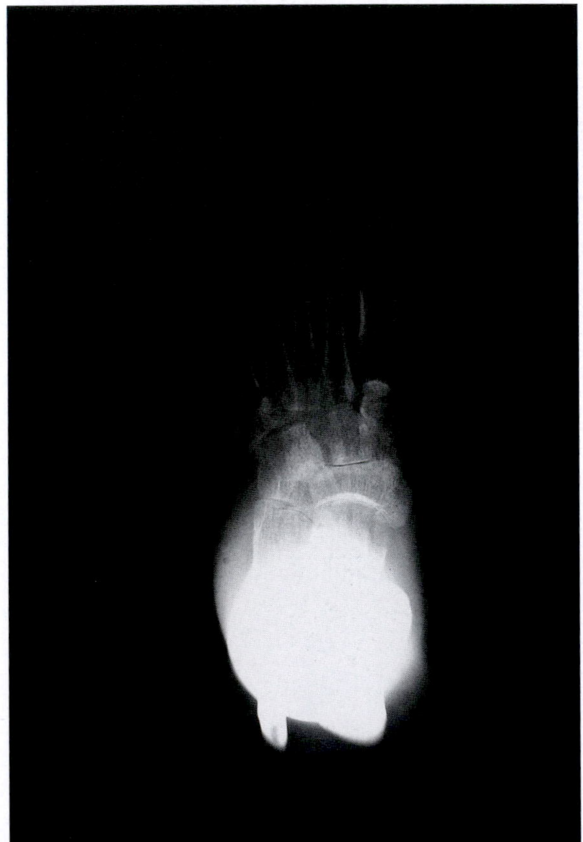

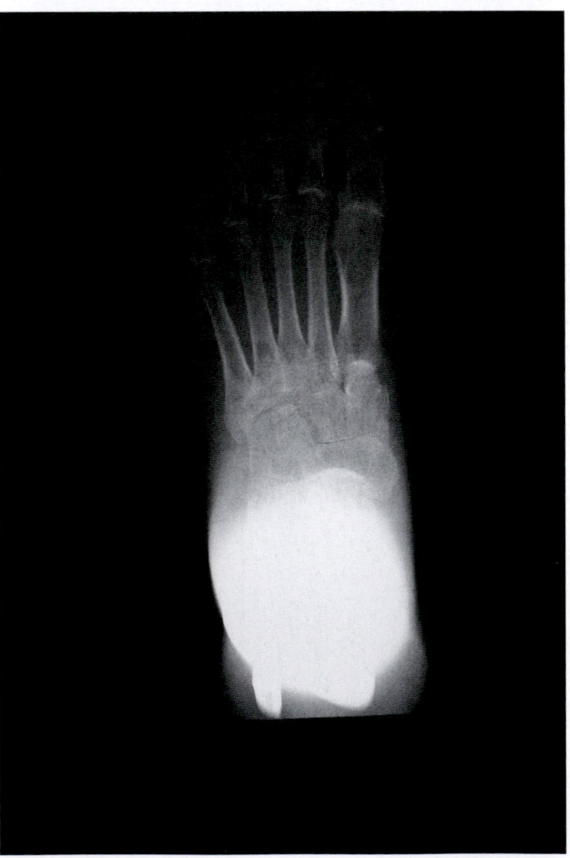

FIGURE 10-4. (A) Normal AP foot. (B) The use of a compensating wedge filter for an AP foot.

Total Filtration

Total filtration is equal to the sum of inherent and added filtration and does not include any compound or compensating filters that may be added later. The thickness of the added filtration varies depending on the anticipated uses of the equipment. The percentage of photons attenuated decreases as photon energy increases, even when filtration is increased (Table 10-2). Note that aluminum filters of 1–3 mm absorb significant percentages of photons below the diagnostic range while permitting the vast majority to pass. The National Council on Radiation Protection and Measurements (NCRP) recommends minimum total filtration levels for diagnostic radiography, as shown in Table 10-3. These filtration levels are commonly used in the United States and correspond to International Council on Radiation Protection (ICRP) recommendations. The importance of the reduction in patient dose, as shown in Table 10-4, must not be overlooked.

TABLE 10-2. Percent Attenuation of Monochromatic Radiation by Various Thicknesses of Aluminum Filtration

Photon Energy (keV)	Photons Attentuated (%)			
	1 mm	2 mm	3 mm	10 mm
10	100	100	100	100
20	58	82	92	100
30	24	42	56	93
40	12	23	32	73
50	8	16	22	57
60	6	12	18	48
80	5	10	14	39
100	4	8	12	35

Reproduced with permission from T. Curry, J. Dowdey, & R. Murry, 1990, *Christensen's Physics of Diagnostic Radiology*, 4th ed. Philadelphia: Lea and Febiger.

TABLE 10-3. Recommended Minimum Total Filtration Levels

Operating kVp	Total Filtration
Below 50 kVp	0.5 mm aluminum
50 to 70 kVp	1.5 mm aluminum
Above 70 kVp	2.5 mm aluminum

Adapted by permission from Table 3–1, National Council on Radiation Protection and Measurement, 1989, *NCRP Report No. 102, Medical X-Ray, Electron Beam and Gamma-Ray Protection for Energies Up to 50 MeV (Equipment Design, Performance and Use).* Bethesda, MD: NCRP.

EFFECT ON OUTPUT

Not only does filtration reduce the patient exposure dose by eliminating low-energy photons from the primary x-ray beam, it also removes a portion of the useful beam. This has a visible effect on radiographic film density. To compensate for the loss of exposure **when filtration is increased, technical factors must be increased to maintain the same image receptor exposure.**

Note that in Table 10-4 the decrease in patient dose compares very favorably with the increase necessary to maintain image receptor exposure. In other words, although the exposure needs to be increased to maintain exposure, there is a greater decrease in overall exposure to the patient.

Beyond 3.0-mm/Al filtration a point of diminishing returns is reached. The reduction in entrance skin exposure (ESE) does not warrant the tube loading increase.

TABLE 10-4. Comparison of Patient Exposure with Filtration

Aluminum Filtration in mm	Entrance Skin Exposure in mR	Decrease in Exposure Dose	Increase in Exposure Required to Maintain Same Exposure
60 KVP, 18 CM PELVIS			
none	2,380		
0.5	1,850	22%	14%
1.0	1,270	47%	17%
3.0	465	80%	52%
85 KVP, 18 CM PELVIS			
none	1,225		
0.5	860	30%	0%
1.0	684	44%	12%
3.0	287	77%	34%

From E. Dale Trout, J. P. Kelley, & G. A. Cathey, 1952, "The Use of Filters to Control Radiation Exposure to the Patient in Diagnostic Roentgenology," *American Journal of Roentgenology* 67, 942.

SUMMARY

Filtration is the process of eliminating undesirable x-ray photons by the insertion of absorbing materials into the primary beam. Any material designed to selectively absorb photons from the x-ray beam is called a filter. Aluminum is the most common filter material used. It is considered the standard filter material and all filtering in diagnostic radiography can be expressed in terms of the thickness of aluminum equivalency (Al/Eq). The half-value layer (HVL) is that amount of absorbing material that will reduce the intensity of the primary beam to one-half its original value.

Filtration occurs at various points between the x-ray tube and the image receptor. It is either inherent in the design of the x-ray tube or added between the tube and the image receptor. Filtration that is the result of the composition of the tube and housing is often called inherent filtration because it is a part of these structures. Any filtration that occurs outside the tube and housing and before the image receptor is considered added filtration. The collimator device adds approximately 1.0 Al/Eq to the beam.

The compound filter uses two or more materials that complement one another in their absorbing ability. A compensating filter is usually designed to solve a problem involving unequal subject density. Two common compensating filters are the wedge and the trough. Total filtration is equal to the sum of inherent and added filtration.

Not only does filtration reduce the patient exposure by eliminating low-energy photons, it also removes a portion of the useful beam and can therefore affect image receptor exposure. ■

REVIEW QUESTIONS

1. What is filtration?
2. What is the standard filter material used in diagnostic radiography?
3. Define half-value layer.
4. What is inherent filtration?
5. When more than one filtering material is used, as in a compound filter, how are the materials arranged in relationship to the x-ray source?
6. What are the two most common compensating filters?
7. What is total filtration?
8. How does filtration affect patient dose and beam intensity?

REFERENCES AND RECOMMENDED READING

Burns, C. B., & Renner, J. B. (1994). Molybdenum/aluminum filters perform effectively. *Radiologic Technology, 64*(4), 216–219.

Bushberg, J. T., Seibert, J. A., Leidholdt, E. M., & Boone, J. M. (2003). *The essential physics of medical imaging* (2nd ed.). Philadelphia: Lippincott, Williams & Wilkins.

Bushong, S. C. (2008). *Radiologic science for technologists: Physics, biology, and protection* (9th ed.). St. Louis, MO: Elsevier Mosby.

Carroll, Q. B. (2007). *Practical radiographic imaging (Fuch's radiographic exposure processing & quality control)* (8th ed.). Springfield, IL: Charles C Thomas.

Curry, T. S., Dowdey, J. E., & Murry, R. C. (1990). *Christensen's introduction to the physics of diagnostic radiology* (4th ed.). Philadelphia: Lea and Febiger.

Dendy, P. P., & Heaton, B. (1999). *Physics for diagnostic radiology* (2nd ed.). Bristol, England: Institute of Physics.

Dilella, D., & Albert, H. (1964). Variable thickness filters for use with 14 × 36 inch film. *Radiologic Technology, 36*(1), 1.

Ekstrand, K. E. (1979). The inverse compensating filter. *Radiology,* 201.

Feczko, P. J. (1983, December). Compensation filtration for decubitus radiography during double-contrast barium enema examination. *Radiology,* 848.

Geissberger, H. (1966). Wedge-shaped filters for improved radiography of the thoracic vertebrae and the foot. *Medical Radiography and Photography, 42*(1), 6.

Gray, J. E., Stears, J. G., & Frank, E. D. (1983). Shaped, lead-loaded acrylic filters for patient exposure reduction and image-quality improvement. *Radiology, 146,* 825–828.

Hart, J. D., Drake, P. A., & Schmugge, M. L. (1986). Plexiglas filtration in cervicocerebrae. *Applied Radiology, 15*(6), 148.

Irvin, R. (1962). Selective filtration: Effect on patient dose and radiographic quality. *Radiologic Technology, 34*(2), 51.

Jacobi, C. A. (1968). Radiation safety: More than filtration. *Radiologic Technology, 40*(2), 97.

James, N. (1983). High kilovoltage radiography using the Cincinnati filter. *Radiography, 49* (585), 210.

Jones, R., & McKenna, A. (1989). The use of saline as a compensating filter. *Radiologic Technology, 62*(2), 134–138.

Kassebaum, M. K. (1949). The use of compensating filters. *Radiologic Technology, 20*(4), 209.

Kelsey, C. A. (1986). Chest radiographs obtained with shaped filters: Evaluation by observer performance test. *Radiology,* 653.

McEnerney, P. (1951). The value of compensating filters in roentgenography including the double filter technique. *Radiologic Technology, 23*(1), 29.

National Council on Radiation Protection and Measurements (NCRP). (1989). *NCRP Report No. 102: Medical X-ray, electron beam and gamma-ray protection for energies up to 50 MeV (equipment design, performance and use).* Bethesda, MD: Author.

Stears, J. G., Gray, J. E., Webbles, W. E., & Frank, E. D. (1986). The variable filter dial. *Radiologic Technology, 57*(6), 542.

Trout, E. D., Kelley, J. P., & Cathey, G. A. (1952). The use of filters to control radiation exposure to the patient in diagnostic roentgenology. *American Journal of Roentgenology, 67,* 946–963.

United States Department of Health and Human Services, Food and Drug Administration, Code of Federal Regulations Title 21 CFR 1020.30.

Wilks, R. J. (2003). *Principles of radiological physics* (4th ed.). Edinburgh: Churchill Livingstone.

Wolbarst, A. B., & Cook, G. (2005). *Physics of radiology* (2nd ed.). Madison: Medical Physics Publishing.

CHAPTER 11

The Prime Factors

KEY TERMS

15 percent rule
direct square law
exposure maintenance formula
milliamperage (mA)
milliamperage-second (mAs)
penetrability
prime factor
reciprocity law
x-ray quality
x-ray quantity

> X-ray technic, like x-ray equipment, has passed through an evolutionary stage from the beginning, in 1896, to the present time, and the end is not yet in sight.
>
> *E. C. Jerman, 1926*

OBJECTIVES

Upon completion of this chapter, the student should be able to:

- Explain the relationships between milliamperage (mA), exposure time, mAs, and x-ray emission.
- State the reciprocity law.
- Calculate mAs when given mA and exposure time, mA when given mAs and exposure time, and exposure time when given mAs and mA.
- Explain the relationship between kVp and x-ray emission.
- State the 15 percent rule.
- Calculate the new kVp value needed to maintain density/ image receptor exposure when changes are made in mAs, using the 15 percent rule.
- Explain the relationship between distance and x-ray emission.
- State the inverse square law.
- Calculate x-ray emission (mR) when distance is changed.
- Calculate the mAs needed to maintain density/ image receptor exposure when changes are made in distance, using the exposure (density) maintenance formula.

THE PRIME FACTORS

The emission of x-ray photons from an x-ray tube is controlled by a number of factors. Those factors related to tube design and construction have been covered in previous chapters and include tube housing, target material, filtration, and voltage waveform. Three principal factors that affect x-ray emission are under the direct control of the radiographer. These are called the **prime factors**. They are milliamperage-second (mAs), kilovoltage (kVp), and distance (d).

The x-ray beam can be described in terms of both its quantity and its quality. **X-ray quantity** is a measure of the number of x-ray photons in the useful beam. It is also called x-ray output, intensity, or exposure. Recall that the unit of measurement of x-ray quantity is the *roentgen (R)*. The factors that directly affect x-ray quantity are milliamperage-second (mAs), kilovoltage (kVp), distance (d), and filtration. **X-ray quality** is a measurement of the penetrating ability of the x-ray beam. Penetrability describes the distance an x-ray beam travels in matter. High-energy x-ray photons travel farther in matter than low-energy photons and are therefore more penetrating. Highly penetrating x-rays are termed hard x-rays and low-penetrating x-rays are called soft x-rays. X-ray quality is numerically represented by the half-value layer (HVL). The half-value layer of an x-ray beam is that thickness of absorbing material needed to reduce the x-ray intensity (quantity) to half its original value. The factors that directly affect x-ray quality are kilovoltage and filtration.

The factors that control the quantity and/or quality of x-ray emission are the prime factors and filtration (Table 11-1). Filtration is not something the radiographer controls from exposure to exposure.

TABLE 11-1. Factors Affecting X-Ray Emission

Quantitative Factors	Qualitative Factors
Milliamperage-second	Kilovoltage
Kilovoltage	Filtration
Distance	
Filtration	

MILLIAMPERAGE-SECOND (MAS)

Milliamperage (mA) is a measurement of x-ray tube current—the number of electrons crossing the tube from cathode to anode per second. Recall that an ampere is equal to an electric charge of 1 coulomb flowing through a conductor per second. The coulomb is equal to 6.3×10^{18} electron charges. Therefore, an ampere equals a flow of 6.3×10^{18} electrons per second and a milliampere would equal 6.3×10^{15} electrons per second. As mA increases, so does the number of electrons that are able to cross the tube to reach the x-ray target. **Milliamperage is directly proportional to tube current.** As the mA doubles, so does the number of electrons able to cross the tube. The number of electrons reaching the target is also controlled by the length of time the tube is energized. Remember that mA is the number of electrons **per second.** This means that changes in the length of time of exposure will affect the total number of electrons flowing from cathode to anode. X-ray exposure time is measured in *seconds*. Generally, exposure times are less than one second and these values may be expressed in decimals, fractions, or milliseconds (ms). Like mA, **exposure time is directly proportional to the number of electrons crossing the tube and is therefore directly proportional to the number of x-rays created.** This is the x-ray quantity.

The number of x-rays that will be created at the target is a product of the number of electrons crossing the tube (tube current) and how long the electrons are allowed to cross (exposure time). **Milliamperage-second (mAs)** is the unit used to describe the product of tube current and exposure time. This simple relationship is described by the equation mA $\times$ s = mAs. Milliamperage-second (mAs) is the primary controller of x-ray quantity. X-ray quantity is directly proportional to mAs. This means that as mAs doubles, x-ray exposure (measured in roentgens) doubles; as mAs triples, x-ray exposure triples, and so forth.

If an x-ray control panel is set at 100 mA and 0.05 (1/20 or 50 ms) second, the mAs would be 100 $\times$ 0.05 or 5 mAs. If either the mA or the exposure time is doubled, the mAs will double, that is, 200 mA at 0.05 second equals 10 mAs, as does 100 mA at 0.1 (1/10 or 100 ms) second. This means that numerous possible settings on the x-ray control can all yield the same x-ray exposure. For example, 10 mAs can be set using any of the following technical factors:

50 mA × 0.2 (1/5 or 200 ms) second = 10 mAs
100 mA × 0.1 (1/10 or 100 ms) second = 10 mAs
200 mA × 0.05 (1/20 or 50 ms) second = 10 mAs

Obviously, numerous other possibilities exist as well. Because mA and exposure time can be manipulated to achieve the same mAs, **it is best to think in terms of mAs when establishing technical factors.** It is important, for technical factor conversions, that the technologist be able to manipulate the mA and time to arrive at the proper mAs for a particular examination.

EXAMPLES: Given the following mA and exposure time values, calculate the mAs.

200 mA × 0.083 second = ____ mAs
100 mA × 2/5 second = ____ mAs
300 mA × 200 ms = _____ mAs

Answers:

200 mA × 0.083 second = 16.6 mAs
100 mA × 2/5 second = 40 mAs
300 mA × 200 ms = 60 mAs

EXAMPLES: Given the following mAs and mA values, calculate the exposure time.

75 mAs = 100 mA × ______ second
15 mAs = 300 mA × ______ second

Answers:

75 mAs = 100 mA × 0.75 (3/4 or 750 ms) second
15 mAs = 300 mA × 0.05 (1/20 or 50 ms) second

EXAMPLES: Given the following mAs and exposure time values, calculate the mA.

60 mAs = 0.3 (3/10 or 300 ms) second × _____ mA
75 mAs = 0.15 (3/20 or 150 ms) second × ______ mA

(continues)

(continued)

Answers:

60 mAs = 0.3 (3/10 or 300 ms) second × 200 mA
75 mAs = 0.15 (3/20 or 150 ms) second × 500 mA

Density/Image Receptor (IR) Exposure Relationship to mAs

Radiographic density is the degree of blackening of an x-ray film. It is created by deposits of black metallic silver within the emulsion of an x-ray film that has been exposed to light or x-ray and then processed. On the resulting radiographic image, the densities are the direct result of an x-ray exposure to the film and intensifying screens (image receptors). In a film/screen imaging environment, density was the term that was routinely used to express the impact of IR exposure to the film. In a digital imaging environment, film is not the receptor of the image. A digital image receptor is a filmless way of recording the image that is then displayed on a monitor for viewing. Although the term *density* might be used to describe the level of brightness on the monitor (how light or dark the image is), the relationship of this brightness level does not correspond to the IR exposure. Brightness on the monitor is controlled separately and is the better term to use when describing how light or dark an image on a monitor appears. When film is not used, the key relationship becomes simply the IR exposure and the term *density* is better used when discussing the amount of silver deposited in a hard-copy film image.

With a digital imaging system, exposure to the IR must be assessed by reviewing a numeric exposure value. These values vary from vendor to vendor (i.e., S number, exposure index), and it is critical to understand and assess these values for every image. There is a definite relationship between these exposure value numbers and the IR exposure. If these numbers are outside of the acceptable range provided by the vendor then the image has been under- or overexposed and most vendors recommend repeating exposures when images are not within the acceptable ranges. Digital systems do not automatically correct for a radiographer's error in selecting an appropriate mAs. Recall that as mAs is increased, x-ray exposure will increase proportionally. Regardless of the type of image receptor being used, insufficient mAs will result in an underexposed image and excessive mAs will cause an overexposed image.

Most radiography departments have moved or will most likely move to a digital imaging environment in the future. Because film/screen systems are still in use, there is still a need to understand both systems. Details of both systems are presented in future chapters.

Whereas the relationship between mAs and IR exposure (mR) is a directly proportional one, the relationship of these two factors to film density is much more complex. Film density is determined by the amount of silver deposition in the emulsion due to the film type, exposure conditions, exposure (mR), and processing. It is measured numerically using a densitometer. A DlogE sensitometric curve expresses the relationship between exposure and density, with log relative exposure plotted on the x-axis and density (D) plotted on the y-axis. The relationship between exposure and density determines the shape and position of the DlogE curve for a given film under specific processing conditions. This relationship is described in detail in Chapter 21, Film Sensitometry.

If the exposure to a film is increased, the density to that film will increase until the point where the film reaches its maximum density (D_{max}). Because density is primarily determined by the amount of exposure a film receives, and because exposure is directly proportional to mAs, **mAs is used as the primary controller of radiographic film density and image receptor exposure.** As mAs increases, x-ray exposure increases proportionally and radiographic density also increases. The direct proportional relationship between mAs and exposure is used to calculate mAs changes necessary to maintain consistent film density/IR exposure when one or more technical factors are altered.

The relationship of a film's reaction to exposure was described in 1875 by Bunsen and Roscoe, who studied the reaction of photographic film to light and stated that the reaction of a photographic film to light is equal to the product of the intensity of the light and the duration of the exposure. This concept is known as the **reciprocity law**. When applied to x-rays, the reciprocity law can be restated as the density/IR exposure should remain unchanged as long as the intensity and duration of the x-ray exposure (controlled by mAs) remains unchanged.

Radiographic film density should remain unchanged as long as the total exposure to the film remains unchanged. If the mAs used to create one image is the same as the mAs used to create a second image of the same structure, then both images should have the same film density. As long as mAs is constant, any combination of mA and exposure time values will create the same density/IR exposure. The radiographs in Figures 11-1A and 11-1B illustrate this point. Remember, accurate results will depend on using equipment that is properly calibrated. Equipment testing is an important part of a quality control program for the radiology department.

Radiographic film density will increase to D_{max} when mAs increases and will decrease to near zero when mAs decreases. Either the mA or the exposure time or both may be increased or decreased to cause an increase or decrease in the mAs. The radiographs in Figure 11-1B and Figure 11-1C illustrate this point. When mAs is increased, the density on the film is increased. The resulting film is darker than the original. If the mAs is reduced by half, the resulting film will be lighter than the original image. Using a digital imaging system, these changes would not likely be evident on the monitor; post-processing can adjust the image so that it will display on the monitor as if the image were properly exposed. Post-processing is not designed to be used to correct poor exposures. This is why evaluating the numeric exposure value is critical.

Whether in a digital or film/screen environment, milliamperage-second (mAs) is the primary controlling factor that will affect the x-ray quantity and the resultant density/IR exposure. The appropriate mAs should be selected to achieve an acceptable radiographic image. The radiographer is usually in control of the mAs selection. However, the equipment may exert automatic control when the radiographer is using an automatic exposure control system, a computerized exposure system, or falling-load generators.

60 kVp	3.2 mAs	40" SID
No grid	400 RS	5.10 mR

A

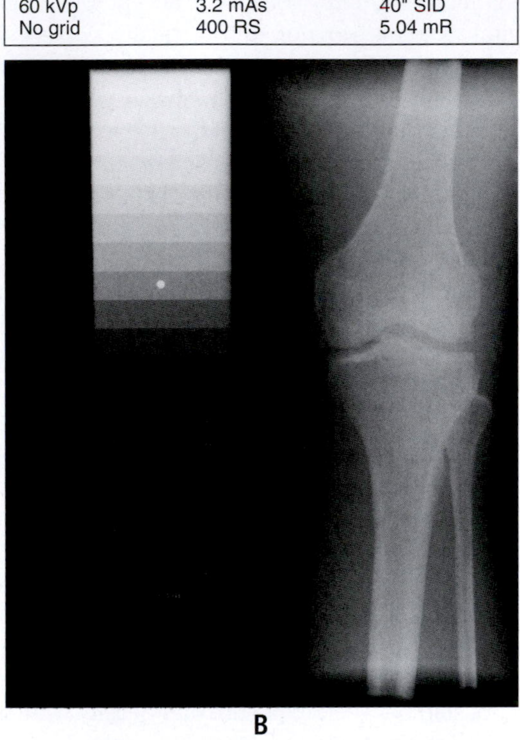

C

60 kVp	6.4 mAs	40" SID
No grid	400 RS	10.20 mR

FIGURE 11-1. These three radiographs demonstrate the effect of mAs on radiographic film density. Although the mA and time may vary, if the mAs remains unchanged, then radiographic film density will be the same. A and B have the same mAs although A was exposed at 80 mA and 0.04 sec, whereas B was exposed at 160 mA and 0.02 sec. When the mAs is doubled, the exposure to the film doubles (C). *(Radiographs courtesy of Arlene Adler and Richard R. Carlton.)*

KILOVOLTAGE (KVP)

Kilovoltage (kVp) controls both the quantity and quality of the x-ray beam. **Increasing the kilovoltage on an x-ray control panel will cause an increase in the speed and energy of the electrons applied across the x-ray tube.** The space charge compensator corrects for the increase in speed of the electrons to maintain a constant number of electrons/second. The increased energy of the electrons results in the production of x-ray photons with greater energy. As x-ray photon energy increases, the penetrating ability of the photon increases. Kilovoltage affects the *quantity* of the x-ray beam because **more** interactions occur at the target as kVp increases, and it affects the *quality* of the x-ray beam because each electron has more energy, resulting in a beam with greater **penetrability**.

The quantity (intensity) of x-ray photons increases very quickly with increases in kVp. X-ray quantity is **approximately** directly proportional to the square of the ratio of the change in kVp. This means that as kVp is doubled, the amount of x-ray photons increases approximately four times. Although this can be mathematically expressed, this formula would have no practical application because it does not take into account the fact that changes in kVp have a significant effect on the penetrability of the beam.

Density/IR Exposure Relationship to kVp

Both the quantity and quality of the x-ray beam will vary significantly with changes in the kilovoltage applied across the x-ray tube. As a result, kVp has a tremendous impact on radiographic density (Figures 11-2A and 11-2B). In addition, because changes in kilovoltage create changes in beam penetrability, kVp is the primary controller of the differences in densities/IR exposures. This is known as contrast. An increase in kVp causes an increase in penetrability, which will result in an image with less contrast. For the present discussion, the effect of kVp on density/IR exposure will be detailed. Contrast is discussed in Chapter 27.

Research was done to determine a practical formula to take into account kVp's effect on both x-ray quantity and quality. This resulted in the **15 percent rule**. The intent of this rule was to provide a guide for radiographers to maintain exposure to the image receptor when kVp is changed. For film/screen image receptors, this will maintain radiographic film density. **The 15 percent rule states that an increase in kVp by 15 percent will cause a doubling in exposure, the same effect as doubling the mA or doubling exposure time.** The reverse is also true. If kVp is decreased by 15 percent, exposure will be reduced by one-half. If maintaining the exposure is desired, decreasing the kVp by 15 percent should be accompanied by a doubling of the mAs (see Figure 11-2B and Figure 11-2C), and increasing kVp should be accompanied by cutting the mAs in half. Because both the amount and penetrability of x-ray photons increase with increases in kVp, the effect of changes in kVp will vary from low kVps to high kVps. In other words, a smaller change in kVp will have a greater impact on x-ray emission in the lower-kVp ranges than in the higher-kVp ranges. For example, 15 percent of 40 kVp is 6, whereas 15 percent of 80 kVp is 12. Exposure will nearly double when kVp is changed from 40 to 46 kVp. At 80 kVp, an increase in 12 kVp is needed to approximately double the exposure.

EXAMPLE: A radiograph of the pelvis is produced using 25 mAs at 70 kVp. What kVp would be needed to double the exposure?

Answer:

15 percent of 70 kVp = 10.5 kVp
70 + 10.5 = 80.5 or 81 kVp

EXAMPLE: An acceptable radiograph of the knee is produced using 10 mAs at 60 kVp. If the kVp is increased by 15 precent to 69 kVp, what mAs would be needed to maintain the exposure?

Answer:

Half of 10 mAs, or 5 mAs

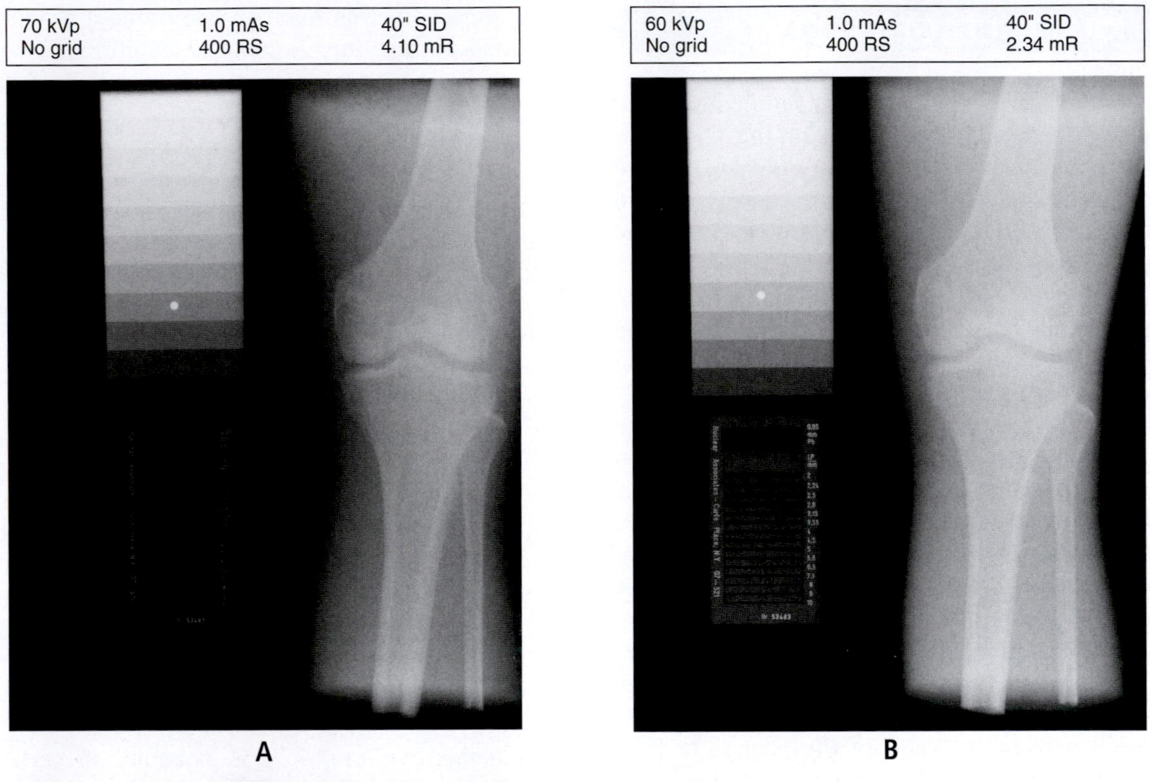

C

60 kVp No grid 2.0 mAs 400 RS 40" SID 4.42 mR

FIGURE 11-2. These three radiographs demonstrate the effect of decreasing kVp on radiographic film density. A and B show the effect of increasing kVp on film density. In C, density and exposure are maintained by applying the 15 percent rule.

Because kVp is expressed as a whole number, answers should be rounded to the nearest whole number.

Although kVp has a tremendous impact on exposure to the image receptor and therefore on film density, **kVp adjustments should not be used to control density/IR exposure.** The selection of a kVp range for specific radiographic procedures is determined by the desired contrast for the image. This is discussed in Unit IV.

DISTANCE

The intensity of x-rays varies greatly with changes in distance. Just as the intensity of light from a light bulb will decrease the further one moves from the source, so will x-ray photons spread out from their source at the x-ray tube target. As a result, the x-ray intensity will decrease as the distance from the tube is increased. The measurement of the x-ray intensity is obtained using a dosimeter. X-ray intensity (exposure) is measured in roentgens (R) or, more commonly in diagnostic radiology, in milliroentgens (mR).

From the point of origin of the x-ray beam at the tube target, the beam begins to diverge. The x-ray photons are most concentrated at the target and from there they spread out in all directions. Those photons that exit the tube port constitute the primary, useful beam. As the useful beam spreads and widens, x-ray intensity or quantity begins to diminish. The actual number of photons created remains unchanged but the distribution of the photons varies with the distance. The farther from their source, the lower will be the quantity of photons within a given area.

The relationship of x-ray quantity to distance is described in the inverse square law. **The inverse square law states that the intensity of radiation at a given distance from the point source is inversely proportional to the square of the distance.** The inverse square law requires an understanding of some basic rules of geometry. In Figure 11-3 the diverging lines represent the x-ray beam diverging from a collimated source. At a distance of 36 inches (D_1), the x-ray beam covers a square area (abcd). Each side has a given dimension (x) so the area of square abcd would equal x times x, or x^2. If the distance is increased to 72 inches (D_2), the sides of the second square (ABCD) are now twice as long, or 2x. The area of square ABCD would be 2x times 2x, or $4x^2$. A doubling of the distance has increased the area of the square by four times.

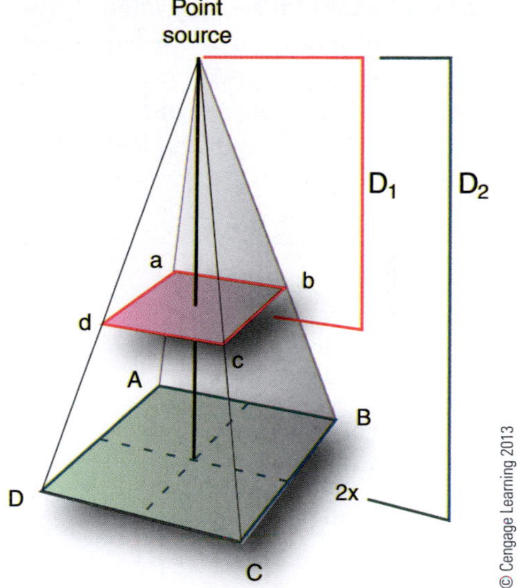

FIGURE 11-3. The inverse square law states that the intensity of radiation at a given distance from a point source is inversely proportional to the square of the distance. The lower surface area (ABCD) is twice as far from the source of radiation and is four times (2^2) the surface area of the upper surface area (abcd).

X-ray photons falling in square abcd are spread out over an area four times as large by the time it reaches square ABCD. The number of photons remains the same, but they are now spread over an area four times larger. A dosimeter in square abcd would measure four times more than a dosimeter in square ABCD. For example, if a dosimeter in square abcd measures 100 mR, a dosimeter in square ABCD would measure 25 mR, or four times less.

Thus, the intensity or quantity of photons decreases with increased distance for a given area, which is an inverse relationship. More specifically, the relationship is inversely proportional to the square of the distance change. If the distance increases by a factor of three, the intensity, in mR, would decrease by a factor of 3^2, or nine times.

The inverse square law can be used to calculate changes in intensity that occur as a result of changes in distance. The mathematical expression of the law is:

$$\frac{I_1}{I_2} = \frac{D_2^{\,2}}{D_1^{\,2}}$$

where: I_1 = original intensity (mR)
I_2 = new intensity (mR)
D_1 = original distance
D_2 = new distance

The formula can also be expressed as:

$$I_1D_1^{\,2} = I_2D_2^{\,2}$$

In order to calculate any of the four factors, three of the four must be known. The equation can then be rearranged to place the unknown factor alone on one side of the equal sign.

EXAMPLE: An x-ray exposure of 240 mR is recorded at a distance of 20 inches. If the same technical factors are used, what will the exposure be if the distance is increased to 40 inches?

Answer:

$$\frac{240}{I_2} = \frac{40^2}{20^2}$$

$$I_2 = \frac{240 \times 20^2}{40^2}$$

$$I_2 = \frac{240 \times 400}{1{,}600}$$

$$I_2 = 60 \text{ mR}$$

EXAMPLE: An x-ray exposure of 400 mR is recorded at a distance of 72 inches. If the same technical factors are used, what will the exposure be if the distance is decreased to 40 inches?

(continues)

(continued)

Answer:

$$\frac{400}{I_2} = \frac{40^2}{72^2}$$

$$I_2 = \frac{400 \times 72^2}{40^2}$$

$$I_2 = \frac{400 \times 5{,}184}{1{,}600}$$

$$I_2 = 1{,}296 \text{ mR}$$

The inverse square law should be used when calculating the relationships between distance and x-ray intensity (mR).

Density/IR Exposure Relationship to Distance

Because distance has an effect on x-ray intensity, it will in turn affect density/IR exposure. **As the distance increases, intensity decreases, which causes a decrease in IR exposure** (Figures 11-4A and 11-4B). For film/screen image receptors, this will decrease film density. The reverse is also true. As the distance decreases, intensity and IR exposure increases, which in turn causes an increase in film density.

A practical application of the inverse square law is found in a formula that is used to compensate for the IR exposure changes that occur when distance is changed. The formula is sometimes known as the **exposure maintenance formula** and is based on the principle of the inverse square law. This formula is a **direct square law**. A direct relationship is necessary to compensate for the changes in intensity and IR exposure.

Because mAs is the primary controller of x-ray intensity and IR exposure, mAs can be adjusted to compensate for changes in distance. For example, an acceptable chest image results from an exposure taken using four mAs at 100 kVp at a 72-inch distance. A second image must be taken supine at a 36-inch distance. If the same technical factors are used, the inverse square law tells us that when the distance is decreased by a factor of 2, the intensity (exposure) will increase by a factor of 4. The second image

60 kVp	2 mAs	36" SID
No grid	400 RS	5.64 mR

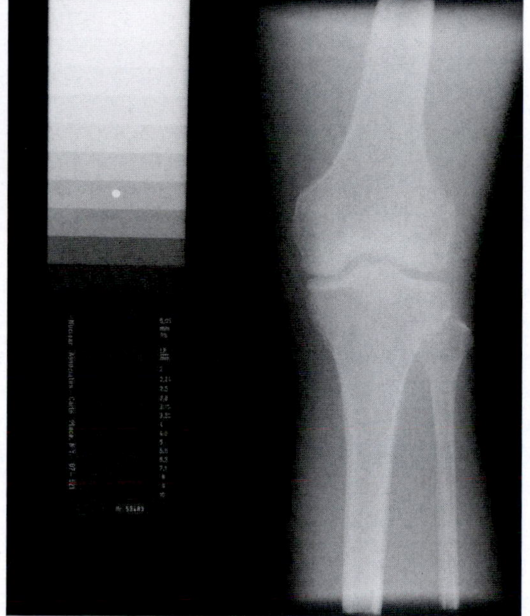

A

60 kVp	2.0 mAs	72" SID
No grid	400 RS	1.21 mR

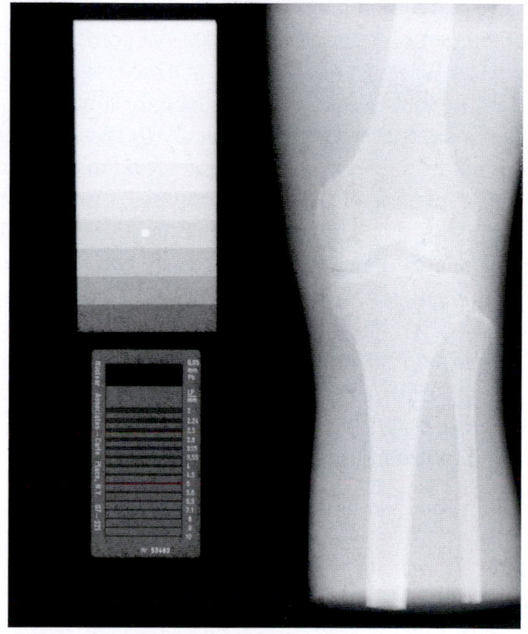

B

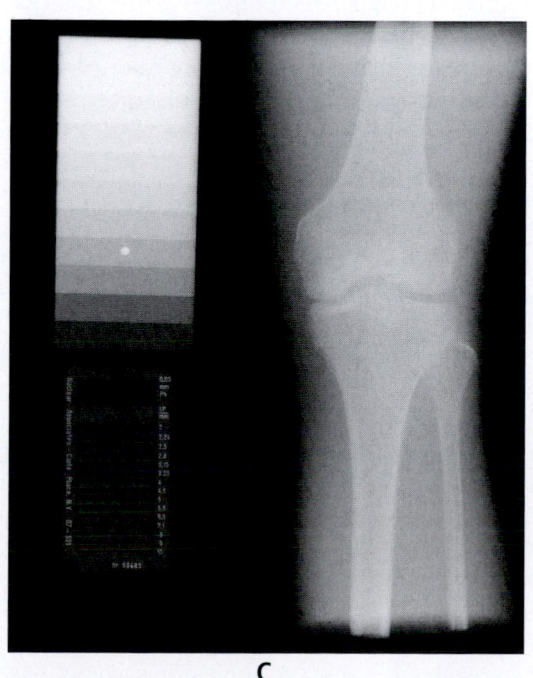

C

60 kVp	8 mAs	72" SID
No grid	400 RS	6.02 mR

FIGURE 11-4. These three radiographs demonstrate the effect of distance on radiographic film density. A and B show the effect of increasing distance on film density. In C, density and exposure are maintained by applying the exposure (film density) maintenance direct square law. *(Radiographs courtesy of Arlene Adler and Richard R. Carlton.)*

will be overexposed if the technical factors are not adjusted. The mAs can be adjusted to compensate for the distance change. The exposure maintenance formula can be used to determine the compensation necessary for any change in distance (see Figure 11-4B and Figure 11-4C). It is a direct square law because mAs should increase proportionally to the square of the change when distance increases, and mAs should decrease proportionally to the square of the change when distance is decreased. In the previous example, if the distance decreases by a factor of two (72 inches to 36 inches), the mAs should be reduced by a factor of 2^2, or 4. The new mAs would be 1/4 the original, or one mAs. Four mAs at 72 inches will produce the same exposure as 1 mAs at 36 inches, provided all other factors remain the same.

The exposure maintenance formula is:

$$\frac{mAs_1}{mAs_2} = \frac{D_1^2}{D_2^2}$$

where: mAs_1 = original mAs
mAs_2 = new mAs
D_1 = original distance
D_2 = new distance

The same formula can be expressed as:

$$mAs_2 = \frac{mAs_1 \times D_2^2}{D_1^2}$$

These formulas have very direct applications to radiography because they provide the radiographer with a means for adjusting mAs to maintain density/IR exposure when changes are made in distance for a given radiographic procedure. Remember that there is no relationship between distance and mAs; changes in distance do not cause changes in mAs. The radiographer must adjust the mAs to compensate for distance changes.

EXAMPLE: An acceptable radiograph of the abdomen is taken using 25 mAs at 80 kVp at a distance of 40 inches. A second radiograph is requested to be taken at 56 inches. What mAs should be used to produce an acceptable radiograph if the distance is increased to 56 inches?

(continues)

(continued)

Answer:

$$mAs_2 = \frac{25 \times 56^2}{40^2}$$

$$mAs_2 = \frac{25 \times 3{,}136}{1{,}600}$$

$$mAs_2 = 49 \text{ mAs}$$

Changes in distance will create changes in the x-ray intensity and the image receptor exposure. The exposure maintenance formula can be used to compensate for the effect that changes in distance will have on the image receptor exposure of the radiographic image. The radiographs of Figures 11-4A and C demonstrate the application of the direct square law for exposure maintenance.

IMAGE QUALITY FACTORS

With digital image detector systems, the traditional relationship that existed with film/screen imaging between the image quality properties of density and contrast to mAs, kVp, and distance does not exist. It is possible to change the mAs, kVp, and distance and have no effect on the brightness or contrast on the display monitor. This topic is covered in more detail in Unit IV that discusses image analysis. In digital image receptor systems, density and contrast are controlled primarily through post-processing parameters.

Despite the ability to control density and contrast through post-processing parameters, it is still critical to provide the digital image receptor with an appropriate exposure for a given procedure. Digital image receptors can respond to a wide range of exposures, from as low as 0.01 mR up to 100 mR. Extremely low and extremely high exposures do not produce acceptable image quality. Most acceptable images can be produced using approximately 1-mR exposure to the receptor. Manufacturers often establish exposure indicator systems based on this fact.

Setting the appropriate mAs, kVp, and distance is the responsibility of the radiographer.

These prime factors control the exposure to the image receptor. The radiographer should select the kVp based on the desired contrast, and adjust mAs to provide the appropriate total exposure to the receptor. Appropriate kVp selection is just as important with digital systems because the selected kVp will control subject contrast (signal differences to the digital detector). Distance is generally set based on the desired beam geometry. It can be used to adjust exposure but this is not generally done. Once a distance is selected based on a given procedure (e.g., chest radiography done at 72 inches and rib radiography done at 40 inches distance), mAs can be appropriately adjusted to maintain an acceptable exposure to the image receptor.

SUMMARY

Prime factors are under the direct control of the radiographer and have a significant impact on x-ray photon emission from the tube. The prime factors are milliamperage-second (mAs), kilovoltage (kVp), and distance (d). X-ray emission can be described in terms of both its quantity (amount) and quality (penetrability). X-ray quantity is affected by mAs, distance, kVp, and filtration. X-ray quality is affected by kVp and filtration.

Milliamperage-second (mAs) is directly proportional to the number of x-ray photons created in the tube. Kilovoltage affects both quantity and quality, and its relationship to x-ray emission is not as easily described. Kilovoltage is approximately proportional to the square of the ratio of the change in kVp. Therefore, if kVp is doubled, the x-ray quantity would increase by a factor of four. This does not, however, take into account the increased penetrability of the beam with increasing kVp. As a result, density/IR exposure is more significantly affected. To maintain exposure with changes in kVp, the 15 percent rule can be applied. The 15 percent rule states that an increase in kVp by 15 percent will cause an approximate doubling of the exposure. To maintain density/IR exposure, if kVp is increased by 15 percent, the mAs must be reduced to one-half its original value. The distance from the actual focal spot to the image receptor is the third prime factor. The quantity of x-ray photons is inversely proportional to the square of the distance. As distance increases, exposure will decrease in an inverse proportion to the square of the change in the distance. ■

REVIEW QUESTIONS

1. What are the three prime factors that affect x-ray emission?
2. What is the unit of measurement for x-ray quantity?
3. Define an ampere.
4. What is the relationship between mAs and density/IR exposure?
5. What effect does increased kVp have on the speed and energy of the electrons in the x-ray tube?
6. What is the relationship between kVp and density/IR exposure?
7. State the inverse square law.
8. What is the relationship between distance and density/IR exposure?

REFERENCES AND RECOMMENDED READING

Ball, J. L., & Moore, A. D. (2008). *Essential physics for radiographers* (4th ed.). Oxford: Wiley-Blackwell Scientific.

Bushberg, J. T., Seibert, J. A., Leidholdt, E. M., & Boone, J. M. (2003). *The essential physics of medical imaging* (2nd ed.). Philadelphia: Lippincott, Williams & Wilkins.

Bushong, S. C. (2008). *Radiologic science for technologists: Physics, biology, and protection* (9th ed.). St. Louis, MO: Elsevier Mosby.

Carroll, Q. B. (2007). *Practical radiographic imaging (Fuch's radiographic exposure processing & quality control)* (8th ed.). Springfield, IL: Charles C Thomas.

Dendy, P. P., & Heaton, B. (1999). *Physics for diagnostic radiology* (2nd ed.). Oxford: Institute for Physics.

Fuchs, A. W. (1950). The rationale of radiographic exposure. *Radiologic Technology, 22*(2), 62.

Jerman, E. C. (1926). An analysis of the end-result: The radiograph. *Radiology, 6*, 59–62.

Johns, H. E., & Cunningham, J. R. (1983). *The physics of radiology* (4th ed.). Springfield, IL: Charles C Thomas.

Selman, J. (2000). *The fundamentals of x-ray physics and radiobiology for the radiologic technologist* (9th ed.). Springfield, IL: Charles C Thomas.

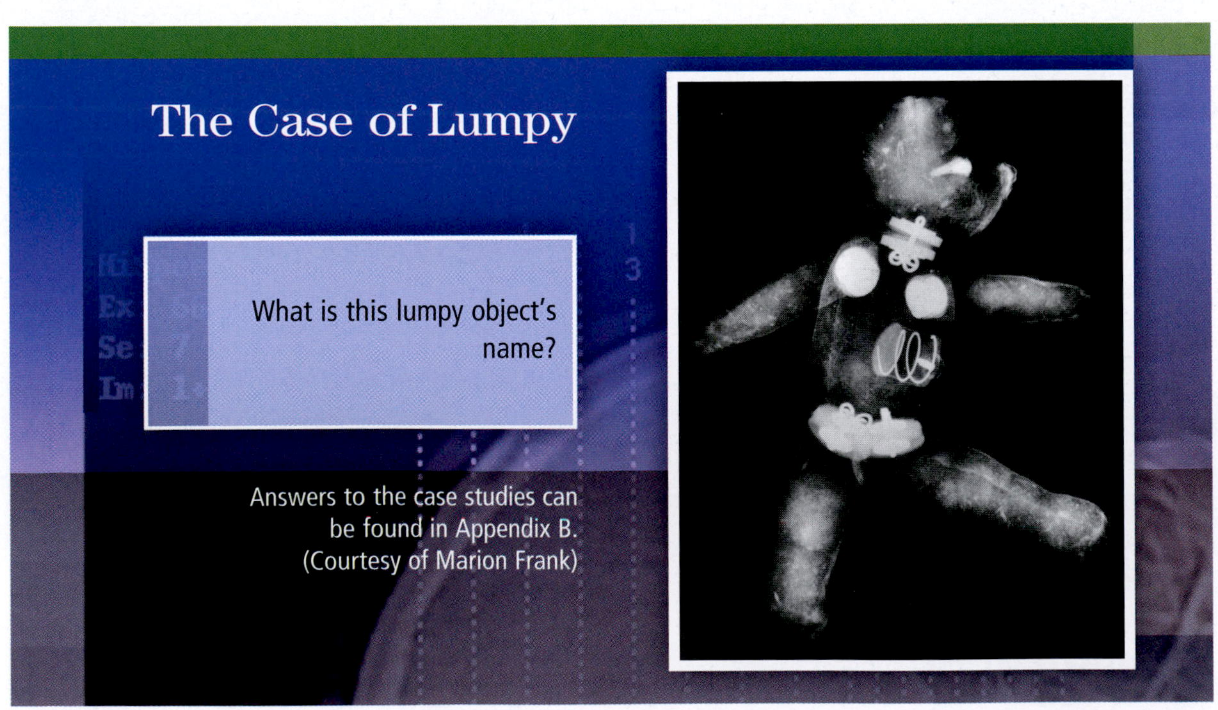

CHAPTER 12

X-Ray Interactions

KEY TERMS

annihilation reaction
attenuation
backscatter radiation
characteristic cascade
characteristic photon
coherent scatter
Compton effect
Compton (or recoil) electron
Compton scattered photon
Compton scattering
negatron
pair production
photodisintegration
photoelectric absorption
photoelectron
positron
radiation fog
scattering
secondary radiation

> Perhaps no single field of investigation has contributed more to our knowledge of atomic structure than has the study of x-rays.
>
> *Arthur H. Compton, preface to the first edition of X-Rays and Electrons*

OBJECTIVES

Upon completion of this chapter, the student should be able to:

- Define attenuation.
- Explain the interactions between x-rays and matter in the following:
  - photoelectric absorption
  - coherent scattering
  - Compton scattering
  - pair production
  - photodisintegration
- Describe the relationship between x-ray interactions and technical factor selections.

X-RAY INTERACTION WITH MATTER

When an x-ray beam passes through matter, it undergoes a process called **attenuation**. Attenuation is the reduction in the number of x-ray photons in the beam, and subsequent loss of energy, as the beam passes through matter (Figure 12-1).

Attenuation is the result of x-ray photons interacting with matter and losing energy through these interactions. Although some photons will pass through matter and not interact, an x-ray photon can interact with the whole atom, an orbital electron, or directly with the nucleus. This will depend on the energy of the photon. Low-energy photons are most likely to interact with the whole atom, intermediate-energy photons generally interact with orbital electrons, and very-high-energy photons, such as those used for radiation therapy, are capable of interacting with the nucleus. In the diagnostic x-ray range, the interactions are most commonly with orbital electrons.

To fully understand x-ray interactions with matter, it is important to recall the structure of the atom. The center of the atom is a positively charged nucleus containing protons and neutrons. The negatively charged electrons are in orbital paths around the nucleus. The energy required to remove an electron from a shell is termed the binding energy of the shell. The K-shell electrons possess the highest binding energy for a given atom and binding energies decrease progressively for successive shells. Not only is the binding energy characteristic of a given shell, it is also specific to a given atom. K-shell electrons are more tightly bound to the nucleus in

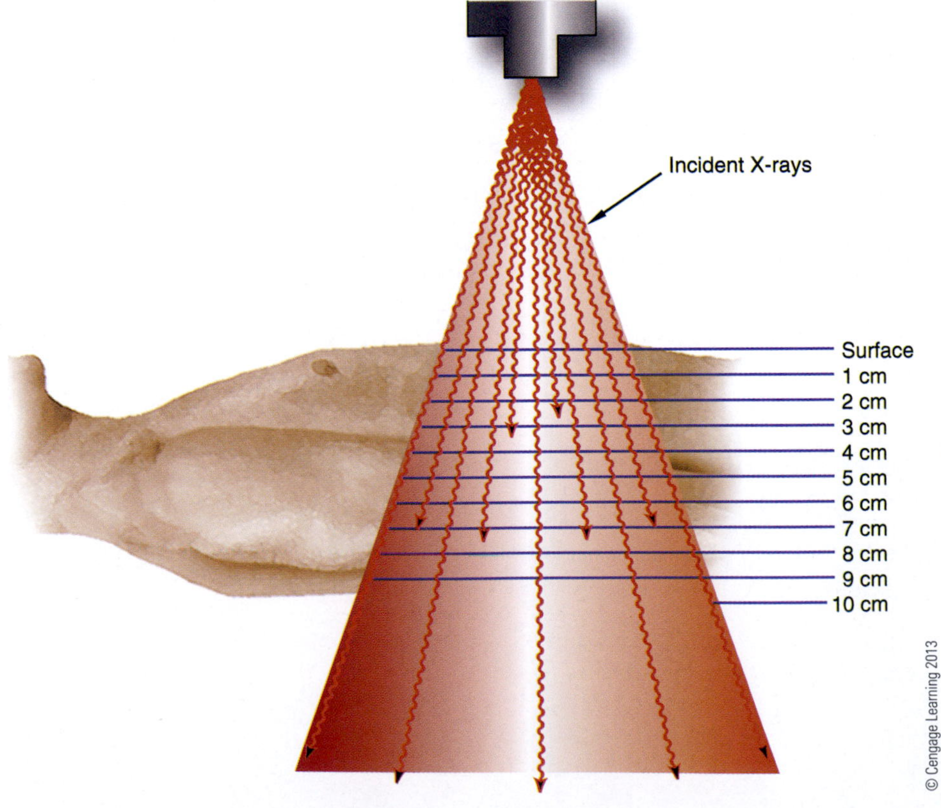

FIGURE 12-1. An x-ray beam undergoes attenuation as it passes through matter.

high-atomic-number elements. For example, the binding energy for the K-shell of tungsten (Z = 74) is approximately 70 keV, whereas the binding energy for the K-shell of calcium (Z = 20) is only about 4 keV. The average atom in the soft tissue of the body has an approximate K-shell binding energy of only 0.5 keV. Therefore, **the higher the atomic number of an element, the more energy will be required to remove a K-shell electron from the atom.**

Because electrons that are further from the nucleus are not bound as tightly, they require less energy to remove them from their orbit. Therefore, they possess a greater total energy. Electrons that are closer to the nucleus are bound more tightly and require more energy to remove them from their position. If a free (unbound) electron is assumed to possess a total energy (ability to do work) of zero, then a bound electron would have a total energy of zero minus the binding energy. **The farther an electron is from the nucleus, the higher the total energy of the electron will be.** This means that K-shell electrons possess less (more negative) total energy than outer-shell electrons. As a result, when an outer-shell electron moves into an inner shell, it will release energy equal to the difference between the binding energies of the two shells.

Electrons in the K-shell have the lowest energy total with the highest binding energy, and with each successive shell, **total electron energies increase and binding energies decrease.** These concepts are particularly important to the understanding of x-ray interactions with matter.

There are five basic interactions between x-rays and matter:

1. Photoelectric absorption
2. Coherent scattering
3. Compton scattering
4. Pair production
5. Photodisintegration

With each of these interactions the x-ray photons either interact and change direction, a process called **scattering**, or are absorbed by the atom. When a photon is absorbed, all of the energy of the photon is transferred to the matter and the photon no longer exists. If a photon interacts and scatters, the photon still exists but usually possesses less energy than before the interaction. Partial energy from the photon is transferred to the matter during the interaction and the lower-energy photon then continues along its new path until again it either interacts and scatters or is absorbed. One photon may scatter several times before it is finally absorbed completely by the matter. The likelihood of one interaction occurring over another varies, depending on the incident photon's energy and the atomic number of the matter. Certain interactions, pair production and photodisintegration, for example, occur only at very high photon energy ranges, while coherent scatter is most predominant in very low photon energy ranges.

PHOTOELECTRIC ABSORPTION

Photoelectric absorption results when an x-ray photon interacts with an inner-shell electron. This interaction is most likely to occur when the incident x-ray photon possesses a slightly greater energy than the binding energy of the electrons in the inner (K or L) shells. The incident photon ejects the electron from its inner shell and is totally absorbed in the interaction (Figure 12-2). The result is an ionized atom, because of the missing inner-shell electron, and an ejected electron, called a **photoelectron**. The photoelectron travels with kinetic energy, which is equal to the difference between the incident photon and the binding energy of the inner-shell electron. This is mathematically expressed in the equation:

$$E_i = E_b + E_{ke}$$

where: E_i = energy of the incident photon
E_b = binding energy of the electron
E_{ke} = kinetic energy of the photoelectron

The incident photon needs an energy that is slightly greater than the binding energy of the electron for the interaction to occur. Because most of the atoms of the body are elements with a very low atomic number, the binding energies of the K-shell electrons are very low. For example, the K-shell binding energy for carbon is approximately 0.28 keV and oxygen is 0.53 keV. The K-shell binding energies of elements that are important in

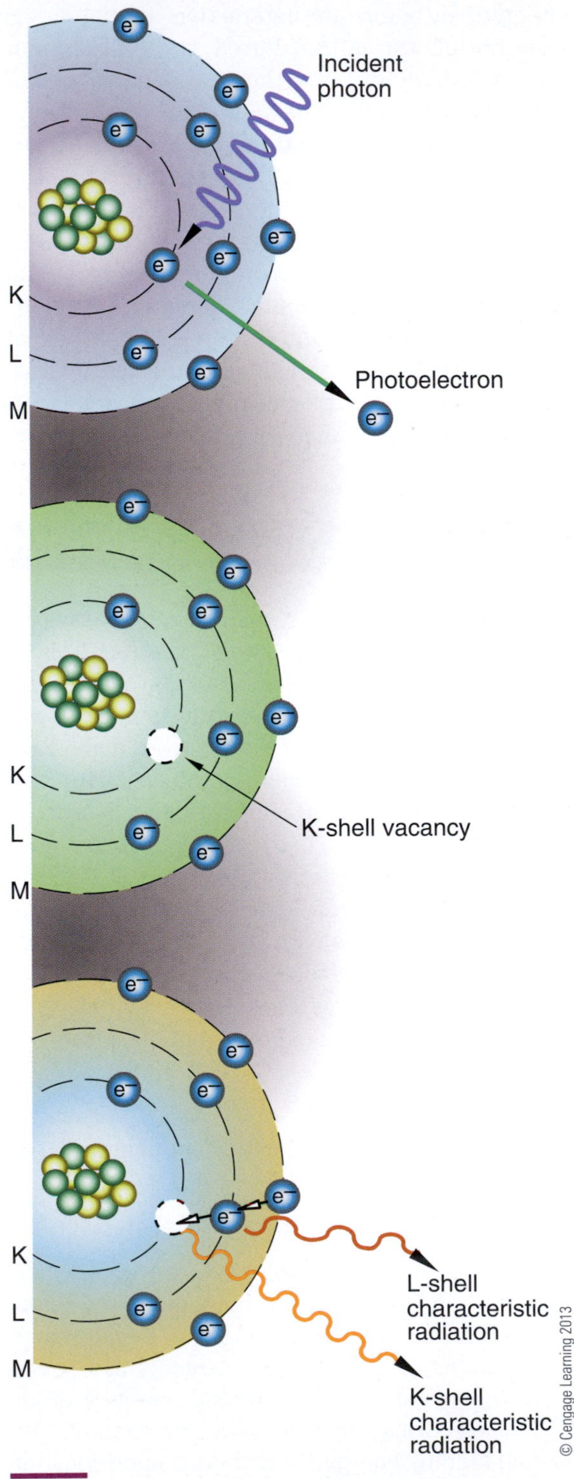

FIGURE 12-2. The photoelectric absorption interaction.

diagnostic radiology are listed in Table 12-1. Most photoelectric interactions in the body result in the majority of the incident photon energy being given to the kinetic energy of the photoelectron. The photoelectron is matter, not just energy, and therefore will not travel far. It is usually absorbed within 1 to 2 mm in soft tissue. Despite the localized absorption, this is still a significant way in which x-ray energy can create biological changes.

The ionized atom is in an unstable state with an inner-shell electron missing. The vacancy is instantly filled by an electron from the L-shell or, less commonly, from an M-shell or free electron. In the vast majority of cases the electron transfers from an outer shell to an inner shell and, as it does, it releases energy in the form of a **characteristic photon**, known as **secondary radiation**. This secondary radiation is produced in the same manner as characteristic radiation is produced at the x-ray target—electron transfer from one shell to another. When it is created at the x-ray target it is considered primary radiation. When characteristic radiation is produced in irradiated matter outside of the x-ray target it is termed secondary radiation. Remember that outer-shell electrons possess a higher energy level than inner-shell electrons. Therefore when an outer-shell electron moves into an inner shell it has excess energy to release. This electron transfer process continues from shell to shell until the atom returns to a normal state and is no longer a positive ion. This process of each

TABLE 12-1. K-Shell Binding Energies of Radiologically Significant Elements

Atom	Atomic Number	K-Shell Binding Energies (keV)
Hydrogen	1	0.016
Carbon	6	0.284
Oxygen	8	0.53
Aluminum	13	1.56
Calcium	20	4.04
Molybdenum	42	20.0
Iodine	53	33.2
Barium	56	37.4
Tungsten	74	69.5
Lead	82	88.0

shell filling lower shells with a corresponding emission of photons is called a characteristic cascade. The energy of each photon of a **characteristic cascade** will be characteristic of the difference in energy in the two shells between which it dropped.

Because of the predominance of low-atomic-number elements comprising the human body, the secondary radiation produced is of extremely low energy, and is therefore often absorbed in the body. Secondary radiation energies are significantly higher for elements such as iodine and barium, which are commonly used as contrast agents in radiology.

There are three basic rules that govern the possibility of a photoelectric interaction:

1. **The incident x-ray photon energy must be greater than the binding energy of the inner-shell electron.** A 30-keV x-ray photon will not be able to remove the K-shell electron from an atom of iodine, which has a binding energy of 33.2 keV, or barium, which has a binding energy of 37.4 keV.
2. **A photoelectric interaction is more likely to occur when the x-ray photon energy and the electron binding energy are nearer to one another.** Of course, the x-ray photon energy must always be greater, but a 40-keV photon is more likely to interact by way of the photoelectric effect with an atom of iodine (K-shell E_b = 33.2 keV) or barium (K-shell E_b = 37.4 keV) than would a 100-keV x-ray photon. As photon energy increases, the chance of a photoelectric interaction decreases dramatically. The actual relationship is expressed as an inverse proportion to approximately the third power of the photon energy (photoelectric effect = $1/[\text{energy}]^3$). A significant change is therefore seen in the percentage of photoelectric interactions that will occur when using low-kVp techniques versus high-kVp techniques. Table 12-2 demonstrates that at 50 kVp, the percent of photon interactions that undergo photoelectric absorption is 50.45 percent, with scatter interactions occurring at 49.55 percent. As the kVp increases, the percent of photon interactions by photoelectric absorption decreases. At 130 kVp, photoelectric absorption accounts for only 24.78 percent of the interactions with matter. These concepts become very important to the radiographer when establishing appropriate technical factors for specific body tissues.

TABLE 12-2. Percentage of Photon Interactions, Attenuation, and Transmission Characteristics in Soft Tissue Based on Effective Photon Energies

kVp	50	70	80	90	110	130
HVL (mm Al)	1.59	2.11	2.35	2.60	3.12	3.67
Mean Photon Energy (keV)	31.3	40.0	41.1	44.2	49.7	54.5
Effective Photon Energy (keV)	27.0	30.0	31.0	33.0	35.0	38.0
% of Photon Interactions by						
—Scattering (with coherent)	49.55%	62.70%	63.95%	66.70%	69.77%	75.22%
—Photoelectric	50.45%	37.30%	36.05%	33.30%	30.23%	24.78%
% Attenuation						
5 cm Tissue	91.45%	84.28%	83.45%	81.67%	79.70%	76.34%
10 cm Tissue	99.27%	97.53%	97.26%	96.64%	95.88%	94.40%
15 cm Tissue	99.94%	99.61%	99.55%	99.38%	99.16%	98.67%
20 cm Tissue	99.99%	99.94%	99.93%	99.89%	99.83%	99.69%
% Transmission						
5 cm Tissue	8.55%	15.72%	16.55%	18.33%	20.30%	23.66%
10 cm Tissue	0.73%	2.47%	2.74%	3.36%	4.12%	5.60%
15 cm Tissue	0.06%	0.39%	0.45%	0.62%	0.84%	1.33%
20 cm Tissue	0.01%	0.06%	0.07%	0.11%	0.17%	0.31%

Courtesy of Raymond P. Rossi, University of Colorado Health Science Center.

3. **A photoelectric interaction is more likely to occur with an electron that is more tightly bound in its orbit.** Binding energies of the electrons are greater in high-atomic-number elements than in low-atomic-number elements. In addition, inner-shell electrons have higher binding energies than outer-shell electrons in a given atom. With low-atomic-number elements, most interactions will occur with the K-shell electron. Because high-atomic-number elements bind their electrons more tightly, interactions will occur with the K-, L-, and M-shells. In fact, the incident x-ray photon often does not possess sufficient energy to remove a K-shell electron. For example, the K-shell binding energy for lead is 88 keV. X-ray photons below this level are incapable of removing the K-shell electrons but can be absorbed through photoelectric interactions with L- or M-shell electrons. The probability of a photoelectric interaction increases dramatically as the atomic number increases. The relationship is approximately proportional to the third power of the atomic number (photoelectric effect = [atomic number]^3). Because bone has an effective atomic number that is higher than that of soft tissue, photoelectric interactions are more likely to occur in bone than in soft tissue. **It is for this reason that radiography is so spectacularly useful in demonstrating the bones of the body.**

COHERENT SCATTERING

Coherent scatter is an interaction that occurs between very-low-energy x-ray photons and matter. It is also called classical scatter or unmodified scatter. There are actually two types of coherent scattering: Thomson scattering and Rayleigh scattering. Thomson scattering involves a single electron in the interaction, whereas Rayleigh scattering involves all of the electrons of the atom in the interaction. Both types have the same basic interaction results.

When a very-low-energy photon, below approximately 10 keV, interacts with the electron(s) in an atom, it may cause the electron(s) to vibrate at the same frequency as the incident photon. The vibrating or excited atom immediately releases this excess energy by producing a secondary photon that has the same energy and wavelength as the incident photon but that travels in a direction different from the initial photon (Figure 12-3). The

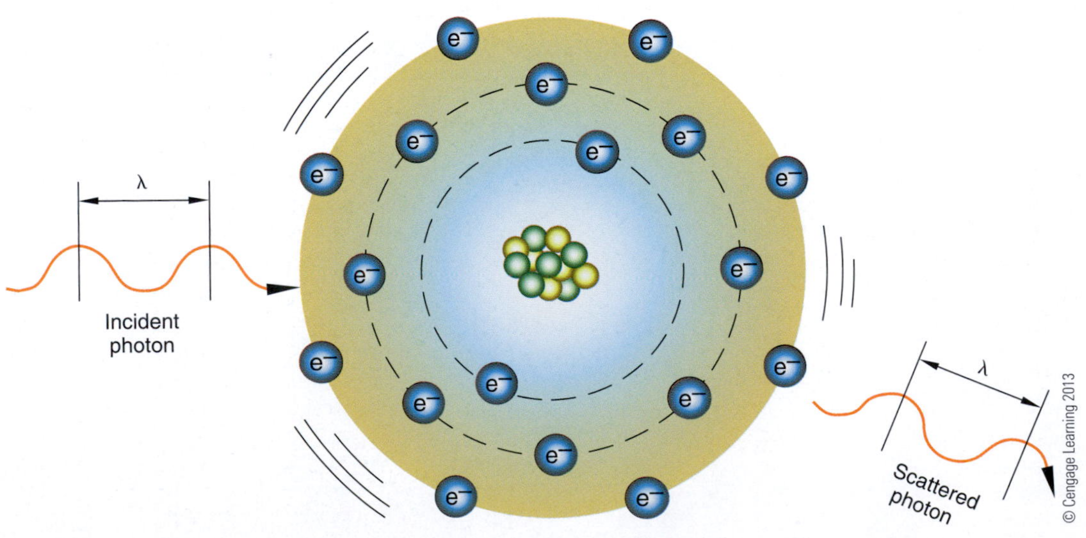

FIGURE 12-3. The coherent scatter interaction.

result is a scattered photon that possesses the same energy, frequency, and wavelength as the initial photon but that is traveling in a different direction. Because there is no energy transferred in the interaction, the atom is not ionized in the process.

Coherent scattering occurs in a very low x-ray energy range, which is generally outside the usual range for diagnostic imaging. A very small amount of the scatter radiation reaching the receptor is produced by this process and, as a result, this interaction has little significance to diagnostic imaging.

COMPTON SCATTERING

Compton scattering occurs when an incident x-ray photon interacts with a loosely bound outer-shell electron, removes the electron from its shell, and then proceeds in a different direction as a scattered photon (Figure 12-4). This interaction was described by the American Nobel laureate physicist Arthur H. Compton (1892–1962) in 1922 and is known as the **Compton effect**. Part of the energy of the incident photon is used to remove the outer-shell electron and impart kinetic energy to it. The dislodged electron is called a **Compton** or **recoil electron**. The photon that exits the atom in a different direction is called a **Compton scattered photon**. It possesses less energy than the incident photon and therefore has a lower frequency and longer wavelength.

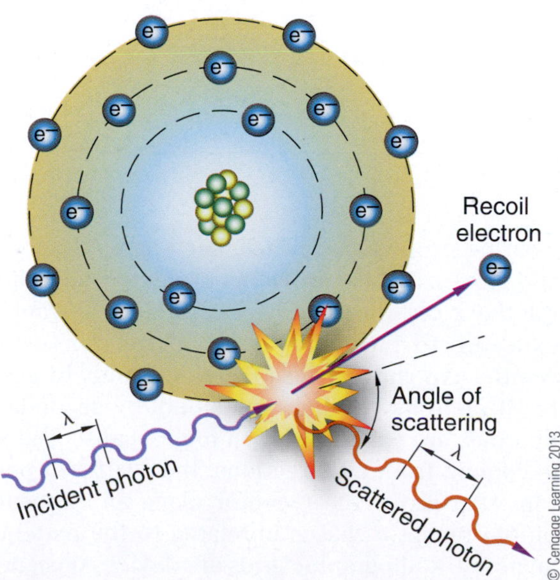

FIGURE 12-4. The Compton scatter interaction.

The energy transfer in the Compton effect is mathematically expressed in the equation:

$$E_i = E_s + E_b + E_{ke}$$

where: E_i = energy of the incident photon
E_s = energy of the Compton scattered photon
E_b = electron binding energy of the Compton electron
E_{ke} = kinetic energy given to the Compton electron

The incident photon energy is divided between the ejected electron and the scattered photon. The scattered photon retains most of the energy because little energy is needed to eject an outer-shell electron, due to its low binding energy. The scattered photon will continue to interact with atoms until it is eventually absorbed photoelectrically. The recoil electron is available as a free electron to fill a shell "hole" created by another ionizing interaction.

The amount of energy retained by the scattered photon is dependent on the initial energy of the photon and its angle of deflection from the recoil electron. The higher the initial energy of the photon, the greater the energy of the scattered photon. Scattered photons can be deflected at any angle from the recoil electron, just as a cue ball is deflected after it strikes a second ball in a game of billiards. At a deflection of 0°, no energy is transferred because the photon is proceeding in its original direction. As the angle of deflection increases to 180°, more energy is imparted to the recoil electron and less energy remains with the scattered photon (Figure 12-5).

When a scattered photon is deflected back toward the source, it is traveling in the direction opposite to the incident photon. These photons are called **backscatter radiation**. Most photons will scatter in a more forward direction, especially when incident photon energy increases.

In Figure 12-5, the innermost ring represents the highest energy level and the scattered photons are all deflected in a forward direction. The third

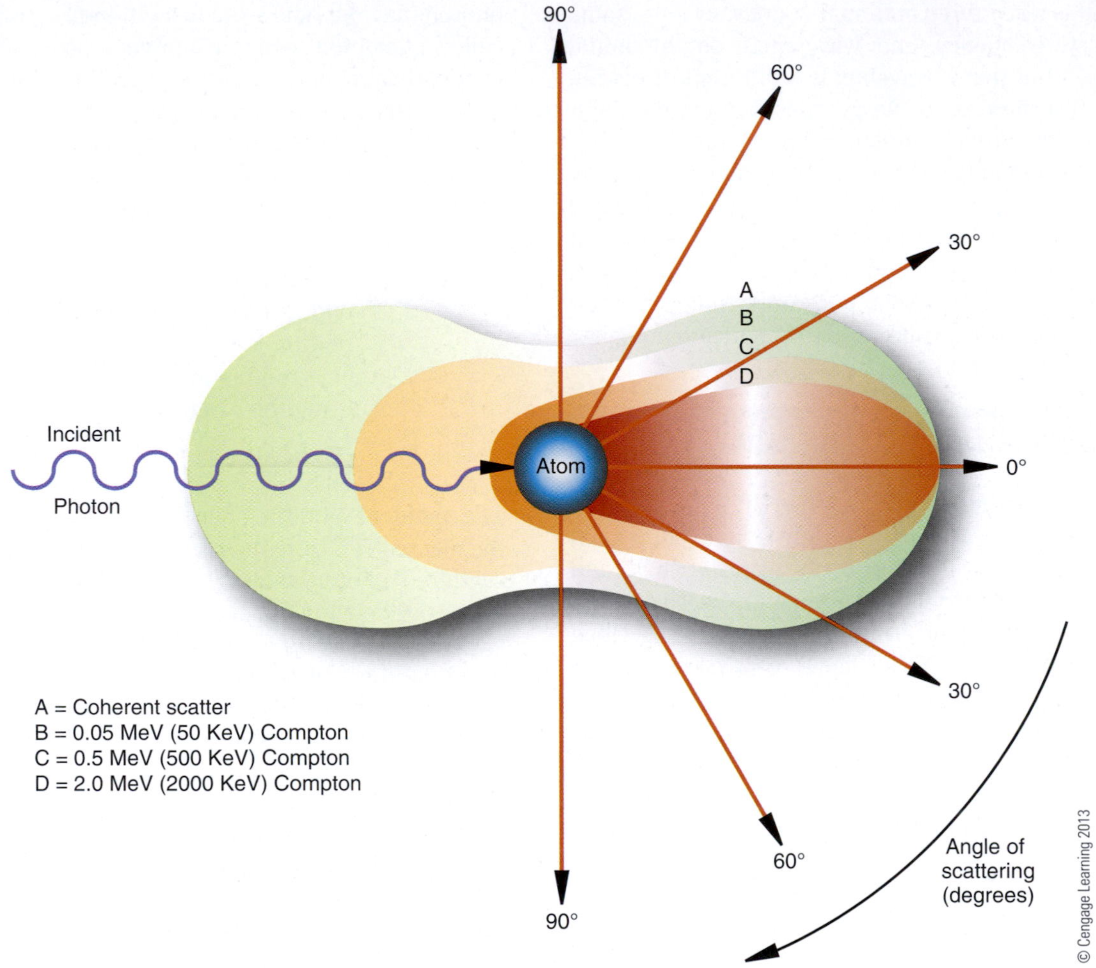

FIGURE 12-5. The distribution of photons in Compton scatter, along with various angles of deflection.

inner ring represents a typical x-ray exposure with an average effective photon energy of 50 keV. Although small numbers of photons are undergoing backscatter, the majority of the scatter is projected in a forward direction toward the image receptor. For this reason, scatter has a serious impact on image quality.

Scattered Compton photons possess an energy high enough to create a radiation hazard and to impair image quality. Scatter radiation emitted from the patient is the primary cause of occupational radiation exposure to the radiographer and is therefore the primary reason for wearing protective devices, such as lead aprons and gloves, and for providing protective shielding for the x-ray room. Scatter also adds unwanted exposure to the radiographic image. These unwanted exposures, caused predominantly by scattered photons and less commonly by secondary photons, are called **radiation fog**. Because scatter is coming from all directions, the scattered photons that strike the receptor place an exposure on the receptor that is unrelated to the patient's anatomy. Radiographic grids are devices designed to remove unwanted scatter and improve radiographic image quality.

PAIR PRODUCTION

In a **pair production** interaction the energy of the x-ray photon is converted to matter in the form of two electrons. For this interaction to occur, a very-high-energy photon with an energy of at least 1.02 MeV is required. This is because the energy equivalent of the mass of one electron at rest is equal to 0.51 MeV. During this interaction, a high-energy incident photon comes close to the strong nuclear field and loses all its energy in the interaction. This energy is used to create a pair of electrons, one with a negative charge, a **negatron**, and the other with a positive charge, a **positron** (Figure 12-6). Because a negative electron is common in nature it is quickly absorbed by other nearby atoms. A positron, because of its unique configuration, with some of the characteristics of a proton, is extremely volatile. It comes to rest and combines with a negative electron nearly instantaneously. When these two particles combine, they disappear and give rise to two photons moving in opposite directions and each possessing energies of 0.51 MeV. This process is called the **annihilation reaction** because matter is being converted back to energy. Pair production requires a minimum incident photon energy of 1.02 MeV but doesn't become a significant interaction until approximately 10 MeV. Therefore, it does not occur in the diagnostic x-ray imaging range.

PHOTODISINTEGRATION

Photodisintegration is an interaction between an extremely high-energy photon, above approximately 10 MeV, and the nucleus. In this interaction, the high-energy photon strikes the nucleus and all of its energy is absorbed by the nucleus, thereby exciting it. The excited nucleus responds by emitting a nuclear fragment (Figure 12-7). Because of the high-energy level needed to cause this interaction, it is not relevant to diagnostic imaging.

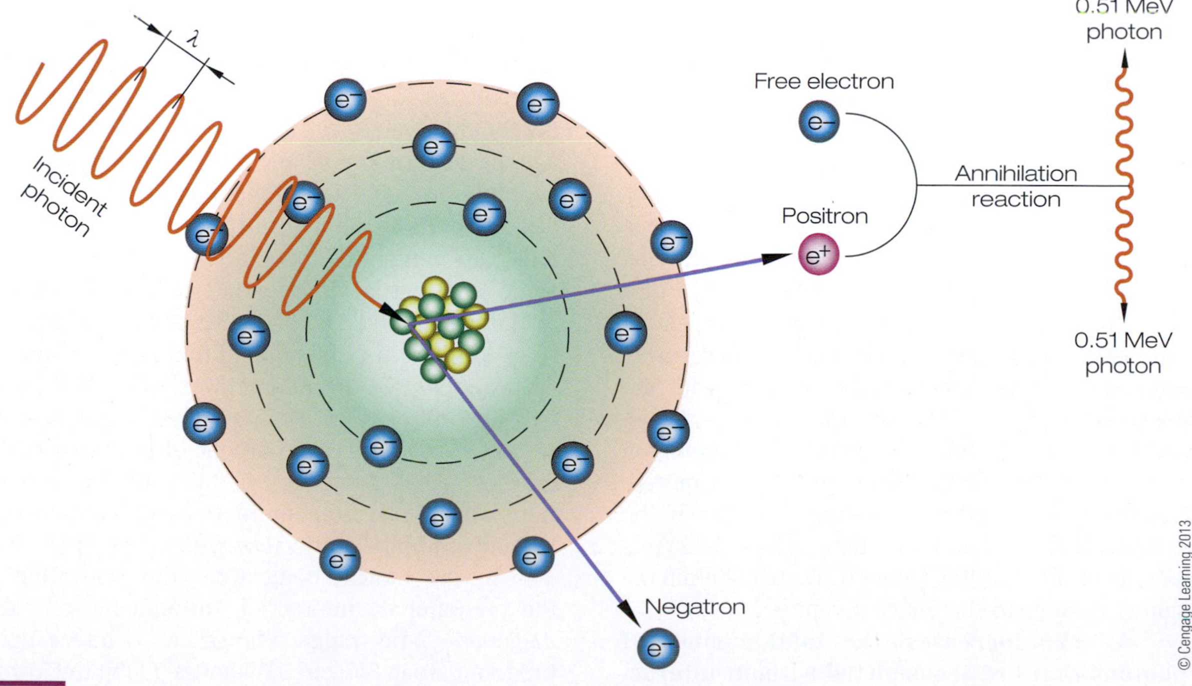

FIGURE 12-6. The pair production interaction.

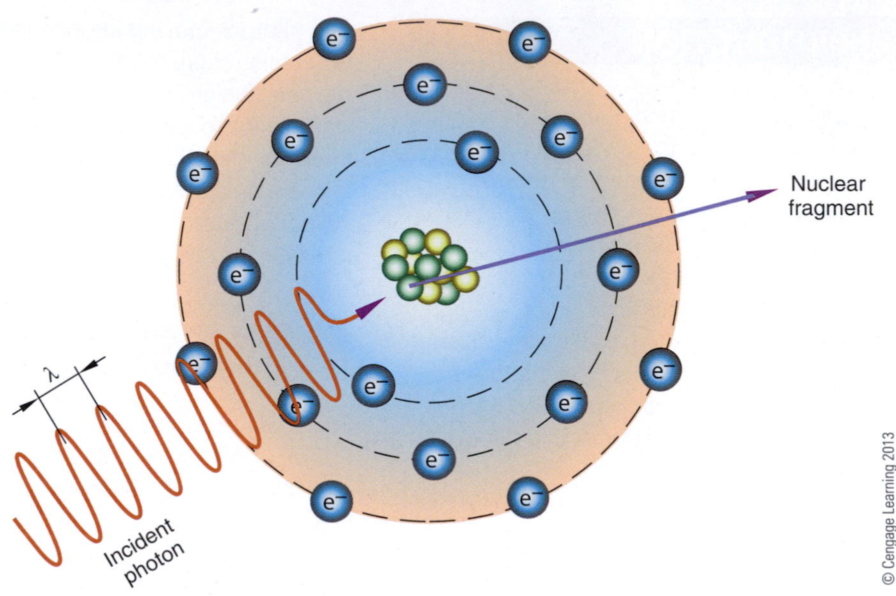

FIGURE 12-7. The photodisintegration interaction.

EFFECT ON TECHNICAL FACTOR SELECTION

Of the five interactions between x-ray and matter, only two have a significant impact on an x-ray image. These two interactions, photoelectric absorption and Compton scattering, must be considered by the radiographer when technical factors are selected.

It is important to remember that in the diagnostic x-ray range the majority of the x-ray beam is attenuated and only a small percentage of photons exit to create the image. Refer to Table 12-2. For a 10-cm tissue exposed at 50 kVp, 99.27 percent of the beam will be attenuated and 0.73 percent of the beam will be transmitted to interact with the image receptor. At 130 kVp, the same 10-cm tissue will attenuate only 94.40 percent of the beam and 5.60 percent of the beam will be transmitted. Obviously, it would be necessary to reduce the overall number of photons (mAs) when the kVp is increased, if the radiographer wants to maintain the same exit dose to the image receptor.

As kVp increases, the total number of photons that are transmitted without interaction increases. This means that the probability of photoelectric and Compton interactions decreases with increasing kVp. A shift does occur, however, in the percentages of photoelectric versus Compton interactions with increased kVp. **The percentage of photoelectric interactions decreases with increased kVp and the percentage of Compton interactions increases with increased kVp.** As a result, as kVp increases, there is an increased percentage of scatter and a decreased percentage of absorption of the attenuated beam. For example, in Table 12-2, for a 5-cm tissue exposed at 50 kVp, 91.45 percent of the beam is attenuated and 8.55 percent is transmitted. At 130 kVp, the same 5-cm tissue will attenuate only 76.34 percent of the beam and 23.66 percent will be transmitted. At 50 kVp, of the 91.45 percent that was attenuated, 50.45 percent of the interactions were photoelectric absorption and 49.55 percent were scatter. At 130 kVp, the overall percent of attenuation decreases (76.34 percent), but most of the interactions are now scatter interactions (75.22 percent) instead of photoelectric absorption (24.78 percent).

In the human body, Compton scattering is the predominant interaction through most of the diagnostic x-ray range. Photoelectric interactions predominate in two circumstances: (1) in the lower-energy ranges (25–45 keV) produced by 40–70 kVp, and (2) when high-atomic-number elements are introduced, such as the contrast agents iodine and barium. Iodine and barium serve as useful contrast agents because they absorb a greater percentage of the photons through photoelectric interactions. These differences in absorption between the contrast agents and the soft tissues are responsible for creating the visible radiographic image.

Figure 12-8 shows the percent attenuation by photoelectric absorption on the scale on the left and the percent attenuation by Compton scatter on the scale on the right. In the diagnostic x-ray range, for bone and soft tissue, photoelectric absorption predominates at lower energies and then Compton scatter begins to predominate. For high-atomic-number materials, such as sodium iodine (NaI), barium, and lead, photoelectric absorption is the predominant if not exclusive interaction. For this reason, as stated, iodine and barium serve as useful contrast agents and lead serves as a useful material for radiation protection.

When just comparing body tissues, in soft tissue (water), interactions are about 50/50 photoelectric absorption versus Compton at approximately 26 keV. In bone, interactions are about 50/50 photoelectric absorption versus Compton at approximately 45 keV (Figure 12-9).

When the photoelectric effect is more prevalent, the resulting radiographic image will possess high contrast. High-contrast images have great differences in densities from white to black, with fewer gray shades in between. This high contrast is the result of the complete absorption of the incident photons without the creation of undesirable scatter to fog the image. High-contrast images can be created by selecting low-kVp/high-mAs technical factors and through the introduction of contrast agents. In both of these instances, the photoelectric effect will be more predominant. Remember that as the percentage of photoelectric interactions increases, so does the absorption of radiation by the

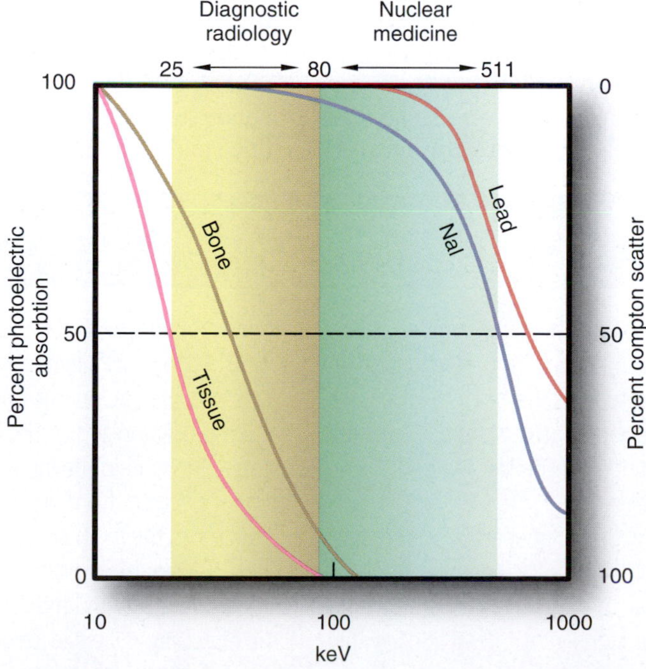

FIGURE 12-8. Percent contribution of photoelectric (left scale) and Compton (right scale) attenuation processes for various tissue as a function of energy. When diagnostic energy photons interact with low-Z materials (e.g., soft tissue), the Compton process dominates. *(Reprinted with permission from J. T. Bushnerg, J. A. Seibert, E. M. Leidholdt, & J. M. Boone, 2002, The Essential Physics of Medical Imaging [2nd ed.]. Baltimore: Lippincott Williams & Wilkins.)*

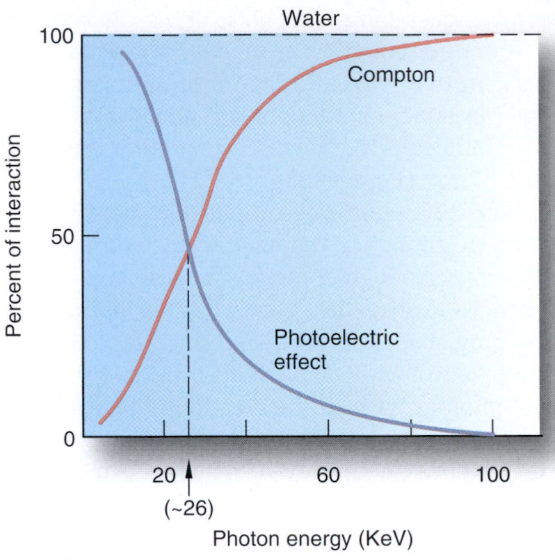

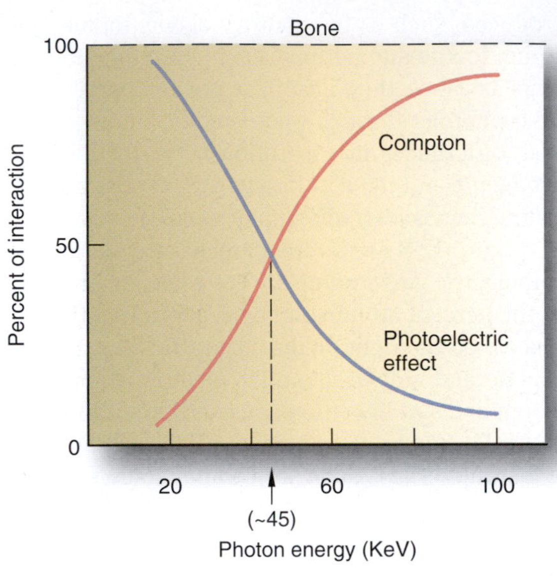

FIGURE 12-9. The relative percentages of photoelectric absorption and Compton scatter in water and bone.

patient. This increases the likelihood of biological effects. Therefore, high-contrast, low-kVp/high-mAs techniques tend to result in higher patient doses.

When Compton interactions prevail, the resulting radiographic image will possess lower contrast. Low-contrast images have very small differences between densities, with more gray shades in between. Low-contrast images can be created by using high-kVp/low-mAs techniques because Compton interactions predominate as kVp increases. Scatter from Compton interactions is a significant cause of the lower-contrast images. However, low-contrast, high-kVp/low-mAs techniques tend to reduce patient dose.

SUMMARY

As an x-ray beam passes through matter it undergoes attenuation, which is the reduction in the number of x-ray photons in the beam as it passes through a given thickness of matter. Attenuation is the result of x-rays interacting with matter by way of one of five types of interactions.

The five basic interactions between x-ray and matter are photoelectric absorption, coherent scattering, Compton scattering, pair production, and photodisintegration. Only two are significant interactions within the diagnostic range of x-rays. These are photoelectric absorption and Compton scattering. Photoelectric absorption results when an x-ray photon interacts with an inner-shell electron. The incident photon is completely absorbed by the ejection of the electron, which then possesses kinetic energy and is called a photoelectron. The atom is ionized in the process and extremely unstable. The void in the inner shell is filled by the transfer of an electron from an outer shell. As the electron moves into the inner shell it releases a photon, which is characteristic for a given atom. Characteristic photons created in irradiated material by way of the photoelectric effect are called secondary radiation.

Compton scattering is an interaction between an x-ray photon and an outer-shell electron. The incident photon ejects the outer-shell electron

SUMMARY (continued)

(Compton or recoil electron). The incident photon loses energy and as a result changes direction or scatters. The scattered photons have sufficient energy to interact again and again. Scatter radiation is the reason for wearing radiation protection devices and for shielding x-ray rooms. Scatter also adds unwanted exposures to the receptor, which impairs image quality.

Image contrast is affected by the most predominant x-ray interaction. High-contrast images will result when the photoelectric effect is prevalent, and low-contrast images will result when Compton scatter is more common. In addition, patient dose is increased when photoelectric interactions prevail. As kVp increases, more photons are transmitted without interaction, and patient dose decreases as a result. ■

REVIEW QUESTIONS

1. Define attenuation.
2. Describe the photoelectric absorption interaction.
3. Describe the coherent scatter interaction.
4. Describe the Compton scatter interaction.
5. What is backscatter?
6. What are the two interactions that have a significant impact on the radiographic image?
7. What type of radiographic contrast will result if the prevalent interaction is photoelectric absorption?
8. What type of radiographic contrast will result if the prevalent interaction is Compton scatter?

REFERENCES AND RECOMMENDED READING

Bushberg, J. T., Seibert, J. A., Leidholdt, E. M., & Boone, J. M. (2003). *The essential physics of medical imaging* (2nd ed.). Philadelphia: Lippincott, Williams & Wilkins.

Bushong, S. C. (2008). *Radiologic science for technologists: Physics, biology, and protection* (9th ed.). St. Louis, MO: Elsevier Mosby.

Compton, A. H., & Allison, H. K. (1935). *X-rays in theory and experiment* (2nd ed.). New York: Van Nostrand.

Curry, T. S., Dowdey, J. E., & Murry, R. C. (1990). *Christensen's introduction to the physics of diagnostic radiology* (4th ed.). Philadelphia: Lea and Febiger.

Dendy, P. P., & Heaton, B. (1999). *Physics for diagnostic radiology* (2nd ed.). Oxford: Institute for Physics.

Fewell, T. R., & Shuping, R. E. (1977). Photon energy distribution of some typical diagnostic x-ray beams. *Medical Physics*, *4*(3), 187–197.

Glasser, O., Quimby, E. H., Taylor, L. S., Weatherwax, J. L., & Morgan, R. H. (1961). *Physical foundations of radiology* (3rd ed.). New York: Paul B. Hoeber, Division of Harper & Brothers.

Hay, G. A., & Hughes, D. (1972). *First-year physics for radiographers*. London: Bailliere Tindall.

Herman, M. W. (1980). A comparative study of scattered radiation levels from 80 kVp and 240 kVp x-rays in the surgical ICU. *Radiology*, 552.

Johns, H. E., & Cunningham, J. R. (1983). *The physics of radiology* (4th ed.). Springfield, IL: Charles C Thomas.

Meredith, W. J., & Massey, J. B. (1977). *Fundamental physics of radiology* (3rd ed.). Chicago: Yearbook Medical.

Selman, J. (2002). *The fundamentals of x-ray physics and radiobiology for the radiologic technologist* (9th ed.). Springfield, IL: Charles C Thomas.

van der Plaats, G. J. (1980). *Medical x-ray techniques in diagnostic radiology* (4th ed.). The Hague: Martinus Nijhoff.

Wilks, R. J. (2003). *Principles of radiological physics* (4th ed.) Edinburgh: Churchill Livingstone.

Wolbarst, A. B., & Cook, G. (2005). *Physics of radiology* (2nd ed.). Madison: Medical Physics Publishing.

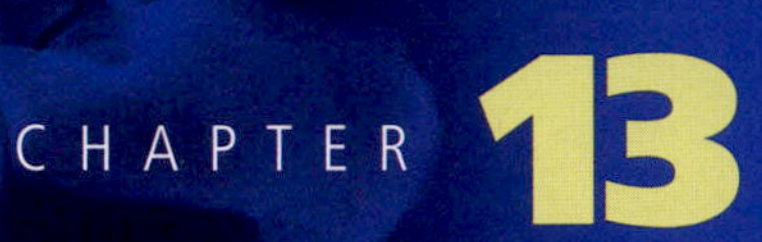

CHAPTER 13 Minimizing Patient Dose

KEY TERMS

approximate entrance skin exposure
entrance skin exposure

> I became acquainted very early with the destructive effect of roentgen rays upon living tissue. In fact, it was only a few months after the announcement of Röntgen's discovery that I required medical care for a roentgen burn covering most of the back of one hand.
>
> *W. D. Coolidge, "Experiences with the Roentgen-ray tube"*

OBJECTIVES

Upon completion of this chapter, the student should be able to:

- Explain the relationship of entrance skin exposure to other measurement points.
- Calculate mR/mAs from a calibration exposure total.
- Calculate total entrance skin exposure when given subject part thickness, SID, kVp, mAs, and an mR/mAs chart.
- Describe typical entrance skin exposures for common radiographic procedures.
- Discuss methods of reducing patient dose through effective communication.
- Describe various methods of reducing patient dose through effective positioning.
- Explain the interrelationship of the prime factors.
- Evaluate various exposure factors for the most effective methods of reducing patient dose under various clinical conditions.
- Describe an effective method of minimizing patient dose by considering radiation risk factors.
- Describe an effective method of maximizing patient diagnostic information by emphasizing radiation benefit factors.
- Analyze various approaches to discussing radiation risk versus benefit with patients, physicians, and radiologists.

A predominant concern of radiographers is how to reduce the radiation dose to the patient. This concern is reflected in every decision made, especially when choosing exposure factors. The conscientious radiographer can reduce the patient dose by at least 50 percent in most examinations by choosing appropriate exposure factors.

Although exposure and dose are often used interchangeably, exposure (roentgen) refers to radiation intensity in air, whereas dose (rad) is a measure of the radiation absorbed as a result of a radiation exposure. Dose is used to identify the irradiation of patients. Exposure (R) is used to calculate entrance skin exposure (ESE) in irradiated patients. Patient dose is usually estimated by conducting phantom experiments.

One of the most important characteristics of the professional is the ability to decide when it is appropriate to tip the radiation benefit versus risk issue in favor of the risk by reducing the patient dose while compromising the diagnostic quality of the image, and when to tip the issue in favor of the benefit by increasing the patient dose while maintaining the diagnostic quality of the image. There are circumstances that dictate when each choice should be made, and this chapter attempts to lay the foundation necessary to make these decisions.

ESTIMATING APPROXIMATE ENTRANCE SKIN EXPOSURE

Figure 13-1 illustrates a typical radiographic examination with the exposure indicated at various points. It is obvious that the maximum exposure received by the patient is not at the area of interest but at the skin entrance to the body. This is known as the **entrance skin exposure** and is calculated at the minimum SOD. Note that the minimum SOD is not equal to the SOD of the area

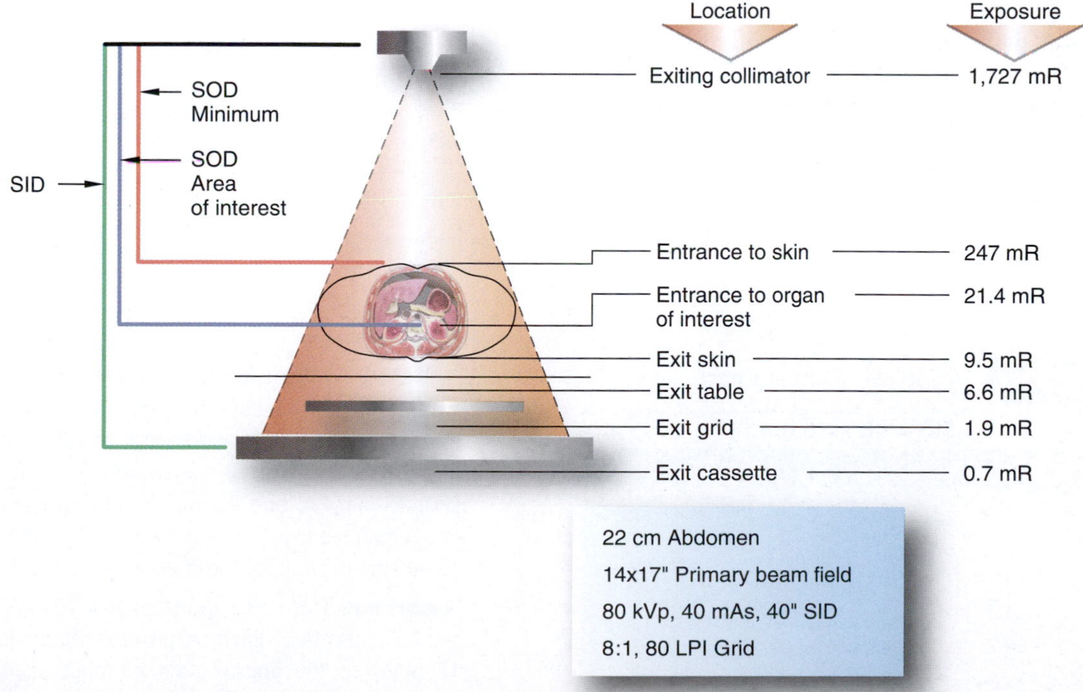

FIGURE 13-1. Exposures at various locations in the imaging process.

of interest and that the entrance skin receives a greater exposure. Although radiobiologists and physicists often discuss organ doses and gonadal doses, the entrance skin exposure is the most common expression to approximate patient exposure because it is safer to assume a maximum effect when attempting to minimize exposure to ionizing radiation.

Diagnostic Radiography mR/mAs Charts

Exposure to patients can be estimated by recording mR/mAs when the x-ray unit is calibrated. This is calculated by recording a reading for any average exposure and then dividing the reading in mR by the total mAs used. The expression mR/mAs represents the formula itself. The mR/mAs measurements are usually recorded for an SID of 40″ (100 cm). To estimate the entrance skin exposure, the inverse square law must be applied to determine the exposure for the source-to-entrance skin distance.

The mR/mAs readings vary according to the kVp used, with higher kVp producing greater mR/mAs. Consequently, mR/mAs readings should be recorded for each kVp range within the normal expectations of the unit. A typical mR/mAs chart is shown in Table 13-1.

A quick estimate of entrance skin exposure can be made from this chart, as shown in the following example.

TABLE 13-1. A Typical mR/mAs Chart

SID = 40″ (100 cm)	
kVp	**mR/mAs**
50	0.9
60	1.7
70	2.5
80	3.5
90	4.5
100	5.6
110	6.9
120	7.9

EXAMPLE: What is the approximate entrance skin exposure for a 20-cm AP abdomen produced at 80 kVp and 20 mAs on the unit for the chart in Table 13-1?

Answer: Table 13-1 indicates that 80 kVp = 3.5 mR/mAs. The exposure required 20 mAs, so the exposure at 100 cm = 3.5 mR/mAs × 20 mAs and the exposure at 100 cm = 70.0 mR.

$$\text{SID} = \text{SOD} + \text{OID}$$

$$100 \text{ cm} = \text{SOD} + 20 \text{ cm}$$

$$\text{SOD} = 100 \text{ cm} = 20 \text{ cm}$$

$$\text{SOD} = 80 \text{ cm}$$

$$\frac{\text{mR}_1}{\text{mR}_2} = \frac{\text{SOD}^2}{\text{SID}^2}$$

$$\frac{70 \text{ mR}}{\text{mR}_2} = \frac{(80 \text{ cm})^2}{(100 \text{ cm})^2}$$

$$\frac{70 \text{ mR}}{\text{mR}_2} = \frac{6{,}400 \text{ cm}}{10{,}000 \text{ cm}}$$

$$\text{mR}_2 \times 6{,}400 \text{ cm} = 70 \text{ mR} \times 10{,}000 \text{ cm}$$

$$\text{mR}_2 = \frac{70 \text{ mR} \times 10{,}000 \text{ cm}}{6{,}400 \text{ cm}}$$

$$\text{mR}_2 = \frac{700{,}000}{6{,}400}$$

$$\text{mR}_2 = 109.4$$

EXAMPLE: What is the total approximate entrance skin exposure for an intravenous pyelogram of a 24-cm abdomen if an AP preliminary scout; 5-min AP; 10-min AP, RPO, and LPO; 15-min PA; and 30-min AP radiographs of the abdomen were produced at 70 kVp and 15 mAs on the unit for the chart in Table 13-1?

Answer: Table 13-1 indicates that 70 kVp = 2.5 mR/mAs. Each exposure required 15 mAs, so the approximate entrance skin exposure = 2.5 mR/mAs × 15 mAs and

(continues)

(continued)
the approximate entrance skin exposure = 37.5 mR per exposure; 37.5 per exposure × 7 exposures = 262.5 mR = 0.2625 R.

SID = SOD + OID

100 cm = SOD + 24 cm

SOD = 100 cm – 24 cm

SOD = 76 cm

$$\frac{mR_1}{mR_2} = \frac{SOD^2}{SID^2}$$

$$\frac{262.5\ mR}{mR_2} = \frac{(76\ cm)^2}{(100\ cm)^2}$$

$$\frac{262.5\ mR}{mR_2} = \frac{5,776\ cm}{10,000\ cm}$$

$$mR_2 \times 5,776\ cm = 262.5\ mR \times 10,000\ cm$$

$$mR_2 = \frac{262.5\ mR \times 10,000\ cm}{5,776\ cm}$$

$$mR_2 = \frac{2,625,000}{5,776}$$

$$mR_2 = 454.5$$

Fluoroscopic R/min Charts

Approximate entrance skin exposure for fluoroscopic equipment is measured in R/min. Estimation of approximate entrance skin exposure is calculated in the same manner.

EXAMPLE: What is the approximate entrance skin exposure for a fluoroscopic examination of the abdomen performed for 5.5 minutes at 110 kVp at 1.7 R/min?

Answer: The exposure required 5.5 min, so the approximate entrance skin exposure = 1.7 R/min × 5.5 min and the approximate entrance skin exposure = 9.35 R = 9,350 mR.

EXAMPLE: What is the total approximate entrance skin exposure for a fluoroscopic examination of an 18-cm abdomen performed for 7 min and 45 sec at 110 kVp at 1.7 R/min and then followed by an AP at 10 mAs, left lateral at 25 mAs, and LPO projection at 20 mAs of the stomach at 120 kVp on the unit for the chart in Table 13-1?

Answer: The exposure required 7.75 min, so the approximate entrance skin exposure = 1.7 R/min × 7.75 min and the approximate entrance skin exposure = 13.175 R = 13,175 mR. The total mAs for the three projections = 10 + 25 + 20 mAs = 55 mAs. Table 13-1 indicates that 120 kVp = 7.9 mR/mAs, so the approximate entrance skin exposure = 7.9 mR/mAs × 55 mAs and the approximate entrance skin exposure = 434.5 mR; 13,175 fluoro mR + 434.5 diagnostic mR = 13,609.5 mR = 13.61 R.

SID = SOD + OID

100 cm = SOD + 18 cm

SOD = 100 cm – 18 cm

SOD = 82 cm

$$\frac{mR_1}{mR_2} = \frac{SOD^2}{SID^2}$$

$$\frac{13,609.5\ mR}{mR_2} = \frac{82\ cm^2}{100\ cm^2}$$

$$\frac{13,609.5\ mR}{mR_2} = \frac{6,724\ cm}{10,000\ cm}$$

$$mR_2 \times 6,724\ cm = 13,609.5\ mR \times 10,000\ cm$$

$$mR_2 = \frac{13,609.5\ mR \times 10,000\ cm}{6,724\ cm}$$

$$mR_2 = \frac{136,095,000}{6,724}$$

$$mR_2 = 20,240 = 20.24\ R$$

TYPICAL ENTRANCE SKIN EXPOSURE

Numerous studies have been done regarding the exposure delivered to patients during diagnostic radiographic examinations. Diagnostic radiography is by far the greatest source of ionizing radiation exposure for the public. It is estimated that 15 percent of the radiation exposure received by the general public is a result of diagnostic radiographic examinations. Table 13-2 shows the average patient exposure guides for entrance skin exposure as published by the Conference of Radiation Control Program Directors. Within an acceptance range of ±20 percent, this guide is considered to be the standard for current practice in the United States.

Radiography of the lumbar spine, pelvis, and hip has the highest ESEs. These examinations deserve special attention from radiographers because careful consideration of the need for the examination, positioning, patient instructions, technical factors, and shielding can result in significant reduction in the total dose to the patient.

Flouroscopic systems in the United States are under a limit set by the Food and Drug Administration (FDA) for entrance exposure (kerma in the SI system) at 10 centigrays per minute (10 cGy/min), which is 11.5 R/min. High-level control mode fluoroscopy is limited to an entrance exposure (kerma) of 20 cGy/min, which is 23 R/min.

TABLE 13-2. Medical ESE Values for Selected Radiographic Exams

Projection	Patient Thickness (cm)	Grid	SID (cm)	Median ESE (mR)	3rd Quartile ESE (mR)
Chest (P/A)	23 23	No Yes	183 183	9 13	13 18
Pediatric Chest (P/A)	15-month-old/ 11-kg infant	No Yes		4 8	5 10
Pediatric Chest (A/P)	15-month-old/ 11-kg infant	No Yes		5 8	9 14
Abdomen (A/P)	23	Yes	102	271	396
Lumbar Spine (A/P)	23	Yes	102	342	477
Full Spine (A/P)	23	Yes	183 145 (400 Speed)	260 (200 Speed)	
Cervical Spine (A/P)	13	Yes	102 95 (400 Speed)	135 (200 Speed)	
Skull (Lat)	15	Yes	102 70 (400 Speed)	145 (200 Speed)	

NOTES:

- Patient thickness corresponds to the dimensions of the average adult patient as clinically validated by the NEXT program.
- All measurements were made in air, without backscatter.
- The ESE values may be converted to entrance air kerma (mGy) by multiplying by 0.00876 mGy/mR.
- Chest data source: 1994 NEXT Chest Radiography Survey.
- Pediatric Chest data source: 1998 NEXT Pediatric Chest Survey (preliminary data).
- Abdomen and Lumbar Spine data source: 1995 NEXT Abdomen and Lumbosacral Spine Survey (hospital data only).
- Full spine, cervical spine, and skull projections are based on data for manual mode techniques only collected by the H-7 Committee prior to the 1992 edition of this manual. ESEs are not necessarily inversely proportional to imaging system speed.
- For the full spine projection, if the facility used a wedge filter, the exposure was measured in the center of the x-ray field with the filter in the beam.

(Reprinted with permission from *Patient Exposure and Dose Guide–2003.* Conference of Radiation Control Program Directors, Inc., Frankfort, KY: CRCPD Publication E-03-2, 2003.)

REDUCING PATIENT DOSE WITH COMMUNICATION

Radiographers often overlook the importance of gaining the trust and confidence of the patient. This is accomplished by a professional approach that includes technical competence, empathy for the patient, and effective communication and questioning skills. When the patient has confidence in the radiographer there is a higher probability that detailed instructions will be followed, which helps to reduce motion and degradation of positioning.

REDUCING PATIENT DOSE WITH POSITIONING

An effective method of reducing patient dose is through accurate and effective positioning. Avoidance of repeated exposures far outweighs all other methods. However, once positioning skills have been developed to a degree of competence, several positioning details may further reduce the total dose.

Radiographic Projection

Some organs are especially sensitive to the effects of radiation, for example, the thyroid, the female breast, the kidneys, and the lens of the eye. Increased recorded detail and decreased distortion result when the area of interest is placed as close to the image receptor as possible. In most instances, a significant reduction in the total dose is achieved because this positioning also places the organ as far from the entrance exposure as possible. For example, a PA chest reduces the dose to the breast, an AP abdomen reduces the dose to the kidneys, and a PA skull reduces the dose to the lens of the eye. Deviation from these projections should occur only when unusual circumstances dictate an alternate projection.

Immobilization

Proper immobilization is a necessary part of achieving satisfactory recorded detail and diminishing the need for repeat exposures. Elimination of motion and decreased tissue density through compression both contribute to a reduction of patient dose.

REDUCING PATIENT DOSE WITH TECHNICAL FACTORS

The radiographer can significantly reduce the approximate entrance skin exposure to the patient by judicious selection of technique exposure factors. Studies have shown that over 50 percent of repeated exposures are the result of improper technical factor selection. Table 13-3 illustrates the effect each of the major technical factors has on patient dose. In most instances when a technical factor is varied, other factors will be modified to maintain image receptor exposure. Therefore, the important information is not the direct result of the technical factor change, but the result of compensation to maintain image receptor exposure or other components of image quality.

Interrelationship of the Prime Factors

The radiation intensity from a diagnostic x-ray unit will vary in a direct relationship with mAs, directly with the square of kVp, and inversely with the square of the distance. This total relationship is often expressed as:

$$\frac{(\text{mAs})(\text{kVp})^2}{\text{d}^2}$$

At the image receptor the kVp is more likely to be kVp^3 or kVp^4. Although this formula includes only the three primary factors, it is useful to understand that they are interrelated and can all be used to influence the total dose.

Kilovoltage Range

When kVp is increased without compensating for other factors, patient dose is increased. Therefore, a decrease in kVp is desired when attempting to reduce patient dose. However, when an increase in kVp is compensated for by a decrease in mAs to maintain image receptor exposure, a significant reduction in patient dose is achieved. **Selection of the highest possible kilovoltage consistent with image quality is the best method of using exposure factors to reduce patient dose.** With fixed kilovoltage systems, care must be taken to achieve an optimal kVp that is within acceptance limits. Because fixed kVp technique systems tend to utilize higher optimal kVp levels, they usually reduce patient entrance skin exposures. A comparison of approximate ESE levels with the two systems is illustrated in Table 13-4.

TABLE 13-4. Comparison of Approximate Entrance Skin Exposures with Fixed and Variable kVp Technique Systems

Variable—56 kVp, 5 mAs = 12.8 mR Fixed—65 kVp, 2.5 mAs = 9.5 mR
Variable—68 kVp, 40 mAs = 175.1 mR Fixed—80 kVp, 20 mAs = 135.4 mR
Variable—102 kVp, 20 mAs = 222.0 mR Fixed—120 kVp, 10 mAs = 156.3 mR

These examples would produce equivalent receptor exposures.

TABLE 13-3. Effects of Radiographic Exposure Variables on Patient Dose

	Effect of Patient Dose When:		
		Variable Is Increased but Image Receptor Exposure Is Maintained by Compensating	
Variable	Variable Is Increased without Compensation	with kVp Only	with mAs Only
Kilovoltage	+	NA	–
Milliamperage	+	+	0
Time	+	+	0
Distance			
SID	–	–	0
SOD	–	–	0
OID	+	+	+
Focal spot size	0	NA	NA
Filtration	–	–	+
Field size	1	varies	varies
Gonadal shielding	–	NA	NA
Subject part density	+	+	+
Grid ratio	0	+	+
Intensifying screens	0	–	–
Film speed	0	–	–
Film processing			
Developer time	0	–	–
Developer temperature	0	–	–
Developer replenishment	0	–	–

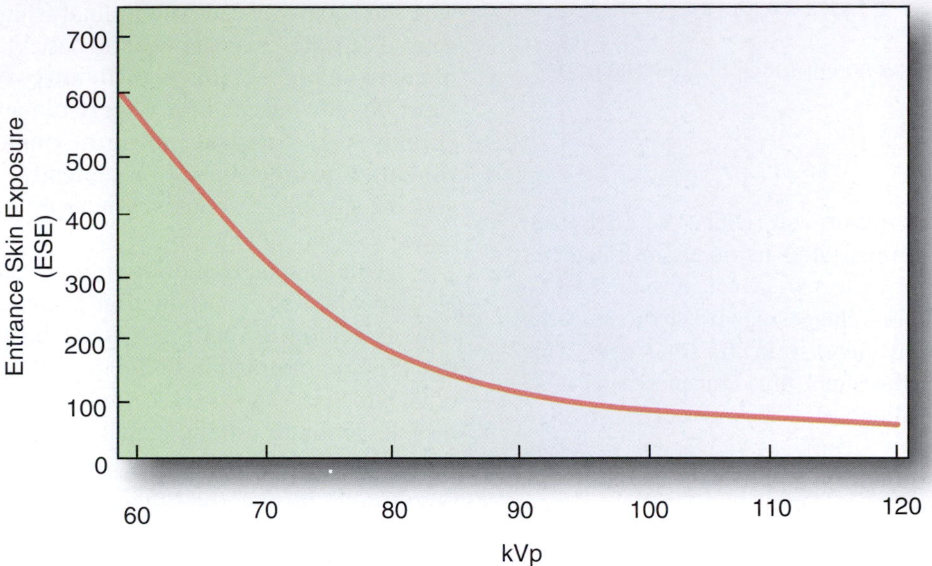

FIGURE 13-2. The effect of kVp on entrance skin exposure. This graph clearly illustrates that increased kVp causes photon energy to be carried through the object. *(Courtesy of Barry Burns, University of North Carolina.)*

Remember that generator phase also has an effect on kilovoltage output. Although an increase in the number of pulses from the generator would seem to increase the patient dose because of the increased average photon energy, there is actually a substantial decrease in patient ESE (from 40 to 60 percent) because of the decrease in the percentage of lower-energy photons from the x-ray tube. The lower-energy photons tend to be absorbed in the body instead of being transmitted to the image receptor, thus contributing to patient ESE without adding any information to the image receptor. This is clearly shown in Figure 13-2.

Milliamperage and Time

When mAs is decreased, patient dose is also decreased. When an increase in mAs is compensated by a decrease in kVp, patient dose will increase. An inverse relationship exists between mAs and kVp in maintaining image receptor exposure. To decrease patient dose, mAs should be maintained at the lowest possible level because there is a direct relationship between mAs and exposure. Because variable kVp technique systems tend to utilize lower kVp levels with higher mAs, the result can be higher average patient ESE than with fixed kVp systems.

Distance

Distance cannot be discussed alone because SID, SOD, and OID have differing relationships to patient ESE. When SID or SOD is increased, patient ESE decreases. One study found a 10 percent decrease in patient ESE between an SOD of 40 and 50 inches. When kVp is used to compensate for image receptor exposure, the ESE will decrease but the use of mAs for compensation will usually increase the total ESE. In most instances, when OID decreases, SOD increases, and this will reduce patient ESE. This holds true regardless of whether kVp or mAs is used to compensate for the air-gap technique and exposure changes. Because patient ESE decreases when SID increases, it is now recommended that 44–48-inch distances become standard.

Focal Spot Size

Focal spot size has no appreciable effect on patient dose.

Filtration

An increase in filtration will reduce the ESE, even when kVp is compensated to maintain image receptor exposure. However, when mAs is used to compensate for lost image receptor exposure, the result is often an increase in the total ESE. This applies only to the small filtration increases used in diagnostic radiography, usually not more than 0.5 mm Al/Eq. Any significant increase in filtration (1.0 mm Al/Eq or more) would have an overall ESE reduction effect.

Field Size

When the primary-beam field size decreases, the patient dose also decreases. An increased field size will increase the total dose even when mAs or kVp is adjusted to compensate for image receptor exposure changes because a greater tissue area is irradiated. An increase in the primary technical factors is necessary to compensate for lost scatter radiation exposure when the field size is decreased. Although this appears to increase dose, the elimination of a greater percentage of tissue from the beam is a greater protective method than the increased factors. Modern x-ray tube collimators utilize two sets of shutters or leaves to eliminate most of the off-focus radiation.

Gonad Shielding

Gonad shielding is extremely effective in reducing dose to the gonads. There are three major types of gonad shields: flat contact, shadow contact, and shaped contact. Flat contact shields are positioned over the gonads at the skin surface. Shadow shields are positioned in the primary beam immediately below the collimator. Shaped contact shields are worn by the patient to surround the gonads. Gonadal shielding is one of the fine arts of radiography. The radiographer who is competent in the specifics of gonadal anatomy can easily satisfy the concerns of the radiologist or supervisor who has experienced suboptimal shielding that caused repeated exposure to the patient. **Properly placed gonadal shields significantly reduce patient dose, whereas improperly placed gonadal shields can increase patient dose through repeated projections.** Consequently, consistent gonadal shielding becomes a measure of the competency of the radiographer.

Gonadal shields should be used routinely for all patients with reproduction capabilities. The only exception to this rule should be projections that require information in the gonadal region. It is critical to locate the exact location of the ovaries or testicles prior to using gonadal shields. Most projections of the pelvic region do not permit the use of gonadal shields. This includes IVP, abdominal, colon, and bony pelvic projections. Hip projections do permit careful gonadal shielding.

Subject Part Density

A decrease in subject part density will decrease scatter production and reduce the patient dose. When compensation for lost scatter is made by increasing mAs or kVp, a reduction in total dose holds true.

Grids

Using grids results in an increase in patient dose as opposed to non-grid procedures, in order to maintain image receptor exposure. When the grid ratio is decreased, and exposure is maintained by decreases in mAs or kVp, a significant dose reduction can be achieved. The use of a grid of unnecessarily high ratio causes routine increases in patient dose as mAs or kVp is increased to maintain exposure.

Film/Screen Image Receptor Systems

Intensifying Screens. Using intensifying screens results in a decrease in patient dose as opposed to non-screen procedures. Whenever the screen speed is increased, a significant reduction in mAs or kVp can be achieved while maintaining image receptor exposure. An effective method of reducing patient dose is to use the highest possible film/screen combination.

Film. Using higher-speed film results in a decrease in patient dose as opposed to slower-speed film, in order to maintain image receptor exposure. Base plus fog is a factor that should not be related to patient dose reductions. If base plus fog becomes too high, the detrimental effect on image quality will result in repeated exposures. However, a decrease in patient dose can be accomplished when a higher-speed film is used and mAs or kVp is reduced to maintain image receptor exposure. Because higher-contrast images also exhibit greater speed, the same effect is achieved with a higher-contrast film. Film latitude becomes wider as speed and contrast decrease. Consequently, a narrow latitude film is desirable when attempting to reduce patient dose. This approach requires radiographers to be extremely accurate in selecting technical factors.

Film Processing. The compensations that are required to overcome reductions in developer time, temperature, or replenishment can result in unnecessarily high patient dose. Developer time, temperature, and replenishment cannot be effectively increased to reduce patient dose. Film processing is a system that must be maintained at an optimal level to ensure satisfactory image quality. Failure to do so can result in increased dose rates, but success in maintaining the system cannot be considered a direct cause of decreased dose.

Digital Image Receptor Systems

With digital image receptor systems, it is still critical to provide the digital image receptor with an appropriate exposure for a given procedure. Digital image receptors can respond to a wide range of exposures from as low as 0.01 mR up to 100 mR. Extremely low and extremely high exposures do not produce acceptable image quality. Most acceptable images can be produced using approximately 1-mR exposure to the receptor. Setting the appropriate technical factors is the responsibility of the radiographer. These prime technical factors control the exposure to the image receptor. The radiographer should select the kVp based on the desired contrast and adjust mAs to provide the appropriate total exposure to the receptor. Because of the wide exposure latitude allowed with digital systems, radiographers should be especially careful not to use higher exposure doses than necessary even though these exposures may produce an acceptable image through the post-processing parameters.

DISCUSSING RADIATION RISK VERSUS BENEFIT WITH PATIENTS

The radiographer is often in the position of discussing radiation risk versus benefit with patients. To the attending physician, and sometimes even to the radiologist, the radiographer must represent the patient's interest in reducing dose. At the same time the radiographer must represent, to the patient, the physician's interest in maximizing diagnostic information. These points of view generally oppose one another. One exception is the use of higher kVp to produce a lower contrast. In this example, patient dose is decreased and the diagnostic information is increased.

Minimizing Patient Dose by Emphasizing Risk

The patient's interest in reducing the total dose must be represented even when the patient does not express such an interest. Some patients even express an opposite interest, as often occurs with minor complaints, such as lung congestion or a sprained ankle, when the patient arrives in the physician's office, a clinic, or an emergency room with a request for an x-ray examination. When patients assume this attitude, the physician may prescribe an x-ray examination as a placebo. Most medical ethicists consider the prescription of a procedure for the purpose of deceiving the patient, or a procedure known to be without specific efficacy, to be unethical. This includes unnecessary radiographic examinations, which are known to be potentially detrimental.

In such a situation, the radiographer should perceive an obligation to act in such a way as to eliminate the request for the examination or at least to reduce the number of exposures. Through demonstration of professional competence, the radiographer can obtain the stature necessary to permit consultation regarding modification or elimination of examination requests.

Part of gaining this type of respect is the ability to make well-considered judgments on when to advocate reductions in patient dose and when to advocate additional examinations. These judgments require all the radiographer's knowledge of anatomy, physics, radiation biology, positioning, pathology, imaging equipment, and, especially, clinical experience. For example, a radiographer should advocate an additional projection of the abdomen when an erect radiograph for an abdominal obstruction series fails to demonstrate the top of both hemidiaphragms. Conversely, the radiographer is acting professionally when advocating the elimination of separate wrist projections when both hand and wrist examinations have been requested but there is visible trauma only to the hand, the patient has no complaint of wrist pain, and the clinical history does not indicate a high probability of referred stress to the wrist joint.

For examinations that are of questionable need, the radiographer is within professional rights to inform the patient of his or her right to refuse an examination. Under no circumstances should this be perceived by the radiographer as cause to inform the patient that an examination is not needed or to give a personal opinion regarding medical treatment or diagnosis. The radiographer must have an introductory background in medical law in order to make judgments of this type. For example, minors, persons who have had their civil rights suspended (such as persons in the custody of law enforcement officers), mentally incompetent persons, and some other categories of patients do not have the right to refuse examinations.

The selection of patients for x-ray examinations has been the focus of considerable study, particularly when the chest, lumbar spine, and skull are involved. Patients can be divided into asymptomatic and symptomatic groups when determining which should be exposed to radiation. Asymptomatic patients should be examined only when there is significant cause, after considering the incidence and severity of the condition, the detection reliability of the examination, and the usefulness of the examination in treatment. The most common examples of asymptomatic patients are those undergoing screening procedures. Although mass chest and lumbar spine screening are now discouraged, mammography screening is encouraged for women of certain age groups. Symptomatic patients are more likely to require x-ray examination but should fit two major criteria: the examination must be capable of providing the desired information, and the information, even if negative, is expected to contribute to the management of the patient. The radiographer has a responsibility to contribute to these criteria whenever possible, primarily through history-taking. When circumstances that appear to routinely violate these principles are encountered, the radiographer should consider withdrawing from participation in the examinations.

Maximizing Diagnostic Information by Emphasizing Benefit

While advocating a reduction of patient dose, the radiographer must simultaneously impress on the patient the physician's primary concern of maximizing diagnostic information. This includes establishing credibility with the patient by demonstrating competence in answering questions, taking a medical history, manipulating the x-ray equipment, exhibiting a professional demeanor, and myriad other details. Established credibility permits the radiographer to convince the patient to follow breathing instructions, endure an additional uncomfortable projection, or permit a repeated exposure.

The benefit of radiographic procedures has been an unquestionable aspect of medicine since Röntgen's discovery in 1895. Although this is generally accepted by the public, some patients have a heightened anxiety about exposure, and there are periodic increases in publicity that cause concern over medical radiation exposures. These issues must be addressed by the radiographer as the primary professional contact with the patient. The radiographer has a responsibility to advocate medically necessary examinations and to assure the patient that the benefit outweighs the risk.

The primary duty of the radiographer on this issue is to provide the patient with sufficient information to permit the patient to make an informed decision regarding the examination. This can be a very sensitive topic and must be approached in a thorough and professional manner. One of the best accepted methods of providing this information to the patient is through comparison of relative radiation risks. Table 13-5 illustrates comparative risks of chest x-ray examinations to other radiation risks that are common public knowledge. Another effective method of illustrating relative radiation risk is through a catalog of risks, such as the extract shown in Table 13-6.

When a patient requests information about the exact dose for a particular examination, the radiographer has an obligation to attempt to provide that information. However, it is important that the patient have a basic understanding that only an **approximate entrance skin exposure** can be provided. The radiographer should inform the patient that the entrance skin exposure is the maximum exposure and that the actual dose to the area of interest would be significantly less.

The Center for Devices and Radiological Health of the United States Food and Drug Administration has advocated the use of radiation record cards for patients. Proposals have been

TABLE 13-5. Gross Comparison of Relative Radiation Levels*

	Scaled Relative Dose†
Natural background	50–100 chest examinations/year
Diagnostic radiology	0.1–500 chest examinations/study‡
Nuclear imaging	50–1,000 chest examinations/study¶
Start of acute radiation syndrome	30,000 chest examinations in one day
Lethal dose ($LD50_{30}$)	300,000 chest examinations in one day
Radiation therapy (small volumes of tissue)	100,000–1,000,000 chest examinations in a few weeks
Ultrasound	This scale does not apply
NMR	This scale does not apply

*Due to differential tissue distributions and sensitivities, such estimates are intended to be rough comparisons (50–100 chest examinations will have different biologic effects from that resulting from 100–200 mrads of natural background).

†1 PA chest examination = 5 millirad average tissue dose in thorax, which corresponds to a whole-body equivalent dose of 2 millirads.

‡Dependent on examination types and techniques.

¶Does not properly account for doses received in those tissues in which the radionuclide concentrates.

(Reprinted with permission from Joseph P. Whalen & Stephen Balter, 1984, *Radiation Risks in Medical Imaging,* Chicago: Yearbook Medical Publishers, Inc.)

TABLE 13-6. Estimated Loss of Life Expectancy Due to Various Causes*

Lifestyle	Estimated Loss in Days
Being unmarried—male	3,500
Cigarette smoking—male	2,250
Being unmarried—female	1,600
Cigarette smoking—female	800
Dangerous job	300
Motor vehicle accidents	207
Alcohol (U.S. average)	130
Accidents at home	95
Average job	74
Radiation job	40
Accidents to pedestrians	37
Safest job	30
Natural radiation	8
Medical x-rays	6
Individual Action	**Estimated Loss in Minutes**
Buying a small car	7,000
Coast-to-coast drive	1,000
Coast-to-coast flight	100
Smoking a cigarette	10
Calorie-rich dessert	50
Non-diet soft drink	15
Diet soft drink	0.15
Crossing a street	0.4
Extra driving	0.4/mile
Not fastening seat belt	0.1/mile
1 mrem of radiation	1.5

*Adapted from permission from Bernard L. Cohen & I-Sing Lee, 1979," A Catalog of Risks," *Health Physics* 36, 707–722. Used by permission of the Health Physics Society.

made for credit-card-style cards with magnetic record tapes for running totals of approximate entrance skin exposures. There are currently x-ray units available with printout capability so this information can be given to patients upon request. As the public becomes more informed about the potential risks of medical radiation exposure, additional developments in this arena can be expected.

The patient has the right to refuse radiographic examination. The radiographer is bound by professional duty to respect this right and to advocate it to physicians, including radiologists, if necessary. As long as the patient has the right to refuse treatment, proceeding with an examination under protest from the patient may place the radiographer at risk of malpractice action (usually as assault and battery).

SUMMARY

A predominant concern of radiographers is how to reduce the radiation dose to the patient. This concern is reflected in every decision that is made, especially when choosing technique exposure factors. The conscientious radiographer can reduce the patient entrance skin exposure by at least 50 percent in most examinations by choosing appropriate exposure factors.

The maximum dose received by the patient is not at the area of interest but at the skin entrance to the body. This is known as the entrance skin exposure and is calculated at the minimum SOD. Exposure to patients can be estimated by recording mR/mAs when the x-ray unit is calibrated. This is calculated by recording a reading for any average exposure and then dividing the reading in mR by the total mAs used. The expression mR/mAs represents the formula itself. The mR/mAs measurements are usually recorded for an SID of 40″ (100 cm). To estimate the entrance skin exposure, the inverse square law must be applied to determine the exposure for the source-to-entrance skin distance. For fluoroscopy, the estimated exposure is calculated in R/min instead of mR/mAs.

Radiographers can reduce the dose to the patient through their communication skills, their positioning skills, and through proper selection of technical exposure factors. Technical factors include the kilovoltage, mA, exposure time, distance, filtration, field size, gonadal shielding, subject part density, grids, and film/screen and digital image detector systems.

The radiographer is often in the position of discussing radiation risk versus benefit with patients. To the attending physician, and sometimes even to the radiologist, the radiographer must represent the patient's interest in reducing the dose. At the same time the radiographer must represent to the patient the physician's interest in maximizing diagnostic information. ■

REVIEW QUESTIONS

1. What is the relationship between entrance skin exposure and other measurement points?
2. What is the mR/mAs for a calibration exposure of 80 kVp at 40 mAs that produces a total exposure of 86 mR?
3. What is the total exposure for a patient measuring 26 cm when the SID is 40″ for an exposure of 70 kVp and 35 mAs and the mR/mAs at 70 kVp is 2.6 at 40″?
4. How can patient dose be reduced through effective communication?
5. How can patient dose be reduced through effective positioning?
6. What changes should be made in kVp, mA, time, and distance if each is the only factor changed to reduce patient dose?
7. What are the variables, other than the prime factors, that can be used to reduce patient dose?
8. What risk factors could be mentioned to answer a patient's inquiry about the dose for an examination?
9. What diagnostic benefits could be mentioned to answer a patient's inquiry about the need for an examination?
10. Describe an approach to discussing radiation risk versus benefit with patients, physicians, and radiologists.

REFERENCES AND RECOMMENDED READING

Anderson, P. E., Anderson, P. E., & Van-der-Kooy, P. (1982). Dose reduction in radiography of the spine for scoliosis. *Acta Radiological*, *23*, 251–253.

Baker, D. G. (1989). How significant are the risks from occupational exposure to ionizing radiation? *Applied Radiology*, *18*(9), 19.

Ball, J. L. (1978). Does high kV reduce the dose? *Radiography*, *64*(523), 163.

Bednorck, D. R., Rozenfeld, M., Lanzl, L. H., & Sabau, M. (1981). A protocol for exposure limitations in radiography. *Radiologic Technology*, *53*(3), 229.

Brown, R. F., Shaver, J. W., & Lamel, D. A. (1980). *The selection of patients for x-ray examinations* (HEW Publication [FDA] 80–8104). Rockville, MD: U.S. Department of Health, Education, and Welfare, Public Health Service, Food and Drug Administration, Bureau of Radiological Health.

Burkhart, R. L. (1983). *Patient radiation exposure in diagnostic radiology examinations: An overview* (HEW Publication [FDA] 83–8217). Rockville, MD: U.S. Department of Health, Education, and Welfare, Public Health Service, Food and Drug Administration, Bureau of Radiological Health.

Bushong, S. C. (2004). Radiation protection. In Philip W. Ballinger (Ed.), *Merrill's atlas of radiographic positions and radiologic procedures* (10th ed., pp. 39–56). St. Louis, MO: Elsevier/C. V. Mosby.

Butler, P., Thomas, A. W., Thompson, W. E., Wollerton, M. A., & Rachlin, J. A. (1986). Simple methods to reduce patient exposure during scoliosis radiography. *Radiologic Technology*, *57*(5), 411.

Butler, P. F. (1985). Chest radiography: A survey of techniques and exposure levels currently used. *Radiology*, 533.

Cohen, B. L., & Lee, I. (1979). A catalog of risks. *Health Physics*, *36*, 707–722.

Committee to Assess Health Risks from Exposure to Low Levels of Ionizing Radiation. (2006). *Health risks from exposure to low levels of ionizing radiation. BEIR VII Phase 2*. Washington, DC: The National Academies Press.

Conference of Radiation Control Program Directors, Inc., Committee on Quality Assurance in Diagnostic Radiology. (1993). *Average patient exposure guides*. Frankfort, KY: Author.

Dowd, S. B., & Tilson, E. R. (1999). *Practical radiation protection and applied radiobiology* (2nd ed.). Philadelphia: Elsevier/W. B. Saunders.

Fazel, R., Krumholz, H. M., Wang, Y., Ross, J. S., Chen, J., Ting, H. H., Shah, N. D., Nasir, K., Einstein, A. J., & Nallamothu, B. K. (2009). Exposure to low-dose ionizing radiation from medical imaging procedures. *New England Journal of Medicine*, *361*(9), 849–857.

Frank, E., Stears, J., Gray, J., Winkler, N. T, & Hoffman, A. D. (1984). Use of the P. A. projection: A method of reducing x-ray exposure to specific radiosensitive organs. *The Canadian Journal of Medical Radiation Technology*, *15*(2), 63.

Frank, E. D. (1983). Use of the posteroanterior projection: A method of reducing x-ray exposure to specific radiosensitive organs. *Radiologic Technology, 54*, 343–347.

Godderidge, C. (1981). A radiology department's response to consumer concerns regarding the hazards of low-dose radiation. *Radiology Management, 4*(3), 1.

Goldman, L. W. (2007). Principles of CT: Radiation dose and image quality. *Journal of Nuclear Medicine Technology, 35*(4), 213–228.

Hall, E. J. (2005). *Radiobiology for the radiologist* (6th ed.). Philadelphia: J. B. Lippincott.

Joseph, L. P., & Wollerton, M. A. (1984). *Extremity radiography following trauma: An overview* (HEW Publication [FDA] 84–8232). Rockville, MD: U.S. Department of Health, Education, and Welfare, Public Health Service, Food and Drug Administration, Bureau of Radiological Health.

Light, M. C., Molloi, S. Y., Yandouo, D. R., & Ranallo, F. N. (1987). Scatter radiation exposure during knee arthrography. *Radiology*, 867.

Maillie, H. D., Segal, A., & Lemkin, J. (1982). Effect of patient size on doses received by patients in diagnostic radiology. *Health Physics, 42*, 665–670.

McGlone, W. E. (1970). Radiation protection of the reproductive organs during radiography of the hip joints. *Radiologic Technology, 41*, 277–279.

National Council on Radiation Protection and Measurements (NCRP). (1987). *Ionizing radiation exposure of the population of the United States* (NCRP Report No. 93). Bethesda, MD.

National Council on Radiation Protection and Measurements (NCRP). (1989). *Medical x-ray, electron beam and gamma-ray protection for energies up to 50 meV (equipment design, performance and use)* (NCRP Report No. 102). Bethesda, MD.

National Council on Radiation Protection and Measurements (NCRP). (1990). *Implementation of the principle of ALARA for medical and dental personnel* (NCRP Report No. 107). Bethesda, MD.

Ng, K. H., & Bardley, D. A. (1998). *Subject dose in radiological imaging*. Saint Louis: Elseiver.

Nickoloff, E. L., Lu, Z. F., Dutta, A. K., & So, J. C. (2008). Radiation dose descriptors: BERT, COD, DAP, and other strange creatures. *RadioGraphics, 28*(5), 1439–1450.

Novitch, M. (1983). Evaluation of radiation exposure in diagnostic radiology examinations. *Radiology Management, 5*(4), 33.

Rosenstein, M. (1988). *Handbook of selected tissue doses for projections common in diagnostic radiology* (HEW Publication [FDA] 89–8031). Rockville, MD: U.S. Department of Health, Education, and Welfare, Public Health Service, Food and Drug Administration, Bureau of Radiological Health.

Schrimpton, P. C. (1988). Monitoring the dose to patients undergoing common x-ray examinations. *Radiography Today, 54*, 619.

Seeram, E., & Travis, E. L. (1997). *Radiation protection*. Baltimore: Lippincott Williams and Wilkins.

Shleien, B., Tucker, T. T., & Johnson, D. W. (1977). *The mean active bone marrow dose to the adult population of the United States from diagnostic radiology* (HEW Publication [FDA] 77–8013). Rockville, MD: U.S. Department of Health, Education, and Welfare, Public Health Service, Food and Drug Administration, Bureau of Radiological Health.

Sidhu, M., Coley, B. D., Goske, M. J., Connolly, B., Racadio, J., Yoshizumi, T. T., Utley, T., & Strauss, K. J. (2009). Image gently, step lightly: Increasing radiation dose awareness in pediatric interventional radiology. *Pediatric Radiology, 39*(10), 1135–1138.

Uffmann, M., & Schaefer-Prokop, C. (2009). Digital radiography: The balance between image quality and required radiation dose. *European Journal of Radiology, 72*(2), 202–208

U.S. Department of Health, Education, and Welfare. (1984). *Nationwide evaluation of x-ray trends (NEXT)—Eight Years of Data (1974–1981)* (HEW Publication [FDA] 84–8229). Rockville, MD: Author.

Watkins, G. L. (1988). Public health risks from low dose medical radiation. *Radiologic Technology, 59*(2), 160.

Wesenberg, R. L., Blumhagen, J. D., Rossi, R. P., Hilton, S. W., Gilbert, J. M., & Nedeau, D. J. (1980). Low-dose radiography of children. *Radiologic Technology, 51*(5), 641.

Whalen, J. P., & Balter, S. (1984). *Radiation risks in medical imaging*. Chicago: Yearbook Medical.

Yanch, J. C., Behrman, R. H., Hendricks, M. J., & McCall, J. H. (2009). Increased radiation dose to overweight and obese patients from radiographic examinations. *Radiology, 252*(1), 128–139.

Unit III

Creating the Image

14 Vision and Perception / 220

15 Beam Restriction / 233

16 The Patient as a Beam Emitter / 240

17 The Pathology Problem / 246

18 The Grid / 257

19 Radiographic Film / 273

20 Film Processing / 283

21 Film Sensitometry / 294

22 Intensifying Screens and Film/Screen Combinations / 308

23 Digital Radiography / 323

24 Picture Archiving and Communications Systems (PACSs) / 362

Creating the image that appears on the radiograph occupies the majority of the radiographer's time and requires a great deal of skill. The ability of the radiologist to make a diagnosis depends on the radiographer's ability to create a diagnostic-quality image. This ability is predicated on a thorough knowledge of the scientific basis by which the image is produced as well as clinical experiences.

This unit introduces the important aspects of **vision and perception.** Understanding how the information from the radiographic image will be transmitted to the brain of the viewer is critical to understanding exactly how to manipulate the image to maximize the diagnostic information it conveys. Producing quality images requires knowledge of x-ray **beam restriction,** the concept of **the patient as a beam emitter,** the **pathology problem** inherent in many examinations, the proper use of the **grid, radiographic film,** and **film processing. Sensitometry** is necessary to evaluate films and monitor their quality, and an understanding of **intensifying screens and film/screen combinations** is required to permit minimum patient exposure while maximizing diagnostic information on the film. Creating the image using **digital radiography** image detector systems requires an understanding of digital image processing, digital radiography, and digital image management. Finally, the use of **picture archiving and communication systems (PACS)** is essential for maintaining the images for diagnosis. The diagnostic image is created only when all of these factors are applied with professional skill.

CHAPTER 14

Vision and Perception

KEY TERMS

cone cells
contrast perception
edge enhancement
Mach effect
rod cell
threshold detection
visual acuity

She is so tall, so slender, and her bones—
Those frail phosphates, those carbonates of lime—
Are well produced by cathode rays sublime,
By oscillations, amperes and by ohms.
Her dorsal vertebrae are not concealed
By epidermis, but are well revealed.
Around her ribs, those beauteous twenty-four,
Her flesh a halo makes, misty in line,
Her noseless, eyeless face looks into mine,
And I but whisper, "Sweetheart, je t'adore."
Her white and gleaming teeth at me do laugh.
Ah! Lovely, cruel, sweet (radio)graph!

Lawrence K. Russell, Life, 1896

OBJECTIVES

Upon completion of this chapter, the student should be able to:

- Draw a cross-sectional image of a human eye with appropriate anatomical structures identified.
- Explain the physiological function of the eye during photopic and scotopic vision.
- Discuss the inefficiency of the medical imaging process.
- Describe the boundary effect, Mach effect, eye motion, veil glare, and the effect of viewing distance on visual perceptions.
- State why pattern recognition is the domain of the radiologist.

OBJECTIVES (continued)

- Discuss the concept of controlling the radiographic image in space.
- Apply the concept of three-dimensional thinking to clinical practice.
- Identify numerous creative uses of radiography in medicine, technology, and art.

IMAGE PERCEPTION

At one time or another we have all been fooled by visual misperceptions. A common example is shown in Figure 14-1. Misperceptions of any type can be dangerous in clinical radiography. An important method of overcoming misperception is the elimination of preconceived ideas about an image. A mental erasing of these opinions is necessary to permit high-quality viewing of radiographic images. This is a skill that is cultivated by radiologists until it becomes part of their routine diagnostic procedure. Radiographers observe the diagnostic reporting of images by radiologists with amazement at first, but with increasing confidence as experience adds knowledge about the potential pathological meaning of various radiologic signs. Radiographers should strive toward developing an understanding of the perceptual problems that radiologists encounter when attempting to interpret radiographic images. Through this understanding the radiographer can work toward producing images with patterns that provide maximum assistance to the radiologist in the diagnostic process.

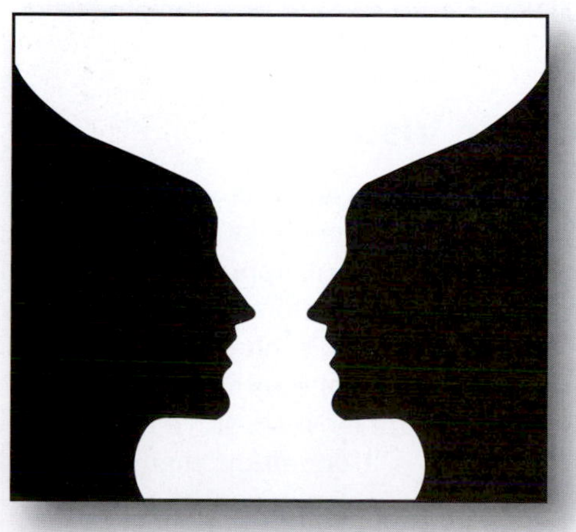

FIGURE 14-1. "The Lady and the Chalice" can be seen either as a pair of black faces in silhouette or as a white vase. This picture was devised by E. Rubin in 1915 and remains popular as a method of demonstrating perceptual differences.

Visual Anatomy

Because radiography depends entirely on images, it is helpful to be introduced to the complexities of visual perception. The mechanics of image perception are mostly unknown. It is little understood exactly how the eye perceives images and transmits them to the brain. Even less is known about how the brain neurologically processes the information.

The human eye is anatomically designed to gather light, focus it, convert it to nervous impulses, and transmit it to the brain for processing. The aqueous humor, cornea, iris, and lens gather and focus the light (Figure 14-2). The specialized cells of the retina, especially the fovea centralis (or macula lutea), convert the image to nervous impulses, and the optic nerve transmits the impulses to the brain for processing. With corneal malfunction, such as myopia and hyperopia, the most common problems requiring corrective lenses, a distinct loss of detail is perceived because the incoming light is not properly focused on the retina. This is easily perceived and well-established means are available for correction. Image conversion and processing problems are not as easily perceived and these deserve some elementary study.

Visual Physiology

It is often uncertain whether conversion and processing problems are caused by the light-sensitive cells located in the retina or by mental misperceptions due to neurological processing. Sufficient research has been done at least to outline some of the factors that may cause misperceptions. Understanding that these factors exist and how they can prejudice perception can assist greatly in reducing visual problems.

An excellent example of misperception is the tendency to stare at an object that is difficult to

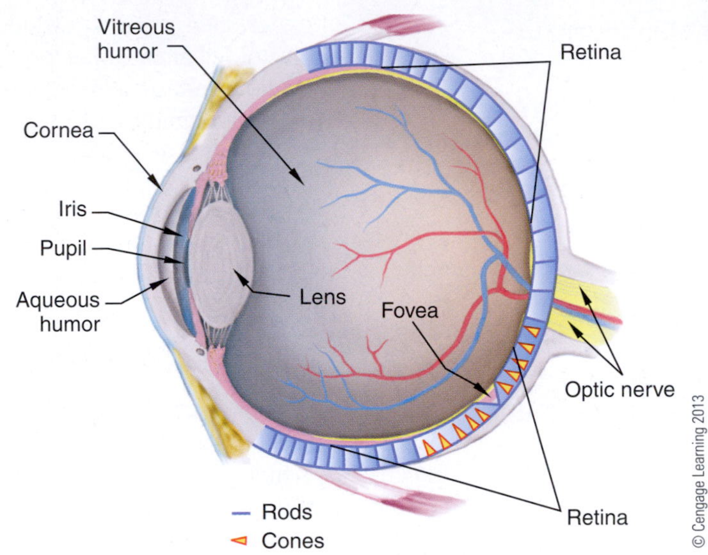

FIGURE 14-2. The human eye.

see. Although this may be a good method of mental concentration, it does nothing to improve the visual quality of the image. In fact, it does the opposite. The length of time the human visual system can integrate (acquire information) is only 0.2 second. If the image does not provide enough information to be converted and processed in that time, the visual system will reset itself and reacquire information for the next 0.2 second. Therefore, when insufficient information is provided to the radiologist due to improper illumination, or distracting reflected light, only an improvement in the quality and quantity of light photons available will improve the visual image. The image does much to resolve the integration time problem. Because the monitor or film can integrate information for a considerable length of time and then hold that information, it permits the human brain to integrate much more visual information than if the image were viewed as it was acquired from the patient.

Rod and Cone Cells

Human image conversion occurs in the **rod** and **cone cells** located in the retina. Both of these types of cells contain photosensitive pigments that will respond to light by sending an electrical potential to specialized nerve cells. These bipolar cells emit neurological impulses when excited by light photons. The two types of cells are so different in their receiving and sending abilities that neurophysiologists tend to consider them as two separate visual systems. The cells are only about 1 μm in diameter and are concentrated to 100,000 per mm^2. There are approximately 7,000,000 cones, which are located only at the fovea centralis. There are approximately 120,000,000 rods covering the remainder of the retina.

Photopic Vision

Photopic (daylight) vision is controlled by the cones. Cone cells require relatively bright light to function (a minimum of approximately 100 light photons). Cone cells contain one of three different light-sensitive pigments, each of which is sensitive to a different range of photon wavelength (color of light). The cones are most sensitive to yellow light. Color blindness is a condition that occurs when there is a lack of cones sensitive to a particular color or colors.

Because most of the cones are located at the fovea centralis in high concentration, daylight vision is sharply focused. Therefore, **visual acuity** is improved in daylight. The sparse concentration of cones in the retina outside the fovea centralis accounts for poor

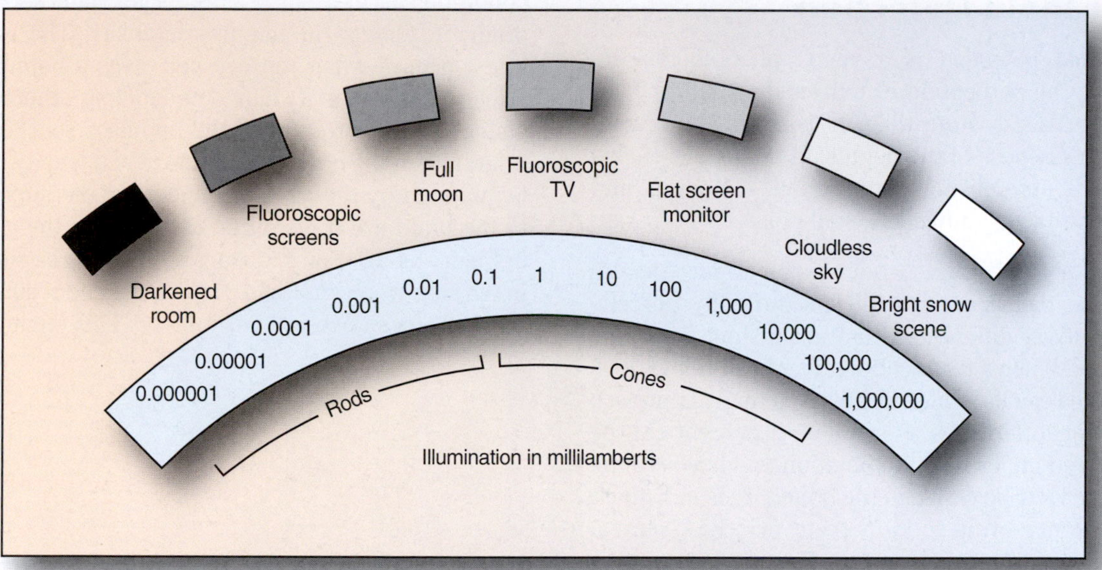

FIGURE 14-3. Human visual ability.

peripheral vision in daylight. Cones are also able to detect changes in brightness far better than rod cells. This permits much greater recognition of gray-scale differences, or contrast, and results in what is called greater **contrast perception** (Figure 14-3).

Scotopic Vision

Scotopic (night) vision is controlled by the rods. Rod cells are sensitive to low light levels (they may respond to as few as 15 photons) but cannot function in bright light. Rod cells cannot distinguish wavelength, although they are more sensitive to green light. As a result, humans are unable to perceive colors in extremely low-light situations. Rod cells function by photosensitization of rhodopsin, also known as "visual purple," because it is most sensitive to blue-green wavelengths. When exposed to vast quantities of light photons, rhodopsin is oversensitized and becomes bleached out. The rod cells then regenerate rhodopsin at the rate of 50 percent each 7 minutes. This is the reason a bright light causes temporary blindness in both humans and animals. Because there are no rods in the fovea centralis, dim-light vision is entirely peripheral and therefore difficult to bring into sharp focus. In addition, rods are not as concentrated because they are spread over a much greater area than cones. For these reasons, radiologists realize that dim objects are best viewed peripherally. Rods function better when the image information is changing. Slow scanning with an old fluoroscopic unit, night binoculars, or when walking in a dark room will increase visual acuity.

Inefficiency of the Medical Imaging Process

Few radiographers realize exactly how inefficient the entire imaging process is. An early fluoroscopic image study showed that although the x-ray tube was emitting 5,000,000 photons per second per mm^2 amplified over 5,000 times by the fluoroscopic intensification screen, only 65 photons contributed to the final impulses received by the brain. This is a conversion efficiency of 0.00005 percent (1 out of 2,000,000 photons) from the fluoroscopic screen and 0.001 percent (1 out of 100,000 photons) from the tube output.

Threshold Detection

Threshold detection is a visual phenomenon involving the perception of extremely small or faint details. This is more than an issue of the resolution, or fineness of the details, in the image. It also involves minimizing background exposure and other artifacts, known as visual noise.

Boundary Effect. A boundary effect occurs because the visual system has difficulty perceiving contrast differences that are distant from one another. When a distinct boundary between various densities can be achieved (this is actually contrast), adjacent differences as small as 2 percent can be perceived under high illumination (such as a radiographic view box). When the boundary is indistinct, a difference of up to 20 percent may be required. Less intense light levels also affect this perception ability.

There is a rule of thumb in radiography that density/image receptor exposure changes should be at least 25–33 percent to be visible. This is because two radiographs of differing densities are seen quite distant from one another. If a change of this magnitude formed an adjacent boundary, it would be strikingly apparent. Surrounding densities have an effect on the perception of nearby densities. This results in confusion when judging absolute and relative levels of density/image receptor exposure and contrast from one image to another.

Another aspect of the boundary effect concerns the length of the boundary line. A subtle exposure difference along the length of a long boundary may be perceived but when it is shortened the boundary may no longer be perceived. As yet there is no explanation for this phenomenon but radiologists can best observe extremely subtle exposure differences when they form a long boundary. They may fail to see diagnostic information when exposure differences are widely separated or form short boundaries. In these instances it is important for the radiographer to attempt to provide better perception through higher contrast.

Mach Effect. Part of the boundary effect may be explained by a phenomenon called the Mach effect. The retina contains neural connections that inhibit impulses under certain conditions. One of these conditions is extremely bright light; another is a dramatic change in impulse intensity. The Mach effect occurs when the eye perceives a boundary. Each time there is a change in exposure, there is a change in the intensity of the impulses sent to the brain. When the beginning of the new intensity level is inhibited by the neural connectors, the impulses to the brain are transmitted as shown in the graph in Figure 14-4B. For exposure differences as shown in the step wedge in Figure 14-4A, the end result is a response as shown in Figure 14-4C. This creates an

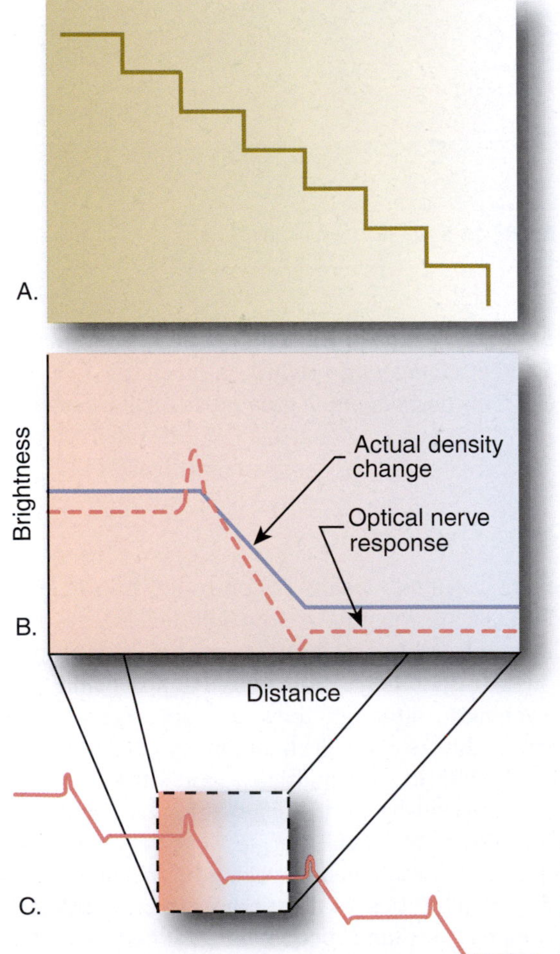

FIGURE 14-4. The Mach effect: (A) actual density differences, (B) comparison of actual density changes to optical nerve response, and (C) optical nerve response from A.

FIGURE 14-5. Optical step wedges. Note the prominent Mach effect through the lighter densities of the upper step wedges.

FIGURE 14-6. A continuous grayscale produced with a continuous sloping aluminum step wedge.

effect known as **edge enhancement**. Edge enhancement compresses the entire grayscale while making the boundary appear more distinct than it really is. For example, in Figure 14-5 many of the lighter steps appear to be lighter just before the edge of the next darker step. This perceptual illusion is the Mach effect. Although this makes it easier to perceive the edges, radiologists are concerned about the possibility of a small detail being lost because its exposure is overwritten by edge enhancement. Figures 14-5 and 14-6 have the same light-to-dark grayscale. Note that the lack of a distinct boundary line causes a difference in perception of the range of visible exposures.

Eye Motion. Contrast perception is dramatically increased when the eye uses a scanning motion, as when reading a book. Because the photosensitive cells in the eye can integrate a limited amount of information, eye movement maintains a constantly changing neurological signal, thus avoiding saturation of the optical nerves.

Veil Glare. Veil glare occurs when the intensely bright light from a view box floods the eye directly. This occurs in unexposed areas of the image and between images. The bright light scatters inside the eye and reduces contrast perception, much as Compton scatter does within the patient.

Viewing Distance. Data concerning threshold detection indicate that results change when the viewing distance is changed. This occurs because of the changes in intensity due to the inverse square law and because the physiological processing of the image changes when the angle of the incident light photons changes. In addition, the fovea centralis creates a blind spot at a viewing distance of about 9 inches. Therefore, radiologists often vary their viewing distances when addressing areas of perceptual difficulty.

Pattern Recognition

Pattern recognition involves perceiving combinations of details that can be defined and classified toward a diagnosis. This is the area radiologists often study the hardest. Just as it is difficult to identify a picture of a familiar face when it is shown upside down, so it is important that radiologists be presented with images in a routine manner. For example, radiographs are universally viewed as if the viewer were facing the patient (the patient's left is on the viewer's right, etc.).

Pattern recognition involves comparing mental images of patterns—anatomical, physiological, pathological, and histological—to arrive at a diagnostic opinion. Because of the complexities between the visual system and the mental capability to store and recall image patterns from memory, and because of the lack of scientific knowledge about how the brain processes information, pattern recognition is a weak area of research and no data can be provided to help the radiographer assist the radiologist. Pattern recognition is the true domain of the radiologist, who has the requisite medical knowledge to be competent in this area.

CONTROLLING THE IMAGE IN SPACE

One of the challenges to the radiographer is to place the patient so that the area to be imaged is in a position that will enhance the quality of the image. It is helpful to visualize the object of radiographic interest (kidney, scapula, sinus, etc.) as floating in space within the body of the patient. The skill of the radiographer lies in manipulating the object to the correct position in relationship to the x-ray beam and image receptor (film). This is the art of controlling the image in space.

Thinking Three-Dimensionally

The radiographer must be capable of controlling the image in space in an artistic manner. This is one of the critical elements of professionalism. It is important to view images from a perspective of thinking three-dimensionally. This concept is extremely valuable in forming perceptual ability. The experienced

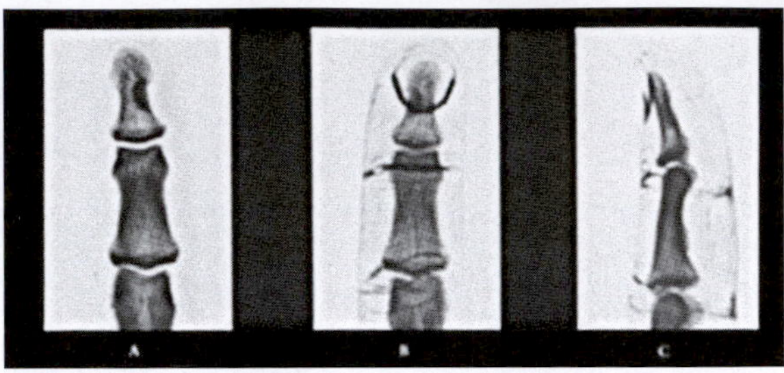

FIGURE 14-7. A three-dimensional effect. *Reprinted by permission of the publisher from* Squires Fundamentals of Radiology, *Fifth Edition, edited by Robert A. Novelline, p. 12, Cambridge, MA: Harvard University Press, (Copyright © 1975, 1982, 1988, 1997 by the President and Fellows of Harvard College.)*

radiographer can see an incredible amount of beauty in the radiographs that are produced every day. Just as the barium-coated finger (Figure 14-7) is easily perceived in three dimensions, so are most radiographs viewed in this manner by radiographers. The magnification of structures some distance from the receptor places them further away in perspective; finely detailed structures seem to move closer, and each image assumes a three-dimensionality usually not noticed by the novice.

Radiographic positioning requires a solid knowledge of the shape and location of skeletal and soft tissue structures and an in-depth understanding of their anatomical relationship to one another.

The human body is a three-dimensional object, but radiographic images possess only two dimensions—length and width. Consequently, conventional radiographic images are missing a critical diagnostic element—the dimension of depth. This can only be compensated for by never settling for a single radiographic view of any structure. **At least two images, as close to 90° angles to one another as possible, are required to view all three dimensions.** Although computed tomography is capable of creating three dimensional images, these take time, special processing procedures, and are expensive to create.

The dimensional views required for all radiographic examinations are **anterior-posterior, medial-lateral, and superior-inferior.** All radiographic images will demonstrate two, but never all three, of these perspectives. For example, a posteroanterior (PA) chest radiograph demonstrates the medial-lateral dimension and the superior-inferior dimension, but not the anterior-posterior dimension. The dimension that describes the entrance and exit of the central ray, which is used to describe the projection, is the dimension not visualized. In situations where superimposition makes PA and lateral projections useless, two oblique positions at 90° angles from one another can be used to achieve the same effect.

An important skill that must be developed by the radiographer is the ability to mentally visualize the changing and moving of overlying anatomical structures from any angle in order to provide an image free of superimposition. Artistic techniques should be understood, such as making exposures while the patient is breathing, thus using patient motion to blur superimposing structures from the image (i.e., to blur ribs from the lateral projection of the thoracic vertebral column).

RADIOGRAPHY AS AN ART FORM

Radiography is an art form. In the century since its discovery it has been used to investigate an incredible variety of animals and objects. Examples of radiography as a technical and purely creative art form abound. Numerous radiographers have not only taken pride in the quality of their clinical abilities but have extended their technical skills into artistic expressions of creativity.

Radiographers can become technically artistic; innovative adaptations of routine procedures should be considered technical artistry. For example, it is technically artistic to reverse angles to produce a diagnostic-quality modified image of a fractured clavicle on a trauma patient who cannot be moved due to thoracic injuries, or to lower the tube and support an image receptor under a wheelchair patient's foot so that it is unnecessary to move a weak patient with a full leg cast onto a radiographic table.

Artistic Radiography

William Conklin, a South Carolina radiographer artist, achieved national acclaim for his radiography/

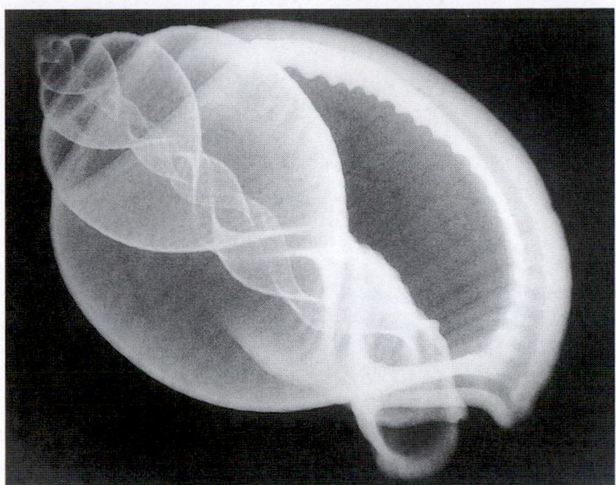

FIGURE 14-8. "Scotch Bonnet," by William A. Conklin, RT FASRT. *(With permission of William A. Conklin, Inner Dimension, 1571 Marshall Avenue, Orangeburg, SC 29115.)*

photography of sea shells (Figure 14-8). Conklin's work has appeared in *National Geographic* and is in the permanent collection of the Smithsonian Institution. Radiography has often been used to produce a unique perspective of flowers, fruit, and other plants, as well as of shells and fish.

Nondestructive Testing

The entire industrial radiography field, known as nondestructive testing (NDT) radiography, is unknown to many medical radiographers. The intent of NDT radiography is to assist in the examination and assessment of materials such as castings, welds, and others through noninvasive techniques.

Biological Research

Radiography has proven an invaluable tool in biological research, not only in medical studies, but also in monitoring animal functions. For example, the study of birds and bats in flight is greatly enhanced by high-speed radiography.

Veterinary Radiography

Veterinary medicine and dentistry also use radiography to accomplish many diagnoses. Figure 14-9, a canary with an egg, is an example of veterinary radiography. This type of radiography is also used in

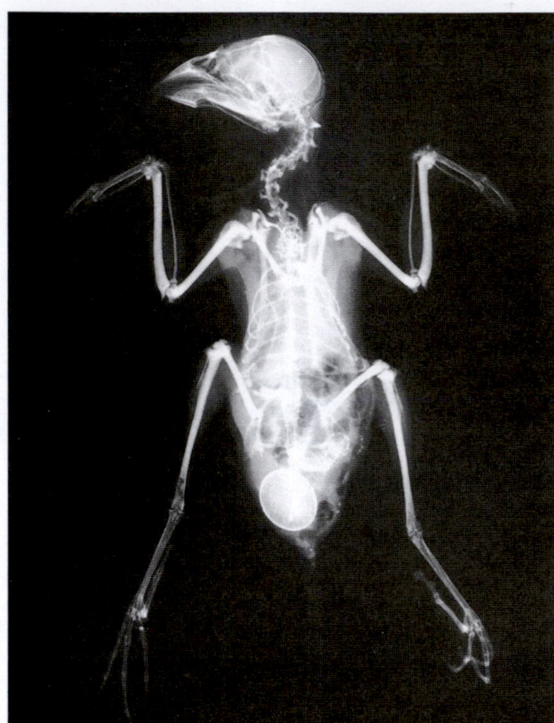

FIGURE 14-9. Canary with an egg. *(Courtesy of Dr. Marion Frank.)*

zoos. Radiographers have been called on to examine all types of animals, from live venomous snakes to passive house pets to million-dollar race horses

Forensic Radiography

Forensic medicine uses radiography in a wide variety of ways. Grenz rays (5–30-kVp x-rays) are used, as are diagnostic x-rays. Grenz rays are emitted by specially designed tubes with minimal inherent filtration. They are useful for demonstrating objects as diverse as the ink on money when counterfeiting is suspected, the contents of envelopes and packages, fingerprints, and art forgery.

Art Restoration

Grenz ray radiography has also proven useful during restoration of paintings and other art objects. Radiography can detect images under existing paint, frame, and canvas construction and different types of paint and brush styles (Figures 14-10A and 14-10B).

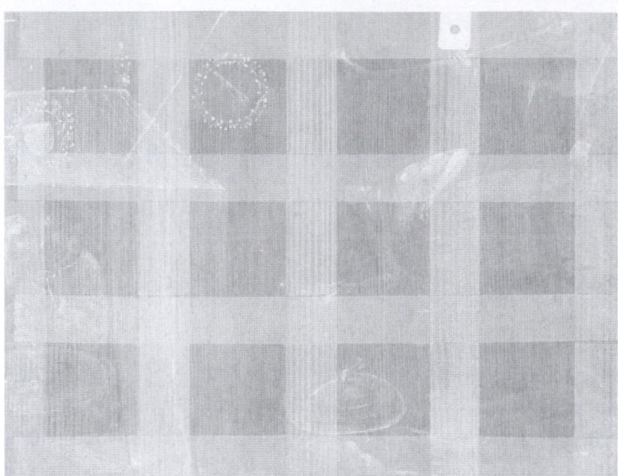

FIGURE 14-10A. A Grenz ray radiograph of a section of "Intemperance" by Hieronymus Bosch. *(Courtesy of Gerald Conlogue, Gulf Coast Community College.)*

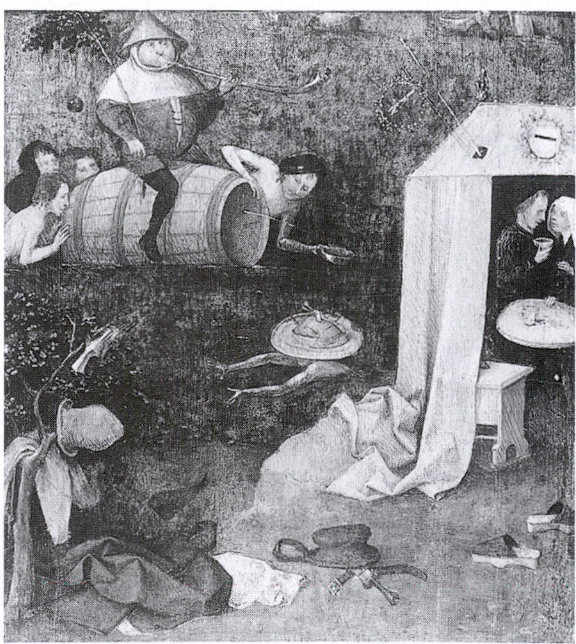

FIGURE 14-10B. "Intemperance" by Hieronymus Bosch. *(Reprinted with permission from Yale University Art Gallery, The Rabinowitz Collection.)*

Archaeological Radiography

Radiography has become a useful archaeological tool, especially in the examination of fragile mummified remains. Numerous reports of such investigations have been published. Among these publications are reports of radiographic discoveries of jewelry, diseases, murders, dietary habits, and the remains of a baboon that had been assumed to be a royal child (Figure 14-11) at the National Museum in Cairo; Peruvian mummies with ceramic pots in the chest; computed tomography images of the royal mummies in Egypt that reveal pathologies previously unsuspected; and many other aspects of imaging of ancient artifacts.

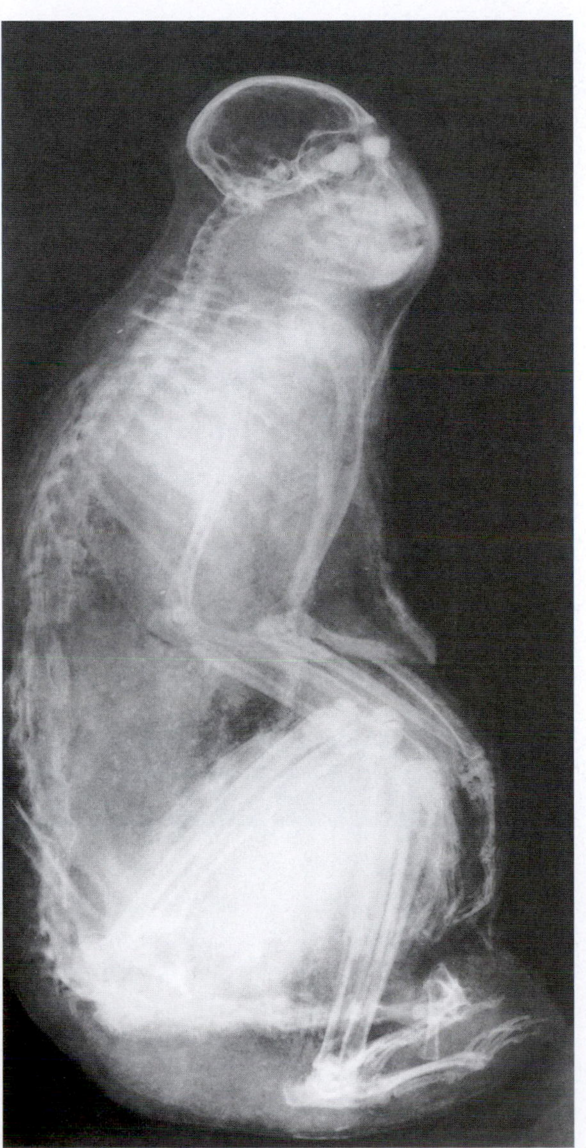

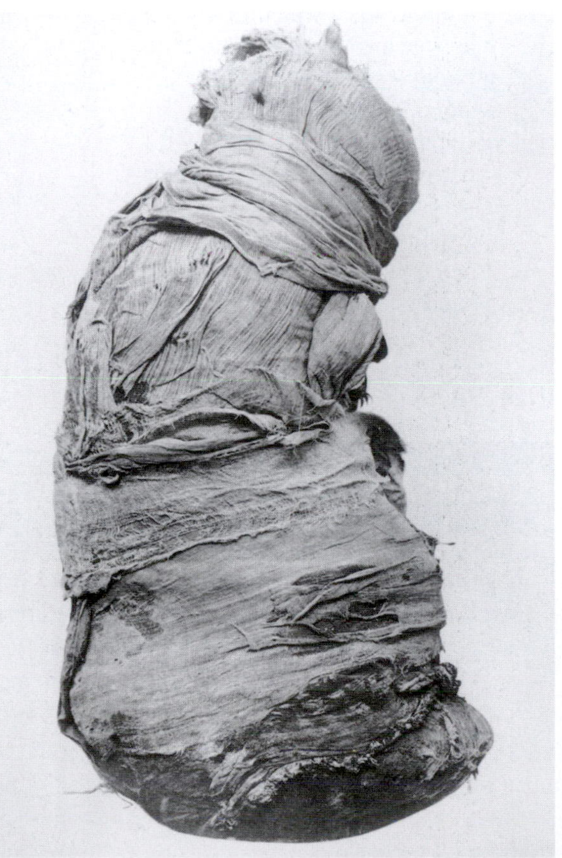

FIGURE 14-11. A female hamadryas baboon mummy found buried with MAkare, a member of an ancient Egyptian priesthood family, who was pregnant at the time of her death. *(Reprinted with permission from "X-Raying the Pharoahs," by James E. Harris and Kent R. Weeks.)*

Poetry

Radiographic images themselves inspire many of us. The physician poet Jack Coulehan was inspired by a chest radiograph to compose this poem:

The Old Man with Stars Inside Him

I look at the X-ray,
a shadow of pneumonia
deep in this old man's chest,
and watch Antonio shake
with a cough that traveled here
from the beginning of life.
As he pulls my hand to his lips
and kisses my hand,
Antonio tells me, for a man
whose death is gnawing at his spine,
pneumonia is a welcome friend
who reaches in between his ribs
without a sound and puff!
a cloud begins to squeeze
so delicately
the great white image of his heart.
The shadow advances
every time Antonio moves—
when a nurse positions his body,
when he takes a sip of ice,
when he shakes with a cough,
moist and diminished.
I see in that delicate shadow
a cloud of gas
at the galaxy's center,
a cloud of cold stunned nuclei
beginning to spin,
spinning and shooting
a hundred thousand
embryos of stars.
I listen to Antonio's chest
where stars crackle from the past
and hear the boom
of blue giants newly caught.
I hear the snap
of white dwarves coughing, shooting.
The second time Antonio
kisses my hand
I feel his dusky lips
reach out from everywhere in space.
I look at the place
his body was
and see inside Antonio, the stars.

(*Reprinted with permission from* Midwest Poetry Review, © *Jack Coulehan 1988*)

SUMMARY

Understanding visual perception is an important aspect of clinical radiography. This understanding helps overcome misperceptions about an image.

The human eye is designed to gather light, focus it, convert it to nerve impulses, and transmit it to the brain for processing. Image conversion occurs in the rod and cone cells, which contain photosensitive pigments that will respond to light. Photopic (daylight) vision is controlled by the cones, and scotopic (night) vision is controlled by the rods.

Threshold detection is a visual phenomenon involving the perception of extremely small or faint details. The boundary effect occurs because the visual system has difficulty perceiving contrast differences that are distant from one another. When densities are adjacent, small differences can be perceived. Part of the boundary effect can be explained by the Mach effect. When the eye perceives a boundary, a change occurs in the intensity of the impulses sent to the brain. This change in intensity creates an effect known as edge

SUMMARY (continued)

enhancement, which makes the boundary appear distinct. Contrast perception is dramatically increased by eye motion or scanning the image. Veil glare occurs when bright lights, such as a view box, flood the eye. Viewing distance has an effect on threshold detection.

Pattern recognition involves perceiving combinations of details that can be defined and classified toward a diagnosis. It helps the radiologist compare mental images of patterns with medical knowledge.

Radiographers need to think three-dimensionally. Radiographic images possess two dimensions and, as a result, at least two images as close to 90° angles to one another as possible are required to view all three dimensions. It is considered technical artistry when radiographers use innovation to adapt a routine procedure.

Radiography is an art form that has been used to investigate a wide array of animals and objects. It is used in nondestructive testing, biological research and veterinary and forensic radiography, art restoration, and archeological radiography, and has even been the subject of poetry. ■

REVIEW QUESTIONS

1. What is the anatomical function of the human eye?
2. What is the difference between photopic and scotopic vision?
3. Explain the boundary effect.
4. What is the Mach effect?
5. How is pattern recognition used by the radiologist in making a diagnosis?
6. Why is it important for the radiographer to produce two images as close to 90° angles to one another as possible?
7. Name three examples of the use of radiography as an art form.

REFERENCES AND RECOMMENDED READING

Abildgaard, A., & Notthellen, J. A. (1992). Increasing contrast when viewing radiographic images. *Radiology, 185*(2), 475–478.

Adrian-Harris, D. (1979). Aspects of visual perception in radiography. *Radiography, 45*(539), 237–243.

Arnold, M. (1993). The importance of spatial ability in the selection of student radiographers. *Radiography Today, 59*(679), 20–22.

Bruce, V., Georgeson, M. A., & Green, P. R. (2003). *Visual perception: Physiology, psychology and ecology.* London: Psychology Press.

Chester, M. S. (1982). Perception and evaluation of images. In P. T. N. Wells (Ed.), *Scientific basis of medical imaging.* Edinburgh: Churchill Livingstone.

Cornsweet, T. N. (1970). *Visual perception.* New York: Academic Press.

Curry, T. S., Dowdey, J. E., & Murry, R. C. (1990). *Christensen's introduction to the physics of diagnostic radiology* (4th ed.). Philadelphia: Lea and Febiger.

Fuchs, A. W. (1932). Radiography of the entire body employing one film and a single exposure. *Radiography and Clinical Photography, 10*, 9–14.

Gibbs, S. J., Price, R. R., & James, A. E. (1981). Image perception. In C. M. Coulam, J. J. Erickson, F. D. Rollo, & A. E. James (Eds.), *The physical basis of medical imaging* (pp. 295–302). New York: Appleton-Century-Crofts.

Graham, D., & Thomson, J. (1980). *Grenz rays: An illustrated guide to the theory and practical applications of soft x-rays.* Oxford: Pergamon Press.

Hendee, W. R. (1988). The human visual system and its application to perception of radiographic images. *Investigative Radiology, 24*, 25.

Hendee, W. R. (1988). Image analysis and perception. In C. E. Putnam & C. E. Ravin (Eds.), *Textbook of diagnostic imaging.* Philadelphia: W. B. Saunders.

Hendee, W. R. (1989). The perception of visual data. *American Journal of Roentgenology, 152*, 1313–1317.

Hendee, W. R., & Ritenour, R. (1993). *Medical imaging physics* (3rd ed.). St. Louis, MO: Elsevier/C. V. Mosby.

Hendee, W. R., & Wells, P. T. N. (1994). *Perception of visual information.* New York: Springer-Verlag.

Jaffe, C. C. (Ed.). (1981). *Second international conference on visual psychophysics and medical imaging.* Piscataway, NJ: Institute of Electrical and Electronic Engineers (Catalog #81CH) 1676–6.

Jaffe, C. C. (1984). Medical imaging, vision, and visual psychophysics. *Medical Radiography and Photography, 60*(1), 1–48.

Manning, D., & Cooper, A. (1993). Chest x-ray image quality: Relationships between physical measurements and observer grading. *Radiography Today, 59*(678), 12–15.

Moore, H. D. (Ed.). (1981). *Materials and processes for NDT technology.* Columbus, OH: American Society for Nondestructive Testing.

Neisser, U. (1964). Visual search. *Scientific American, 210*(6), 94–102.

Novelline R. (2004). *Squire's fundamentals of radiology* (6th ed.). Cambridge, MA: Harvard University Press.

Richardson, H. D. (1968). *NDT radiography manual.* Washington, DC: U.S. Government Printing Office, U.S. Department of Health, Education, and Welfare.

Rose, A. (1948). The sensitivity performance of the human eye on an absolute scale. *Journal of the Optical Society of America, 38*(2), 196–208.

Schnitzler, A. D. (1973). Image-detector model and parameters of the human visual system. *Journal of the Optical Society of America, 63*(11), 1357–1368.

Schwartz, S. (2009). *Visual perception: A clinical orientation* (4th ed.). New York: McGraw-Hill Medical.

Tuddenham, W. J. (1957). The visual physiology of Roentgen diagnosis. *American Journal of Roentgenology, 78*(1), 116–123.

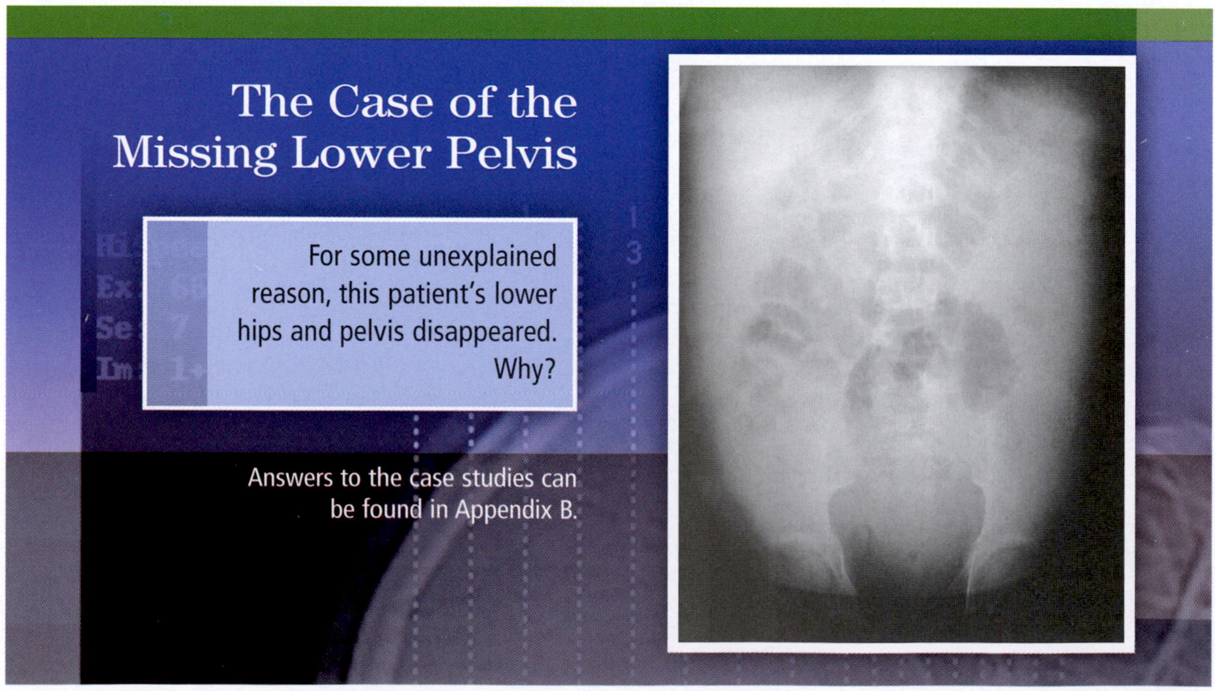

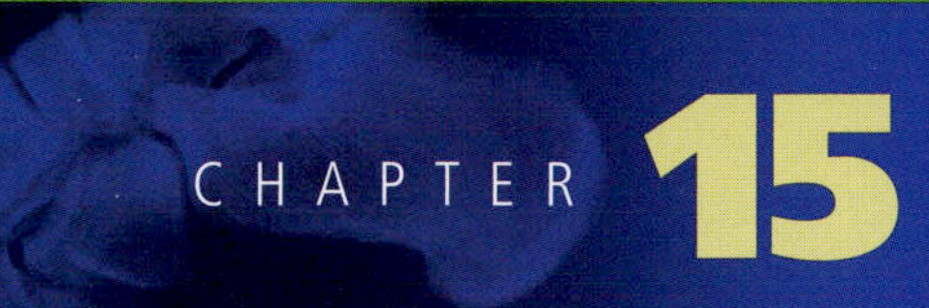

CHAPTER 15 Beam Restriction

KEY TERMS

collimator

penumbra

positive beam limitation (PBL) device

> Tell the world to wait
> till we set the record straight
> x-ray vision
> baby, I can see thru you
>
> *Moon Martin, Pete Sinfield, and Terry Taylor, "X-Ray Vision," from Mystery Ticket*

OBJECTIVES

Upon completion of this chapter, the student should be able to:

- Identify the factors that affect the amount of scatter radiation produced.
- Discuss the primary methods used by radiographers to control the amount of scatter radiation reaching the image receptor.
- Explain the purpose and construction of beam-restricting devices.
- Compare the advantages and disadvantages of the various beam-restricting devices.
- Describe the effect of beam restriction on image quality and patient dose.

CONTROLLING SCATTER

Scatter radiation is produced during a Compton interaction. In this interaction, a primary photon interacts with an outer-shell electron and changes direction, thereby becoming a scattered photon. Scattered photons are not a part of the useful beam and will impair image quality by placing exposures on the image receptor that are unrelated to patient anatomy. In order to provide the best possible image, the radiographer must try to minimize the amount of scatter radiation reaching the image receptor. **This can best be accomplished by restricting the x-ray beam and by using a grid.** Proper beam restriction will keep the total amount of tissue irradiation to a minimum and has great importance in both improving image quality and reducing patient dose.

As the beam is restricted, fewer primary photons are emitted from the tube and collimator and fewer scattered photons are created. Additionally, the decrease in the number of primary photons results in a decrease in the dose to the patient. The only way to improve image quality once scattered photons have been created is to try to decrease the numbers that are allowed to interact with the image receptor. Grids are devices that are placed between the patient and the image receptor to absorb scatter radiation.

The principal factors that affect the amount of scatter produced are (1) kilovoltage and (2) the irradiated material. In order to control the amount of scatter produced, it is important to understand how kilovoltage and the irradiated material affect scatter production.

Kilovoltage

Kilovoltage affects the penetrability of the beam. As kVp increases, fewer photons undergo interaction with matter and more pass through the patient to interact with the image receptor. For the photons that undergo an interaction, photoelectric absorption and Compton interactions are predominant in the diagnostic x-ray range. Although the total number of photons that undergo interaction decreases with increased kVp, a shift is seen in the percentage of photoelectric versus Compton interactions as kVp increases. As the kilovoltage increases, the percentage of x-rays that undergo a Compton interaction increases and the percentage of photons that undergo photoelectric absorption decreases. Because Compton interactions create scatter, as kilovoltage increases, the percentage of primary photons that will undergo scattering also increases. At the same time, the percentage of primary photons that are absorbed photoelectrically decreases, resulting in a reduction in patient dose.

If kilovoltage is increased with no other change in the technical factors selected for a given exposure, the end result will be an increase in the transmission of photons and therefore an increase in the exit dose from the patient. More radiation will reach the image receptor. This increase in kilovoltage will also result in an increase in the percent and amount of scatter radiation produced. Table 12-2 illustrates this point. At 50 kVp with a 10-cm tissue, for every 1,000 photons, 990 photons (approximately 99 percent) will be attenuated and 10 photons (approximately 1 percent) will be transmitted. Of the 990 attenuated photons, approximately one-half interact by photoelectric absorption and one-half by Compton scatter (495 interactions each). At 130 kVp with a 10-cm tissue, for every 1,000 photons, 940 photons (approximately 94 percent) will be attenuated and 60 photons (approximately 6 percent) will be transmitted. Of the 940 attenuated photons, approximately 25 percent (235 photons) interact by photoelectric absorption and 75 percent (705 photons) by Compton scatter.

In radiography, the kilovoltage level is selected based predominantly on the size of the part being examined and the radiographic contrast desired for the image. When kilovoltage is increased without any other changes in technical factors, more scatter will result. If, however, the increase in kilovoltage is accompanied by a reduction in mAs to maintain the same exit dose, the overall result will be a decrease in the amount of scatter produced. Overall less photons are needed to create an acceptable image.

An x-ray image is created when some photons pass through the patient unaffected and others are absorbed photoelectrically. This difference is the basis for varying levels of image receptor exposure. When more photons pass through unaffected, the result is greater image receptor exposure. When more photons are absorbed photoelectrically, the result is less image receptor exposure. Scattered photons from Compton interactions are of no use in demonstrating the structures of interest. They merely add unwanted exposure to the image receptor that does not correspond to any particular structure. Much of the overall image receptor exposure is created by scattered photons. Image quality is improved when the amount of scatter reaching the image receptor is reduced.

Irradiated Material

The amount of scatter created during an interaction is affected by the volume and atomic number of the material being irradiated. The volume of irradiated material is controlled by field size and patient thickness (Figure 15-1).

As the volume of irradiated tissue increases, the amount of scatter increases. Volume increases as the field size increases or as the patient thickness increases. Larger field sizes, such as with 14″ × 17″ (35 × 43 cm) film, allow for more photons to interact with tissue, thereby creating more scatter. Larger body parts have more tissue to interact with the photons, resulting in greater scatter production. In order to decrease scatter, the smallest possible field size should be used. It is for this reason that beam restriction is an important part of scatter reduction and, of course, of patient protection. Patient thickness cannot be significantly altered by the radiographer, but certain techniques, such as the use of compression bands, can be useful in slightly reducing patient thickness.

The atomic number of the irradiated material also has an impact on the amount of scatter produced because higher-atomic-number materials have a greater number of electrons within each atom and photons have a greater chance of striking an electron, creating an absorption interaction. Therefore, the higher the atomic number of a material, the greater will be the number of photoelectric absorption interactions and the less scatter. Bone absorbs more radiation and scatters less than soft tissue. For this same reason, high-atomic-number materials, such as iodine, barium, and lead, absorb more radiation through the photoelectric interaction

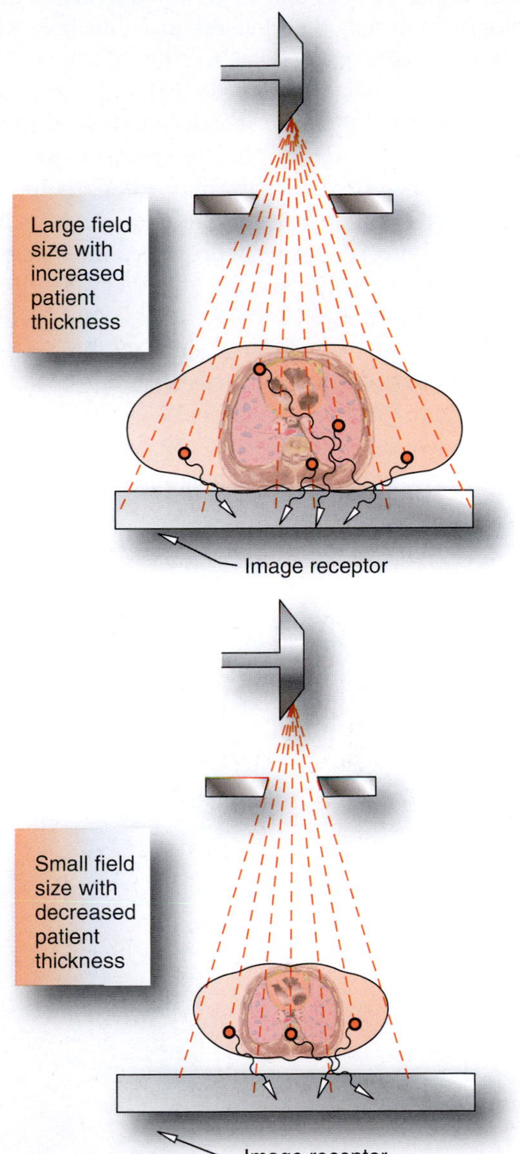

FIGURE 15-1. The amount of scatter increases with increased field size and patient thickness.

than low-atomic-number materials do. These photoelectric absorption interactions create the high contrast seen when contrast media are used.

Of the factors affecting the amount of scatter produced, the kilovoltage and the field size are under the direct control of the radiographer. Kilovoltage levels must be selected based on the area being radiographed, and the smallest possible field size should always be used. Beam restriction is therefore important to image quality. Remember, however, that **when the beam is restricted, less scatter radiation will reach the image receptor and, as a result, technical factors may need to be increased to compensate for the reduction in the overall image receptor exposure.** For example, the technical factors used for an AP projection of the abdomen using a 14″ × 17″ (35 × 43 cm) film would be insufficient to produce a good image of the same patient's bladder imaged on an 8″ × 10″ (18 × 24 cm) receptor. Technical factors would typically need to be increased 25 to 50 percent to compensate for this type of reduction in the field size.

BEAM RESTRICTORS

The foremost method of restricting the primary beam field size is the use of a device known as a **collimator**. Aperture diaphragms and cones/cylinders are also devices that historically were used to restrict the beam but are not in common use today.

Collimator

The collimator is the most commonly employed beam restrictor in radiography. A collimator permits an infinite number of field sizes (Figure 15-2). It also has the advantage of providing a light source for the radiographer as an aid in properly placing the tube and central ray.

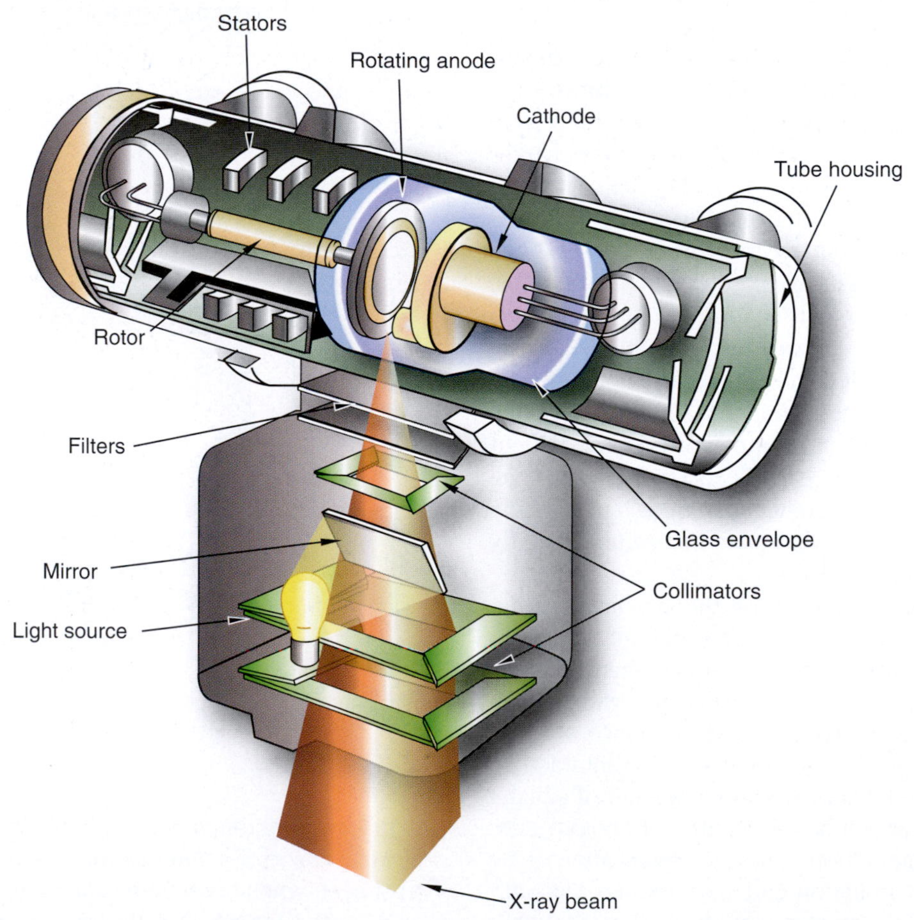

FIGURE 15-2. Schematic drawing of an x-ray tube and collimator. *(Courtesy of Siemens Medical Systems, Inc., Iselin, NJ.)*

A collimator consists of sets of lead shutters at right angles to one another that move in opposing pairs. Each set moves symmetrically from the center of the field. These lead shutters can be adjusted to correspond to an infinite number of square or rectangular field sizes.

The shutters serve to regulate the field size and, in addition, have two other purposes. The bottom shutters reduce penumbra along the periphery of the beam because of their greater distance from the focal spot. **Penumbra** is a geometric unsharpness around the periphery of the image, also known as edge unsharpness. It is the result of x-ray photons being created in all areas of the focal spot rather than at just a single point. Primary photons diverge from the tube at varying angles and intersect with the structures of interest at varying angles when creating the image. Reducing penumbra will improve the sharpness of the recorded image edge. This concept is described in further depth in Chapter 28. The upper shutters of the collimator help in reducing the amount of off-focus (stem) radiation reaching the image receptor by absorbing this radiation before it exits the tube. Recall that off-focus radiation originates within the x-ray tube but not at the focal spot. Off-focus radiation can result in images, similar to shadows of the patient, beyond the exposed field of radiation (see Figure 6-23). These shadows are often believed to be caused by scatter radiation. However, scatter will never create an image of a specific anatomical structure.

The collimator offers the radiographer a light field that outlines the exposure field and provides a crosshair to identify the center of the beam. Some units also provide an outline of the automatic exposure control (AEC) chambers' size and location. The light field is provided by mounting a mirror in the path of the x-ray beam at a 45° angle. A light source is then placed opposite the mirror and the light is projected through the collimator. The light source and the x-ray source must be equidistant from one another to ensure that the light field and the x-ray field are the same size. Improper positioning of the mirror or the light can result in improper alignment of the light field to the exposure field. Collimator accuracy should be checked on a regular basis as a part of the department's quality control program.

Most collimators are equipped with an accessory known as a **positive beam limitation (PBL) device**. PBL automatically collimates the beam to the size of the cassette. When a cassette is placed in the Bucky tray and secured in position, sensing devices determine the size and placement of the cassette. The sensing devices activate an electric motor that drives the collimator lead shutters into proper position. When operating properly, automatic collimators should leave a small unexposed border on all four sides of the exposed image. However, it is possible to override the PBL devices so that the field size can be controlled by the radiographer. This allows the radiographer to collimate to a field that is less than the cassette size. The field size should never be greater than the size of the cassette.

The use of a collimator results in some filtration of the x-ray beam because the primary beam is passing through the mirror in the collimator. The added filtration is usually equivalent to approximately 1 mm of aluminum. Because collimators result in increased filtration of the x-ray beam, their use during low-kVp radiography (such as mammography) is restricted.

Proper collimation is the responsibility of the radiographer. Under no circumstances should the exposure field exceed the size of the image receptor. Automatic collimation helps to ensure that the exposure field does not exceed the size of the image receptor, but the radiographer should always limit the field to the part being examined. By so doing, image quality can be improved and patient dose can be minimized.

Aperture Diaphragm and Cones/Cylinders

The aperture diaphragm is a flat sheet of metal, usually lead, with an opening cut in the center and attached to the x-ray tube port. This is the simplest of all beam-restricting devices and different diaphragms are needed to accommodate different receptor sizes and different distances. Cones and cylinders are essentially circular aperture diaphragms with metal extensions. A cone has an extension that flares or diverges, with the upper diameter smaller than the bottom flared end, and a cylinder does not flare. Although rarely used, cones remain the most effective means of scatter control. Aperture diaphragms and cones/cylinders have the principal disadvantage of a fixed field size and are rarely used today.

ANCILLARY DEVICES

Beam restrictors may be made for a very specific purpose. Ancillary devices are generally designed with a special need in mind. Examples include lead blockers and lead masks. These devices are tailored for a specific use during a given procedure. They are designed to restrict the beam to a specific shape for a particular examination.

A lead blocker is simply a sheet of lead-impregnated rubber that can be cut to any size or shape. Placement of a lead blocker on the radiographic table during radiography of the lower spine in the lateral position will help to absorb the scatter that is produced in the soft tissue of the patient's back (Figure 15-3). A lead blocker may also be helpful when placed on the radiographic table above the level of the shoulder during positioning for AP projections of the shoulder joint. Lead blockers are most helpful when examining large patients, because the amount of scatter increases with increases in the size of the patient. Early digital imaging systems would often have problems processing images created with lead blockers. Most digital systems now can avoid these problems. However, it is wise to check the vendor's information for recommendations prior to attempting to use a lead blocker with a digital image receptor.

A lead mask is usually cut to correspond to the particular field size desired and is then secured to the end of the collimator. Lead masks in the shape of a keyhole were sometimes used during cerebral angiography to help improve image quality by reducing scatter

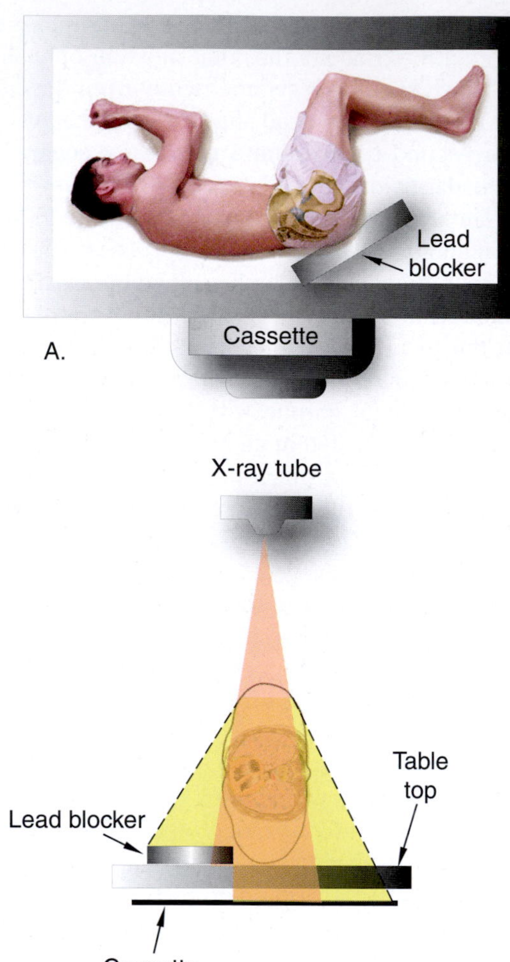

FIGURE 15-3. The use of a lead blocker for radiography of the lower spine (A), and cutaway view of absorption of scatter (B).

SUMMARY

In order to provide the best possible image, the radiographer must try to control the amount of scatter radiation reaching the image receptor. The principal factors that affect the amount of scatter produced are: (1) kilovoltage and (2) the irradiated material. As kilovoltage increases, the percentage of primary photons that will undergo scattering also increases. As the volume of irradiated tissue increases, the amount of scatter produced is increased. Volume will increase as the field size increases or as the patient thickness increases. The atomic number of the irradiated material also has an impact on the amount of scatter produced. Higher-atomic-number materials have a greater number of electrons within each atom. Photons have a greater chance of being absorbed by these materials.

The collimator is the most commonly employed beam restrictor in radiography because it permits an infinite number of field sizes using only one device. It also has the advantage of providing a light source for the radiographer as an aid in properly placing the tube.

Proper collimation is the responsibility of the radiographer. Under no circumstances should the exposure field ever exceed the size of the image receptor. In addition, the radiographer should always limit the field to the part being examined. By so doing, image quality will be improved and patient dose will be minimized. ■

REVIEW QUESTIONS

1. Why does beam restriction reduce scatter radiation production?
2. What are the two principal factors that affect the amount of scatter produced?
3. How does the atomic number of a material affect the amount of scatter produced?
4. How does a collimator restrict the primary beam field size?
5. What is PBL?
6. How does beam restriction affect patient dose?

REFERENCES AND RECOMMENDED READING

Bushberg, J. T., Seibert, J. A., Leidholdt, E. M., & Boone, J. M. (2003). *The essential physics of medical imaging* (2nd ed.). Baltimore: Lippincott, Williams & Wilkins.

Carroll, Q. B. (2003). *Fuchs's radiographic exposure, processing, and quality control* (7th ed.). Springfield, IL: Charles C Thomas.

Crooks, H. E., & Ardran, G. M. (1976). Checking x-ray beam field size. *Radiography, 42*(503), 239.

Curry, T. S., Dowdey, J. E., & Murry, R. C. (1990). *Christensen's introduction to the physics of diagnostic radiology* (4th ed.). Philadelphia: Lea and Febiger.

Mitchell, F. (1991). Scattered radiation and the lateral lumbar spine part 1: Initial research. *Radiography Today, 57*(644), 18–20.

Mitchell, F., Leung, C., Ahuja, A., & Metreweli, C. (1991). Scattered radiation and the lateral lumbar spine part 2: Clinical research. *Radiography Today, 57*(645), 12–14.

Seeram, E., & Travis, E. L. (1997). *Radiation protection.* Baltimore: Lippincott, Williams & Wilkins.

Thomas, S. R., Freshcorn, J. E., Krugh, K. B., Henry, G. C., Kereiakes, J. G., & Kaufman, R. A. (1983). Characteristics of extrafocal radiation and its potential significance in pediatric radiology. *Radiology, 146*, 793–799.

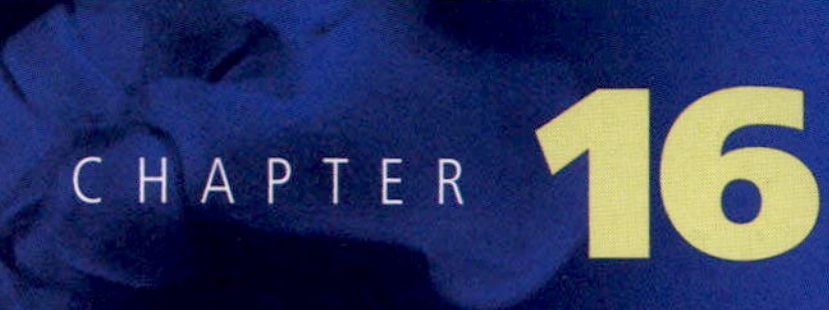

CHAPTER 16 The Patient as a Beam Emitter

KEY TERMS

subject contrast
subject density
subject detail
subject distortion

> . . . the patient . . . would shape up into something that called for attention, his peculiarities, her reticences or candors. And though I might be attracted or repelled, the professional attitude . . . would steady me and dictate the terms on which I was to proceed.
>
> *By William Carlos Williams, from* The Autobiography of William Carlos Williams, *copyright © 1951 by William Carlos Williams. Reprinted with permission of New Directions Publishing Corp.*

OBJECTIVES

Upon completion of this chapter, the student should be able to:

- Explain the process of attenuation.
- Describe the basic composition of the human body.
- Describe the effect of the human body on the attenuation of the x-ray beam.
- Explain the relationship of the subject (patient) to the density/image receptor exposure, contrast, recorded detail, and distortion of the recorded image.

ATTENUATION

Attenuation is the reduction in the total number of x-ray photons remaining in the beam after passing through a given thickness of material (see Figure 12-1). It is the result of x-rays interacting with matter and being absorbed or scattered. The amount of attenuation is determined by the amount and type of irradiated material. X-rays are attenuated exponentially. This means that they are reduced by a certain percentage for each given thickness of material they pass through. Theoretically, then, the number of x-rays passing through an absorber will never reach zero. This is because each succeeding thickness of material reduces the number of photons by only a fraction of the previous amount.

As an x-ray beam passes through a patient, the beam is attenuated. The thicker the body part being radiographed, the greater the attenuation will be. In order to provide a sufficient number of x-ray photons for interaction with the image receptor, the original quantity and quality of the photons must be increased with increased body part thickness. The incident beam is significantly altered as it passes through the patient. **The beam emitted from the patient contains the radiologically significant information needed by the radiologist to make a diagnosis.**

In the diagnostic x-ray range, attenuation is the result of either photoelectric absorption or Compton scattering. Photoelectric absorption provides radiologically significant information, whereas Compton scatter contributes no useful information. Scatter is the primary contributor to personnel exposure when in the radiographic or fluoroscopic room.

Attenuation is also affected by the type of absorber. **Higher-atomic-number materials** (such as lead and barium) **attenuate a greater percentage of the beam than low-atomic-number materials** (such as hydrogen, carbon, and oxygen). This is due to the presence of a greater number of electrons with which photons may interact. Bone produces less image receptor exposure because it attenuates the x-ray beam more than soft tissue. This is predominantly because of the presence of calcium in bone, which has a higher atomic number than the majority of the elements found in the human body. The effective atomic numbers of the important materials comprising the human body are listed in Table 16-1.

TABLE 16-1. Basic Substances Comprising the Human Body

Substance	Effective Atomic Number	Density (kg/m^3)
Air	7.78	1.29
Fat	6.46	916
Water	7.51	1000
Muscle	7.64	1040
Bone	12.31	1650

The density of the absorbing material also has an impact on attenuation. **Density is the quantity of matter per unit of volume measured in kilograms per cubic meter.** It describes how tightly the atoms of a given substance are packed together. For example, the molecules in most solids are more tightly packed than the same molecules when they are in their liquid state. Bone tissue is a denser substance than lung tissue. Table 16-1 lists the densities of the important materials comprising the human body. Because density and atomic number affect attenuation, it is important to understand the basic composition of the human body, particularly in terms of the average atomic number and density of the major substances.

THE HUMAN BODY AS AN ATTENUATOR

The patient is the greatest variable the radiographer faces when performing a radiographic procedure. The human body is comprised of a variety of organic and inorganic substances. At the atomic level, the body consists primarily of hydrogen, carbon, nitrogen, and oxygen. These elements have atomic numbers of 1, 6, 7, and 8, respectively. Calcium, found in concentrated amounts in bones and teeth, has an atomic number of 20.

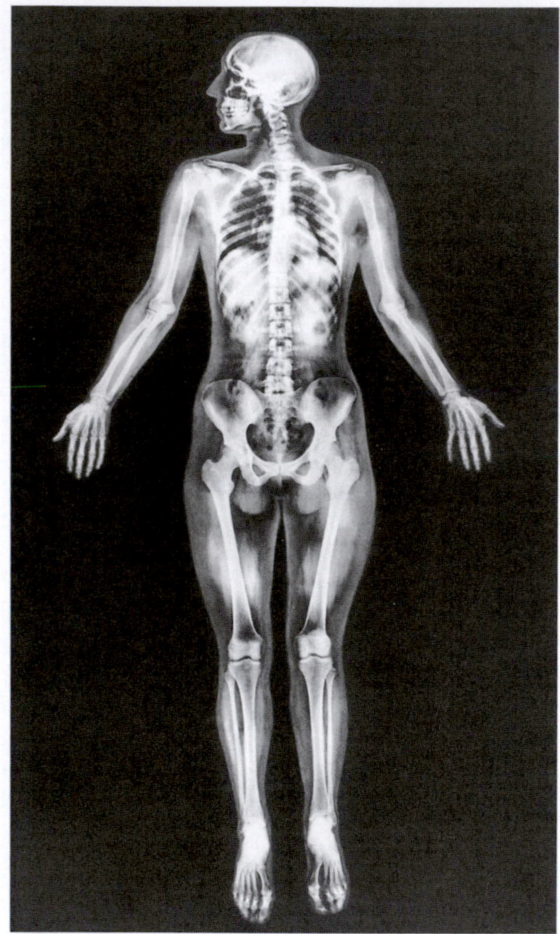

FIGURE 16-1. An antique full-body radiograph. *(Reprinted with permission of Dr. Marion Frank.)*

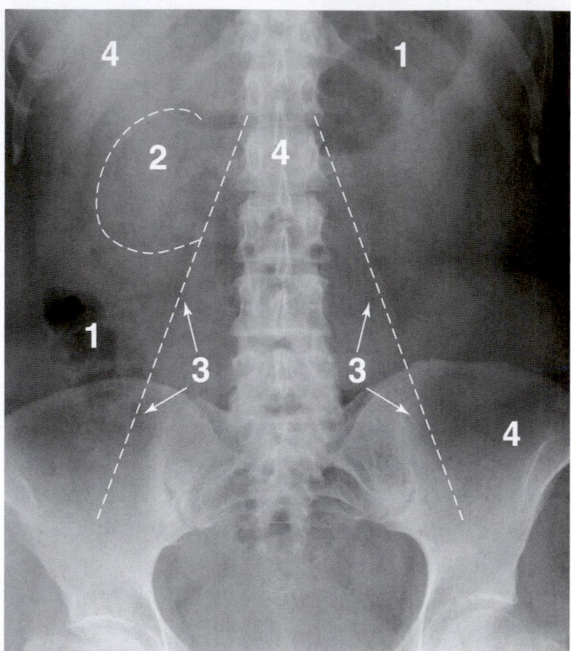

FIGURE 16-2. A radiograph of the abdomen demonstrating (1) air in the stomach and colon; (2) fat around the kidneys; (3) muscle to the right and left of the spine (psoas muscle); and (4) ribs, spine, and pelvis. *(Radiographs courtesy of Arlene Adler and Richard R. Carlton.)*

The composition of the human body determines its radiographic appearance (Figure 16-1). Although human anatomy and physiology are quite complex, when studying the absorption characteristics of the body, four major substances account for most of the variations in x-ray absorption: air, fat, muscle, and bone (Figure 16-2).

Air

Air has an effective atomic number of 7.78, which is greater than either fat or muscle. Despite the slightly higher effective atomic number, air has a significantly lower tissue density. As a result, air will absorb fewer photons as they pass through it. Because air absorbs fewer photons than other body substances, more photons reach the image receptor, thus producing a greater image receptor exposure. Air is naturally present in the lungs, the sinuses, and, in small amounts, in the gastrointestinal tract. On a typical image of the abdomen, air can usually be seen in the stomach and colon.

Fat

Fat is similar to muscle in that they are both among the soft tissue structures in the body. The soft tissue structures have effective atomic numbers and tissue densities that are very similar to those of water. For this reason, water is sometimes used to simulate soft tissue for experimental purposes. Fat has an effective atomic number that is slightly less than muscle's. In addition, fat has less tissue density than muscle. Muscle cells are more closely packed than fat cells. The amount of fatty tissue varies considerably between patients. Although this is also true of muscle tissue, the variations are generally less pronounced and therefore have less effect on the overall attenuation of the beam. On a radiograph of the abdomen, the kidneys can often be outlined because of the perirenal fat capsule that surrounds them.

Muscle

Like fat, muscle is a soft tissue. Muscle, however, has a slightly higher effective atomic number and a greater tissue density than fat. As a result, muscle is a greater attenuator of the beam. On an image of the abdomen, it is often easy to distinguish the psoas muscle on each side of the spine because of the increased absorption of radiation by these muscles.

Bone

The skeletal anatomy is easily seen radiographically because of the calcium content of bone. Calcium has a higher atomic number than most of the elements found in the human body. As a result, bone has the highest effective atomic number of the four basic substances. It also has the greatest tissue density and, as a result, absorbs radiation at a greater rate than any of the soft tissues or air-filled structures. This absorption means that fewer photons will reach the image receptor and less image receptor exposure will be produced. On an image of the abdomen, the lower ribs, spine, and pelvis are all very easily distinguished because of the increased x-ray absorption that occurs in bone.

THE PATIENT'S RELATIONSHIP TO IMAGE QUALITY

The patient has an impact on all properties affecting radiographic quality: density/image receptor exposure, contrast, recorded detail, and distortion. These are described in detail in Chapters 26–30. The relationships between these factors and the patient (subject) are termed **subject density**, **subject contrast**, **subject detail**, and **subject distortion**.

Subject Density

The various tissues in the human body are responsible for the differing exposures to the image receptor. Subject density refers to the impact the subject (patient) has on the resultant radiographic density/image receptor exposure. **Image receptor exposure will be altered by changes in the amount and/or type of tissue being irradiated.** In other words, thicker and denser body parts absorb more radiation, thus producing less image receptor exposure, and vice versa.

Subject Contrast

Radiographic contrast is the difference in densities of a recorded image. The differences in image receptor exposure are the result of differences in the absorption of the x-ray beam as it passes through the patient. **Subject contrast is the degree of differential absorption resulting from the differing absorption characteristics of the tissues in the body.** Subject contrast is dependent on the specific characteristics of an individual patient's tissues.

When there is little difference in the absorption characteristic of the given body tissues within a part being examined, as in mammography, subject contrast will be low. When there is a greater difference in the absorption characteristics of the body tissues within a part being examined, as in the chest with the lungs, heart, and spine, subject contrast is high.

Subject Detail

One of the primary factors that affects the sharpness or detail of an image is the distance between the structure of interest and the image receptor. Because anatomical structures are located at varying distances from the image receptor, **the recorded detail of the structures is dependent on their position within the body and also on the body's placement in relationship to the receptor**. The overall size and placement of the patient have a great impact on the recorded detail. The larger the patient, the greater the distance between the anatomical structures and the image receptor will be. This results in less sharpness in the recorded details. Conversely, greater sharpness will result when the anatomical part is closer to the image receptor, as is the case with thinner patients. Specific positions have been established to place the anatomical structures of interest in as close proximity to the image receptor as possible. For example, chest radiography is typically performed in the PA projection and in the left lateral position to place the heart closer to the image receptor.

Subject Distortion

Distortion is the misrepresentation of the size or shape of the structure of interest. Because of the way in which certain structures lie within the body, **unless the patient is positioned specifically to demonstrate a particular structure, it may not be accurately represented on the image receptor.** For example, to properly demonstrate the apophyseal joints of the lumbar spine, the patient should be in the oblique position. In the AP projection of the lumbar spine, these joints will be distorted. Distortion, in the form of magnification, also occurs because various anatomical structures sit at varying levels.

SUMMARY

Attenuation is the reduction in the total number of x-ray photons remaining in the beam after passing through a given thickness of material. It is the result of x-rays interacting with matter and being absorbed or scattered. The amount of attenuation will be determined by the amount and type of irradiated material.

The patient is the greatest variable that the radiographer faces when performing a radiographic procedure. The composition of the human body determines its radiographic appearance. When studying the absorption characteristics of the body, four major substances account for most of the variations in x-ray absorption: air, fat, muscle, and bone.

The patient has an impact on all of the properties that affect radiographic quality: density/image receptor exposure, contrast, recorded detail, and distortion. The relationships between these factors and the patient (subject) are termed subject density, subject contrast, subject detail, and subject distortion. ■

REVIEW QUESTIONS

1. How does atomic number affect attenuation?
2. How does tissue density affect attenuation?
3. What elements comprise the majority of those found in the human body?
4. What are the differences between air, fat, muscle, and bone with respect to their attenuation and the resultant image?
5. How does the patient affect each of the factors of image quality?

REFERENCES AND RECOMMENDED READING

Bower, R. (1989). Stripes in the abdomen. *Radiologic Technology, 60*(6), 511.

Bushberg, J. T., Seibert, J. A., Leidholdt, E. M., & Boone, J. M. (2003). *The essential physics of medical imaging* (2nd ed.). Baltimore: Lippincott Williams & Wilkins.

Carroll, Q. B. (2003). *Fuchs's radiographic exposure, processing, and quality control* (7th ed.). Springfield, IL: Charles C Thomas.

Cohen, M. (1971). Attenuation of x-rays in the human body. *Radiography, 37*(436), 88–90.

Fuchs, A. W. (1948). Relationship of tissue thickness to kilovoltage. *Radiologic Technology, 19*(6), 287.

Handbook of chemistry and physics (78th ed.). (1998). Boca Raton, FL: CRC Press.

Haynes, W. M. (2010). *CRC handbook of chemistry and physics* (91st ed.). Boca Raton, FL: CRC Press.

Lindsay, R., & Anderson, J. B. (1978). Radiological determination of changes in bone mineral content. *Radiography, 44*(517), 21–26.

Seeram, E., & Travis, E. L. (1997). *Radiation protection.* Baltimore: Lippincott Williams & Wilkins.

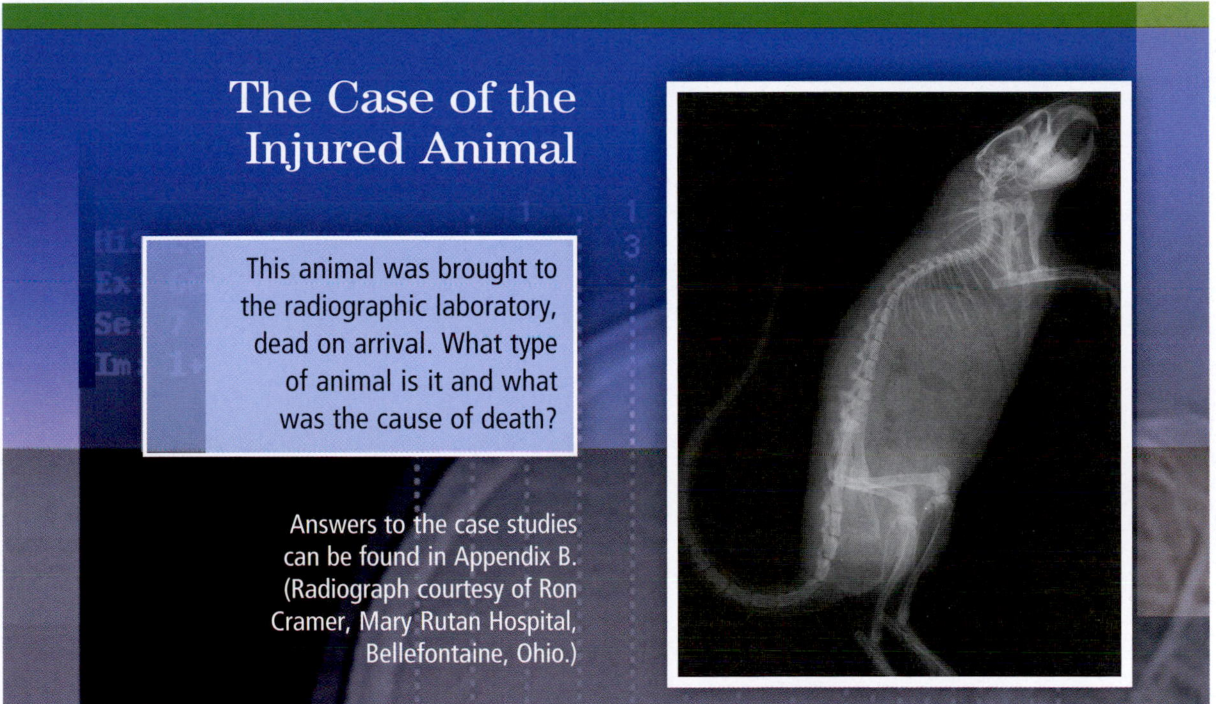

The Case of the Injured Animal

This animal was brought to the radiographic laboratory, dead on arrival. What type of animal is it and what was the cause of death?

Answers to the case studies can be found in Appendix B. (Radiograph courtesy of Ron Cramer, Mary Rutan Hospital, Bellefontaine, Ohio.)

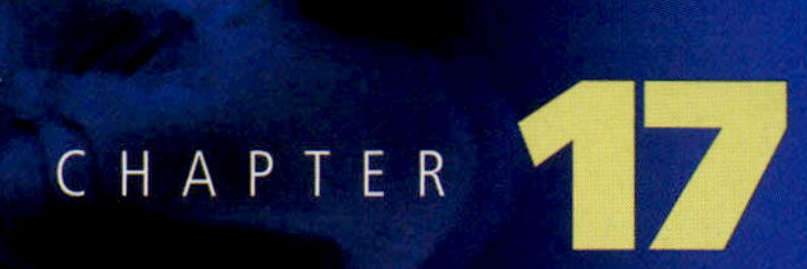

The Pathology Problem

KEY TERMS

abscess
acromegaly
active osteomyelitis
additive condition
aerophagia
anorexia nervosa
aortic aneurysm
ascites
aseptic necrosis
atelectasis
atrophy
bowel obstruction
bronchiectasis
calcified stones
carcinoma
cardiomegaly
chronic osteomyelitis
cirrhosis
congestive heart failure
degenerative arthritis
destructive condition
edema
emaciation
emphysema
empyema
fibrosarcoma
gout

You don't look different but you have changed.
I'm looking through you you're not the same

John Lennon and Paul McCartney "I'm Looking Through You," from Rubber Soul (Provided by Rockmine, the Internet's largest rock music resource www.rockmine.com)

OBJECTIVES

Upon completion of this chapter, the student should be able to:

- Explain the effect that a pathological condition can have on radiation absorption.
- Describe the effect of pathology on the radiographic image.
- Differentiate between pathological conditions that result in increased attenuation versus those that result in decreased attenuation of the x-ray beam.
- Identify pathological conditions that result in an increased attenuation of the x-ray beam.
- Identify pathological conditions that result in a decreased attenuation of the x-ray beam.

KEY TERMS (continued)

hemothorax
hydrocephalus
hydrothorax
hyperparathyroidism
multiple myeloma
osteitis deformans
osteoblastic metastases
osteochondroma
osteolytic metastases
osteomalacia
osteoporosis
Paget's disease
pathology
pleural effusions
pneumoconiosis
pneumonectomy
pneumonia
pneumonitis
pneumothorax
pulmonary edema
sclerosis
tuberculosis
tumor

PATHOLOGY AND RADIATION ABSORPTION

As radiation passes through the patient it undergoes attenuation or absorption of the x-ray photons. The patient is the greatest variable the radiographer faces when trying to select adequate exposure factors for a specific procedure. Attenuation will vary, depending on the thickness and the composition of the patient's tissues. As an added dilemma, the radiographer must also realize that pathological conditions can affect the overall thickness and composition of the patient's tissues. The radiographer must first be aware of the variations between normal body tissues and then be concerned about possible additional variations as a result of a specific disease process.

Pathology is the medical science that is concerned with all aspects of disease, including the structural and functional changes caused by a disease process. Disease will often bring about changes in body tissues that can be viewed radiographically and interpreted by the radiologist. If this were not true, radiography would be of no use in diagnosing disease. These changes may be structural and/or functional in nature and they may or may not have an impact on the degree of radiation absorbed by the patient. Certain diseases can increase or decrease tissue thickness or alter tissue composition (change the effective atomic number or density of the tissue). When this occurs, the disease will affect the degree of radiation absorption for that specific body tissue. Two common pathologies of the chest demonstrate the differences in radiation absorption (Figures 17-1A and 17-1B). In Figure 17-1A, the patient has pneumonia, which causes air-filled lung tissue to fill with fluid. Fluid will absorb more radiation than air. In Figure 17-1B, the patient has emphysema. With emphysema, normal lung tissue is destroyed and the air sacs become enlarged. A greater amount of air is then present in the lungs, which results in less attenuation of radiation.

Radiographers must have an understanding of pathology in order to properly select the technical factors for a procedure. Properly reading the x-ray requisition, taking an adequate patient history, and close observation of the patient are the essential responsibilities of the radiographer. Fulfilling these responsibilities reduces the need to repeat an image, due to the patient's condition. For example, it may be necessary to adjust the technical factors if a chest x-ray is requested for a patient with emphysema. By taking a good history, the radiographer can determine how long the patient has had the condition and what signs and symptoms the patient has exhibited. By observing signs,

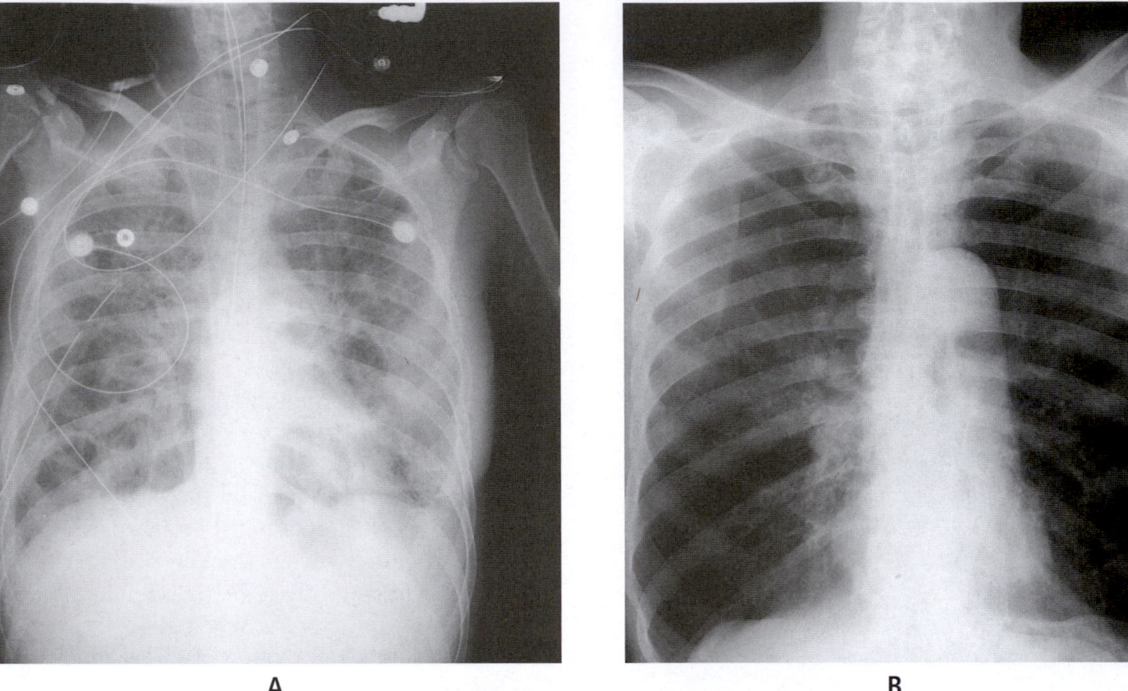

FIGURE 17-1. (A) The patient has bilateral pneumonia, resulting in an increase in radiation absorption. (B) The patient has severe emphysema, resulting in a decrease in radiation absorption. *(Radiographs courtesy of Arlene Adler and Richard R. Carlton.)*

such as shortness of breath or prolonged exhalation, the radiographer can assess the extent of the disease. Of course, disease conditions are not always known prior to performing the examination. This is one of the primary reasons that a repeat exposure may be necessary, even though there was no error in judgment on the part of the radiographer. As an individual gains clinical experience, his or her assessment skills improve and he or she is able to make better judgments concerning the presence and extent of disease.

If a disease causes the affected body tissue to increase in thickness, effective atomic number, and/or density, there will be a greater attenuation of the x-ray beam. As more photons are absorbed by the body tissues, fewer will be available to reach the image receptor to create an adequate exposure. These diseases are harder to penetrate and are called **additive conditions** because they require increasing technical factors to achieve the proper image receptor exposure. There is an inverse relationship between additive conditions and image receptor exposure. This means that when additive conditions are present, image receptor exposure will decrease as the extent of the disease increases.

If a disease causes the affected body tissue to decrease in thickness, effective atomic number, and/or density, there will be less attenuation of the x-ray beam. As more photons are able to pass through the body tissues, more will be available to reach the image receptor. These diseases are easier to penetrate and are called **destructive conditions**. They require decreasing the exposure to achieve the proper image receptor exposure. There is a direct relationship between destructive conditions and image receptor exposure. This means that when destructive conditions are present, the image receptor exposure will increase as the extent of the disease increases.

A disease influences radiation absorption when it alters the overall number or types of atoms comprising the affected tissue. For example, if a person sprains an ankle, one of the body's responses to the injury is swelling or edema at the site. The ankle becomes enlarged because there is an increase in blood and serous fluid around the ankle joint. The body tissue increases in thickness, but, in this example, the opacity of the tissue is generally the same. Blood and serous fluid have approximately the same opacity as the soft tissue around the ankle. What is occurring at the molecular and atomic level is an increase primarily in the number of water molecules (hydrogen and oxygen atoms), which comprise most of blood and serous fluid. If there are more water molecules present around the ankle, a greater number of x-ray photons will interact with that tissue, resulting in increased radiation absorption and decreased exposure to the image receptor. Technical factors must be increased to compensate for an increase in the thickness of the part. Proper measurement of the body part and the use of technique charts will ensure that the correct technical factors are selected.

The extent to which a body part is affected by disease will determine if technical factors must be adjusted. For example, no change in technical factors is necessary to visualize a small, localized tumor in the lung or a small kidney stone. If, however, the tumor is large and diffuse, or the kidney stone causes severe hydronephrosis, adjustments in the technical factors may be required to adequately visualize the pathology (Figures 17-2A and 17-2B). It is important to remember that the degree or extent of the pathology is critical in determining the technical factor adjustments. If the technical factors must be adjusted, the change must be enough to make a noticeable difference in image receptor exposure. **To produce a visible difference requires a minimal change of 25–50 percent in the overall exposure to the image receptor.** This issue is more complex with digital image detector systems, where the traditional relationship between image receptor exposure and mAs, kVp, and distance no longer exists. It is possible to change the mAs, kVp, and the

A

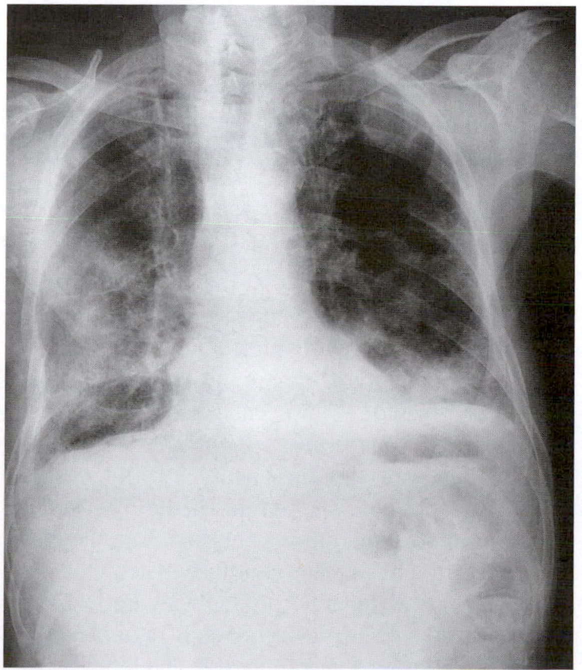

B

FIGURE 17-2. (A) When a tumor is smaller and more localized, there is less need for technical factor adjustments. (B) Tumors that are larger and more diffuse throughout both lungs require greater technical factor adjustments. *(Radiographs courtesy of Arlene Adler and Richard R. Carlton.)*

distance and have no effect on the brightness on the display monitor. A wider range of patient exposures can be displayed as acceptable images, and it is the radiographer's responsibility to keep the patient dose for a given exam as low as possible without compromising image quality.

Many diseases do not affect the thickness or opacity of body tissues but can be diagnosed by way of radiography simply because of the structural or functional changes that they produce. These diseases generally do not require an adjustment in the selected technical factors. Examples include ulcers, diverticula, and simple fractures (provided there is minimal swelling). There are many diseases that do not affect the thickness or alter the composition of the body tissues and therefore cause no radiographically evident structural or functional changes. These conditions generally do not require radiography; they are usually diagnosed through laboratory testing. Diseases such as diabetes mellitus, anemia, and meningitis are examples.

INCREASED ATTENUATION (ADDITIVE) CONDITIONS

Many disease processes will result in an increase in thickness, effective atomic number, and/or density of the body tissue. Recall that the body tissues vary in thickness (the femur is thicker than the humerus) and in composition (bone has a higher effective atomic number and greater tissue density than muscle). These diseases absorb more radiation and require the radiographer to increase technical factors to compensate for the changes in the body tissues. The extent of the disease also plays an important role in technical factor adjustment. The technical factor adjustments will vary, depending on the degree to which the body tissues are affected. Because of this, each patient will be different and must be examined individually.

No magic formula exists to adjust technical factors to compensate for a pathological problem. The radiographer must carefully review the requisition, obtain a patient history, and then examine the patient. By following these steps, the radiographer can make a judgment concerning the necessary technical adjustment to be made. Experience is particularly valuable in determining the proper changes to be made. As a general rule, additive conditions will require an increase in kilovoltage to adequately penetrate the thicker, more opaque body parts. Remember that an increase of 15 percent in kVp will approximately double the exposure to the image receptor. An increase of 5–15 percent in kilovoltage will compensate for most additive pathological conditions. Automatic exposure control (AEC) systems will compensate for most pathological changes by adjusting the exposure automatically. However, the compensation will be the result of increased mAs rather than increased kVp.

Some of the common conditions that cause an increase in attenuation and may therefore require an increase in technical factors are outlined. A summary of the conditions is provided in Table 17-1.

Conditions Affecting Multiple Systems

Certain diseases can occur in a wide variety of body systems and, as a result, they may be present at various sites. Whenever an x-ray requisition indicates the presence of any of the following conditions, it may be necessary to increase technical factors for the procedure.

Abscess—an encapsulated infection increases tissue thickness and may alter composition, particularly in the lungs.

Edema—swelling causes an increase in tissue thickness and may alter composition if it occurs in the lungs.

Tumor—an abnormal new growth in tissue results in an increase in tissue thickness and may alter composition, particularly in the lungs or bones or when calcification results.

Conditions of the Chest

The chest is a common site for pathological conditions, and chest radiography is a common diagnostic procedure. It may be necessary to increase

TABLE 17-1. Summary of Pathology Problems

Increased Attenuation Conditions	Decreased Attenuation Conditions
Multiple Sites	**Multiple Sites**
Abscess Edema Tumors	Anorexia Nervosa Atrophy Emaciation
The Chest	**The Chest**
Atelectasis Bronchiectasis Cardiomegaly Congestive Heart Failure Empyema Pleural Effusions Pneumoconiosis Pneumonia Pneumonectomy Pulmonary Edema Tuberculosis (advanced/ miliary)	Emphysema Pneumothorax
The Abdomen	**The Abdomen**
Aortic Aneurysm Ascites Cirrhosis Calcified Stones	Aerophagia Bowel Obstruction
The Extremities and Skull	**The Extremities and Skull**
Acromegaly Chronic Osteomyelitis Hydrocephalus Osteoblastic Metastases Osteochondroma Paget's Disease Sclerosis	Active Osteomyelitis Aseptic Necrosis Carcinoma Degenerative Arthritis Fibrosarcoma Gout Hyperparathyroidism Multiple Myeloma Osteolytic Metastases Osteomalacia Osteoporosis

technical factors for a procedure whenever an x-ray requisition indicates the presence of any of the following conditions.

Atelectasis—a collapse of the lung results in airlessness of all or part of the lung tissue. This causes lung tissue density to increase.

Bronchiectasis—the chronic dilatation of the bronchi can result in peribronchial thickening and small areas of atelectasis. This causes an increase in lung tissue density.

Cardiomegaly—an enlargement of the heart causes an increase in thickness of the part.

Congestive Heart Failure—when the heart is in failure, the cardiac output is diminished. This results in backward failure, or increased venous congestion in the lungs. Lung tissue density is increased and the heart is enlarged as well.

Empyema—pus in the thoracic cavity causes an increase in tissue density.

Pleural Effusions (Hemothorax, Hydrothorax)—when the pleural cavity fills with either blood or serous fluid, it displaces normal lung tissue. This results in an increased tissue density within the thoracic cavity.

Pneumoconiosis—the inhalation of dust particles can cause fibrotic (scarring) changes. When healthy lung tissue becomes fibrotic, the density of the tissue increases.

Pneumonectomy—the removal of a lung will cause the affected side to demonstrate an increase in density because normal air-filled lung tissue is removed.

Pneumonia (pneumonitis)—inflammation of the lung tissues causes fluid to fill in the alveolar spaces. Fluid has much greater tissue density than the air normally present.

Pulmonary Edema—when fluid fills the interstitial lung tissues and the alveoli, tissue density increases. This is a typical complication of congestive heart failure.

Tuberculosis (advanced and miliary)—an infection by a mycobacteria causes the inflammatory response, which results in an increase in fluid in the lungs. If the mycobacteria were inhaled, it generally begins as a localized lesion (usually upper lobes), which can spread to a more advanced stage. If the infection reaches the lungs by the bloodstream, it has a more diffuse spread (miliary TB). Increased tissue density results in both advanced and miliary TB (Figure 17-3).

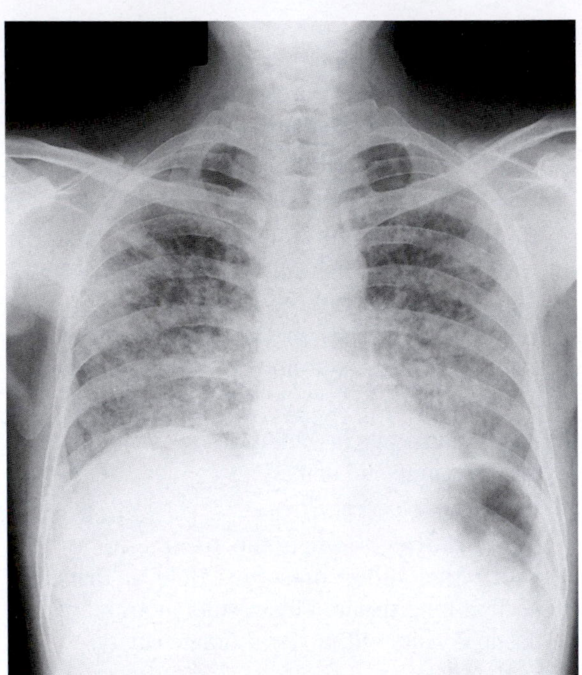

FIGURE 17-3. This patient has military tuberculosis with bronchopneumonia. These are both additive conditions, resulting in increased radiation absorption. *(Radiographs courtesy of Arlene Adler and Richard R. Carlton.)*

Conditions of the Abdomen

Abdominal conditions usually cause the abdomen to distend. It may be necessary to increase technical factors for a procedure when an x-ray requisition indicates the presence of any of the following conditions. Most technical factor changes, however, will be the natural result of the noted increase in abdominal size when measuring patient thickness.

Aortic Aneurysm—a large dilatation of the aorta will result in increased thickness of the affected part.

Ascites—fluid accumulation within the peritoneal cavity causes an increase in tissue thickness. The free fluid has a unique "ground glass" appearance radiographically.

Calcified stones—stones are most commonly found throughout the abdomen in such organs as the gallbladder and the kidney. Calcium may be deposited, which causes an increase in the effective atomic number of the tissue.

Cirrhosis—fibrotic changes in the liver cause the liver to enlarge and ascites can result. The result is an increase in the thickness of the liver and the entire abdomen.

Conditions of the Extremities and Skull

Conditions that result in new bone growth are termed osteoblastic. These conditions generally require an increase in technical factors. It may be necessary to increase technical factors for a procedure whenever an x-ray requisition indicates the presence of any of the following conditions.

Acromegaly—an overgrowth of the hands, feet, face, and jaw as a result of hypersecretion of growth hormones in the adult will result in an increase in bone mass.

Chronic Osteomyelitis—a chronic bone infection results in new bone growth at the infected site.

Hydrocephalus—a dilatation of the fluid-filled cerebral ventricles causes an enlargement of the head, resulting in an increased thickness.

Osteoblastic Metastases—the spread of cancer to bone can result in uncontrolled new bone growth.

Osteochondroma—a tumor arising in the bone and cartilage will result in an increased thickness of the bone.

Paget's Disease (**osteitis deformans**)—an increase occurs in bone cell activity, which leads to new bone growth. The result is increased bone thickness, with the pelvis, spine, and skull most often affected (Figure 17-4).

Sclerosis—an increase in hardening as a result of a chronic inflammation in bone. This increases the density of the bone tissue.

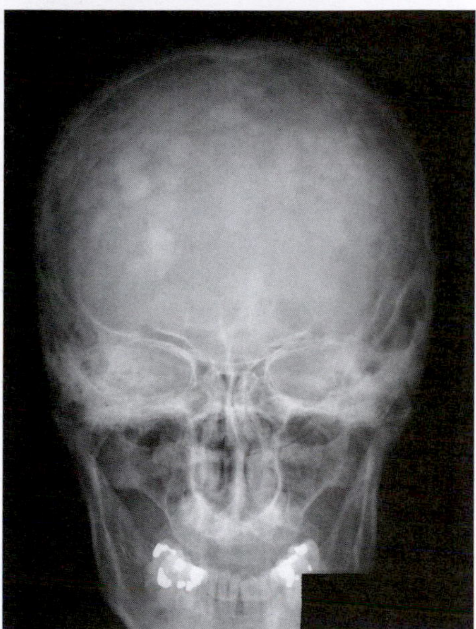

FIGURE 17-4. Paget's disease is an additive condition, resulting in increased radiation absorption. *(Radiographs courtesy of Arlene Adler and Richard R. Carlton.)*

DECREASED ATTENUATION (DESTRUCTIVE) CONDITIONS

Various disease processes can result in a decrease in thickness, effective atomic number, and/or density of the body tissue. These conditions cause the absorption of less radiation and require the radiographer to decrease technical factors to compensate for the changes in the body tissues. Recall also that the extent of the disease plays an important role in technical factor adjustment. As a general rule, compensations for destructive conditions can be made by decreasing the mAs. Remember that a decrease of 50 percent in mAs will reduce the exposure to the image receptor by half. A decrease of 25–50 percent in mAs will compensate for most of these pathological conditions. AEC systems will compensate for most pathological changes by adjusting the exposure automatically.

Some of the common conditions that cause a decrease in attenuation and may therefore require a decrease in technical factors are outlined. A summary of the conditions is provided in Table 17-1.

Conditions Affecting Multiple Sites

Certain diseases can occur in a wide variety of body systems and, as a result, they may be present in various sites. Whenever an x-ray requisition indicates the presence of any of the following conditions, it may be necessary to decrease technical factors for the procedure.

Anorexia Nervosa—a psychological eating disorder that results in an extreme weight loss. Overall body thickness is reduced.

Atrophy—a wasting away of body tissue with diminished cell proliferation, resulting in reduced thickness of a specific part or the entire body.

Emaciation—a generalized wasting away of body tissue, resulting in reduced thickness of the body.

Conditions of the Chest

The chest is a common site for pathological conditions and chest radiography is a common diagnostic procedure. It may be necessary to decrease technical factors for a procedure when an x-ray requisition indicates the presence of the following conditions.

Emphysema—the overdistention of the lung tissues by air will result in a decrease in lung tissue density.

Pneumothorax—free air in the pleural cavity displaces normal lung tissue and results in decreased density within the thoracic cavity (Figure 17-5).

Conditions of the Abdomen

Abdominal conditions usually cause the abdomen to distend. This distention may be the result of the accumulation of fluid (in which case technical factors need to be increased) or air. Distention of the abdomen from air will require a decrease in technical factors. Whenever an x-ray requisition indicates the presence of the following conditions, it may be necessary to decrease technical factors for the procedure because of the presence of air.

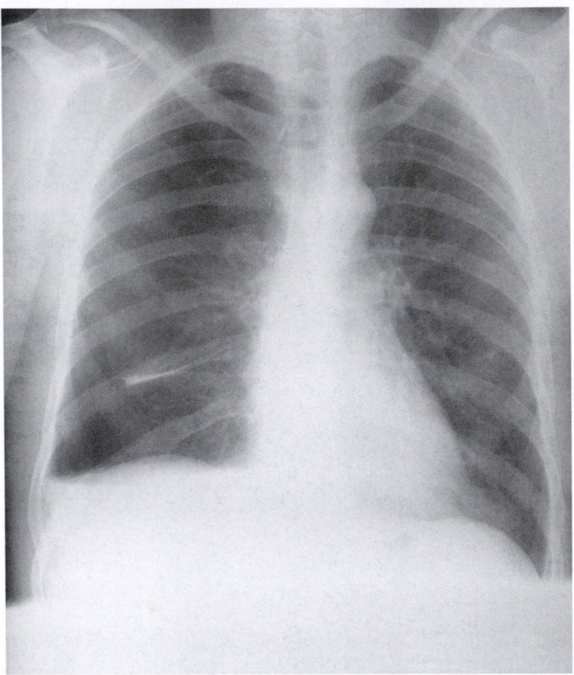

FIGURE 17-5. A large, right-sided pneumothorax is a destructive condition, resulting in decreased radiation absorption. *(Radiographs courtesy of Arlene Adler and Richard R. Carlton.)*

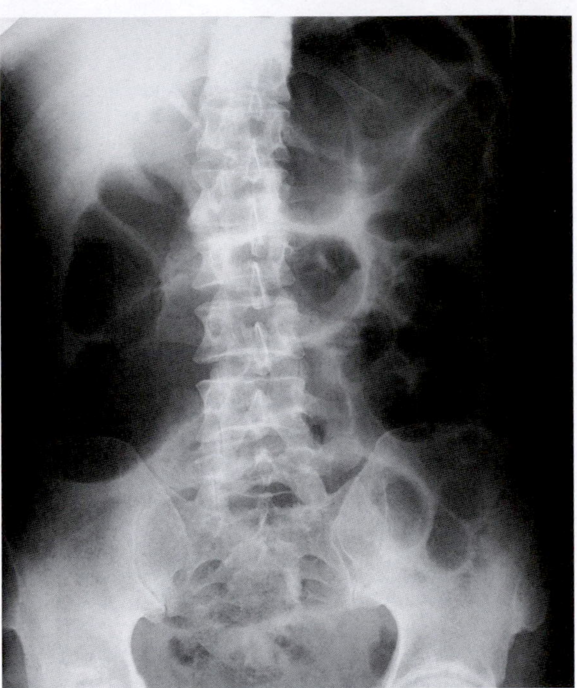

FIGURE 17-6. An obstruction of the large bowel is a destructive condition, resulting in decreased radiation absorption. *(Radiographs courtesy of Arlene Adler and Richard R. Carlton.)*

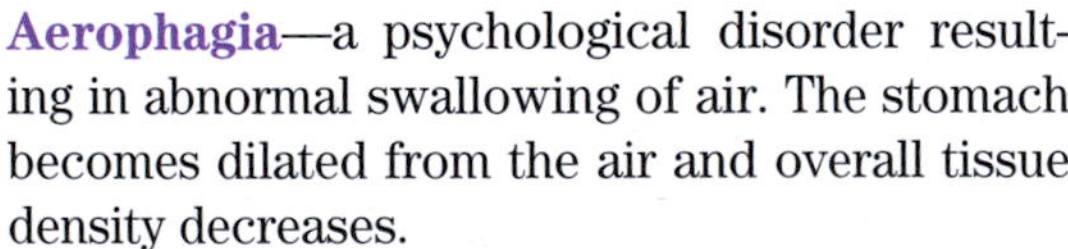

Aerophagia—a psychological disorder resulting in abnormal swallowing of air. The stomach becomes dilated from the air and overall tissue density decreases.

Bowel Obstruction—an obstruction in the bowel results in the abnormal accumulation of air and fluid. If a large amount of air is trapped in the bowel, the overall density of the tissues is decreased (Figure 17-6).

Conditions of the Extremities and Skull

Conditions that result in the destruction of bone tissue are termed osteolytic. These conditions result in a loss of bone mass or calcium within the bone. They alter the composition of the bone by decreasing the effective atomic number and/or the tissue density. The result is areas of radiolucency, which are easier to penetrate than normal bone. Approximately 50 percent of the bone substance must be lost before changes can be seen radiographically. As a result, these conditions must generally be extensive before technical factor changes are necessary.

Active Osteomyelitis—with a bone infection, there is initially a loss of bone tissue (containing calcium), resulting in a decrease in the thickness and composition of the part.

Aseptic Necrosis—death of bone tissue results in a decrease in composition and thickness of the part.

Carcinoma—malignancies in bone can cause an osteolytic process, resulting in decreased thickness and composition of the part.

Degenerative Arthritis—inflammation of the joints results in a destruction of adjoining bone tissue, which decreases the composition of the part.

Fibrosarcoma—this malignant tumor of the metaphysis of bone causes an osteolytic lesion with a "moth-eaten" appearance. The result is reduced bone composition.

Gout—during the chronic stages of this metabolic disease, areas of bone destruction result in punched-out lesions that reduce the bone composition.

Hyperparathyroidism—oversecretion of the parathyroid hormone causes calcium to leave bone and enter the bloodstream. The bone becomes demineralized and composition is decreased.

Multiple Myeloma—this malignant tumor arises from plasma cells of bone marrow and causes punched-out osteolytic areas on the bone. Often many sites are affected and reduced bone tissue composition results.

Osteolytic Metastases—when some malignancies spread to bone they produce destruction of the bone, resulting in reduced composition.

Osteomalacia—a defect in bone mineralization results in decreased composition of the affected bone.

Osteoporosis—a defect in bone production due to the failure of osteoblasts to lay down bone matrix results in decreased composition of the affected bone (Figure 17-7).

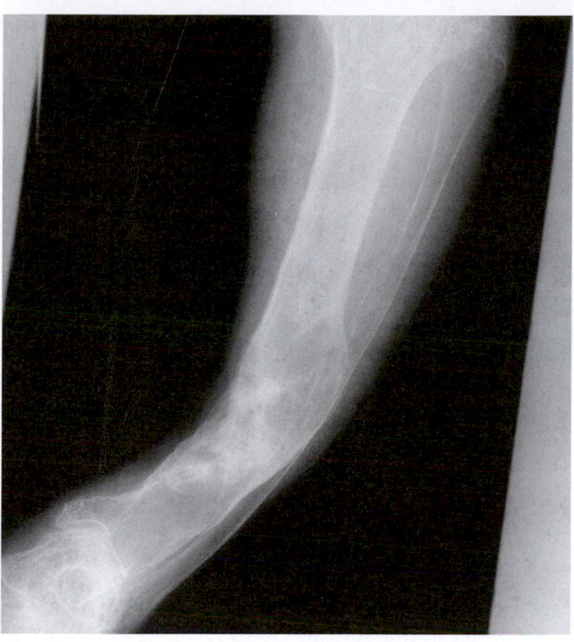

FIGURE 17-7. This patient has a severe bone deformity from a fracture that resulted in chronic osteomyelitis and diffuse osteoporosis. The chronic osteomyelitis is an additive condition (seen around the fracture site) and the osteoporosis is a destructive condition, resulting in a decrease in radiation absorption throughout the remaining bone. *(Radiographs courtesy of Arlene Adler and Richard R. Carlton.)*

SUMMARY

The presence of a pathological condition can greatly affect the degree of radiation absorption. Radiographers must have an understanding of pathology in order to properly select the technical factors for a procedure. Properly reading the x-ray requisition and taking an adequate patient history are essential responsibilities of the radiographer. Fulfilling these responsibilities reduces the need to repeat an image, due to the patient's condition.

If a disease causes the affected body tissue to increase in thickness, effective atomic number, and/or density, which disease will result in a greater attenuation of the x-ray beam. As more photons are absorbed by the body tissues, fewer will be available to reach the image receptor to create adequate exposure. These diseases are harder to penetrate and are called additive conditions because they require adding to the exposure to achieve the proper image receptor exposure.

If a disease causes the affected body tissue to decrease in thickness, effective atomic number, and/or density, that disease will result in less attenuation

SUMMARY (continued)

of the x-ray beam. As more photons are able to pass through the body tissues, more will be available to reach the image receptor to create the required exposure. These diseases are easier to penetrate and are called destructive conditions. They require decreasing the technical factors to achieve the proper image receptor exposure. ■

REVIEW QUESTIONS

1. Why do some pathological conditions affect the attenuation of the x-ray beam?
2. Why is it important that radiographers have an understanding of pathological conditions?
3. What is the relationship between additive conditions and attenuation? Destructive conditions and attenuation?
4. Why should the radiographer take a good clinical history and closely observe the patient?
5. Describe how the following additive conditions may affect the radiographic image:
   a. edema
   b. congestive heart failure
   c. pneumonia
   d. ascites
   e. Paget's disease
6. Describe how the following destructive conditions may affect the radiographic image:
   a. atrophy
   b. emphysema
   c. pneumothorax
   d. degenerative arthritis
   e. osteoporosis

REFERENCES AND RECOMMENDED READING

Eisenberg, R. L., & Johnson, N. M. (2007). *Comprehensive radiographic pathology* (4th ed.). St. Louis, MO: Elsevier/Mosby.

Gould, B. F., & Dyer, R. (2010). *Pathophysiology for the health professions.* St. Louis, MO: Elsevier/Saunders.

Hiss, S. S. (2003). *Understanding radiography* (4th ed.). Springfield, IL: Charles C Thomas.

Mace, J. D., Kowalczyk, N. M., & Evans, K. D. (2008). *Radiographic pathology for technologists* (5th ed.). St. Louis, MO: Elsevier/Mosby.

McPhee, S. J., & Hammer, G. D. (2009). *Pathophysiology of disease:* An introduction to clinical medicine (6th ed.). New York, NY: McGraw-Hill.

CHAPTER 18

The Grid

KEY TERMS

criss-cross grid
cross-hatched grid
focused grid
grid
grid cutoff
grid frequency
grid ratio
linear grid
parallel grid

> We . . . hope that roentgenologists . . . may become convinced of the serious role played by object-secondary rays, to the end that it will soon be practicable for every roentgenologist to rid himself of their nuisance in his every-day work.
>
> *Hollis E. Potter, "The Bucky Diaphragm Principle Applied to Roentgenography"*

OBJECTIVES

Upon completion of this chapter, the student should be able to:

- Describe the purpose of the grid.
- Explain the construction of a grid, including grid materials, grid ratio, grid frequency, and lead content.
- Describe the various grid patterns.
- Differentiate between parallel and focused grids.
- Differentiate between the uses of a stationary and a moving grid.
- Explain the process of grid selection for specific radiographic procedures.
- Explain the relationship of grid selection to patient dose and image receptor exposure.
- Calculate changes in technical factors to compensate for changes in grid selection.
- Describe methods for evaluating the performance of a grid.
- Discuss common errors that are made when using a grid and the effects of these errors on the radiographic image.
- Describe other scatter reduction methods.

PURPOSE OF THE GRID

A **grid** is a device used to improve the contrast of the radiographic image. It does this by absorbing scatter radiation before it can reach the image receptor. When an x-ray beam passes through the body, one of three things will occur with the primary photons that originated at the target. They will: (1) pass through the body unaffected, (2) be absorbed by the body, or (3) interact and change direction (Figure 18-1).

The photons that pass through the body unaffected will interact with the image receptor to create the image. These are the photons responsible for creating the contrast (differences in the image receptor exposures or densities) on the image. These differences exist because some photons pass through the body while others are absorbed. Absorption of photons occurs as the result of photoelectric interaction. This interaction results in the complete absorption of the primary photon and the production of a secondary photon. The secondary radiation created by this interaction is, with few exceptions, very weak and is quickly absorbed in the surrounding tissues.

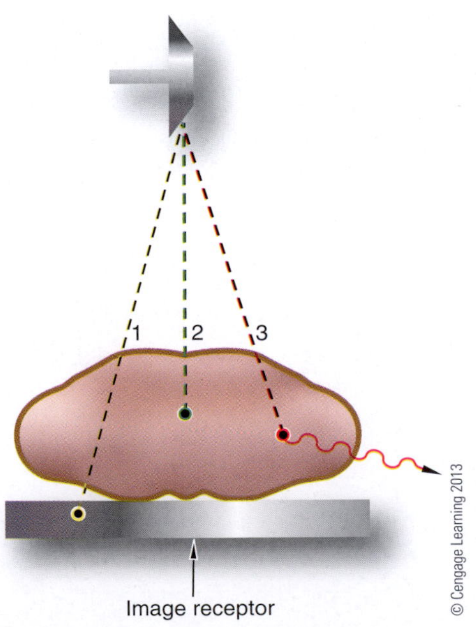

FIGURE 18-1. When x-rays interact with the patient, they will either (1) pass through unaffected; (2) be absorbed; or (3) interact and change direction (scatter).

Primary radiation that interacts and, as a result of this interaction, changes direction is known as scatter radiation. The interaction that produces scatter radiation is known as a Compton interaction. These interactions can result in photons that are strong enough to be emitted by the patient and interact with the image receptor. Because these photons have changed direction, they are no longer able to record exposures on the image receptor that relate to the patient's anatomy. The exposures that they add to the image receptor are of no diagnostic value. Scattered photons add an overall exposure to the image receptor and, as a result of this overall graying of the image, contrast is lowered. An important point to remember is that the percentage of Compton interactions increases with increased kVp. Therefore, **scatter increases and contrast is further impaired as kVp increases**.

Because the patient is the source of the scatter that is degrading the image, it is logical to assume that the patient will also control the quantity of scatter produced. Scatter increases with increases in the volume of the tissue irradiated and decreases with increased atomic number of the tissue. The volume of tissue that is irradiated is controlled by the thickness of the patient and the exposure field size. Although the thickness of the patient is predetermined (but can sometimes be reduced by compression), the field size can be kept to a minimum by collimation. The atomic number of the tissue will also affect the quantity of scatter. The greater the atomic number of the tissue, the less will be the quantity of scatter created. For example, less scatter is produced in bone than in soft tissue, because bone absorbs more photons photoelectrically. This is the result of changes in the number and types of atoms that are present for interaction. In summary, **the amount of scatter radiation increases with (1) increases in patient thickness, (2) larger field sizes, and (3) decreases in atomic number of the tissue.** (This is discussed in further detail in Chapter 15.)

Because a grid is designed to absorb the unwanted scatter radiation, it is necessary to use a grid with thicker, larger body parts and with procedures that require higher-kVp techniques. As a general rule, a grid is employed when:

1. body part thickness exceeds 10 cm
2. kVp is above 60

A grid is a thin, flat, rectangular device made by placing a series of radiopaque lead strips side by side and separating the strips by an interspace material that is radiolucent. The lead strips are of very thin foil and the interspace material is thicker and usually made of aluminum. These strips are then encased in a plastic or aluminum cover to protect them from damage.

The very first grid was made in 1913 by the American radiologist Gustav Bucky (1880–1963). Dr. Bucky's first grid consisted of wide strips of lead spaced 2 cm apart and running in two directions, along the length of the image and across the image (Figure 18-2). This crude design created an image of the grid that was superimposed on the patient's image. Despite having to view the anatomy through this checkerboard pattern, the original grid did remove scatter and improve contrast.

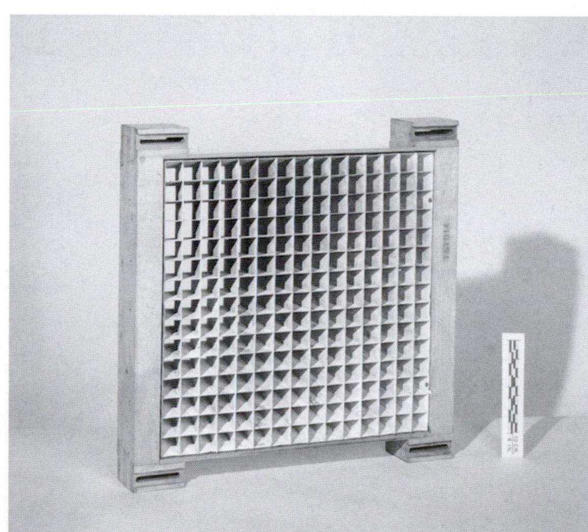

FIGURE 18-2. Dr. Bucky's original grid. *(Courtesy of Smithsonian Institution's Division of Science, Medicine, & Society.)*

In 1920 Hollis Potter (1880–1963), a Chicago radiologist, improved Dr. Bucky's grid design. Dr. Potter realigned the lead strips so they would run in only one direction, made the lead strips thinner and therefore less obvious on the image, and then designed a device (now known as the Potter-Bucky diaphragm) that allowed the grid to move during the exposure. By moving the grid, the lead strips became blurred and were no longer visible on the image. All these improvements resulted in a practical grid device, which significantly improved contrast without impairing the view of the patient's anatomy.

GRID CONSTRUCTION

Various grids are available today (Table 18-1). The choice of the proper grid for a particular clinical procedure requires an understanding of a grid's function. Grid construction involves the selection of materials, grid ratio, and grid frequency.

Grid Materials

A grid is a series of radiopaque strips that alternate with radiolucent interspace strips. These strips are bonded firmly together and then sliced into flat sheets. The radiopaque strips are needed to absorb the scatter radiation and must therefore be made of a dense material with a high atomic number. Lead is the material of choice because it is relatively inexpensive and is easy to shape into very thin foil.

The interspace material must be radiolucent. In other words, it allows radiation to pass easily through it. Several organic and inorganic materials have been tried but only two are commercially available—aluminum and plastic fiber. Ideally, this material should not absorb any radiation. However, in reality, it does absorb a small amount. Aluminum is more commonly used than plastic fiber because it is easier to use in manufacturing and is more durable. Also, because it has a higher atomic number than fiber, it can provide additional absorption of low-energy scatter. With its higher atomic number, aluminum also increases the absorption of primary photons. This can be a disadvantage, especially with low-kVp techniques where

TABLE 18-1. Grids for Use in Digital Imaging

Ratio	Linear	Focused/ Parallel	Interspacer Material	Lines Inch/ cm	Weight (g/cm^2)	Thickness (mm)	Use	Positioning latitude
17:1	L	F/P	AL	178/70	0.97	3.1	Chest	Very narrow
12:1	L	F/P	AL	200/80	0.67	1.6	General	Narrow
12:1	L	F/P	AL	178/70	0.72	1.6	General	Narrow
10:1	L	F/P	AL	200/80	0.58	1.4	General	Moderate
10:1	L	F/P	AL	178/70	0.61	1.4	General	Moderate
8:1	L	F/P	AL	200/80	0.48	1.2	Portables	Wide
8:1	L	F/P	AL	178/70	0.51	1.2	Portables	Wide
6:1	L	F/P	AL	200/80	0.39	1.0	Portables	Very wide
6:1	L	F/P	AL	178/70	0.41	1.0	Portables	Very Wide
Grids for Analog (Film) and Reciprocating Buckys								
15:1	L	F/P	AL	103/40	1.30	3.4	Chest	Very narrow
12:1	L	F/P	AL	103/40	1.06	2.8	General	Narrow
12:1	L	F/P	AL	85/34	1.26	3.4	General	Narrow
10:1	L	F/P	AL	103/40	0.90	2.4	General	Moderate
10:1	L	F/P	AL	85/34	1.07	2.9	General	Moderate
8:1	L	F/P	AL	103/40	0.74	2.0	Portables	Wide
8:1	L	F/P	AL	85/34	0.88	2.4	Portables	Wide
6:1	L	F/P	AL	103/40	0.58	1.6	Portables	Very wide
6:1	L	F/P	AL	85/34	0.68	1.9	Portables	Very Wide
Grids For Mammography Use								
5:1	L	F	Fiber	31 lines cm			Reciprocating mammo Bucky	

Courtesy of Leo Reina, Reina Imaging, Inc., Crystal Lake, IL.

this absorption would be greater. Fiber interspace grids are preferred when using low-kVp techniques where their application can contribute to lower patient dose, such as in mammography.

Grid Ratio

Grid ratio has a major influence on the ability of the grid to improve contrast. It is defined as the ratio of the height of the lead strips to the distance between the strips (Figure 18-3). This is expressed in the formula:

$$\text{Grid ratio} = \frac{h}{D}$$

where: h = lead strip height
D = interspace width

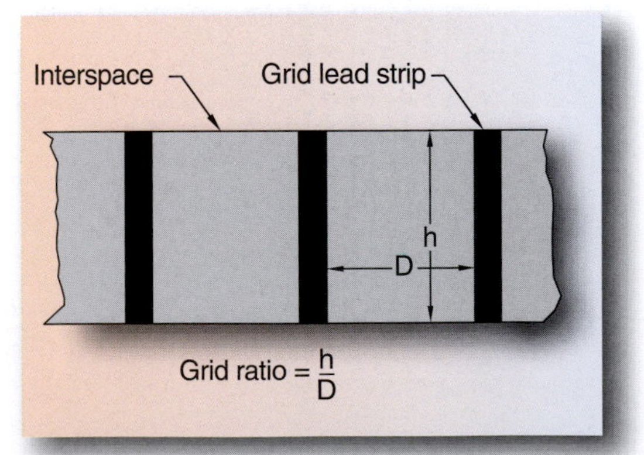

FIGURE 18-3. Grid ratio is the height of the lead strips divided by the width of the interspace.

EXAMPLE: If the lead strips are 3 mm high and are separated by an interspace of 0.25 mm, what is the grid ratio?

Answer:

$$\text{grid ratio} = \frac{3.0}{0.25}$$

$$\text{grid ratio} = 12{:}1$$

If the height of the grid is a constant, decreasing the distance between the lead strips would result in an increase in the grid ratio. Conversely, if the height of the grid is a constant, increasing the distance between the lead strips would result in a decrease in grid ratio. **An inverse relationship exists between the distance between the lead strips and grid ratio when the height of the grid strips remains the same.**

Higher grid ratios allow less scatter radiation to pass through their interspace material to reach the image receptor. Figure 18-4 demonstrates the effect of grid ratio on the maximum angle possible for a scattered photon to pass through the grid. The higher the grid ratio, the straighter the scattered photon has to be in order to pass through the interspace material. Scattered photons, therefore, have to be more closely aligned to the direction of the primary photons in order to reach the image receptor. This means that higher grid ratios are more effective at removing scatter. For the same reason, higher-ratio grids require greater accuracy in their positioning and are more prone to grid errors.

Grids are sometimes rated according to their weight instead of ratio. This is usually expressed in terms of grams per square centimeter (g/cm^2) or occasionally in the United States as grams per square inch (g/in^2).

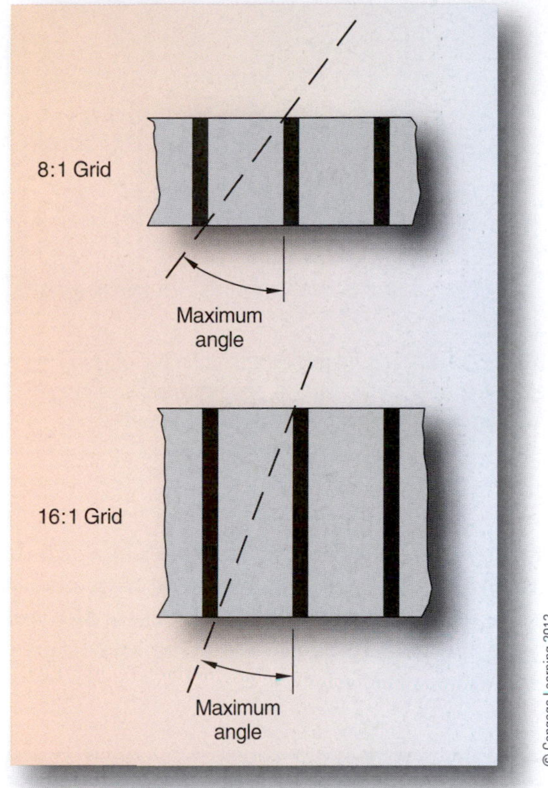

FIGURE 18-4. Grid ratio affects the amount of scatter absorbed by determining the maximum angle of a scattered ray that can get through the grid. The smaller the angle, the less scatter reaches the image receptor.

Grid Frequency

Grid frequency is defined as the number of grid lines per inch or centimeter. Grids are made with a range in frequency from 60–200 lines/inch (25–80 lines/cm). Most commonly used grids have a frequency of 85–103 lines/inch (33–41 lines/cm). In general, grids with higher grid frequencies have thinner lead strips (Figure 18-5). Very-high-frequency grids of approximately 178 to 200 lines/inch (70–80 lines/cm) are recommended for stationary grids used with digital image receptor systems to minimize the possibility of seeing the grid lines on the image.

By combining information about grid ratio and frequency, one can determine the total quantity of lead in the grid. It is the grid's lead content that is most important in determining the grid's efficiency at cleaning up scatter. Lead content is measured in mass per unit area, or grams per square centimeter.

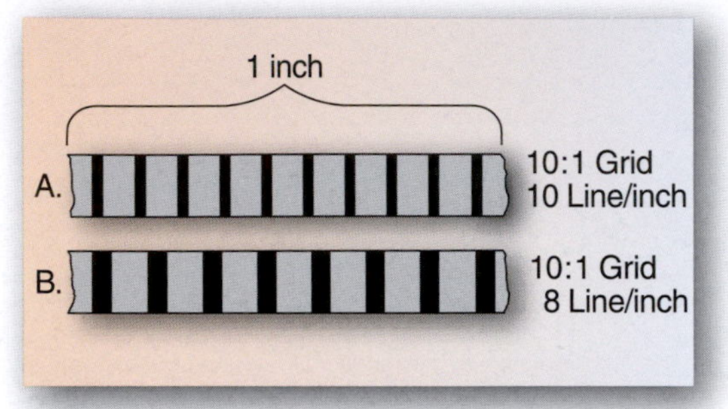

FIGURE 18-5. Grid frequency is the number of grid lines per inch or centimeter. Grids A and B have the same grid ratio, but A has a higher grid frequency than B.

In general, the lead content is greater in a grid that has a higher grid ratio and lower grid frequency. **As the lead content of a grid increases, the ability of the grid to remove scatter and improve contrast increases.**

GRID PATTERNS

Grid strips can be made to run in one or two directions. Grids with lead strips running in only one direction are called linear grids. Grids may also made by placing two linear grids on top of one another so the grid lines are running at right angles. These grids are termed **criss-cross** or **cross-hatched** (Figure 18-6). Dr. Bucky's original grid was made using this pattern.

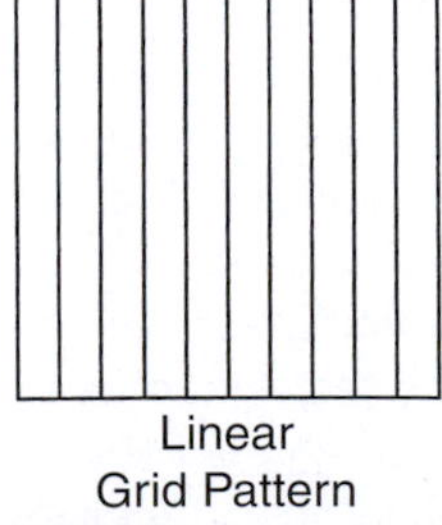

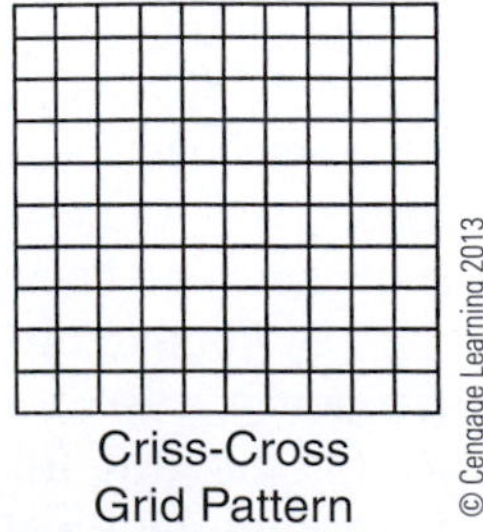

FIGURE 18-6. A linear versus a criss-cross grid pattern.

Linear grids are more commonly used in clinical practice because they can be used when performing procedures that require tube angulation. Linear grids allow the radiographer to angle the tube only *along* the direction that the lines are running. For most grids, this is along the long axis. In a grid located in a typical x-ray table, the grid strips run along the long axis of the table, which allows for angling the tube toward the head or feet of the patient. Angulation *across* the long axis (toward the patient's right or left side) would result in the primary beam being directed into the lead strips. If the primary beam is angled into the lead, the lead will absorb an undesirable amount of primary radiation, resulting in a problem known as **grid cutoff**. When criss-cross grids are used, no tube tilt is permitted, as any angulation would result in grid cutoff because lead strips are running in both directions. As a result, criss-cross grids have limited applications in radiography.

Grids are also sometimes classified according to the direction the grid lines run within the grid. Most grid lines run in the direction of the long axis of the grid, but it is possible to obtain short-axis grids, which have grid lines running across the short axis of the grid. Short-axis grids are useful for portable chest procedures to decrease the change of grid cutoff when the cassette is placed crosswise.

GRID TYPES

Grids are manufactured with either a parallel or a focused design. **Parallel grids** are made with the lead and interspace strips running parallel to one another. This means that if the grid lines were extended into space they would never intersect. **Focused grids** are designed so that the central grid strips are parallel and as the strips move away from the central axis they become more and more inclined (Figure 18-7).

The focused design results in a grid with lead strips designed to match the divergence of the x-ray beam. If these lead strips were extended, the strips would intersect along a line in space known as the convergence line. The distance from the face of the grid to the points of convergence of the lead strips

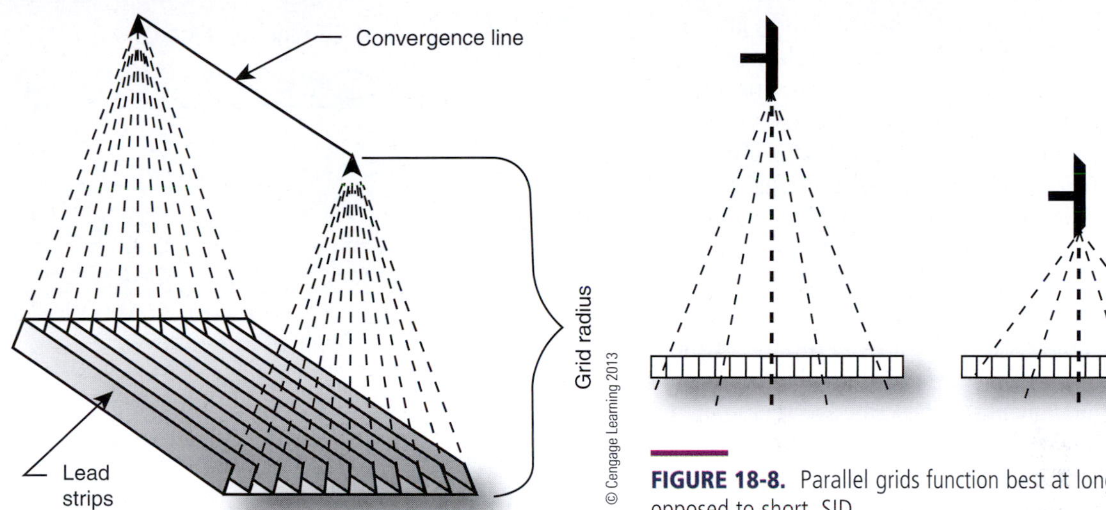

FIGURE 18-7. A focused grid is designed to match the divergence of the x-ray beam. The grid radius is the distance from the face of the grid to the points of convergence of the lead strips.

FIGURE 18-8. Parallel grids function best at long, as opposed to short, SID.

is called the grid radius. **For the grid to be properly focused, the x-ray tube must be located along the convergence line.** Each focused grid will identify the focal range within which the tube should be located. For example, grids are made with short, medium, or long focal ranges, depending on the distance for which they are designed. Short-focal-range grids (14–18 inches or 36–46 cm) are made for use in mammography; long-focal-range grids (60–72 inches or 152–183 cm) are used for chest radiography. Focused grids with lower grid ratios allow for greater latitude in the alignment of the tube with the grid. With higher grid ratios, proper alignment of the grid with the tube is more critical.

Parallel grids are less commonly employed than focused grids. Because the strips do not try to coincide with the divergence of the x-ray beam, some grid cutoff will occur along the lateral edges, especially when the grid is employed at short SIDs. The parallel grid is best employed at long SIDs because the beam will be a straighter, more perpendicular one (Figure 18-8).

GRID USES

A grid is used either in a stationary position or mounted in a Potter-Bucky diaphragm to move it during exposure. Most radiology departments have a supply of stationary grids, in various sizes, that can be mounted to the front of a cassette. These are generally made approximately one inch larger than the image receptor size they are intended to cover. Stationary grids are used primarily in portable procedures or for upright or horizontal beam views. Some departments may also purchase a special cassette with a grid built into it. This design, called a grid cassette, requires reloading between exposures using the grid. This may be an inconvenience in situations where multiple images are needed. When grids are used in a stationary fashion, grid lines on the image will usually be noticed on close inspection. This is especially true with low-frequency grids. High-frequency grids, like those used for digital imaging, have a minimal visual effect.

The most common use of the grid is for procedures using the Potter-Bucky diaphragm (usually called the Bucky). This device is mounted below the tabletop of radiographic and radiographic/fluoroscopic tables and holds the cassette in place below the grid. It can move the grid during the exposure so that grid lines will be blurred and therefore not evident on the image. These grids are approximately 17″ × 19″ (43 × 48 cm), large enough to cover a 14″ × 17″ (35 × 43 cm) cassette placed either lengthwise or crosswise in the cassette tray. The direction in which the grid moves is important if it is to accomplish the job of blurring the grid lines. The lead strips of the grid run along the long axis of the table. To blur the lead lines, the grid must move at a right angle to the direction of the lines. This means that it will be moving back and forth across the table and not from top to bottom.

There are two movement mechanisms used today. The movements are described as reciprocating and oscillating. With the reciprocating grid, a motor drives the grid back and forth during the exposure for a total distance of no more than 2–3 cm. With the oscillating grid, an electromagnet pulls the grid to one side and then releases it during exposure. The grid oscillates in a circular motion within the grid frame.

GRID SELECTION/ CONVERSIONS

Selecting the best grid to use for a specific radiographic procedure is a complex process. Most procedures that are done with a grid use a moving grid mounted in a table or upright holder. Grid choice must be made in the equipment purchase phase of quality control. Once a grid is selected and mounted in the Potter-Bucky diaphragm, it is not easily changed. Purchase decisions are generally made by the department administrator in collaboration with the radiologist.

Grids absorb scatter and scatter adds exposure to the image receptor. The more efficient a grid is at absorbing scatter, the less exposure will be received by the image receptor. Therefore, compensations must be made to increase this exposure. This is generally accomplished by increasing mAs, which, in turn, results in greater patient dose. The better the grid cleans up scatter, the greater will be the dose given to the patient to achieve an adequate exposure. The amount of mAs needed can be calculated using the following formula:

$$\text{Grid Conversion Factor (GCF)} = \frac{\text{mAs with the grid}}{\text{mA}}$$

TABLE 18-2. Grid Conversion Factors

Grid Ratio	60 kVp	85 kVp	110 kVp
No grid	1	1	1
5:1	3	3	3
8:1	3.75	4	4.25
12:1	4.75	5.5	6.25
16:1	5.75	6.75	8

Adapted with permission from *Characteristics and Applications of X-Ray Grids*, Liebel-Flarsheim division of Sybron Corporation, Cincinnati, Ohio. Approximate values based on clinical tests of pelvis and skull.

This formula is referred to as the Bucky factor as well as the grid conversion factor. **Grid-conversion factors (GCFs) increase with higher grid ratios and increasing kVp.** Because grids vary in respect to their ratio, frequency, and lead content, it would be useful to check the grid conversion factor for each of the common grids used in a department. Table 18-2 offers a guide of grid conversion factors for commonly purchased grids.

EXAMPLE: A satisfactory chest radiograph is produced using 5 mAs at 85 kVp without a grid. A second image is requested using a 12:1 grid. Using Table 18-2, what mAs is needed to produce a second satisfactory image?

Answer:

$$\text{GCF} = \frac{\text{mAs with the grid}}{\text{mAs without the grid}}$$

$$5.5 = \frac{X}{5}\text{ mAs}$$

$$X = 5.5 \times 5\text{ mAs}$$

$$X = 27.5\text{ mAs}$$

When converting from one grid ratio to another, the following formula is used:

$$\frac{mAs_1}{mAs_2} = \frac{GCF_1}{GCF_2}$$

where: mAs_1 = original mAs
mAs_2 = new mAs
GCF_1 = original grid conversion factor
GCF_2 = new grid conversion factor

EXAMPLE: A satisfactory abdominal image is produced using an 8:1 grid, 35 mAs, and 85 kVp. A second image is requested using a 12:1 grid. Using Table 18-2, what mAs is needed to produce a second satisfactory image?

Answer:

$$\frac{mAs_1}{mAs_2} = \frac{GCF_1}{GCF_2}$$

$$\frac{35}{X} = \frac{4}{5.5}$$

$$4X = 192.5$$

$$X = 48 \text{ mAs}$$

GRID PERFORMANCE EVALUATION

The efficiency of a grid in cleaning up or removing scatter can be quantitatively measured. The International Commission on Radiologic Units and Measurements (ICRU) Handbook 89 defines two criteria for measuring a grid's performance: selectivity and contrast improvement ability.

Selectivity

Although grids are designed to absorb scatter, they also absorb some primary radiation. Grids that absorb a greater percentage of scatter than primary radiation are described as having a greater degree of selectivity. Selectivity is identified by the Greek sigma (Σ) and is measured by using the following formula:

$$\text{Selectivity} = \frac{\text{\% primary radiation transmitted}}{\text{\% sca}}$$

The better a grid is at removing scatter, the greater will be the selectivity of the grid. **This means that a grid with a higher lead content would have a greater selectivity.**

Contrast Improvement Ability

The best measure of how well a grid functions is its ability to improve contrast in the clinical setting. The contrast improvement factor is dependent on the amount of scatter produced, which is controlled by the kVp and volume of irradiated tissue (see Chapter 27). As the amount of scatter radiation increases, the lower will be the contrast and the lower the contrast improvement factor. The contrast improvement factor (K) can be measured using the following formula:

$$K = \frac{\text{Radiographic contrast with the grid}}{\text{Radiographi}}$$

If K = 1, then no improvement in contrast has occurred. Most grids have contrast improvement factors between 1.5 and 3.5. This means that contrast is 1.5–3.5 times better when using the grid. **The higher the K factor, the greater the contrast improvement.**

GRID ERRORS

Poor images can result from improper use of the grid. Errors in the use of the grid occur mainly with grids that have a focused design. This is because focused grids are made to coincide with the divergence of the x-ray beam. The tube must be centered to the focused grid and aligned at the correct distance. Additionally, a focused grid has a tube side and a receptor side based on the angulation of the grid strips. Proper tube/grid alignment is essential to prevent the undesirable absorption of primary radiation known as grid cutoff.

Off-Level

An off-level grid error occurs when the tube is angled across the long axis of the grid strips. This can be the result of improper tube or grid positioning (Figure 18-9). Improper tube positioning results if the central ray is directed across the long axis of the radiographic table. Recall that

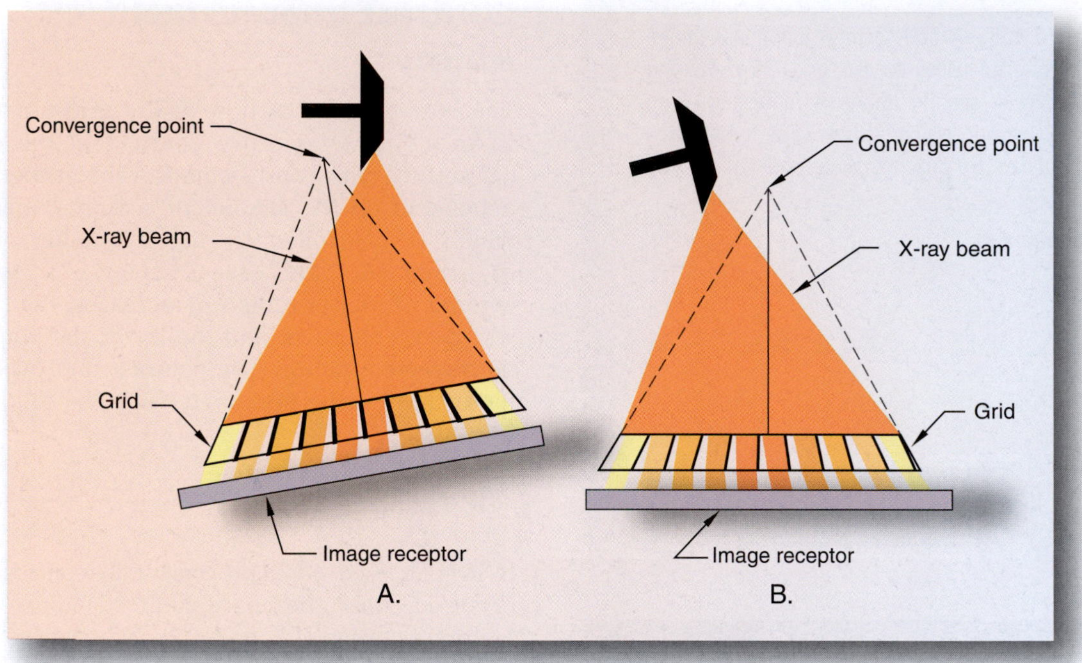

FIGURE 18-9. An off-level grid error can occur with a parallel or focused grid. A linear grid can be off-level in one direction, whereas a criss-cross grid can be off-level in both directions (across and along the grid).

it is only possible to angle along the long axis of the table with a linear grid and it is not possible to angle at all with a criss-cross grid. Improper grid positioning most commonly occurs with stationary grids being used for mobile procedures or decubitus views. If, for example, a patient is lying on a grid for a mobile abdominal procedure and the patient's weight is unevenly distributed on the grid, the grid may not be properly aligned to the tube.

An off-level grid error can occur with a focused grid and it is the only positioning error possible with a parallel grid. Care must always be taken when aligning the tube to the grid, especially when using stationary grids, to avoid this error. When this error occurs, there is an undesirable absorption of primary radiation, which results in a radiograph with a decrease in exposure across the entire image (Figure 18-10).

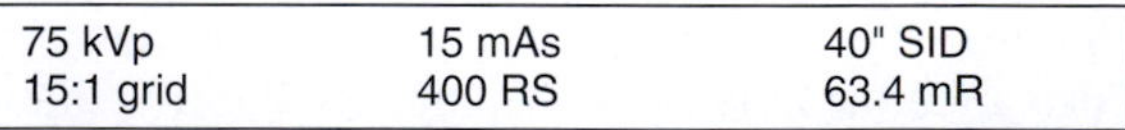

75 kVp	15 mAs	40" SID
15:1 grid	400 RS	63.4 mR

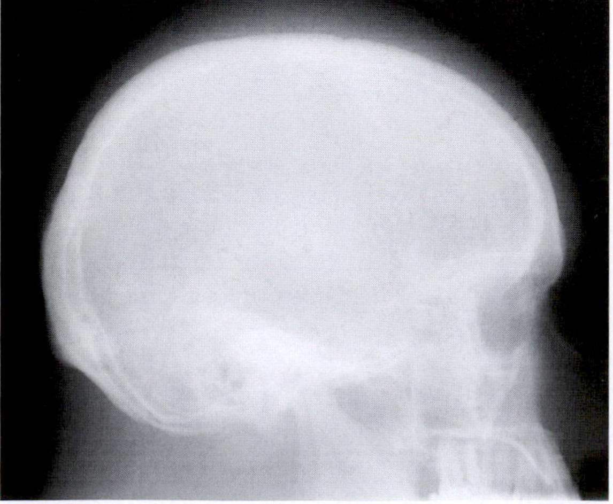

FIGURE 18-10. A radiograph illustrating an off-level grid error. *(Arlene Adler and Richard R. Carlton.)*

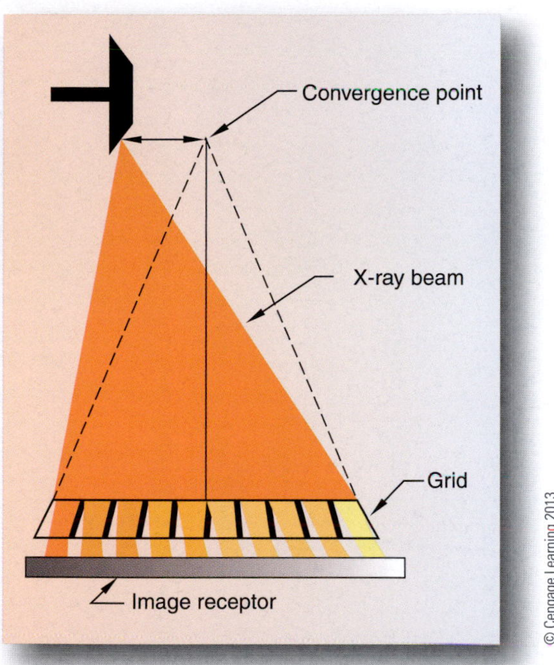

FIGURE 18-11. An off-center grid error.

75 kVp	15 mAs	40" SID
15:1 grid	400 RS	66.1 mR

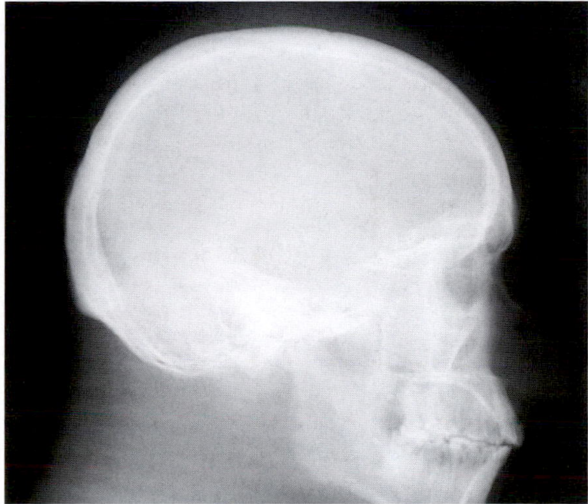

FIGURE 18-12. A radiograph illustrating an off-center grid error. *(Arlene Adler and Richard R. Carlton.)*

Off-Center

The x-ray tube must be centered along the central axis of a focused grid to prevent an off-center (off-axis or lateral decentering) grid error (Figure 18-11). The center grid strips are perpendicular and become more and more inclined away from the center. This design coincides with the divergence of the x-ray beam from the tube. If the central ray is off-center, the most perpendicular portion of the x-ray beam will not correspond to the most perpendicular portion of the grid. The result is a decrease in exposure across the entire image (Figure 18-12).

The greater the degree of lateral decentering, the greater the grid cutoff.

Off-Focus

A focused grid is made to be used at very specific distances identified as the focal range labeled on the front of the grid. When a grid is used at a distance other than that specified as the focal range, an off-focus error results (Figure 18-13). For example, if a grid has a focal range of 36–44 inches (91–112 cm) and it is used at 72 inches, severe grid cutoff will occur. Off-focus errors result in grid cutoff along the peripheral edges of the image (Figure 18-14). Higher grid ratios require greater positioning accuracy to prevent grid cutoff.

Upside-Down

A focused grid has an identified tube side based on the way the grid strips are angled. If the grid is used upside-down, severe peripheral grid cutoff will occur (Figure 18-15). Radiation will pass through the grid along the central axis where the grid strips are most perpendicular and radiation will be increasingly absorbed away from the center (Figure 18-16). It is important that the technologist check the tube side prior to using a focused grid.

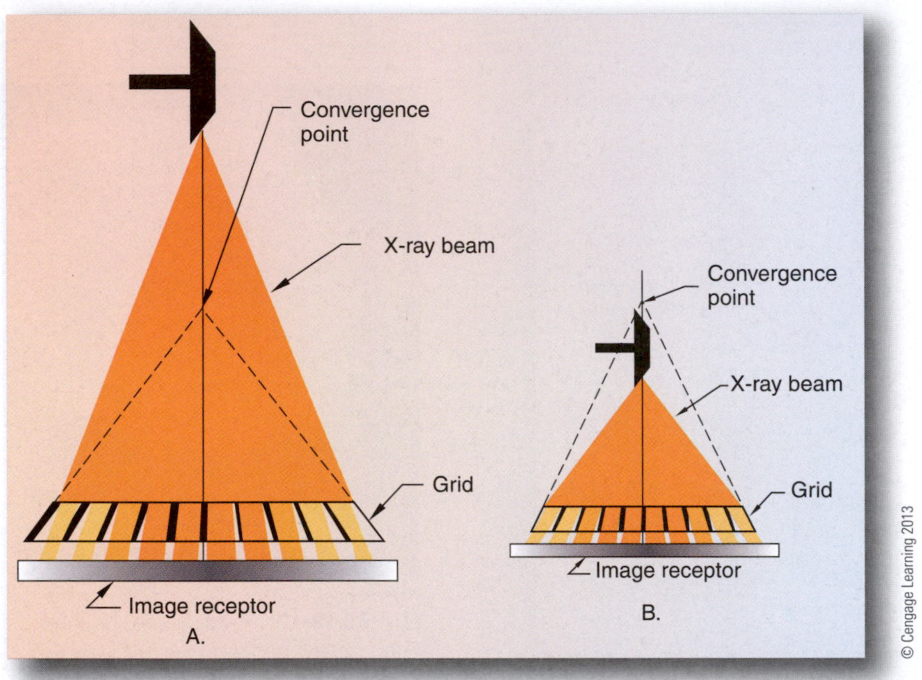

FIGURE 18-13. An off-focus grid error occurs when the grid is used at distances less than or greater than the focal range.

75 kVp	15 mAs	40" SID
15:1 grid	400 RS	69.3 mR

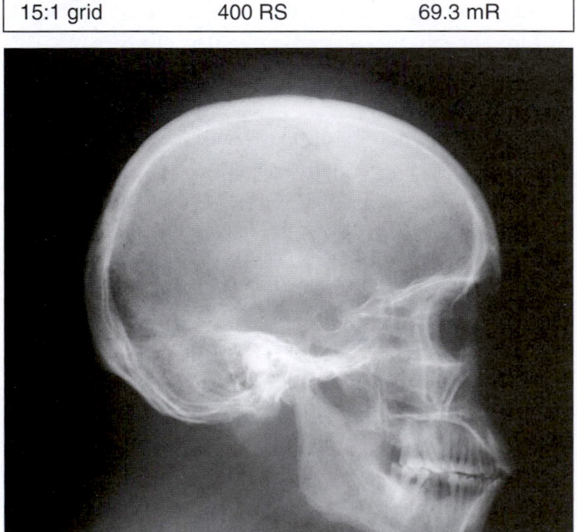

FIGURE 18-14. A radiograph illustrating an off-focus grid error taken at less than the recommended focal range distance. *(Arlene Adler and Richard R. Carlton.)*

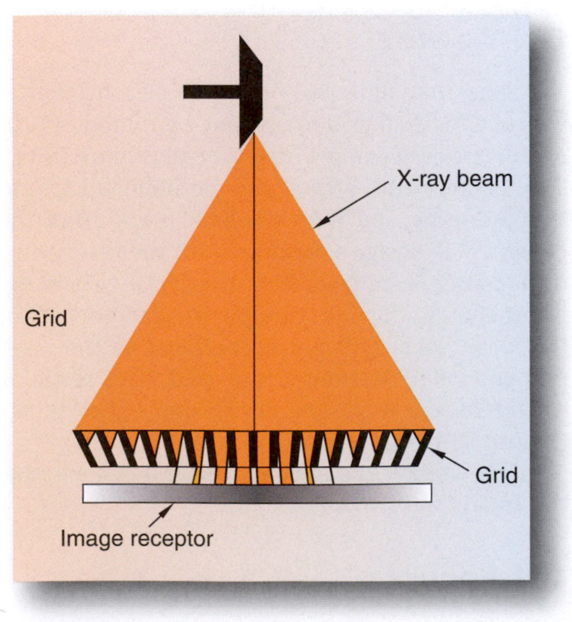

FIGURE 18-15. An upside-down grid error.

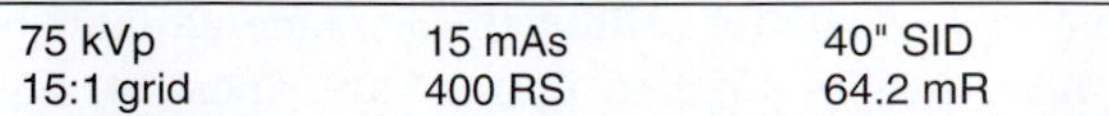

75 kVp	15 mAs	40" SID
15:1 grid	400 RS	64.2 mR

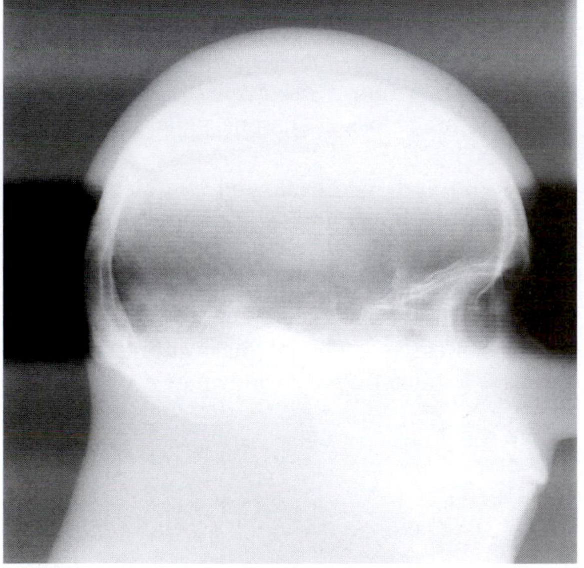

FIGURE 18-16. A radiograph illustrating an upside-down grid error. *(Arlene Adler and Richard R. Carlton.)*

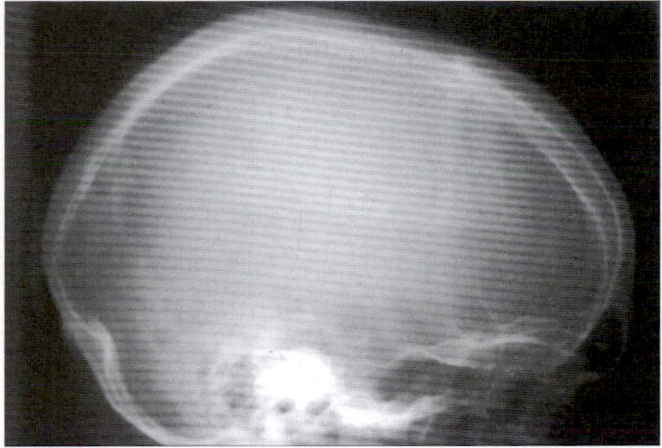

FIGURE 18-17. The Moire effect. *(Courtesy of Barry Burns, MS.R [R], DABR, UNC, Division of Radiographic Science.)*

The Moire Effect

The Moire effect is a grid error that occurs with digital image receptor systems when the grid lines are captured and scanned parallel to the scan lines in the imaging plate readers. This error occurs with grids used in a stationary fashion for examinations such as portable radiography or translateral hip images. In order for the Moire pattern to demonstrate on the image, the grid lines must be running in the same direction as the movement of the laser beam that is scanning the imaging plate (Figure 18-17). Most imaging plates are scanned across the short axis of the plate, and, most often, grid lines run parallel to the long axis of the imaging plate. In these instances, the Moire pattern will not demonstrate. To prevent this grid error, it is recommended that high-frequency grids of 103 lines per inch or greater be used for digital image receptor systems when a stationary grid is needed.

AN ALTERNATE SCATTER REDUCTION METHOD—THE AIR-GAP TECHNIQUE

In addition to the use of a grid, there are a number of other methods that can be employed to reduce the amount of scatter reaching the image receptor. Remember, the most important way to improve image quality is to decrease the amount of scatter initially being created. This is best done by restricting the primary beam. Collimating to the size of the area being examined is critical to image quality. Even with the use of close collimation, it is still necessary to reduce scatter reaching the image receptor when radiographing larger body parts or when using higher kVps. The grid is the primary device employed to reduce scatter. The body part may also be compressed to decrease the amount of scatter created.

The air-gap technique is an alternative to the use of a grid. It has primary applications in magnification radiography and, to a lesser extent, in chest radiography. The technique involves placing the patient at a greater object image receptor distance (OID), thus creating an air gap between the patient and the image receptor. By moving the patient away from the image receptor, the amount of scatter reaching the image receptor will be reduced. As stated earlier, the patient is the source of the

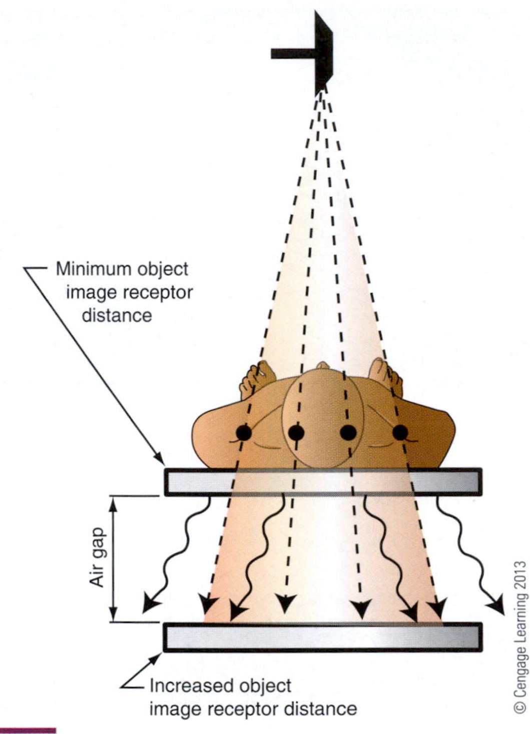

FIGURE 18-18. The air-gap technique reduces the amount of scatter reaching the image receptor.

majority of scatter. Although the same amount of scatter will be created during the exposure, less of the scatter will reach the image receptor if the patient is moved farther away (Figure 18-18). The result is improved contrast without the use of the grid. The primary disadvantage of the air-gap technique is the loss of sharpness that results from increased OID.

Gould and Hale evaluated contrast improvement between the use of a grid and the air-gap technique, showing that a 10-inch (25-cm) air gap has the same degree of clean-up of scatter as a 15:1 grid for a 10-cm body part. This same grid was shown to be more effective at eliminating scatter than the air gap with a thicker (20-cm) body part.

SUMMARY

A grid is a tool used by the radiographer to improve image contrast. Grids are made of lead strips alternating with an interspace material, which is usually made of aluminum. Grids are constructed with a specific grid ratio and frequency. The grid ratio and frequency are important in determining the total lead content of the grid. Generally, grids with higher grid ratios and lead content are more efficient at removing scatter. This can be quantitatively studied by measuring the selectivity and contrast improvement ability of the grid.

Grids absorb scatter and scatter adds exposure to the image receptor. The more efficient a grid is at absorbing scatter, the less image receptor exposure. Therefore, compensation must be made to increase exposure. This is generally accomplished by increasing the mAs, which, in turn, results in greater patient dose. The better the grid is at cleaning up scatter, the greater is the dose given to the patient to achieve adequate exposure.

Grids are manufactured in either a linear or crisscross pattern, with either a parallel or focused design. They can be used in either a stationary manner or may be placed in a device that moves the grid and thereby blurs the grid lines.

An alternative to the use of a grid is the air-gap technique. ■

REVIEW QUESTIONS

1. Why does a grid improve contrast?
2. As a general rule, when should a grid be used?
3. How is a grid constructed?
4. Define grid ratio.
5. What type of grid pattern has lead strips running in only one direction?
6. How is a focused grid designed?
7. As the ability of a grid to clean up scatter increases, what is the effect on patient dose and image receptor exposure?
8. How is the contrast improvement of a grid measured?
9. How does an off-level grid error occur?
10. How does the air-gap technique improve contrast?

REFERENCES AND RECOMMENDED READING

Bednarek, D. P., Rudin, S., & Wong, R. (1983, April). Artifacts produced by moving grids. *Radiology*, 255.

Bell, N., Erskine, M., & Warren-Forward, H. (2003). Lateral cervical spine examinations: An evaluation of dose for grid and non-grid techniques. *Radiography*, *9*(1), 43–52.

Bushberg, J. T., Seibert, J. A., Leidholdt, E. M., & Boone, J. M. (2003). *The essential physics of medical imaging* (2nd ed.). Philadelphia: Lippincott, Williams & Wilkins.

Chan, H. P. (1985, March). Ultra-high-strip-density radiographic grids: A new antiscatter technique for mammography. *Radiology*, 807.

Coleman, N. J., Cowen, A. R., & Parkin, G. J. S. (2000). Effect on mammographic CR image quality of removing the anti-scatter grid. *Radiography*, *6*(3), 199–204.

Cullinan, A., & Cullinan, J. (1994). *Producing quality radiographs* (2nd ed.). Philadelphia: J. B. Lippincott.

Curry, T. S., Dowdey, J. E., & Murry, R. C. (1990). *Christensen's introduction to the physics of diagnostic radiology* (4th ed.). Philadelphia: Lea and Febiger.

Doi, K., Frank, P. H., Chan, H. P., Vyborny, C. J., Makino, S., Iida, N., et al. (1983). Physical and clinical evaluation of new high-strip-density radiographic grids. *Radiology*, *147*(2), 575–582.

Fry, O. E., & Cesare, G. (1960). Bedside radiography reduction of patient exposure and orientation of grid cassettes. *Radiologic Technology*, *31*(4), 387.

Gould, R. G., & Hale, J. (1974). Control of scattered radiation by air gap techniques: Applications to chest radiography. *American Journal of Roentgenology*, *122*, 109–118.

Harlow, C. (1993). Off-centering secondary radiation grids. *Radiography Today*, *59*(674), 11–13.

Heriand, J., & Varma, D. G. K. (1986). A lung opacity caused by grid artifact. *Radiologic Technology*, *58*(2), 147.

Hufton, A. P., Crosthwaite, C. M., Davies, J. M., & Robinson, L. A. (1987). Low attenuation material for table tops, cassettes, and grids: A review. *Radiography*, *53*(607), 17.

Jensen, G., & Scheid, C. (1980). The performance of radiographic grids. *Optimization of chest radiography* (HHS Publication [FDA] 80–8124). Rockville, MD: U.S. Department of Health and Human Services.

Lehrer, R. (2010, January/February). *Minimizing grid cutoff. Radiologic Technology*, *81*(3), 280–281.

Partridge, J., McGahan, G., Causton, S., Bowers, M., Mason, M., Dalby, M., & Mitchell, A. (2006, April). Radiation dose reduction without compromise of image quality in cardiac angiography and intervention with the use of a flat panel detector without an antiscatter grid. *Heart*, *92*(4), 507–510.

Potter, H. E. (1920). The Bucky diaphragm principle applied to roentgenology. *The American Journal of Roentgenology*, *7*, 292.

Potter, H. E. (1931). History of diaphragming roentgen rays by the use of the Bucky principle. *The American Journal of Roentgenology*, *25*, 396.

Seeman, H. E., & Splettstosser, H. R. (1954). The physical characteristics of Potter-Bucky diaphragms. *Radiology*, *62*, 575–583.

Seeman, H. E., & Splettstosser, H. R. (1955). The effect of kilovoltage and grid ratio on subject contrast in radiography. *Radiology*, *64*, 572–580.

Stanford, R. W., Moore, R. D., & Hills, T. H. (1959). Comparative performance of grids in relation to their stated ratio. *British Journal of Radiology*, *32*(374), 106–113.

Stears, J. G., Gray, J. E., & Frank, E. D. (1986). Grids are not created equal. *Radiologic Technology*, *57*(4), 345.

Stober, E. V. (1947). Off-distance cut-off. *Radiologic Technology, 19*(3), 111.

Stober, E. V. (1951). The term "ratio" as applied to an x-ray grid. *Radiologic Technology, 23*(3), 180.

Switzer, D. (1981). The use of grids in diagnostic radiography. *The Canadian Journal of Medical Radiation Technology, 12*(2), 60.

Trout, E. D., Kelley, J. P., & Cathey, G. A. (1952). The use of filters to control radiation exposure to the patient in diagnostic roentgenology. *American Journal of Roentgenology, 67*(6), 946–963.

Warner, R. (1998). Focus on quality. Grid cutoff as a result of improper FFD . . . focal film distance. *Radiologic Technology, 69*(3), 265–266.

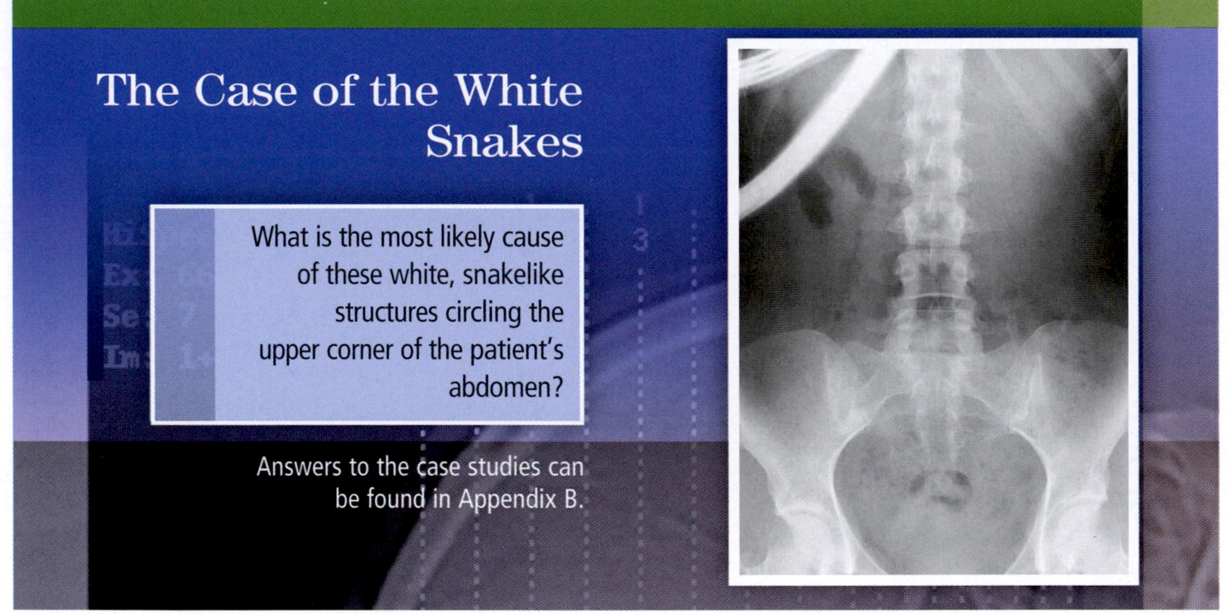

CHAPTER 19

Radiographic Film

KEY TERMS

adhesive
antihalation coating
base
coating
crossover effect
crystal production
duplication film
duplitized
emulsion with crystals
halation
mixing
orthochromatic
panchromatic
ripening
sensitivity speck
silver bromide
silver chloride
silver iodide
silver iodobromide
supercoat

Any discussion relating to the rationale of radiographic exposure should begin with the understanding that the characteristics and the exposure response of x-ray film are the foundations of an exposure system.

Arthur W. Fuchs, from the Jerman Memorial Lecture at the 1950 Annual Meeting of the American Society of X-Ray Technicians

OBJECTIVES

Upon completion of this chapter, the student should be able to:

- Describe the components of radiographic film.
- Explain the production of silver halide crystals.
- State the purpose of various additives to radiographic film.
- Describe latent image formation.
- Discuss the differences between direct exposure film, screen film, and films for various special applications, such as duplication.
- Explain the fundamentals of proper film storage and handling.
- Identify common radiographic film artifacts.
- Discuss automated film systems.
- Explain the responsibilities involved in proper radiograph identification.

Photosensitive film is no longer the most common radiographic image receptor. By the turn of the twenty-first century, digital imaging began to predominate throughout radiography. Film was the first image receptor chosen by Röntgen and it continues to be used for some applications, including its predominance outside developed nations, where it remains useful for nearly all types of medical imaging. Knowledge of film information continues to be required of all radiographers.

Radiographic and photographic film are very similar in nature and both derive from early experiments in recording light images. The discovery of photography cannot be assigned to one person. A permanent photographic process was discovered about 1816 by the French inventor Joseph Nièpce (1765–1833). Nièpce eventually collaborated with the French artist Louis Daguerre (1787–1851), who improved the process and sold it to the French government, which released it to the public in 1839. Simultaneously, between 1835 and 1840, the English photographer William Fox Talbot (1800–1877) developed the now common negative-to-positive process that was given the name photography. Many photographers contributed to the scientific understanding of the process, and by the 1850s the process was similar to, although more primitive than, the process that was utilized through the turn of the twenty-first century.

Photographic materials are photosensitive, or capable of responding to exposure by photons. Both radiographic and photographic film are sensitive to the wavelengths and energies that comprise most of the electromagnetic spectrum of both light and x-rays (see Figure 2-12), although it is possible to manufacture film that is insensitive to portions of the spectrum. Proper use of photosensitive materials requires an understanding of how film is constructed and how the image is formed.

CONSTRUCTION

Diagnostic radiographic film is manufactured by coating both sides of a base material with an emulsion containing photosensitive crystals. Several other materials are also used to improve the performance and permanence of the film. The complete construction of diagnostic radiographic film includes the **base**, **adhesive**, **emulsion with crystals**, and **supercoat** (Figure 19-1). The total thickness of the film varies with the manufacturer, from 175 to 300 μm (0.007″ to 0.012″).

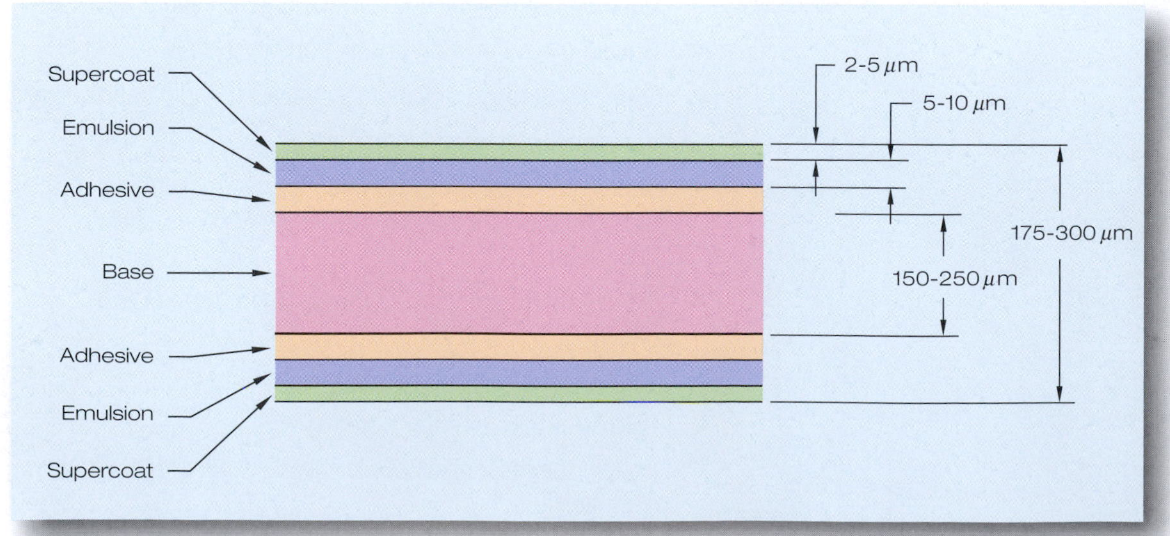

FIGURE 19-1. Cross-sectional view of diagnostic radiographic film.

Base

The film base was originally composed of a glass plate. Glass plates coated with emulsion were used in photography from soon after its discovery until World War I (circa 1914) (Figure 19-2). Modern radiography has retained in the professional jargon an old-fashioned term, *flat plate of the abdomen*, from this period. Of course, the physician requesting such an image intends the image to be digital or a film base to be of polyester plastic, not a glass plate.

During World War I a shortage of the good, optical-quality glass needed for the film base caused film manufacturers to switch to cellulose nitrate. Because of its flammable nature (which caused several tragic hospital fires), nonflammable cellulose triacetate was introduced in the 1920s. Radiographic film base is polyester, which was introduced in the 1960s. It is usually 150–200 µm (0.006″–0.008″) thick.

The film base must be flexible yet tough, stable, rigid, and uniformly lucent. It must be flexible to permit easy handling in the darkroom and to make good contact with the cassette pressure pads. It must be stable so that it does not change its dimensions during the heating and immersion in chemicals required for processing. It must be rigid enough to be conveniently placed onto a viewbox (radiographic illuminator). Most important, it must be uniformly lucent so that it permits the transmission of light without adding artifacts to the diagnostic image.

The film base usually includes a blue dye to tint the film and reduce eyestrain for the interpreting radiologist, thereby increasing the diagnostic accuracy available from the image. The film base is also often coated with a special substance to prevent light from one screen crossing over to the other, causing blurring of the image. This reflection of light is called the **crossover effect**. Some manufacturers use an ultraviolet emission from the intensifying screen to reduce the crossover effect. **Halation** is a different effect caused by light being reflected from the air interface on the back of the base material (Figure 19-3). An **antihalation coating** may be applied to the back of single-emulsion film. This coating is designed to absorb the light coming from the emulsion and prevent backscatter, visible light, or reflected light from degrading the image. The coating is removed by the processing chemicals to permit light to be

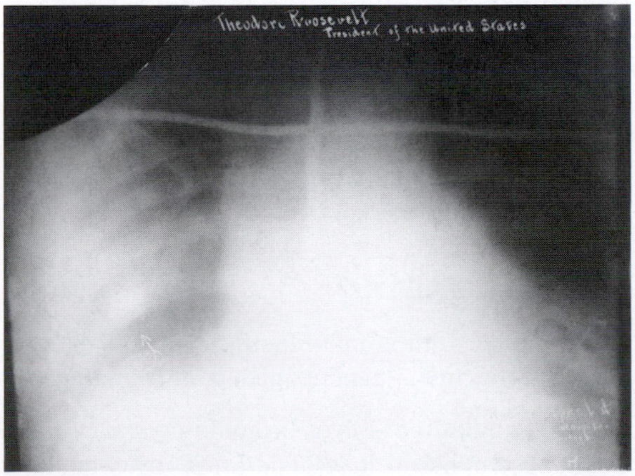

FIGURE 19-2. Glass plate radiograph of Theodore Roosevelt taken at Mercy Hospital in Chicago on October 15, 1912, after he was shot in the chest during an assassination attempt in Milwaukee. *(Reprinted with permission from the American College of Surgeons, Chicago, IL.)*

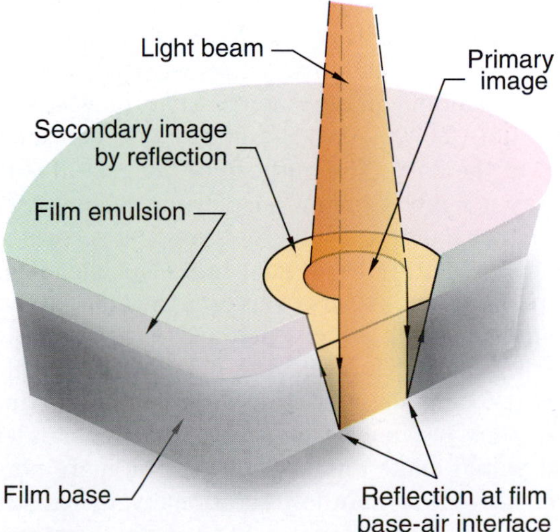

FIGURE 19-3. The halation effect. *(Reprinted with permission of David Jenkins from Radiographic Photography and Imaging Processes, MTP Press, Lancaster, England.)*

transmitted through the film for viewing. Antihalation layers contribute to patient dose and are often used only in extremity systems.

If a single-emulsion film is loaded into a cassette with the antihalation coating toward the intensifying screen (the source of the light photons), most of the light will be absorbed. **Single-emulsion film must be loaded with the emulsion toward the intensifying screen.** The emulsion side of the film always appears dull, the nonemulsion side shiny. In addition, single-emulsion films have an identifying notch cut in the lower left corner. The mnemonic double L (LL) for the lower-left corner makes this easy to remember.

Adhesive

A thin coating of adhesive is applied to the base material before it is coated with the emulsion. This substratum coating is designed to glue the emulsion to the base and prevent bubbles or other distortion when the film is bent during processing or handling, or when it is wet and heated during development.

Emulsion

The emulsion is composed of gelatin in which photosensitive silver halide crystals are suspended. It is spread in an extremely even coating that, depending on the manufacturer, ranges from 5–10 μm (0.0002″–0.0004″) of thickness on each side of the base. The purpose of the gelatin is to act as a neutral lucent suspension medium for the silver halide crystals that must be separated from one another to permit processing chemicals to reach them. Gelatin serves as a nonreactive medium through which chemicals can diffuse to reach the silver halides. The gelatin also distributes the crystals evenly over the surface of the film, thus preventing clumping of silver halides that would make one area of the film more photosensitive than another. Additionally, the gelatin must be clear, to permit light to travel through it uniformly, and flexible enough to permit bending without distorting the recorded image. The gelatin that is used for film is of extremely high quality.

The photosensitive agents suspended in the emulsion are silver halide crystals (or grains). The silver halides used in radiographic film are **silver bromide**, **silver iodide**, and **silver chloride**. Although the exact formula of each company is a closely guarded trade secret, film manufacturers agree that modern silver halides are 95–98 percent silver bromide, with the remainder usually consisting of silver iodide. This has led to the term **silver iodobromide** as a generic specification of the silver halide crystals.

Because photographic film normally has emulsion on a single side, diagnostic radiographic film is sometimes called **duplitized**, double-emulsion, or double-coated film. Not all radiographic film is duplitized, though. There are special radiographic films (such as duplication, mammography, and fine-detail extremity films) that are coated on a single side.

Supercoat

The supercoat is a layer of hard, protective gelatin designed to prevent the soft emulsion underneath from being physically or chemically abused by scratches, abrasions from stacking, and skin oils from handling. It is usually designed to be antistatic as well. The supercoat is extremely strong and, when combined with the tough base material, makes it nearly impossible to tear a radiograph.

The only items routinely used during film handling that are capable of permanently damaging the surface of a radiograph are a paper clip and a staple. To avoid this problem, a properly designed radiograph envelope has a separate compartment for the consultation report.

Manufacturing

Radiographic film is manufactured in four stages: **crystal production**, **ripening**, **mixing**, and **coating**.

Crystal Production. Silver bromide crystal production is accomplished, in total darkness, by combining silver nitrate and potassium bromide in the presence of gelatin. The silver bromide will precipitate out and the potassium nitrate can be washed away as a waste product. The gelatin must be present as a medium to permit the crystals to form. The gelatin functions to limit oxidation and reduce crystal surface energy tension, as well as to facilitate other chemical reactions. This process is described by the formula:

$AgNO_3$ + KBr		→ AgBR ↓ + KNO_3	
silver +	potassium →	silver +	potassium
nitrate	bromide	bromide	nitrate
		(precipitate)	

The silver halide crystals are flat and roughly triangular in shape. Although different types of film emulsions require different size crystals, they are all very small, about 1 μm (0.00004″) on each side. A cubic millimeter contains over half a billion (>500,000,000) crystals.

Each crystal is a cubic lattice (or matrix) of silver, bromide, and iodine atoms (Figure 19-4). A conventional crystal contains approximately 10^{10} (10,000,000,000) atoms. They are bound together by moderately strong ionic bonds with the silver positive (Ag^+) and the bromine or iodine negative (Br^- or I^-). The crystal structure permits both free silver atoms and free electrons to drift through the lattice. This ability is the key to the formation of the latent image.

It is thought that the halide ions (bromine and iodine) tend to cluster on or near the surface of the crystal while the silver ions form the center. This results in silver halide crystals having negatively charged surfaces and positively charged interiors.

The silver halide crystals must have an impurity added, usually gold-silver sulfide, to form **sensitivity specks**. The gold-silver sulfide may adhere to the surface of the crystal or even be partially incorporated into its structure. There can be a few or many specks, but they must be present to provide film sensitivity. During latent image formation the sensitivity specks serve as electrodes to attract the free silver ions. During development, the bromide concentrations will serve as ion pumps to assist in the deposition of silver, thus amplifying the image.

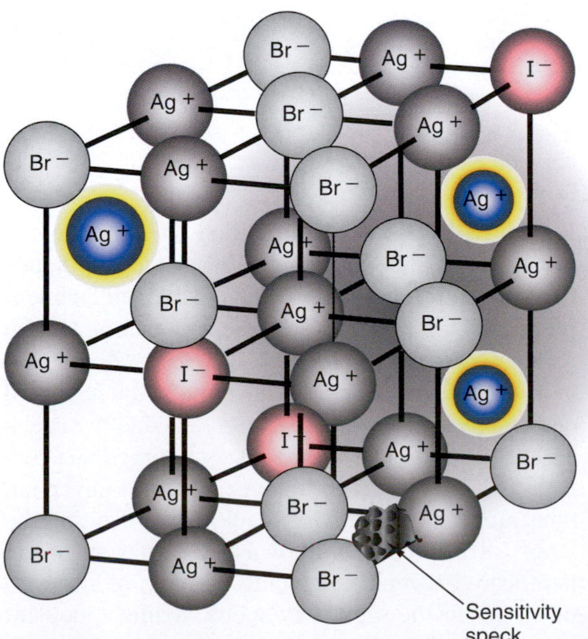

FIGURE 19-4. Cubic lattice arrangement of ions in a silver halide crystal. The surfaces are primarily negative bromine and iodine halides, whereas the interior is primarily positive silver. Note the free silver atoms and the sensitivity speck.

Ripening. Ripening is the period during which silver halides are allowed to grow. The size of the crystals determines their total photosensitivity, so the longer the ripening period, the larger the crystals (or grains) and the more sensitive the emulsion. The relationship of crystal size and emulsion thickness to various film factors is shown in Table 19-1. At the proper time, the emulsion is cooled, shredded, and washed to remove the potassium nitrate.

Mixing. The mixing process follows ripening. The shredded emulsion is melted at a precise temperature to properly sensitize the crystals. Numerous additives are then mixed into the emulsion. Usually included among these are:

colored dyes that improve the sensitivity of the silver halides to match the wavelengths of

TABLE 19-1. Relationship of Film Crystal and Emulsion to Film Factors

	Crystal Size		Emulsion Layer	
	Small	Large	Thin	Thick
Resolution	high	low	high	low
Speed	slow	fast	slow	fast

photons that will be striking the emulsion during exposure,

hardeners to prevent physical trauma,

bactericides and fungicides to inhibit the growth of these organisms (especially in warmer climates or where water supplies are not chemically treated), and

antifogging agents to decrease sensitivity to environmental factors, such as heat.

Films are often classified as **panchromatic** or **orthochromatic**, according to their sensitivity to the color of light. Panchromatic films are sensitive to all colors, whereas orthochromatic films are not sensitive to the red spectrum. This sensitivity is controlled by the dyes that are added during this stage.

Coating. The coating process requires extremely precise and expensive coating equipment. First, the adhesive layer is applied to the base, then the emulsion, and, finally, the supercoat. The emulsion is applied to 40-inch-wide (102-cm) sheets of film, which are stored on rolls, cut to size, and packaged for the consumer. Standard film sizes are shown in Table 19-2. All film manufacturing, packaging, transport, exposure, and processing must be accomplished in total darkness.

TABLE 19-2. Standard Radiographic Film Sizes

SI	U.S. Customary
35 × 91 cm	14 × 36 inches
40 × 40 cm	
35 × 43 cm	**14 × 17 inches**
35 × 35 cm	14 × 14 inches
30 × 40 cm	
30 × 35 cm	
28 × 35 cm	11 × 14 inches
25 × 30 cm	**10 × 12 inches**
24 × 30 cm	
24 × 24 cm	9.5 × 9.5 inches
20 × 40 cm	
20 × 25 cm	**8 × 10 inches**
18 × 24 cm	
18 × 43 cm	7 × 17 inches
	5 × 12 inches
15 × 30 cm	6 × 12 inches
	6.5 × 8.5 inches

Bold sizes are in routine use at most institutions.

NOTE: In most cases the metric and English sizes are not equivalent; they are similar but not exactly interchangeable.

LATENT IMAGE FORMATION

The photons that reach the emulsion are primarily light photons from the intensifying screens that are in contact with the film. However, x-ray photons are also involved in the production of the image. This deposits energy from the photon within the lattice of the silver halide crystals.

The latent image is the unseen change in the atomic structure of the crystal lattice that results in the production of a visible image. Although there is still much that is unknown about the exact mechanisms that control the formation of the latent image, the theory proposed by Gurney and Mott in 1938 remains almost unchallenged. Their theory accounts for sensitivity specks being essential to the image formation process.

The arrangement of the silver and halide ions, free silver ions, and sensitivity specks (see Figure 19-4) has been simplified to illustrate the Gurney-Mott theory (Figure 19-5) of latent image formation. The process begins when an incident photon (light or x-ray) interacts with one of the halides (bromine or iodine). The ejected electron is freed to wander and may eventually be attracted and trapped by a sensitivity speck, giving the speck a negative charge. The negatively charged sensitivity speck attracts a free silver ion. The silver ion neutralizes the sensitivity speck (thus resetting the "trap"). This process is known as the ionic stage and is repeated several times until a clump of silver atoms rests at the sensitivity speck. A single incident photon may free thousands of electrons for deposition at sensitivity specks. However, not all freed silver is deposited at sensitivity specks. At least three silver atoms must be deposited for a visible clump of black metallic silver to be formed by chemical development of the image.

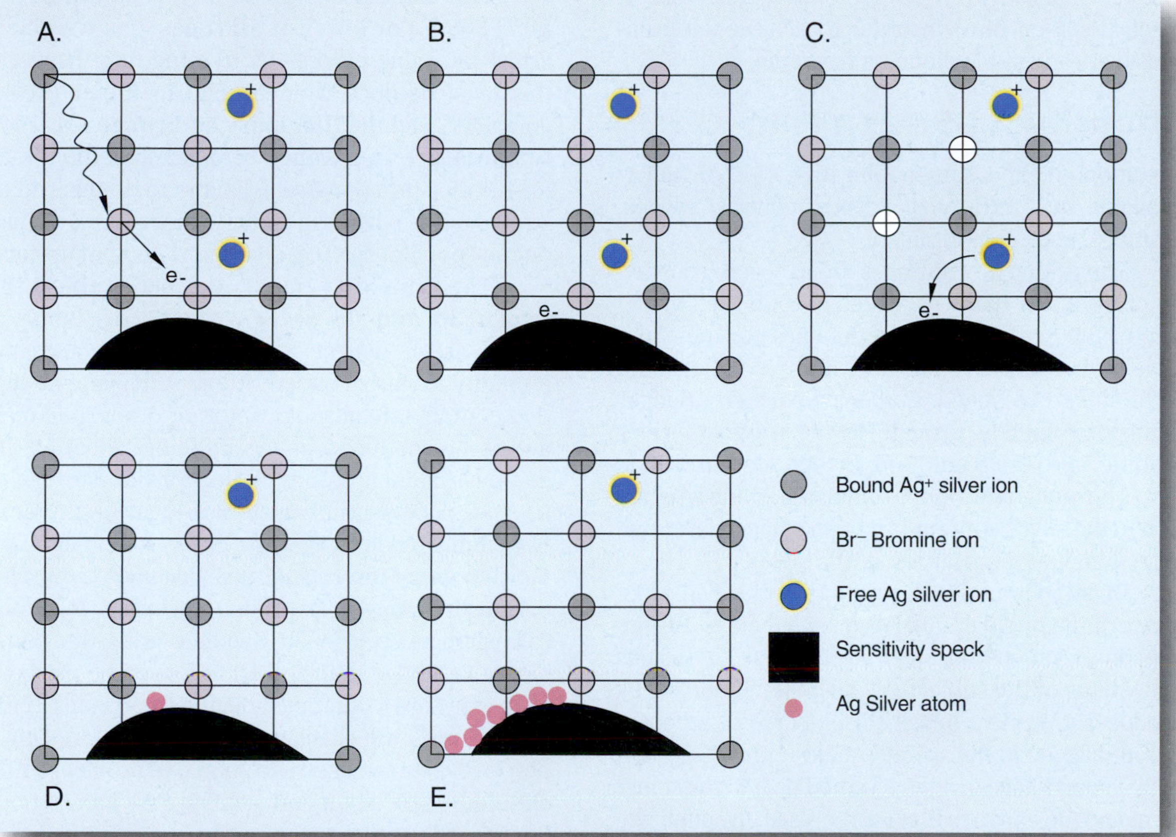

FIGURE 19-5. Latent image formation according to the Gurney-Mott theory.

A–A bromine ion absorbs an incident light photon and frees an electron.
B–The freed electron is trapped at the sensitivity speck, giving it a negative charge.
C–The negatively charged sensitivity speck attracts a free silver ion.
D–The silver ion neutralizes at the sensitivity speck.
E–Repetition of the process deposits several silver atoms at the sensitivity speck.

TYPES OF FILM

The first radiographs were exposed to x-ray photons only. Once the technology had been developed to use the x-rays to produce light at the intensifying screen, the dose reduction resulted in intensifying-screen film (usually called screen film) becoming predominant in medical radiography. In addition, numerous special application films were developed, such as mammography, detail-extremity, laser-exposed, duplication, and fluoroscopic films.

Direct Exposure or Nonscreen Film

Although used primarily for industrial nondestructive testing (NDT) radiography, occasionally its use was justified for patients when extremely fine detail was critical to the diagnostic quality of the image. Because of the extremely high radiation exposure that results from the use of nonscreen film, this was unusual. Direct exposure film has a single emulsion, extremely fine-grain silver halide crystals, and a much greater silver content. It also requires a much thicker emulsion layer (two or three times that of medical screen film) in order to achieve sufficient sensitivity and still maintain a fine grain.

Intensifying-Screen Film

Commonly called screen film, this type of film is available in a variety of speeds, contrast ranges, latitudes, and resolutions.

The primary differences are in speed (sensitivity of the silver halides), which is controlled by the size of the crystals and the thickness of the emulsion layer. Contrast, latitude, and resolution tend to be linked to speed. Larger crystals and thicker emulsions usually provide lower contrast, wider latitude, and less resolution. Screen films are made faster through their double emulsion, while a reduction in the silver content has been achieved through more efficient distribution of the silver.

Duplication film is designed to provide an exact image of the original film. Diagnostic radiographs are actually negatives because they reverse the blacks and whites of the subject (white-bone). Fluoroscopy produces a positive image (black-bone). If an unexposed diagnostic film is laid under a processed film with a good image, a light is turned on for a brief moment and the exposed film is processed, the duplicate film will have densities opposite from the original (i.e., the white-bone image will be converted to black-bone). Duplicating film is pre-exposed to permit it to duplicate the original image (i.e., a white-bone image is recorded as a white-bone image). It is sensitive to the ultraviolet light used in duplicating machines.

FILM STORAGE AND HANDLING

Proper storage and handling of film is an important part of radiography if film is part of the operation.

Basic Storage and Handling

Attention must be given to the **age** of the film, heat, **humidity, light**, radiation, and **handling**. All film is sold with an expiration date stamped on the box. Photosensitive materials are constantly absorbing photons of both heat and background radiation and, over time, this exposure can reach a level where the fog on the film interferes with image quality. Rotation of new stock must be established to observe expiration dates.

Film should be stored at a temperature of 20°C (68°F) or lower at all times. It is possible to arrest the aging process by freezing film. However, this must be done with the film in vacuum-sealed containers and the **film must be brought to room temperature in advance of use** and before breaking the moisture-proof seal. Failure to do this will destroy the film when atmospheric moisture condenses on the cool film surface, creating waterspot artifacts.

The humidity must be maintained between 30 and 60 percent. Static discharge artifacts are a danger at low humidity, and high humidity causes condensation. A basement area that contains steam, cold water, or other fluid pipes and is not included in the building's heating and cooling system is a poor choice for film storage.

All photosensitive materials must be protected from unfiltered light. Because film is sold in light- and moisture-proof packaging, this becomes a problem only with damaged or opened packages. Darkroom safelighting permits film handling with the convenience of limited visibility. All film must be protected from exposure to ionizing radiation. Lead lining of film storage areas will eliminate this problem. Handling of film is often overlooked as a source of problems. **Film should be stored on end,** not flat. Film boxes should be opened carefully, and under no circumstances should a film, paper interleaf, or cardboard insert be removed quickly. Abrasion artifacts can occur from quick movement over film and under pressure. Even at the proper humidity, quick movement can cause static discharge with artifact exposure from the resulting light (see Figure 3-5). Chemical fumes can also cause film fog. Film should not be stored near cleaning solutions, formaldehyde, or other strong chemicals.

Automatic film handling systems involve a transport mechanism that feeds a single film from a storage unit, transports it into position for exposure between a pair of intensifying screens, and then transports it into a processor after exposure.

FILM IDENTIFICATION

All radiographs should be permanently identified with medical record information. This includes the date of the exposure, the full name of the patient, the institution where the exposure was made, the referring physician, the patient identification number, and any other important information. The identification information is usually added to the film by a light exposure after the radiographic exposure and can be accomplished with a special daylight identification camera and cassette system. It can also be done in the darkroom after the film has been removed from the cassette but before it is processed. Most radiographic cassettes have a lead blocker space in one corner to prevent the film from being exposed to x-rays in that small area. This reserves the space for identification information to be "flashed" by light. This information, like the radiograph, becomes part of the legal medical record and should be treated as such. Additionally, a method of identifying right and left sides of the patient should be required. Many institutions use lead markers, although film punches and blocker placement systems can also be used. The radiographer performing the examination is usually identified through some means, such as initials or number on a lead marker and signature on accompanying paperwork.

Depending on institutional policy, it may or may not be acceptable to change the identification information if it is recorded incorrectly. Some institutions permit changes to be made with wax pencil, stickers, or punches, whereas others require that the radiograph be repeated. The radiographer is nearly always held responsible for recording the identification information correctly.

SUMMARY

Photographic materials are photosensitive, or capable of responding to exposure by photons. Diagnostic radiographic film is duplitized; in other words, the base is coated on both sides with an adhesive, an emulsion with crystals, and a supercoat.

The film base is polyester, the adhesive glues the emulsion to the base to prevent distortion during processing or handling, the emulsion is gelatin in which photosensitive silver halide crystals are suspended, and the supercoat is a protective layer. An antihalation coating is used to decrease light reflections within the base itself.

Radiographic film is manufactured in four stages: crystal production, ripening, mixing, and coating. The silver halides used are silver bromide, silver iodide, and silver chloride. The term *silver iodobromide* best describes the silver halides used in radiographic film. They are produced in total darkness by combining silver nitrate and potassium bromide in the presence of gelatin. The silver halide crystals that are produced are flat and roughly triangular in shape. Each crystal is a cubic lattice of silver, bromide, and iodine atoms with sensitivity specks. Ripening time determines crystal size and sensitivity. During mixing, additives are included in the emulsion. Panchromatic films are sensitive to all colors, whereas orthochromatic films are not sensitive to red. Coating is the final stage before the film is cut and packaged.

The latent image is the unseen change in the atomic structure of the crystal lattice that results in the production of a visible image. At least three silver atoms must be deposited to form a visible clump of black metallic silver.

Direct exposure or nonscreen film can be used when extremely fine detail is critical, although the extremely high radiation exposure requires a careful justification. Intensifying-screen film is the most common radiographic film. Films vary in speed, contrast, latitude, and resolution.

Duplication produces a nearly exact copy of a radiographic image.

Care must be taken in storing and handling film because it is affected by age, heat, humidity, light, radiation, and handling. Some of the handling is avoided by automated systems. All radiographs should be permanently identified with the appropriate medical record information. ■

REVIEW QUESTIONS

1. What are the primary components of radiographic film?
2. Explain the production of silver halide crystals.
3. What is the purpose of various additives to radiographic film?
4. How is the latent image produced?
5. Describe common problems due to improper film storage and handling.
6. What are the radiographer's responsibilities concerning proper radiograph identification?

REFERENCES AND RECOMMENDED READING

Curry, T. S., Dowdey, J. E., & Murry, R. C. (1990). *Christensen's introduction to the physics of diagnostic radiology* (4th ed.). Philadelphia: Lea and Febiger.

Daniels, C., & Halloway, A. F. (1983, January). Comparison and variations of the speed of radiographic film. *Radiology*, 203.

Doi, K. (1981, June). Effect of crossover exposure on radiographic image quality of screen-film systems. *Radiology*, 707.

Frantzell, A. (1950). The practical roentgenographic importance of reciprocity law failure. *Acta Radiologica, 34*, 6–16.

Fuchs, A. (1956). Evolution of Roentgen film. *American Journal of Roentgenology*, 75, 30–48.

Jenkins, D., & Latham, S. M. (1979). The duplication of chest radiographs. *Radiography, 45*(539), 244–248.

Kim, O., Ahn, M., & Bahk, Y. (1992). Use of film duplicator to lighten dark radiographs. *Radiology, 184*(2), 573.

Kofler, J., & Gray, J. (1991). Sensitometric responses of selected medical radiographic films. *Radiology, 181*(3), 879–883.

Mathias, J. L., & Marquis, J. R. (1976). Radiographic duplication: A simple method of minimizing radiation dosage to the patient. *Radiologic Technology, 48*(3), 293.

McKinney, W. (1988). *Radiographic processing and quality control.* Philadelphia: J. B. Lippincott.

Mees, C. E. K., & Sheppard, S. E. (2010). *Investigations on the theory of the photographic process.* Nabu Press. Charleston, SC

Morgan, R. H. (1944). Reciprocity law failure in x-ray films. *Radiology, 42*, 471–479.

Morgan, R. H. (1946). An analysis of the physical factors controlling the diagnostic quality of roentgen images: Part IV. Contrast and the film contrast factor. *American Journal of Roentgenology and Radiation Therapy, 55*(5), 627–633.

Newhall, B. (2010). *The history of photography* (5th ed.). New York: The Museum of Modern Art.

Ramsey, L. J. (1978). Notes on x-ray film speeds. *Radiography, 44*(524), 200.

Rao, G. U. V., Witt, W., Beachley, M. C., Bosch, H. A., Fatouros, P. P., & Kan, P. T. (1981). Radiographic films and screen-film systems. In C. M. Coulam, J. J. Erickson, F. D. Rollo, & A. E. James (Eds.), *The physical basis of medical imaging.* New York: Appleton-Century-Crofts.

Sturge, J., Walworth, V., & Shepp, A. (1989). *Imaging processes and materials: Neblette's 8th edition.* New Jersey: Wiley.

Sweeney, R. J. (1983). *Radiographic artifacts: Their cause and control.* Philadelphia: J. B. Lippincott.

Wilson, P. (1976). Principles of formation of the latent and developed images. *Canadian Journal of Radiography, Radiotherapy, and Nuclear Medicine, 7*(6), 268–278.

CHAPTER 20

Film Processing

KEY TERMS

activator
chemical fog
circulation system
clearing agent
clearing time
developing
dryer system
drying
entrance rollers
fixing
hardener
preservative
reducing agent
replenishment system
restrainer
solvent
superadditivity
temperature control system
transport system
washing

At first it seems to be

a smeared

print: blurred lines and grey flecks

blended with the paper

Excerpt from "This Is a Photograph of Me," from selected poems, 1965–1975, by Margaret Atwood.

OBJECTIVES

Upon completion of this chapter, the student should be able to:

- Explain the process of film developing and fixing.
- Describe the synergistic properties of automatic processor reducing agents.
- Identify the primary chemical and its function for each of the developer and fixer agents.
- Explain the washing and drying processes of film archiving.
- Describe the functions of the subsystems of an automatic processor.
- Discuss the basic function of a radiographic darkroom and the safelights.
- Explain the rationale for the use of silver recovery systems.

The primary purpose of radiographic processing is to deposit enough black metallic silver at the latent image sites in film to permit a permanent visible image to form. The development of the latent image can be accomplished manually or with automatic processing equipment. Due to the predominance of digital imaging with electronic transmission of images, very little wet chemical processing of images occurs in most developed nations. Radiographers can apply their knowledge of both manual and automatic processing with the modifications provided by the manufacturer's information inserts that are packed with the chemicals.

Quality control experts agree that film processing is the most sensitive and variable factor in the production of a radiograph. The radiographer is responsible for monitoring the performance of the processor, troubleshooting problems, and repairing minor malfunctions.

Processing of a radiograph involves four primary steps: **developing**, **fixing**, and two archiving steps—**washing** and **drying**. Developing and fixing are accomplished in solutions that combine numerous chemicals. Archiving involves a two-step process of washing and drying the radiograph for use as a medical record.

DEVELOPING

Developing is the first step in wet processing a film. At this stage silver is deposited at the latent image sites and an image becomes visible. The deposition of silver amplifies the density of the image. X-ray developers are capable of amplifying the image by a factor of 10^8–10^9 within 3 to 4.5 minutes. The silver ions of the latent image are stabilized and more silver is added to the site until a visible silver clump is formed. The primary agents of the developer are two **reducing agents**, although automatic radiographic developer solutions also include an **activator**, **restrainer**, **preservative**, **hardener**, and water as a **solvent** (Table 20-1). The action of the developer is controlled by the immersion time, solution temperature, and chemical activity.

Reducing Agents

Reducing agents provide electrons to the silver ions attached to the sensitivity specks of the silver halide crystals (the latent image). Silver halides have negative exteriors (where bromine and iodine ions are located) and positive interiors (where silver ions are located). This arrangement effectively prohibits the reducing agent from supplying electrons to the silver ions because the bromine and iodine repel electrons. However, when a sensitivity speck has attracted silver ions, a gate exists through which the interior of the crystal can be supplied with electrons. When a silver ion obtains an extra electron, it is converted to a stable black metallic silver atom. Reduction is actually the process of the reducing agents giving up electrons to neutralize the positive silver ions. This reduction process is illustrated in Figure 20-1.

The secret to the production of the various densities is that the sensitivity speck gate will be larger when more silver ions are deposited at the speck during exposure. A larger gate permits faster reduction of the internal silver atoms. When the reduction process is stopped at the appropriate time, the silver halides have accumulated black metallic silver in proportion to the size of the sensitivity speck gate. This produces a film with varying degrees of blackness. Of course, all silver halides with gates will become totally reduced, and the entire film will appear black if the reducing agents are permitted to work for too long a time, if they work too fast due to high temperature, or if the solution has too high a concentration. The term **chemical fog** is used to describe development when these factors cause unexposed silver halides to be reduced.

Those silver halide crystals that have fewer than three silver atoms on their sensitivity specks are unable to open a gate and remain unreduced (undeveloped). Each reduced silver atom is accompanied by a liberated bromine ion with a negative charge. A bromide ion barrier is created when too many liberated bromine ions are permitted to accumulate. They may produce sufficient charge to repel reducing agents and effectively stop silver halide development. This is the same effect that is achieved by using potassium bromide as a "starter" solution to slow down the hyperactivity of newly mixed developer

TABLE 20-1. Automatic Radiographic Processing Chemicals and Their Functions

Solution	Time in 90-Second Processor	Chemical	Function
Developer	20–25 sec		reduces latent image to visible black metallic silver
reducing agent		phenidone	rapidly produces fine detail shades of gray
reducing agent		hydroquinone	slowly produces heavy densities
activator		sodium carbonate	produces alkaline pH, swells gelatin
restrainer		potassium bromide	decreases reducing agent activity, antifogging agent
preservative		sodium sulfite	controls oxidation, buffer agent
hardener		glutaraldehyde	hardens emulsion, reduces gelatin swelling
solvent		water	dissolves chemicals
Fixer	20 sec		stops reduction and removes undeveloped silver halides from emulsion
clearing agent		ammonium thiosulfate	removes undeveloped silver halides from emulsion
activator		acetic acid	provides acidic pH, stops reduction
hardener		potassium alum	hardens emulsion
preservative		sodium sulfite	maintains pH
solvent		water	dissolves chemicals
Wash	20 sec		removes developing and fixing chemicals
solvent		water	removes excess chemicals
Dry	25–30 sec		removes water and seals emulsion
		hot air	evaporates water and hardens emulsion

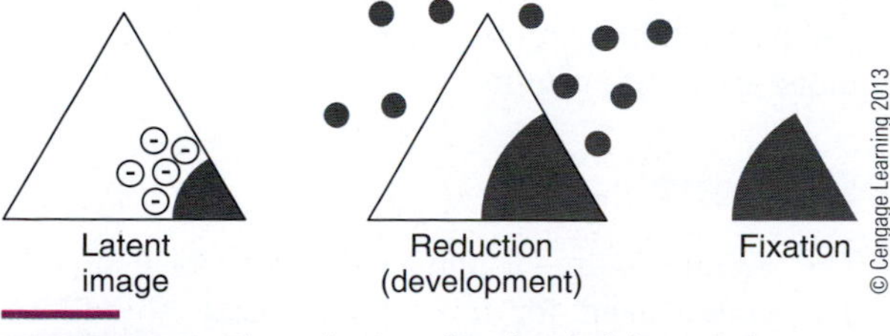

FIGURE 20-1. The reduction of a silver halide crystal through a sensitivity speck gate.

replenisher solutions. The problem is overcome by replenishment of the developer strength at regular intervals. A freshly cleaned automatic processor may require seasoning by running for 20 to 30 minutes to thoroughly mix the starter solution.

The reducing agents used in automatic radiographic processors are phenidone (known as P developer) and hydroquinone (known as Q developer). **Phenidone quickly reduces silver, enhancing fine detail and subtle shades of gray, and works only in areas of light exposure**. It cannot reduce heavily exposed areas. Phenidone replaces the function of metol (often known by the Kodak brand name Elon) in manual processing. **Hydroquinone slowly reduces silver and produces heavy density**. Hydroquinone is ineffective at first but then rapidly increases in action. When the two reducing agents are combined, forming a PQ developer, their reducing ability is greater than the sum of their independent abilities. This is a synergistic phenomenon known as **superadditivity** (Figure 20-2). As can be seen from the graph, phenidone controls the lower part of the curve (the toe), and hydroquinone controls the upper portion (the shoulder).

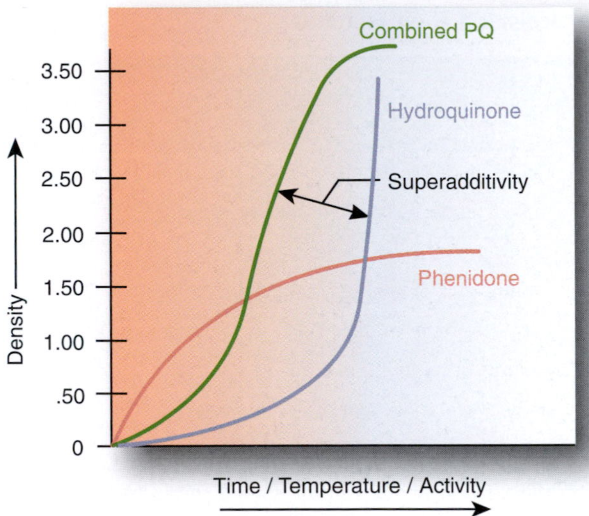

FIGURE 20-2. The superadditivity or synergistic effect of phenidone and hydroquinone combined, as compared to their independent reducing abilities.

Oxidation and reduction are opposite processes. When the reducing agent is oxidized, it gives up electrons. Reduction occurs when a silver halide crystal takes one of the electrons and is changed to black metallic silver. The oxidation/reduction process reduces the strength of the developer solution. As developer oxidizes, it changes color, first to a deep amber, then to brown, and, finally, to a thick, rust red.

Activator

The action of the reducing agents is enhanced by maintaining the developer solution in an alkaline state (around pH 10.0–10.5) by using an activator, usually sodium carbonate. Potassium carbonate, sodium hydroxide, and potassium hydroxide may also be used. The activator also assists the reducers in reaching the silver halides by causing the gelatin to swell and become more permeable. The activator is caustic, and therefore rubber gloves and an apron should be worn when handling developer solutions. Developer solution that is splashed onto clothing and walls is corrosive and should be neutralized with fixer solution or diluted with water.

Restrainer

A restrainer, usually potassium bromide, is also added to the developer to restrict the reducing action to those crystals with sensitivity speck gates. It does this by permitting overactive reducers to attack it, instead of unexposed silver halides.

Preservative

Sodium sulfite is used as a preservative agent to help decrease the oxidation of the reducing agents when they are combined with air. The attraction of air for the reducers is so strong that developer solutions remain effective for only a few weeks after mixing.

Hardener

Glutaraldehyde is the most common developer solution hardener. It controls the swelling of the gelatin to prevent scratches and abrasions to the emulsion during processing. It also maintains uniform film thickness to assist in transport through an automatic processor. Insufficient hardener will cause films to deposit gelatin on processor rollers, which may cause transport and artifact problems for subsequent films. Insufficient hardener may also cause films to exit the processor with moist, softened surfaces. Hot-air drying alone cannot seal the emulsion. Excessive hardener may cause the emulsion to harden prematurely, preventing chemical interactions with the silver halides and trapping moisture in the gelatin.

Solvent

The chemicals are suspended in water as a solvent. The water used for mixing chemistry should be filtered to remove impurities (a 5–10 μm filter is recommended). In tropical climates, it should be treated to eliminate bacteria and fungus that may find the gelatin emulsion an attractive meal.

Contamination

The developer is the only solution that is dramatically affected by contamination. Only 0.1 percent fixer in a developer tank will destroy the ability of the reducing agents (10 ml in a 2.5 gallon [10 liter] tank). Films processed in contaminated developer appear extremely gray (they exhibit extremely low contrast). Because the fixer tank is usually adjacent to the developer, it is easy for splashing to occur. The most common cause of contamination is splashing, which occurs during lifting or when replacing the fixer transport rack. Special splash guards are supplied with automatic processors, and they should always be used. Developer contamination requires total dumping, washing, refilling, and seasoning of the developer tank. When cleaning a processor, the fixer tank should always be filled first. If splashing occurs, it is a simple matter to reclean the developer tank before it is filled.

Evaporation of solutions can also cause contamination. Due to the heat necessary for processing, solutions evaporate and condense on the processor lid. Contamination can occur if fixer condensation drips into the developer tank. Individual evaporation covers for both developer and fixer tanks should be in place at all times. When a processor is shut down, excessive condensation can occur as it cools. To prevent contamination, the processor lid should be propped open whenever the processor is not in use. Splashing or evaporation of developer into the fixer tank does not cause contamination. Developer is regularly carried into the fixer by the films being processed.

FIXING

If a film is exposed to light after development, the unreduced silver halides will open gates and be converted to black metallic silver. This is seen as a slow blackening of the film, which obscures the image. Undeveloped silver halides must be removed from the emulsion to permanently fix the image before exposure to light for viewing. (This was the last reaction to be discovered and delayed development of the photographic process by nearly 25 years.) This important step is accomplished by using a clearing agent that bonds with the unexposed silver halides and removes them from the emulsion. The primary agent of the fixer is the **clearing agent**, although automatic radiographic fixer solutions also include an activator, preservative, hardener, and water as a solvent (see Table 20-1).

Clearing Agent

Nearly all fixer solutions use ammonium thiosulfate as the clearing (fixing) agent (also known by the term "hypo"). Ammonium thiosulfate uses silver in the emulsion to form ammonium thiosilversulfate. Within 5–10 seconds after the clearing agent has begun to function, the film can be exposed to full room light for inspection without damage to the image. If the fixer has not completely cleared the film of unexposed silver halides, the film will have a milky appearance. The **clearing time** is defined as twice the time necessary for the milky appearance to disappear. In a 90-second automatic processor, the clearing time is usually 15–20 seconds, whereas manual processing may take 2–3 minutes.

Activator

Acetic acid is used as the activator in the fixer. It maintains an acidic pH (4.0–4.5) to enhance the functioning of the clearing agent. It also serves as a stop bath to keep the reducing agents from continuing to function when the film is immersed in the fixer. Recall that reducing agents function in an alkaline solution. An acidic solution will neutralize and thereby stop the alkaline developing solution from continuing its reduction of the silver halides.

Preservative

The fixer uses the same preservative as the developer—sodium sulfite. It dissolves silver from the ammonium thiosilversulfate, thus permitting it to continue to remove silver from the emulsion.

Hardener

The hardener in the fixer must function in an acidic environment. Glutaraldehyde is effective only in an alkaline solution, so fixer hardeners are aluminum chloride, chromium alum, or potassium alum. The hardener serves the same purpose as glutaraldehyde in the developer—prevention of scratches and abrasions to the emulsion during processing and maintenance of a uniform thickness of the film during transport. Insufficient hardener will cause films to exit the processor with moist, softened surfaces.

Solvent

Water (which should be filtered and treated) is used as the solvent.

Depletion

After a time, the fixer solution will become saturated with silver ions from the emulsion. The solution slowly becomes unable to accept additional silver and requires a longer clearing time. Automatic processors constantly replenish the fixer solution to eliminate this problem. The silver ions in the fixer can be reclaimed through various silver recovery processes.

ARCHIVING

The archiving process is composed of two steps: washing and drying. Archiving prepares the film for long-term storage as a medical record by protecting it from deterioration by chemicals, fading, and physical forces.

Washing

The washing process uses water to remove as much of the fixer and developer solutions as possible. The water temperature should be slightly lower than the temperature of the other solutions (about 5°F or 3°C lower) because some processors use the water to help control temperature fluctuations in the developer and fixer. The emulsion may reticulate (crack into many pieces) if the temperature is changed too dramatically.

Both fixer and developer solutions contain chemicals that, even in weak concentrations, can damage the image over time. Because most of the developer action is stopped by the acidic pH of the fixer, the main concern is removing the fixer from the emulsion. Failure to provide sufficient agitation or wash time to clear fixer from the film may result in silver stains or a yellowing of the emulsion after a few years.

Warm water will increase the efficiency of the wash. Wash tanks, especially those not made of stainless steel, are susceptible to algae and bacteria growth during periods when the processor is turned off. To eliminate this problem, the wash tank should be drained whenever the processor is shut down.

Drying

Drying is done by forcing hot air over both sides of the film as it begins its exit from the processor. The air temperature ranges from 120–150°F (43–65°C). The hot air sets a final hardening to the emulsion and seals the supercoat. Table 20-1 illustrates all of the automatic processing steps, the processing times, and the functions of the component chemicals.

Storage

Proper storage is a critical part of the archiving process. The length of time an original radiograph is stored is usually 5–7 years, depending on institutional policies and applicable laws. Films taken of minors and cases involved in litigation may be retained much longer (sometimes permanently). Processed radiographs should be stored at about 70°F (23°C) and 60 percent humidity.

AUTOMATIC PROCESSING

Radiographic films were manually processed from the discovery of radiography until Eastman Kodak introduced the first continuous roller automatic processor in 1957. This unit processed a film in 15 minutes and was so large that an overhead winch was required to lift the racks of rollers from the chemical tanks for cleaning. It was a great improvement over manual processing, which required an hour to process and dry a film, and often produced erratic results.

Automatic processors are complex and utilize several subsystems to completely process a radiograph: the **transport system**, **dryer system**, **replenishment system**, **circulation system**, and **temperature control system**.

Transport System

The transport system is designed to move a film through the developer, fixer, wash, and dryer sections of the processor. As it does this, it controls the length of time the radiograph is immersed in each of the solutions and agitates the chemistry to ensure maximum reaction

In most automatic processors, the **entrance rollers** also open a microswitch or laser scanning system that activates the replenishment system.

Dryer System

The final stage of processing is drying the film with the dryer system. The emulsion of a wet film is sticky and may adhere permanently if brought into contact with another film. The dryer system begins with a series of squeegee crossover rollers removing excess wash water from the surface of the film. The film is then driven between a double row of slotted, hot-forced-air tubes. A high-speed fan draws room air past electric heating coils, producing air at 120–150°F (50–65°C). The film emulsion shrinks and seals dry in a single pass and the film is ready for viewing and storing when it exits the processor. The excess air is returned to the room. This is the primary cause for uncomfortable temperatures in processing areas during hot weather. When damp films exit the processor, the cause is more likely to be in the fixer (depletion or lack of hardener) or wash tank (saturation or insufficient fresh water) than in the dryer section.

Replenishment System

The replenishment system replaces chemicals that are depleted through the chemical reactions of processing, oxidation, and evaporation. The developer replenisher solution has a different composition than the solution in the processing tank. Because bromides build up in functioning developer, they tend to restrain the activity of the reducing agents on the silver halides. For this reason, developer replenisher lacks sufficient restrainer. A special starter solution of acetic acid and potassium bromide (the restrainer) must be added to the replenisher solution when starting a fresh tank of developer. Potassium bromide is needed to develop films properly. Potassium bromide gets into the developer solution from the bromide in the emulsion of the film. However, when new developer is mixed and put into the developer tank, no bromide is present because no films have been processed. This is why starter solution needs to be added to fresh developer chemistry. If starter solution is not added to the fresh developer, images will be dark and the sensitometry will be out of control. The tank of fresh solution must then be seasoned by running the processor for 15 to 20 minutes to permit adequate mixing of the solutions.

The replenishment rate can be adjusted so that more fixer is replenished than developer. Although they must be adjusted for specific conditions, procedures, and manufacturersí recommendations, developer replenishment rates often range from 4–5 ml per inch (1.5–2.0 ml per cm) of film feed. This is about 55–70 ml per 14-inch (36-cm) length of film. Fixer rates range from 6–8 ml per inch (2.5–3.0 ml per cm). This is about 85–110 ml per 14-inch (36 cm) length of film. Some processors provide a digital display of this information on the front panel.

All mixing should be done strictly according to the manufacturer's recommendations regarding temperature and the proper sequence of additives (for example, solution A, then B, then C, etc.). Always mix additives to water. Adding water to additives will cause splashing of corrosives and a decrease in solution strength. There are occasions when the chemicals react in undesirable ways with one another, the water, and air. For example, if hardener is added to fixer replenisher too rapidly, it may precipitate sulfur and aluminum, leaving the solution with insufficient hardener.

Processing solutions are hazardous materials and are covered by several federal agencies in the United States. Since 1986 the Occupational Health and Safety Administration (OSHA), the Environmental Protection Agency (EPA), and the Department of Transportation have all implemented regulations affecting processing chemicals. Users of the chemicals are required to have material safety data sheets (MSDSs) on hand, policies regarding handling, a teaching program, and safety equipment, particularly an eyewash station.

Radiographic solutions are not available to the general public in the United States. When developer solution is mixed on-site, the concentrated solution containing hydroquinone and the preservative and activator (usually the first part mixed) has a pH of about 12.0, which is extremely destructive to the eyes if splashed. For this reason, protective eyeglasses should always be worn when mixing solutions. Additionally, hydroquinone can be absorbed through the skin, and glutaraldehyde is a tanning agent that will work on human skin just as it works in leathermaking.

Circulation System

The circulation system is designed to stabilize temperatures, agitate solutions, mix the chemistry, and filter the solutions. Temperatures are maintained in conjunction with the temperature control system. Constant mild agitation of the developer and fixer solutions is required so the chemicals will enter and exit the emulsion. The fresh chemistry added by the replenishment system must be constantly mixed throughout the tanks to avoid overdevelopment, underdevelopment, and underfixation.

The fixer circulation lines are usually fitted with a 100-µm wire mesh filter to trap dirt or bits of gelatin that have been washed from films.

Fixer overflow should be considered toxic and under no circumstances should it be dumped directly into an open drain.

The wash tank uses a constant flow of fresh water, which is pumped in at the bottom ends of the tank and overflows from the top to a drain. Most manufacturers recommend 4 to 8 liters per minute (1–2 gallons [U.S.] per minute). It is environmentally unsound to drain wash tank water into sewer lines. Increasing concern over heavy metal pollution may place liability on persons or institutions responsible for dumping processing chemicals, especially silver. Although expensive, storage of processing overflow and disposal by hazardous materials professionals is advisable.

Temperature Control System

The temperature control system maintains all three solutions at compatible temperatures. A 90-second automatic processor will usually require a developer temperature of 92–96°F (33–35°C), whereas a 2-minute processor will operate at 83–86°F (28–30°C).

The developer temperature is especially critical. A difference is visible with a fluctuation of only 0.5° (F or C). Some processors provide a digital display of this information on the front panel. The optimal reducing agent temperature is 68°F (20°C) for an immersion time of 4–8 minutes. High temperature developers reduce immersion time to 20–22 seconds, thus permitting 90-second or less processing. Specific developing temperatures vary with manufacturer and can be adjusted with an adjustable thermostat, which is part of an automatic processing system.

DARKROOM

The darkroom is the lightproof laboratory used for loading and unloading cassettes and feeding film into the automatic processor. Film is twice as sensitive after exposure and must be handled carefully to avoid trauma to the film surface.

Safelights

Radiographic film is designed to be insensitive to specific wavelengths of orange-red light. This permits the use of low-level illumination within this wavelength to make work in the darkroom easier. The amount of light is controlled by the type of filter, wattage of the light source, and distance from the working surface. Not all films are insensitive to the same wavelengths, and some may require special lighting or no-light conditions.

Direct illumination for most radiographic films is possible with a Kodak GBX filter (dark red) over a low-intensity (7–15-watt) bulb that is 4 feet (1.25 meters) from the working area. Films that are sensitive only to blue emitting phosphor light (blue-violet) may be handled with a Kodak Wratten Series 6B filter (orange-brown) at the same intensity and distance. Light-emitting diode (LED) safelights are also available. They emit light in the 660-nm range. A safelight test calculates how long a film may be handled before fogging becomes a problem. Darkroom walls and floors should be light colored to increase the amount of light in the darkroom. If light is safe at its first reflection, it loses intensity and remains safe on additional reflections. When benches and flooring are light colored, it is much easier to locate films and other objects.

Pass Box

Film cassettes are passed into the darkroom through a pass box, or cassette hatch, which is a lightproof container set in the darkroom wall. Most pass boxes have two sides, one labeled "exposed," the other "unexposed," and both have interlocking lightproof doors. The interlocking doors are designed to prevent both doors from being opened at once, allowing light into the darkroom.

Darkroom ventilation should be a primary concern. Chemical fumes must be vented directly to the outside of the building. Failure to do so can result in toxic fumes being picked up by ventilation systems.

SILVER RECOVERY SYSTEMS

As mentioned in the fixer and circulation system sections, sufficient silver is dissolved in the fixer solution to make recovery before discarding feasible from a financial standpoint and to prevent toxic heavy metal pollution of the environment. In the United States, the Water Control Act of 1972, Resources Conservation-Hazardous Waste Act of 1976, Clean Water Act of 1984, and Resource Conservation and Recovery Act of 1986 all affect the disposal of heavy metals into the public environment. In essence, these laws require that the best available methods be used to clear silver from fixer overflow solutions prior to disposal. In addition, they limit liquid waste to a toxic level of 5 parts per million (ppm). A permit is required for dumping more than 27 gallons (U.S.) per month into a public sewer and any amount into the ground. Even shipping the waste to a treatment plant requires a permit. Compliance with these regulations is the reason commercial firms are usually employed to handle silver recovery.

The fixer may accumulate silver at the rate of as much as 100 mg/m^2 of film processed. This is well above the dumping limits allowed by law in the United States. In fact, **the fixer is as valuable, if not more valuable, after processing than before**.

About half of the silver in the film remains in the emulsion after processing. The other half is dissolved into the fixer solution. Much of this silver may be removed from the fixer by diverting the overflow through a silver recovery system before discarding. It is estimated that about 10 percent of the purchase price of film may be recovered, depending on the type of recovery system used and the market price for silver.

There are several types of silver recovery units, including electrolytic, metallic replacement, chemical precipitation, and resin. All of these units operate by providing electrons that can be used by the silver in the fixer solution to form black metallic silver. They differ in the method by which the electrons are provided and by the process used to refine the metallic silver.

All silver recovery methods require that the fixer sit within the unit for some time to permit the chemical interactions to occur. This dwell time is the single most important factor in unit effectiveness. Agitation of the fixer solution during this time is also important because it enhances the ability of electrons and silver to contact each other.

Electrolytic

Electrolytic units pass a current from a cathode to an anode through the fixer. The ionized silver in the fixer solution is attracted to the negatively charged cathode. It then plates onto the cathode as metallic silver. Electrolytic units should not be run when the processor has not been used for a long period of time (such as overnight).

Film

The film itself retains half the silver (about 0.1 troy ounce per pound [0.45 kg]) and this can also be recovered. Unexposed (green) film has twice the amount of silver as processed film.

SUMMARY

The primary purpose of radiographic processing is to deposit enough black metallic silver at the latent image sites to permit a permanent visible image to form. Quality control experts agree that the radiographic film processor is the most sensitive and variable factor in the production of a radiograph. Processing of a radiograph involves developing, fixing, washing, and drying.

During development, silver is deposited at the latent image sites and an image becomes visible. The primary agents of the developer are the two reducing agents, phenidone and hydroquinone; an activator, sodium carbonate; a restrainer, potassium bromide; a preservative, sodium sulfite; a hardener, glutaraldehyde; and water as the solvent. The action of the developer is controlled by immersion time, solution temperature, and chemical activity.

Fixing removes the undeveloped silver halides from the emulsion. This is necessary before exposure to light for viewing. The primary agent is the clearing agent, ammonium thiosulfate. Fixer solutions also include an activator, acetic acid; a preservative, sodium sulfite; a hardener, aluminum chloride; and water as the solvent.

The archiving process prepares the film for long-term storage as a medical record. Archiving involves washing the film with water to remove the processing chemicals and drying to harden and seal the radiograph.

Automatic processors utilize several subsystems to completely process a radiograph: (1) the transport system, (2) the dryer system, (3) the replenishment system, (4) the circulation system, and (5) the temperature control system.

The darkroom is the lightproof laboratory used for loading and unloading cassettes and feeding them into the automatic processor. Safelights use low-level illumination within this wavelength to make work in the darkroom easier.

Sufficient silver is dissolved into the fixer solution to make recovery before discarding feasible from a financial standpoint and desirable for environmental reasons. ■

REVIEW QUESTIONS

1. What are the four primary steps in wet chemistry film processing?
2. What is the purpose of fixing?
3. What are the two steps of the archiving process?
4. How does an electrolytic silver recovery unit operate?

REFERENCES AND RECOMMENDED READING

Ball, J., & Price, T. (1995). *Chesneys' radiographic imaging* (6th ed.).Oxford: Blackwell Scientific.

Carroll, Q. B. (2003). *Fuchs's radiographic exposure, processing, and quality control* (7th ed.). Springfield, IL: Charles C Thomas.

Curry, T. S., Dowdey, J. E., & Murry, R. C. (1990). *Christensen's introduction to the physics of diagnostic radiology* (4th ed.). Philadelphia: Lea and Febiger.

Dohms, J. (1992). OSHA safety requirements for hazardous chemicals in the workplace. *Radiology Management, 14*(4), 76–80.

Gordon, M. (1988). Chemical hazards in film processing. *International Society of Radiographers and Radiological Technicians Newsletter, 24*(1), 9–12.

Haus, A. G. (Ed.). (1993). *Film processing in medical imaging.*Madison, WI: Medical Physics.

Jenkins, D. (1980). *Radiographic photography and imaging processes.*Lancaster, England: MTP Press Limited.

McKinney, W. (1988). *Radiographic processing and quality control.* Philadelphia: J. B. Lippincott.

Newhall, B. (2010). *The history of photography* (5th ed.). New York: The Museum of Modern Art.

Sturge, J., Walworth, V., & Shepp, A. (1989). *Imaging processes and materials: Neblette's eighth edition.* New Jersey: Wiley.

Wolbarst, A. B. (1993). *Physics of radiology.* Norwalk, CT: Appleton & Lange.

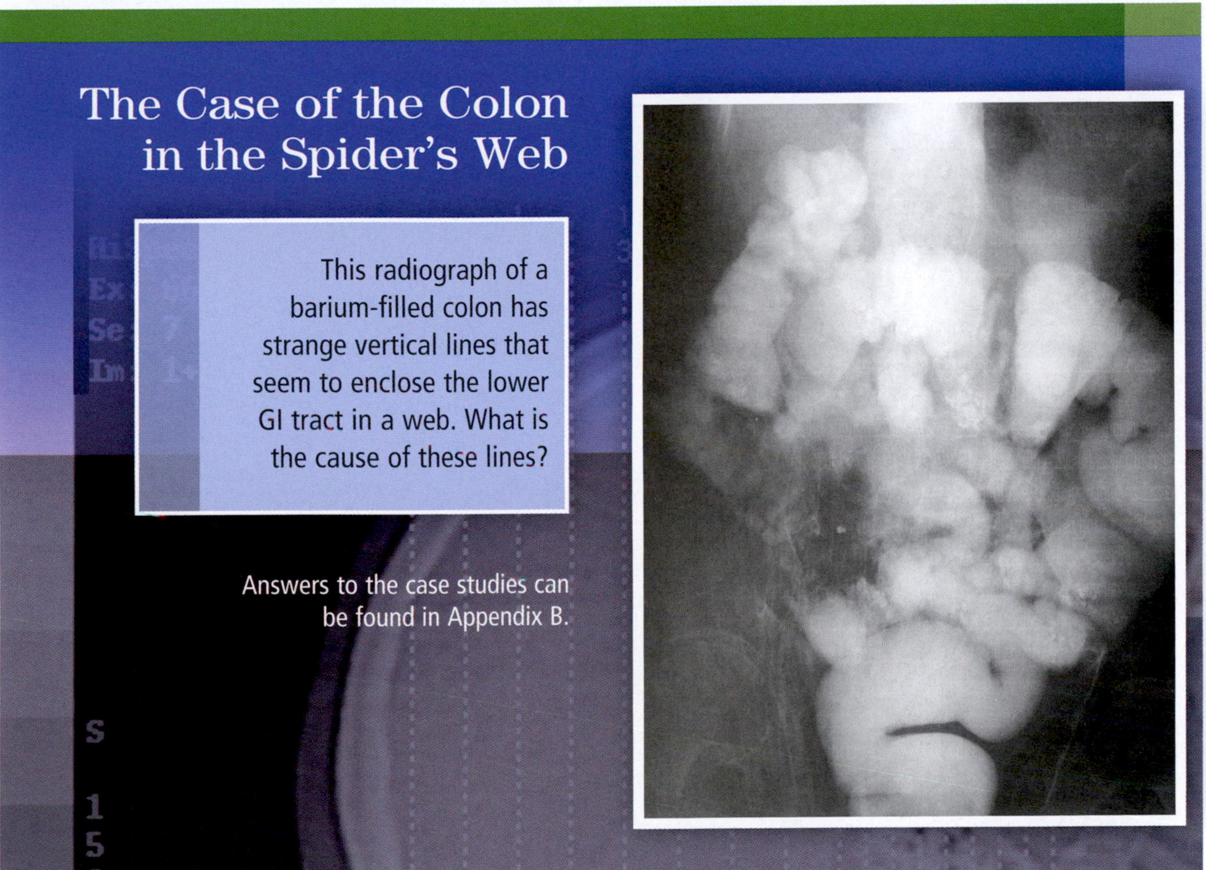

The Case of the Colon in the Spider's Web

This radiograph of a barium-filled colon has strange vertical lines that seem to enclose the lower GI tract in a web. What is the cause of these lines?

Answers to the case studies can be found in Appendix B.

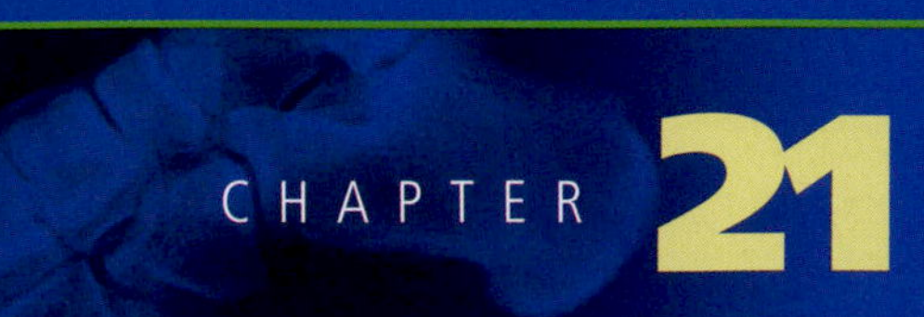

Film Sensitometry

KEY TERMS

average gradient
base plus fog
calibrate
characteristic curve
contrast
D log E curve
definition
densitometer
detail
D_{max}
gamma
gradient point
Hurter and Driffield (H&D) curve
latitude
opacity
optical density numbers
penetrometer
resolution
resolving power
reversal
sensitometer
sensitometric curve
sensitometry
sharpness
solarization
speed exposure point
speed point
step wedge
straight-line portion

You lie on a turning table cold as snow.
Down press the camera's praying-mantis arms,
Avid to embrace your negative below;
Your inner organs light their secret farms
Not even lovers come close enough to know.

Howard Moss, "In the X-Ray Room"

OBJECTIVES

Upon completion of this chapter, the student should be able to:

- Define *sensitometry* as it is applied to radiography.
- Describe the production of a step wedge on radiographic film through the use of a penetrometer and a sensitometer.
- Explain the function of a densitometer.
- Estimate the percentage of light transmitted by a radiograph according to optical density logarithms.
- Construct a D log E curve from sensitometric data.
- State acceptable base-plus-fog and diagnostic-range optical density numbers.
- Describe the effect of automatic-processor reducing agents on the shape of a D log E curve, especially with relation to speed and contrast.
- Define resolution, speed, contrast, and latitude.
- Explain the effect of silver halide crystal size on image resolution.

OBJECTIVES (continued)

- Discuss the physical and processing factors that affect film speed.
- Calculate speed points, speed exposure points, and relative speeds from D log E curves.
- Calculate gamma, gradient point, average gradient, and latitude from D log E curves.
- Analyze D log E curves to determine speed, contrast, and latitude relationships.
- Discuss the relationships between speed, contrast, and latitude.

Sensitometry is the measurement of the characteristic responses of film to exposure and processing and it is accomplished by exposing and processing a film and then measuring and evaluating the resulting densities. Sensitometric methods are useful to evaluate technical factor exposure systems, films, intensifying screens, and processing equipment, and to maintain technical exposure factor charts.

SENSITOMETRIC EQUIPMENT

Either a **penetrometer** or a **sensitometer** is required to produce a uniform range of densities on a film, and a **densitometer** is required to provide an accurate reading of the amount of light transmitted through the film.

Penetrometer

A penetrometer is a series of increasingly thick, uniform absorbers. They are usually made of aluminum steps, although tissue-equivalent plastic is sometimes used (Figure 21-1). A penetrometer is referred to as a **step wedge** because of its shape. It is used to produce a step wedge on radiographic film by exposure to x-rays (Figure 21-2). Because of the vast number of variables in x-ray-generating equipment, the use of a penetrometer is not recommended for quality control monitoring of film processors. However, it is an excellent method for monitoring both x-ray equipment and film/intensifying-screen combinations because it reproduces the variables associated with a clinical situation.

Sensitometer

A sensitometer is designed to expose a reproducible, uniform, optical step wedge onto a film (Figure 21-3). It contains a controlled-intensity light source (a pulsed stroboscopic light is best) and a piece of film with a standardized optical step wedge image (a step tablet). The controlled light source reproduces the same amount of light each time it is triggered. Voltage fluctuations and other factors that might cause the intensity to vary are controlled by circuits that supply an exact quantity of power to a capacitor that discharges to the stroboscopic light

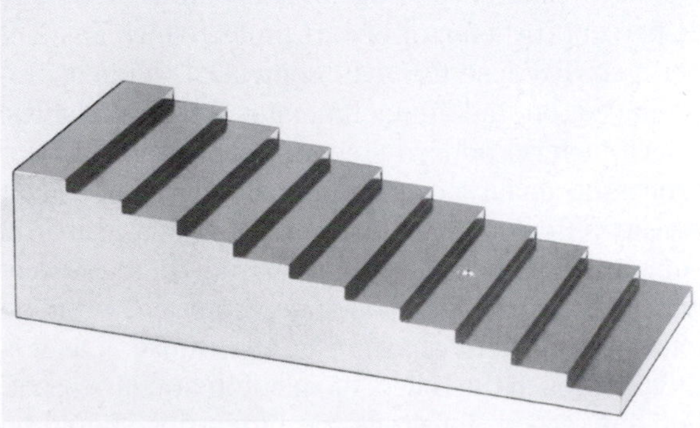

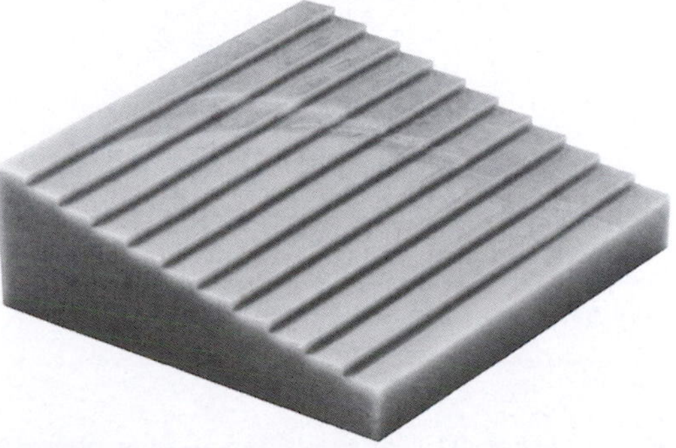

FIGURE 21-1. Two basic types of penetrometers or step wedges: (A) aluminum and (B) tissue equivalent plastic. (*Courtesy of Fluke Biomedical.*)

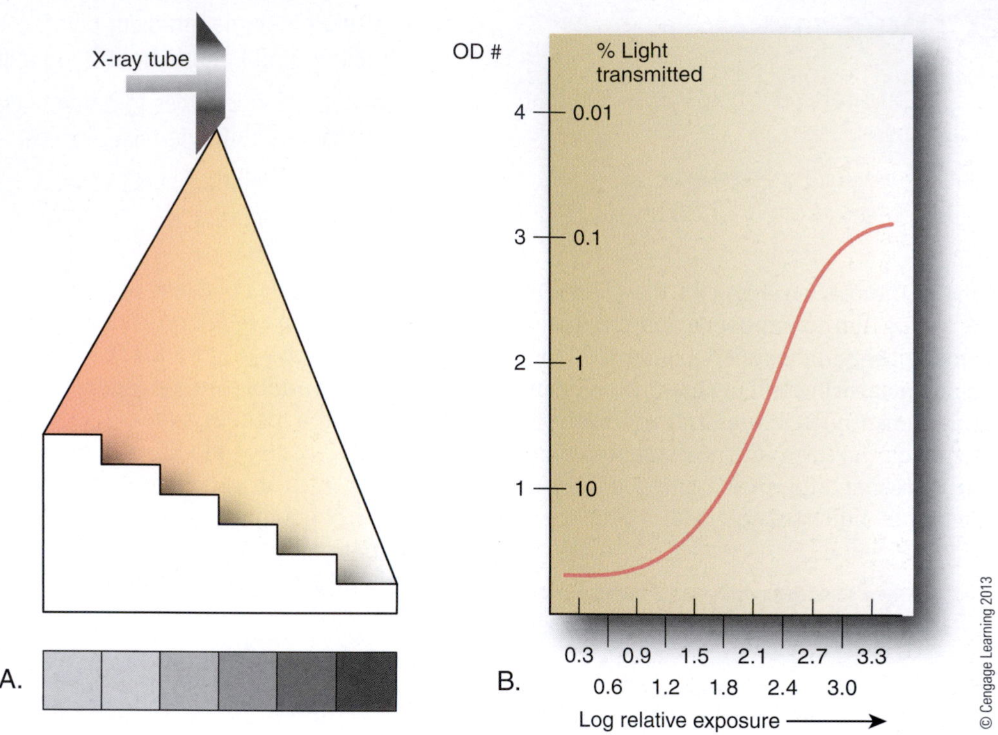

FIGURE 21-2. A density curve produced from graphing the exposures of a penetrometer exposure. (A) The exposure. (B) The graph.

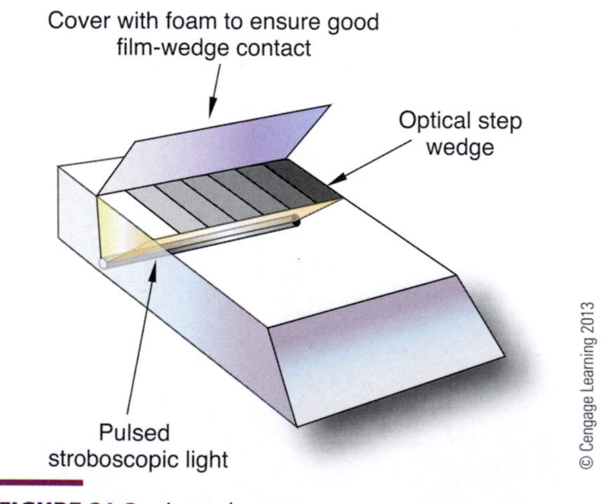

FIGURE 21-3. A sensitometer.

when triggered. The optical step wedge absorbs a calibrated amount of this light, leaving a uniform and reproducible "light penetrometer" to expose any film placed in the sensitometer over the optical step wedge. The optical step wedge should not be touched because hands leave a film of oil that interferes with the light intensity.

Optical step wedges (step tablets) are available in 11- and 21-step versions. The 11-step wedges usually increase density 100 percent (by a factor of two) per step. The 21-step wedges usually increase density 41 percent (by a factor of 1.41 times [which is $\sqrt{2}$]) per step. Because the rigid control of the densities produced on the film eliminates other variables, sensitometer-produced step wedges are perfect for processor quality control monitoring. Very slight density differences can be detected by sensitometric equipment. When a film is processed, there is a tendency for exhausted reducing agents and bromine ions to be carried backward on the emulsion as it is driven through the rollers of an automatic processor. For this reason, sensitometric film strips should be fed into automatic processors with either the long axis of the step wedge parallel to the entrance rollers or with the light edge entering the processor first.

Sensitometric strips are also produced electronically by most laser and dry imaging systems (when images are transferred to film) as well as by most Picture Archiving and Communications Systems PACS systems for use in calibrating the sensitometric response of flat-panel monitors.

Densitometer

A densitometer is an instrument that provides a readout of the amount of blackening (density) on a film. A densitometer consists of a calibrated uniform light source, a stage for placing the film to be measured, a light aperture to control the amount of light from the source, a sensor arm with an optical sensor, a readout display, and a calibration control (Figure 21-4). Density readings are accomplished by comparing the amount of light emitted by the light source with the amount of light transmitted through the film. To do this, the densitometer must be calibrated before each reading by recording the amount of light the light source is emitting. This is done by pushing the sensor arm so that the sensor is in contact with the light source (this eliminates the inverse square law factor) and by using the calibration control to set the readout display at zero. This **calibrates** or zeroes the densitometer and prepares it for a reading. When a film is placed on the stage and the sensor arm is pushed down into contact with the film, the densitometer can calculate the difference between the calibration intensity and the intensity of light the film is transmitting.

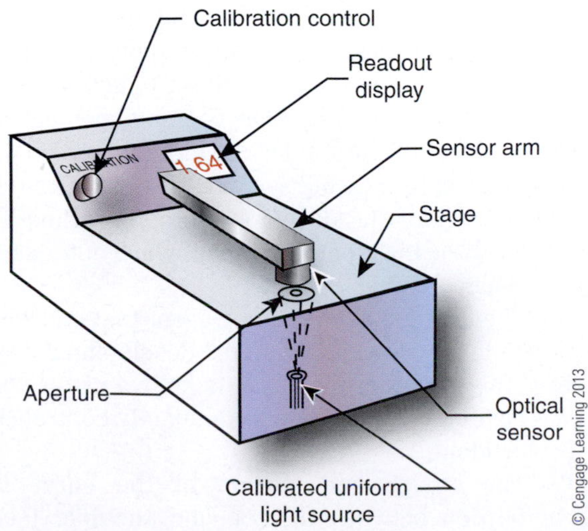

FIGURE 21-4. A densitometer.

Because films are sensitive to a wide range of exposures, their densities are best visualized if the range is compressed into a logarithmic scale. When using a logarithmic scale with a base of 10, an increment of 0.3 represents a doubling of exposure. This is because the log of 2 is 0.3. The numbers that are displayed by a densitometer are known as **optical density numbers.** They can be expressed with the term OD in front of the number (e.g., OD 1.5). They are calculated using the following formula:

$$\text{OD} = \log_{10} \frac{I_o}{I_t}$$

where: OD = optical density number
I_o = intensity of the incident light
I_t = intensity of the transmitted light

This formula can be stated as the log of the intensity of the incident light divided by the intensity of the light transmitted through the film. Radiographic film densities range from OD 0.0 to 4.0.

The ability of a film to stop light is termed **opacity.** Opacity is calculated using the following formula:

$$\text{opacity} = \frac{I_o}{I_t}$$

where: I_o = intensity of the incident light
I_t = intensity of the transmitted light

Note that density is the $\log_{10}$ of opacity (density = $\log_{10}$ of opacity). Table 21-1 shows both the opacity and optical density numbers for various percentages of light transmitted within the radiographic film density range of 0.0 to 4.0. For example, if a region of a radiograph has an OD of 1.0, this means only 10 percent or 1/10 of the incident light is transmitted through the radiograph in this region. The opacity of the region would be 10. If the OD number is increased to 1.3, the opacity is doubled (to 20) and the percentage of light transmitted through the film is halved (to 5 percent or 1/20). Increments of 0.3 changes in OD numbers represent a doubling or halving of opacity.

TABLE 21-1. Example Opacities, Optical Density Numbers, and Light Transmission Percentages

Opacity	OD Number	Percentage of Light Transmitted through Film
1	0.0	100
2	0.3	50
4	0.6	25
8	0.9	12.5
10	1.0	10
20	1.3	5
40	1.6	2.5
80	1.9	1.25
100	2.0	1
200	2.3	0.5
400	2.6	0.25
800	2.9	0.125
1,000	3.0	0.1
2,000	3.3	0.05
4,000	3.6	0.025
8,000	3.9	0.0125
10,000	4.0	0.01

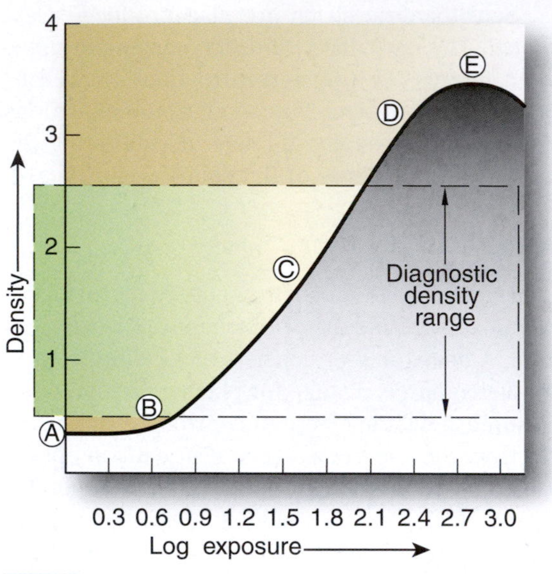

FIGURE 21-5. A typical D log E (characteristic, sensitometric, or H&D) curve. (A) Base plus fog; (B) toe; (C) straight-line portion; (D) shoulder; (E) D_{max}.

THE D LOG E CURVE

Sensitometry is normally shown as a graphic relationship between the amount of exposure and the resultant density on the film (Figure 21-5). The horizontal exposure axis (x axis) is compressed into a logarithmic scale and the vertical optical density axis (y axis) is shown as a logarithmic scale (OD numbers are logarithmic). Consequently, the curves are known as density log exposure, or **D log E curves.** They are also called **characteristic, sensitometric,** and **Hurter and Driffield (H&D) curves** after the two photographers who first described the relationships in 1890. The important elements of a typical D log E curve are the base plus fog, toe, straight-line portion (gamma), shoulder, and maximum density (D_{max}).

The **base plus fog** (b+f) (see Figure 21-5A) is the density at no exposure, or the density that is inherent in the film. It includes the density of the film base, including its tints and dyes, plus any fog the film has experienced. Radiographic film base density ranges around OD 0.05–0.10. Processing the film usually adds about OD 0.05–0.10 in fog density. The total base plus fog is seldom below OD 0.10 but should not exceed OD 0.22. Fog may be caused by heat, chemical fumes, light, and x-radiation. Over time, the natural amounts of these radiations will produce a slight density that is sometimes called age fog. Most of the fog level will be produced by the chemical processing system. This includes the hyperactivity of the developer solution, primarily caused by the high temperature at which automatic processors operate.

Phenidone is the reducing agent that controls the subtle gray tones early in the development process. This region of the curve is known as the toe (see Figure 21-5B) and is predominantly controlled by phenidone.

The **straight-line portion** of the curve is that portion between the toe and shoulder (see Figure 21-5C). It is usually fairly straight because the film is reacting in a linear fashion to exposure in the range of its primary sensitivity, which is in this region. The range of diagnostic densities varies from a low of OD 0.25–0.50 to a high of OD 2.0–3.0. The majority of diagnostic-quality information on a radiograph will measure between OD 0.5 and OD 1.25. These densities are within the straight-line portion of the curve.

Hydroquinone is the reducing agent that controls the heavy black tone later in the development process. This region of the curve is known as the shoulder (see Figure 21-5D) and is entirely controlled by hydroquinone.

D_{max} is the maximum density the film is capable of recording (see Figure 21-5E). It is the highest point on the D log E curve. It represents the point where all the silver halides have a full complement of silver atoms and cannot accept more. Additional exposure beyond D_{max} will result in less density because silver atoms attached to sensitivity specks will be ionized again, reversing their charge and causing them to be repelled from the speck. This process of **reversal,** or **solarization,** reduces the intensity of the latent image and will produce less density. The true D log E curve is bell-shaped (Figure 21-6). Duplication film is actually film that is pre-exposed to D_{max} so that additional exposure will cause a reversed, duplicated image instead of a negative one.

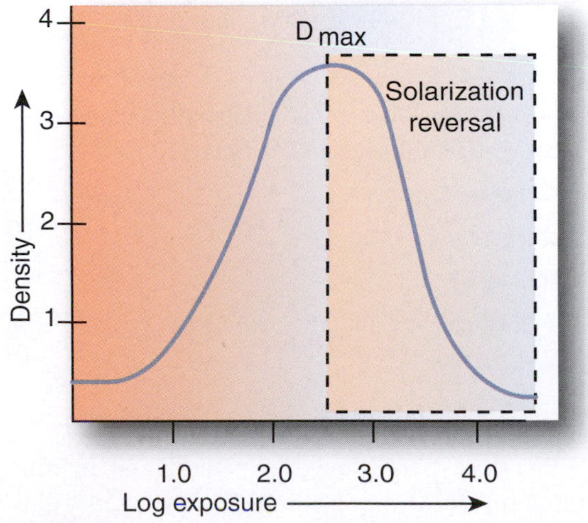

FIGURE 21-6. Solarization or reversal of duplicating film.

FILM CHARACTERISTICS

The primary characteristics of film are classified as **resolution,** speed, **contrast,** and **latitude.** Sensitometry permits analysis of speed, contrast, and latitude within the normal exposure ranges of the film. Extremely long or high-intensity exposure can overload the silver halide crystals and cause a phenomenon known as reciprocity failure. Although films are designed to handle a wide range of exposures, when unusual circumstances require large exposures, films may deviate from their expected performance.

Resolution

Resolution is the ability to accurately image an object. It is also called **detail, sharpness, definition,** and **resolving power.** Resolution is measured by the ability to see pairs of lines. The unit of resolution is line pairs per millimeter, expressed as lp/mm.

Film resolution is determined by the **size of the silver halide crystals**. Smaller crystals will darken a smaller area of the film, whereas larger ones will darken larger areas. Information that is smaller than an individual silver halide crystal cannot be visualized. **An inverse relationship exists between film resolution and crystal size** (the smaller the crystals, the higher the resolution; the larger the crystals, the lower the resolution). Silver halide crystals are sometimes called grains, thus the term *graininess* for poor resolution. Although film graininess can sometimes be seen, radiographic film/screen system resolution is generally controlled by the size of the intensifying-screen phosphors, not the size of the silver halide crystals in the film emulsion.

Speed

The amount of density (degree of blackening) a film produces for a given amount of exposure is the film speed. It is determined by the film's sensitivity to exposure. Speed is controlled by the activity of the phenidone because it affects the toe of the D log E curve. The position of the toe determines how soon the straight-line portion will begin, and this indicates the overall speed of the film. Figure 21-7

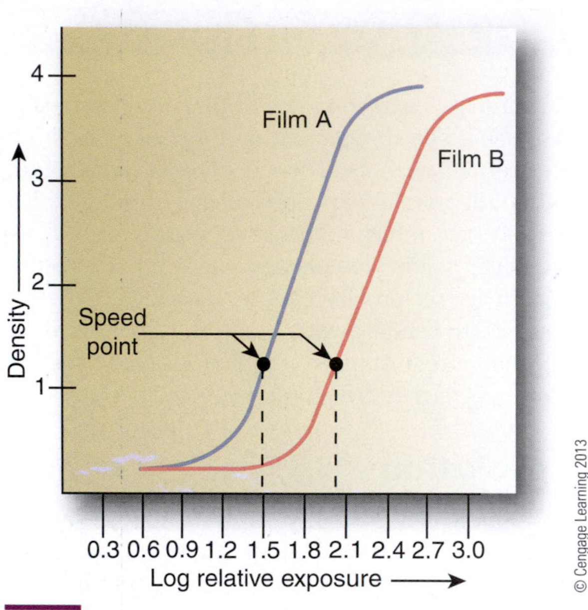

FIGURE 21-7. The effect of film speed on D log E curves.

illustrates the effect of the toe and shoulder on the overall position of the curve.

Film sensitivity is determined primarily by the **size of the silver halide crystals**. However, **the number of sensitivity specks and the thickness of the emulsion layer** also have an effect. Larger crystals will receive more photons because of the greater area they cover. Larger crystals will darken a greater area of the film than smaller crystals with the same exposure. Therefore, **film speed and crystal size are directly related** (the larger the crystals, the faster the film speed; the smaller the crystals, the slower the film speed). **Film speed and the number of sensitivity specks are also directly related** for the same reason.

A thicker emulsion layer will place more crystals in a given area. Each incoming photon may interact with more than one crystal, so when more crystals are stacked on top of one another in the same area, the same number of photons will produce more film density. Therefore, **film speed and thickness of emulsion layer are directly related** (the thicker the emulsion, the faster the film speed; the thinner the emulsion, the slower the film speed).

Screen films are capable of responding to (producing visible densities for) exposures as low as 1 mR and as high as 1,000 mR. In Figure 21-7, film A produces all density levels with less exposure than film B requires for the same density. This demonstrates that film A is more sensitive to exposure, or faster. Film B is less sensitive, or slower.

The **speed point** of a film is that point on the D log E curve where a density of OD 1.0 + b+f is achieved. The American National Standards Institute (ANSI) specifies x-ray film speed as the exposure required to reach OD 1.00. However, many users add base plus fog to this standard. The **speed exposure point** is the log exposure that will produce the speed point for a given film. Film A in Figure 21-7 has a speed exposure point of 1.5, and film B has a speed exposure point of 2.0.

In clinical radiography it is important to be able to adjust technical factors from one film to another. The radiographer must be able to calculate the difference in exposure that will produce a diagnostic-quality image on a new film when the proper factors are known for a previous one. In Figure 21-7, film B would require a log exposure of 2.0 to produce OD 1.0. Film A would require a log exposure of 1.5 to produce the same density. The difference in film speed is calculated as:

antilog ($\log E_1 - \log E_2$)

where: $\log E_1$ = log exposure of 1st film
$\log E_2$ = log exposure of 2nd film

EXAMPLE: What is the difference in speed between film A and film B in Figure 21-7?

Answer:

antilog($\log E_1 - \log E_2$) =

antilog(2.0 − 1.5) =

antilog(0.5) = 3.16

Film A is 316 percent faster than film B.

Relative speeds have been assigned by film manufacturers to assist radiographers in relating films to one another as they are used in film and intensifying-screen combinations (film/screen combinations). Relative film/screen speed can be determined by using the reciprocal of the exposure required to produce a given density:

$$\text{relative speed} = \frac{1}{\text{exposure in R needed to produce speed point density (OD 1.0 + b + f)}}$$

EXAMPLE: What is the relative speed for a film that requires an exposure of 5 mR to produce the speed point density?

Answer:

$$\text{relative speed} = \frac{1}{\text{exposure in R needed to produce speed point density (OD 1.0 + b + f)}}$$

$$\text{Relative speed} = \frac{1}{5\text{ mR}}$$

$$\text{Relative speed} = \frac{1}{0.005\text{ R}} = 200$$

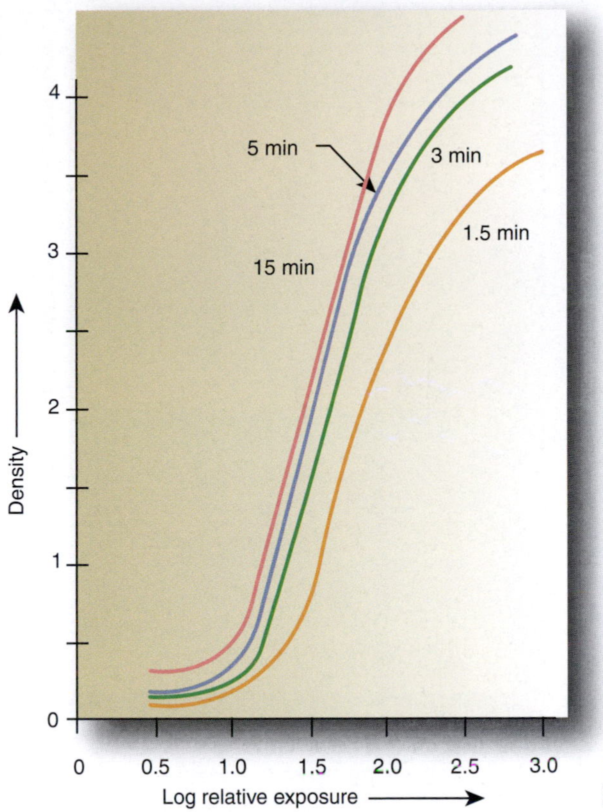

FIGURE 21-8. The effect of developer solution immersion time on film speed.

Film speed is affected by immersion time, solution temperature, and chemical activity. The immersion time in a high-speed automatic processor may be as short as 20–25 seconds. The longer the film is subjected to the chemical action of the developer solution, the greater is the amount of black metallic silver deposited on the latent image sites through the reduction process (Figure 21-8). Film speed is most affected by developer solution temperature (Figure 21-9). Only 0.5° will cause a visible change in film density. Higher temperature increases the activity level of the reducing agents in the developer, and this produces greater density on the film. High-speed automatic processors use high temperatures to permit sufficient development to occur in the 20–25 seconds the film is immersed in the developer. The chemical activity of the developer solution will also increase the development of density. Film speed is affected when the bromide ion barrier has not formed properly (due to insufficient restrainer or overreplenishment) or when it is too strong (due to excess restrainer or underreplenishment). Determination of the proper time, temperature, and activity for a particular developer and film is done by graphing speed, contrast, and base plus fog levels for various activity concentrations (Figure 21-10). This is how the manufacturer arrives at the recommended time and temperature for optimal results.

Contrast

Contrast is the difference between adjacent densities. This concept can be confusing when one tries to understand the difference between density and contrast. There is a relationship between contrast and density because contrast consists of the difference between adjacent densities. For the same film type, **a change in density will affect contrast only when above or below the straight-line portion of the D log E curve**.

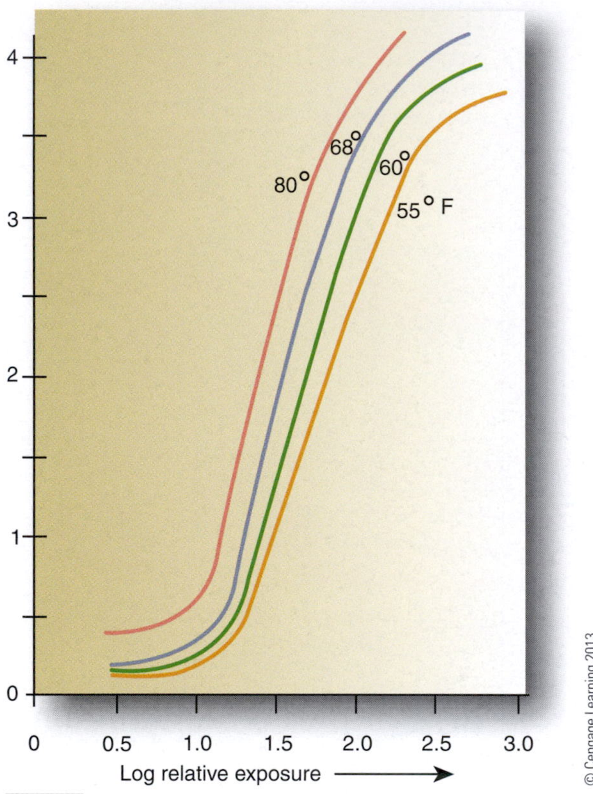

FIGURE 21-9. The effect of developer solution temperature on film speed.

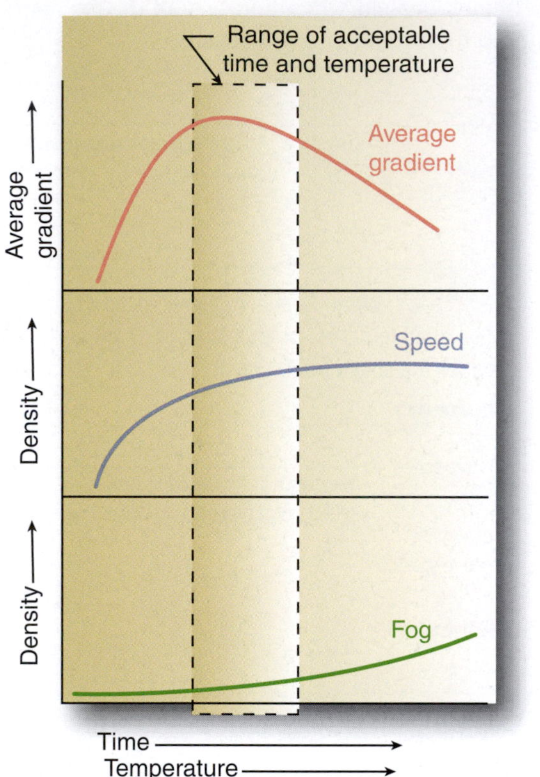

FIGURE 21-10. Determination of optimal development time and temperature for a particular film by comparison of contrast, speed, and base plus fog for a particular developer solution concentration.

Contrast is controlled by the level of activity of the hydroquinone. Hydroquinone establishes the shoulder of the D log E curve and the position of the shoulder affects the slope of the straight-line portion of the curve (Figure 21–11).

Contrast is defined by the slope of the straight-line portion of the D log E curve, but, because the straight-line portion is actually a curve, it is important to define the point at which the slope is measured. **Gamma** is simply a measure of the slope of the straight line portion of the curve at the speed point (OD 1.0). In practice, a gamma may be read with the speed point in the center, top end, or bottom end, as long as all comparative readings are done from the same reference point. Contrast differences cannot be appreciated unless they are measured from identical reference points.

The slope can be read as "rise over run" (Figure 21-12). More sophisticated measurements, such as the trigonometric tangent of the slope, are also used. The slope of any portion of the D log E curve can be calculated, and this is known as a **gradient point.** Gradient points must have their OD values stated—for example, a gradient of 1.75 at OD 0.80. Gradient points are sometimes known by their location: toe gradient, middle gradient, and upper gradient. The toe gradient is calculated between OD 0.25 and OD 1.00. The middle gradient is calculated between OD 1.00 and OD 2.00. The upper gradient is calculated between OD 2.00 and OD 2.50. Overall radiographic film contrast is more commonly defined by the **average gradient** of the straight-line portion of the D log E curve between OD 0.25 + b + f and

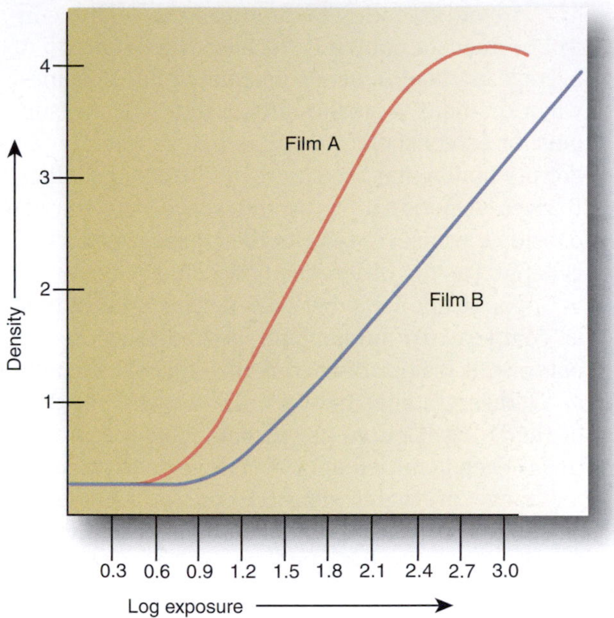

FIGURE 21-11. Comparison of film contrast.

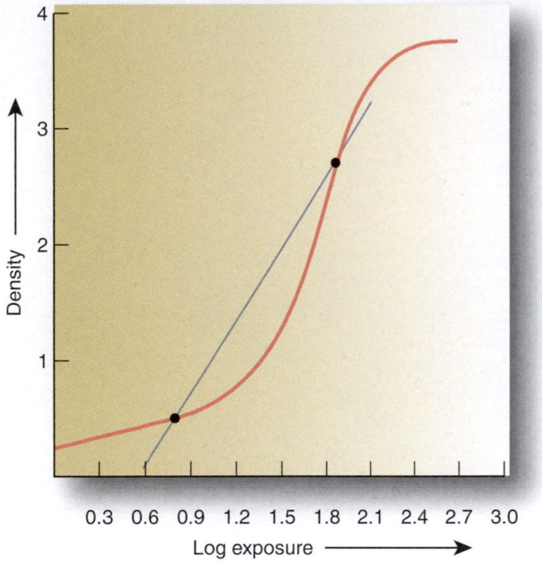

FIGURE 21-12. Average gradient from a D log E curve.

OD 2.50 + b + f. Opinions differ on whether b + f should be added to average gradient calculations. The average gradient is calculated as:

$$\text{average gradient} = \frac{\Delta D}{\Delta E} \text{ or}$$

$$\text{average gradient} = \frac{D_2 - D_1}{E_2 - E_1}$$

where: D_1 = OD 0.25 + b + f,
D_2 = OD 2.50 + b + f,
E_1 = exposure that produces D_1
E_2 = exposure that produces D_2

Note: ΔD is a constant of OD 2.25 (OD 2.50 – 0.25).

Figure 21-13 illustrates the difference between various gradient points and the average gradient. Most radiographic film average gradients are between 2.5 and 3.5.

The important part of the D log E curve is that portion between the toe and the shoulder (the diagnostic range of the film). In this central straight-line portion, the density is approximately proportional to the log relative exposure. This is because a straight line will always have a constant ratio. If the slope of the straight-line portion is at a 45° angle, the average gradient will measure 1.0. In this example, a doubling of exposure will result in a doubling of the opacity. (Note that the term *doubling of density* is not used because density is a log number. A change of 0.3 in density reflects a doubling or halving of opacity.) **A common misnomer in radiography is that doubling the exposure will double the density.** This is not true for typical radiographic film/screen systems.

Radiographic films have a slope steeper than 45°. In these films, when exposure is doubled, opacity is increased by more than a factor of 2. Because of the steepness of the slope (and the average gradient above 1.0), radiographic films amplify exposure by producing a greater proportion of density per exposure increase. **Doubling the radiographic exposure will produce more than a doubling of radiographic opacity.**

Toe and shoulder gradients are less than a 45° angle ($<$1.0) and therefore not only fail to amplify the contrast but actually decrease it. This is one reason why extremely light or dark areas on radiographs are not acceptable for diagnosis.

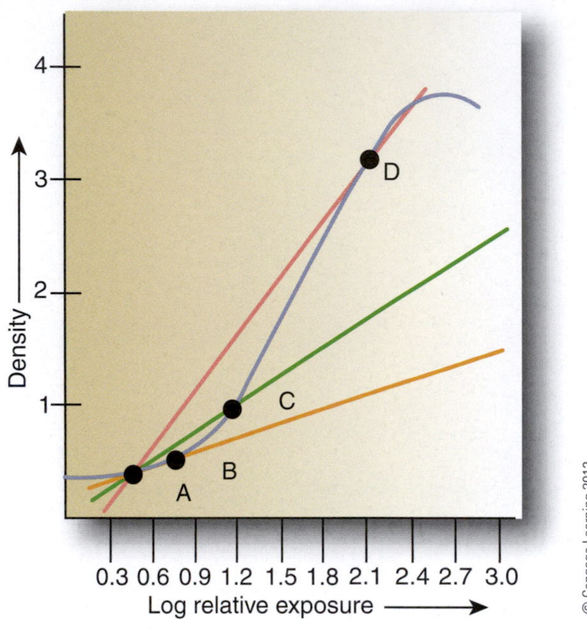

FIGURE 21-13. Average gradient and gradient point calculations from a D log E curve. The slopes of points A-B, A-C, and A-D are quite different.

A contrast index is often used in quality control to indicate contrast. Because the definition of average gradient depends on comparable densities, when the density itself shifts, a different measure must be established. A contrast index is simply two density points that are subtracted from each other. It gives a measure of the difference between set densities, which represents the contrast. (Contrast is defined as the difference between densities.)

The relationship between density and contrast is complex. To understand how density affects contrast, it is important to realize that the changes in average gradient between the toe and shoulder of the D log E curve are actually changes in contrast. When insufficient or excessive density causes the range of visible densities on the radiograph to change, contrast is affected. For example, the film used for the data in Figure 21-14 achieved a maximum optimal contrast with an OD of 1.2–1.5. For OD measurements above or below this range, contrast is decreased. For radiographic films under most conditions, contrast is maximized when

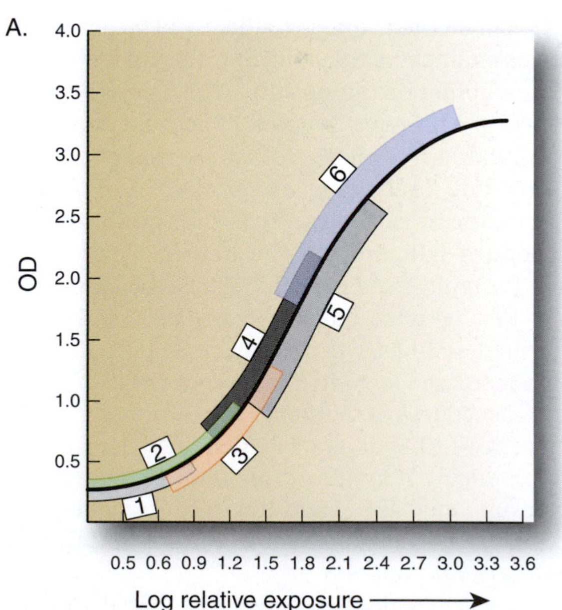

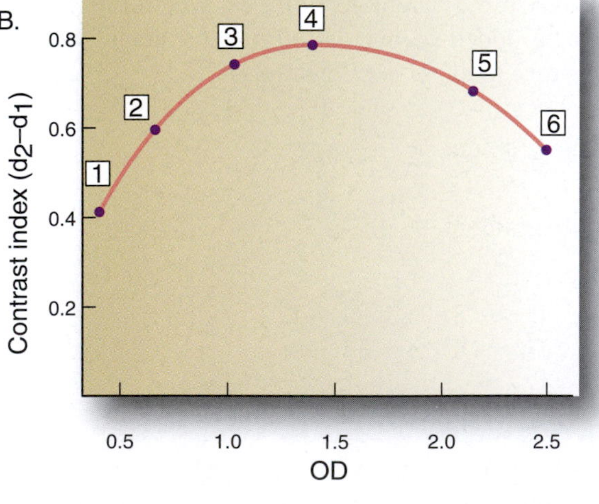

FIGURE 21-14. (A) Density ranges (1–6) from D log E curve of film measured for contrast index. (B) Contrast index for the density ranges (1–6) measured from Figure A. Note that the maximum contrast (range 4) is essentially the straight-line portion of the curve. Contrast is decreased for toe and shoulder measurements but is maximized for the straight-line portion of the D log E curve (OD 1.2–1.5). (Also note this range corresponds to the speed point [OD 1.2].) *(Courtesy of Barry Burns, UNC Division of Radiologic Science.)*

the density range is within the range of diagnostic densities (a low of OD 0.12–0.50 and a high of OD 2.0–3.0). When the diagnostic densities are below or above this range, the contrast will be decreased. This occurs because the slope of the range of diagnostic densities has moved into the toe or shoulder of the D log E curve.

The contrast must exist within the diagnostic range of the film if it is to be visualized; in other words, within the straight-line portion of the curve.

Latitude

For clinical radiographic purposes, latitude is the range of exposures that will produce densities within the diagnostic range (Figure 21-15). Latitude can be recorded as the width of the range of exposures that will produce diagnostic-range densities according to the following formula:

latitude = $E_h - E_1$

where: E_h = OD 2.50 exposure point
E_1 = OD 0.25 exposure point

when: E_h = high exposure point
E_1 = low exposure point

> ***EXAMPLE:*** What is the latitude for film A in Figure 21-15?
>
> ***Answer:***
>
> latitude = $E_h - E_1$
>
> latitude = 1.8 – 1.1
>
> latitude = 0.7

The latitude for film B can be calculated to be 1.0. Film A has a narrow latitude, whereas film B has a wider latitude. Because a wide-latitude film permits considerable variation in the exposure while still exhibiting densities within the diagnostic range, it is sometimes called a forgiving film. The use of a narrow-latitude film for routine radiography requires greater exposure accuracy.

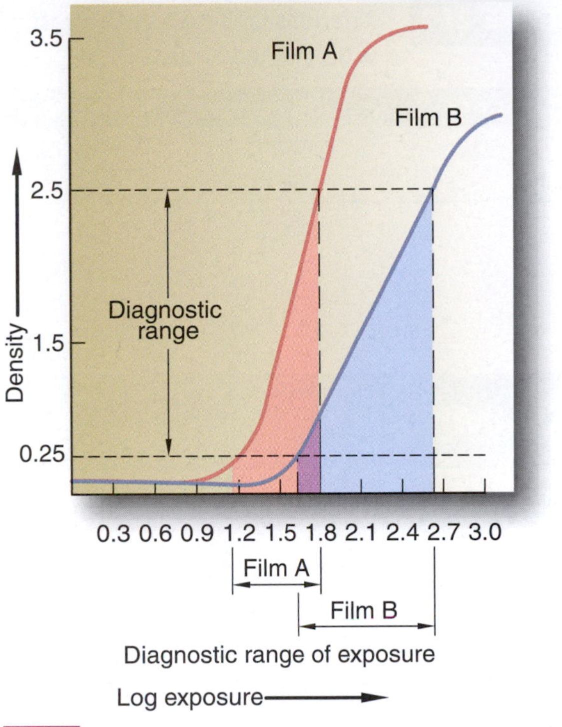

FIGURE 21-15. Comparison of film latitude. The range of relative exposure is indicated for each film.

Latitude and contrast are inversely related. As contrast increases, latitude tends to decrease. This affects the overall shape of the D log E curve. Latitude changes whenever there is a change in the average gradient of the D log E curve. Speed could change without altering the average gradient and latitude. A difference in film speed usually results in different contrast and latitude because it is rare for the entire D log E curve to shift the same degree. Usually the toe and shoulder will not shift exactly the same amount and this causes a change in the slope of the straight-line portion of the curve (which changes contrast and latitude). The relationships of speed, contrast, and latitude to patient dose are listed in Tables 21-2 and 21-3.

TABLE 21-2. Relationship between Contrast, Latitude, and Patient Dose

Contrast	Latitude	Patient Dose
high	narrow	high
low	wide	low

TABLE 21-3. Relationship between Speed and Patient Dose

Speed	Patient Dose
slow	high
fast	low

SUMMARY

Sensitometry is the measurement of the characteristic responses of a film to exposure and processing. It is accomplished by exposing and processing a film and then measuring and evaluating the resulting densities. Either a penetrometer or a sensitometer is required to produce a uniform range of densities on the film. A densitometer is required to provide an accurate reading of the amount of light transmitted through the film.

Because films are sensitive to a wide range of exposures, their densities are best visualized if the range is compressed into a logarithmic scale. When using a logarithmic scale with a base of 10, an increment of 0.3 represents a doubling of exposure. This is because the log of 2 is 0.3.

Sensitometry is normally shown as a graphic relationship between the amount of exposure and the resultant density on the film. The horizontal axis (exposure) of the graph is compressed into a logarithmic scale and the vertical axis (density) is a linear scale. Consequently, the curves are known as density log exposure, or D log E, curves. They are also called characteristic, sensitometric, and Hurter and Driffield (H&D) curves. The important elements of the D log E curve are the base plus fog, toe, straight-line portion (gamma), shoulder, and maximum density (D max).

The primary characteristics of film are resolution, speed, contrast, and latitude. Resolution is the ability to accurately image an object and is measured by the ability to see line pairs. The amount of density a film produces for a given amount of exposure is the film speed. The film speed is determined by the size of the silver halide crystals, the number of sensitivity specks, and the thickness of the emulsion. Relative speeds have been assigned by film manufacturers to assist radiographers in relating films to one another as they are used in film/screen combinations. Contrast is the difference between adjacent densities. It is defined as the slope of the straight line portion of the D log E curve. Latitude is the range of exposures that will produce densities within the diagnostic range. As contrast increases, latitude tends to decrease. ■

REVIEW QUESTIONS

1. What is the purpose of sensitometry?
2. Explain the design of a penetrometer.
3. Why is a logarithmic scale used for describing optical densities?
4. Describe the five important elements of the D log E curve.
5. What is the relationship between film resolution and the size of the silver halide crystals?
6. What is the relationship between film speed and emulsion layer thickness?
7. State the formula for relative speed.
8. How is the average gradient calculated?
9. What is the relationship between contrast and latitude?

REFERENCES AND RECOMMENDED READING

Carroll, Q. B. (2003). *Fuchs's radiographic exposure, processing, and quality control* (7th ed.). Springfield, IL: Charles C Thomas.

Chow, M. F. (1988). The effect of a film's sensitivity to its speed, contrast, and latitude. *The Canadian Journal of Medical Radiation Technology, 19*(4), 147.

Eastman Kodak Co. *Sensitometric properties of x-ray films*. Rochester, NY: Eastman Kodak Company Radiography Markets Division.

Haus, A. G. (Ed.) (1993). *Film processing in medical imaging.* Madison, WI: Medical Physics.

McKinney, W. (1988). *Radiographic processing and quality control.* Philadelphia: J. B. Lippincott.

Thompson, M. A., Hattaway, M. P., Hall, J. D., & Dowd, S. B. (1994). *Principles of imaging science and protection*. Philadelphia: W. B. Saunders.

Wolbarst, A. B. (1993). *Physics of radiology.* Norwalk, CT: Appleton & Lange.

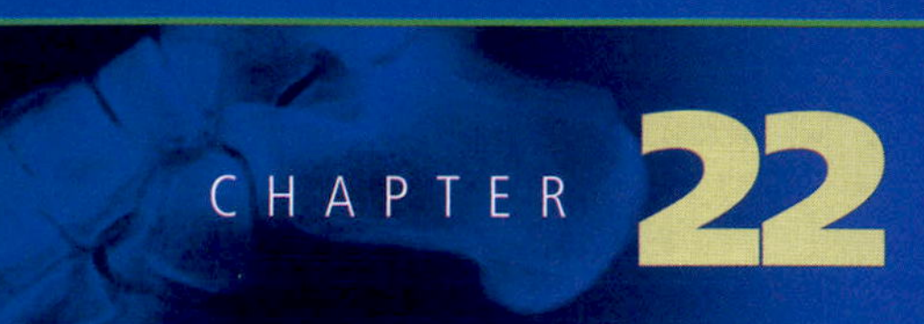

CHAPTER 22

Intensifying Screens and Film/Screen Combinations

KEY TERMS

afterglow
base
conversion efficiency
fluorescence
intensification factor
intensifying screen
K-shell absorption edge
line pairs per millimeter (lp/mm)
line spread function (LSF)
luminescence
modulation transfer function (MTF)
phosphorescence
phosphor layer
protective coat
reflective layer
relative speed
screen lag
spectral emission

> Mr. Edison has discovered … tungstate of calcium … [with which] you can see other people's bones with the naked eye … . On the revolting indecency of this there is no need to dwell. But what we seriously put before the attention of the Government is that the moment tungstate of calcium comes into anything like general use, it will call for legislative restriction of the severest kind.
>
> *Pall Mall Gazette*, March 1896

OBJECTIVES

Upon completion of this chapter, the student should be able to:

- Explain the purpose of radiographic intensifying screens.
- Describe the function of each layer of an intensifying screen.
- Evaluate the desirability of phosphor materials according to atomic number, conversion efficiency, spectral emission, and fluorescence.
- Describe luminescence.
- Analyze the effect of phosphor crystal size, layer thickness, and concentration on intensifying-screen resolution.
- Explain the effect of film/screen contact on resolution.
- Describe how to remedy quantum mottle.
- Classify intensifying screens according to intensification factor, descriptive rating, and relative speed number.
- Describe the effect of K-shell absorption edges on intensifying-screen efficiency.

OBJECTIVES (continued)

- Describe the components of a radiographic cassette.
- Describe the proper cleaning and care of radiographic cassettes and screens.
- Evaluate film/screen combinations for specific clinical uses.
- Relate the emission spectra of various intensifying screens to specific types of radiographic film.
- Explain radiographic film/screen combination relative speed numbering systems.
- Calculate relative speed conversions from one film/screen combination to another.
- Describe various methods of measuring resolution, including a basic description of line pairs per millimeter, line spread function, and modulation transfer function.
- Relate film/screen contrast to latitude.
- Determine appropriate film/screen combinations for various clinical situations.

Intensifying screens are used to amplify the incoming x-ray beam and reduce patient radiation dose. Introduced in 1896 by the American inventor Thomas Edison (1847–1931), intensifying screens produce large quantities of light photons when struck by x-rays. In this manner they intensify the latent imaging power of the beam, even though less than 33 percent of the x-ray photons that strike the cassette interact with the intensifying screen. Over 99 percent of the latent film image is formed by this light, with less than 1 percent contributed by x-ray photons. This permits a great reduction in the amount of radiation necessary to produce a diagnostic-quality image. Intensifying screens are normally used in pairs with duplitized film, although there are specialized cassettes that are designed for a single screen with single-emulsion film.

CONSTRUCTION

Intensifying screens are composed of radiolucent plastic, coated with phosphors that will emit light when struck by x-ray photons. They are designed to be mounted in pairs inside the top and bottom of a lightproof cassette so that a sheet of radiographic film can be sandwiched tightly between them. A screen consists of a **base**, a **reflective layer**, a **phosphor layer**, and a **protective coat** (Figure 22-1).

Base

The base is usually made of polyester plastic 1 mm thick, although cardboard and metal have been used. Its requirements are similar to those for a film base. It must be flexible yet tough, rigid, chemically inert, and uniformly radiolucent. It must be flexible to permit it to achieve good contact with the film. It must be rigid enough to stay in place in the top and bottom of a cassette. It must be chemically inert so that it does not react with the phosphor and interfere with the conversion of x-ray photons to light. It also must not react with air or chemicals in a manner that would cause discoloration. Discoloration filters and changes the wavelengths of the light emitted by the screen by absorbing wavelengths that could be used to create the radiographic image. Because films are designed to be most sensitive to the particular wavelength of light emitted by the screen, discoloration may require more light, and consequently more patient radiation dose, to form the latent image. Most important, base material must be uniformly radiolucent so that it permits the transmission of x-ray photons without adding artifacts to the diagnostic image.

Reflective Layer

The base material is not transparent to light. In fact, a special layer of reflective material, such as magnesium oxide or titanium dioxide, about 25 µm thick, is used to reflect light toward the film. When

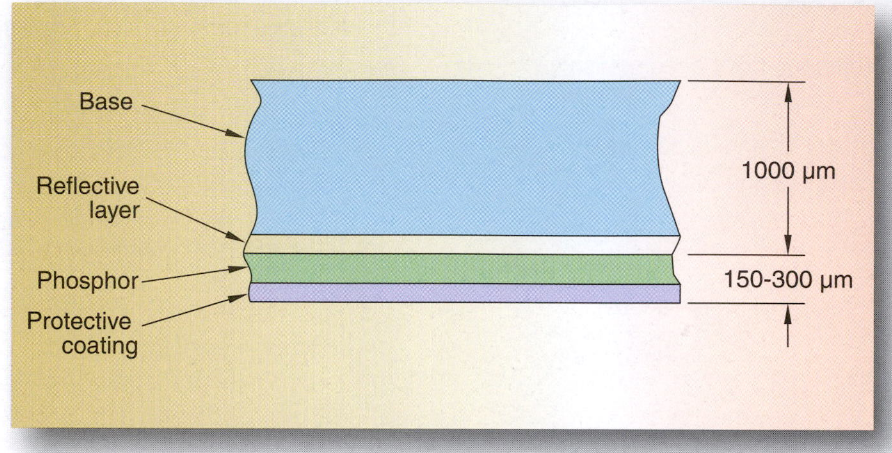

FIGURE 22-1. Cross-sectional view of a typical radiographic intensifying screen.

a phosphor is struck by an x-ray photon, it will emit light isotropically (in all directions) (Figure 22-2A). When a reflective layer is added (Figure 22-2B), nearly twice as much light is reflected toward the film. This increase in light striking the film assists in creating the latent image and decreases the radiation dose to the patient.

Light that is emitted at a large angle from the direction of the incident x-ray photon will have a slightly longer wavelength. Some intensifying screens use dyes in the reflective layer to selectively absorb this longer-wavelength light. This assists in reducing the scattering of light that would decrease the resolving ability of the screen. Scattered light of this type causes a large area of penumbra, which reduces the sharpness of the image.

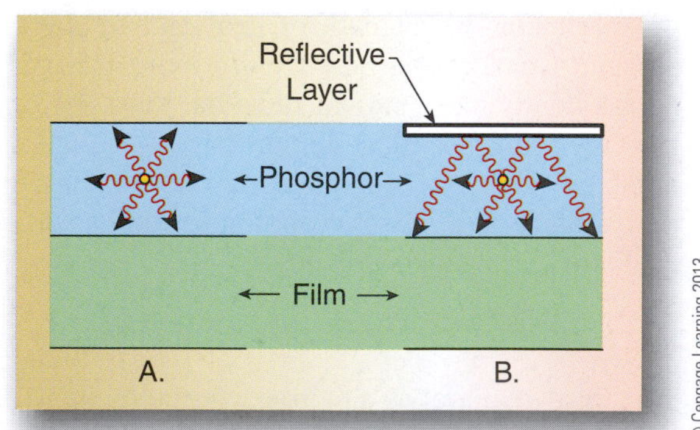

FIGURE 22-2. Intensifying-screen reflective layer redirection of isotropic light emission to film.

Phosphor Layer

The active layer of the intensifying screen is the phosphor layer. Phosphors are materials that are capable of absorbing the energy of an incident x-ray photon and then emitting light photons. Röntgen discovered x-rays when he observed the luminescence of the phosphor barium platinocyanide from a piece of cardboard in his laboratory. This phosphor layer varies from 150 to 300 μm, depending on the speed and resolving power of the screen.

Protective Coat

A coating of protective plastic about 25 μm thick is applied on top of the phosphor layer. The coating protects the phosphor layer from abrasions and stains during the loading and unloading of films. Fingernails and jewelry are the prime trauma to screens in the darkroom. Although the protective coating will prevent scratching of the phosphor layer during normal handling, repeated trauma can remove the coating. When intensifying screens are scratched, phosphor crystals may be removed, creating unexposed white-line artifacts on the radiographic image.

PHOSPHORS

Phosphors must have a high atomic number, high **conversion efficiency**, appropriate **spectral emission**, and minimal **phosphorescence**.

Atomic Number

A high atomic number is desirable to increase the probability of an incident x-ray photon interaction. Because x-ray photons are of high energy, a high atomic number is required to permit photoelectric and Compton interactions.

Conversion Efficiency

The ability of the phosphor to emit as much light per x-ray photon interaction as possible is a measurement of the screen speed. As this **conversion efficiency** increases, the radiation dose to the patient decreases. A typical conversion efficiency would produce 1×10^3 light photons per incident 50-keV x-ray photon for a rare-earth screen.

Spectral Emission

The spectral emission is an indication of the precise wavelength of light emitted by the phosphor. It is important that the spectral emission match the sensitivity of the film to ensure maximum latent image formation.

Luminescence

Luminescence is the ability of a material to emit light in response to excitation (usually by increased outer-electron-shell energy levels). Because of the narrow energy band within which these interactions occur, luminescent materials emit light with wavelengths that are characteristic of the particular luminescent material. This results in light emissions of a characteristic color. **Fluorescence and phosphorescence are the two types of luminescence**. **Fluorescence** occurs when the light is emitted within the time it takes an electron to complete one orbit of the affected shell electrons (within 1 nanosecond). Phosphorescence occurs when the light is emitted for a period longer than that necessary for one orbit of the affected shell electrons. In other words, **fluorescence is instantaneous emission whereas phosphorescence is delayed emission**, sometimes considerably delayed. Phosphorescence occurs when the phosphor continues to emit light after the incident x-ray photon energy has dissipated. Maximum fluorescence and minimal phosphorescence are desirable because delayed emission of light may permit the film to be removed from the cassette before the maximum latent image formation has occurred. Additionally, if another film is loaded into the cassette it may be faintly exposed to a previous image.

Delayed phosphorescent emission is called **screen lag** or **afterglow** and is common in older intensifying screens with exhausted phosphors. The normal life of intensifying-screen phosphors is 5 to 7 years.

Roughly 50,000 photons per mm^2 must exit the object being examined to produce a radiographic image. The intensifying screens must produce enough light from these photons to create the latent image in the film emulsion.

Several phosphors have been used in radiography since Röntgen's discovery: zinc sulfide, barium lead sulfate, calcium tungstate ($CaWO_4$), and a family of hybrid rare earths, including gadolinium, lanthanum, and yttrium. Calcium tungstate was used by Edison and it predominated as the best phosphor until the late 1970s, when the rare earths were introduced.

Rare Earths

Rare earths are the preferred phosphor materials because they have greater absorption abilities, intensification factors, and conversion efficiency. Older calcium tungstate screens had an x-ray-to-light conversion efficiency of about 5 percent, as compared to rare-earth conversion efficiencies of 15–20 percent. The rare-earth screens use phosphors with atomic numbers of 57–71. These elements are known as rare earths because they are difficult to isolate. Gadolinium and lanthanum were the most common rare earths used for radiographic intensifying screens.

CHARACTERISTICS

Intensifying screens exhibit the same types of characteristics as films. Consideration must be given to screen **resolution, speed, contrast**, and **latitude**.

Resolution

Resolution is the ability to accurately image an object. Intensifying-screen resolution is controlled by the size of the phosphor crystals, the thickness of the layer, and the concentration (packing density) of the crystals, exactly as silver halide size and distribution affect film resolution. Smaller crystals and a thinner layer increase resolution but decrease screen speed. Larger crystals and a thicker layer decrease resolution but increase screen speed (Figure 22-3). **Phosphor crystal size and layer thickness are both inversely related to resolution and directly related to screen speed**. A greater concentration of crystals will increase both resolution and screen speed. Phosphor concentration is directly related to resolution and screen speed. Intensifying-screen phosphor crystals are much larger than the silver halide crystals in the film emulsion. In radiographic film and intensifying-screen combinations, **the screen resolution always predominates over the film resolution**.

Measurement. Under ideal conditions, the naked eye can resolve approximately 10–20 lp/mm. Direct exposure nonscreen radiographic film can resolve up to 100 lp/mm, detail-speed screens about 15 lp/mm, par-speed screens about 10 lp/mm, and high-speed screens about 7 lp/mm.

Film/Screen Contact. One of the most common screen resolution problems is caused by poor contact between the film and the intensifying screen in the cassette (Figure 22-4). Poor film/screen contact also decreases the image density. There are numerous possible causes of poor film/screen contact, including foreign objects in the cassette and warped or damaged cassettes.

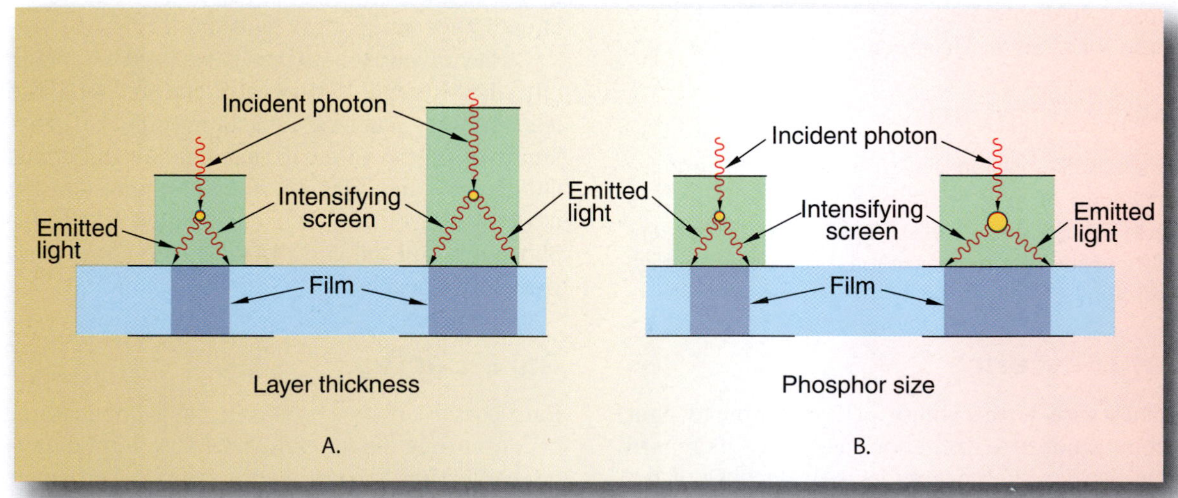

FIGURE 22-3. The effect of intensifying-screen phosphor layer thickness and crystal size on film resolution.

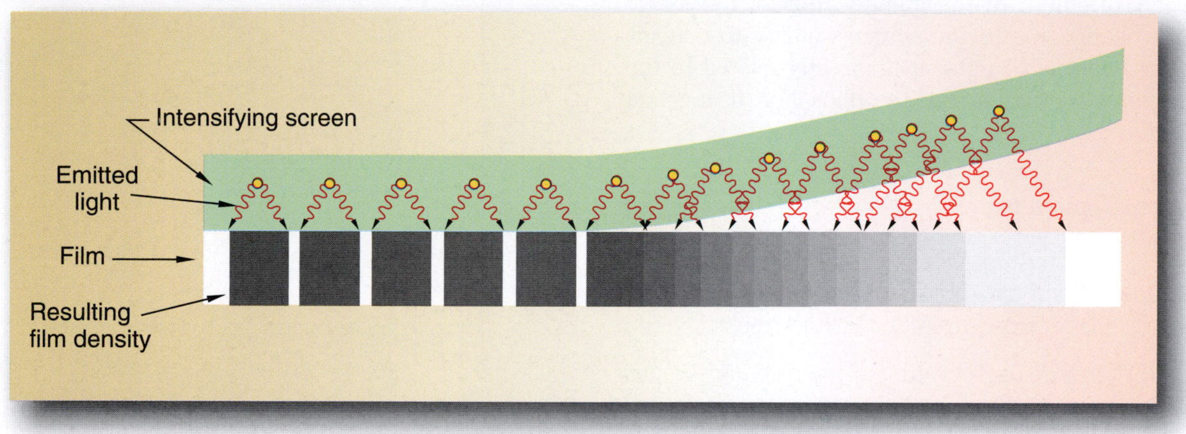

FIGURE 22-4. Poor resolution and decreased image density due to loss of film/screen contact.

Quantum Mottle. Each phosphor crystal emits light that exposes a corresponding area of silver halide crystals in the film emulsion. When insufficient phosphor crystals emit light to expose a coherent expanse of film, the resulting image will appear grainy (Figure 22-5). [Quantum mottle is caused by an insufficient quantity of photons striking the intensifying screen. Although film graininess may appear mottled, radiographic mottle is nearly always a result of intensifying-screen quantum mottle. The radiographer controls the quantity of photons with the mAs setting, so an increase in this factor will eliminate quantum mottle. Fluoroscopic tubes normally operate at very-low-mA levels. For this reason, quantum mottle is more commonly seen in fluoroscopy.

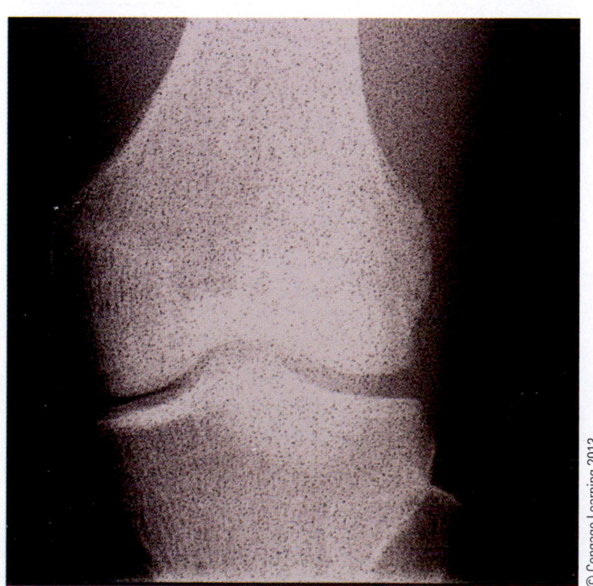

FIGURE 22-5. Quantum mottle.

Speed

The speed or sensitivity of the intensifying screen is determined by the same factors that control resolution. Increasing phosphor size and layer thickness increase speed. An increase in phosphor concentration also increases speed. In addition, there are factors that affect speed but not resolution. As kVp is increased, the efficiency of the intensifying screen will also increase. **An increase in kVp will cause an increase in screen speed**. Intensifying-screen phosphors have relatively high atomic numbers, so higher kVp will increase the probability of light-producing interactions within the phosphors. Temperature increases (over 100°F [38°C]) will decrease screen speed significantly.

Screen Speed Classifications. The most accurate factor that measures the speed or sensitivity of an intensifying screen is the **intensification factor**. It is a measurement of the amplification of the image that occurs due to the screen's ability to convert x-ray photons to light. It is directly related to the conversion efficiency of the phosphor. It is calculated as:

$$\text{intensification factor} = \frac{D_n}{D_s}$$

where: D_n = exposure in mR nonscreen
D_s = exposure in mR with screens

The most useful rating of intensifying screens is the **relative speed**. Relative speed is expressed with par-speed screens, and film, being arbitrarily assigned a relative speed (RS) number of 100, as a control point. High-speed screens are usually rated RS 200–1,200, whereas fine-detail screens are usually rated RS 20–80.

K-shell Absorption Edge. Calcium tungstate screens will absorb about 20–40 percent and rare-earth screens will absorb about 50–60 percent of the incident beam. These percentages vary depending upon the keV level of the incident photons. Nearly 100 percent of the absorption occurs through photoelectric interactions. Because photoelectric interactions produce characteristic photons, when the incident x-ray photons match the K-shell binding energy of the phosphor, there is a dramatic increase in characteristic production within the screen. This is the **K-shell absorption edge** (Figure 22-6). The K-shell edges for screen phosphors can result in a dramatic increase in light emission. This causes problems for the radiographer who uses a variable-kVp technical factor system. If the kVp selected happens to be on or slightly above the K-shell edge, a slight decrease in kVp can cause a tremendous decrease in light emission, greatly reducing film density, instead of the slight decrease intended. In the reverse situation, if the original kVp happens to be slightly below the K-shell edge and a slight increase is desired, if the increase activated the K-shell peak, the resulting increase in density might be excessive. On a repeated examination, these situations could require third exposures. Table 22-1 provides the K-shell edges for the most common phosphors. **The kVp level should not be varied around screen-phosphor K-shell edges.** Note that the K-shell edges are stated in keV levels. About 5–6 percent higher kVp levels would be required to produce the maximum number of K-shell edge-level photons for single-phase generators.

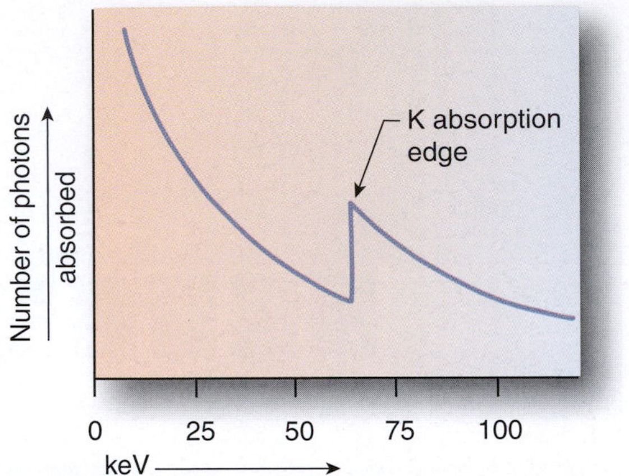

FIGURE 22-6. The K-shell absorption edge effect for calcium tungstate phosphors.

TABLE 22-1. K-Shell Edges for Intensifying-Screen Phosphors

Phosphor	K-Shell Edge	Atomic Number
lanthanum	39 keV	57
gadolinium	50 keV	64
tungsten	70 keV	74

Contrast and Latitude

Intensifying-screen contrast and latitude are insignificant factors because most phosphors have a relatively linear conversion efficiency except for their K-shell edges. Film contrast and latitude are much more critical because of the nonlinear shape of the D log E curve. A slight improvement in screen contrast is achieved by the use of anti-halation crossover dyes in the screens, but their use remains primarily with film base and emulsion. However, the effect of intensifying screens on image contrast is so slight as to be negligible.

CASSETTES AND HOLDERS

Cassettes and holders are designed to create a portable, lightproof case for film to utilize the intensifying screens to best advantage and to attenuate the residual x-ray beam as much as possible (Figure 22-7). Various sizes and types of cassettes are available. Originally, direct exposure film was exposed in a cardboard holder, which is simply a lightproof container. There are numerous specialty cassettes available, such as curved cassettes and cassettes designed for specialty equipment, such as panoramic facial units.

Characteristics

The front of the cassette must be uniformly radiolucent to eliminate artifacts, rigid to provide good support for body parts, and lightweight. The intensifying screens are attached to the inside of the front and back of the cassette. At least one must be mounted on a foam pressure pad to provide good contact between the screens and the film. The back must be rigid and lightweight and may also include a sheet of lead foil to reduce the residual beam and absorb backscatter. Backscatter is a significant problem with large body parts, especially in hypersthenic chest and abdomen examinations. It is caused when the incident beam is of such magnitude that enough backscatter is produced from behind the cassette to form a second image (Figure 22-8). The lead sheet must be minimal in cassettes designed to be used with automatic exposure controls (AECs).

Extremely low-attenuation graphite carbon fiber materials are sometimes used for cassettes, grid interspaces, and tables when low-energy photons may be carrying critical information.

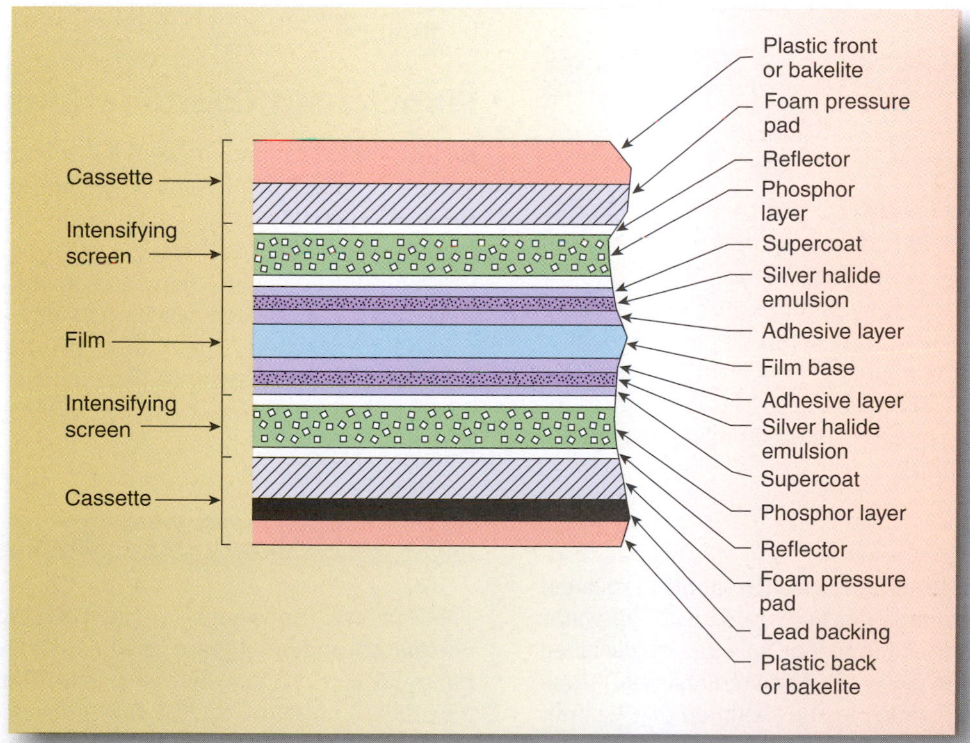

FIGURE 22-7. Cross section of a typical radiographic cassette.

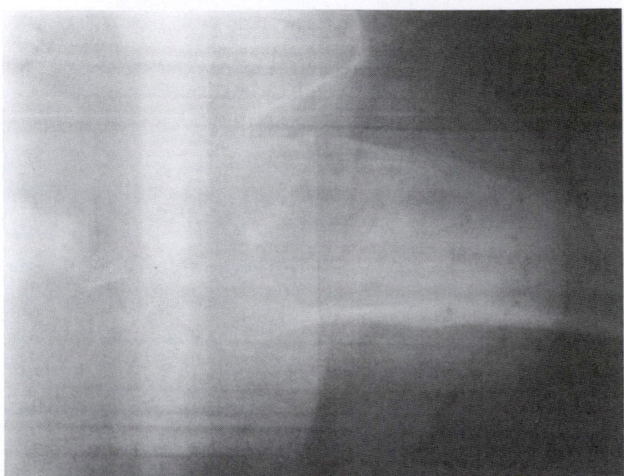

FIGURE 22-8. Backscatter forming an image of a cassette hinge. This resulted from lack of collimation, which permitted the remnant beam to strike a wall and backscatter through the back of the cassette onto the film. *(By permission of Mayo Foundation for Medical Education and Research. All rights reserved.)*

CARE

Loading and Storage

When loading cassettes, the tops should never be fully open in order to prevent dust and condensation from accumulating and to prevent the formation of the artifacts they cause on the radiograph. The cassette top should be opened slightly; 2–3 inches, or 6–8 cm, is enough for the radiographer to unload and load any cassette.

Cassettes should be stored on end like a book and empty of film.

Cleaning

Intensifying screens and cassettes should be cleaned regularly. They must not be cleaned with tap water or any cleaning solution not specifically designed for intensifying screens. Most commercial firms offer an electrostatic cleaning solution that will not leave mineral stains, will not become sticky (resulting in damage when screens stick to film or to one another after cleaning), and discourages static electricity that could discharge and expose film.

Never close a wet cassette because the screens may adhere to one another, permanently damaging their surfaces.

Artifacts

A loaded cassette that is stored near heat, bright sunlight, or in an ionizing radiation area may fog the film as the heat, light, or ionizing radiation activates the screen phosphor slightly. Always store cassettes away from any type of radiation.

A white spot (low density) represents an area where an artifact blocked the transmission of light between the screen and film or prohibited the ionizing radiation from activating the intensifying screen. Pitted screens or dust on the film or screen in the cassette are common causes of white spots. Cleaning the screens will often remove the artifacts.

Poor contact between the film and screens can produce lack of detail. A screen contact quality control test may be performed to verify the artifact diagnosis, but often the cassette and screens must be discarded.

Film/Screen Combinations

Radiographic film and intensifying screens are designed to complement each other and to produce the highest-quality image with the lowest patient radiation dose. Film and screens must be matched to each other to achieve diagnostic-quality images. If the screens have been designed to emit a specific wavelength, then the film must be designed to have enhanced sensitivity to the same wavelength. Mismatching of film and screens often increases patient dose.

EMISSION SPECTRA

The spectral emissions of intensifying screen phosphors and radiographic films are shown in Figure 22-9. Note that blue sensitive film will not respond to most of the wavelengths emitted by the rare-earth phosphors. However, green sensitive film is more sensitive to the entire range of phosphor emissions, including the yellow-green wavelengths. Note also that green sensitive film is

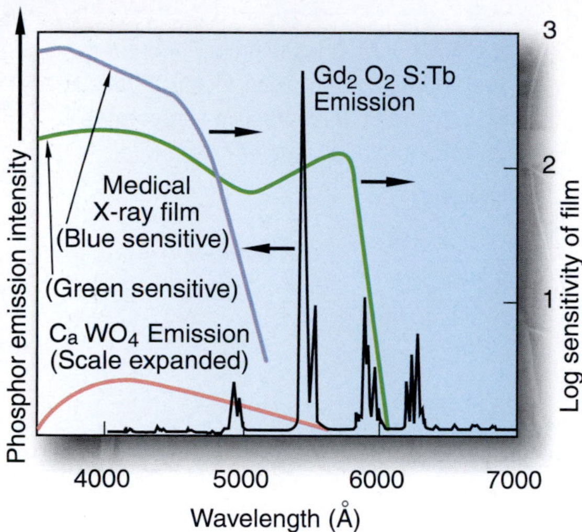

FIGURE 22-9. Light sensitivity of various films and intensifying screens. Note that blue sensitive screens are not sensitive to the major rare-earthlight emissions. *Note.* from "An Improved X-Ray Intensifying Screen," by Robert A. Buchanan, New York, New York. 1971, *IEEE Transactions on Nuclear Science. Copyright 1971 by the IEEE. Reprinted with permission.*

not quite as sensitive to the blue-violet wavelengths as the blue sensitive film.

The appropriate film/screen combination for a specific clinical situation must be selected based on the combined qualities of the film and the screen. Clinical selection cannot be accomplished by evaluating film and intensifying screens separately. The qualities that must be considered are **speed, resolution, contrast**, and **latitude**. Film/screen combination relationships are the same as the interrelationships of these factors for film (see Tables 21-2 and 21-3). The most common decision that must be made when selecting film/screen combinations is image resolution versus patient dose.

CHARACTERISTICS

The important characteristics of film/screen combinations are **speed, resolution, contrast, and latitude**.

Speed

The speed of an imaging system depends on the **thickness of the layer** of phosphor or silver halide, the **crystal/phosphor** size, and the **efficiency** of the crystal/phosphor in emitting (in the case of intensifying screens) or capturing (in the case of silver halides) photons.

Commercial firms use relative speed (RS) numbers to rate film/screen combinations. The numbers are not quantitative and represent no units. They are based on a relative value of 100 for calcium tungstate intensifying screens used with a medium contrast and latitude blue sensitive film. This was the standard film/screen combination known as par or medium speed before the advent of rare-earth screens. Each manufacturer tends to calibrate film/screen combinations to its own brands. However, it has been suggested that the base RS 100 be calibrated equal to 1.28 mR to produce the film speed point (OD 1.00 + base + fog). Relative speed numbers are usually established at 70–80 kVp, with 80 kVp preferred. When kVp values below 70 or above 100 are used, RS numbers may be less consistent. Therefore, the relationship between the RS number and the sensitivity of the film/screen combination is established by the following formula:

$$\text{Sensitivity in mR} = \frac{128}{\text{RS}}$$

Table 22-2 shows the relationship of RS number to the sensitivity in mR to produce the film speed point.

RS numbers are accurate enough to be used by radiographers to convert exposure technique settings from one situation to another. The formula for converting mAs from one relative speed to another is:

$$\frac{mAs_1}{mAs_2} = \frac{RS_2}{RS_1}$$

where: mAs_1 = old mAs
mAs_2 = new mAs
RS_1 = old relative speed
RS_2 = new relative speed

TABLE 22-2. Relationship between Relative Speed Number and Exposure Sensitivity

RS Number	Exposure Sensitivity in mR
1200	0.10
800	0.16
400	0.32
200	0.64
100	1.28
50	2.56
25	5.00
12	10.00

Note: From *Physical Principles of Medical Imaging,* by P. Sprawls, 1987, Rockville, MD: Aspen. Reprinted with permission.

The most common problem is to determine a new mAs for use with a relative speed that is different from the one for which an acceptable technique is known. To determine a new mAs, the following version is used:

$$mAs_2 = \frac{RS_1 \times mAs_1}{RS_2}$$

EXAMPLE: What is the proper mAs for use with a 400-RS system when technical factors of 80 kVp and 50 mAs produce an acceptable image with a 200-RS system?

Answer:

$$\frac{mAs_1}{mAs_2} = \frac{RS_2}{RS_1}$$

$$\frac{50}{mAs_2} = \frac{400}{200}$$

$$mAs_2 \times 400 = 50\text{ mAs} \times 200$$

$$mAs_2 \times 400 = 10{,}000\text{ mAs}$$

$$mAs_2 = \frac{10{,}000\text{ mAs}}{400}$$

$$mAs_2 = 25\text{ mAs}$$

EXAMPLE: What is the proper mAs for use with a 250-RS system when technical factors of 80 kVp and 50 mAs produce an acceptable image with an 800-RS system?

Answer:

$$\frac{mAs_1}{mAs_2} = \frac{RS_2}{RS_1}$$

$$\frac{50}{mAs_2} = \frac{250}{800}$$

$$mAs_2 \times 250 = 50\text{ mAs} \times 800$$

$$mAs_2 \times 250 = 40{,}000\text{ mAs}$$

$$mAs_2 = \frac{40{,}000\text{ mAs}}{250}$$

$$mAs_2 = 160\text{ mAs}$$

Film/screen combinations are available from RS 20 to RS 1,200. An RS combination of 400 is the most common compromise between patient dose and resolution in hospital settings. Although not an absolute relationship, for the most part, higher RS numbers reduce patient dose, decrease latitude, and decrease resolution.

Resolution

Recorded detail, sharpness, and resolution are measured as **line pairs per millimeter (lp/mm**, or cycles per mm), **line spread function (LSF)**, and **modulation transfer function (MTF)**.

Line Pairs per Millimeter. Line pairs per millimeter, or cycles per millimeter, measures the minimum size and space between objects that can be visualized on the final image.

Line Spread Function. The line spread function (LSF) measures the ability of a film/screen system to accurately measure the boundaries of an image. It is calculated by using a microdensitometer to measure the ability of the image receptor to record a line from a 10-mm wide beam of radiation. A typical film/screen system might display densities from a 10-mm line over 600–800 mm.

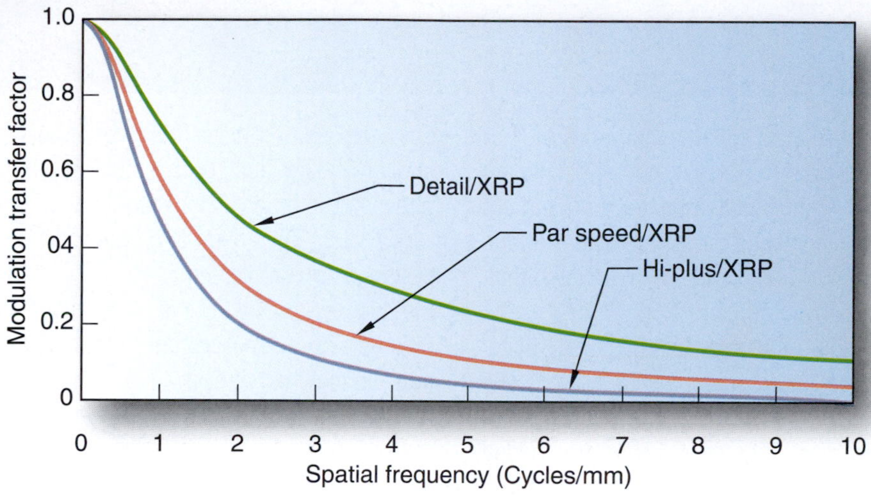

FIGURE 22-10. MTF versus lp/mm for several different film/screen combinations. *(Note: Reprinted from MTF's and Wiener Spectra of Radiographic Screen-Film Systems [HHS Publication FDA 82-8187], by Doi Kunio, G. Holje, L. Loo, and H. Chan, 1982, FDA 82-0187, Rockville, MD: U.S. Department of Health and Human Services, Public Health Service, Food and Drug Administration, Bureau of Radiological Health.)*

Modulation Transfer Function. The modulation transfer function (MTF) provides the best measurement of the resolving ability of a film/screen combination. It measures the information lost between the subject and the image receptor. There are no units of MTF. The MTF is determined primarily by the amount of light diffusion that occurs between the screens and the film. The MTF is primarily controlled by the chemical composition of the screen, phosphor size, thickness of the phosphor layer, absorbing dye, and, most important, by film/screen contact. Therefore, MTF is a function of the screens because the resolving power of film is far superior to that of the intensifying screens. The intensifying screens impose the resolution limitations on the film/screen system.

The MTF is sometimes presented as a formula:

$$\text{MTF} = \frac{\text{Recorded Detail (Resolution)}}{\text{Available Detail (Resolution)}}$$

A perfect MTF would be 1.0. Therefore, MTFs are less than 1.0 because more information cannot be recorded than what is available. An MTF curve plots MTF against resolution (lp/mm) (Figure 22-10). Faster film/screen combinations exhibit an obvious decrease in resolution when compared to the detail combinations.

Contrast

Contrast is primarily the contrast of the film, although intensifying screens, especially the rare earths, also exhibit contrast. The effect of higher contrast that is achieved when lower kVp can be used due to higher speed screens is often overlooked. In addition, the rare-earth phosphors often exhibit slightly higher contrast.

Latitude

The film/screen system latitude is primarily dependent upon the latitude of the film, which is directly related to the contrast. Narrow-latitude film/screen systems exhibit high contrast. High-speed film/speed systems tend to have lower resolution (decreased detail).

SUMMARY

Intensifying screens produce large quantities of light photons when struck by x-rays, thereby amplifying the incoming x-ray beam and reducing patient radiation dose. Over 99 percent of the latent image is formed by light from the screens, with less than 1 percent being contributed by x-ray photons.

An intensifying screen consists of a base, reflective layer, phosphor layer, and protective coat. The base is usually made of polyester plastic and serves to hold the phosphor layer. The reflective layer is added to increase the amount of light reaching the film. The phosphor layer is the active, light-emitting layer of the screen, and the protective coat protects the phosphor layer from abrasions.

The phosphors used in intensifying screens must have a high atomic number, high conversion efficiency, appropriate spectral emission, and minimal phosphorescence. Luminescence is the ability of a material to emit light in response to excitation. The two types of luminescence are fluorescence and phosphorescence.

Various phosphor materials have been used in radiography. The most popular of the phosphors are the rare earths.

Intensifying screens exhibit the same characteristics as film: resolution, speed, contrast, and latitude. Resolution and speed are affected by phosphor crystal size, layer thickness, and the concentration of the crystals. Contrast and latitude are relatively insignificant factors.

Cassettes and holders are designed to create a portable, lightproof case for the film, to utilize the intensifying screens to best advantage, and to attenuate the residual x-ray beam as much as possible. Cassettes should never be fully open when loading and unloading film. Both cassettes and intensifying screens should be cleaned regularly.

Radiographic film and intensifying screens are designed to complement each other and to produce the highest-quality image with the lowest patient radiation dose. To accomplish this, film and screens must be matched to each other, especially with regard to their emission spectra. Mismatching of film and screens increases patient dose.

The qualities that must be considered in a film/screen combination are speed, resolution, contrast, and latitude. The most frequent decision that must be made when selecting film/screen combinations is image resolution versus patient dose.

Commercial firms use relative speed (RS) numbers to rate film/screen combinations. The formula for converting mAs from one relative speed to another is:

$$\frac{mAs_1}{mAs_2} = \frac{RS_2}{RS_1}$$

Recorded detail, sharpness, and resolution are measured as line pairs per millimeter (lp/mm, or cycles per mm), line spread function (LSF), and modulation transfer function (MTF). Contrast is primarily the contrast of the film, although intensifying screens, especially the rare earths, also affect contrast. The film/screen system latitude is primarily dependent upon the latitude of the film. The selection of appropriate film/screen combinations requires consideration of the various film and screen characteristics and of the clinical situation for which they are to be used. ■

REVIEW QUESTIONS

1. How do intensifying screens reduce patient dose?
2. What are the four basic components of an intensifying screen?
3. What characteristics should an intensifying screen phosphor possess?
4. What is the difference between fluorescence and phosphorescence?
5. What is the relationship between resolution and phosphor crystal size, layer thickness, and phosphor concentration?
6. What is quantum mottle?
7. What is the purpose of a cassette?
8. What is the formula used to calculate a relative speed conversion from one film/screen combination to another?
9. What are the three methods of measuring resolution?
10. How is film/screen contrast related to latitude?

REFERENCES AND RECOMMENDED READING

Ardran, G. M., Crooks, H. E., & James, V. (1969). Testing x-ray cassettes for film-intensifying screen contact. *Radiography, 35*(414), 143.

Burgess, A. E., & Hicken, P. (1982, May). Comparative performance of x-ray intensifying screens. *Radiology,* 55.

Bushberg, J. T., Seibert, J. A., Leidholdt, E. M., & Boone, J. M. (2003). *The essential physics of medical imaging* (2nd ed.). Baltimore: Lippincott, Williams & Wilkins.

Carroll, Q. B. (2003). *Fuchs's radiographic exposure, processing, and quality control* (7th ed.). Springfield, IL: Charles C Thomas.

Cullinan, A., & Cullinan, J. (1994). *Producing quality radiographs* (2nd ed.). Philadelphia: J. B. Lippincott.

Curry, T. S., Dowdey, J. E., & Murry, R. C. (1990). *Christensen's introduction to the physics of diagnostic radiology* (4th ed.). Philadelphia: Lea and Febiger.

Doi, K., Holje, G., Loo, L., & Chan, H. (1982). *MTF's and Wiener spectra of radiographic screen-film systems* HHS Publication FDA 82-8187. Rockville, MD: United States Department of Health and Human Services, Public Health Service, Food and Drug Administration, Bureau of Radiological Health.

Doi, K., Loo, L., Anderson, T. M., & Frank, P. H. (1981). Effect of crossover exposure on radiographic image quality of screen-film systems. *Radiology, 139,* 707–714.

Fuchs, A. W. (1947). Edison and röntgenology. *The American Journal of Röntgenology and Radium Therapy, 57*(2), 145–156.

Fuchs, A. W. (1956). Evolution of Röntgen film. *The American Journal of Röntgenology and Radium Therapy, 75*(1), 30–48.

Haus, A. G., & Cullinan, J. E. (1989). Screen film processing systems for medical radiography: A historical review. *Radiographics, 9*(6), 1203–1224.

Higashida, Y., Frank, P. H., & Doi, K. (1983, November). High-speed, single-screen/single-emulsion film systems: Basic imaging properties and preliminary clinical applications. *Radiology,* 571.

Jenkins, D. (1980). *Radiographic photography and imaging processes.* Lancaster, England: MTP Press Limited.

Kodera, Y., Doi, K., & Chan, H. (1984). Absolute speeds of screen-film systems and their absorbed-energy constants. *Radiology, 151,* 229–236.

McKinney, W. (1988). *Radiographic processing and quality control.* Philadelphia: J. B. Lippincott.

Morgan, R. H. (1953). Röntgenoscopic screen intensification. *Radiologic Technology, 25*(2), 80.

Rao, G. U. V., & Fatouros, P. P. (1978). The relationship between resolution and speed of x-ray intensifying screens. *Medical Physics, 5,* 205–208.

Rao, G. U. V., Fatouros, P. P., & James, A. E. (1978). Physical characteristics of modern radiographic screen-film systems. *Investigative Radiology, 13,* 460.

Schmidt, R. A. (1983, March). Evaluation of cassette performance: Physical factors affecting patient exposure and image contrast. *Radiology,* 801.

Shearer, D. R., & Moore, M. M. (1986). Lag in radiographic imaging systems: Simple methods for evaluation. *Radiology, 159*(1), 259–263.

Sklensky, A. F., Buchanan, R. A., Maple, T. G., & Bailey, H. N. (1974). Quantum utilization in x-ray intensifying screens. *The Institute of Electrical and Electronics Engineers Transactions on Nuclear Science, 21,* 685–691.

Skucas, J., & Gorski, J. (1980). Application of modern intensifying screens in diagnostic radiology. *Medical Radiography and Photography, 56*(2), 25–36.

Sprawls, P. (1987). *Physical principles of medical imaging.* Rockville, MD: Aspen.

Sprawls, P. (1990). *Principles of radiography for technologists.* Rockville, MD: Aspen.

Sturm, R. E., & Morgan, R. H. (1949). Screen intensification systems and their limitations. *The American Journal of Röntgenology and Radium Therapy, 62*(5), 617–634.

Sweeney, R. J. (1983). *Radiographic artifacts: Their cause and control.* Philadelphia: J. B. Lippincott.

Taylor, K. W., McLeich, B. P., Hobbs, B. B., & Hughes, T. J. (1980). Selection of screen-film combinations. *The Canadian Journal of Medical Radiation Technology, 11*(3), 154.

Thompson, M. A., Hattaway, M. P., Hall, J. D., & Dowd, S. B. (1994). *Principles of imaging science and protection.* Philadelphia: W. B. Saunders.

Trout, E. D., & Kelley, J. P. (1973). The effect of the temperature of intensifying screens on radiographic exposure. *Radiologic Technology, 45*(2), 70–72.

U.S. Department of Health, Education, and Welfare, Food and Drug Administration. (1976). Bureau of Radiological Health. *First Image Receptor Conference: Film/screen combinations* (HEW Publication [FDA] 77-8003). Washington, DC: Authors.

Venema, H. W. (1979). X-ray absorption, speed, and luminescent efficiency of rare earth and other intensifying screens. *Radiology, 130,* 765–771.

Vyborny, C. J. (1980, August). Relative efficiencies of energy to photographic density conversions in typical screen-film systems. *Radiology,* 465.

Wilson, P. (1977). Principles of intensifying screens in image formation. *Canadian Journal of Radiography, Radiotherapy, and Nuclear Medicine, 8*(3), 134–140.

Wolbarst, A. B. (1993). *Physics of radiology.* Norwalk, CT: Appleton & Lange.

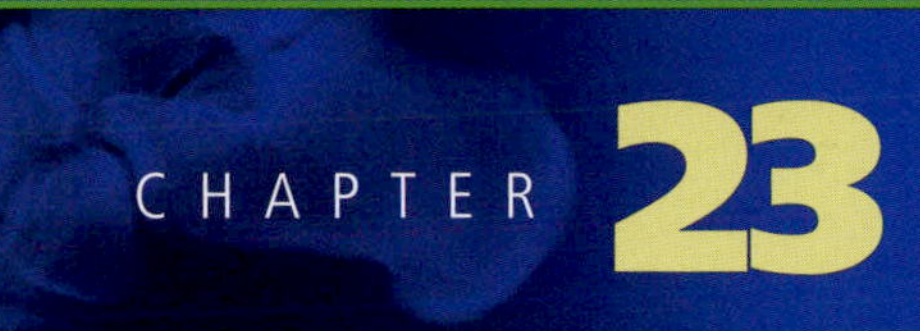

Digital Radiography

Barbara Smith,
Richard R. Carlton,
Arlene Adler

KEY TERMS

bit
byte
computed radiography (CR)
detective quantum efficiency (DQE)
deviation index (DI)
digital radiography (DR)
direct conversion
edge enhancement
flat panel detector
grayscale bit depth
high-pass filtering
histogram
indirect conversion
look-up table (LUT)
low-pass filtering
matrix
photostimulable storage phosphor imaging plate
pixel
pixel pitch
rescaling
signal-to-noise ratio
spatial resolution
windowing

My body is the frame wherein 'tis held,
And perspective it is the painter's art.
For through the painter must you see his skill,
To find where your true image pictured lies;

Shakespeare, Sonnet XXIV

OBJECTIVES

Upon completion of this chapter, the student should be able to:

- Discuss the various types of digital radiography systems.
- Describe the process of digital image data formation.
- Explain the types of digital image processing operations.
- Describe the process by which the histogram is acquired and the look-up table (LUT) is applied to the collected data.
- Explain the function of digital image window level and width controls.
- Describe the factors that affect digital image quality.
- Describe various digital radiography image receptor and detector systems.
- Explain critical elements used in the different digital radiography systems.
- Explain why digital radiography systems have significantly greater latitude than conventional film/screen radiography systems.

OBJECTIVES (continued)

- Analyze elements of digital radiography systems that make them prone to violation of ALARA radiation protection concepts.
- Explain the causes of several digital radiography artifact problems.

HISTORICAL DEVELOPMENT

The future of medical imaging continues to be driven by computer applications in the numerous modalities that currently exist, as well as in the integration of new systems now on the horizons of research and development. The explosion of the imaging sciences that took place between the early 1970s and the 1990s was caused by the first wave of digital computerization in computed tomography (CT) and ultrasound. Computed tomography captured the imagination of the public. Digital processing has now been successfully applied to nuclear medicine, cardiovascular imaging, and magnetic resonance imaging (MRI) and predominates in diagnostic imaging and mammography as well.

The method by which these imaging modalities handle the digital processing of imaging information requires radiographers to understand anatomy from transverse, sagittal, and coronal perspectives. Those who work in the radiologic and imaging sciences must often visualize anatomy as a dynamic three-dimensional tilting, rotating, and tumbling process due to computer manipulation of imaging data in four dimensions. This is especially true in order to correlate CT and MRI with radiographic images in the diagnostic process.

Digital radiography imaging systems replace traditional film with a reusable detector. These systems are divided into two types generally known as **computed radiography (CR)** and **digital radiography (DR).** Computed radiography systems uses a **photostimulable storage phosphor imaging plate** (PSP or IP) typically inside a cassette. This cassette can be used in a bucky or for portable exams, similar to traditional film/screen systems. Once the PSP is exposed, the cassette is taken to a reader to process the plate and create the image. With these systems, there is a two-step process because the radiographer must move the detector between image acquisition and display. There are some PSP systems that are permanently fixed in units that do not require this two-step process; however, they are not the norm. Digital radiography (DR) systems typically have the detector and reader that are a permanent part of a table or wall unit; therefore, a cassette is not needed. Newer technology has now made some of these systems wireless and they can resemble a sealed cassette that can be moved around a room from a table bucky to an upright unit. With these systems, great care must be taken in moving the wireless DR unit as it is a very expensive device. With DR systems, the image is acquired and sent directly to the display monitor without the need for the radiographer to physically move the detector for the image to be processed. This makes these systems faster and more efficient at creating an image.

There are a number of detector configurations used in DR that employ either **direct conversion** (without scintillator) or **indirect conversion** (with scintillator). Indirect conversion detectors use a two-part process involving a scintillator (which converts incoming x-ray photons to light) and a photodetector (which converts light into an electronic signal). Indirect systems include those used in CR (PSP technology) and those used in DR, including either a charged coupled device (CCD) or amorphous silicon with a thin film transistor (TFT) array. Direct conversion detectors directly convert incoming x-ray photons to an electronic signal. These systems use amorphous selenium and a TFT. The term **flat panel detector** is also being used to describe both the indirect amorphous silicon and the direct amorphous selenium plates that are being used in some digital systems, and although CCDs are not technically flat panel detectors, they will be discussed under this header.

DIGITAL IMAGE FORMATION

A digital image is one that has been converted into numerical values for transmission or processing. Digital radiography systems have replaced traditional film with a reusable detector. In order to understand digital systems you must have some understanding of how computers manage data.

Computers operate from a binary machine language. Just as English has a 26-letter-symbol alphabet, the binary system operates with a two-symbol alphabet. Because electrical currents are most easily understood as being either on or off, the binary system consists of information recorded as either a 0 for off or a 1 for on. Each binary number is called a **bit,** for binary digit. Nominal numbers function on a base 10 system instead of base 2. Table 23-1 illustrates how the numbers 1 through 10 are written in binary code. An 8-bit word is required to form the 26 letters of the English alphabet. As a convenience, an 8-bit word is called a **byte.** Computer memory is often rated in terms of the total byte memory (rounded off). For example, a 10-megabyte magnetic hard disk will store over 10,000,000 bytes (80,000,000 bits) of information.

TABLE 23-1. Binary Code Numbers

Arabic	Binary
1	1
2	10
3	11
4	100
5	101
6	110
7	111
8	1000
9	1001
10	1010
.	.
.	.
.	.
.	.
16	10000
.	.
.	.
.	.
32	100000
.	.
.	.

Digital Image Characteristics

Computerized digital images are described in terms of the number of values displayed per image. A **matrix** is a series of boxes laid out in rows and columns that gives form to the image (Figure 23-1A). The matrix in Figure 23-1A would be described as a 4 × 4 matrix. Each box of an image matrix will display a numerical value that can be transformed into a visual brightness or density level (Figures 23-1B and C). The individual matrix boxes are known as picture elements or **pixels.** Each pixel location is determined by its address. (For example, in Figure 23-1A the address of the labeled pixel is 4,3.)

The total number of pixels in the matrix would be calculated by multiplying the number of boxes in the row by the number of boxes in the column. For example, a matrix of 512 × 512 would have a total of 262,144 pixels that form the image. In medical imaging, each pixel represents a three-dimensional volume of tissue known as a voxel.

The overall dimension of the image matrix is called the field of view (FOV). In digital radiography systems, the FOV is determined by the size of the detector, whereas in other modalities, such as CT and MRI, the operator can select the FOV for a particular study. If the FOV remains the same, then as matrix size increases, the pixels must get smaller, creating a sharper image. For example, if the overall dimensions of the matrix are 400 × 400 mm and the matrix size is 200 × 200, then every pixel would be 2 mm in size. If the overall dimensions of the matrix remains unchanged at 400 × 400 mm and the matrix size is increased to 400 × 400, then every pixel would be smaller, only 1 mm in size. The greater the matrix size for the same FOV, the better the **spatial resolution** because a larger matrix provides smaller pixels. Spatial resolution or image sharpness is a critical image quality factor that is determined by pixel size. Spatial resolution is measured in line pairs per millimeter (lp/mm) and in digital imaging it can be no better than the size of the pixel (Figure 23-2).

Each pixel in the matrix is capable of representing a wide range of different shades of gray from pure white through total black. The

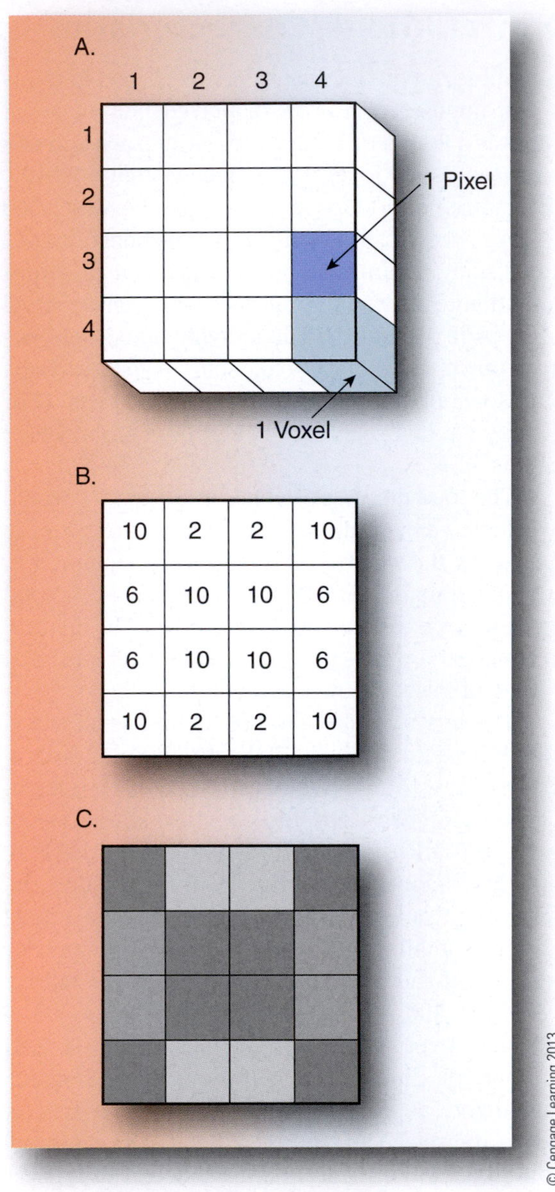

FIGURE 23-1. Digital image matrix expressions: (A) a matrix; (B) a matrix with numerical values; and (C) a matrix with visual density values corresponding to the numerical values in B.

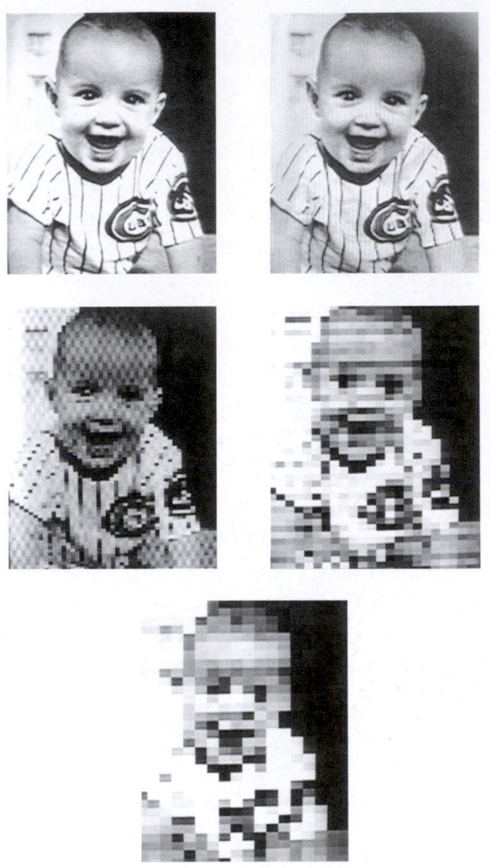

FIGURE 23-2. The effect of matrix size on resolution. *(Photographs courtesy of Richard R. Carlton.)*

number of shades of gray is determined by the **grayscale bit depth**. Grayscale bit depth ranges from 8 bits to 32 bits. A grayscale bit depth of 8–32 equals a range of 1–4 bytes of storage that would be required per pixel in the image matrix. A grayscale bit depth of 12 produces 2^{12} gray levels. This represents 4,096 different shades of gray that are available, a spectacular diagnostic range that is far beyond the range of the human visual system. This is also known as density resolution.

The radiologic community has promulgated a digital standard for imaging known as the Digital Imaging and Communication in Medicine (DICOM) standard. It is designed to ensure that all equipment from all manufacturers who choose to adhere to the standard is speaking the same computer language that can be understood across manufacturer and device lines. This also allows images to be transferred between institutions.

Spatial Domains

Digital images are represented in two domains, based on how the image is acquired. Images in the spatial location domain are based on a matrix that has specific locations for each pixel. The spatial location is usually described as the pixel location, with the x coordinate representing the location of the pixel on a horizontal line from left to right followed by the y coordinate representing the location of the pixel on a vertical line from top to bottom. Images in the spatial frequency domain are based on the number of cycles per unit length (which is the definition of frequency). The spatial frequency is usually described as the resolution (object size) and the contrast. Small structures produce high frequency and high contrast. Low frequency is produced by larger structures and low contrast. The Fourier transformation (FT) is the mathematical algorithm that is applied to change an image from the spatial location domain to the spatial frequency domain, and an inverse FT can be used to return an image back to the spatial location domain. Physicians and radiographers view images in the spatial location domain, whereas physicists and engineers can extract information from the mathematical representations of the image in the spatial frequency domain.

IMAGE PROCESSING OPERATIONS

There are a number of computer operations that can occur to process the image. These image processing operations are primarily intended to change the input values of the pixels to improve the diagnostic quality of the output image. They include (1) point processing, (2) local processing, and (3) geometric processing. Of these, point processing operations are the most important to understand for digital radiography systems.

Point Processing Operations

Point processing operations are those that are performed between the receipt of the input image from the image receptor and the output image that is viewed on the monitor. Point processing operations involve adjusting the value of an input pixel (point) to the corresponding output pixel and are the most common processing operations in digital radiography. One common point processing operation is called grayscale processing, which then allows for adjustments to image brightness and contrast. This process involves the creation of a **histogram** and the application of the **look-up table (LUT)** and **windowing**.

A histogram is generated during initial processing from the image data that allows the digital system to find the useful signal by locating the minimum and maximum signal within the anatomical regions of interest in the image. To generate a histogram, the scanned area is divided into pixels and the signal intensity for each pixel is determined. An example of pixel values with the corresponding bar graph and histogram are shown in Figure 23-3.

The shape of a histogram will correspond to the specific anatomy and technique used for an exam. The system will perform a histogram analysis to determine the values of interest (VOI) and the exposure index. (Figure 23-4 shows the histogram with VOI). The VOI is used to locate the minimum and maximum exposure values for the body part. This histogram is compared to a reference histogram stored in the computer. Each body part has a reference histogram that was obtained using the correct exposure factors. If the exposure is outside the range from underexposure or overexposure then the computer will correct the image by shifting or **rescaling** the histogram to the correct area (Figure 23-5). This is referred to as histogram modification or stretching. A wide histogram demonstrates higher contrast, whereas a narrow histogram shows lower contrast. If the histogram values are concentrated in lower comparative values the image appears dark or dim. If the histogram values are concentrated in higher comparative values the image appears bright or light.

The next step is to adjust the contrast. The digital detector has a linear response that would result in a low-contrast image if it is displayed without this step. An LUT is applied to the data that has the standard contrast for that exam to give the desired image contrast for

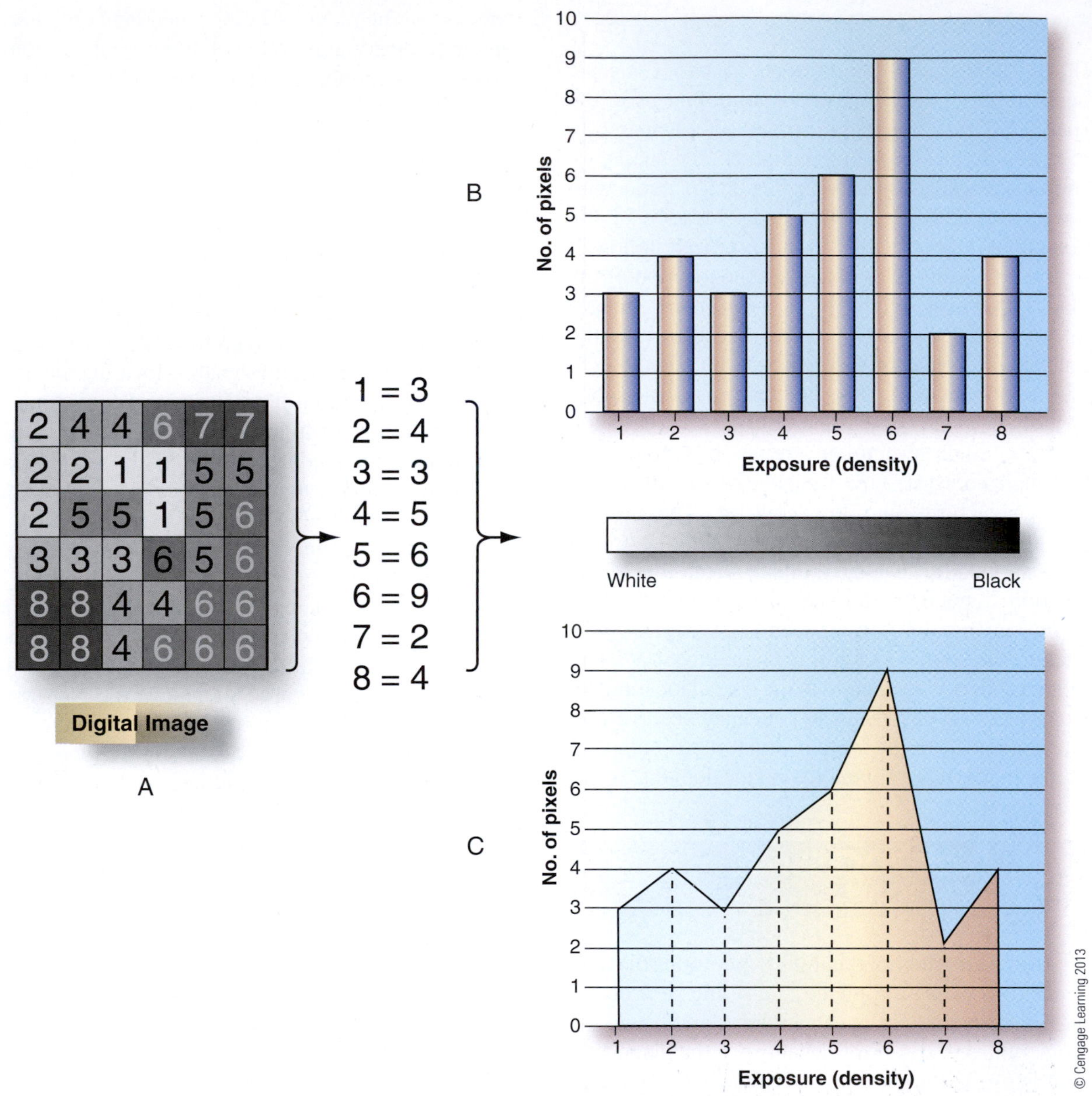

FIGURE 23-3. (A) Matrix with pixel values for radiation exposure; (B) pixel values displayed as a bar graph. The vertical axis represents the number of pixels. The horizontal axis represents the quantity of information (image density). Low density is to the left, high density to the right. (C) The same information displayed as a histogram.

display (Figure 23-6). Selecting the proper projection by informing the processing system of which projection it is to process ensures that the proper LUT will be applied when the image is processed. The LUT contains stored data to substitute new values for each pixel during processing. The proper LUT will provide the proper grayscale, regardless of variations in kVp and mAs, resulting in consistent images. However, **if the exposure values are far outside the normal range, the system cannot compensate and produce a diagnostic image**. This is why radiographers must set exposure factors that will produce images

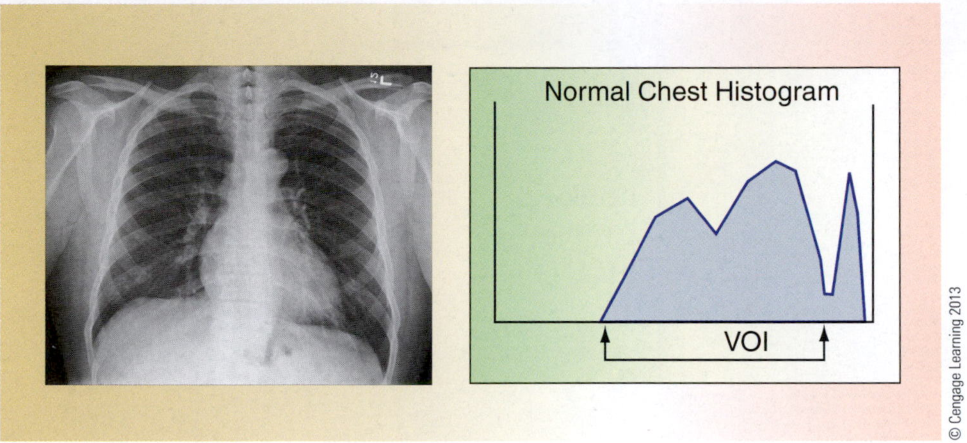

FIGURE 23-4. Histogram of the chest with VOI identified.

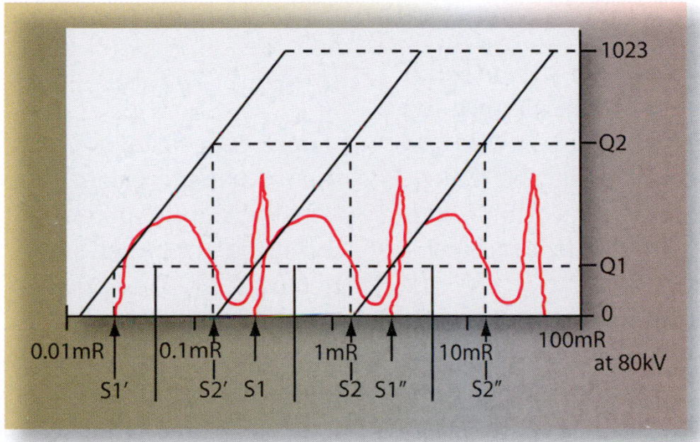

FIGURE 23-5. Digital systems compensate for over- or underexposures by automatically rescaling based on histogram data. The center graph illustrates appropriate data with over- and underexposure to the right and left, repectively. *(Courtesy of FUJIFILM Medical Systems USA.)*

within normal exposure ranges for specific projections if a digital system is to function properly.

Windowing is a point processing operation that changes the contrast and brightness of the image on the monitor. The brightness (density) and contrast of the digital image depends on the shades of gray, which are controlled by varying the numerical values of each pixel. The human visual range encompasses 32 or fewer shades of gray, whereas the photon beam that exits the patient encompasses over 1,000 different variations. Most digital image detectors are sensitive to the majority of these 1,000 differences. Remember that a 12-bit depth will have 4,096 shades of gray from white to black. Because the range of stored densities is so much wider than the visual range, any digital image is only a small part of the total data obtained by the computer. Each image is only a "window" on the total range of data. The window width (WW) is the range of densities that will be displayed; a narrow width will have few densities, so the image will have high contrast, whereas a large width will have a lot of densities, resulting in low contrast. The window level is the center of the window

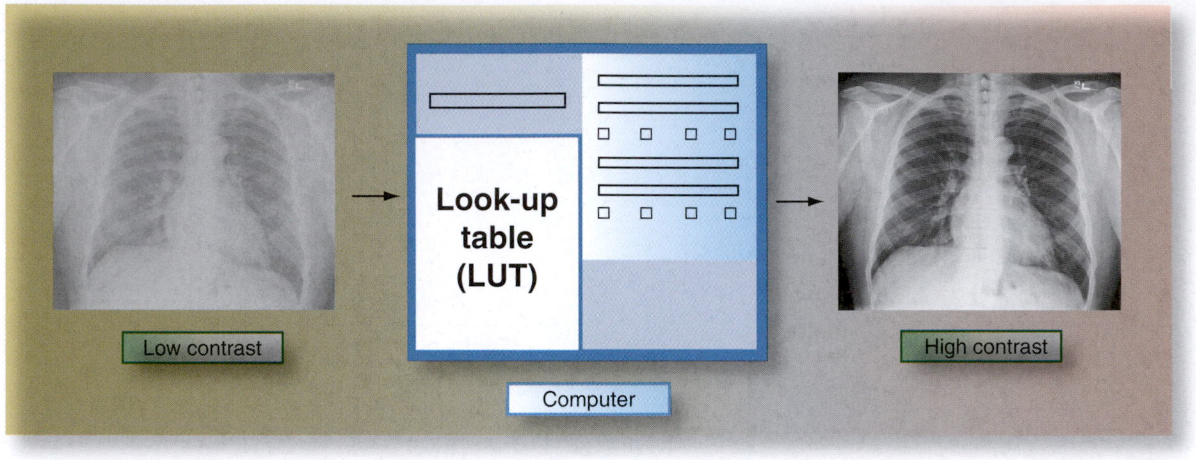

FIGURE 23-6. A chest image before and after the LUT has been applied to adjust the brightness and contrast.

width and controls the brightness of the image; if the level is set at the low end of the scale then the overall image will be light, whereas a setting at the high end would cause the image to be darker. The computer can easily change the level and width of the display window by mathematical recalculations (Figure 23-7).

The quantity of information stored for each pixel varies depending on the grayscale (bit depth) imaging abilities of the system. The radiographer controls which portion of this vast amount of information will be seen by manipulating the data prior to sending it to PACS, affecting the image that the radiologists will use to diagnose. Radiologists can manipulate the data that is sent to them; however, the more the technologist changes the original data before it is sent to PACS, the less information the radiologist has to work with. It is critical that radiographers who are required to produce digital images be familiar with the manner in which the computer determines what portion of the image information will be displayed. Careful image processing is critical to avoid obscuring diagnostically critical information.

In addition, both image subtraction and temporal averaging are considered to be point processing operations. These functions are used primarily in digital subtraction angiography.

Local Processing Operations

Local processing operations are those in which mathematical calculations are applied to only a small group of pixels, although the operation will often be continued until all pixels have been subjected to it. This process is often referred to as a kernel. A kernel is processing code that is mandatory and common to the computer system. It is normally applied over and over to the entire set of data being processed. Local processing is also called area or group processing.

Spatial frequency filtering is considered a type of local processing operation. It is used to sharpen, smooth, blur, reduce noise, or pull elements of interest from an image. It can occur in the spatial location domain or in the spatial frequency domain. When spatial frequency filtering is done in the spatial frequency domain the Fourier transform is used. When it is done in the spatial location domain the pixel values themselves are used.

High-pass filtering (which is also referred to as **edge enhancement** or sharpness) uses a Fourier transform algorithm to convert the image into the spatial frequency domain. Then a high-pass filter is applied to remove low spatial frequency and produce a sharper output image (Figure 23-8). When the frequencies that represent structures of interest can

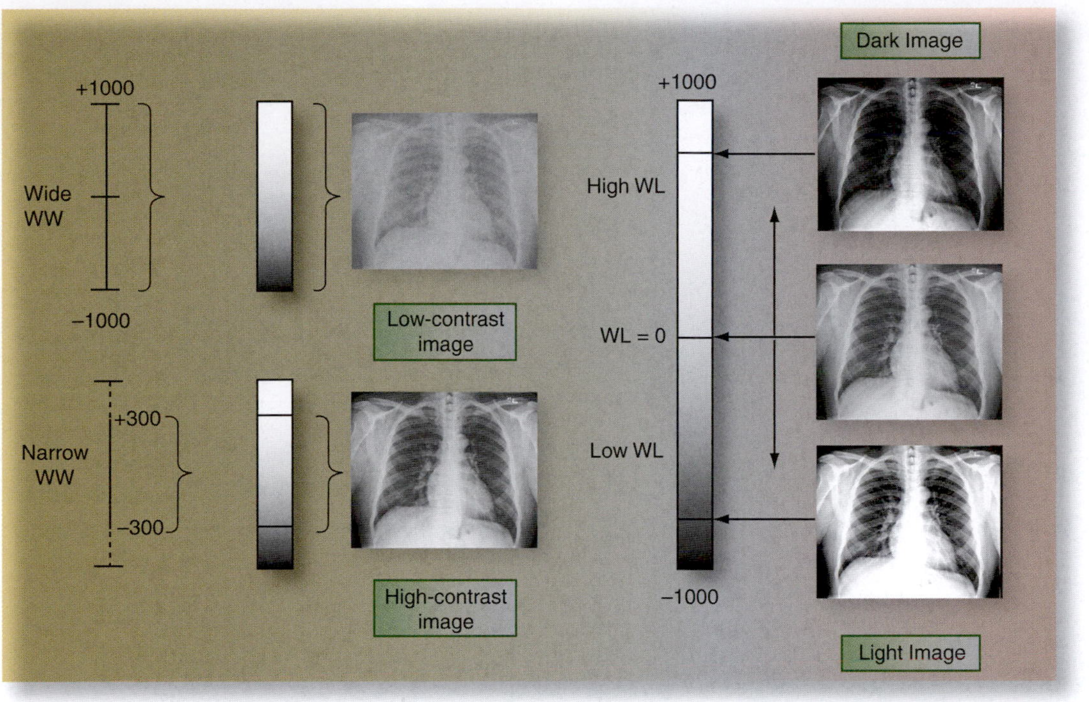

FIGURE 23-7. The effect of windowing the width for contrast and windowing the level for brightness.

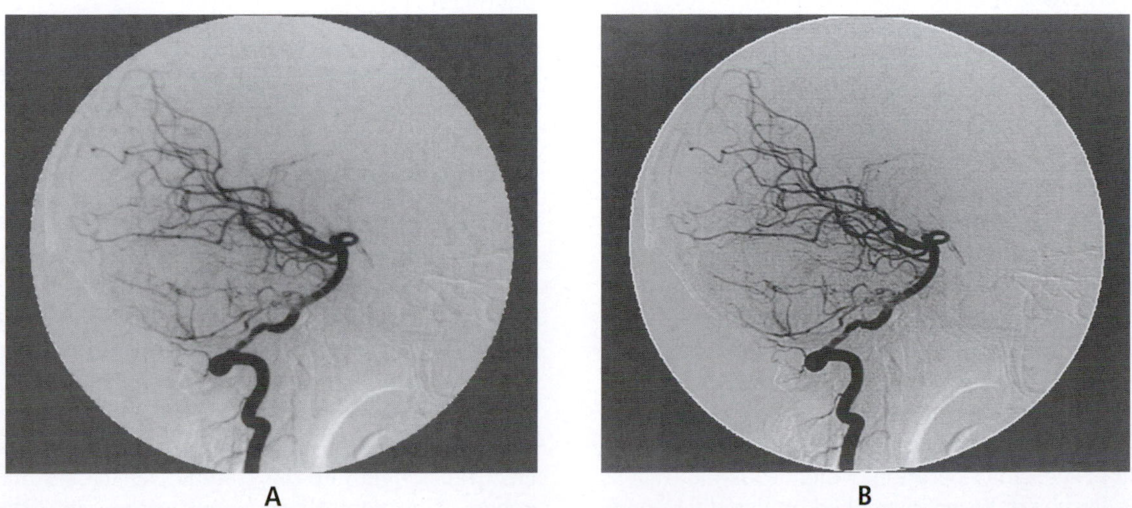

FIGURE 23-8. High-pass filtering or sharpening. Edge enhancement is demonstrated on these digital subtraction angiograms: (A) normal image and (B) with high-pass filtering. *(Courtesy of Rick Halker, Lima Memorial Hospital, Lima, OH.)*

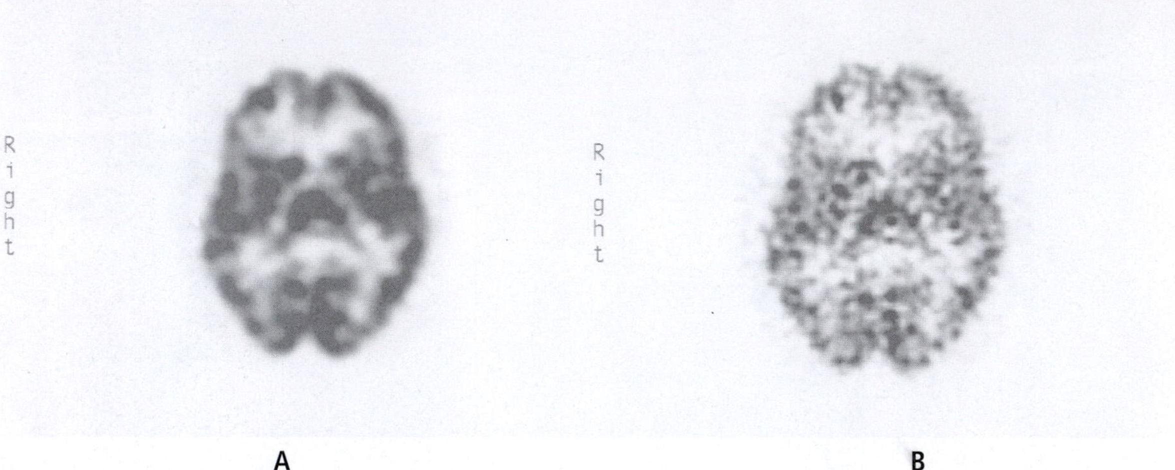

FIGURE 23-9. Low-pass filtering or smoothing. Transverse brain sections from a nuclear medicine study: (A) smoothed and (B) noisier filter. *(Courtesy of Mike Ballistrea, Department of Nuclear Medicine, Meridia Hillcrest Hospital, Mayfield Heights, OH.)*

be identified, as in contrast-medium–filled vessels, amplification of their frequencies can produce an edge enhancement effect while other frequencies are actually suppressed. The result is an image with edge enhancement and greatly increased contrast. This type of high-pass filtering is useful in digital vascular imaging and in digital mammography. However, extremely small structures can sometimes be buried in an edge, and undesirable edges are usually enhanced as well as those that are of diagnostic value.

Low-pass filtering (which is also referred to as smoothing) uses a similar process to intentionally blur the image, thus reducing noise and the displayed brightness level of the pixels (Figure 23-9). This process also decreases image detail, which is not good. Therefore, low-pass filtered images should also be viewed in a normal or high-pass mode.

Unsharp masking (which is also referred to as blurring) subtracts a low-pass filtered (blurred) image from the original image, thus producing a new subtracted and sharper image.

Spatial location filtering is another type of local processing operation, which is also known as convolution. A kernel is applied repeatedly to each pixel in a matrix in order to weigh the values or to apply a coefficient across the matrix. Application of convolution kernels usually works better when array processors can be used to rapidly apply them.

Geometric Processing Operations

Geometric processing operations are used to change the position or orientation of the pixels in the image. This allows rotation, magnification, and other operations similar to those used in digital photographs.

DIGITAL IMAGE QUALITY

Resolution

Spatial resolution is controlled by the matrix size and how many pixels can be displayed by the monitor. There is a direct relationship between matrix and pixel size and spatial resolution. When matrix size is increased and pixel size goes down, spatial resolution increases. Matrix size is not typically variable within a system. It is controlled by the design of image detectors and the accompanying electronics built into the system. Density resolution is part of bit depth (how much information can be held by each pixel in terms of the number of gray-scale levels that can be displayed). High-resolution mammography systems with a matrix of 4096 × 4096 can provide 12-bit depth. Greater bit depth

TABLE 23-2. Typical Memory Requirements for Various Imaging Modalities

Imaging Modality	Typical Image Matrix	Grayscale Bit Depth	Images per Typical Exam	Approximate Storage Requirements
Digital Mammography	4096 × 4096	12	4	80 Mb
Computed Radiography	3520 × 4280	12	4	50 Mb
Digital Fluoroscopy	1024 × 1024	8	24 sec × 5 min	7.5 Gb
Computed Tomography	512 × 512	16	120	60 Mb
Computed Tomography—MSCT	512 × 512	16	2,000	1 Gb
Ultrasound	512 × 512	32	50	50 Mb
Magnetic Resonance Imaging	256 × 256	16	2,000	1 Gb
Nuclear Medicine	128 × 128	8	100	25 Mb

provides better density resolution. Typical matrix sizes and bit depths for various imaging modalities along with typical storage requirements are shown in Table 23-2.

Noise

Noise can be classified as either electronic system noise or quantum mottle noise. Electronic system noise is a result of undesirable signals from the digital system itself, often through normal functioning. Electronic system noise is random background information that is detected but does not contribute to image quality. It is congruent with audio noise, such as the static "white noise" heard on frequencies between radio stations (although most modern radios suppress the sound between stations). It is measured as the **signal-to-noise ratio** (S/N). A high S/N indicates little noise in the image. Image noise has an inverse relationship to contrast. Increased noise decreases image contrast. Conversely, increased image contrast tends to obscure or decrease noise. The effect of image noise on density is irrelevant in digital imaging, because the computer can easily compensate for lack of density as long as sufficient contrast exists to differentiate diagnostic data from noise.

Quantum mottle noise results from an insufficient quantity of photons from improperly set exposure factors (mAs and kVp). This produces a grainy image that is easily corrected by increasing mAs or kVp, depending on which is appropriate for the clinical situation. Although these increases produce better-quality images, they also increase patient exposure. The correct exposure is a combination of image quality achieved with reasonable patient exposure.

Detective Quantum Efficiency (DQE)

Detective quantum efficiency (DQE) is a measure of the sensitivity and accuracy by which the image receptor converts the incoming data to the output viewing device. A perfect device would perform this task with 100 percent efficiency (no loss of information) or with a DQE of 1, so DQEs are lower than 1. Digital radiography systems have DQEs of 0.3–0.7 or 30–70 percent.

EXPOSURE INDICATORS

Exposure Index

It is important for the radiographer to understand the exposure indicator numbers provided by most manufacturers on each image produced, as well as how to use this data to assess image quality. Digital radiography processing systems use exposure indicators to provide information regarding the exposure to the image receptor, which is useful to indirectly determine patient exposure. The correct exposure factors will deliver an exposure indicator that is within an acceptable range and will give the best image quality. There is no universal system at this time, and different manufacturers use different systems for this information.

The American Association of Physicists in Medicine (AAPM) released preliminary information on its attempts to quantify exposure index information in the summer of 2009. The International Electrotechnical Commission (IEC) has also released information in this regard. The most important concept detailed in these early reports is the definition of the term **deviation index (DI),** which is defined as an "indicator as to whether the detector response of a specified image K_{IND} agrees with K_{TGT}." K_{IND} is defined as the indicated equivalent air Kerma, which is essentially the radiation dose measurement for the incoming photon beam at the detector surface. K_{TGT} is defined as the target equivalent air Kerma, which is essentially the radiation dose measurement for a proper exposure to the detector. **Therefore, the DI is essentially a comparison between the actual exposure and the proper exposure received by the image detector**.

Exposure indicators reflect the amount of x-ray exposure to an imaging plate, which looks at the quantity of photons that strike the detector. Exposure indicator numbers can be used as a quality control tool for image quality and radiation protection.

Different manufacturers calibrate the response of their systems with different beam qualities and report the results using parameters that have different dependencies on exposure. Therefore, it is extremely difficult to compare the sensitivity of one system with that of another. In addition, as manufacturers improve their systems they sometimes introduce entirely new image receptors and software enhancements that also cause sensitivity measures to change.

The exposure sensitivity of imaging detectors ranges from a minimum of 0.1 mR up to a maximum of 100 mR, a range of approximately 1,000:1 (Table 23-3). If soft tissue and bone densities are required, one exposure will give the information owing to the ability to change window levels. In order to evaluate the exposure for an image, most manufacturers have an exposure indicator that provides information on the average amount of radiation used to produce an ideal diagnostic image.

The Fuji, Konica, and Philips computed radiography systems use a sensitivity number (S number) to assist in evaluating exposure. It is inversely proportional to the exposure reaching the imaging plate. For example, an S value of 200 indicates that the imaging plate received about 1 mR (approximately the same exposure necessary to produce a diagnostic density image with a typical 200-RS film/screen combination). A higher S value indicates that the imaging plate (IP) was underexposed, whereas a lower S value indicates overexposure of the IP. Fuji's sensitivity numbers are calculated by the formula: S = 200/(exposure in mR). Generally with these systems the S values relate back to film/screen speed systems; in other words, 400-speed film/screen systems used lower exposure factors than 200-speed systems, so an S number of 400 means less exposure was used. Properly exposed imaging plates should produce S values of 150–250 (Figure 23-10).

The Carestream (formerly Kodak) CR indicator system is called the exposure index (EI), which is directly proportional to the radiation striking the imaging plate. An exposure of 0.1 mR has an

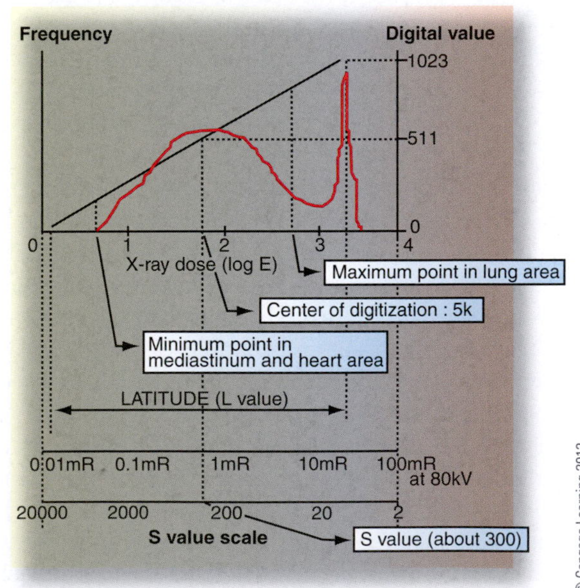

FIGURE 23-10. Graph showing relationship between x-ray exposure and S number. (*Courtesy of FUJIFILM Medical Systems USA.)*

TABLE 23-3. Exposure Index Numbers Relative to Imaging Plate Exposure

Agfa LgM Index		>2.95	2.15	<1.45	
Fuji S Value	2	20	200	2,000	20,000
Carestream Exposure Index		>2750	2,000	<1,250	
mR	100	10	1	0.1	0.01

EI of 1,000, whereas 1 mR in this system gives an EI of 2,000, and 10 mR results in an exposure index of 3,000. This is calculated by the formula EI = Log (exposure in mR) × 1,000 + 2,000. Properly exposed images should have an exposure index that ranges from 1,800 to 2,200. When exposure changes by a factor of 2, then the EI will change by 300; for example, if the EI is 2,500, reducing the mAs by ½ (divided by 2) will lower the EI to 2,200. Conversely, if the EI is 1,500, then doubling the mAs will result in an EI of 1,800.

Agfa uses an exposure indicator called the log median exposure LgM; it compares the exposure level of an image to a baseline established for the department. Because it is based on a log system, a change of 0.3 means the dose changed by a factor of 2, analogous to doubling or halving the exposure. Agfa systems use the scanned average level (SAL), which is the average grayscale value as represented by the formula: SAL 200 = 1,214 × (exposure in mR). Agfa also has a "speed class" that is similar to film/screen, such as 50, 100, 200, and 400, that is programmed into the algorithm that is selected before the plate is put in the reader. Exposure factors selected by the radiographer will also need to reflect the speed class selected, though the technologist may be able to change the speed class prior to running the plate. Choosing the speed for the imaging plate will direct the system to prepare for the relative amount of light to be read from the plate. This will allow the electronics in the system to be optimized to the appropriate range and result in a better image data set.

Exposure Factor Selection

Kilovoltage for computed radiography will control subject contrast similar to film radiography. However, some computed radiography manufacturers recommend avoiding the use of more than 80 kVp for non-grid imaging because higher kVp levels produce excessive fog due to Compton scatter that will decrease contrast significantly more than the same increase with a film/screen imaging receptor.

One advantage to digital imaging is the wide dynamic range response of the detectors. Rather than the characteristic curve of film/screen systems, the response of an imaging plate to x-ray is linear. This linear response gives the detector increased exposure latitude over film/screen (Figure 23-11). This means that areas that receive very little radiation can be enhanced by the computer instead of all the densities clumping around the toe of the D log E curve as they do when using a film receptor. Conversely, areas receiving greater exposure can be separated and brought down into the visible density range by the computer instead of all clumping around the shoulder of the D log E curve.

An important extension of the density range occurs when using digital radiography with areas of much greater exposure because the detector does not have a D_{max}. Instead it has a straight line that far surpasses the D log E curve of a film emulsion. This creates a dangerous radiation safety problem because digital radiography systems have an extremely high toleration for patient overexposure. When film is exposed beyond D_{max}, it actually reverses and begins to get lighter (as with duplicating film). The digital imaging detector continues to record the exposure and the computer can bring these densities down into the visible range. This is why a digital system can compensate for gross overexposure. This is also why the radiographer using system must realize that **there is great danger**

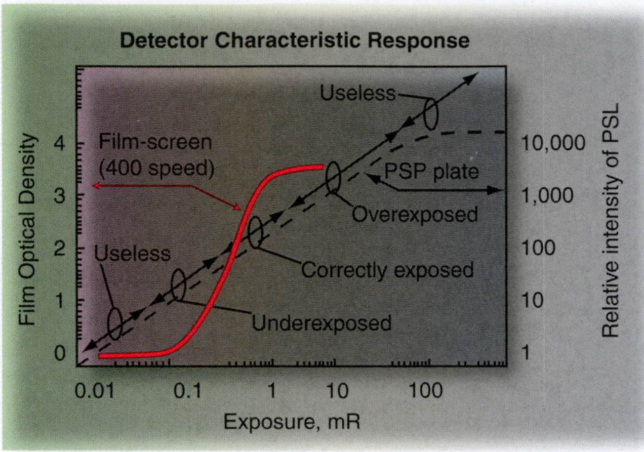

FIGURE 23-11. Graph demonstrating the linear response of a digital receptor along with a typical characteristic curve for film. Digital receptors provide a much wider exposure latitude between over- and underexposure areas. *(Adapted from AAPM Report 93, American Association of Physicists in Medicine [AAPM]. Reproduced by permission.)*

in permitting personal professional standards to relax and routinely overexposing all patients with the intention of the system adjusting the histogram to correct the exposure. Figure 23-12 demonstrates a full range of over- and underexposed skull images. This practice is unethical, violates ALARA radiation protection guidelines, and is to be avoided at all times.

Digital processing requires the technologist to be knowledgeable in the details of digital image acquisition as well as post-processing parameters and procedures. For example, many manufacturers state in their technical usage information that mAs has little effect on the visualization of image density. This can be a confusing statement for radiographers who are knowledgeable about the relationships between mAs and kVp and clearly understand how to control them when creating an optimal diagnostic image. What manufacturers are trying to convey is that the extended range of the straight-line portion of the image receptor response curve allows a system to digitally process the image after exposure to rescale the density into the visible range, even when the image receptor is grossly overexposed. This does not change the fact that changes in mAs will increase or decrease the quantity of photons received by the image receptor. These changes directly affect the quantity of information the image receptor passes on to the post-processing system and what is used to determine the exposure indicator. Many image post-processing systems may not require mAs settings as high as film-based image receptors did in the past, but this is why diagnostic-quality images may now be produced with less mAs—not a reason to overexpose patients so the post-processing system can adjust the display density downward.

Another important quality factor in digital processing is better known and tends to receive more attention because the results are immediately visible on the images: adequate mAs is required to activate any digital image receptor. Failure to use a high enough mAs setting produces quantum mottle, which produces a grainy, reticulated image for which digital post-processing cannot compensate. This is why a minimum sensitivity number is required by many radiologists to ensure they are diagnosing from an image that meets the minimum data requirements of the digital system.

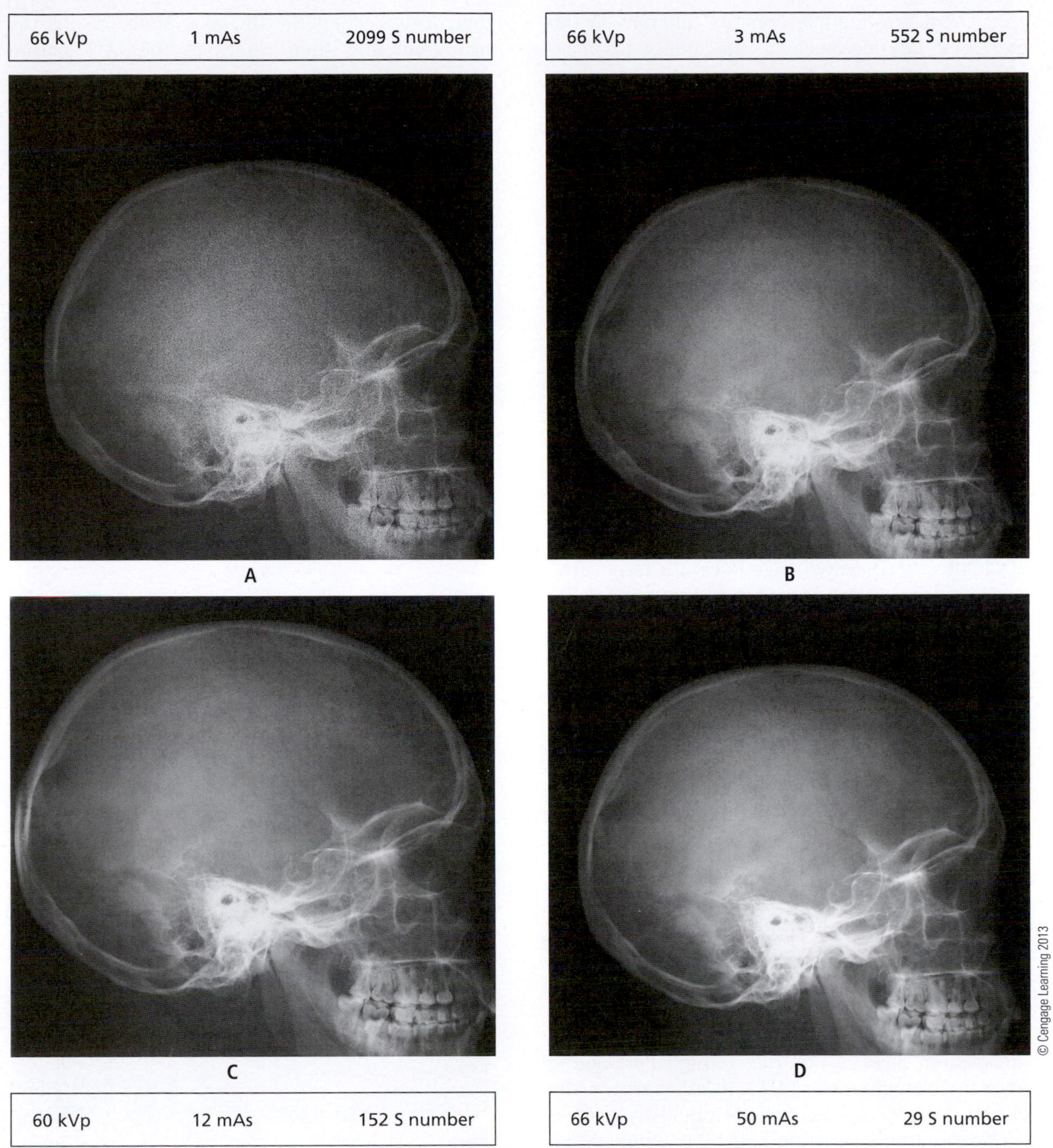

FIGURE 23-12. A demonstration of over- and underexposure with a CR system. While it may appear that all four CR images have appropriate density ranges, a careful inspection will show that with the exception of image C, the Fuji S numbers are outside the optimal range of 150–250. Image A has an S number of 2099, which indicates that it was grossly underexposed, As a result, it exhibits excessive loss of detail and graininess. Image D has an S number of 29, which indicates that patient exposure was probably close to 10 times more than it should have been.

There are multiple benefits inherent in this increased latitude, such as the ability to image structures of widely different attenuation values, such as the chest, on the same image without loss of visibility of structures with widely different densities (such as lung vasculature and the mediastinum). (See Figure 23-7.) Another benefit is the increased margin for error in over- and underexposure to the receptor. Digital radiography can maintain a useful density over a wider latitude than allowable with film/screen. However, even though density can be maintained, the overall image quality may be poor if exposures are too far from optimal. **Images that are underexposed will show quantum mottle, even though the density is acceptable, whereas overexposed images will tend to suffer from low contrast.**

The issue of how to select proper technical factors for digital systems requires clear understanding. Although this will be discussed in detail in Chapter 26 (Density/Image Receptor Exposure), it is important to understand that the term *density* was descriptive of the result of image receptor exposure. It is now appropriate to think of this factor as the actual image receptor exposure. From that perspective, it must be clear that mAs and kVp can no longer be assessed by viewing the difference between adjacent densities or brightness levels. Because the response curve of the image receptor is now linear and much greater than with conventional film/screen systems, the initial contrast that is received from the detector is extremely low. Some digital radiography systems allow display of this information as it is collected from the detector, and these images clearly demonstrate the low-contrast nature of this initial information. As soon as the programmed processing algorithm is applied, the image is displayed with the desired level of contrast (which is acquired from the histogram and LUT). In other words, the display image contrast is determined by a great extent from the histogram and LUT, although the kVp level does have an impact. This impact is in the differential attenuation (or signal difference or subject contrast). This means that the proper selection of the kVp is a required preliminary step that must be achieved prior to the post-processing that occurs when the digital system creates the histogram and then refers to the LUT before displaying the final viewing image.

When setting kVp levels for digital systems, the most important thing to remember is that when higher kVp levels are used, the width of the acquired data is less (becomes narrower). (See Figure 23-13.) Note how the difference between the minimum to maximum incoming radiation is dramatically reduced. This is a desirable effect because it displays more anatomical data while reducing patient dose (Figure 23-14). It is recommended that kVp levels not exceed 80 for any non-grid radiography, including the chest. It is recommended that when scatter ratios approach 50 percent, grids should become mandatory. Failure to do so greatly reduces image contrast due to the scatter radiation reaching the image receptor. Table 23-4 lists suggested kVp levels for various procedures when using digital radiography imaging systems.

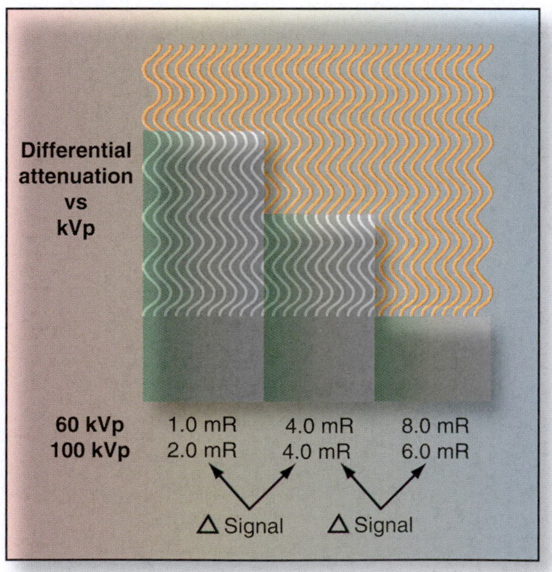

FIGURE 23-13. Different attenuation resulting from large kVp changes. With higher kVp the signal difference between maximum and minimum exposure is lowered, thereby reducing the width of the acquired data.

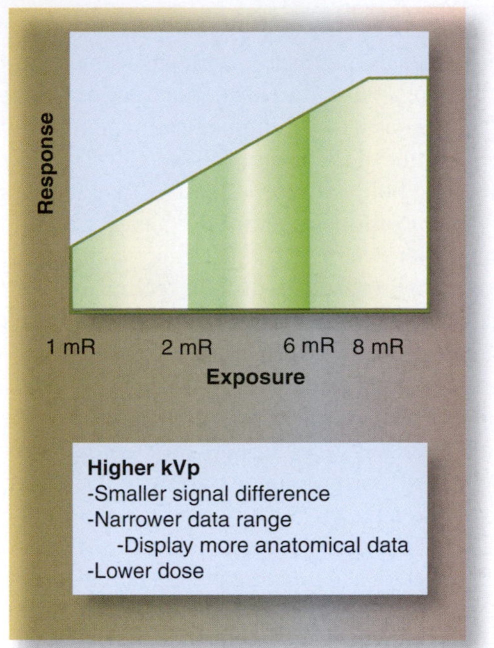

FIGURE 23-14. Relation of kVp to dose. Higher kVp reduces dose and although the data width is narrowed more anatomical information is displayed for a given display setting.

TABLE 23-4. Suggested kVp Ranges for Digital Imaging Systems

Infant extremities	50–60 kVp
Adult extremities	65–75 kVp
Bucky extremities	75–90 kV
AP spine	85–95 kVp
Lateral spine	
Cervical	85–100 kVp
Dorsal	85–100 kVp
Lumbar	85–100 kVp
Chest	110–130 kVp
Skull	80–90 kVp

COMPUTED RADIOGRAPHY (PSP) SYSTEMS

Computed radiography (CR) uses a photostimulable storage phosphor imaging plate (PSP or IP), typically inside a cassette. This cassette can be used in a bucky or for portable exams, similar to traditional film/screen. CR first became available in the early 1980s when it was introduced by Fuji, but, as happens with many new technologies, there were problems with high cost and poor image quality. As computer technology has advanced, so too has the ability of CR to produce images comparable to, and in many instances better than, film. Currently, a number of manufacturers produce CR plates and processor systems. Many of them have Internet websites with a considerable amount of information on the advantages of their particular systems. (Commercial websites with information on computed radiography include *www.fujifilm.com*, *www.carestreamhealth.com*, *www.konicaminolta.us*, and *www.agfaus.com*.) The cassette-based CR with the PSP requires a reader to process the plate and create the image and is a two-step process because the radiographer must move the detector between image acquisition and display.

Photostimulable Imaging Plates

A photostimulable phosphor imaging plate is a rigid sheet with several layers that are designed to record and enhance transmission of the image from a beam of ionizing radiation. The layers include a protective layer, a phosphor layer, a support layer made of polyester, a conductor layer, and a light-shield layer (Figure 23-15). The protective layer simply insulates the imaging plate from handling trauma. The phosphor layer holds the photostimulable phosphor, which is the active component in the plate. The support layer is simply a base on which to coat the other layers. The conductor layer grounds the plate to eliminate electrostatic problems and absorb light to increase sharpness. Finally, the light-shielding layer prevents light from erasing data on the imaging plate or leaking through

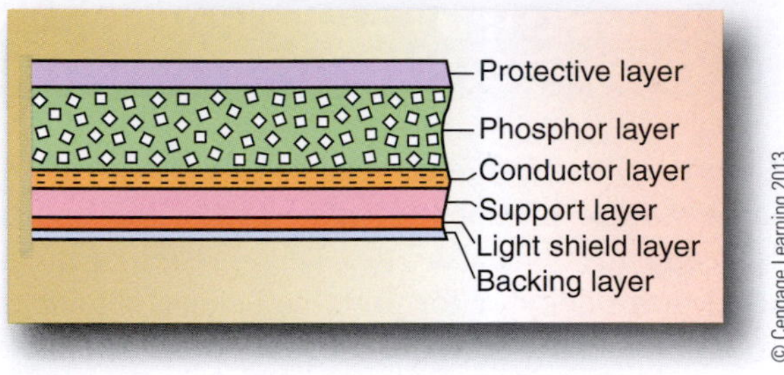

FIGURE 23-15. Photostimulate phosphor imaging plate showing layers.

the backing, decreasing the spatial resolution. The imaging plate is loaded into a cassette that looks much like a radiographic film and intensifying-screen cassette. Consequently, computed radiography cassettes are sometimes referred to as "filmless cassettes."

In order for CR to function, the imaging plate material must have the ability to store and release the image information in a usable form. The most common phosphors with characteristics favorable for CR are barium fluorohalide bromides and iodides with europium activators (BaFBr:Eu and BaFI:Eu). The halides are approximately 85 percent bromide and 15 percent iodide. Due to the lower atomic number of barium, the K-edge attenuates best between 35 and 50 keV, somewhat lower than the typical K-edge for rare-earth intensifying screens, but well within the diagnostic range (35 keV is a typical average energy production from an exposure of 80 kVp). However, **the absorption efficiency above and below 35 to 50 keV is below that of rare-earth intensifying screens.** This means that more exposure may be needed in order to have similar quantum noise outside the optimal energy range. Also, the imaging plate phosphor will absorb more low-energy scatter than the rare-earth phosphor and film, which means appropriate kVp, collimation, and masking must be used to achieve optimal images. **This also makes the imaging plate more sensitive to scatter both before and after it is sensitized through exposure to the x-ray beam.**

Some other compounds that may be used in the PSP are BaSrFBr:Eu, RbBr:T1, RbCl, and CsBr:Eu.

Image Acquisition

Image acquisition begins with x-ray exposure to the imaging plate. Because the imaging plate is placed in a cassette, it can be used tabletop or with a grid, similar to the use of film/screen. The rules of positioning hold true for CR; areas that are clipped or poorly positioned cannot be corrected with this or any other system. It is the responsibility of the radiographer to select proper technique; chronic overexposure should be avoided. Radiation exposure causes fluorescence of the imaging plate but some of the energy of the beam is also stored in the plate. It is this stored energy that is used to create an image during reading and processing. Some of the electrons, which are excited by the absorbed energy, are trapped in the crystal structure of the phosphor at higher energy levels. Thus a latent image is stored in the imaging plate, similar to a latent image on film, but with wider latitude. The imaging plate then needs to be read to release the stored information, which can be manipulated by the computer and used in either soft- or hard-copy form.

Latent Image Production

The incident x-ray beam produces a latent image within the photostimulable fluorohalides that comprise the active layer of the imaging plate (IP) in the cassette. When the fluorohalides luminesce, they do not release all the energy absorbed from the incident x-ray beam. Although some light is emitted, the phosphors retain sufficient energy in the form of a latent image. It is this latent image that will be used to create a digital image for the computer to record and display.

This latent image is actually created by energy transfer during photoelectric interactions. The photoelectrons that are produced then excite a number of low-energy electrons to create "holes" in the crystal phosphor. Although about half of the electron holes will recompose and emit light photons, the fluorohalides will hold or trap the other half of the electrons, thus creating the "holes" at the europium sites. These europium electron holes are the actual latent image (Figure 23-16). **The latent image will lose about 25 percent of its energy in 8 hours, so it is important to process**

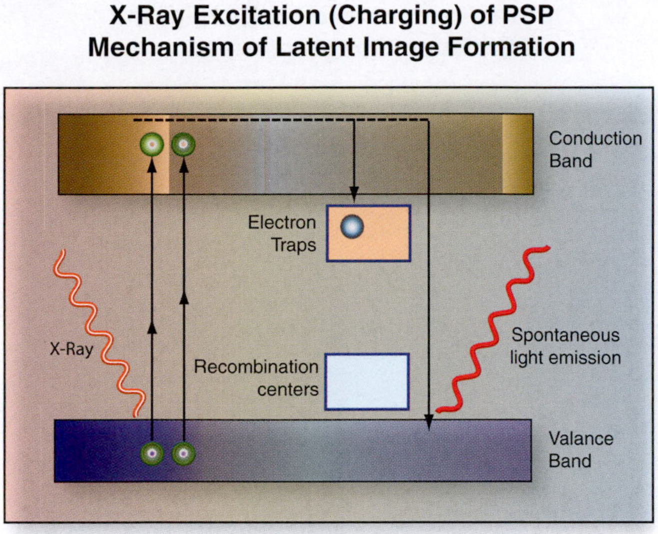

X-Ray Excitation (Charging) of PSP
Mechanism of Latent Image Formation

FIGURE 23-16. Latent image formation on a PSP. X-rays interact with the phosphor causing electrons to be raised to a higher energy level where they are trapped in proportion to the exposure received to the plate. In addition some light is emitted spontaneously during the interaction. *(Courtesy of Andrew Woodward, M.A., R.T.[R][CT][QM], University of North Carolina at Chapel Hill.)*

the cassette shortly after exposure. Cassettes stored for several days after exposure and before processing lose most of their latent image.

The latent image is processed by loading the cassette into an image reader device (IRD) where the imaging plate is scanned by a helium-neon laser beam. These laser beam scans cause the phosphors to emit the stored latent image in the form of light photons, which are detected by photosensitive receptors and converted to an electrical signal, which is in turn converted to a unique digital value for that level of luminescence. Once the plate is read, it is erased to remove all vestiges of the latent image. When a plate is grossly overexposed it may not erase completely. This results in a ghosting artifact on the next image.

Reading CR Data

Reading the imaging plate involves a finely focused red laser beam (670–690-nm wavelength) that frees the trapped electrons, allowing them to return to a lower-energy state, referred to as photostimulated luminescence (PSL). Electrons moving from a high-energy state to a lower-energy state release blue-purple light photons (415-nm wavelength) in proportion to the absorbed radiation (Figure 23-17). The laser light beam is directed to the imaging plate through a series of light guides; this beam must be monitored because the intensity of the blue light from the imaging plate is dependent on the power of the laser beam. Scanning of the imaging plate by the laser occurs in a raster pattern as the plate is fed through the processor. A raster pattern is the method by which the data are collected from the imaging plate. Data collection begins in the upper left corner, proceeds in a line to the upper right corner, then drops down a line and repeats. You are reading this book in a raster pattern, from top left, line by line, until you finish the page at the bottom right. The plate can be scanned by a point scan reader, which moves from side to side. Newer readers use a line scan reader, which has reduced scan time. The light liberated from the imaging plate is emitted in all directions and is collected by an optical system that directs it to one or more photodetectors, commonly photomultiplier (PM) tubes or linear CCD array, which are sensitive to the blue

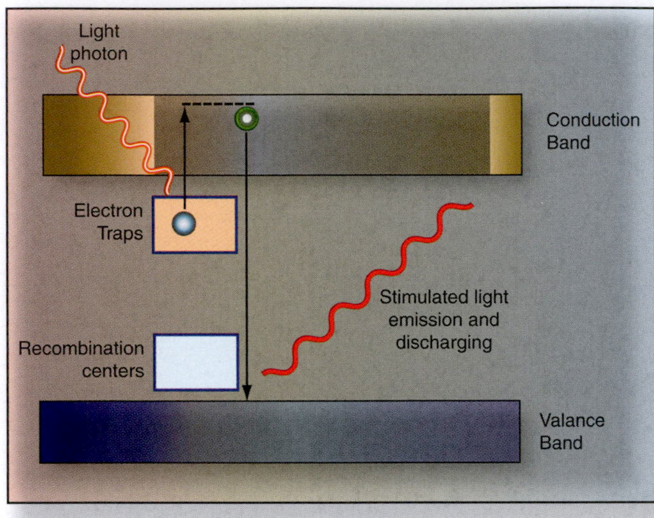

FIGURE 23-17. During readout of the plate, a laser light releases the trapped electron from the higher energy state to a lower state causing the emission of a bluish-purple light. *(Courtesy of Andrew Woodward, M.A., R.T.[R][CT][QM], University of North Carolina at Chapel Hill.)*

light. The photodetectors convert the visible light into an electronic signal whose output is in analog form. This analog signal must be converted into a digital signal before the computer can work with the image information. This is accomplished with an analog-to-digital converter (ADC). The entire reading process is illustrated in Figure 23-18. The photodetectors adjust the output signal range so it can be optimally handled during the digitization process. Any residual image left on the imaging plate is erased by exposure to an intense light to release any remaining trapped electrons.

Another way to speed up the process and at the same time obtain more information is to use a dual-sided PSP, which has a screen on both sides that can be scanned and read simultaneously. The primary advantage of dual-sided reading is that more signal is obtained, which improves image quality.

The reading and erasing of an imaging plate can occur in a single processor unit, as shown in Figure 23-19. The larger units typically allow stacking and loading of multiple cassettes for use in a large department, whereas a small processor will only process one plate at a time and is typically used in an office or single room. Plate readers are also used with some mobile units. Plate throughput can average anywhere from 30 plates/hour to over 200 plates/hour depending on the type of processor used. Workload and cost will determine which unit will best serve department requirements. There are also tables and upright bucky units that contain multiple PSP plates and a reader in the unit, so no cassette handling is required. The units move and process plates after each exposure, allowing the radiographer to view images in a monitor within the control booth. Fuji offers these combined units, which can process over 200 images per hour.

The finely focused laser beam that scans each line of the imaging plate correlates to one line spacing or **pixel pitch**. Pixel pitch is defined as the physical distance between pixels and is

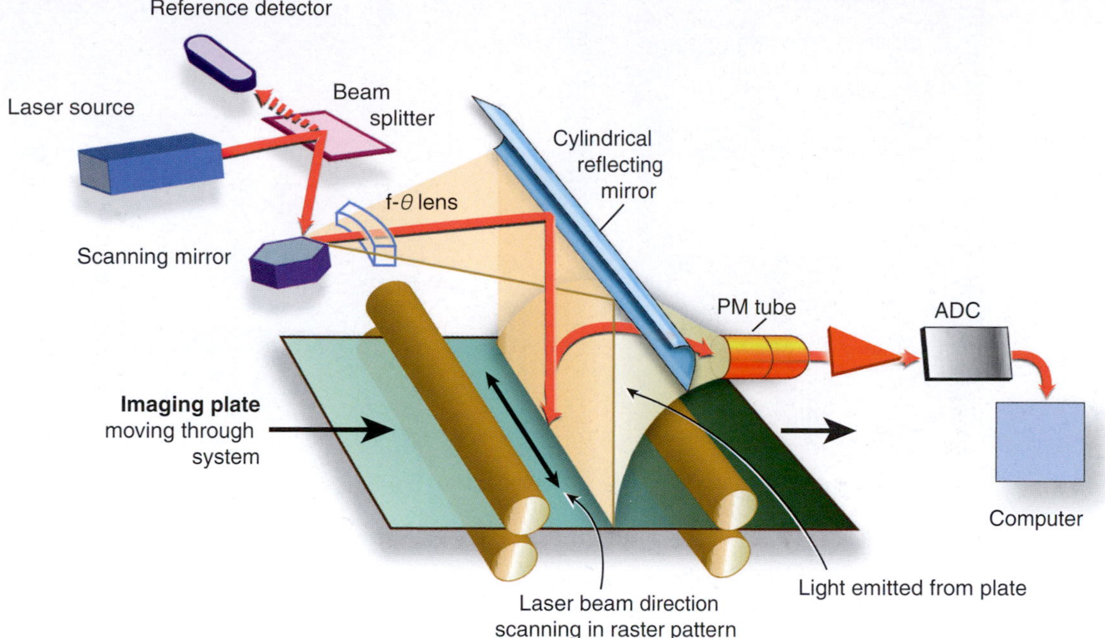

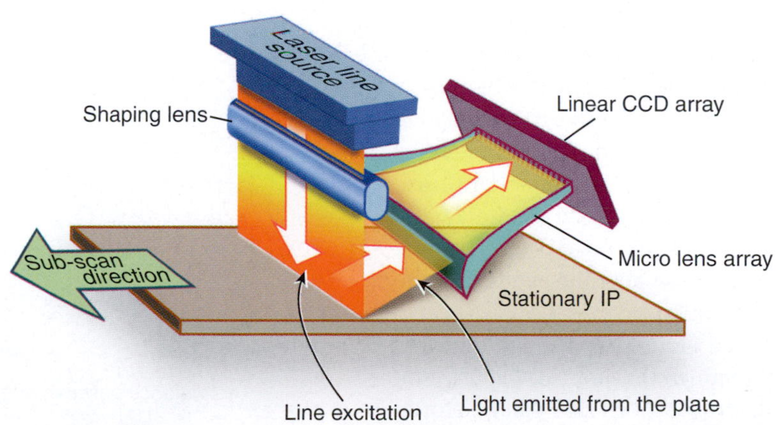

FIGURE 23-18. Photostimulable phosphor imaging plate readers. The top drawing illustrates a point scan reader. The plate is moved through the system while a focused laser scans the surface in a raster pattern. When the laser strikes the surface of the imaging plate, the emitted light is detected by the PM tube, which sends an analog signal to the ADC for conversion into a digital signal, which is then sent to the computer for processing and display. The bottom illustrates a line scan reader. The plate remains stationary while a laser scans an entire line at once. *(Source: Seibert, J. A. (2004). Computed radiography technology. In L. W. Goldman & M. V. Yester (Eds.),* Specifications, performance, and quality assurance of radiographic and fluoroscopic systems in the digital era. *College Park, MD: American Association of Physicists in Medicine (AAPM). Reproduced by permission.)*

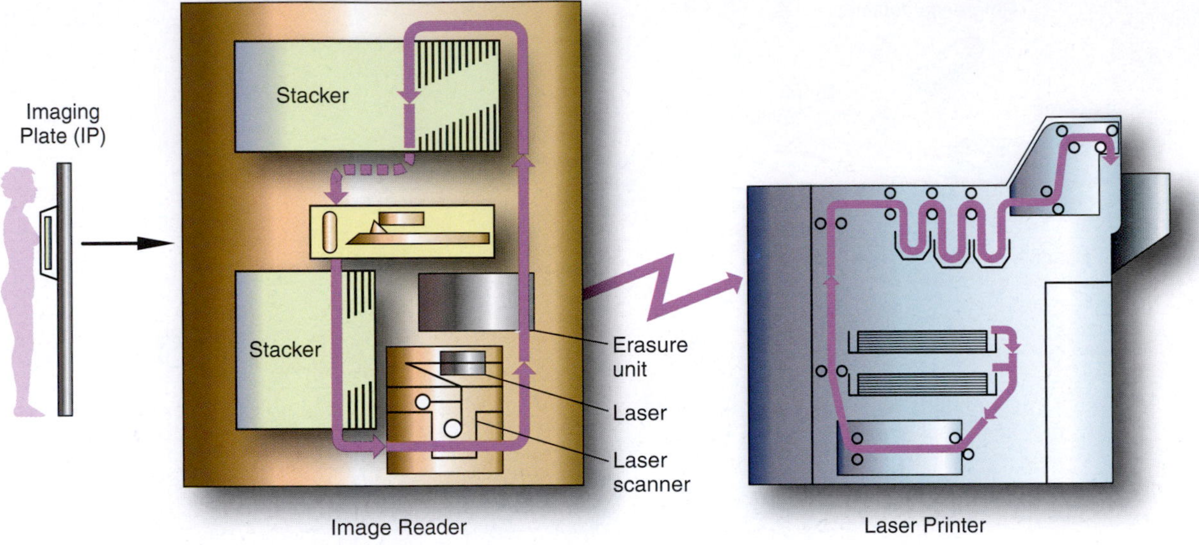

FIGURE 23-19. Internal view of image reader and stacker with relationship to a chest unit and laser printer. Image can also be sent to a PACS. *(Courtesy of FUJIFILM Medical Systems USA.)*

generally measured from center to center. In CR, it is dependent on the sampling frequency, or Nyquist frequency, which is related to how the laser scans the plate. The more the signal is sampled, the more information is obtained and the smaller the pixels can be, but this increases scan time. This sampling frequency is expressed as pixels/mm. Pixel pitch for DR is determined by the detector element (DEL) size (discussed in the DR section). (See Figure 23-20.) Another important variable related to pixels is spatial resolution. Recall that the smaller the pixel pitch, the higher the spatial resolution.

The analog signal emitted by the PM tube has an infinite range of values that the ADC must convert into limited discrete values that can be stored as digital code. Pixel bit depth or the number of bits that represent an analog signal will determine the number of density values. Typically, there are 10 bit (2^{10} = 1,024), 12 bit (2^{12} = 4,096), and 16 bit (2^{16} = 65,536) ADCs, which will determine the density values for the analog signal and thus the grayscale of the system. Therefore, the number of bits/pixels will determine how many density values can be present, which will affect the density and contrast of an imaging system. The matrix size for

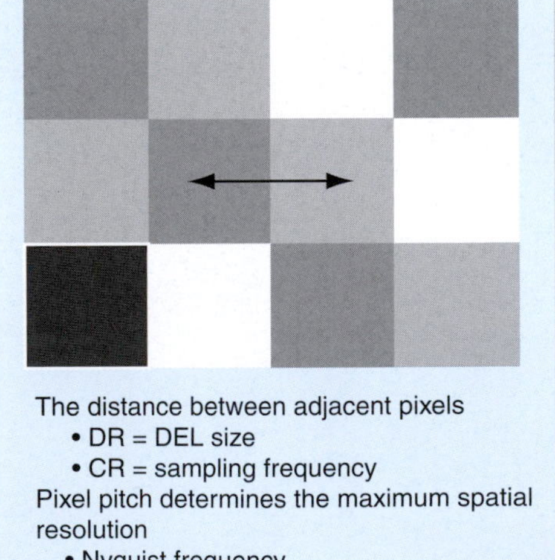

FIGURE 23-20. A diagram of pixel pitch or sampling pitch, which is the principal factor that determines spatial resolution. In CR, this is determined by the sampling frequency and in DR it is controlled by the DEL size.

CR is dependent on the sampling frequency, and for some systems the image receptor size. At 10 pixels/mm a 14″ × 17″ (35 cm × 43 cm) plate would have a matrix of 3,500 × 4,300, whereas at 5 pixels/mm the 14″ × 17″ would have a matrix of 1,750 × 2,150. Pixel size, matrix, and bit depth determine the size of the computer file for a given image.

To accomplish the task of changing the analog signal into the correct components for digital manipulation, the analog signal must be sampled in order to find the location and size of the signal. It must then be quantified to determine the average value of the signal in the sample. Quantization is the process that will determine the brightness levels or grayscale for the pixels.

Data Manipulation

After the plate has been scanned and the data are sent to the computer it undergoes preprocessing or initial image processing, which is where the raw image data are prepared according to the proprietary algorithms of the manufacturer. These are complex operations and only the basics will be covered here. The CR system must determine the orientation of the part on the plate as well as the number of projections present per plate. Locating the image data on the plate allows the system to sample and manipulate only the clinically useful information. This raw data from scanning will have a range of values related to how much radiation the plate received. Areas outside the lines of collimation will have the lowest exposure, and therefore the lowest values. The highest values will lie within the collimated field, allowing the system to locate the useful information or data and disregard the data outside these lines. This is why markers placed outside the collimated field may not appear in the processed image. The method used by Fuji for this preprocessing is known as exposure data recognition (EDR); for Carestream, it is called segmentation. During preprocessing the following will occur: exposure field recognition, histogram analysis, and grayscale analysis. Exposure recognition therefore is used to recognize the clinically useful area on the imaging plate so it is the only data that will be manipulated, and it eliminates the signals from outside the collimated field. The best image will result when the part is parallel to the sides of the cassette and collimation is used on at least two sides (Figure 23-21). Also, there are certain expectations that need to be met when placing more than one image per plate. The beam and part should be centered within each pattern, and collimation should be parallel and equidistant from the edges of the imaging plate.

The appropriate anatomical menu is selected by body part by the radiographer when the imaging plate is loaded into the reading unit. The histogram is also used to eliminate unnecessary information outside the collimated field, such as scatter radiation, which degrades the final image. Once the true patient image data are identified, that information is rescaled and the LUT is applied to stabilize image density and contrast (Figure 23-22). This is when exposure errors are corrected. Algorithms, which are unique to each manufacturer, process the data once the exposed area is determined and the signal

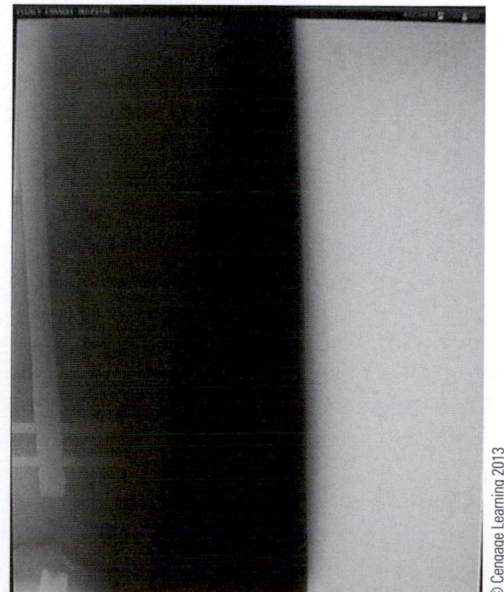

FIGURE 23-21. Distal femur, collimation on only one side, part is not centered. An S# 504 indicates underexposure; however, the image does not display that way.

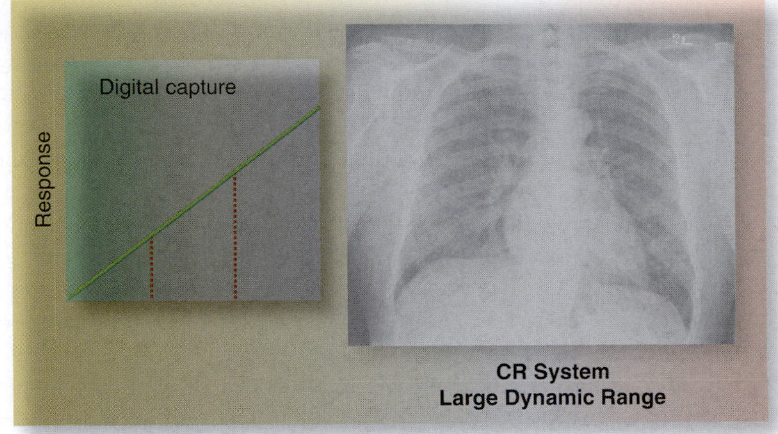

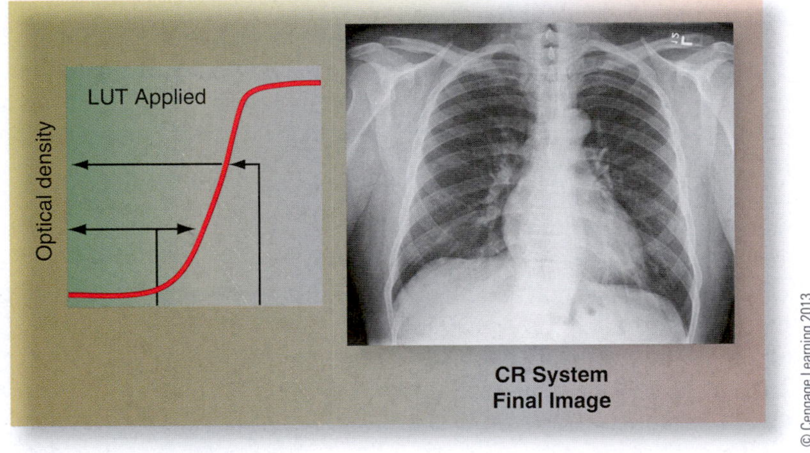

FIGURE 23-22. (A) Chest with linear digital response showing an initial display with very low contrast; (B) chest with look-up table applied to correct contrast.

histogram is established. Fuji uses MFP (multi-objective frequency), tonescaling is used by Carestream, and Agfa is using a MUSICA (multi-scale image contrast algorithm) system.

The correct anatomical menu should be selected prior to processing the imaging plate; otherwise the image will not process the correct density and contrast. Figure 23-23 is an example of a typical chest histogram with the various anatomical areas annotated on the histogram. Figure 23-24 illustrates how a computed radiography system can analyze a pediatric chest histogram and then display regions of interest outside the lung. Finally, it is critical to adhere to uniform positioning and collimation procedures when using a computed radiography system. The reading system must be given consistent data to analyze if it is to provide consistent diagnostic-quality results.

The knee images in Figure 23-25 illustrate the ability of a CR system to adjust the histogram into the visible diagnostic density range. Look carefully at Figures 23-25A and B as compared to C and D and then to E and F. Although it may appear that all three CR images (B, D, and F) have appropriate

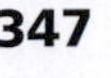

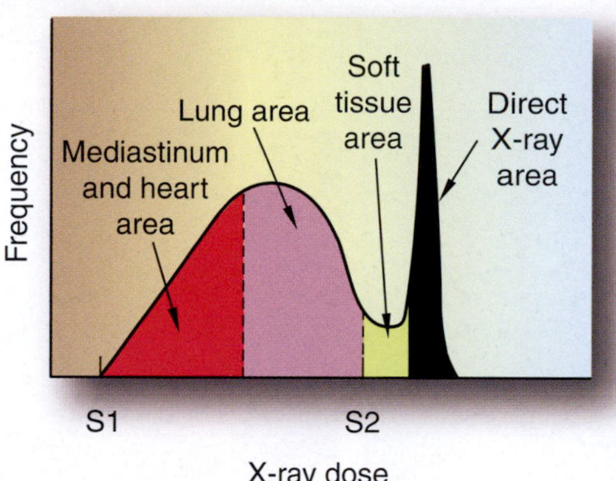

FIGURE 23-23. Example of a histogram that would be produced by a normal chest radiograph. *(Courtesy of FUJIFILM Medical Systems USA.)*

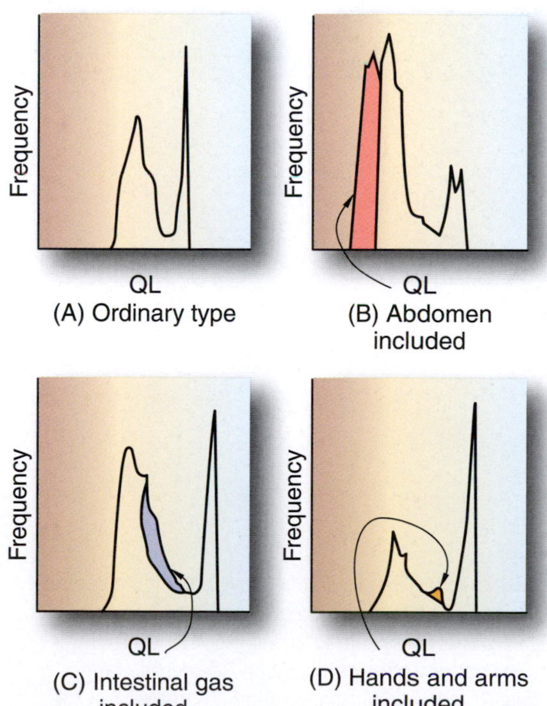

FIGURE 23-24. Example of a histogram that would be produced by a pediatric chest with potential computerized enhancements possible by displaying density ranges typical of other regions of interest outside normal lung densities. *(Courtesy of FUJIFILM Medical Systems USA.)*

density ranges as compared to the conventional radiography images, a careful inspection will show that the CR image in Figure 23-25B is extremely grainy and as a result is outside the acceptable range for detail. This is an example of the CR histogram adjusting for density but lacking adequate data to fill in an acceptable level of detail.

In the past, most CR systems relied completely on the technologist's accuracy of selecting the correct anatomical menu before the imaging plate was processed. This means that if an image of a knee was processed as a chest, or a pediatric chest was processed under the adult chest histogram, the resulting image may not be of diagnostic quality (Figure 23-26). New-generation CR readers store the "raw" data (pre-histogram analysis) in the workstation. This feature allows images that were processed with an incorrect anatomical menu to be re-processed using the correct anatomical menu with no loss of its original quality. However, once the image data are sent to PACS it cannot be re-processed; only the original data on the workstation can be re-processed.

Spatial frequency processing is a post-processing function and is used when it is necessary to increase image sharpness. Edge enhancement is obtained with an unsharp mask technique. In this technique the original image is blurred by a low-pass filter, which is subtracted from the original to leave only a high-spatial-frequency signal. This signal is amplified and added back into the exam data to produce an image with higher frequencies or edge enhancement. It is important to understand that edge enhancement techniques usually increase noise and as a result may produce lower-quality images with higher base fog levels and lower contrast.

Fuji allows the plate reader to be programmed for a number of different scanning detection patterns (Figure 23-27). It has three modes—automatic (auto), semiautomatic (semi), and fixed—which allows the user more control when processing the plate and image data. Automatic mode adjusts latitude and sensitivity for the image automatically and works well when the correct parameters are used for an exam. It is also used when placing more than one image on a cassette.

The semi mode automatically adjusts only sensitivity, while the reading latitude is fixed, so

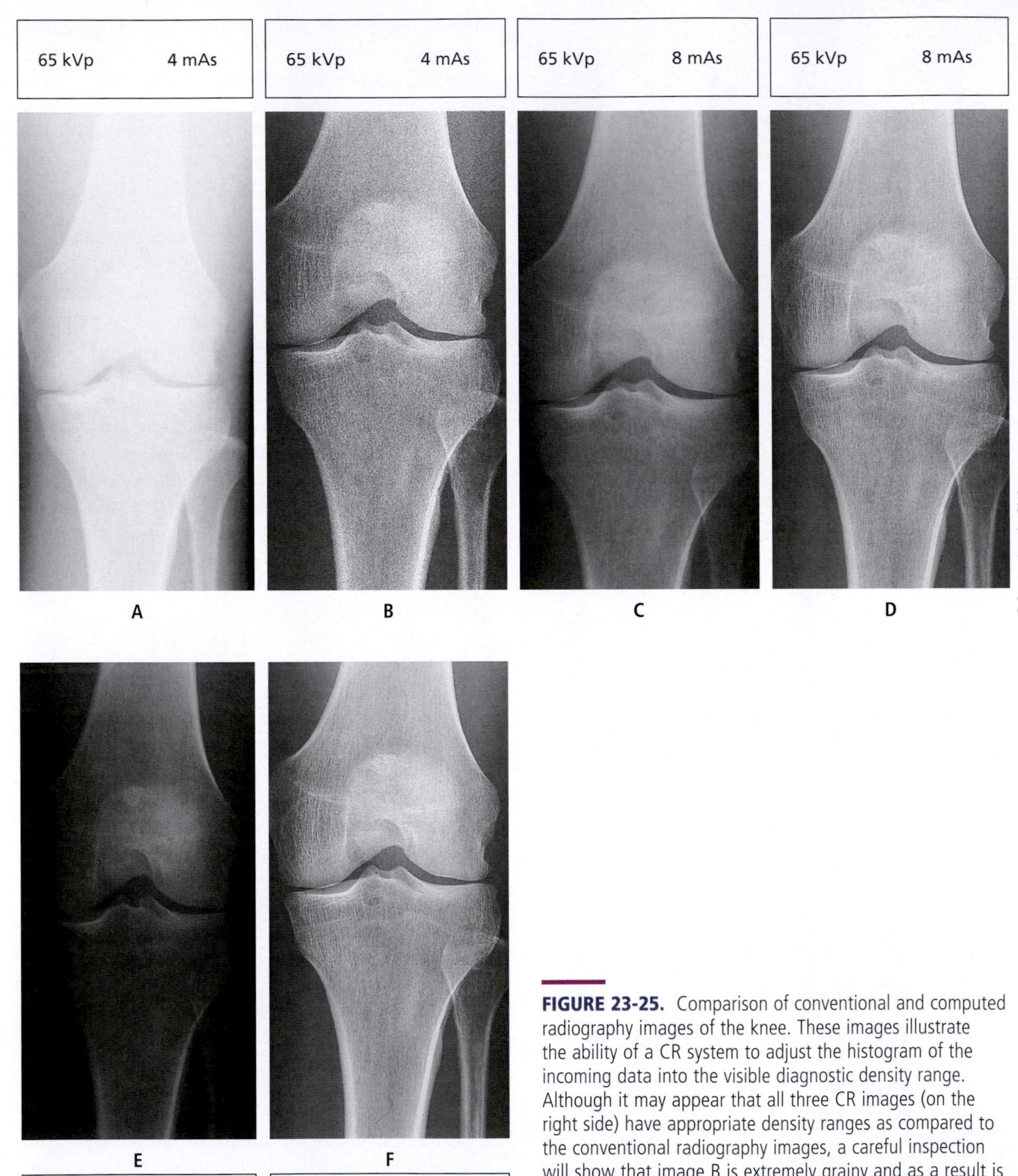

FIGURE 23-25. Comparison of conventional and computed radiography images of the knee. These images illustrate the ability of a CR system to adjust the histogram of the incoming data into the visible diagnostic density range. Although it may appear that all three CR images (on the right side) have appropriate density ranges as compared to the conventional radiography images, a careful inspection will show that image B is extremely grainy and as a result is outside the acceptable range for detail. This is an example of the CR histogram adjusting for density but lacking adequate data to fill in an acceptable level of detail.

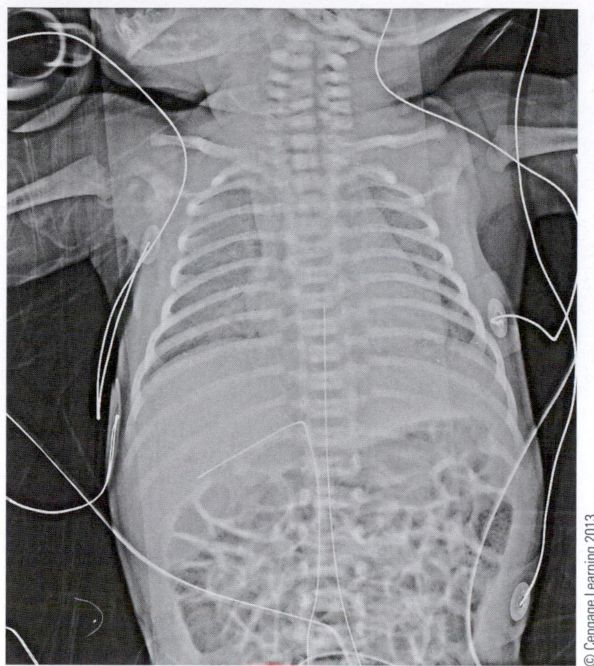

FIGURE 23-26. Histogram error artifact. Selection of an adult histogram used on a pediatric chest.

the correct kVp must be used in this mode. It is used when the image is centered, but the collimation borders are not parallel or equidistant from the plate edges. This mode works well for areas using tight collimation, such as navicular or odontoid projections or a closely collimated view of the knee joint (Figure 23-28). Semi-x mode divides the plate into nine areas and allows the user to select the area where the anatomy of interest is located. This mode works well when the anatomy is not located in the center of the plate. Fixed mode is similar to film/screen processing in that latitude and sensitivity are fixed, requiring correct technique factors to be used to obtain a diagnostic image because this mode will not correct density problems. Fixed mode will display the image similar to what you would see with film/screen systems.

Histogram Analysis. As mentioned earlier, the data in the imaging plate is located within the collimated edges in order to develop a histogram. Most CR systems do not send all the data acquired by the image receptor to the post-acquisition system

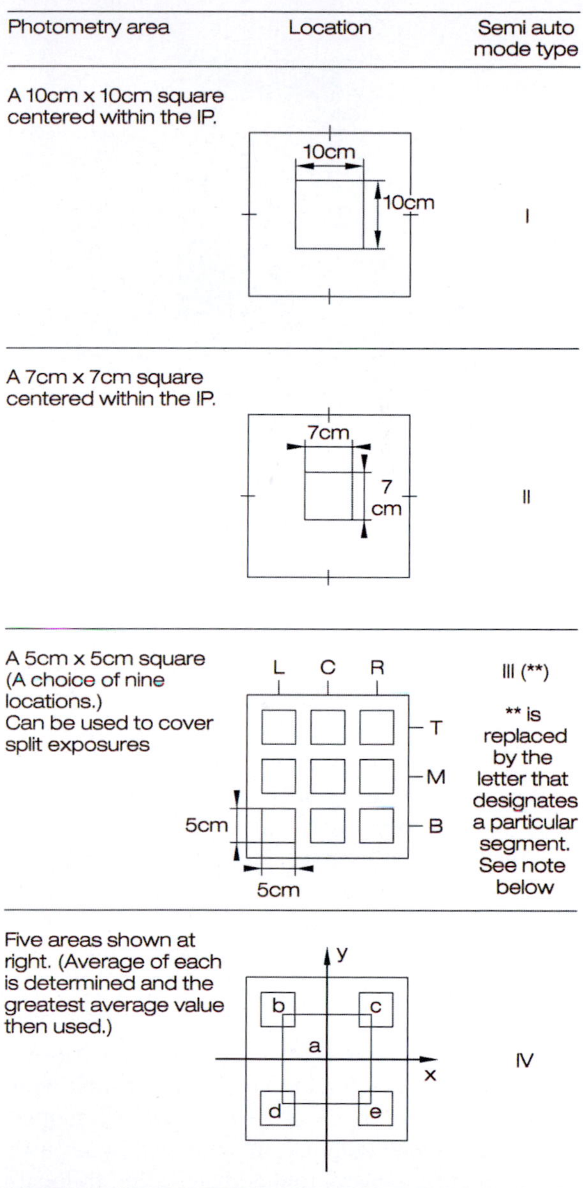

Photometry area	Location	Semi auto mode type
A 10cm x 10cm square centered within the IP.	10cm, 10cm	I
A 7cm x 7cm square centered within the IP.	7cm, 7 cm	II
A 5cm x 5cm square (A choice of nine locations.) Can be used to cover split exposures	L C R; T M B; 5cm, 5cm	III (**)
Five areas shown at right. (Average of each is determined and the greatest average value then used.)	y; x; a b c d e	IV

** is replaced by the letter that designates a particular segment. See note below

FIGURE 23-27. An example of different scanning detection patterns available on a Fuji system set for semiautomatic exposure data recognition (EDR) mode. *(Courtesy of FUJIFILM Medical Systems USA.)*

because the quantity of data is far greater than the display system can provide for viewing. This element of CR is called data clipping because the software processing the data coming from the image receptor

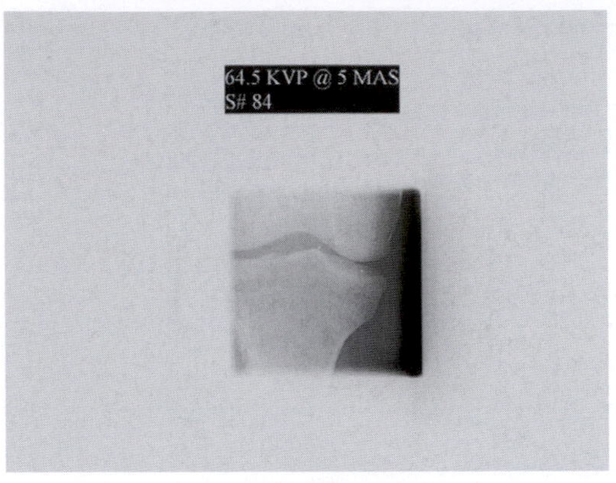

A

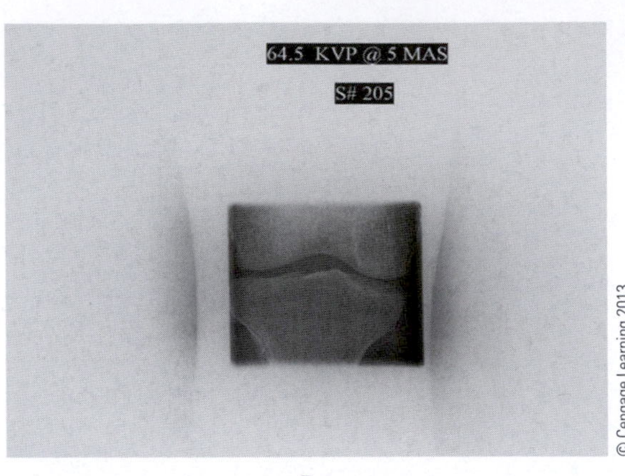

B

FIGURE 23-28. (A) Using auto mode for a closely collimated (cone down) view of the knee joint; (B) using semi mode.

is programmed to recognize that some data represents exposure below the diagnostic imaging range, whereas other data represents exposure far above the diagnostic range. Essentially, the algorithm eliminates data that is clinically irrelevant to a particular examination. The information that is important on the histogram will be determined by the values of interest (VOI), which will be different for each body part. The algorithm also has an LUT that has the appropriate contrast for each body part. Therefore the algorithm will vary, depending on the body part. This is why CR systems demand to know what examination is being performed before the image can be acquired, processed, and displayed.

Histogram Analysis Error. The computer has reference histograms for the body parts, which were developed using appropriate exposure techniques, positioning, and collimation. The computer uses the shape of the histogram and algorithm to locate the VOI and determine the exposure indicator. When an image is obtained that does not fit the parameters that were used for the reference histogram, it may result in a histogram analysis error. When a histogram analysis error occurs the image will not display appropriately. The appropriate density and contrast will not be displayed because the computer does not recognize the data. It can also give an incorrect exposure indicator number.

Most CR systems include algorithms designed to detect abrupt edges of exposure and non-exposure, which are assumed to represent collimator edges. If the computer has a field recognition error, where it cannot find the edges of collimation, it can include off focus and scatter in the histogram. This can lead to dark, light, or low-contrast images. It can also cause an inaccurate exposure indicator number. If there is no collimation then there will be too much exposure in the histogram, and that will also cause a histogram analysis error and will cause the exposure indicator to reflect a large exposure to the plate. If the histogram has excess exposure from poor collimation techniques, this could cause an error in locating the VOI, which can cause rescaling errors that result in poor density and contrast on the image. Likewise, too much collimation can also cause histogram analysis errors and lead to poor image quality (Figure 23-29).

It is also possible to have an abrupt straight line of tissue density when there are prosthetic devices or other parts with large density differences that may lead to a histogram analysis error such as an adult hand visible on an image of a neonate leg (Figure 23-30). Most CR systems have been developed to the point where it is rare for this to occur; nevertheless it is useful for the knowledgeable CR operator to remember that this algorithm functions during most post-acquisition processing.

Another histogram analysis error will occur when an area of increased or decreased attenuation is located in the body where it is not normally

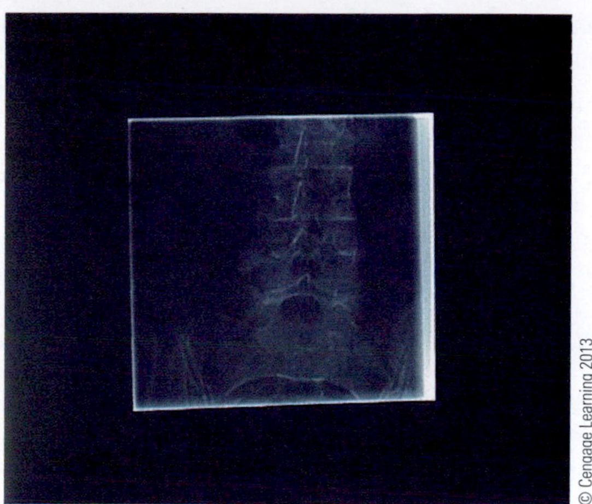

FIGURE 23-29. Lumbar spine with too much collimation. The S# 2005 indicates underexposure; however, the image is dark due to the fact that the computer put all the density for a lumbar spine in a smaller space.

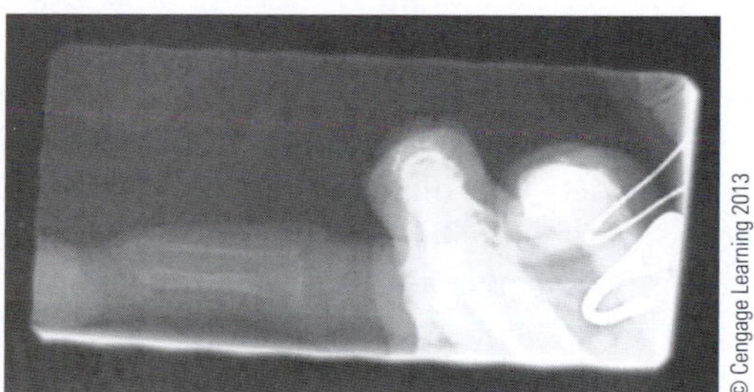

FIGURE 23-30. Neonate leg that has poor density and contrast due to the adult hand that causes a large difference in part density, the result is a histogram analysis error.

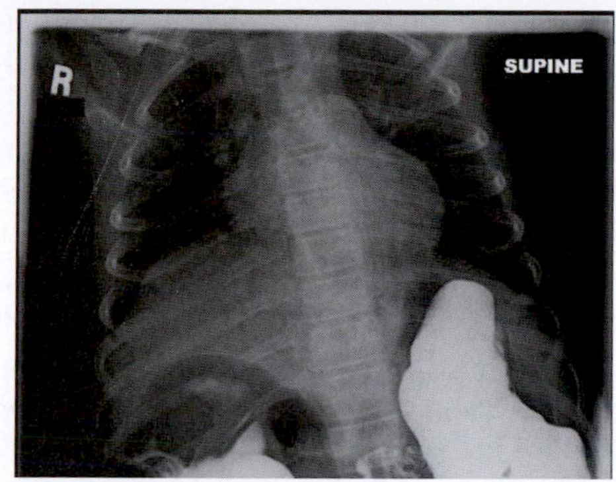

A

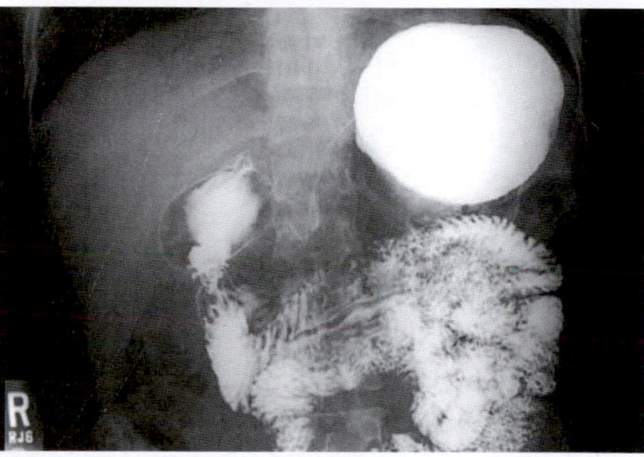

B

FIGURE 23-31. (A) and (B). Barium in chest image. This is not expected and is not included in histogram analysis; however, the UGI has barium displayed correctly because it is expected and included in the histogram analysis for this exam. *(Courtesy of Andrew Woodward, M.A., R.T.[R][CT][QM], University of North Carolina at Chapel Hill.)*

located. An example of this is barium in the stomach on a chest or an uneven border of a lead shield. The exposure field recognition portion of the software will not function correctly and the area corresponding to the lead or barium will be included in the histogram. This makes the system think the image was underexposed and the low-density area will be included in the VOI, which results in a rescaling error that produces a dark image (Figure 23-31).

When multiple exposures are done on one plate, symmetric part placement and exposure field borders will give the best results. Lack of symmetry may result in poor image quality due to histogram analysis errors if the computer has exposure field recognition errors. Each exposure of multiple exposures must also have the appropriate technique, because the computer will average the density and contrast between all exposures. This is why most exams only use one exposure per plate. Another problem is that when obtaining cross-table images, often the part is close to one side of the plate, which can also cause exposure field recognition errors and lead to rescaling errors.

Look-up Table Adjustments. The CR system look-up table is a graph of the processed pixel values (for image display) derived from the original image receptor pixel values (from image acquisition). All CR systems allow the display to be adjusted from the LUT. This permits changes in optical density or contrast that are often compared to adjusting the D log E curve of a film emulsion to enhance a particular portion of the image. Unfortunately, some manufacturers set their systems so that only authorized persons can access the LUT adjustments. When used this way, the LUT becomes a system calibration tool. However, accomplished CR users can use this feature to enhance pathologies such as fractures that are difficult to visualize—for example, periosteal tears in infants who have been abused.

Histogram Equalization. Some CR systems that are in dedicated environments, such as a chest unit, may have the histogram of the image receptor data modified to enhance a particular element. Chest CR systems can stack histogram-equalized images behind the normal image. This allows radiologists to view a normal display of a chest along with a bone-enhanced histogram image, a soft-tissue-enhanced image, and so forth. An image that is often cited for this process is a PA chest with a lung neoplasm hiding behind a rib. Although this lesion would be missed by most physicians, when a soft-tissue-enhanced image is viewed (which essentially removes all bony trabeculae from the ribs), the neoplasm is seen clearly. Because these are modified images, they should never be viewed for diagnosis without comparative images from the same data set in an unmodified state. This feature of CR creates a major imaging dilemma for radiologists because there is no end to the number of modified and enhanced images that can be created from a single image data set. Medical malpractice liability that assumes a radiologist is responsible for viewing all possible enhancements would require physicians to read from dozens of images for each standard projection and literally bring the practice of radiology to a halt. The American College of Radiology addresses this issue by issuing standard procedure guidelines that clearly indicate that digitally enhanced images are not routine. This permits radiologists to view them as needed, much the same way that an angiogram might be recommended as a follow-up study to acquire more information after a CT of the brain.

Image Stitching. It is possible to stitch together multiple images from some CR systems. This is especially useful for scoliosis studies of the spine, long bone studies, or angiographic imaging of peripheral vasculature. The algorithms that accomplish these images rely on overlapping exposures to verify registration marks and image contrast edges to align multiple exposures into a single image.

Grid Use

Grid use in CR occurs more often due to the sensitivity of the imaging plate to scatter. When performing chest radiography, a grid should be used when chest measurements exceed 24 to 26 cm for optimum images. Even when using a grid, if a substantial overexposure (>2X) occurs, enough scatter may be generated to degrade the image. Selecting the proper grid will depend on part size, kVp desired, scatter cleanup desired, and grid frequency (lines per cm or inch). The imaging plate is scanned line by line; **if the scan frequency and the grid frequency are similar and oriented in the same direction, a moire effect will be observed.** High-frequency grids (178–200 lines/inch) are often recommended for digital imaging systems. Grid cutoff occurs with CR; however, it is more difficult to identify because the computer will often not display the lines observed with film/screen. Rather, the image will suffer from poor detail, contrast, and density (Figure 23-32).

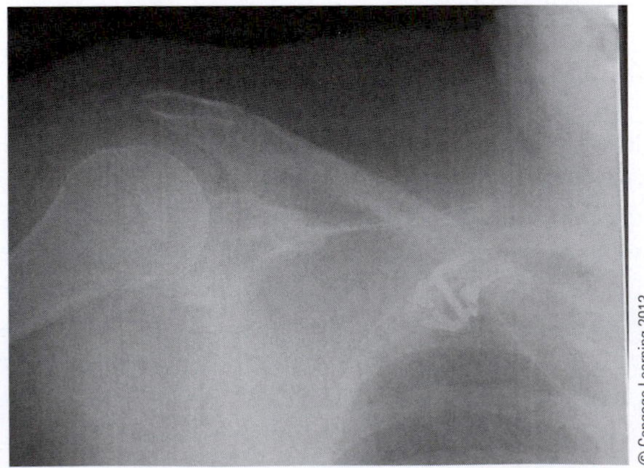

FIGURE 23-32. Grid cutoff error.

FLAT PANEL DIGITAL RADIOGRAPHY

Although CR has allowed a wider dynamic range for imaging and reduced some repeats due to technique, it still requires multiple steps for the technologist. Manufacturers continued to look for a more streamlined approach to imaging and produced flat panel detector digital systems generally referred to as DR. These systems eliminated cassettes and have reduced the number of steps required to perform exams. Initially these image receptors were built into the table or wall units, but there are now wireless DR cassettes. DR systems use either direct or indirect detectors. Direct detectors use a photoconductor, whereas indirect detectors use a scintillator (Figure 23-33).

Direct Detectors

Direct conversion systems directly convert incoming x-ray photons to an electronic digital signal. These systems use amorphous selenium (a-Se) and a thin film transistor (TFT) and are sometimes referred to as direct DR systems.

The active layer in the imaging plate is amorphous selenium, which is a semiconductor with excellent x-ray photon detection ability. Prior to the exposure, a high-voltage charge is applied from the top surface of the selenium layer. The ionization caused by the x-ray photons results in the selenium atoms freeing electrons for collection by the electrodes at the bottom of the selenium layer. The charges are collected at a TFT and then read out line by line to the computer for processing. This process is illustrated in Figure 23-34.

Indirect Detectors

There are two types of indirect DR detectors; one uses a flat panel TFT detector and the other uses a charged coupled device (CCD). Both systems need a scintillator to change the x-ray photons to light; the main difference is in the way the light is converted to an electrical signal. Amorphous silicon (a-Si:H) cannot directly convert x-rays into an electric charge, but it does work as a light detector (photodiode) to capture fluorescent light. Because the atomic number of silicon is only 14, it requires a relatively thick silicon layer to provide adequate sensitivity to the incoming x-ray photons. Therefore

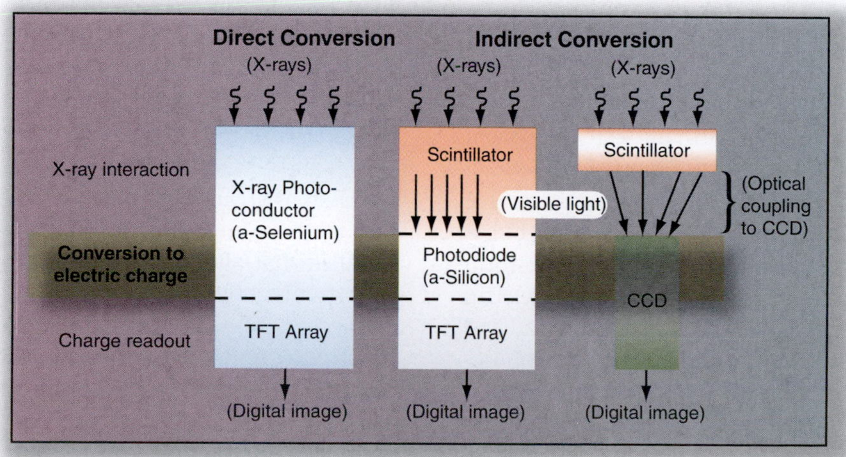

FIGURE 23-33. Direct and indirect flat panel detectors.

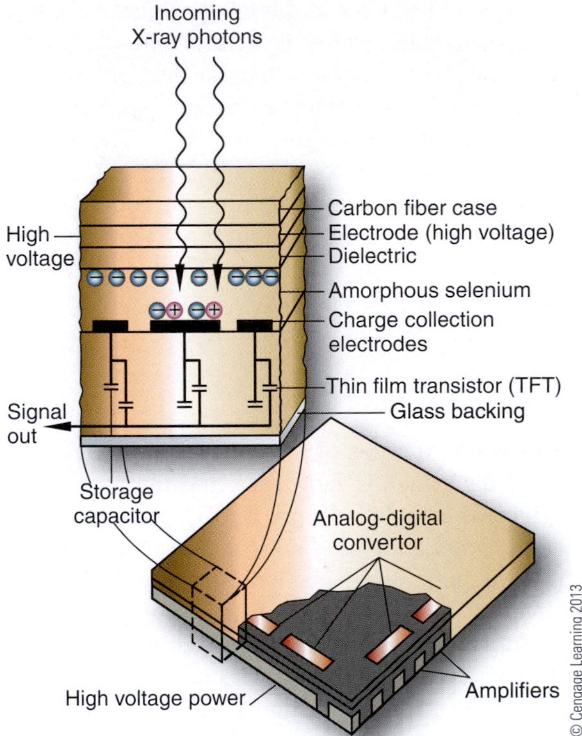

FIGURE 23-34. Direct conversion amorphous selenium flat panel imaging plate. The high-voltage charge at the top surface of the selenium layer results in the ionization caused by the x-ray photons to free electrons for collection by the electrodes at the bottom of the selenium layer. The charge that is collected is then transmitted through thin film detectors (TFTs) to the computer for processing.

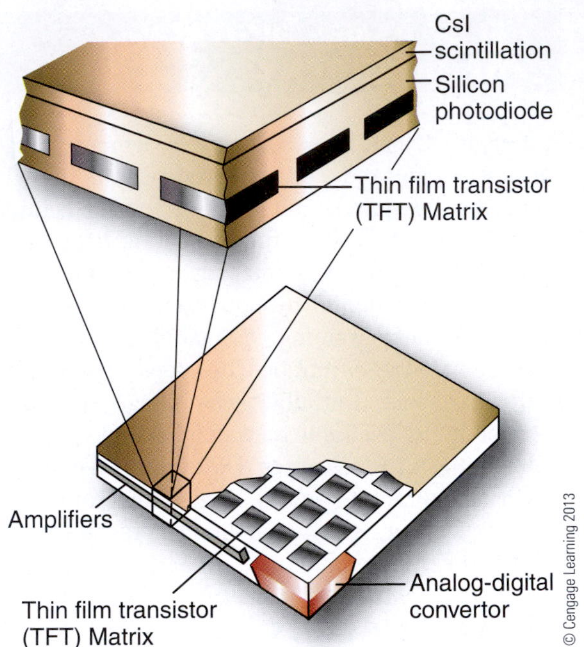

FIGURE 23-35. Indirect amorphous silicon flat panel imaging plate system. When x-ray photons strike the CsI they are converted to light. The columns of CsI reduce the light spread interacting with the amorphous silicon.

amorphous silicon requires a scintillator, such as cesium iodide (CsI), or a rare-earth intensifying screen composed of gadolinium oxysulfide (Gd_2O_2S). Scintillators emit light isotropically, which can reduce spatial resolution. To minimize light spread, CsI is manufactured as structured crystals in the form of needles or columns 10 to 20 micrometers in diameter. This significantly reduces light spread and channels light toward the amorphous silicon photodiode. The Gd_2O_2S is considered a turbid phosphor where the crystals are deposited as fine powdered particles. Once the light reaches the amorphous silicon, it is converted into electrical charges that are then deposited on a TFT. Figure 23-35 illustrates the design of an amorphous silicon system.

Flat Panel Thin Film Transistors (TFTs). Both the amorphous silicon and amorphous selenium flat plate detectors use thin film transistors (TFTs) for electronic readout. The TFT collects the electric charges produced by either the selenium or silicon as an array or matrix of pixel-size detector elements (DEL). (See Figure 23-36.) Each DEL has a switch and a sensing/storage area. When the switch for each DEL in a row is activated the signal is sent to the computer. The DELs are positioned in a matrix that allows the charge pattern to be read out on a pixel-by-pixel and column-by-column basis (Figure 23-37). Pixel size is related to the DEL, which affects pixel pitch and resolution. Detector electronics that are not sensitive to charge take up a certain amount of space. The *fill factor* refers to the sensing area compared to the non-sensing area and can be expressed as a percentage. If a detector has a fill factor of 80 percent, then the other 20 percent would be covered by the electronics. Currently

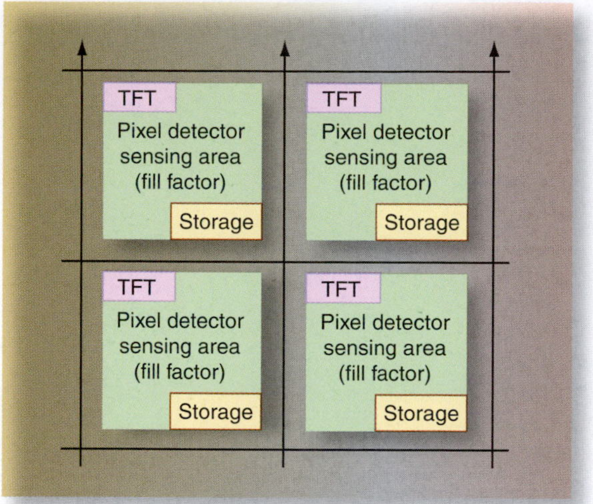

FIGURE 23-36. Portion of TFT array, with a capacitive storage element and switching element.

Thin Film Transitor (TFT)

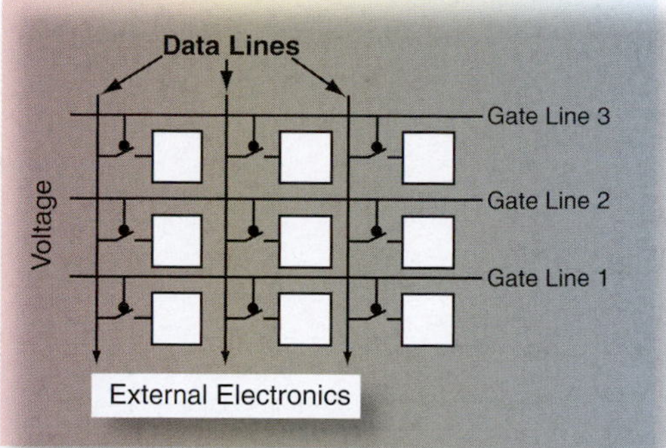

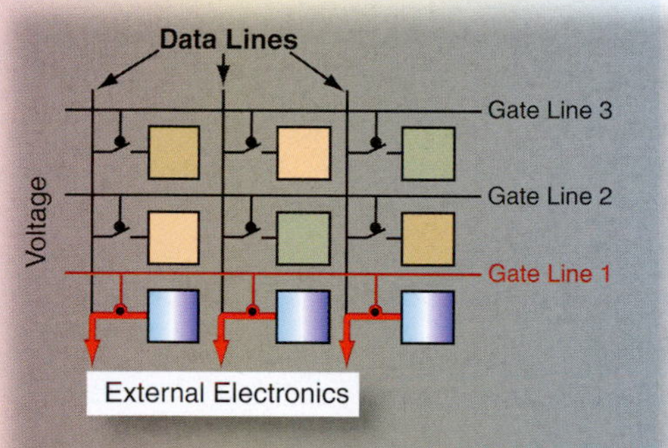

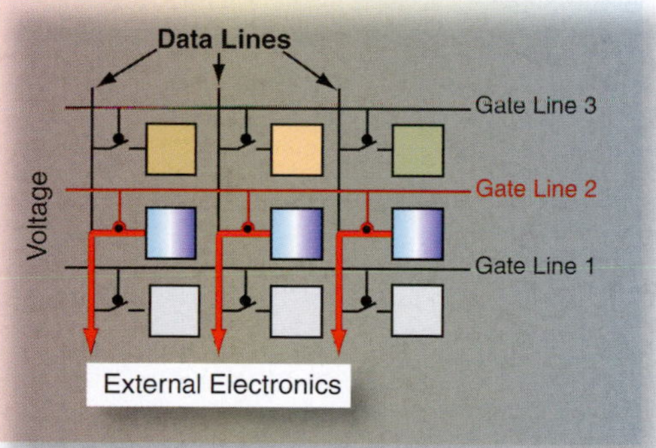

FIGURE 23-37. TFT—first array ready for exposure; middle has been exposed and first line is switched on to allow electron signal to leave; last image is next line being read. *(Adapted from RSNA 2003 Syllabus, "Digital Radiographic Technology," by John Yorkston, Ph.D., page 29.)*

most systems are at the smallest DEL possible, because trying to have a smaller pixel pitch will increase the electronics and lower the fill factor, resulting in less sensitivity.

Charge Coupled Device (CCD). The CCD is a photodetector, a device that is capable of converting visible light into an electric charge and storing it in a sequential pattern. This stored charge can then be released line by line to the ADC. A gadolinium oxysulfide (Gd_2O_2S) or a cesium iodide (CsI) screen is used as a scintillator, and the light produced from x-ray interactions must be optically coupled to the CCD sensor chip by lenses or fiber optics. The electrical signal produced by the CCD is then sent to the computer for image processing.

DR Image Processing

The processing principles for DR are similar to those for CR, as mentioned earlier in this chapter, with a few differences. Most flat field detectors have some bad detector elements, which would create artifacts if not corrected. The computer has a program to adjust for any deficiencies in the rows or columns of the TFT (Figure 23-38). The image is processed in a similar fashion as that in CR, where an algorithm is selected that will use exposure field recognition, histogram analysis, and the application of LUT. One difference in DR is that the entire image receptor is not read as it is when processing a CR plate. Only the exposed detector elements are used for the image data.

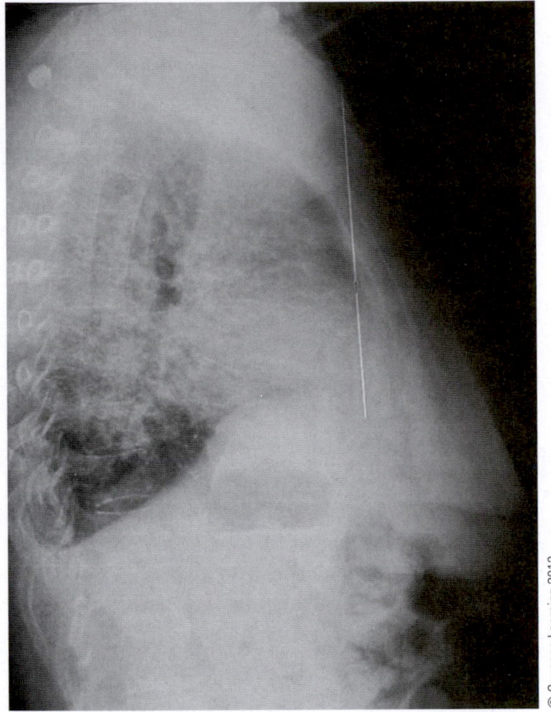

FIGURE 23-38. Note the white line, which is caused by a column of bad detector elements in the TFT. This requires a correction program and then it can be used again.

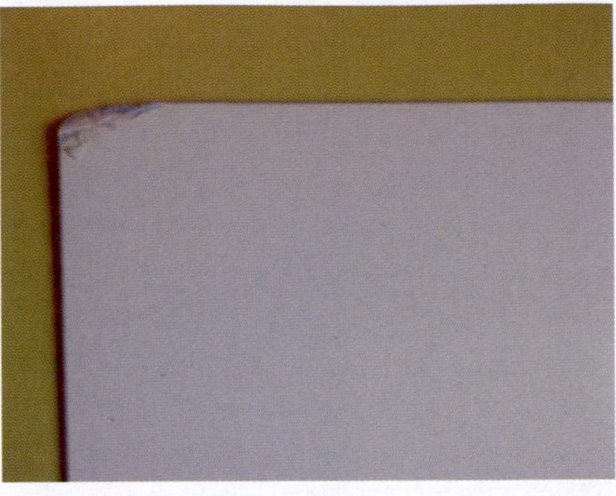

A

B

FIGURE 23-39. Note the peeling CR plate (A), which caused the artifacts at the bottom of the abdomen image (B).

DIGITAL RADIOGRAPHY ARTIFACTS

Just as there were artifacts in film/screen imaging, CR and DR also have unique artifact patterns in digital radiography systems. Generally, an artifact is an error of some sort on the image. Most artifacts are related to the following imaging system or operator errors, though this list is by no means inclusive of all artifact problems.

- Phantom or ghost images may appear as a result of incomplete image plate erasure. This artifact requires troubleshooting of both the CR plate preparation system and the display systems (laser imagers and/or display monitors). Extreme overexposure may require two erasure cycles to completely remove the image.
- Scratches or tears are permanent artifacts caused by damage to CR plates. Replacement of CR plates is expensive, but it is the only solution because these artifacts cannot be repaired (Figures 23-39A and B).
- Light spots are usually caused by dust or other foreign material on the imaging plate. CR plates can be cleaned, but this must be done carefully according to the manufacturer's recommendations to avoid permanent damage.
- A white line along the length of travel on the image is due to dust on the light guide (Figure 23-40).

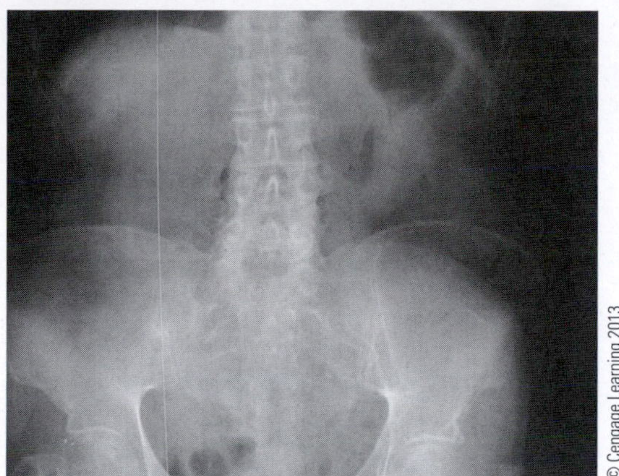

FIGURE 23-40. White line is from dust on the light guide blocking the light from CR plate.

- Dropout artifacts are reductions in resolution either overall or in specific areas of the image. They tend to be accompanied by contrast scale reductions, but this is difficult to assess because there are so many ways to modify image contrast and display monitors have inherent contrast deterioration over time. Dropout artifacts are a result of dust accumulation in the CR or laser imaging unit components (polygonal mirror, light gate, or other reflective surfaces). Cleaning of these units on a regular quality assurance schedule may avoid both image deterioration and early replacement of both CR and laser imaging equipment.
- Fogging from background radiation is due to imaging plates being much more sensitive than film (Figures 23-41A and B).
- Quantum mottle (or reticulation) is caused by inadequate exposure (usually insufficient mAs).
- Algorithm artifacts cover a wide range of image problems that correspond to the post-acquisition processing functions that are available on a specific CR system. To control these artifacts, manufacturers restrict access or provide preset values in order to provide a reasonable level of consistency between images for diagnostic comparisons.

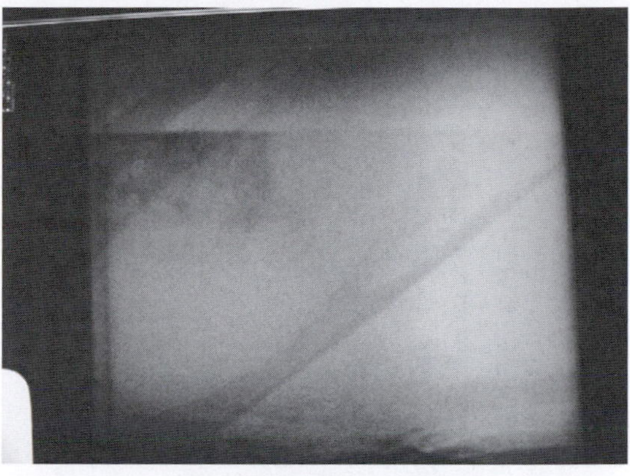
A

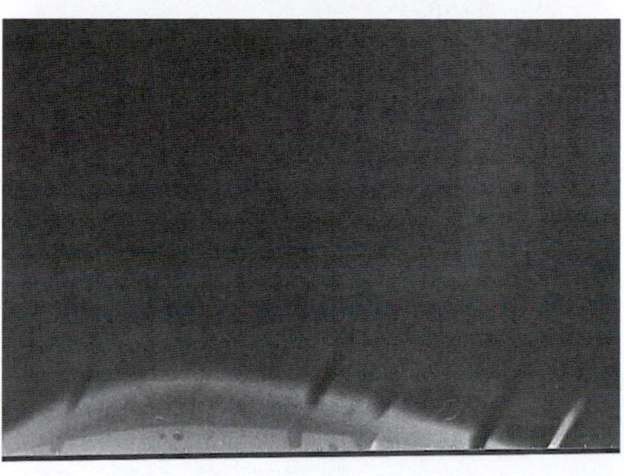
B

FIGURE 23-41. (A) Background radiation on plate was that not used for a week. (B) Scatter on a plate left propped up in room.

- Laser film transport artifacts, including uneven scanning, distortion, and overlapping shading, are all caused by uneven transport of film material through a laser imaging system.
- Histogram analysis error may be due to any of the following: improper collimation, improper technique, beam alignment, scatter, and extreme density differences (Figure 23-42).
- Nonparallel collimation—histograms require that collimation edges be parallel to the sides of imaging plate.
- Poor grid alignment may result in grid lines or poor image quality, as the computer may not display the grid lines (Figure 23-43).

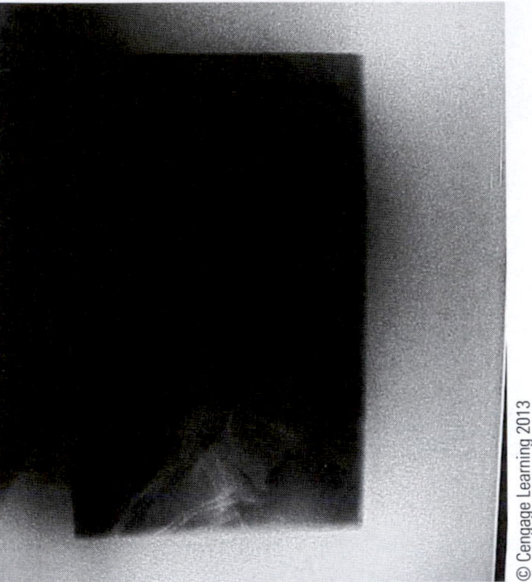

FIGURE 23-42. Improperly collimated and centered lumbar spine. S# 5396 indicates extreme underexposure; however, the image does not display that way.

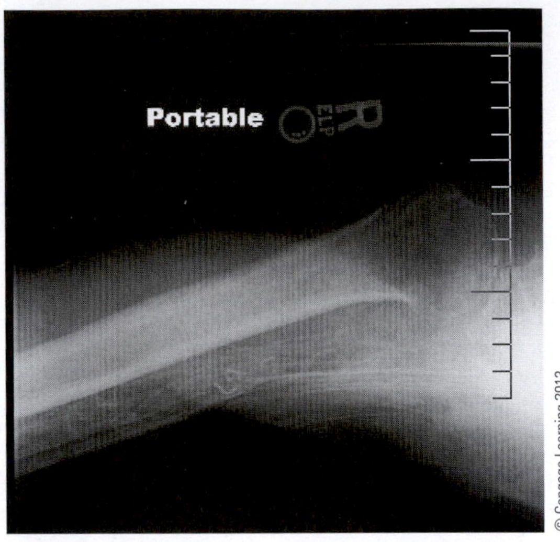

FIGURE 23-43. Axial shoulder with grid lines from a misaligned grid.

SUMMARY

Digital radiography imaging systems replace traditional film with a reusable detector. These systems are divided into two types generally known as computed radiography (CR) and digital radiography (DR). Computed radiography systems use a photostimulable storage phosphor imaging plate (PSP or IP), typically inside a cassette. Digital radiography (DR) systems typically have the detector and reader as a permanent part of a table or wall unit; therefore, a cassette is not needed. With DR systems, the image is acquired and sent directly to the display monitor without the need for the radiographer to physically move the detector for the image to be processed. There are a number of detector configurations used in DR that employ either direct conversion (without scintillator) or indirect conversion (with scintillator).

A digital image is one that has been converted into numerical values for transmission or processing. A matrix is a series of boxes laid out in rows and columns that gives form to the image. The individual matrix boxes are known as picture elements or pixels. Each pixel in the matrix is capable of representing a wide range of different shades of gray from pure white through total black. The number of shades of gray is determined by the grayscale bit depth.

There are a number of computer operations that can occur to process the image. These image processing operations are primarily intended to change the input values of the pixels to improve the diagnostic quality of the output image. They include (1) point processing, (2) local processing, and (3) geometric processing.

SUMMARY (continued)

Digital image quality factors include resolution, noise, and DQE. When matrix size is increased and pixel size goes down, spatial resolution increases. Noise can be classified as either electronic system noise or quantum mottle noise. Detective quantum efficiency (DQE) is a measure of the sensitivity and accuracy by which the image receptor converts the incoming data to the output viewing device.

Digital radiography processing systems use exposure indicators to provide information regarding the exposure to the image receptor, which is useful to indirectly determine patient exposure. The correct exposure factors will deliver an exposure indicator that is within an acceptable range and will give the best image quality. There is no universal system at this time, and different manufacturers use different systems for this information.

Computed radiography (CR) uses a photostimulable storage phosphor imaging plate (PSP or IP), typically inside a cassette. Currently, a number of manufacturers produce CR plates and processor systems. The cassette-based CR with the PSP requires a reader to process the plate and create the image and is a two-step process because the radiographer must move the detector between image acquisition and display. In order for CR to function, the imaging plate material must have the ability to store and release the image information in a usable form. The most common phosphors with characteristics favorable for CR are barium fluorohalide bromides and iodides with europium activators (BaFBr:Eu and BaFI:Eu). The latent image is processed by loading the cassette into an image reader device (IRD) where the imaging plate is scanned by a helium-neon laser beam. Once the plate is read, it is erased to remove all vestiges of the latent image. DR systems use either direct or indirect detectors. Direct conversion systems directly convert incoming x-ray photons to an electronic digital signal. These systems use amorphous selenium (a-Se) and a thin film transistor (TFT) and are sometimes referred to as direct DR systems. There are two types of indirect DR detectors; one uses a flat panel TFT detector and the other uses a charged coupled device (CCD). Both systems need a scintillator to change the x-ray photons to light; the main difference is in the way the light is converted to an electrical signal.

Digital radiography has unique artifacts as a result of errors in the systems, including phantom images, quantum mottle, and histogram errors. ■

REVIEW QUESTIONS

1. Give an example of the types of image receptors used for both a direct and indirect conversion digital radiography system.
2. Name the image receptors used in one of the flat panel detector systems.
3. Explain the function of two of the layers of a photostimulable phosphor imaging plate.
4. Why are imaging plates more sensitive to radiation than radiographic film?
5. Why do digital radiography cassettes stored for several days after exposure and before processing lose most of their latent image?
6. How is digital radiography spatial resolution controlled?
7. What data are collected during the creation of the histogram from a digital radiography exposure?
8. Why do digital radiography systems have significantly greater latitude than conventional film/screen radiography systems?

9. What elements of computed radiography systems make them prone to violations of ALARA radiation protection concepts?
10. Name as many digital radiography artifacts as you know.

REFERENCES AND RECOMMENDED READING

Bell, J. (1999). A direct image capture system: The future of digital x-ray. *Medical Imaging Technology, 17*(2), 105–109.

Burns, C. (1993). Using computed digital radiography effectively. *Seminars in Radiologic Technology, 1*(1), 24–35.

Bushberg, J., Seibert, J., Leidholdt, E., & Boone, J. (2011). *The essential physics of medical imaging* (3rd ed.) Baltimore, MD: Williams & Wilkins.

Cesar, L. (1997). Computed radiography: Its impact on radiographers. *Radiologic Technology, 68*(3), 225–232.

Choatas, H., Dobbins, J., & Ravin, C. (1999). Principles of digital radiography with large-area electronically readable detectors: A review of the basics. *Radiology, 210*(3), 595–599.

Cowen, A. R., Kengyelics, S. M., & Davies, A. G. (2008). Solid-state, flat-panel, digital radiography detectors and their physical imaging characteristics. *Clinical Radiology, 63*(5), 487–498.

Floyd, C., Warp, R., Dobbins, J. III, et al. (2001, March). Imaging characteristics of an amorphous silicon flat-panel detector for digital chest radiography. *Radiology, 218*, 683–688.

Fuji Photo Film Co., Ltd. (1996). *Fujifilm imaging and information: Chapter 2: Information capacity of FCR images.* (Ref. No. CR-008040C2 [CR-96-9]). Tokyo: Author.

Fuji Photo Film Co., Ltd. (1996). *Fujifilm imaging and information: Chapter 3: Auto density control (EDR).* (Ref. No. CR-008040C3 [CR-96-9]). Tokyo: Author.

Fuji Photo Film Co., Ltd. (1996). *Fujifilm imaging and information: Chapter 4: Image processing.* (Ref. No. CR-008040C4 [CR-96-9]). Tokyo: Author.

Fuji Photo Film Co., Ltd. (1996). *Fujifilm imaging and information: Chapter 5: Special image processing.* (Ref. No. CR-008040C5 [CR-96-9]). Tokyo: Author.

Fuji Photo Film Co., Ltd. (1996). *Fujifilm imaging and information: Appendix 1: Clinical effects of FCR.* (Ref. No. CR-008040A1 [CR-96-9]). Tokyo: Author.

Fuji Photo Film Co., Ltd. (1996). *Fujifilm imaging and information: Appendix 2: Case studies.* (Ref. No. CR-008040A2 [CR-96-9]). Tokyo: Author.

Hillman, B., & Fajardo, L. (1989). Clinical assessment of phosphor-plate computed radiography: Equipment, strategy, and methods. *Journal of Digital Imaging, 2*(4), 220–227.

Honey, I. D., & Mackenzie, A. (2009). Artifacts found during quality assurance testing of computed radiography and digital radiography detectors. *Journal of Digital Imaging, 22*(4), 383–392.

International Electrotechnical Commission (IEC). (2008). Medical electrical equipment: Exposure index of digital x-ray imaging systems—part 1: Definitions and requirements for general radiography. Geneva, Switzerland: Author.

Koenker, R. M. (2007). Digital radiography quality assurance: A technique for standardizing image appearance across CR and DR platforms. *Applied Radiology, 36*(6), 22, 24–28.

Krupinski, E. A., Williams, M. B., Andriole, K., Strauss, K. J., Applegate, K., Wyatt, M., Bjork, S., & Seibert, J. A. (2007, June). Digital radiography image quality: Image processing and display. *Journal of the American College of Radiology, 4*(6), 389–400.

Lança, L., & Silva, A. (2009). Digital radiography detectors—a technical overview: Part 1. *Radiography*, 15(1): 58–62.

Lança, L., & Silva, A. (2009). Digital radiography detectors—a technical overview: Part 2. *Radiography, 15*(2), 134–138.

Lim, A. (1996). Image quality in film digitizers: Testing and quality assurance. In *Syllabus: A course in physics* (pp. 183–193). Chicago, IL: Radiological Society of North America.

Long, B. W. (1989). Computed radiography: Photostimulable phosphor image plate technology. *Radiologic Technology, 61*(2), 107–112.

Mixdorf, M., & Tortorici, M. (1993). Practical considerations in computed radiography. *Seminars in Radiologic Technology, 1*(1), 16–23.

Neitzel, U. (1999, July). Integrated digital radiography with a flat electronic detector. Retrieved from www.de.ms.philips.com/sections/rad/digbucky/news/html/neitzel.htm.

Oakley, J. (2004). Digital imaging: A primer for radiographers, radiologists and health care professionals. Cambridge, UK: Greenwich Medical Media Cambridge University Press.

Prieto, C., Vano, E., Ten, J. I., Fernandez, J. M., Iñiguez, A. I., Arevalo, N., Litcheva, A., Crespo, E., Floriano, A., & Martinez, D. (2009). Image retake analysis in digital radiography using DICOM header information. Digital imaging and communications in medicine. *Journal of Digital Imaging, 22*(4), 393–399.

Reiner, B. I., Siegel, E. L., & Carrino, J. A. (Eds.). (2002). *Quality assurance: Meeting the challenge in the digital medical enterprise.* Great Falls, VA: Society for Computer Applications in Radiology (SCAR).

Samei, E., & Flynn, M. J. (Eds.). (2003). *Advances in digital radiography: Categorical course in diagnostic radiology physics.* Oak Brook, IL: Radiological Society of North America.

Samei, E., Seibert, J., Willis, C., Flynn, M., Mah E., & Junck, K. (2001). Performance evaluation of computed radiography systems. *Medical Physics, 28*(3), 361–371.

Seeram, E. (2011). *Digital radiography, an introduction.* Clifton Park, NY: Delmar Cengage Learning.

Seibert, J., Bogucki, T., & Ciona, T. (1998). *Acceptance testing and quality control of photostimulable storage phosphor imaging systems* (Report of Task Group #10). College Park, MD: American Association of Physicists in Medicine.

Seibert, J. A. (2004). Performance testing of digital radiographic systems: Computed radiography. In L. W. Goldman & M. V. Yester (Eds.), Specifications, performance, and quality assurance of radiographic and fluoroscopic systems in the digital era. College Park, MD: American Association of Physicists in Medicine.

Seibert, J. A. (2009). Digital radiography: The bottom line comparison of CR and DR technology ... computed radiography ... digital radiography. *Applied Radiology, 38*(5), 21–28.

Shepard, J., Wang, J., Flynn, M., Gingold, E., Goldman, L., & Krus, K. (2009). An exposure indicator for digital radiography: AAPM Task Group 116 (Executive Summary). *Medical Physics, 36*(7), 2898–2914.

Solomon, S., Jost, R., Glazer, H., Sagel, S., Anderson, D., & Molina, P. (1991). Artifacts in computed radiography. *American Journal of Roentgenology, 157,* 181–185.

Uffmann, M., & Schaefer-Prokop, C. (2009). Digital radiography: The balance between image quality and required radiation dose. *European Journal of Radiology, 72*(2), 202–208.

Williams, M. B., Krupinski, E. A., Strauss, K. J., Breeden, W. K., Rzeszotarski, M. S., Applegate, K., Wyatt, M., Bjork, S., & Seibert, J. A. (2007). Digital radiography image quality: Image acquisition. *Journal of the American College of Radiology, 4*(6), 371–388.

Willis, C. E. (2008). Digital radiography: CR versus DR? Sometimes recognizing the distinction in technologies makes a difference. *Applied Radiology, 37*(1), 25–28.

Wilson, P. (1984). Digital imaging: An introduction. *Radiography, 50*(590), 449.

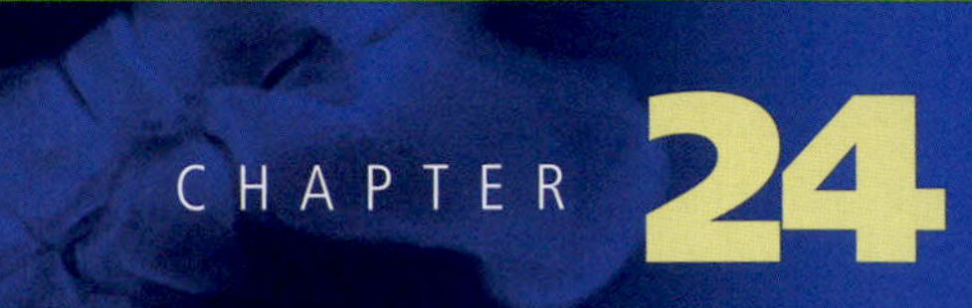

Picture Archiving and Communications Systems (PACSs)

Rick Hay, PhD, MD, FAHA

KEY TERMS

biomedical informatics (BMI)
digital imaging and communication in medicine (DICOM)
electronic health-care (or health) record
electronic medical record (EMR)
hard copy
hospital information system (HIS)
informatics
picture archiving and communication system (PACS)
radiology information system (RIS)
soft copy

> It is a very sad thing that nowadays there is so little useless information.
>
> *Oscar Wilde (1854–1900)*

OBJECTIVES

Upon completion of this chapter, the student should be able to:

- Describe various platforms used in biomedical informatics.
- Discuss the advantages of using a PACS in a medical imaging department.
- Explain why a PACS network may require a separate computer network from the one used throughout an institution.
- Discuss the necessity for DICOM in medical imaging.
- Describe the various types of laser printers that can be used for digital images.
- Explain soft-copy monitor display parameters.
- Identify types of storage available for digital images.

INFORMATICS

Informatics describes the body of ideas, devices, and processes related to handling multiple types of information. In the early twenty-first century, electronic devices (computers, computer-based instruments, and electronic storage media) are de facto workhorses for pursuing informatics. A particular configuration of informatics devices and processes is called a *platform*.

Biomedical informatics (BMI) refers to platforms that are used for medical purposes, such as patient care, and for biological applications and activities related to health care, including both preclinical research (studying disease or treatments in cells and animals) and clinical research (e.g., testing new drugs on patients or analyzing health-care statistics). Although some BMI platforms are better suited for patient-oriented applications and others for research activities, their underlying features overlap sufficiently to make BMI a popular and useful term.

A **picture archiving and communication system (PACS)** denotes a BMI platform configured in a manner that facilitates storing, retrieving, and distributing medical images. Although images need not be originally acquired in a digital format (e.g., they could be photographs of skin lesions or before-and-after pictures of plastic surgery), they must be converted to digital format in order to be accessed by a PACS.

A **hospital information system (HIS)** and **radiology information system (RIS)** encompass BMI platforms used in a health-care facility and in a radiology department, respectively. There has been a proliferation of similar BMI platforms (with proprietary acronyms) tailored for smaller health-care facilities such as individual medical (or dental, optometric, or veterinary) practices. These systems now render electronic a wide range of functions that were formerly done by hand or via separate electronic programs, including scheduling patient appointments and issuing reminders, tracking staffing assignments, submitting invoices to health-care insurers and patients, monitoring different insurance coverage provisions and updating them, filing and locating patient medical records, printing and mailing letters and reports, ordering prescriptions, and so on.

Finally, **electronic (or enterprise) medical record (EMR)** and **electronic health-care (or health) record (EHR)** are synonyms for an electronic version of an individual patient's collection of medical documents. Within a single health-care facility (such as a primary care provider's office), the EHR serves in lieu of or in addition to a hard-copy paper file (medical chart) as a medicolegal record. Most health-care facilities maintain separate records but may communicate all or part of that record to other facilities.

A PACS platform usually begins with the process of gathering and organizing the images after their acquisition. Post-processing may be helpful if the images were not all acquired in the same proprietary format. There must be a designated place for processed image storage, as well as a backup archive. There should be a reliable procedure for retrieving the stored images and displaying them in a format meaningful to the viewer. Finally, there should be some means for distributing or communicating the content of the images to intended viewers (but not to unintended ones).

The DICOM Standard

In the highly competitive market of biomedical imaging, each instrument and its computer platform typically use proprietary, vendor-unique software and formatting for image acquisition and display. As PACSs became more common, some proprietary platforms did not communicate smoothly with PACS platforms, requiring some studies to be specially read at one or more specific acquisition terminals. Some imaging equipment manufacturers began to provide programs that would translate files into a format so they could be read at different manufacturers' PACS reading stations.

DICOM is an acronym for the **Digital Imaging and Communications in Medicine** standard. It originated in the 1980s as a collaborative effort between the American College of Radiology (ACR) and the National Electrical Manufacturers' Association (NEMA) to establish a universal, standardized public format and protocol for communicating biomedical imaging files, and it is periodically upgraded. A current DICOM reader utility program may be downloaded for free, and most manufacturers provide a utility program to convert their proprietary image files into DICOM format. Once an image has been converted to DICOM format, it may be shared with anybody else in the world who has a DICOM reader, regardless of what proprietary imaging acquisition and display platform.

Each image has many files attached to it, which contain data such as patient and image information. There is a large amount of raw data that needs to travel through the system, which needs to be converted, especially when traveling to equipment from different vendors.

DICOM is an object-oriented standard that designates real-world objects that it models and the information objects used to achieve that modeling. There are two classes of information: the object class, which contains information about the study and patient, and the service class, which describes what to do with objects. The service class includes image storage, image query, image retrieval, image print, storage resource, and examination. The object class includes normalized and composite information. The normalized object can contain information in areas such as patient, study, results, storage resource, and image annotation. The composite object will have the modality used, such as CR, DR, CT, MR, digitized film, US, and NM. (See Table 24-1.)

The object class and service class combine to form units, or service object pairs (SOPs). The combination of a service, such as image storage, with an object, such as a CT exam, would constitute an SOP. Equipment can either use or provide a service, leading to the terms service class user (SCU) and service class provider (SCP). Whether equipment is a user or provider depends on how it is asked to function. For example, if the CT scanner wants to send an image to the workstation for storage, the CT scanner is the SCU (user) and the workstation is the SCP (provider). The CT scanner must know how to send the image data and the workstation must know how to receive it. Then the workstation can become a user when it wants to send the image for storage, while the storage is the provider. In this case the workstation can be either a provider or user depending on how it is asked to function. DICOM is an extremely complex software; this is only a simple explanation of how it can work.

TABLE 24-1. DICOM Information Classes

Service Class	Object Class
Image storage	Normalized
Image query	• Patient, study, results, storage resource, image annotation
Image retrieval	Composite
Image print	• CR
Storage resource	• CT
Examination	• MR
	• Digitized film
	• NM
	• US

Other Standards

In addition to the DICOM standard, there are several official acronyms for standards or regulations that affect how BMI or its individual components operate. Those of greatest importance are:

HIPAA is the acronym for the Health Insurance Portability and Accountability Act of 1996. This federal law requires that all communications concerning health-care information must have features to safeguard both the identity of an individual and the confidentiality of the information being communicated. For BMI, this means that any medical information that is handled electronically must either be encrypted, have all patient identifiers removed, or be scrubbed of all except the relevant data fields.

HL-7 or HL7 refers to Health Level Seven International, an organization that "provides standards for interoperability that improve care delivery, optimize workflow, reduce ambiguity and enhance knowledge transfer among all of our stakeholders, including healthcare providers, government agencies, the vendor community, fellow SDOs and patients." The standards concern computer-related communications involving health-care information, and are widely adopted throughout the BMI community.

When using BMI, or its PACS component, there are personal practices that should be adopted. These are not law or regulation. Instead, many clinical and research institutions have internal policies that reflect them. Two good common-sense practices to implement are:

- Always observe all employer-mandated personal computer or network terminal workstation precautions and etiquette. In particular, adhere to password protection and log-in and log-out requirements, such as logging out of a terminal (or locking it) whenever you leave it, however briefly.
- Do whatever else you possibly can to protect patients' health-care information from unauthorized access. For example, health-care personnel should never carry or keep patient-specific or patient-traceable information on portable media (laptops, CDs, flash drives, tapes, hard copies) unless explicitly authorized to do so for a specific purpose. Ironically, sometimes patients are their own worst security threats, carrying confidential information with them as they travel to get a second opinion. Whenever possible, health-care information should be transmitted electronically in encrypted form directly from one health-care provider to another rather than by physical courier or the patient.

IMAGE ACQUISITION

Computers were used early on for computed tomography, magnetic resonance imaging, ultrasound, and nuclear medicine to capture, display, and move images between workstations and printers. These configurations are sometimes called mini PACS. This development was followed by digital fluoroscopy and angiography, where the video signal from the image intensifier was converted into a digital signal. Finally, radiographic images were converted to digital through the use of computed radiography and film digitizers.

A film digitizer is used to convert an analog film image to a digital image that can then be used in a PACS. Film digitizers also allow images to be sent to outside institutions through teleradiology.

IMAGE DISTRIBUTION

Network infrastructure and file management have a tremendous impact on how image data travels or is distributed. Once images are obtained they need to be transmitted over a network. Just as film images need to be sent to a radiologist to be read, stored, and often sent to clinicians, so do digital images. A PACS allows digital images to be sent from their acquisition point to a radiologist or other clinician to be diagnosed and then stored for retrieval. In order to move digital information, a network is required to allow computers in the system to communicate with one another.

Each digital acquisition system (CR, DR, CT, etc.) has a computer workstation that holds the images in files for the technologist to check for quality before sending them for diagnosis. The size of an image file will depend on matrix size and bit depth.

Grayscale bit depth ranges from 8 bits to 32 bits. A byte is equal to 8 bits, so the file size of a pixel is multiplied by the bit depth divided by 8. A grayscale bit depth of 8–32 equals a range of 1–4 bytes of storage that would be required per pixel in the image matrix. A grayscale bit depth of 12 produces 2^{12} gray levels. This represents 4,096 different shades of gray that are available, a spectacular diagnostic range that is far beyond the range of the human visual system.

Image file size is determined by the formula XY (B/8)

where: X = x-axis pixel matrix size
Y = y-axis pixel matrix size
B = gray scale bit depth

EXAMPLE: What is the anticipated image file size for a computed radiography digital image comprised of a 2,500 × 2,500 matrix with a 12-bit depth?

Answer:

XY (B/8)

2,500 × 2,500 (12/8) =

6,250,000 (12/8) =

6,250,000 (1.5) =

9,375,000 = 9.375 Mb

EXAMPLE: What is the anticipated file storage necessary for a computed tomography examination comprised of 2,500 images, each with a 512 × 512 matrix at 16-bit depth?

Answer:

XY (B/8)

512 × 512 (16/8) =

262,144 (16/8) =

262,144 (2) =

524,288 = 524.288 Kb

524.288 Kb × 2,500 images = 1,310,720 = 1.31072 Gb

Diagnostic radiography has a large matrix size for each image to increase resolution, whereas a CT image has a lower matrix for each image, but many more images are obtained for each exam. A PACS transmits large amounts of data to a wide range of processing, storage, and display units.

To move image data from one place to another in a PACS requires a network with bandwidth capable of handling large data files. Bandwidth is measured in bits per second (bps) and describes how much data can be moved. Usually a PACS network is separate from other hospital information systems because the data files are large and need to move quickly. A local area network (LAN) connects all the computers in a system and often uses a special wiring system such as an ethernet that can have a bandwidth of 10 Mbps. When information leaves the system to go to another location far away, such as in teleradiology, it is over a wide area network (WAN), which often operates at much slower speeds. Many institutions are establishing wireless networks, which, although convenient, may operate even slower. Slower transmission systems require more time to display images with extremely large files, such as multiple detector CT or 3D echocardiography. Display times for these modalities may be too long to allow reasonable use via some of the networks. This factor, along with the special language and operating systems used by PACSs, often causes problems in interfacing with patient HIS.

IMAGE DISPLAY

Image display devices are dependent on the purpose of the user. Traditionally, film was displayed on an illuminator viewbox. Digital images can still be produced on film (**hard copy**) with a laser printer. However, in a filmless environment the images are viewed on a flat screen monitor (**soft copy**). Digital images need to be displayed for the technologist to review and for the radiologist to read. They can also be displayed for clinicians throughout a hospital or clinic. There are numerous advantages to soft-copy display: multiple viewing of the same image, variation of image display parameters (such as density/brightness/sensitivity and contrast), and reduced numbers of lost films.

Hard-copy Display

Hard-copy display refers to images that are visualized on film. Hard-copy images are typically produced using laser printers or dry processors.

Laser Printers. Laser printers were introduced in 1983 as part of the Fuji CR system. Since that time many manufacturers and types of laser printers have been developed. There are three light sources for laser printers: infrared (780–820 nm), solid-state diode (~670–680 nm), and helium-neon (HeNe: 633 nm). The printers produce transilluminated hard-copy film images from computerized digital information. Printers work with either wet or dry processors and often have a bit depth or grayscale of 8 bits, whereas some detectors may have 10, 12, 15, or 16 bits. This requires a calibration from the larger bit size of the detector to the lower 8 bits for the printer. Calibration films can be printed to check the optical density range of the printer (Figure 24-1).

Generally, a laser printer, regardless of the manufacturer, has the following components: a laser source, collimator lens or beam-shaping optics, a beam modulator, deflecting mirror-shaping lenses, and a cylindrical reflection mirror (Figure 24-2). The printer also has an unexposed film storage with a mechanical transport to move the film through the printer as it is exposed line by line in a raster scan pattern by the laser. After passing through the

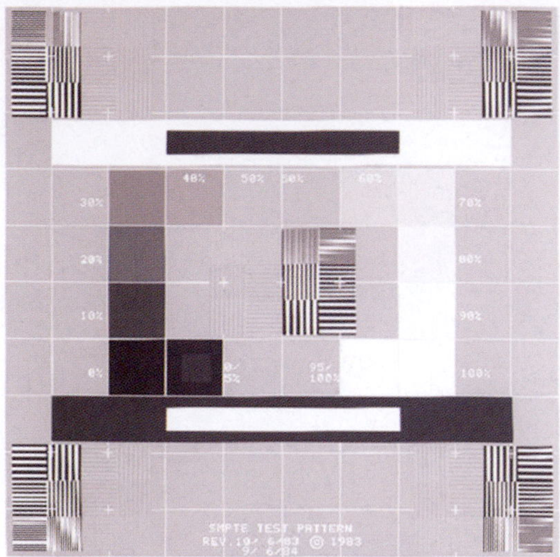

FIGURE 24-1. A laser printer calibration film demonstrates the full range of density and contrast for the unit. *(Courtesy of Jeff Lloyd, Spectrum Health.)*

laser area, the film is processed, either by wet or dry processing methods, and it is deposited into the exposed film receptor bin.

Dry Processors. Dry processors do not use developer, fixer, or wash to process an image on film, eliminating the need for the chemicals and plumbing required by wet processing. This allows more flexibility in printer placement within an imaging department. Medical printers commonly use thermal processing for film-based images. Thermal processing involves the use of heat-sensitive film with silver-based emulsion, dye microcapsules, and carbon-based adherographic printing.

Silver-based dry film contains silver benhate that responds to light from a laser and heat from a thermal head. The laser beam produces latent image centers; only the activated silver halide grains develop when heated by the thermal head. Because the density results immediately after exposure to the laser and heat, it does not require wet processing, which leaves all the chemical compounds on the film. Potentially, the film could continue to develop density if exposed to high-heat conditions, something referred to as "print-up." Manufacturers have developed films that minimize this condition, resulting in a stable film image in most circumstances. Unexposed dry processing laser film has a shorter shelf life than conventional film because it is more sensitive to heat and humidity.

Adherographic processing uses selective adhesion of carbon particles onto a plastic base that is then sealed. The film is composed of multiple layers, which are exposed to a gallium arsenide laser. Wherever the laser exposes the film, carbon particles adhere. This becomes a distinct image when the layers are separated. This process was first developed by Polaroid Medical Imaging Systems in 1993. To protect the image and keep the carbon particles in place, a cover sheet is sealed or laminated onto the finished film.

Soft-copy Display

Soft-copy display refers to images visualized on monitors, usually flat panel technology, although there are still some older cathode ray tube (CRT) monitors.

A great advantage of digital imaging is the ability to manipulate the image without re-exposing the patient. Images are best manipulated when they are displayed on a monitor. Additionally, images can be viewed in multiple locations simultaneously and can be quickly distributed to multiple locations when in digital format.

Monitor characteristics are determined by the requirements of the user. Technologists need to evaluate an image prior to sending it to a PACS, whereas radiologists need to use images for diagnosis. Physicians will look at images either in the hospital or at remote locations. All of these uses will not need the same display quality. Diagnostic viewing by the radiologist requires a monitor with the highest spatial and contrast resolution (along with higher cost), whereas clinical viewing stations for physicians may be acceptable with lower resolution and less cost. Radiographers require monitors that will allow adequate visualization of contrast and resolution to determine if the image is of diagnostic quality for the physician.

There are two types of monitors on the market that are found in most imaging departments: the cathode ray tube (CRT) monitor and the liquid crystal display (LCD) flat panel monitor. The

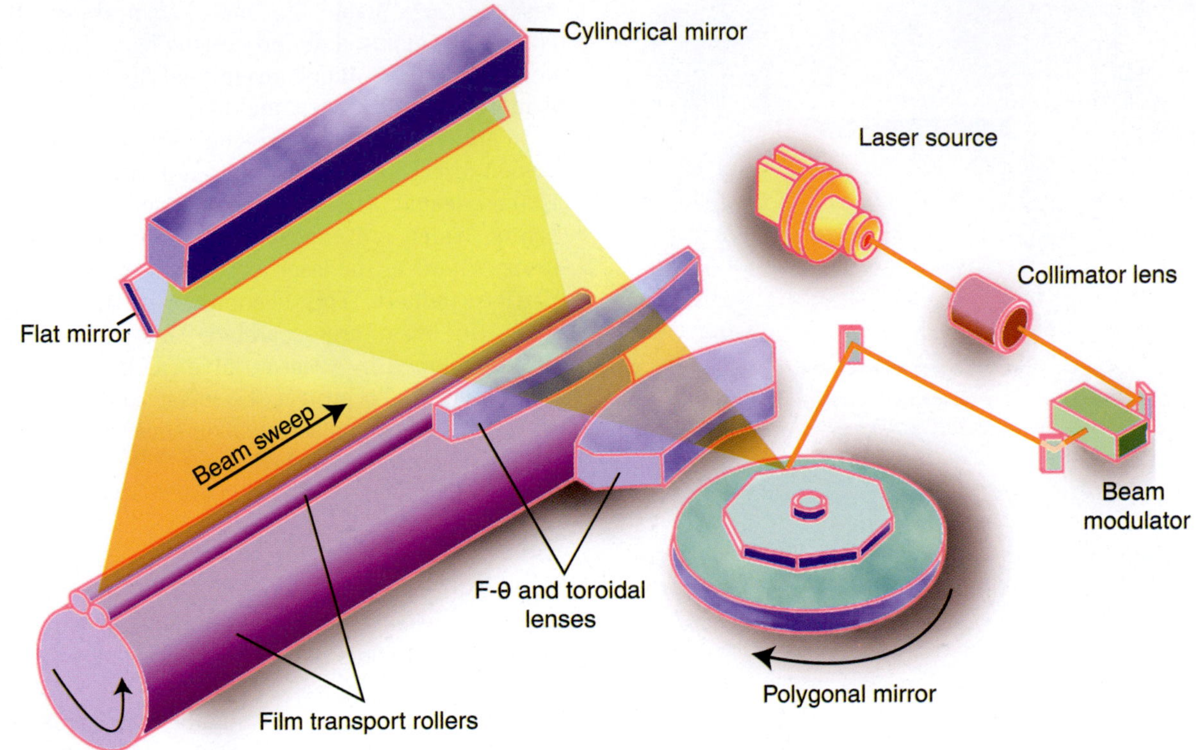

FIGURE 24-2. Schematic diagram of a film laser camera. A constant-intensity laser source is focused by a collimator lens, modulated according to the digital value of the image pixel, and directed at the film. The F-theta/toroidal lenses and the cylindrical mirror modify the shape of the beam to minimize distortion toward the periphery of the image. [*Used with permission from Bushberg, J., Beth, J., Landholt, K., and Boone, J. (2002). The Essential Physics of Medical Imaging (2nd ed.). Philadelphia: Lippincott, Williams, Wilkins, Fig. 17-12.*]

resolution of a monitor is based on how many pixels can be displayed in the horizontal and vertical dimensions. A 1-K CRT monitor would display 1,280 × 1,024 pixels, and a 2-K CRT monitor would display 2,048 × 2,560 pixels. The higher the number of pixels, the higher the resolution. LCD monitors may have resolutions as high as 3–5 megapixels. Typically, radiographers and physicians use lower-resolution monitors, whereas the radiologist workstations provide higher resolution.

Image quality on a monitor is affected by resolution, luminance, contrast, uniformity, and glare. Because these areas can affect the technologist and radiologist when viewing images, a quality control (QC) program needs to be performed on a regular basis to ensure high quality is maintained. Acceptance testing of new equipment will establish a baseline for QC measurements that will be a reference for annual testing. There are phantoms available for QC testing, and a photometer for measuring luminance will be needed. All monitors in a workstation should have the same level of luminance.

Resolution is related to the number of pixels in the horizontal and vertical dimensions. However, detail of a monitor with a large matrix may still be poor due to electron spot size changing or "blooming," causing pixel size to become larger than the nominal or state size. This blooming is affected by luminance and monitor age. A SMPTE test pattern can be used for a visual inspection of resolution, or more complex tests can be run (refer to Figure 24-1).

Contrast should be set the same on all monitors so that the same grayscale is consistent throughout the department. Ambient light reflections on a monitor will have a negative impact on contrast. Monitors have design features to reduce this effect; however, it cannot be eliminated. Therefore, monitors should not be used in rooms with bright lighting. Acceptance testing will allow an acceptable test pattern image to be stored that can be retrieved for testing annually. Contrast is also a function of luminance, and the monitor must have adequate amounts of light from all areas. A luminance uniformity test uses a photometer to test the light from the center and outer corners of the monitor. This will pick up any deviation across the display.

Soft-copy veiling glare, often referred to as "glare," results from the internal process of a monitor, rather than the external light causing reflection off the monitor screen. Glare will also cause a decrease in contrast, producing lower image quality. There are a number of factors that cause glare, for example, light scattering on the faceplate, light leakage, and electron backscattering. All of these actions will cause light spread, which will decrease contrast. Veiling glare is discussed in detail in Chapter 14, Vision and Perception.

The use of monitors requires a consistent power source because fluctuations in voltage will affect the electron gun and image display. Ambient room light must be reduced so as to maximize image contrast. Placing workstations with the corresponding monitors and control panels requires a different environment from using hard-copy film illuminator viewboxes.

Flat panel LCD monitors are much thinner than CRT monitors, which means they use less space on desks and counters. The LCD monitor regulates the image by using a light source behind the screen shining on individual pixels, which control the amount of light transmitted through. Liquid crystal and hydrogenated amorphous silicon (a-Si:H) thin film transistors (TFTs) are contained between glass plates on the front of the monitor, which regulate pixel transparency. This allows rapid changes in voltage to alter a pixel from black (no light transmitted) to transparent (full light transmission). LCD monitors have restricted fields of view. This is the angle from which the display screen can be viewed. A special problem of LCD displays is that the field of view gradually deteriorates as the viewer moves away from the center of the screen. The LCD requires quality testing on a regular basis, starting with acceptance testing and continuing periodically throughout the life of the monitor.

STORAGE

A major problem for all radiology departments is the storage of images as required by local legal precedents. Many institutions store all images for 5 to 7 years, with pediatric and litigation films retained indefinitely. The exact number of years is often determined by state laws regarding statute of limitations. Many hours of staff time and immense amounts of space are required to maintain these files. A PACS eliminates the need for most of the space for storage and reduces the time requirements. Misfiling becomes much less likely and acquisition time can be reduced tremendously. In addition, PACS terminals permit access to images from remote locations (e.g., surgery, emergency units, etc.).

Image storage requires immense amounts of memory. Digital storage of images for a typical large radiology department that does 150,000 examinations per year (with about 100,000 of these diagnostic radiography and the 50,000 divided among CT, ultrasound, MRI, nuclear medicine, mammography, and vascular procedures) has been estimated at about 3.2 terabytes of computer memory per year. Considering a normal 3 to 5 year image storage requirement, a total memory of 10–16 terabytes (Tb) (10,000 Gb or 10,000,000–16,000,000 Mb) would be required for a complete digital PACS. With gigabytes and terabytes of memory now readily available, many radiology departments are beginning digital storage of many procedures.

Consideration must be given to short-term, long-term, and off-site storage for backup due to catastrophic data loss. Short-term storage is often on a local modality hard drive when an exam is completed. Upon completion of the exam, the image is sent to the PACS server and can be stored in a redundant array of independent discs (RAID) for a few weeks or months for quick retrieval. This is similar to keeping films in the radiology department prior to long-term storage. Once the necessity for quick access is not required, the image can be placed in long-term storage. This storage may be in a "jukebox," where either discs or tapes are retrieved by a robotic arm. Off-site storage is used to ensure data integrity if a catastrophic event were to occur that could destroy data at an institution. Transition to digital storage frees up space in the imaging department previously occupied by film storage.

SUMMARY

Informatics describes a body of ideas, devices, and processes related to handling multiple types of information. Biomedical informatics (BMI) refers to platforms that are used for medical purposes, such as picture archiving and communications systems (PACSs), hospital information systems (HISs), and radiology information systems (RISs). The introduction of PACS has changed everything about radiology. When fully implemented, PACS is designed to save time and space by eliminating all areas associated with the use of film. In order that digital image files can be shared, DICOM standards were developed. DICOM allows for easier communication of biomedical information files. Other important standards include HIPAA and HL-7. The digital environment allows faster image acquisition with fewer repeats and faster turnaround time with diagnosis. PACS provides wider and faster availability of images and may shorten hospital stays. Image display devices can be in either hard- or soft-copy format. Digital images are printed to hard copy using laser printers or dry processors. Image storage requires immense amounts of memory. Health-care institutions utilize short-term, long-term, and off-site storage for backup of images. ■

REVIEW QUESTIONS

1. What are some examples of biomedical informatics platforms?
2. What is the difference between object class and service class in DICOM?
3. Why are digital image data files so large?
4. What is the difference between an RIS and an HIS?
5. How does a laser film printer create an image?
6. What are some advantages of using soft-copy display?
7. Why do radiologists' monitors have a higher resolution than the ones used by the technologist?
8. What affects image quality on a CRT monitor?
9. Why can higher ambient light be used with an LCD?
10. Why would an institution consider off-site storage for images?

REFERENCES AND RECOMMENDED READINGS

Alkhalifah, K., Brindhaban, A., Al' Ali, H., & Alhuraibi, A. (2005). The stability of dry and wet laser imaging systems. *Radiologic Technology. 76*(3), 192–196.

Chu, R., Christian, E., & Eaton, B. (1999). Stability of a dry laser imaging system. *Radiologic Technology, 71*(1), 29–34.

DeJarnette, W. T. (1999, September). PACS: The next generation. *Applied Radiology, 28*, 31–35.

Dreyer, K. J., Hirschorn, D. S., Thrall, J. H., & Mehta, A. (Eds.). (2006). *PACS: A guide to the digital revolution* (2nd ed.). New York: Springer.

Graf, B., Simon, U., Eickmeyer, F., & Fiedler, V. (2000). 1K versus 2K monitor: A clinical alternative free-response receiver operating characteristic study of observer performance using pulmonary nodules. *American Journal of Roentgenology, 174*(4), 1067–1074.

Huang, H. (2004). *PACS and imaging informatics.* New York: John Wiley & Sons.

Huang, H. K. (1999). *PACS: Basic principles and applications.* New York: Wiley-Liss.

Huda, W., & Szeverenyi, N., (1999, February). The filmless radiology department: A primer. *Applied Radiology, 28*, 30–34.

Juni, J. E. (1990). NucNet: A single-vendor clinical picture archiving and communication system—description and reflections. *Semin. Nucl. Med., 20*, 193–204.

NEMA. (2004, August 14). DICOM, Digital Imaging and Communications in Medicine. Retrieved from http://medical.nema.org/.

Reiner, B. I., Siegel, E. L., & Carrino, J. A. (Eds.). (2002). *Quality assurance: Meeting the challenge in the digital medical enterprise.* Great Falls, VA: Society for Computer Applications in Radiology (SCAR).

Samei, E., & Flynn, M. J. (Eds.). (2003). *Advances in digital radiography: Categorical course in diagnostic radiology physics.* Oak Brook, IL: Radiological Society of North America.

Seeram, E. (2011). *Digital radiography: An introduction.* Clifton Park, NY: Delmar Cengage Learning.

Seibert, J. A., Filipow, L. J., & Andriole, K. P. (Eds.). (1999). *Practical digital imaging and PACS.* Madison, WI: Medical Physics.

Shortliffe, E. H., & Cimino, J. J. (Eds.). (2006). *Biomedical informatics: Computer applications in health care and biomedicine* (3rd ed.). New York: Springer.

Siegel, E. L., & Kolodner, R. M. (Eds.). (1999). *Filmless radiology.* New York: Springer.

Takahashi, M., Rhodes, D. R., Furge, K. A., Kanayama, H., Kagawa, S., Haab, B. B., & Teh, B. T. (2001). Gene expression profiling of clear cell renal cell carcinoma: Gene identification and prognostic classification. *Proc. Natl. Acad. Sci. U.S.A., 98*, 9754–9759.

www.rsna.org/Technology/DICOM/index.cfm/accessed 10-10-10

www.genome.gov/Pages/PolicyEthics/GeneticDiscrimination/GINAInfoDoc.pdf accessed 10-10-10

www.hipaa.org/ accessed 10-10-10

www.hl7.org/ accessed 10-10-10

Zahriger, M., Wassmer, G., & Kurg, B. (2001). Image quality of digital chest x-ray wet versus dry laser printers. *Journal of Digital Imaging. 314*, 158–162.

Unit IV

Analyzing the Image

25 The Imaging Process / 375

26 Density/Image Receptor Exposure / 386

27 Contrast / 403

28 Recorded Detail / 424

29 Distortion / 442

30 The Art of Image Critique / 458

31 Quality Management / 467

The ability of the radiographer to analyze the image brings his or her professional skills to the highest levels possible. The process of analyzing demands a thorough knowledge of the scientific basis by which the image was produced as well as a significant amount of clinical experience. When these skills are applied via problem-solving techniques, the process of diagnosis results. The radiographer diagnoses the image exactly as the physician diagnoses pathology. This unit is designed to provide the analytical abilities in both diagnosis and treatment that make the radiographer an image expert.

The **imaging process** is remarkably similar for all radiologic and imaging sciences modalities. From conventional film and screen radiography through digital radiography to magnetic resonance imaging and ultrasound, the phases of acquiring, processing, archiving, and displaying the image have common parameters. This unit explores the process of analyzing the image from this common perspective.

Digital radiography acquires the image and then processes, archives, and displays it very differently from conventional radiography. Unit III is devoted to the specifics of these differences. Before attempting to diagnose the quality of the image, it is important that the radiographer understands the imaging process, including a diagnostic problem-solving technique. Then it is important to explore in depth each of the properties that affect radiographic quality to examine the controlling and influencing factors, their effect on the appearance of the image, how to assess them, and how to make adjustments properly.

There are four primary image quality factors. **Density/image receptor exposure** and **contrast** are photographic or visibility of detail quality factors. **Recorded detail** and **distortion** are geometric quality factors.

As an image quality factor, *density* was the term that was used to reflect exposure to the radiographic film. Density is the degree of overall blackening from the deposit of black metallic silver in the film emulsion as a result of exposure. In the digital world this important image quality factor has not changed but can be expressed simply as *image receptor exposure* because film is no longer the primary image receptor. *Brightness* and *density* are not interchangeable terms. Brightness is a monitor control function that does affect the lightness and darkness of the image but is not related to image receptor exposure. It is for this reason that we have renamed the density chapter density/image receptor exposure.

When a diagnostic process is applied to all of the properties together, an artistic skill in image evaluation results. A system that utilizes this process is presented as the **art of image critique**.

Finally, it is the responsibility of the radiographer to monitor and evaluate the performance of all radiographic equipment. This is accomplished through the process of **quality management**.

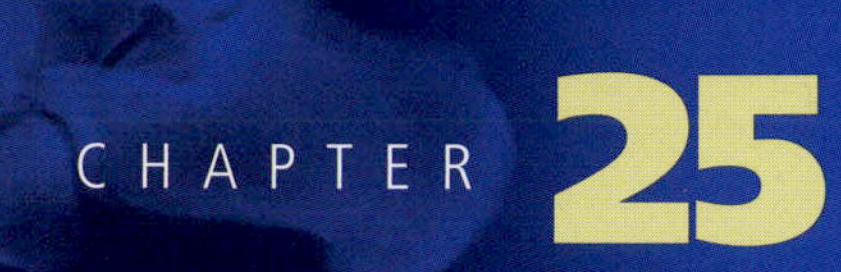

The Imaging Process

KEY TERMS

acceptance limits
pyramid problem

> [a] requirement of radiography when it is to be practiced as a personal art is the deliberate deviation from "average values." The practice of deviating from average values, settings, measurements, etc. is the mark of the successful professional man in almost any field, and is the principal reason for the esteem he enjoys in his community. His services are sought because he knows how and when to deviate from a standard solution of a problem.
>
> *Gerhart S. Schwarz, M.D., inventor of the XVS Unit-Step Radiography System*

OBJECTIVES

Upon completion of this chapter, the student should be able to:

- Describe the five phases of the imaging process.
- Describe the pyramid problem of geometrical progression as it relates to radiographic image quality.
- Apply the four steps of the diagnostic process to a clinical imaging problem.
- Explain how image acceptance limits may fluctuate due to various external factors.

THE IMAGING PROCESS

The imaging process is nearly the same for all radiologic and imaging sciences modalities. All modalities have phases such as where the image is acquired, processed, archived, and, finally, displayed for analysis.

The difference between conventional film/screen radiography and digital radiography is in the specifics of how these five phases are achieved. The parameters of image quality remain the same for the vast majority of factors. This includes image display, which is a major component of digital radiography but was neglected with conventional film/screen radiography because it was a simple process of viewing hard-copy images on an illuminated viewbox. Although considerable research had been done regarding controlling conditions for viewing hard-copy films, it was not until digital radiography required a monitor display that the full technology of viewing the image was pursued with the same scientific rigor.

The five phases of the imaging process occur in a well-established sequence (Figure 25-1). The image begins with acquisition, proceeds through processing, then is archived, followed by display, and is then ready for analysis.

Image Acquisition

The image acquisition process is unique to each imaging modality. Figure 25-2 shows the image acquisition phase for both conventional film/screen imaging and digital imaging as used in this textbook.

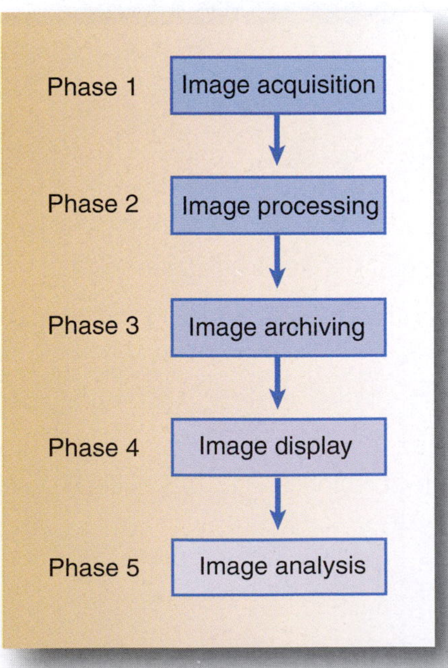

FIGURE 25-1. The imaging process.

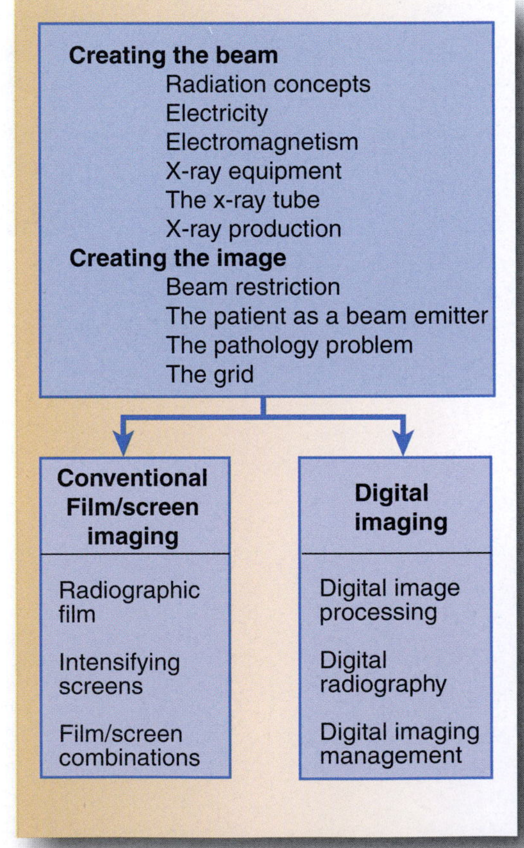

FIGURE 25-2. Image acquisition phase.

The creation of the x-ray beam (see Chapters 2–7) and the creation of the x-ray image (see Chapters 15–18) are common to both conventional film/screen imaging and digital imaging. Conventional film/screen imaging is detailed in Chapters 19 to 22. Digital imaging is detailed in Chapters 23 and 24.

Image Processing

Image processing is divided into film/hard copy and monitor/soft copy. Figure 25-3 shows the image processing phase for both conventional radiographic imaging and digital radiography used in this textbook. Chapters 19–21 detail film hard-copy processing. Chapters 23 and 24 detail digital image processing. Both film/screen and digital imaging can be processed either film/hard copy or monitor/soft copy. Conventional film/screen images can be recorded on film/hard copy or they can be digitized into DICOM-format images that can be processed via monitor/soft-copy methods. Digital images can be processed for monitor/soft copy or they can be produced as film/hard copy by a laser or dry imaging system.

Image Archiving

Image archiving consists of storing images for reference. Film/hard copy can be physically stored (these issues are addressed in Chapters 19 and 20) or digitized and stored electronically. Monitor/soft-copy images can be stored through a variety of electronic storage options (which are detailed in Chapter 24). Figure 25-4 shows the image archiving phase for conventional and digital radiography.

Image Display

Image display is a critical element in both conventional film/screen and digital imaging. Although it was considered a minimal area for investigation and change when all images were viewed as film/hard copy on an illuminated viewbox, the advent of digital imaging required a monitor display and a focus of attention. Figure 25-5 illustrates the components of image display for both film/screen and digital imaging.

Although considerable research had been done regarding controlling conditions for viewing

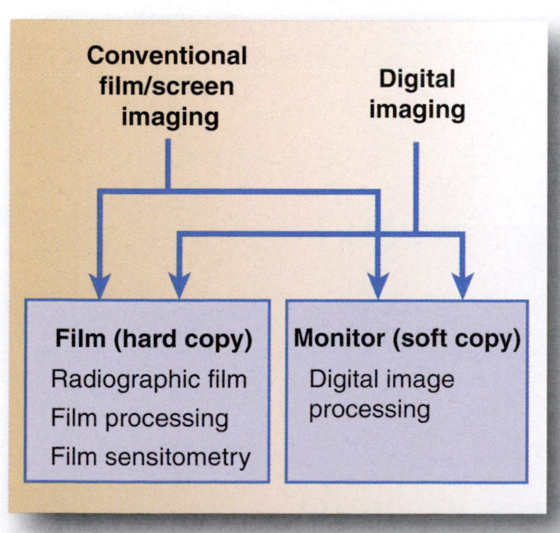

FIGURE 25-3. Image processing phase.

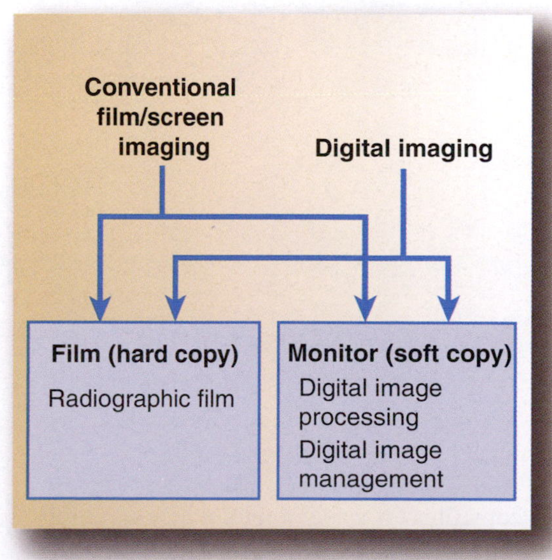

FIGURE 25-4. Image archiving phase.

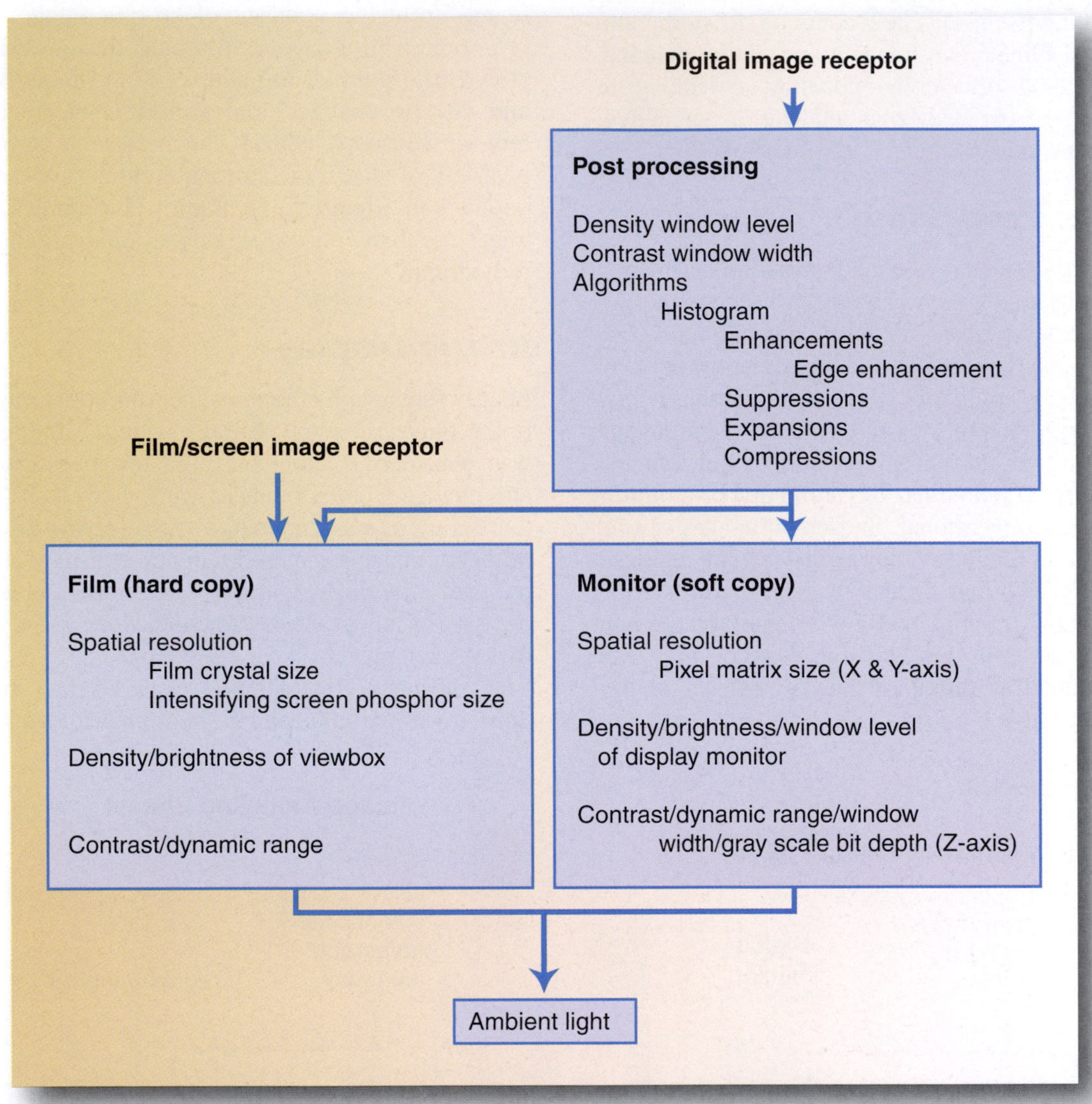

FIGURE 25-5. Image display phase.

hard-copy films, it was not until minor variations in spatial resolution, density/brightness, and contrast/dynamic range became obvious with the new technology that image display became a full phase for consideration.

Image Analysis

Analyzing the image (see Chapters 26–29) includes the traditional image quality factors of density/image receptor exposure, contrast, recorded detail, and distortion. These factors are shown in Figure 25-6. These factors apply to how the x-ray beam is controlled by the radiographer prior to detection by the image receptor. Control of the beam remains the same for both conventional film/screen imaging and digital imaging. Although there are differences in how conventional film/screen and digital imaging acquire the image, these are variations in how the image receptor responds to the incoming data, not fundamental changes in the quality factors of density, contrast, recorded detail, and distortion. For example, just as a high-speed intensifying screen

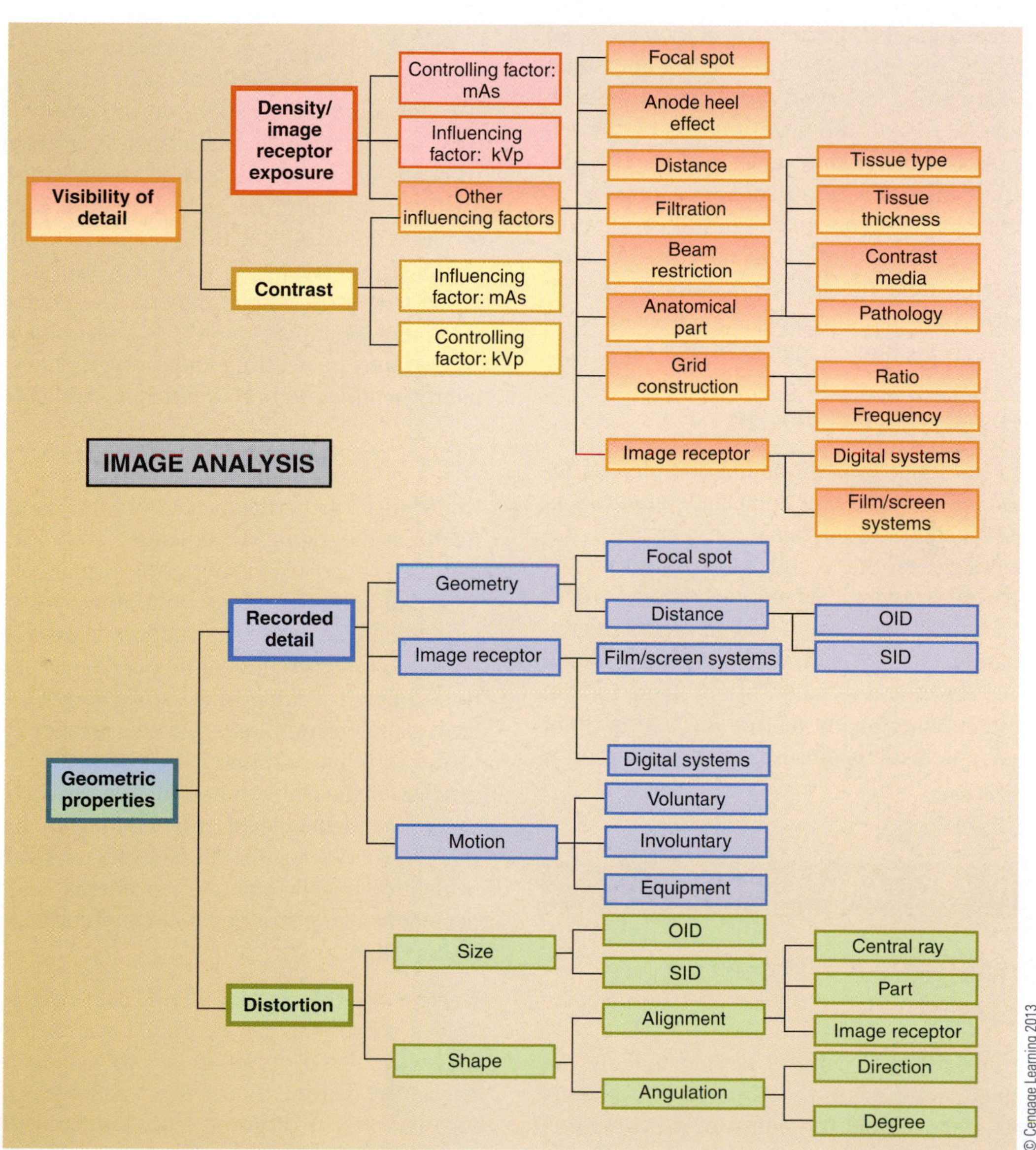

FIGURE 25-6. Image analysis phase.

will respond differently from a wide-latitude phosphor to the incoming x-ray photons, so will a direct digital image receptor.

PROFESSIONAL IMAGING STANDARDS

Just as all professionals are expected to adhere to the technical and ethical standards of their field, so radiographers are expected to establish personal imaging standards that satisfy the diagnostic needs of the radiologist and the quality needs of the supervisor. Additionally, they must not violate the personal ethical standards of radiation protection and patient care. Everyone makes mistakes, but professionals are able to correct their mistakes by using a careful analytical process to determine exactly what went wrong. In radiography, emphasis must be placed on learning how to look at images critically.

The Pyramid Problem

A major roadblock in overcoming complex problems such as establishing imaging standards is sometimes called the **pyramid problem**. An acceptable image is the result of a multitude of factors, including technical factor selection, subject density, contrast, pathology, and film processing. Unfortunately, some factors can act upon each other, thus creating a pyramid of problems for the radiographer. When many factors are acting upon each other, the result is an astronomical number of possibilities.

THE ANALYTICAL PROCESS

Diagnosing and Treating the Image

Anyone working in a clinical setting quickly becomes acquainted with the process of medical diagnosis. Determining the cause of a problem is a fascinating process. Most medical professionals would welcome an opportunity to participate in this process but they are restricted by law unless they hold a license to practice medicine in their state. In fact, the *American Registry of Radiologic Technologists Standards of Ethics* states "The radiologic technologist acts as an agent through observation and communication to obtain pertinent information for the physician to aid in the diagnosis and treatment of the patient and recognizes that interpretation and diagnosis are outside the scope of practice for the profession."

However, the diagnosis of technical problems in the imaging process requires the same skills that a physician uses in medical diagnosis.

Physicians are experts in the science of anatomy and physiology. Radiologists are physicians who are expert in the art of diagnosing through anatomical images as well. But even radiologists are not trained in the finer points of creating and analyzing the image. In this area the radiographer is the true professional expert. The diagnosis and treatment of image quality is the domain of the radiography profession, and radiographers are eminently qualified to practice this art and science.

The Diagnostic Process

Knowledge of the diagnostic process is necessary for the radiographer to diagnose and treat the image. The secret to solving any pyramid problem is a careful and meticulous breakdown of the whole into individual parts. The difference between being good and being great is often only a matter of attention to detail. Taking time to break down and analyze technical problems permits proper diagnosis to occur. When properly followed, the diagnostic process makes the treatment clear. Diagnosis involves the highest level of mental acuity. It requires the use of the skills of analysis, synthesis, and evaluation to solve complex problems. A diagnostic problem-solving strategy includes four major steps, as described next.

Narrowing the Search Field. The first phase involves narrowing the search. Experts begin with a review of the entire image to avoid premature narrowing. During this review a search is made for anything that is different from a diagnostic-quality image. When differences are noticed a pattern is sought, especially when there is more than one cue. These cues focus attention on a suspicious area, thus narrowing the search. An example would be an image that looks light, gray, and blurred. An inexperienced radiographer might jump to the conclusion that the image was too light and there was motion. However, an expert radiographer might notice additional cues, such as the loss of detail confined to a small region and proper image receptor exposure in other areas.

Hypothesis Activation. The second phase requires that the cues be used to seek hypotheses. An effort is made to formulate a hypothesis that will explain all the cues. Cues that do not fit the hypothesis should be held in reserve. In the previous example, the inexperienced radiographer might hypothesize that too little radiation was used and that the patient was breathing. The expert would realize that many hypotheses could account for the image, including several cases of "too little radiation," such as insufficient kVp, mA, or time; excessive distance; and improper film, screens, or processing. The expert would also include several explanations for a blurred image, such as poor film/screen contact, increased object-to-image receptor distance, and tube motion, as well as the patient motion hypothesis.

Information Seeking. The next phase demands that the hypotheses be tested by seeking more information. When stumped, radiographers should use general questioning to produce more cue information. It may be necessary to shift focus to other possible solutions when new cues are discovered. In the example, the novice radiographer might ask the patient if she held her breath. When the patient answers "yes," the novice radiographer might not believe her, rather than reject the hypothesis of patient motion. The expert, on the other hand, might notice during the questioning of the patient that her breast was superimposed over the area of interest. This additional cue could be used to return to the image. A new look at the image might show that the underexposed area was confined to the breast region.

Hypothesis Evaluation. The last phase of the diagnostic process is the evaluation of the final hypothesis. It is critical that the hypothesis used resolves the greatest amount of cue data. At this point the radiographer should be able to predict the solution to the problem. The inexperienced radiographer would apply the "too little radiation and patient motion" hypothesis and increase the mAs while watching the patient closely. The expert radiographer would conclude that the most likely hypothesis was increased subject density, decreased subject contrast, and poor film/screen contact. The expert would then ask the patient to move the breast aside and use a different cassette with good film/screen contact. Of course, the expert would produce a diagnostic-quality image. The novice would be left with an overexposed image of even poorer quality than the first one.

Remember, however, that data shows that novices often do surprisingly well when using the diagnostic process. Diagnosing ability can be improved by:

1. Remembering that cues are not a diagnosis;
2. Being careful to separate observations from inferences;
3. Not jumping to conclusions at the first cue;
4. Looking for competing hypotheses;
5. Trying each cue with each hypothesis;
6. Validating the hypothesis with questioning, when possible;
7. Ruling out hypotheses one by one;
8. Being cautious of premature closure;
9. Being tentative in the diagnosis until experienced; and, most important,
10. **Being confident in your expert knowledge.**

ACCEPTANCE LIMITS

Knowing how to diagnose an imaging problem is not helpful until the knowledge can be applied to radiographic quality analysis. This application involves establishing and adhering to quality imaging standards.

Graphing Acceptance Limits

The main goal must be to fix the limits of the radiographs that will be accepted against those that will not. This is much easier to understand by looking at the concept of **acceptance limits** graphically. The quality of all the radiographs produced by a technologist over a period has been graphed in Figure 25-7.

Although the radiographer's goal is to always produce a diagnostic-quality image, suboptimal images are often accepted for diagnosis. There are many reasons for this practice, the most important being the knowledge that the prime cause of increased patient radiation dose is repeated exposure. Radiologists do not expect textbook results on every patient. They do, however, have the right to expect the radiographer to provide an image that permits them to see all the structures critical to their diagnosis. Figure 25-8 shows where a typical radiologist might draw the line on overexposed or underexposed images. The important thing to remember is that if the radiographer, supervisor, radiologist, or other physician determines that an image is not acceptable, it is outside the acceptance limits of quality. When this occurs, the radiographer is obligated to analyze the image and make a proper decision on what factor or factors caused the error. The technique and procedure must then be adjusted to bring the unacceptable image back to the perfect center of diagnostic quality.

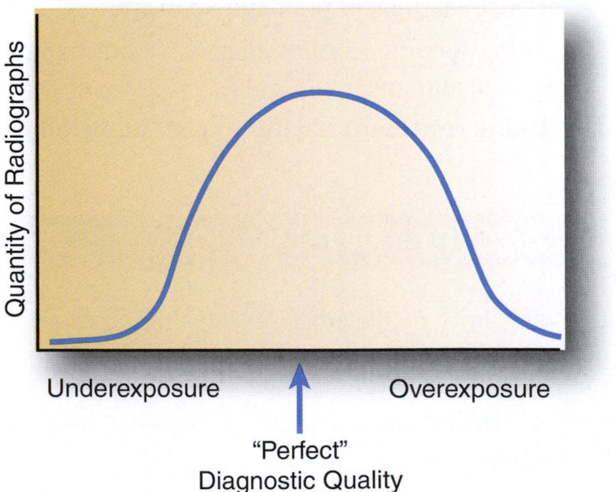

FIGURE 25-7. Radiographic image quality distribution curve. Note that the curve is skewed to the dark side. Standard practice dictates that a dark or low-contrast image is always preferable to one that is too light or high in contrast.

Striving for Perfection

Too often there is a tendency to correct only enough to obtain a passable image (Figure 25-9). All corrections should strive for perfection. Attempting to get by with minimal adjustments contributes to a negative image of the profession. The best radiographer

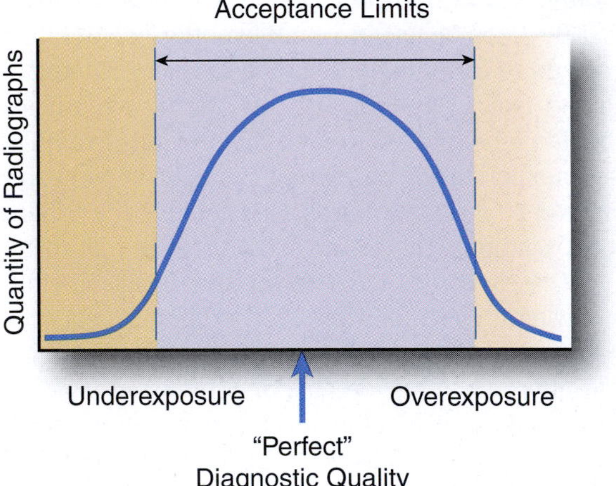

FIGURE 25-8. Typical acceptance limits of radiographic quality.

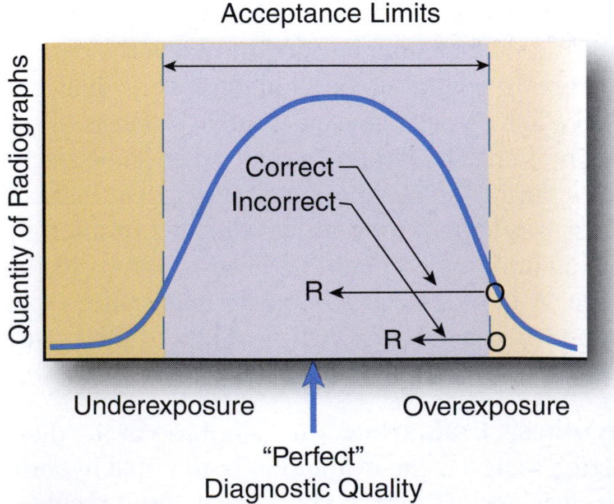

FIGURE 25-9. Correcting image quality.

can miscalculate and produce a poor image once, but competency is questioned when a radiographer is repeatedly unable to correct mistakes. The true professional completes the meticulous analysis by making a competent adjustment and achieves near perfection each time an exposure must be repeated.

Factors Affecting Acceptance Limit Curves

It is interesting to consider the factors that may affect the shape of the acceptance limit curve. Figure 25-7 is skewed to the overexposure side because these errors are more acceptable than underexposure mistakes. A bright light is capable of revealing information that is obscured in an overexposed film image and a digital system is capable of extracting more information from an overexposed detector. However, when an image is underexposed there is no method to see information that is not present on the image receptor. There are many other factors that can modify the shape of the acceptance curve. When acceptance limits are very narrow, a high repeat rate occurs (Figure 25-10). However, if the radiographers are not producing many perfect images, the repeat rate will remain high (Figure 25-11) even when acceptance limits are very wide.

An interesting phenomenon has been observed over the years in many radiology departments.

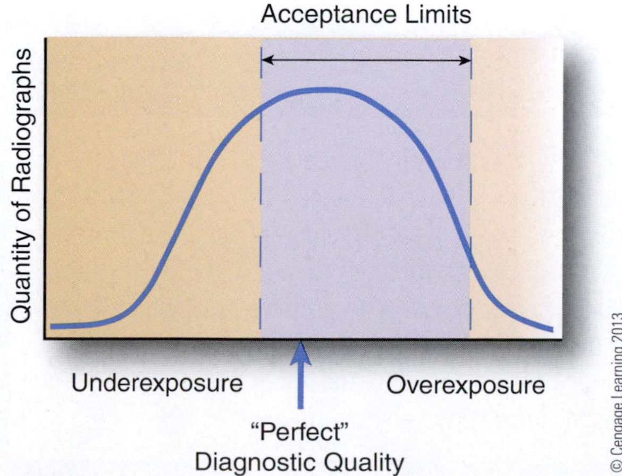

FIGURE 25-10. Narrow acceptance limits may produce a high repeat rate.

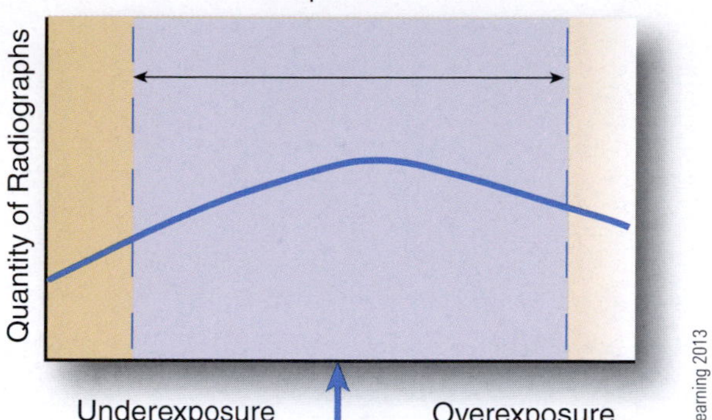

FIGURE 25-11. Wide acceptance limits may produce a high repeat rate by permitting radiographers to become careless and produce fewer images near perfect center.

When a radiograph is hovering near the acceptance limits for the department, radiographers will often attempt to have it approved by a radiologist known to have wide acceptance limits. Departmental acceptance limits are simply a composite of the limits imposed by each radiologist, supervisor, and radiographer in the department. Narrow acceptance limits may cause radiographers to produce more images near perfect center, thus changing the curve shape, as shown in Figure 25-12.

Conversely, wide limits may permit radiographers to become careless and produce fewer images near perfect center, thus changing the curve shape, as shown in Figure 25-11. Many factors can change the shape of the image quality curve. Among them are the positioning and technical abilities of the radiographer, the quality standards of everyone involved in the imaging chain, the condition of the equipment, the stress level of the department, and on and on. Awareness of these factors, combined with high professional standards, can help one's personal curve appear as in Figure 25-13.

Practical Considerations

In actual clinical practice the achievement of a diagnostic-quality image the first time is not as hard as it might at first appear. Each factor must

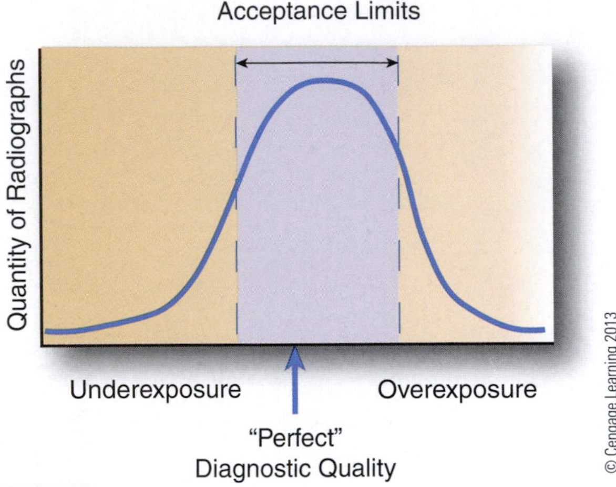

FIGURE 25-12. Narrow acceptance limits may cause radiographers to produce more images near perfect center.

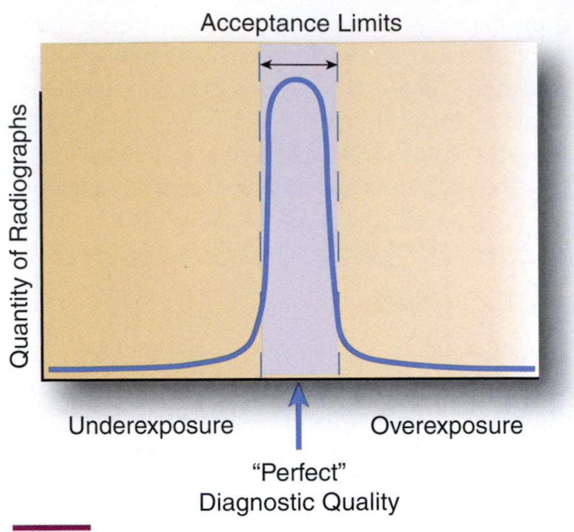

FIGURE 25-13. Ideal acceptance limits.

be varied within set limits to see a noticeable change in the image. It is important not only to learn the rules pertaining to image quality but to be sure they are used in clinical practice. The real problem is in learning to make large enough changes to cause visible differences on the image. Radiographers who are unsure of their ability often make timid changes that cannot be seen in the repeat image. When a decision is made to repeat a procedure (and doubly expose the patient), a change large enough to bring the image to the center of diagnostic quality must be made. Shifting the image from just outside the acceptance limits to just inside them is inexcusable. As professionals, radiographers must always strive toward perfection.

SUMMARY

Professional imaging standards can be established by overcoming the pyramid problem. Evaluating imaging problems is the true professional expertise of the radiographer. The analytical process of diagnosis is appropriate for use in solving these problems. The diagnostic process involves narrowing the search field, hypothesis activation, information seeking, and hypothesis evaluation.

The concept of acceptance limits is helpful in understanding how repeated radiographs must be corrected. All repeated radiographs should strive for perfection by attempting to reach the "diagnostic-quality" center of the acceptance limit curve. When a decision is made to repeat a procedure, a change large enough to bring the image to the center of diagnostic quality must be made. ■

REVIEW QUESTIONS

1. What is the pyramid problem?
2. What are the four steps in the diagnostic problem-solving strategy?
3. What is the purpose of a cue in narrowing the search?
4. When is an image determined to be outside acceptance limits?
5. Why are acceptance limit curves skewed to the dark side?

REFERENCES AND RECOMMENDED READING

American Registry of Radiologic Technologists. (2010). *Standards of ethics as revised August 1, 2010.* Minneapolis, MN: Author.

Berman, L., De Lacey, G., Twomey, E., Twomey, B., Welch, T., & Eban, R. (1985). Reducing the errors in the accident department: A simple method of using radiographers. *British Journal of Radiology, 290*, 421–422.

Bowman, S. (1991). Introducing an abnormal detection system by radiographers into an accident and emergency department: An investigation into radiographers' concerns about the introduction of such a system. *Research in Radiography, I*(I), 2–20.

Carlton, R. R. (1992). Another dimension of quality assurance in radiology. In L. T. Gurley & W. J. Callaway (Eds.), *Introduction to radiologic technology* (3rd ed., pp. 149–166). St. Louis, MO: C. V. Mosby.

Carlton, R. R., & McKenna, A. (1989). Repeating radiographs: Setting imaging standards. In E. Frank (Ed.), *Postgraduate advances in radiologic technology.* Berryville, VA: Forum Medicum.

Carnevali, D. L., Mitchell, P. H., Woods, N. F., & Tanner, C. A. (1984). *Diagnostic reasoning in nursing.* Philadelphia: J. B. Lippincott.

Cheyne, N., Field-Boden, W., Wilson, I., & Hall, R. (1987). The radiographer and the front line diagnosis. *Radiography, 53*(609), 114.

Cullinan, A., & Cullinan, J. (1994). *Producing quality radiographs* (2nd ed.). Philadelphia: J. B. Lippincott.

Cullinan, J. E. (1981). A "perfect" chest radiograph—or a compromise? *Radiologic Technology, 53*(2), 121.

Edwards, J., & Bowman, S. (1994). The expanding role of the radiographer. *Radiologic Science and Education, 1*(1), 14–20.

Goldman, L. W. (1977). Effects of film processing variability on patient dose and image quality. *Second Image Receptor Conference: Radiographic Film Processing: Proceedings of a Conference held in Washington, DC, March 31–April 2, 1977.* (HEW Publication [FDA] 77–8036, 55–63). Rockville, MD: U.S. Department of Health, Education, and Welfare, Public Health Service, Food and Drug Administration, Bureau of Radiological Health.

Hendee, W. R., & Ritenour, R. (2002). *Medical imaging physics* (3rd ed.). New York: Wiley.

Mumford, L. C. (1980). Radiographic quality "a seminar." *The Canadian Journal of Medical Radiation Technology, 11*(1), 10.

Prior, J. A., Silberstein, J. S., & Stang, J. M. (1981). *Physical diagnosis: The history and examination of the patient.* St. Louis, MO: C. V. Mosby.

Singer, B. H. (1971). The aesthetic method in radiographic exposure. *Radiologic Technology, 42*(6), 411.

Swinburn, K. (1971, March 20). Pattern recognition for radiographers. *The Lancet*, 7699, 589–590.

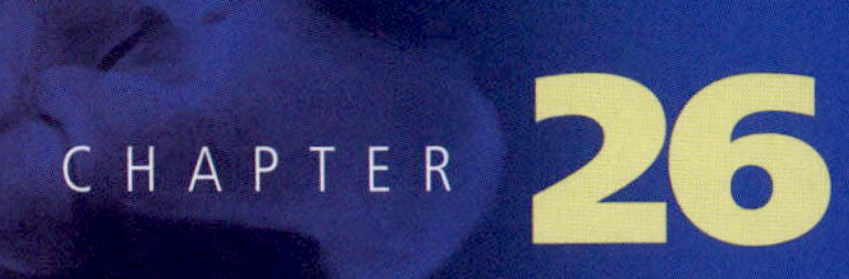

CHAPTER 26

Density/Image Receptor Exposure

KEY TERMS

brightness
density
exposure maintenance formula
IR exposure
window level

Radiographic density and contrast are closely related, but by a careful study of the radiograph they may be readily differentiated and each brought under control.

Ed. C. Jerman, The Father of Radiologic Technology

OBJECTIVES

Upon completion of this chapter, the student should be able to:

- Identify density/image receptor (IR) exposure as a prime component of the photographic properties controlling visibility of detail of radiographic image quality.
- Define density and IR exposure.
- Describe the effects of density/IR exposure changes on image appearance.
- Describe the process of evaluating image density/IR exposure.
- Explain why mA and time are the controlling factors of density/IR exposure.
- Explain how each influencing factor affects image density/IR exposure.
- Assess density/IR exposure on various images.
- Recommend appropriate adjustments to compensate for variation in the controlling and influencing factors that affect density/IR exposure.

ASSESSING DENSITY/ IR EXPOSURE

Density/image receptor (IR) exposure is one of the two photographic properties that comprise visibility of detail. Visibility of detail refers to the fact that the image is visible to the human eye only because sufficient IR exposure/density (and contrast) exists to permit the structural details to be perceived. As an image quality factor, *density* was the term that was used to reflect exposure to the radiographic film. Density has been defined since the 1920s as the degree of overall blackening that is the result of black metallic silver deposited in the emulsion of film. Density was the viewable result of a film's response to exposure. When the IR was primarily film, density was a term that could adequately describe the effects of IR exposure. In the digital environment this important image quality factor has not changed but can be expressed simply as *IR exposure* because film is no longer the primary IR. ***Brightness* and *density* are not interchangeable terms.** **Brightness** is a monitor control function that can change the lightness and darkness of the image on a display monitor but it is not related to IR exposure. Brightness is the proper term for the luminous intensity (measured in candela) of the display monitor's light emission. It is for these reasons that the photographic property of density has been renamed density/IR exposure.

In both film screen and digital imaging, the visibility of the image has always been the result of the proper exposure to the IR. With digital imaging, printing to film is not common, but in both environments the key to a visible image is having the correct IR exposure. **Window level** describes digital post-processing that produces changes in brightness, so it also is appropriate to use when controlling the display of an image.

The physical concept of the result of IR exposure on density is discussed in detail in previous chapters (particularly in Chapter 21, Film Sensitometry). In this chapter the concept of density/ IR exposure is approached in an artistically professional manner aimed at diagnosing the image. The art of radiography is a clinical one and must be practiced as such. It is extremely important that this information be used in a clinical setting concurrently with its study.

The major consideration in assessing density or IR exposure on film is verification that proper densities are visible throughout the anatomical area of interest on the image. Of course, these densities must be well within the range of human visibility (usually OD 0.25–2.50). Much of this ability to verify proper film densities is a result of clinical experience (Figure 26-1). It is obvious that the proper IR

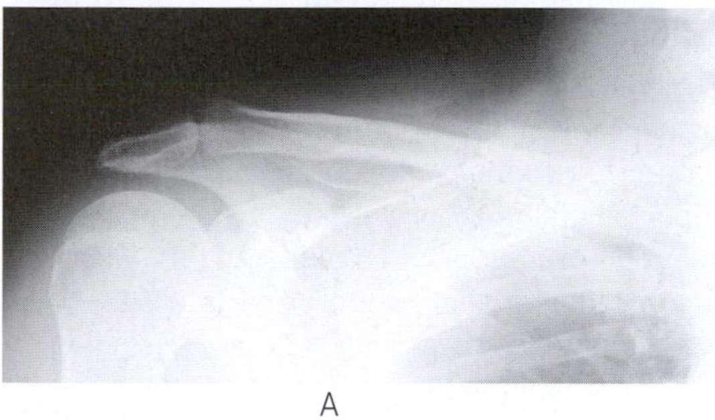

A

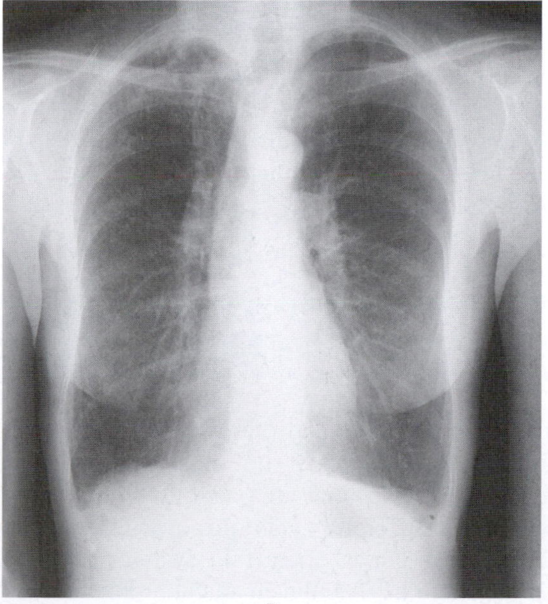

B

FIGURE 26-1. Clinical experience in assessing film density: (A) Although this image is not acceptable for the clavicle, it is a diagnostic-quality image of the acromioclavicular joints. (B) Although this image is not acceptable for the thoracic spine, it is a diagnostic-quality image of the chest.

exposure for lung tissue is not as great as the proper IR exposure for the thoracic spine, even though they are both thoracic structures. Common sense and a trained professional eye are the primary tools of the radiographer when evaluating IR exposure or density. The ability to assess IR exposure is a result of continued conscientious evaluation of images during clinical experiences. The radiographer who becomes professionally interested in the process of diagnosing the image quickly gains and refines this ability.

Information is recorded on an image that is overexposed but may not exist at all on an image that is underexposed. The overexposed IR has received too many photons and, as a result, has recorded too much information. A bright light or proper digital post-processing can eliminate the excess information and reveal details within the range of human visual ability. With a digital imaging system, this is very easily accomplished by adjusting the window level. This is not the case with an image that is underexposed. The underexposed image has not received the information in the first place and is not capable of being manipulated to reveal details that were never recorded. Consequently, whenever a choice must be made between excess and insufficient IR exposure, the wise decision is always the choice that will produce the overexposed image.

EFFECTS ON IMAGE APPEARANCE

The effects of mAs and the other influencing factors on IR exposure are not exact because of the multiple variables that are part of the imaging system. Most digital systems utilize a relatively linear IR response curve. Many film systems affect the IR exposure in a nonlinear fashion. For example, the typical D log E curve is only somewhat linear in the straight-line portion. If exposure conditions push into the toe or shoulder regions of the curve, dramatic film density changes can be seen. Similarly, density changes can sometimes be seen from only a slight nonlinearity in the intensifying-screen phosphor response curve, the film silver halide response, the thermionic emission of the x-ray tube filament, and so on. The reason digital systems are not effected by these factors is because a digital response curve can be preset or adjusted to compensate for these problems.

Fortunately, these variables have a statistical tendency to balance one another. But in cases where conditions cause a majority of the variables to increase or decrease exposure a total of more than 30 percent, an unexpected change in film density may become visible. Even when unexpected density/IR exposure changes exceed the 30 percent necessary to become visible, they seldom place the image outside the acceptance limits.

FACTORS AFFECTING DENSITY/ IR EXPOSURE

A wide variety of factors affect density/IR exposure (Figure 26-2). These factors are classified as either controlling or influencing factors. The controlling factor should be used as the principal method for adjusting for insufficient or excessive exposure.

Milliampere-Seconds as the Controlling Factor

Although the relationship between mAs and IR exposure is a direct proportional one, the relationship of these two factors to density is much more complex. Density is determined by the characteristics of the film. A D log E sensitometric curve expresses the relationship between exposure and density. For digital IR systems, changes in mAs control IR exposure. Image brightness on the display monitor is controlled by window leveling. Setting the correct mAs is still critical in determining proper digital IR exposure.

Despite the ability to control image brightness through post-processing parameters, it is still the responsibility of the radiographer to provide the digital IR with an appropriate exposure for a given procedure. Digital image histograms are graphic representations of the exposure to the IR. They are

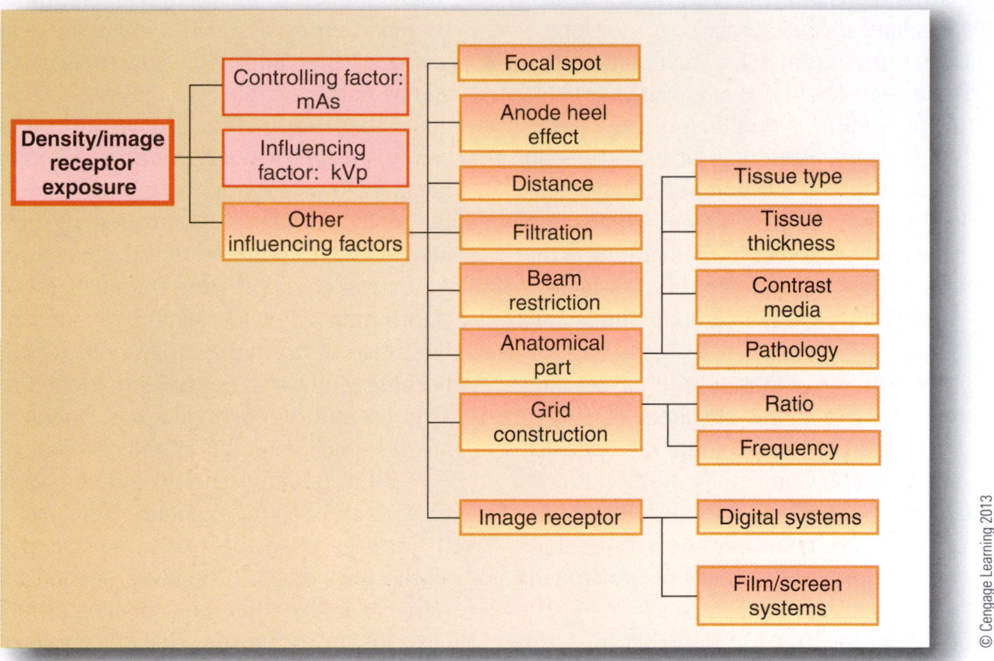

FIGURE 26-2. Image analysis: factors affecting density.

explained and illustrated in Figures 23-23 through 23-25. The manipulation of the histograms during input and output (post-processing) provides opportunities to enhance the image to facilitate diagnosis. These same features also allow information to be obscured and can impede diagnosis. Because the use of the histogram is a dangerous two-edged sword, most manufacturers have elected to restrict most users from manipulating this portion of the digital system. As radiographers become more knowledgeable about digital acquisition and post-processing, some manufacturers are opening portions of this feature to users. There are some digital units that offer preset histograms that either must or may be changed by the radiographer. Advanced users are also provided access to create custom histograms for specific clinical situations, which can then be displayed as presets to all users. There is an increasing tendency for radiographers to assert their professional knowledge base in this area that is well worth the effort for both patient and professional.

For film, the log-relative exposure is plotted on the x axis and density (D) is plotted on the y axis. The relationship between exposure and density determines the shape and position of the D log E curve for a given film under specific processing conditions. This relationship is described in detail in Chapter 21. Recall that film density is the $\log_{10}$ of opacity and opacity is the relationship of incident light to transmitted light. For example, if a region of a radiograph has an OD of 1.0, only 10 percent or 1/10 of the incident light is transmitted through the radiograph in this region. The opacity of the region would be 10. If the OD number is increased to 1.3, the opacity is doubled (to 20) and the percentage of light transmitted through the film is halved (to 5 percent or 1/20). Increments of 0.3 changes in OD numbers represent a doubling or halving of opacity.

The important part of the D log E curve is that portion between the toe and the shoulder (the diagnostic range of the film). In this centr al straight-line portion, the film density is approximately proportional to the log relative exposure. This is because a straight line will always have a constant ratio. If the slope of the straight line portion is at a 45° angle, the average gradient will measure 1.0. In this example, a doubling of exposure will result in a doubling of the opacity. (Note that the term *doubling of film density* is not used because density is a log number. A change of 0.3 in film density reflects a doubling or halving of opacity.) A common misnomer in radiography is that doubling the exposure will double the film density. This is not true for a typical radiographic film/screen system.

If the exposure to a film is increased, density will increase to a point. Because density is primarily determined by the amount of exposure the film receives, and because exposure is directly proportional to mAs, mAs is used as the primary controller of IR exposure and film density. As mAs increases, x-ray exposure increases proportionally and film density also increases (Figure 26-3). The direct proportional relationship between mAs and exposure is used to calculate mAs changes necessary to maintain consistent density/IR exposure when one or more technical factors are altered. By maintaining a specific exposure relative to the speed of the film, consistent density/IR exposure can be achieved.

When applied to x-rays, the reciprocity law can be restated to say film density should remain unchanged as long as the intensity and duration of the x-ray exposure (controlled by mAs) remains unchanged. Remember that the reciprocity law fails for extremely short (less than 0.01 second) or long (more than a few seconds) exposure times. Within the range of normal radiographic exposures, it can become a factor in special situations (such as pediatric extremities or high-speed angiography). This law does not apply to digital systems.

Film density should remain unchanged as long as the total exposure remains unchanged. If the mAs used to create one image is the same as the mAs used to create a second image of the same structure, then both images should have very close to the same film density. As long as mAs is constant, any combination of mAs and exposure time values will create the same film density and

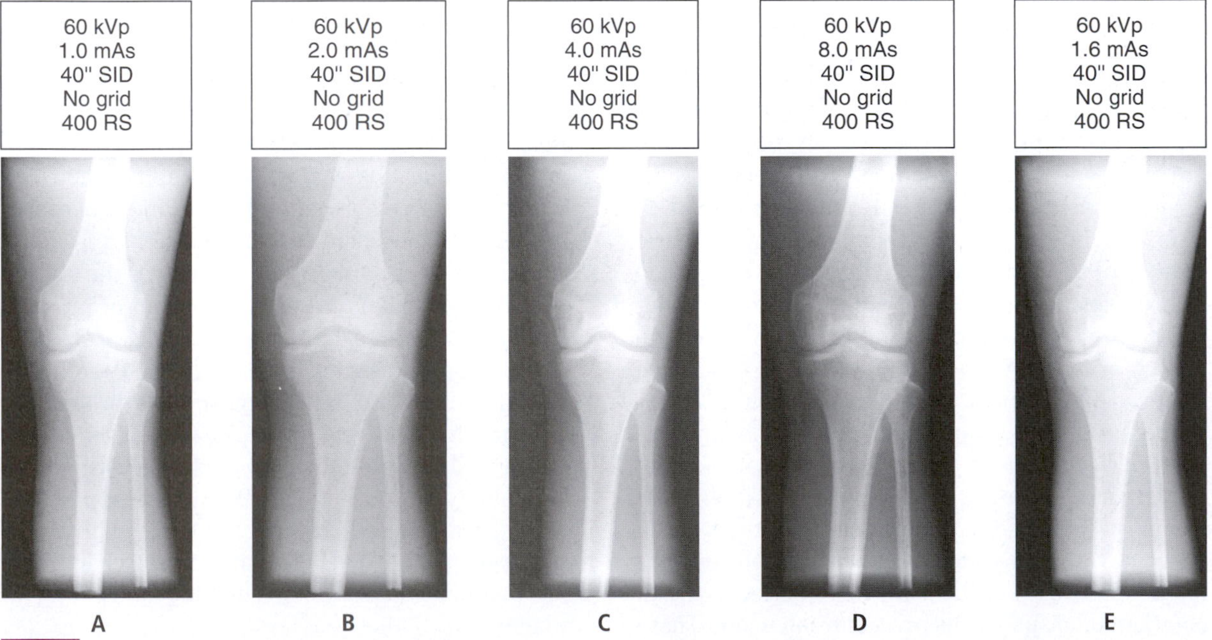

FIGURE 26-3. The effects of mAs change on film density. Images A–D demonstrate the effect of increasing mAs. Each image is double the mAs of the previous one. Image D represents a 20 percent decrease in mAs from image B. *(Radiographs courtesy of Arlene Adler and Richard R. Carlton.)*

IR exposure. This was demonstrated previously by the radiographs in Figure 11-1. Of course, accurate results depend on using equipment that is properly calibrated and maintained through an effective quality control program.

The control of density/IR exposure rests with the radiographer. An appropriate mAs setting may be selected from a technique chart developed for the particular x-ray unit in use. An automatic exposure system will control the time but the mAs and the exact density/IR exposure setting will be decided by the radiographer. Computerized exposure systems will provide a suggested technique setting, which can then either be accepted or modified. Other variables, such as generator phase, may also affect the final decision. The experienced radiographer will adapt the suggested mAs setting for the individual patient. Experience and study of various body habitus, pathologies, positioning, and equipment quickly provide the radiographer with clinical knowledge that can be used for these adjustments.

With film/screen systems the minimum change necessary to cause a visible shift in film density is about 30 percent of mAs, or any other influencing factors that would equal this change. Various authors over the years have set the minimum for a visible density change at values between 25 and 35 percent of mAs. This rule is essentially true for most digital systems as well. In fact, most digital exposure indicator systems are set to incorporate an acceptable range that includes 33 percent on either side of the ideal 1-mR exposure. Regardless of the exposure to the digital receptor, the system will attempt to rescale the histogram to provide a display image that appears acceptable to the eye. It is critical that the radiographer evaluate the exposure indicator for his or her system to assure a proper exposure has been made. Although studies of vision have demonstrated that some people can detect changes in brightness as small as 1 percent, this level of perception is not possible when viewing a complex clinical image with many widely separated densities. Some trained professionals, such as radiologists and radiographers, can perceive as small a change as 10 percent on a radiograph, but this is extraordinary. In clinical practice a change as small as 30 percent is seldom justified. A comparison between Figures 26-3B and E illustrates a 20 percent change in mAs. This change is difficult to see and would not compensate for improper IR exposure.

An image must be outside the acceptance limits to require repeating the exposure. All acceptance limits permit some degree of variation—at least 30 percent over- or underexposed. In these instances the image would have to be significantly more than 30 percent over- or underexposed than a diagnostic-quality image.

The general rule of thumb for mAs changes is to make adjustments in increments of doubles or halves. For example, a repeated image that is underexposed at 10 mAs should be repeated at 20, 40, or 80 mAs, depending on the circumstances. Of course, determining which circumstances require 20 mAs, which require 40 mAs, and which require 80 mAs is something that is acquired only through experience and further study. Figures 26-3A–E illustrate the doubling and halving rule.

Regardless of variations in equipment output, anatomy, physiology, or pathology, the idea is to adjust the intensity to permit the same amount of radiation to reach the IR, thus creating the same density/IR exposure. From this perspective, the art of radiography does not look especially difficult. However, many other factors are yet to be added to the simple task of determining appropriate density/IR exposure.

Essentially, if the image does not require doubling or halving of the exposure, it seldom requires repeating. Exceptions to this rule are special studies where a fine adjustment of barely 30 percent is crucial to demonstrating a small vessel or pathological condition. The radiographer will often adjust his or her technique chart by a 30 percent margin, but will seldom subject the patient to a second exposure for such a minor change. Making exposure adjustments should be a case of taking bold action (at least doubling or halving) or taking no action at all.

Kilovoltage as an Influencing Factor

Kilovoltage alters the intensity of the beam reaching the IR in two ways. Kilovoltage controls the energy and therefore the strength of the electrons striking the target of the x-ray tube for any given mAs. More important, kilovoltage controls the average energy of the x-ray photons produced at the anode target. Therefore, a change in kilovoltage alters the intensity of the beam when the mAs and other factors remain the same. Kilovoltage also affects the production of scatter radiation. Because of this, a change in kilovoltage alters the intensity of the beam after it enters the subject (or object) but before it reaches the IR.

Both the quantity and quality of the x-ray beam will vary significantly with changes in kilovoltage. As a result, kVp has a tremendous impact on density/IR exposure. Research has been done to determine a practical formula that takes both the quantity and quality factors into account. The primary finding is that there are too many variables to be quantified into a reliable formula. A change in film density can usually be detected with a 4–5 percent change in kVp in the lower ranges (30–50 kVp), but an 8–9 percent change is required in the middle ranges (50–90 kVp), and a 10–12 percent change in the higher ranges (90–130 kVp).

Because the radiographer must have a method of using kilovoltage to adjust and compensate for density/IR exposure changes, the rough guide known as the *15 percent rule* has been developed. The 15 percent rule is used as a guide to maintain the same IR exposure/density when kilovoltage changes, as follows:

A 15 percent increase in kilovoltage causes a doubling of exposure to the IR. A 15 percent decrease in kilovoltage causes a halving of exposure to the IR.

EXAMPLE: A radiograph of the elbow is produced using 4 mAs at 60 kVp. What kVp would be required to halve the exposure to the IR?

Answer:

60 kVp − (60 kVp × 15%)

60 kVp − (60 kVp × 0.15)

60 kVp − (9 kVp) = 51 kVp

The 15 percent rule is somewhat accurate within the range of 60 to 100 kVp. Of course, this does not include the entire diagnostic radiography range, which may run from 30 to 150 kVp. The percentage of kVp required to halve the exposure to the IR is always greater as the kVp increases. This is primarily due to the increased scatter radiation produced at higher kilovoltages. However, the greatest variable in the production of scatter is the thickness of the part. Therefore, IR exposure is increased when radiographing a thick subject (Figure 26-4). Consequently, a 20 percent rule may be more accurate when radiographing a 5-cm wrist, whereas a 15 percent rule may be more accurate when radiographing a 20-cm abdomen. Another factor that has a mathematical effect on the 15 percent rule is the starting kVp. The percentage change for doubling or halving decreases slightly as the starting kVp increases. In actual fact, the 15 percent rule may vary from a 15 percent rule to a 25 percent rule within the diagnostic radiography range of kVps and the diagnostic range of IR exposures. The 15 percent rule is commonly applied by radiographers because it can be used without producing images outside the acceptance limits. However, understanding the variability of the rule will do much to increase awareness of potential problems when radiographing extremely large or small objects, or with unusually low or high kVp settings. Changing kilovoltage is the primary method of changing image contrast. Consequently, the 15 percent rule will always change the differential absorption by the tissue and the resultant contrast of the image. When a contrast change is desirable, the 15 percent rule is a useful method of maintaining density/IR exposure. However, when only a density/IR exposure change is desired, the 15 percent rule should not be used because it causes a contrast change as well. When density/IR exposure changes are desired, the method of choice is to vary the mAs because it is the controlling factor for density/IR exposure.

The configuration of the generator is another important consideration in how kVp affects IR exposure/film density. The total number of higher-energy photons in the x-ray tube emission spectrum is controlled by the amount of ripple in the waveform. For example, a single-phase waveform has a significantly lower average photon energy than a high-frequency waveform, resulting in less density/IR exposure (see Chapter 7).

Compensation for the configuration of the generator is most commonly accomplished by considering only the phasing and number of pulses.

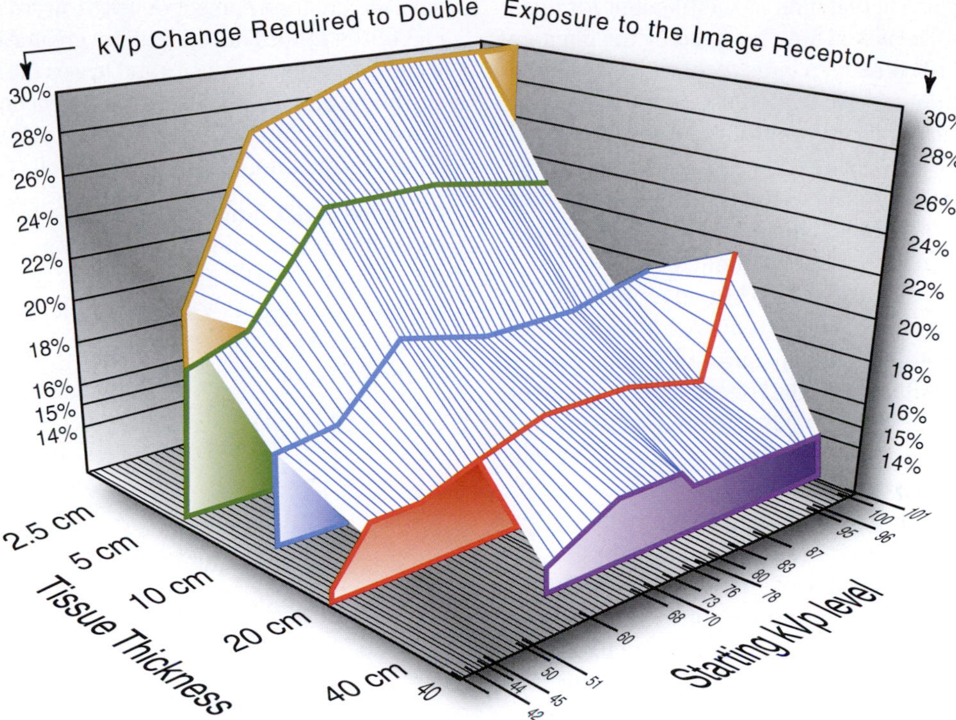

FIGURE 26-4. The relationship of kVp and tissue thickness to image receptor exposure. Note that the line representing a 15 percent increase in kVp is not within the range of some part thicknesses and kVps used in routine diagnostic radiography. It is apparent that the 15 percent rule is not a constant and must be applied with careful consideration of other factors, especially tissue thickness and starting kVp. *(Data extracted from "Kilovoltage Conversion in Radiography," The X-Ray Technician, 32, 373–379, 436, 1960, by Gerhart S. Schwartz, courtesy of the American Society of Radiologic Technologists. Graphics courtesy of Chris Innskeepp, Lima Technical College.)*

The only generator phase conversion currently requiring consideration occurs when changing between single-phase units and high-frequency multiphase units (see Table 26-1).

TABLE 26-1. Conversion Factors Effect of Generator ϕ on IR Exposure

When Converting Generator Phase From:	To:	To Maintain Exposure Multiply mAs by a Conversion Factor of:
1ϕ2p	high frequency	0.5
high frequency	1ϕ2p	2.0

EXAMPLE: If 80 kVp and 20 mAs produce a satisfactory exposure on a 1ϕ2p unit, what mAs should be used with the same patient and examination on a high-frequency unit?

Answer:

mAs × conversion factor

20 mAs × 0.5 = 10 mAs

Other Influencing Factors

Focal Spot Size. Larger focal spots utilize a greater incident electron stream than small focal spots. Most manufacturers carefully compensate for this effect by adjusting the actual mAs at the filament for dual-focus tubes. The actual mAs received by the filament when set at 100 mAs for a large focal spot is less than the actual mAs received when set at 100 mAs for a small focal spot. There should be no difference between large and small focal spots when the unit has been calibrated properly. However, this effect may differ by the 30 percent necessary to alter density/IR exposure in an improperly calibrated unit.

Large focal spots tend to bloom more at higher milliamperages and may occasionally reach a point where they alter the IR exposure. Blooming occurs with large milliamperages because the incident electron beam is not as easily focused by the focusing cup. It is rare for blooming to cause a visible density/IR exposure difference.

Because properly calibrated units will not exhibit density/IR exposure changes when focal spots are changed, differences of this type should be reported as a quality control procedure. If density/IR exposure differences are perceived due to focal spot blooming, replacement of the tube may be indicated.

Anode Heel Effect. The anode heel effect alters the intensity of radiation, and therefore the density, between the anode and cathode ends of the x-ray tube. Depending on the angle of the anode, this effect can cause an IR exposure variation of up to 45 percent between the anode and cathode ends of the image. IR exposure is always greater at the cathode end. The anode heel effect is more pronounced when the collimator is open wide than when it is closed because a greater portion of the peripheral beam, and therefore a greater portion of the intensity difference, reaches the IR when the collimator is wide open. The anode heel effect is also more significant when using extremely small angle anodes (12° or less).

When the anode heel effect becomes apparent, it can be minimized or converted to an advantage. It is minimized by collimating the beam and eliminating as much of the intensity difference at the periphery as possible. If a given film size is required (i.e., 14″ × 17″), collimation may be achieved by using a greater source-to-IR distance (SID).

The anode heel effect may be converted to an advantage in examinations of objects with greater subject density at one end than at another. The advantage is utilized by placing the portion of the object with the greatest subject density toward the cathode end of the tube. This utilizes the greater intensity for the greater subject density and leaves the lesser intensity of the anode end of the tube for the lesser subject density. The anode heel effect can often be used to advantage in a number of examinations (Table 26-2).

Distance (SID and OID). Source-to-IR distance (SID) alters the intensity of the beam reaching the IR, according to the inverse square law. The inverse square law affects exposure in inverse proportion to the square of the distance. This is represented by the formula:

$$\frac{I_1}{I_2} = \frac{D_2^2}{D_1^2}$$

where: I_1 = old intensity

I_2 = new intensity

D_1^2 = old distance squared

D_2^2 = new distance squared

The law states that the intensity (exposure) varies inversely with the square of the distance.

The inverse square law formula expresses the change in intensity when the distance changes. For example, as distance increases, radiation intensity

TABLE 26-2. Projections That May Use the Anode Heel Effect to Advantage

Projection	Body Part to Be Placed Toward	
	Cathode End of Tube	Anode End of Tube
Femur (AP/lateral)	hip	knee
Lower leg (AP/lateral)	knee	ankle
Humerus (AP/lateral)	shoulder	elbow
Forearm (AP/lateral)	elbow	wrist
Thoracic spine (AP)	abdomen	neck
Thoracic spine (lateral)	neck	abdomen
Lumbar spine (AP/lateral)	pelvis	abdomen

and IR exposure decrease. However, the most common situation in radiography is a need to maintain an acceptable IR exposure/density while changing the distance. To maintain IR exposure, mAs (or an influencer) must be changed to compensate for the exposure change. The **exposure maintenance formula** is used for this purpose. This formula is based on the inverse square law but is reversed to a direct square law because mAs must increase when distance increases, and vice versa, in order to maintain IR exposure.

$$\frac{mAs_1}{mAs_2} = \frac{D_1^{\,2}}{D_2^{\,2}}$$

where: mAs_1 = original mAs

mAs_2 = new mAs

$D_1^{\,2}$ = old distance squared

$D_2^{\,2}$ = new distance squared

EXAMPLE: If a satisfactory exposure is obtained with 20 mAs at 72″, what mAs will be required to maintain the same exposure at 40″?

Answer:

$$\frac{mAs_1}{mAs_2} = \frac{D_1^{\,2}}{D_2^{\,2}}$$

$$\frac{20\text{ mAs}}{mAs_2} = \frac{72^2}{40^2}$$

$$\frac{20\text{ mAs}}{mAs_2} = \frac{5{,}184}{1{,}600}$$

$$mAs_2 = \frac{20\text{ mAs} \times 1{,}600}{5{,}184}$$

$$mAs_2 = \frac{32{,}000}{5{,}184}$$

$$mAs_2 = 6.2\text{ mAs}$$

It is more useful when algebraically changed to solve for the new mAs, which is the most common factor that must be calculated in clinical practice:

$$mAs_2 = \frac{mAs_1 \times 3D_2^{\,2}}{D_1^{\,2}}$$

EXAMPLE: If a satisfactory PA chest radiograph is made at 72″ with 4 mAs, what mAs will be required at 56″?

Answer:

$$mAs_2 = \frac{mAs_1 \times D_2^2}{D_1^2}$$

$$mAs_2 = \frac{4\text{ mAs} \times 56^2}{72^2}$$

$$mAs_2 = \frac{4\text{ mAs} \times 3{,}136}{5{,}184}$$

$$mAs_2 = \frac{12{,}544}{5{,}184}$$

$$mAs_2 = 2.5\text{ mAs}$$

The exposure maintenance formula is only accurate within a moderate acceptance range. The nonlinearity of some components in the imaging system makes it impossible to exactly quantify the relationship between radiation beam intensity and IR exposure.

Table 26-3 illustrates the mAs change factors for the most common distances employed in radiography. The vast majority of diagnostic radiography today is done at 40″ to 72″. In addition 56″, which is halfway between 40″ and 72″, is useful in mobile radiography when circumstances do not permit either of the two preferred distances. A useful rule of thumb for doubling and halving distances can be derived from this table by considering the 30 percent range necessary to produce a visible density/IR exposure difference in the image:

> Use only the distances 40″, 56″, and 72″. When increasing distance, double the mAs for each change. When decreasing distance, halve the mAs for each change. For example, halve the mAs when changing from 72″ to 56″ and halve it again when changing from 56″ to 40″.

Distance doubling and halving will bring IR exposure within roughly 50 percent of the original exposure and usually within image acceptance

TABLE 26-3. mAs Change Factors for Approximate Exposure Maintenance When Distance Changes

To calculate the new mAs, multiple the old mAs by the factor in the corresponding box to the distance change.

	New Distance				
	36″ (90 cm)	40″ (100 cm)	48″ (120 cm)	56″ (140 cm)	72″ (180 cm)
36″ (90 cm)	—	1.23	1.77	2.42	4.00
40″ (100 cm)	0.81	—	1.44	1.96	3.24
48″ (120 cm)	0.59	0.69	—	1.36	2.25
56″ (140 cm)	0.41	0.51	0.73	—	1.65
72″ (180 cm)	0.25	0.31	0.44	0.60	—

limits. This is only a rough rule of thumb for clinical practice. The exact conversion factors will produce much better mAs estimates.

Object-to-image-receptor distance (OID) has an effect on density/IR exposure. The air-gap technique uses an increased OID to prevent scatter radiation from reaching the IR. This scatter radiation would normally cause a visible increase in density/IR exposure when radiographing large patients. By increasing OID using the air-gap technique, scatter that would normally strike the IR will miss the receptor, causing a decrease in density/IR exposure. In most instances, however, OID variations are insufficient to cause visible density/IR exposure changes.

Filtration. Filtration and its ability to alter beam intensity affect IR exposure and density/IR exposure. All types of filtration—inherent, added, and total—alter density/IR exposure. Density/IR exposure decreases when filtration is increased.

X-ray units are calibrated with inherent, added, and total filtration in place. When added filtration is changed, which is rare, a half-value layer calculation should be made to permit adjustment of mAs or other factors to maintain exposure levels. When compensating filtration is used, density/IR exposure must be established for both filtered and unfiltered regions. As with any other exposure problem, this is a matter of measurement of part size and clinical experience.

Beam Restriction. Restricting the beam, collimating, or reducing the primary beam field size reduces the total number of photons available. This reduces the amount of scatter radiation and therefore reduces the overall IR exposure and density/IR exposure.

Scatter production is dramatically increased with large anatomical part size and high starting kVp levels (see Figure 26-4). Therefore, these two factors also determine when compensation must occur for beam restriction. However, the effect of beam restriction on density/IR exposure depends on how much scatter reaches the IR, not how much scatter is produced. Some of the scatter that is produced, especially in very large patients or when using high-ratio grids, may not reach the IR and therefore will not affect the density/IR exposure. For example, a high-efficiency grid may be capable of removing as much as 95 percent of the scatter, leaving very little to affect density/IR exposure.

Technical factor compensation for changes in density/IR exposure is required only under the following circumstances:

- large anatomical part
- high kilovoltage
- low grid efficiency
- non-grid examinations

Figure 26-5 demonstrates that only extremely small beam restrictions (4″ × 4″ or smaller) when used with no grid or a low-efficiency grid require mAs compensation to maintain IR exposure. The compensation necessary in mAs for the effect of beam restriction on density/IR exposure is less than 30 percent (a notable difference) for nearly all images produced with grids at 8″ × 10″ or larger beam sizes (Figure 26-6).

Anatomical Part. Because the patient is the prime attenuator of the beam, the anatomical part being examined has a great deal of influence on IR exposure. The amount of attenuation is dependent on the thickness and type of the tissue being

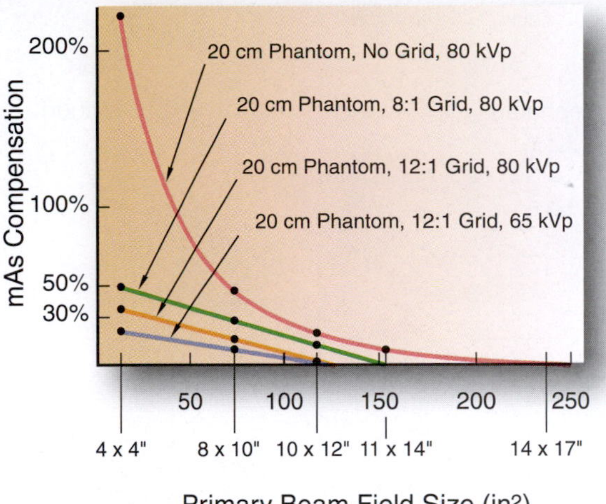

FIGURE 26-5. The effect of beam restriction on mAs compensation required to maintain film density. *(Courtesy of Barry Burns, University of North Carolina, Chapel Hill, NC.)*

imaged. The tissue type is affected by the average atomic number and the density (quantity of matter per unit volume) of the tissue. The use of contrast media will alter the average atomic number of the tissue and can affect density/IR exposure. Pathology can alter tissue thickness and/or type.

There is an inverse relationship between tissue thickness/type and density/IR exposure. In other words, as tissue thickness, average atomic number of the tissue, and/or tissue density increases, density/IR exposure decreases. This is not a linear relationship because of the multitude of variations in tissue composition. Depending on the type of contrast media or the type of pathology, an inverse or a direct relationship may exist.

Adjustments for changes in the anatomical part depend on the radiographer's ability to assess the tissue thickness and tissue type while also considering the pathology and the use of contrast

85 kVp	1.0 mAs	40" SID
12:1 No grid	400 RS	29.8 mR

85 kVp	1.0 mAs	40" SID
12:1 No grid	400 RS	31.6 mR

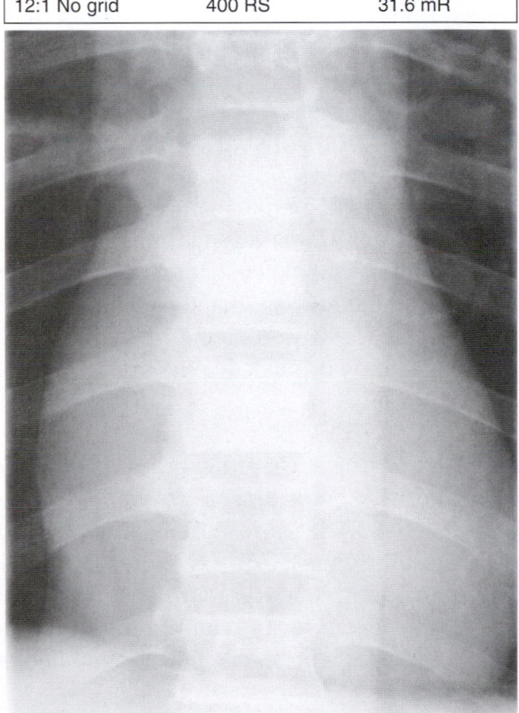

FIGURE 26-6. The effect of beam restriction on film density. Although both radiographs were produced at the same technical factors, A was collimated to 14″ × 17″ whereas B was collimated to 4″ × 8″. *(Radiographs courtesy of Arlene Adler and Richard R. Carlton.)*

media. This ability is achieved only through clinical experience. Technique charts are designed to compensate for most changes in tissue thickness and type. Radiolucent contrast media (such as air) will increase density/IR exposure, whereas radiopaque contrast media (such as barium and iodine) will decrease density/IR exposure. Pathology can have either an additive or a destructive effect. Additive conditions decrease density/IR exposure, whereas destructive conditions increase density/IR exposure.

A special problem related to part thickness occurs whenever severe tube angles (more than 15″) are used. The geometry of a severe tube angle causes a significant difference in tissue thickness between the edges of the image (Figure 26-7). Measurement of body parts for angles must occur at the central ray to average these differences. However, in some instances more than a 30 percent exposure difference may occur between the central ray and both ends of the image (more than a 60 percent difference between the ends of the image). Careful consideration of technical factors and use of the anode heel effect, when possible, may prevent some of these problems.

Casting materials present during orthopedic radiography affect the thickness of the anatomical part. Casting materials differ somewhat in composition but they attenuate the beam in a manner very similar to normal tissue attenuation. Adjustments for cast materials should be made for the increased thickness of the body part exactly as if an uncasted part of the same size were being radiographed. No adjustment should be made for the casting material itself.

Grid Construction. Grids absorb scatter, which would otherwise add exposure to the IR and density to the film. The more efficient the grid, the less will be the density/IR exposure. Grids with high ratios, low frequency, and dense interspace material; moving grids; and improperly used grids (incorrect focal distance, etc.) all reduce density/IR exposure.

Compensation for varying grid ratios is generally accomplished by increasing mAs. The amount of mAs required can be calculated using the grid conversion factors (see Table 18-2). Changing between

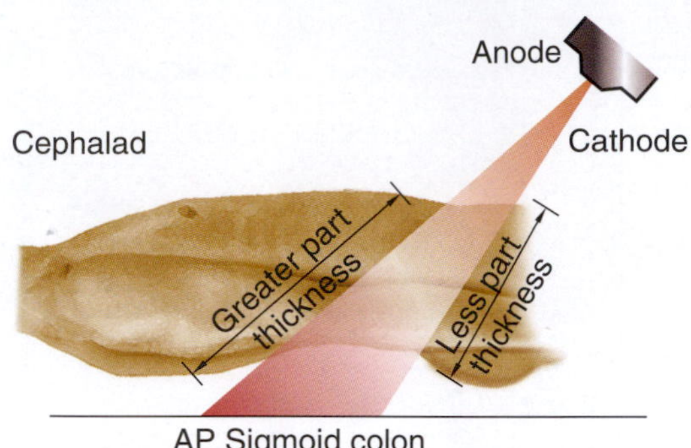

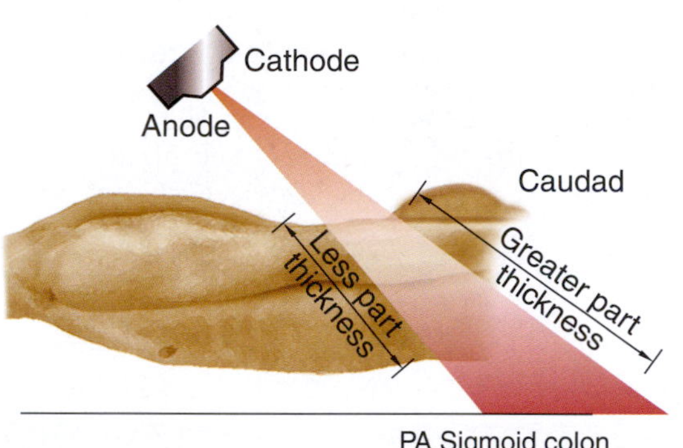

FIGURE 26-7. The effect of severe tube angle on film density. Note the changes in part thickness from the superior to inferior edges of the primary beam field.

grids, which is the most common clinical problem, is accomplished by using the following formula:

$$\frac{mAs_1}{mAs_2} = \frac{GCF_1}{GCF_2}$$

where: mAs_1 = original mAs
mAs_2 = new mAs
GCF_1 = original grid conversion factor
GCF_2 = new grid conversion factor

Because the primary purpose of a grid is the improvement of contrast, compensating for density/IR exposure changes by varying the kVp is not recommended because it may change the contrast in the opposite direction, thus negating the reason for using the grid in the first place.

Image Receptors. Both film/screen systems and digital systems have an impact on density/IR exposure. With film/screen systems, intensifying-screen phosphors convert x-ray photons to the light photons that will expose the silver halides in film. When the silver halide crystals in the film emulsion form latent image centers, they establish the physical foundation for the black metallic silver that is film density. Exposure index (EI) numbers are the most useful parameter for digital imaging systems. Relative speed (RS) numbers are the most useful parameters for film/screen combinations.

RS numbers have been developed by manufacturers to permit easy adjustment of technical factors when changing film/screen combinations (see Chapter 22). As relative speed increases, the amount of exposure required to maintain the same density/IR exposure decreases. Compensations for changes in relative speed can be made by adjusting mAs because exposure is directly proportional to mAs. Density/IR exposure can be maintained by using the following formula:

$$\frac{mAs_1}{mAs_2} = \frac{RS_2}{RS_2}$$

where: mAs_1 = old mAs
mAs_2 = new mAs
RS_1 = old relative speed
RS_2 = new relative speed

Of course, the relative speed conversion formula may also be algebraically expressed as:

$$mAs_2 = \frac{RS_1 \times mAs_1}{RS_2}$$

EXAMPLE: What is the proper mAs for use with an 80-RS system when technical factors of 55 kVp and 5 mAs produce an acceptable image with a 200-RS system?

Answer:

$$\frac{mAs_1}{mAs_2} = \frac{RS_2}{RS_1}$$

$$\frac{5}{mAs_2} = \frac{80}{200}$$

(continues)

(continued)

$$mAs_2\ 80 = 5\ mAs \times 200$$

$$mAs_2 \times 80 = 1{,}000\ mAs$$

$$mAs_2 = \frac{1{,}000\ mAs}{80}$$

$$mAs_2 = 12.5\ mAs$$

The condition of the film processing solutions can dramatically alter film density. Film density will increase when the developer solution temperature increases, immersion time increases, or replenishment rates increase. Film density will decrease when these factors decrease, as well as when contamination decreases solution strength.

Digital radiographic systems can be varied in their sensitivity to the incoming x-ray photons. Because radiographers need a reference point in order to produce quality images, most digital radiography system manufacturers calibrate the sensitivity processing algorithms to both the histogram control features as well as provide a sensitivity index or exposure value for each image.

Digital radiography systems use exposure indicators to provide information regarding the exposure to the IR. The correct exposure factors will deliver an exposure indicator that is within an acceptable range and will give the best image quality. Digital systems exhibit a wide dynamic range. Rather than the characteristic curve of film/screen systems, the response of a digital IR to x-ray exposure is linear. This linear response gives the digital system increased exposure latitude over film/screen systems. This means that areas that receive very little radiation can be enhanced by the computer instead of all the densities clumping around the toe of the D log E curve. Conversely, areas receiving greater exposure can be separated and brought down into the visible density range by the computer instead of all clumping around the shoulder of the D log E curve.

Digital processing requires the technologist to be knowledgeable in the details of image acquisition as well as post-processing parameters and procedures. For example, many manufacturers state in their technical usage information that mAs has little effect on the visualization of density/IR exposure. This can be a confusing statement for radiographers who are knowledgeable about the relationships between mAs and kVp and clearly understand how to control them when creating an optimal diagnostic image. What manufacturers are trying to convey is that the extended range of the straight-line portion of the IR response curve allows a CR system to digitally process the image after exposure to rescale the density into the visible range, even when the IR is grossly overexposed. This does not change the fact that changes in mAs will increase or decrease the quantity of photons received by the IR. These changes directly affect the quantity of information the IR passes on to the post-processing system and what is used to determine the exposure indicator. This information is discussed in detail in Chapter 23.

SUMMARY

Density/IR exposure is one of the two photographic properties that comprise visibility of detail. Visibility of detail refers to the fact that the radiographic image is visible to the human eye only because sufficient density/IR exposure (and contrast) exists to permit the structural details to be perceived.

As an image quality factor, *density* was the term that was used to reflect exposure to the radiographic film. Density has been defined since the 1920s as the degree of overall blackening that is the result of black metallic silver deposited in the emulsion of film. Density was the viewable result of a film's response to exposure. When the IR was primarily film, density was a term that could adequately describe the effects of IR exposure. In the digital environment this important image quality factor has not changed but can be expressed simply as *IR exposure* because film is no longer the primary IR. *Brightness* and *density* are not interchangeable terms. Brightness is a monitor control function that can change the lightness and darkness of the image on a display monitor but it is not related to IR exposure. Brightness is the proper term for the luminous intensity (measured in candela) of the display monitor's light emission. It is for these reasons that the photographic property of density has been renamed density/IR exposure.

In both film screen and digital imaging, the visibility of the image has always been the result of the proper exposure to the IR. With digital imaging, printing to film is not common, but in both environments the key to a visible image is having the correct IR exposure. Window level describes digital post-processing that produces changes in brightness, so it also is appropriate to use when controlling the display of an image.

When mAs is decreased, the resulting density/IR exposure will be decreased and vice versa. The effects of mAs and the other influencing factors on density/IR exposure are not exact because of the multiple variables that are part of the imaging system.

A wide variety of factors affect density/IR exposure. These factors are classified as either controlling or influencing factors. The controlling factor is mAs and it should be used as the principal method for adjusting for insufficient or excessive density/IR exposure. The influencing factors include kilovoltage, focal spot size, anode heel effect, distance, filtration, beam restriction, anatomical part, grids, IRs, and film processing.

When the controlling or any of the influencing factors are altered, some change in density/IR exposure will occur. However, with some of the factors, the effect is often negligible. Table 26-4 illustrates the effect on IR exposure/film density when the various factors are changed. ■

TABLE 26-4. Effect on Density/IR Exposure When Factors Are Changed

+ = increases density/IR exposure
− = decreases density/IR exposure
∅ = negligible effect
Controlling Factor
+ Increasing milliamperage-seconds
− Decreasing milliamperage-seconds
Influencing Factors
+ Increasing kilovoltage
− Decreasing kilovoltage
+ Increasing number of pulses in the generator waveform
− Decreasing number of pulses in the generator waveform
∅ Focal spot size
∅ Anode heel effect
− Increasing distance
+ Decreasing distance
− Increasing filtration
+ Decreasing filtration
− Increasing beam restriction/collimation
+ Decreasing beam restriction/collimation
− Increasing anatomical part thickness or tissue type
+ Decreasing anatomical part thickness or tissue type
+ Using radiolucent contrast media
− Using radiopaque contrast media
− Additive pathological conditions
+ Destructive pathological conditions
− Increasing grid ratio
+ Decreasing grid ratio
+ Increasing film/screen combination relative speed
− Decreasing film/screen combination relative speed
+ Increasing film processing developer time, temperature, and/or replenishment rate
− Decreasing film processing developer time, temperature, and/or replenishment rate

REVIEW QUESTIONS

1. Define density/IR exposure.
2. Explain how density/IR exposure and brightness differ.
3. What is the controlling factor of density/IR exposure and how is it affected?
4. How are density/IR exposure adjustments made for changes in kilovoltage?
5. How do the inverse square law and the exposure maintenance formulas differ from one another?
6. How do variations in the anatomical part affect density/IR exposure?
7. What are the relationships to density/IR exposure of grid ratio, frequency, interspace material, and grid use?
8. What is the relationship to density/IR exposure of relative speed for film/screen combinations?
9. How does film processing affect density?

REFERENCES AND RECOMMENDED READING

Bauer, R. G. (1970). High kilovoltage chest radiography with an air gap. *Radiologic Technology, 42*, 10–14.

Bierman, A., & Boldingh, W. H. (1951). The relation between tension and exposure times in radiography. *Acta Radiologica, 35*, 22–26.

Bryan, G. J. (1970). *Diagnostic radiography: A manual for radiologic technologists.* Baltimore: Williams & Wilkins.

Cahoon, J. B. (1961). Radiographic technique: Its origin, concept, practical application and evaluation of radiation dosage. *The X-Ray Technician, 32*, 354–364.

Carlton, R. R., & McKenna, A. (1989). Repeating radiographs: Setting imaging standards. In E. Frank (Ed.), *Postgraduate advances in radiologic technology.* Berryville, VA: Forum Medicum.

Carroll, Q. B. (1993). *Evaluating radiographs.* Springfield, IL: Charles C Thomas Publishers.

Carroll, Q. B. (2003). *Fuchs's radiographic exposure, processing, and quality control* (7th ed.). Springfield, IL: Charles C Thomas Publishers.

Chow, M. F. (1988). The effect of a film's sensitivity to its speed, contrast, and latitude. *The Canadian Journal of Medical Radiation Technology, 19*(4), 147.

Clark, K. C. (1953). An introduction to high-voltage technique. *Radiography, 19*, 2–33.

Cullinan, A., & Cullinan, J. (1994). *Producing quality radiographs* (2nd ed.). Philadelphia: J. B. Lippincott.

Distance—technique relationship of angulated projections. (1980). *Radiologic Technology, 52*(3), 301.

Eastman Kodak Company. (1980). Health sciences markets division. *The Fundamentals of Radiography* (12th ed.). Rochester, NY: Kodak Publication M1–18.

Eastman, T. R. (1975). Technique charts: The key to radiographic quality. *Radiologic Technology, 46*, 365–368.

Eastman, T. R. (1973). Measurement: The key to exposure with manual techniques. *Radiologic Technology, 45*, 75–78.

Epp, E. R., Weiss, H., & Laughlin, J. S. (1961). Measurement of bone marrow and gonadal dose from the chest x-ray examination as a function of field size, field alignment, tube kilovoltage and added filtration. *British Journal of Radiology, 34*, 85–100.

Fauber T. (2008). *Radiographic imaging and exposure.* St. Louis: Mosby.

Files, G. W. (1935). Maximum tissue differentiation. *The X-Ray Technician, 7*, 17–24.

Files, G. W. (1952). *Medical radiographic technique.* Springfield, IL: Charles C Thomas Publishers.

Fuchs, A. W. (1940). Balance in the radiographic image. *The X-Ray Technician, 12*(3), 81–84, 118.

Fuchs, A. W. (1947). The anode "heel" effect in radiography. *Radiologic Technology, 18*(4), 158.

Fuchs, A. W. (1948). Relationship of tissue thickness to kilovoltage. *The X-Ray Technician, 19*, 287–293.

Fuchs, A. W. (1949). Control of radiographic density. *The X-Ray Technician, 20*, 271–273, 291.

Fuchs, A. W. (1950). The rationale of radiographic exposure. *The X-Ray Technician, 22*, 62–68, 76.

Fuchs, A. W. (1958). *Principles of radiographic exposure and processing.* Springfield, IL: Charles C Thomas Publishers.

Funke, T. (1966). Pegged kilovoltage technic. *Radiologic Technology, 37*, 202–213.

Geiger, J. (1960). The heel effect. *Radiologic Technology, 32*(1), 55.

Gratale, P., Turner, G. W., & Burns, C. B. (1986). Using the same exposure factors for wet and dry casts. *Radiologic Technology, 57*(4), 325–328.

Gratale, P., Wright, D. L., & Daughtry, L. (1990). Using the anode heel effect for extremity radiography. *Radiologic Technology, 61*(3), 195–198.

Hiss, S. S. (2003). *Understanding radiography* (4th ed.). Springfield, IL: Charles C Thomas.

Jenkins, D. (1980). *Radiographic photography and imaging processes.* Lancaster, England: MTP Press Limited.

Jerman, E. C. (1928). *Modern x-ray technic.* St. Paul, MN: Bruce.

Lauer, O. G., Mayes, J. B., & Thurston, R. P. (1990). *Evaluating radiographic quality: The variables and their effects.* Mankato, MN: The Burnell Company.

Mattsson, O. (1955). Practical photographic problems in radiography. *Acta Radiologica Supplementum, 120*, 1-206.

Schwarz, G. S. (1959). Kilovoltage and radiographic effect. *Radiology, 73*, 749–760.

Schwarz, G. S. (1960). Kilovoltage conversion in radiography. *The X-Ray Technician, 31*, 373–379, 436.

Schwarz, G. S. (1961). *Unit-step radiography.* Springfield, IL: Charles C Thomas.

Seeman, H. E. (1968). *Physical and photographic principles of medical radiography.* New York: Wiley & Sons.

Seeram, E. (2011). *Digital radiography: An introduction.* Clifton Park, NY: Delmar Cengage Learning.

Shephard, C. (2003). *Radiographic image production and manipulation.* New York: McGraw Hill.

United States War Department. (1941, July 3). *Technical manual: Roentgenographic technicians* (TM 8–240). Washington, DC: Author.

Wallace, J. E. (1995). *Radiographic exposure: Principles & practice.* F.A. Davis. Philadelphia, PA.

Williams, W. A. (1956). Radiographic effect formula: Its practical application. *The X-Ray Technician, 28*, 1–6, 67.

Wilsey, R. B. (1921). The intensity of scattered x-rays in radiography. *American Journal of Roentgenology, 8*, 328–338.

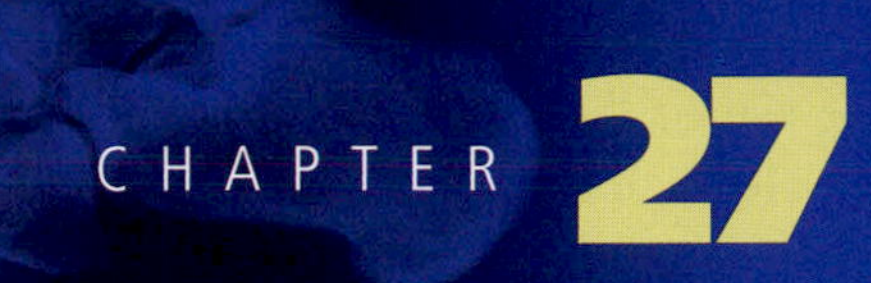

CHAPTER 27 Contrast

KEY TERMS

contrast
differential attenuation
dynamic range
grayscale
image receptor contrast
scale of contrast
subject contrast
window width

> The conclusion drawn from these experiments was that there was no mystery—that, other things being equal, contrast was determined solely by the voltage used. . . .
>
> *W. D. Coolidge, "Experiences with the Roentgen-ray Tube"*

OBJECTIVES

Upon completion of this chapter, the student should be able to:

- Identify contrast as a prime component of the photographic properties controlling visibility of detail of image quality.
- Explain the various terms used to describe contrast/dynamic range.
- Define contrast and the factors that affect it.
- Describe the factors that affect image receptor contrast.
- Describe the factors that affect subject contrast.
- Describe the effect of fog on contrast.
- Describe the effects of contrast changes on image appearance.
- Determine the technical factor changes necessary to achieve optimal contrast.
- Assess contrast on various radiographic images.
- Recommend appropriate adjustments to improve contrast under various conditions.
- Explain why kilovoltage peak is the controlling factor of contrast.
- Explain how each influencing factor affects contrast.

ASSESSING CONTRAST

Contrast is one of the two properties that comprise visibility of detail. Visibility of detail refers to the fact that the image is visible to the human eye only because sufficient contrast (and density/image receptor [IR] exposure) exists to permit the structural details to be perceived. **Image contrast is the difference between adjacent densities/IR exposures.** It can be mathematically evaluated as the percentage or ratio of the differences between densities/IR exposure. These differences can range from clear white through various shades of gray to black.

The term **dynamic range** describes the concept of contrast as it is displayed on a soft-copy monitor for digital images. It is the proper term for the range of brightness of the display monitor light emission. For radiographic images, the term *contrast/dynamic range* can be applied. The term **window width** accurately describes the digital processing that produces changes in the range of brightness, so it also is appropriate to use when controlling image contrast. Finally, the term *contrast/dynamic range/window width* is applied to grayscale bit depth (also known as the z axis). Sufficient differences in exposure to the receptor are necessary for the individual pixels to exhibit different exposure values. These exposure differences are displayed through various bit-depth values along the z axis of the image.

Because contrast consists of various densities/IR exposures, a thorough knowledge of the factors that control density/IR exposure is a prerequisite to understanding it. Although contrast must be considered an independent factor, the fact that it is composed of densities/IR exposures makes it very difficult to separate it from the evaluation of overall density/IR exposure. Any change in overall density/IR exposure will affect contrast. This makes contrast the most difficult of the prime technical factors to evaluate and adjust.

Describing Contrast

When the differences between adjacent densities that comprise contrast are great, the image is described as high contrast. The result is fewer discernible shades of gray. Conversely, when the differences are minimal, the image is described as low contrast. This produces more discernible shades of gray. Figure 27-1F has the fewest shades of gray and therefore has the highest contrast.

In Figure 27-1A-F, there are progressively less discernible shades of gray. Figure 27-1A has the lowest contrast image. This is analogous to a gray scarf on a gray coat, which has low contrast, versus a black scarf on a white coat, which has high contrast. Table 27-1 summarizes the relationships between the various terms used to describe contrast.

As the differences between adjacent densities increase, there are fewer shades of discernible gray and the contrast is increased. Increasing contrast produces a high-contrast image. As the differences between adjacent densities decrease, there are more shades of discernible gray and the contrast is decreased. Decreasing contrast produces a low-contrast image.

The term *good contrast* is often applied to high contrast, but this is a misnomer and should be avoided because high contrast is not necessarily the most desirable. In fact, in most instances low contrast provides more information. Low contrast provides more differences in density/IR exposure even though the difference between densities is less. As long as the differences remain within the visible range of densities, low contrast provides more diagnostic information. Figures 27-2A and B are good examples of how high contrast fails to provide all the information that is obtained from a low-contrast image.

Contrast is a psychovisual perception. In other words, the psychological effects of the relationships between the densities produce a visual perception that we call contrast. The perception problem is greater because not only do individuals have different physiological visual abilities, but individual background experiences also affect the final perception. Perhaps it would be better to think of contrast in terms of an individual's "contrast sensitivity."

Although high-contrast images may be perceived as more pleasing to the untrained eye, radiographers and radiologists realize that although the lower contrast-image is not as dramatic in its presentation, it often demonstrates more information. Without contrast there would be no image because all densities would appear identical. More information is visible simply because more densities are present, thus forming more possibilities for contrast differences.

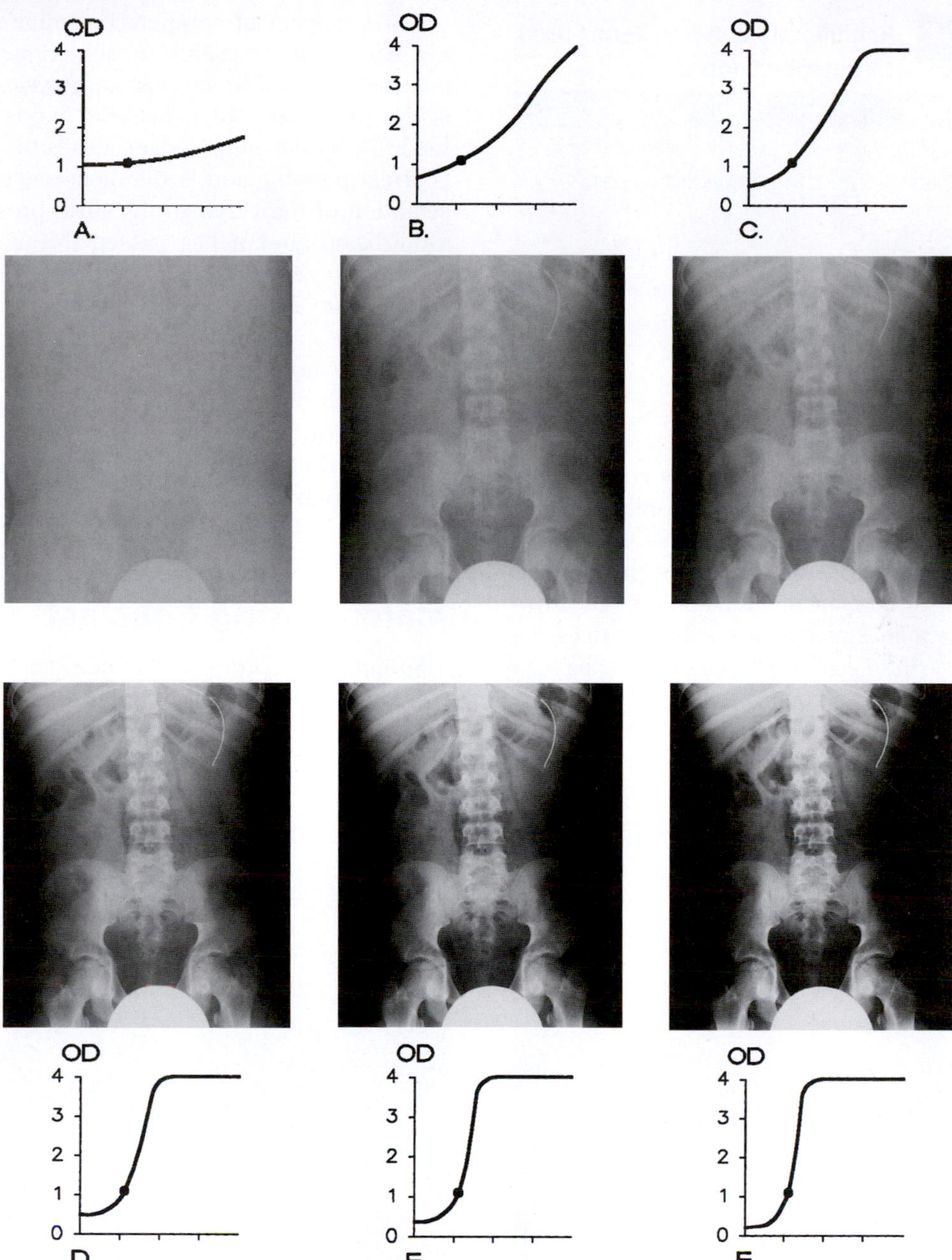

FIGURE 27-1. Pure contrast changes in a digital abdomen image produced with a fixed density point. These computerized images vary only in contrast, as shown in the accompanying D log E curves. From A to F the contrast curve becomes steeper and shorter, but the density point does not move up or down. C is considered optimal contrast for a diagnostic image. *(Computed radiography images courtesy of Bruce Long, Indiana University, Medical Center, Indianapolis.)*

TABLE 27-1. Relationship between Terms Used to Describe Contrast

High Contrast	Low Contrast
Few shades of gray	Many shades of gray
Increased contrast	Decreased contrast
Low kVp	High kVp
Short scale contrast	Long scale contrast
Short (narrow) dynamic range/window width	Large (wide) dynamic range/window width

Scale of contrast is the number of useful visible densities or shades of gray. Short scale contrast refers to an image that demonstrates considerable or maximal differences between densities and has a minimal total number of densities. Conversely, long scale contrast refers to an image that demonstrates slight or minimal differences between densities but has a maximal total number of densities (Figure 27-3). Short scale contrast is also called high contrast, or increased contrast, whereas long scale contrast is called low contrast, or decreased contrast.

The advent of computerized digital processing has made it useful to sometimes describe contrast as physical and visible. Physical contrast is the total range of density/IR exposure values recorded by the image receptor. It is the maximum contrast possible and is the most accurate representation of the varying intensities present in the x-ray beam after it has passed through the subject. Visible contrast is the total range of density/IR exposure values that can be perceived by the human eye in a single image. It is a portion of the physical contrast and comprises the information from which diagnosis is made. Digital imaging allows radiographers access to the entire range of densities available. Radiographers manipulate the physical contrast available into the visible range to produce the diagnostic image.

Manipulating Contrast

The image receptor records many densities that cannot be seen by the human eye. Depending on the desired contrast, the recorded densities

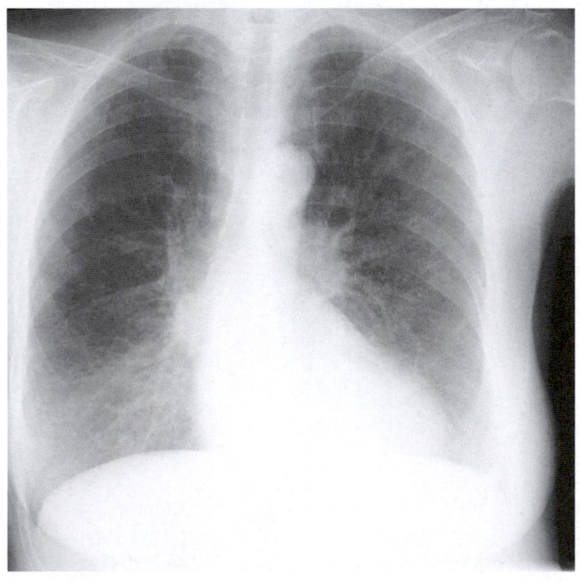

A

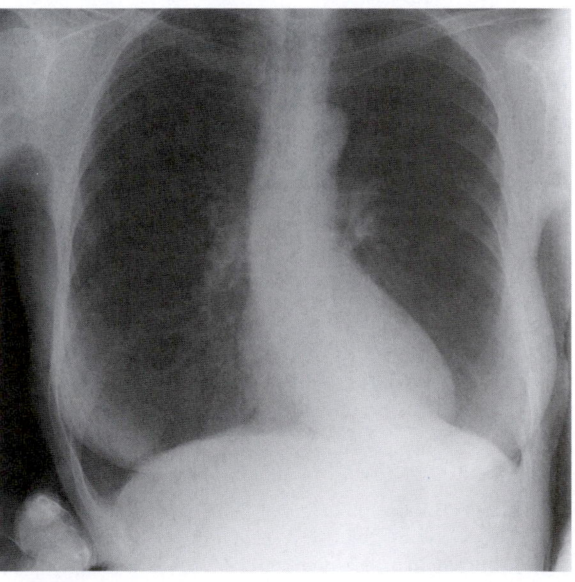

B

FIGURE 27-2. High and low contrast. (A) Chest radiograph produced using 80 kVp. (B) Chest radiograph of same patient using 110 kVp. *(Radiographs courtesy of Arlene Adler and Richard R. Carlton.)*

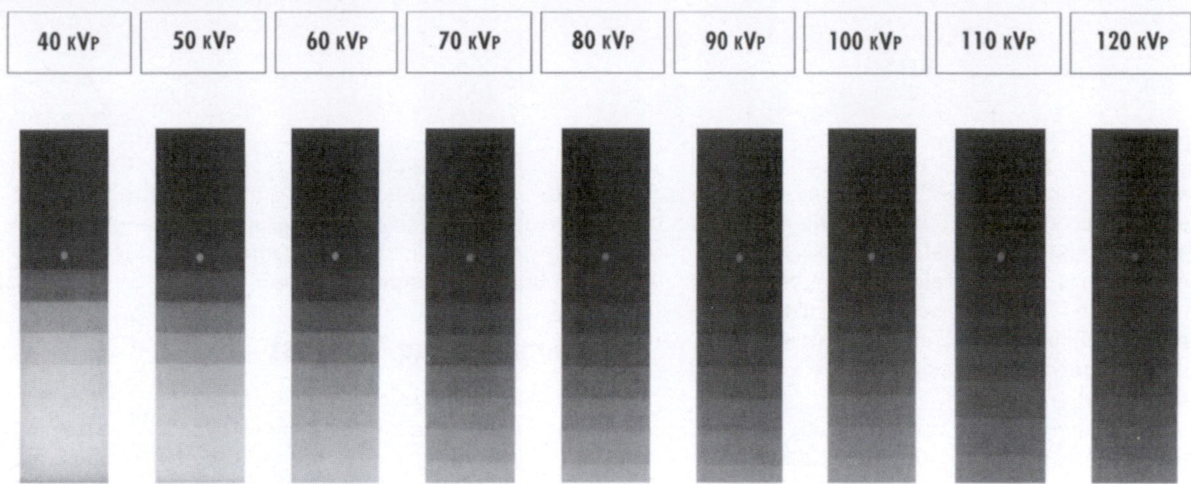

FIGURE 27-3. Variations in scale of contrast. The number of shades of gray, the scale or range of contrast, increases as kVp increases. *(Radiographs courtesy of Arlene Adler and Richard R. Carlton.)*

are compressed or expanded to form a range of visible densities. This can be accomplished by changes in the film's D log E curve, adjustments in kVp, or by the use of digital window width adjustments. Compression or expansion of the range of densities separates the physical contrast that is actually recorded by the image receptor from the visible contrast that can be perceived by the viewer on a single image.

It is important to realize that the digital response curve can be manipulated to make a very slight change in exposure, causing a huge change in contrast/dynamic range/window width/grayscale bit depth. Although it is not normal for a response curve to produce results outside normal usage, it is certainly possible.

IMAGE CONTRAST

Image contrast is the total amount of contrast acquired from both the image receptor and anatomical part. These are described as **image receptor** and **subject contrast**, respectively.

Image Receptor Contrast

Film Contrast. Film contrast is the range of densities that the film is capable of recording. Mathematically, this is expressed as the slope of the D log E curve. Film contrast depends on four factors: the use of **intensifying screens**, **film density**, **the D log E curve**, and **processing**.

Intensifying screens create an inherently higher-contrast image. Although the exact reason is unknown, contrast is always lower for a film exposed to x-rays only than it is for the same film exposed to light from intensifying screens. It is most likely related to the way in which the film responds to the x-ray photons. The D log E curve changes dramatically when a film designed for exposure by light is exposed directly to x-rays. Changing screen speed has a negligible effect on contrast.

Contrast also changes with changes in film density. The exact effect is shown in Figure 27-4. There is an optimal range of densities/IR exposures that permits contrast to be visualized at a maximum. Excessive or inadequate density/IR exposure decreases contrast. This is especially true in the

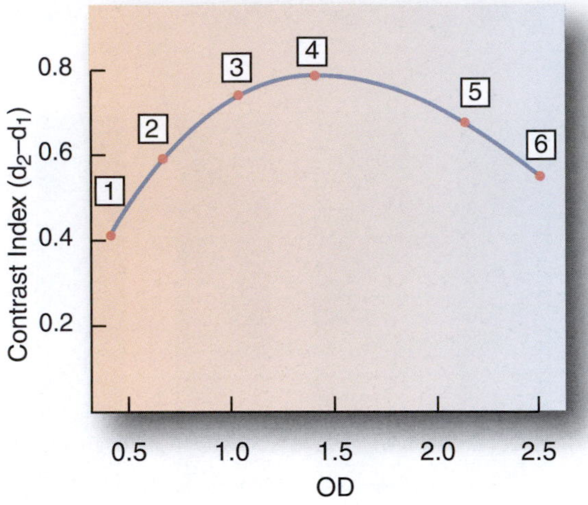

FIGURE 27-4. Contrast index for film density ranges (1–6). Note that the maximum contrast (range 4) is essentially the straight-line portion of the curve. Contrast is decreased for toe and shoulder measurements but is maximized for the straight-line portion of the D log E curve (OD) 1.2–1.5. (Also note that this range corresponds to the speed point [OD 1.2].) *(Courtesy of Barry Burns, University of North Carolina, Division of Radiologic Science.)*

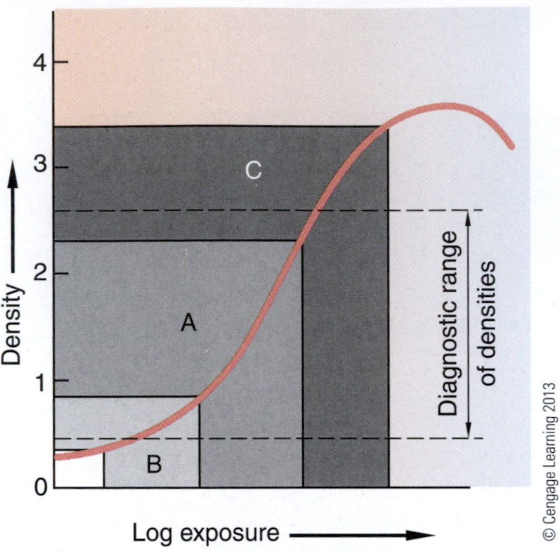

FIGURE 27-5. The effect of film density on contrast. (A) When the film is correctly exposed, the densities fall within the visible range. (B) An underexposed film occurs when the exposure places the developed densities into the toe. (C) An overexposed film occurs when the exposure places the developed densities into the shoulder. The decrease in contrast of underexposed and overexposed films occurs because the slope is not as steep in the toe and shoulder.

toe and shoulder regions of film D log E curves. If the kVp remains constant, mAs and distance will determine the actual value of exposure, thereby determining the location of the exposure on the log relative exposure axis of the curve. If a film is exposed correctly, the film densities will fall within the visible range of the D log E curve. If the exposure places the developed densities on the toe (an underexposed film) or shoulder (an overexposed film), the slope is not as steep, resulting in a decrease in contrast (Figure 27-5).

The primary determinant of the shape of the D log E curve is the physical composition of the film emulsion. As the slope of the curve becomes steeper, contrast is increased. For example, in Figure 27-6, film A possesses higher contrast than film B. Because of the steeper slope of the curve, the visible density range is compressed into a narrower exposure range. Film A is a high-contrast, narrow-latitude film. Film B is a low-contrast, wide-latitude film because the visible density range is expanded across a wider exposure range.

Increasing film developer time, temperature, or replenishment rate will increase the chemical fog on the film. These changes produce a decrease in the slope of the curve, especially in the toe region (Figure 27-7). When any processing factor causes a change in base fog, contrast is affected. Developer temperature and immersion time, replenishment, and developer contamination are the primary processing factors that cause objectionable fog levels. Increased developer temperature, time, and replenishment rates cause increased fog and decreased contrast. As shown in Figure 21-10, film processing has an optimal range and any factor that causes processing to deviate from optimal values will decrease contrast. Developer contamination by fixer causes increased fog and decreased contrast because the chemical ability of the developer reducing agents is seriously impaired by the pH change in the solution.

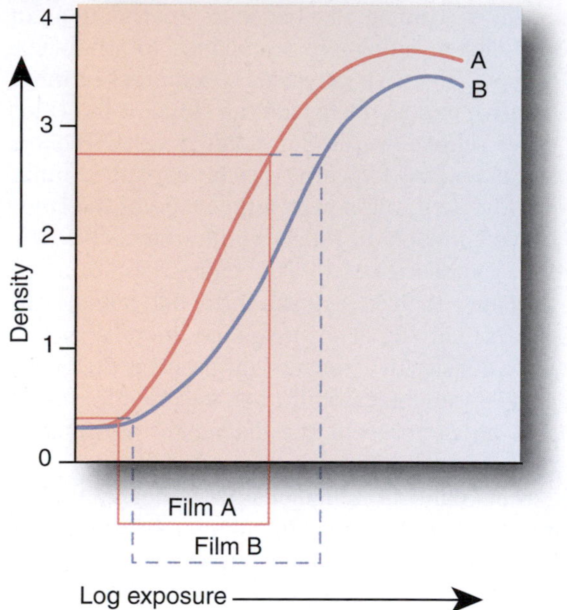

FIGURE 27-6. The effect of the D log E curve on contrast. As the slope of the curve becomes steeper, contrast is increased. Film A possesses higher contrast than Film B, because Film A compresses the visible density range into a narrower exposure range.

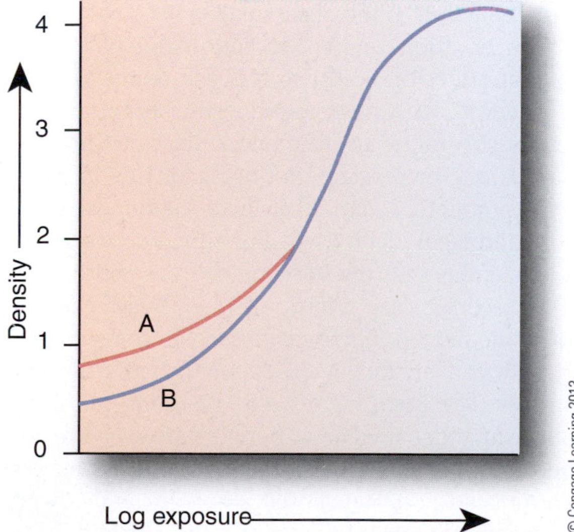

FIGURE 27-7. The effect of processing fog on contrast. In curve A, increased fog raises the toe of curve and decreases its slope, thus decreasing contrast.

Digital Image Receptor Contrast. The primary method for adjusting display contrast with digital imaging systems is through window width manipulations. Digital response curves can be varied in their sensitivity to the incoming x-ray photons and therefore to the range of densities/IR exposures available for acquisition processing and/or display. Because radiographers need a reference point in order to produce quality images, most digital radiography system manufacturers calibrate the sensitivity processing algorithms to provide a reasonable linear range of density/IR exposure for each image. Chapter 23, Digital Radiography, discusses both of these factors at length with the obvious implications for controlling the density/IR exposure and contrast of the image.

As digital images undergo post-processing, both the histogram and look-up table (LUT) that are used may affect the final image contrast that is displayed. Although this information is discussed in Chapter 23, essentially the histogram assesses the range and quantity of image receptor exposures in the digital image matrix. Then the look-up table is applied to the data that has a standard contrast for the selected exam to give the desired image contrast for display. Image processing will provide the proper **grayscale**, regardless of most variations in kVp and mAs. Despite the ability of the digital system to provide a proper contrast, the receptor should receive the correct exposure both in terms of the quantity of photons (mAs) as well as the differences in the energies of the photons (kVP). The proper kVP is important for the desired **differential attenuation** through the patient for a given examination. This differential attenuation causes signal differences to the digital detector.

Subject Contrast

Subject contrast is the range of differences in the intensity of the x-ray beam after it has been attenuated by the subject. This range in differences is the result of the differential attenuation by the tissues in the body. It is dependent on kilovoltage and the amount and type of irradiated material.

Kilovoltage. Kilovoltage peak (kVp) is the primary controller of subject contrast. As kVp increases, a wider range of photon energies is produced

(Figure 7-6). The wider the range of photon energies, the greater will be the ability of the photons to penetrate the body tissues. This leads to a wider range of exposures on the image receptor, which results in an overall lower contrast.

As long as the kVp is adequate to penetrate the part being examined, low kVp will produce high subject contrast. When the kVp is too low, most of the photons do not reach the image receptor because they are absorbed in the patient. Low kVp produces higher subject contrast because most of these low-energy photons are absorbed by thicker parts while more penetrate the thin part. With high kVp, subject contrast is decreased because more uniform penetration occurs between thick and thin parts.

The effect of kVp on subject contrast can be detailed by examining the D log E curve. Figure 27-8 shows the range of transmitted photon intensities forming the exposure to the film for both high- and low-kVp techniques for the same film type. High kVp produces a compressed range of relative exposures, which the slope of the D log E curve reflects within the visible density/IR exposure range. Low kVp produces an expanded range of relative exposures, which the slope of the D log E curve is unable to reflect within the visible density/IR exposure range. This causes some of the lowest and highest exposures to fall outside the visible density/IR exposure range. Increasing kVp causes density/IR exposure differences that were previously undetectable to become visible, resulting in an increase in the diagnostic information provided by the image.

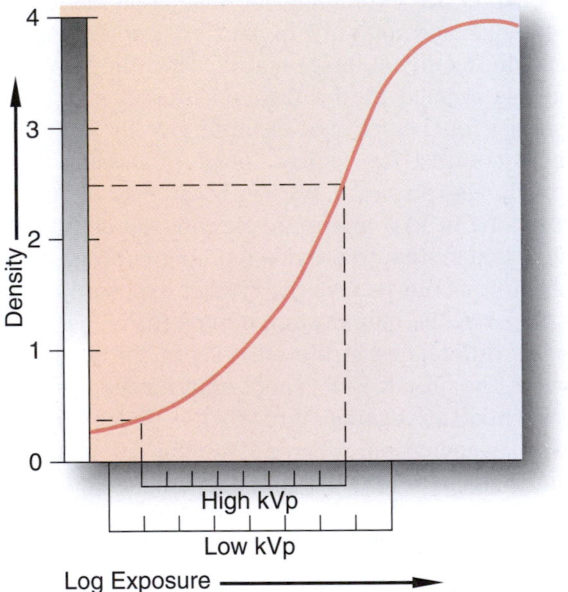

FIGURE 27-8. The effect of kVp on subject contrast. The range of transmitted photon intensities for high kVp produces a compressed range of relative exposures, which is reflected within the visible density range by the slope of the curve. The expanded range of exposures produced by low kVp is too wide for the curve to reflect within the visible density range. This causes some of the lowest and highest photon intensities not to be visible when low kVp is used.

This concept is demonstrated nicely by comparing chest radiographs to radiographs of the ribs. In chest radiography high kVps result in a wide range of image densities that fall within the visible range. Both the air-filled lungs and the bony structures are demonstrated within the visible range. No structures appear under- or overexposed. In rib radiography low kVps are used to enhance the differences between the air-filled lungs and the overlying bony structures. The air-filled lungs demonstrate increased density/IR exposure, whereas the bony structures demonstrate decreased density/IR exposure compared to the chest image.

In addition to kVp, radiation fog has a significant effect on contrast. It is the result of x-ray interactions with matter, primarily Compton scatter. As kVp increases, the percentage of Compton interactions increases. As a result of this increase in the amount of scatter reaching the image receptor, contrast is decreased. For film, scatter raises the base plus fog (the toe) and decreases the slope of the curve (see Figure 27-7). These changes cause the lightest film densities to be "fogged over" so they can no longer be distinguished from one another (see Figure 27-9). The resulting image no longer includes a clear or pure "white" region, and therefore has less contrast. With digital receptors, scatter also adds unwanted exposure and lowers the acquired contrast.

Fog can be caused by factors other than scatter radiation. These include subjecting film to heat, low-level ionizing radiation, or chemical fumes. Developer temperature, replenishment, and contamination may

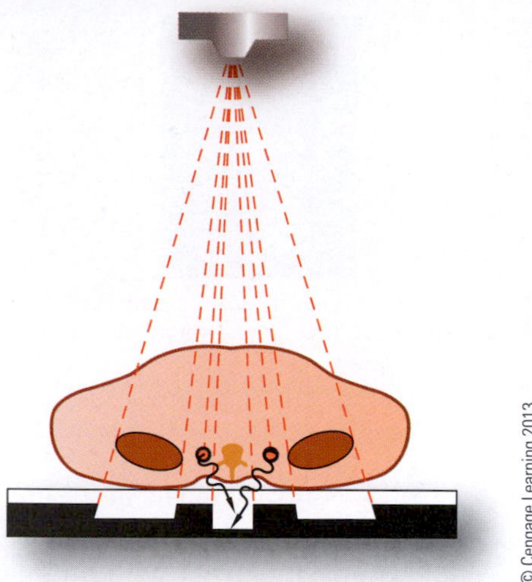

FIGURE 27-9. The effect of scatter radiation on contrast. Scatter radiation producing image density (and incorrect information) in a region of high subject density (under the vertebral column). The scatter interferes with the ability of the bone to cast a light shadow on the image.

also cause objectionable fog levels. The effect of fog on contrast must be considered during clinical radiography because it sets the acceptance limits for contrast regulation. The radiographer should remember that any factor that results in an increase in fog will decrease contrast.

Amount of Irradiated Material. The amount of irradiated material depends on the thickness of the body part and the field size. Both of these factors influence the number of x-rays transmitted to the image receptor. As body part thickness increases, x-ray absorption increases. Conversely, as body part thickness decreases, so does absorption. This difference in absorption between various thicknesses influences subject contrast. When the difference between adjacent thicknesses of various body parts is great, subject contrast is increased. When little difference exists in the thickness of adjacent body parts, subject contrast is decreased.

When the overall thickness of a body part increases, or when field size increases, the amount of scatter created will increase. This results in a decrease in subject contrast. A decrease in overall body part thickness or field size results in increased subject contrast.

Type of Irradiated Material. The type of irradiated material is influenced by the atomic number of the material and its tissue density. Both of these factors influence subject contrast.

Materials with a higher atomic number, such as lead and iodine, absorb a greater percentage of the x-ray beam than low-atomic-number materials, such as hydrogen, carbon, and calcium. This results from the presence of a greater number of electrons, which enables more interactions to occur. When the difference between the average atomic number of adjacent tissues is great, subject contrast is increased. When little difference exists between them, subject contrast is decreased. For example, bone has a higher average atomic number than soft tissue. Therefore, subject contrast between bone and soft tissue is greater than the contrast between adjacent soft tissue structures. Contrast media increase subject contrast by introducing greater differences in atomic-number variations than those that exist naturally.

Tissue density describes how tightly the atoms of a given substance are packed together. When the difference between the densities of adjacent tissues is great, subject contrast is increased. When little difference exists between them, subject contrast is decreased. For example, bone tissue is a denser substance than lung tissue. Therefore subject contrast between bone and lung tissue is greater.

EVALUATING CONTRAST

The major consideration in evaluating visible contrast is verification that a proper range of densities is visible throughout the anatomical area of interest on the image. Proper density/IR exposure alone is not enough. The anatomical structures of interest are visible only when sufficient contrast between the densities exists. Of course, these densities must be well within the range of human visibility.

Unlike the evaluation of density/IR exposure, contrast assessment requires more than just sufficient density/IR exposure within the visibility range. Adequate contrast must demonstrate enough distinctly different densities within the range to satisfy diagnostic-quality requirements for the particular examination. Much of this ability is the result of clinical experience. It is obvious that proper contrast is not the same for all tissues. Knowledge of anatomy and physiology, both normal and abnormal, as well as pathology and technical factors, is critical for proper contrast evaluation. Only when these skills are combined with an experienced and trained professional eye can proper contrast evaluation occur.

Because there is more information recorded on an image than is seen, the diagnostic importance of contrast is a matter of how many densities are included in the visible contrast range. To some extent, it can be said that low-contrast images have more information. However, the critical point is that the various densities must be discernible.

The human eye is limited in its ability to discern light and dark. This essentially establishes a value for the lightest and darkest visible shades of gray. When additional shades of gray are added to the visible range of contrast, they must fit between these two densities. Each additional shade of gray reduces the magnitude of the density/IR exposure difference, or the contrast, between the lightest and darkest grays. Eventually, a point is reached where additional shades of gray do not have enough density/IR exposure difference to be visible (see Figure 27-1A). Of course, this occurs at different points, depending on individual visual abilities. A 30 percent exposure difference has been used as the minimum change to cause a visible difference because this magnitude is discernible by nearly everyone. However, some professionals may be able to discern as little contrast as a 15 percent difference, which means they are capable of seeing twice as many shades of gray as someone who can discern only a 30 percent change.

Discerning contrast can be extremely difficult for even the experienced radiographer when the image exhibits poor density/IR exposure. Contrast evaluation can be made only when sufficient density/IR exposure exists to permit the range of contrast to be seen. The eye tends to consider nearby densities and contrast when evaluating image quality. It is so difficult for the eye to ignore nearby factors that a **contrast mask** is often helpful

FIGURE 27-10. A contrast mask. *(Courtesy of Arlene Adler and Richard R. Carlton.)*

(Figure 27-10). A contrast mask is a simple tool to help focus on the contrast in a selected area. When a contrast mask is used with an image, adjacent information is eliminated. This makes the evaluation much easier as the contrast problem becomes evident as well as easier to evaluate (Figure 27-11). Because of the difficulty in ignoring nearby density/IR exposure problems (either too light or dark), even the experienced radiographer will find a contrast mask useful in making some evaluations.

Selecting the Appropriate kVp

There are no established rules concerning how much contrast is desirable in all situations. Experience and knowledge enable the radiographer to determine when a change in contrast will increase the diagnostic quality of an image. Many radiologists find it desirable to have uniform contrast throughout a single examination to permit comparisons between projections. Low contrast can be achieved to some degree by utilizing a fixed kilovoltage technique system. Other radiologists prefer a higher contrast. This can be achieved to some degree by utilizing a variable kilovoltage technique system.

The radiographs in Figures 27-1 and 27-12 illustrate the effect of contrast on image quality. Notice in Figure 27-12 that the contrast varies as the kVp varies. Also notice that the contrast varies for the same kVp with different body part thickness (different subject densities). The exposure factors for these images used different mAs values to compensate for the differences in scatter radiation as the kVp was changed.

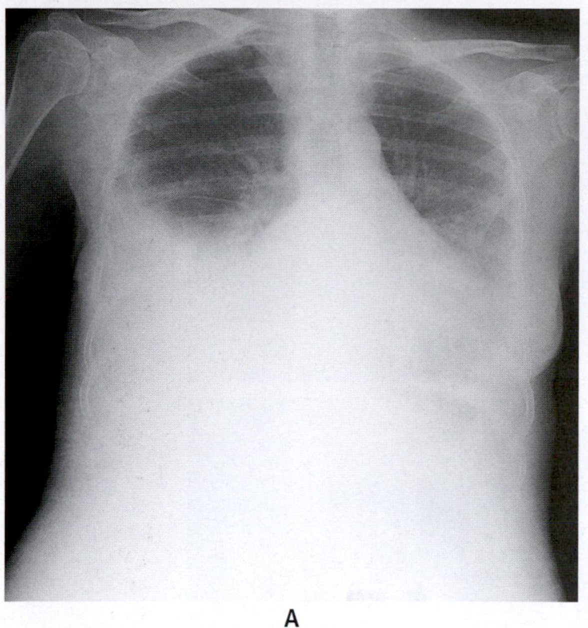

A

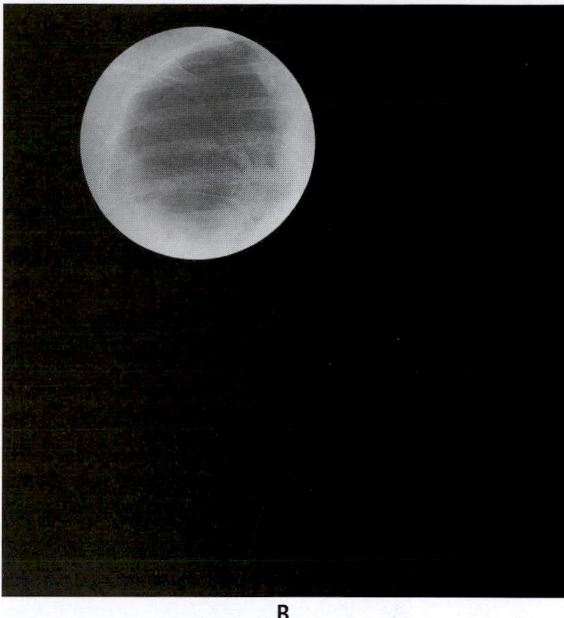

B

FIGURE 27-11. Using a contrast mask. (A) A radiograph of a chest that appears to be too light, making contrast evaluation difficult. (B) The same radiograph with the contrast mask applied to the right upper lobe of the lung, making contrast evaluation easier. *(Radiographs courtesy of Arlene Adler and Richard R. Carlton.)*

The images in Figure 11-2 illustrate the effect of kVp on image density/IR exposure. To perceive a contrast change, density/IR exposure should be maintained at a uniform level. The 15 percent rule is an acceptable method of achieving uniform image receptor exposure/film density/IR exposure when changing contrast. A visible change in contrast will not be perceived until kVp is changed by 4–12 percent, depending on the kVp range (Table 27-2). There is no reason to repeat an exposure for contrast reasons unless at least a 4–5 percent change is made, although higher kVps require even greater changes. The effects of mAs and the influencing factors on image contrast are not exact because of the wide variety of variables that are part of the imaging system. Many of the variables affect the contrast of the image as a side effect of other changes.

Both the quantity and quality of the x-ray beam will vary with changes in kilovoltage. There are too many variables to be quantified into a reliable formula. Because the 15 percent rule is used so much when maintaining exposure, it is convenient to use it as the minimum practical change within the diagnostic range. Remember that the 15 percent rule is a misnomer as the actual changes necessary to maintain exposure vary from 15–25 percent (Figure 26-4).

When a radiograph is outside acceptance limits, it needs to be repeated. All acceptance limits permit some degree of variation, at least 8–15 percent change in contrast. The rule for contrast changes is to make adjustments in increments of 15 or 8 percent. If the radiograph does not require an 8 percent change in kVp and contrast, it seldom requires repeating. Exceptions to this rule are fine adjustments of 8 percent that are crucial to demonstrate small structures. Radiographers may adjust technique charts by an 8 percent margin, but will seldom subject the patient to a second exposure for such a minor change. As with density/IR exposure adjustments, contrast changes require bold action or no action at all.

In some instances it may be desirable to decrease kVp to increase contrast when mAs must

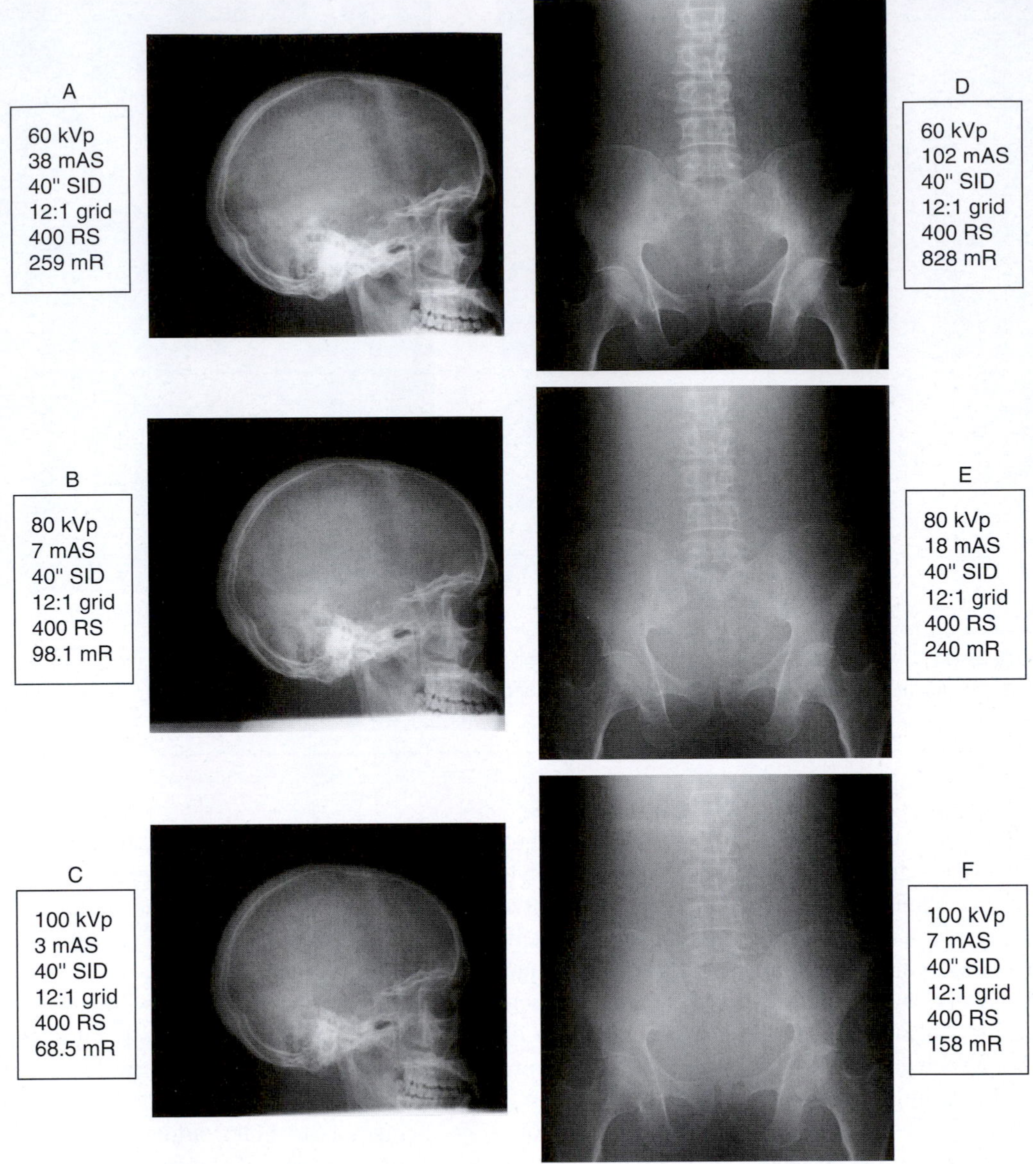

FIGURE 27-12. The effect of contrast on image quality. Skull radiographs produced at (A) 60 kVp; (B) 80 kVp; (C) 100 kVp. Abdomen radiographs produced at (D) 60 kVp; (E) 80 kVp; (F) 100 kVp. Compare these images, noting contrast changes due to anatomical part differences. *(Radiographs courtesy of Arlene Adler and Richard R. Carlton.)*

be increased. A radiograph of a 20-cm abdomen produced at 90 kVp demonstrates a relatively low contrast (Figure 27-13B). When the same abdomen is radiographed at 70 kVp, a significantly higher contrast results (Figure 27-13A). The reduced kVp produced less scatter radiation, thus producing higher contrast. The natural tendency to increase kVp for thicker parts will not produce satisfactory radiographs if the effect of increased Compton scatter on contrast is not considered first.

Radiographic image contrast occurs due to the photoelectric effect's total absorption of photons in the subject. High contrast is directly related to the number of photoelectric effect interactions that occur in the subject. Because Compton interactions produce scatter, low contrast is directly related to the amount of Compton scatter that occurs in the subject. Image contrast can be controlled by adjusting kVp. The kVp controls the relationship between the number of photoelectric versus Compton interactions.

TABLE 27-2. Changes Necessary to Produce Visible Contrast Differences

Level	Change Necessary to Produce Visible Change	Change Equal to Percent Change
30–50 kVp	4–5 percent	1–3 kVp
50–90 kVp	8–9 percent	4–8 kVp
90–130 kVp	10–12 percent	9–16 kVp

Contrast can be determined by matching the average incident photon energy with the average inner-shell binding energy of the predominant subject material, as shown in Figure 12-8. For example, when maximum contrast is desired for bone tissue, technical factors that increase the

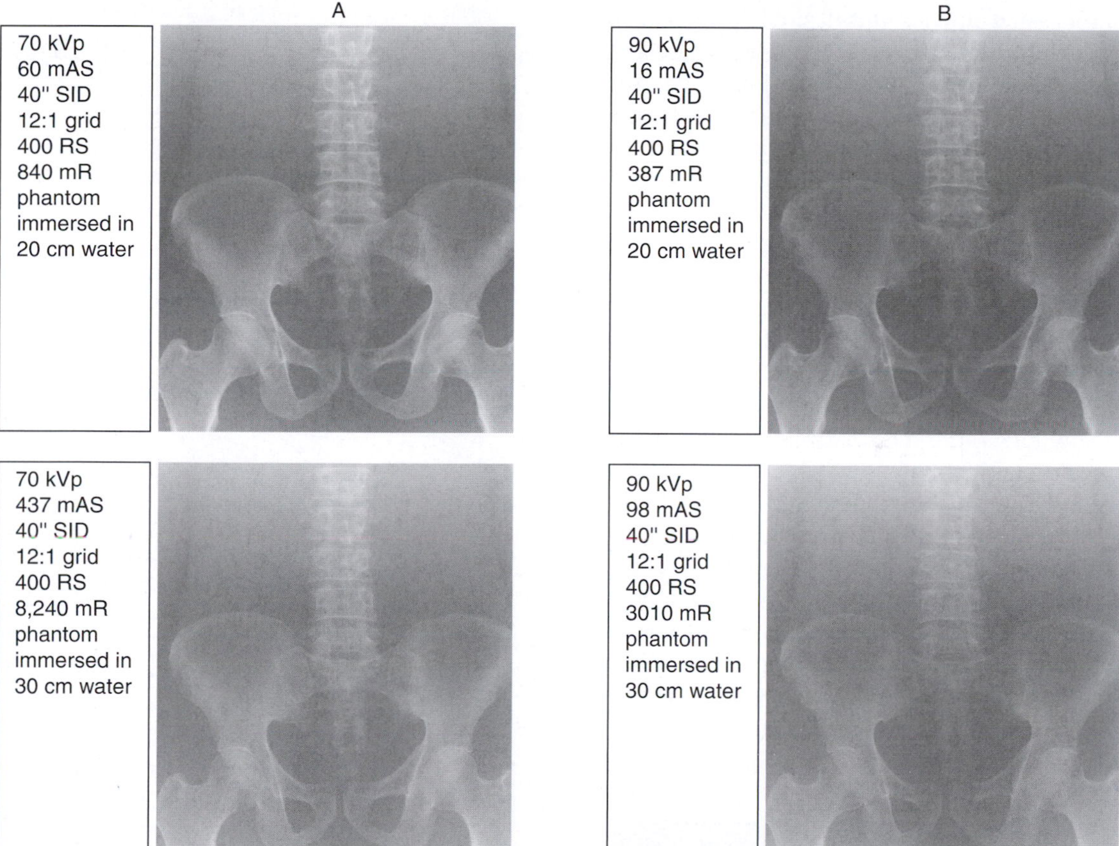

FIGURE 27-13. Increased contrast on 20- and 30-cm abdomens. (A) 20-cm abdomen at 70 kVp; (B) 20-cm abdomen at 90 kVp; (C) 30-cm abdomen at 70 kVp; (D) 30-cm abdomen at 90 kVp. All images were exposed with the same AEC and have the same overall density values. (Note the differences in mAs and mR dose.) *(Radiographs Courtesy of Arlene Adler and Richard R. Carlton.)*

percentage of photoelectric interactions should be used. Photoelectric effect interactions increase as kVp decreases.

The issue of how to select kVp levels for digital systems requires clear understanding. KVp can no longer be assessed by viewing the difference between adjacent densities or brightness levels when it is viewed. Because the response curve of the IR is now linear and much greater than with conventional film/screen systems, the initial contrast that is received from the detector is extremely low. Some digital radiography systems allow display of this information as it is collected from the detector, and these images clearly demonstrate the low-contrast nature of this initial information. Post-processing applies the desired level of contrast based on the histogram analysis and look-up table. In other words, the display image contrast is determined to a great extent from the histogram and look-up table, although the kVp level does have an impact. This impact is the result of differential attenuation (or signal difference). This means that proper selection of the kVp is required prior to post-processing.

When setting kVp levels for digital systems, the most important thing to remember is that when higher kVp levels are used the width of the data acquired is less (becomes narrower) (Figure 27-14). Note how the difference between the minimum to maximum incoming radiation is dramatically reduced. This is a desirable effect because it displays more anatomical data while reducing patient dose (Figure 27-15). It is recommended that kVp levels not exceed 80 for any non-grid radiography, including the chest. It is recommended that when scatter ratios approach 50 percent, grids should become mandatory. Failure to do so greatly reduces image contrast due to the scatter radiation reaching the IR.

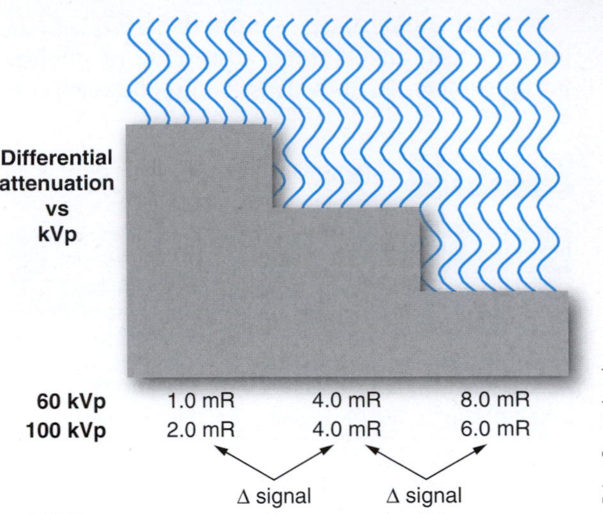

FIGURE 27-14. The differential attenuation resulting from a large kVp changes. As the kVp increases, the differential attenuation decreases and the signal difference from max to min is dramatically reduced.

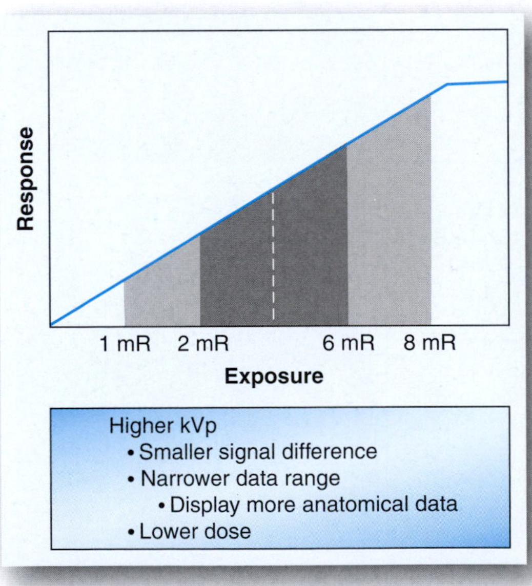

FIGURE 27-15. The values from Figure 27-14 applied to a diagram show that as the kVp increases, the data width acquired is less, so that more anatomical information may be visible on an image without having to change the brightness.

FACTORS AFFECTING CONTRAST

The controlling and influencing factors that affect contrast are shown in Figure 27-16. The controlling factor that affects contrast has the most direct effect on the image. When it is changed, the image

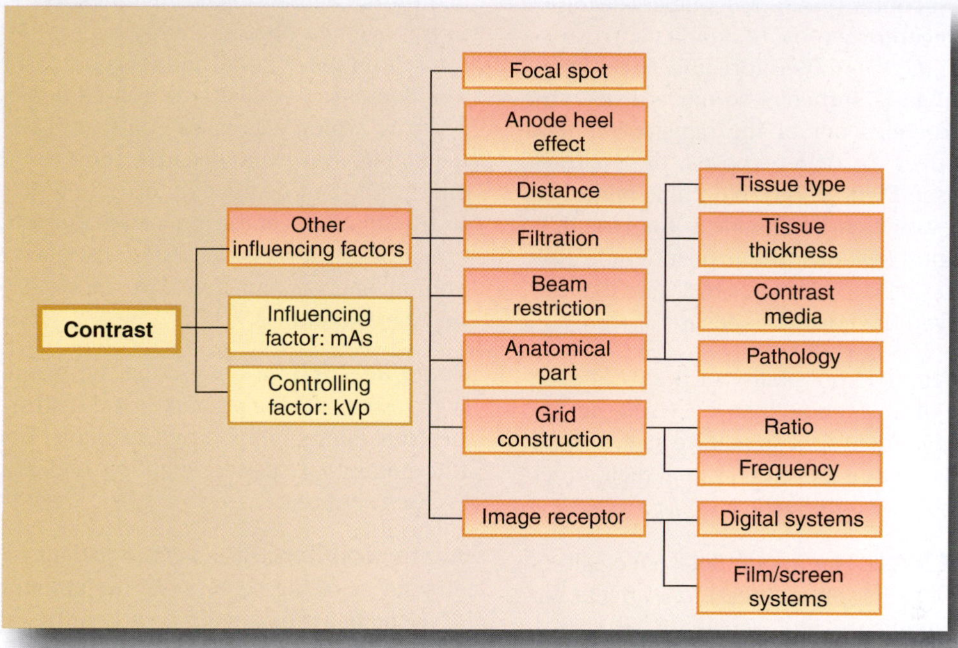

FIGURE 27-16. Image analysis: factors affecting contrast.

will change as a primary result. The influencing factors that control contrast have a less direct effect on the image or change other factors as well as contrast. When the influencing factors are changed the contrast is affected, but not as directly as with the controlling factor. With some of the factors this change is so small that it is essentially negligible.

Kilovoltage as the Controlling Factor

Kilovoltage peak (kVp) is the controller of contrast. As kVp increases, contrast decreases. As kVp decreases, contrast increases. In most instances the control of contrast rests with the radiographer by selecting an appropriate kVp setting from a technique chart developed for the particular x-ray unit in use. Other variables such as generator configuration may also affect the final decision. A generator configuration that increases the effective kVp will result in a decrease in contrast. For example, for a given kVp a multiphase generator will produce a lower contrast than a single-phase unit.

Kilovoltage also controls the amount of scatter radiation produced. Increasing kVp increases the amount of radiation fog, thereby decreasing contrast.

The radiographer must adapt the suggested kVp setting for the individual procedure. Experience and study of various body habitus, pathologies, positioning, and equipment quickly provides the radiographer with clinical knowledge that can be used for these adjustments.

Influencing Factors

Influencing factors include milliampere-seconds (mAs), focal spot size, anode heel effect, distance, filtration, beam restriction, anatomical part, grids, film/screen combinations, and processing.

Milliampere-Seconds (mAs). Milliampere-seconds alters image receptor exposure and density/IR exposure of the image and therefore affects contrast. When the change is sufficient to move density/IR exposure differences out of the range of human vision, either over- or underexposed, the contrast is decreased (see Figure 27-5). With film, under- or overexposure was clearly evident in the resultant image. For digital systems, the exposure indicator should be in the acceptable range to assure that the detector received the correct exposure.

Focal Spot Size. The possibility of the focal spot size altering contrast enough to be visible is extremely unlikely. Focal spot sizes have such a small effect on exposure that it is unlikely that their effect on contrast could be detected.

Anode Heel Effect. The anode heel effect alters the intensity of radiation and therefore affects image receptor exposure and density/IR exposure, which can affect contrast. The intensity of radiation is greater at the cathode end of the tube. This difference would become visible only with open collimation and a small anode target angle (less than 12°). The anode heel has very little effect on contrast.

Distance. Source-to-image-receptor distance (SID) alters the intensity of the beam reaching the image receptor according to the inverse square law. This affects density/IR exposure and therefore contrast. Greater distance decreases density/IR exposure, whereas less distance increases it. As distance alters exposure, it can change the contrast exactly as does mAs.

Object-to-image-receptor distance (OID) also has an effect on density/IR exposure and contrast. An air-gap technique increases OID, and this permits scatter radiation to avoid the image receptor. This scatter radiation would normally contribute radiation fog to the exposure. Removing scatter from the image will increase contrast.

Filtration. Filtration increases the effect of kVp by changing the average photon energy of the beam. All types of filtration—inherent, added, and total—alter density/IR exposure and contrast. Filtration affects contrast by changing the average photon energy and decreasing beam intensity. The increase in the average photon energy causes more Compton scatter production, and this decreases contrast. The decreased intensity decreases densities/IR exposures, which decreases contrast. This change is negligible, however, because most of these low-energy photons do not exit the patient to contribute to the image receptor exposure. The predominant effect of filtration is caused by changes in average photon energy, and therefore increased filtration decreases contrast.

Beam Restriction. Restricting the beam, collimating, or reducing the primary beam field size reduces the total number of photons available. This reduces the amount of scatter radiation and therefore increases contrast.

Anatomical Part. Because the patient is the prime attenuator of the beam, both the amount and type of tissue being examined greatly influence density/IR exposure and contrast. As the anatomical part size increases, the amount of scatter created by the part also increases, resulting in a decrease in contrast. As tissue density increases, the amount of scatter increases, which also results in a decrease in contrast. As average atomic number increases (i.e., using contrast media), there is more photoelectric absorption, resulting in higher or increased contrast.

As with density/IR exposure adjustments, compensation for anatomical part changes depends on an ability to assess tissue type, thickness, pathology, and so on. This ability is achieved only through clinical experience.

Grid Construction. The primary function of a grid is contrast improvement (Figure 27-17). Grids improve contrast by removing scatter before it reaches the image receptor. The contrast improvement factor (K) is the best measure of how well a grid accomplishes this function. The contrast improvement factor is dependent on the amount of scatter produced, which is controlled by the kVp and the amount and type of irradiated tissue. As the amount of scatter radiation that reaches the image receptor increases, the lower the contrast and the lower the contrast improvement factor. The contrast improvement factor K is measured by using

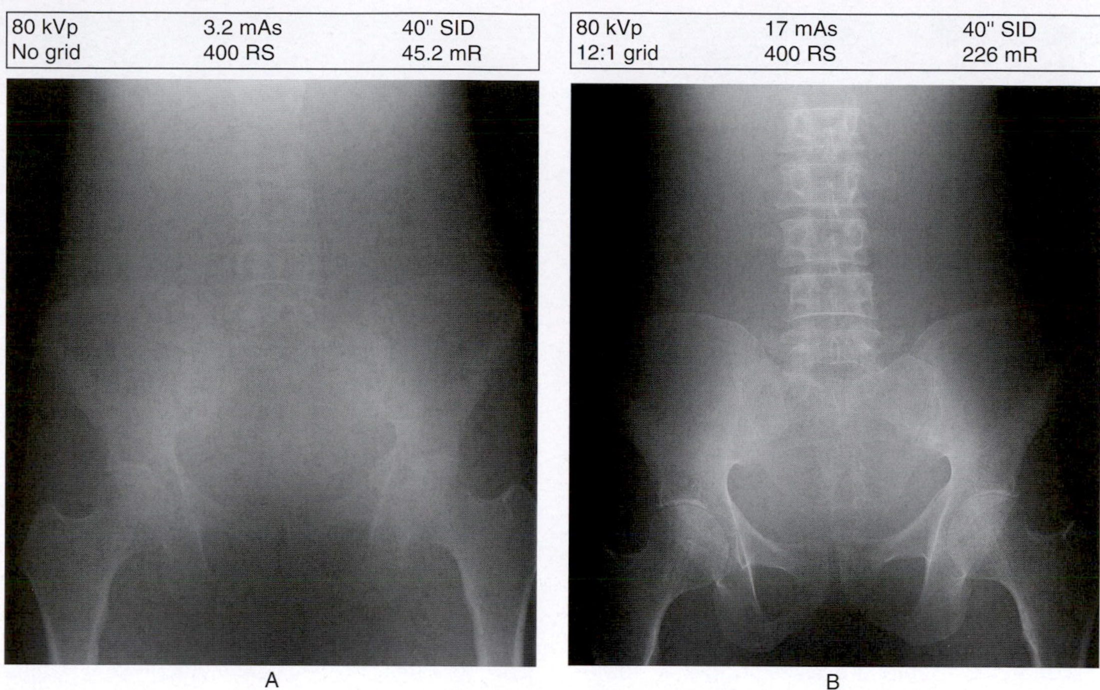

FIGURE 27-17. The effect of a grid on contrast. (A) 80 kVp without a grid; (B) 80 kVp with a grid. Both images were exposed with the same AEC and have the same overall density values. (Note the differences in mAs and mR dose.) *(Radiographs courtesy of Arlene Adler and Richard R. Carlton.)*

the average gradient (or gamma) of the straight-line portion of the D log E curve:

$$K = \frac{\text{average gradient with the grid}}{\text{average gradient without the grid}}$$

If K = 1, then no improvement in contrast has occurred. Most grids have contrast improvement factors between 1.5 and 3.5 so their contrast is 1.5-3.5 times better than an identical non-grid image. The higher the K factor, the greater the contrast improvement.

Higher ratio grids remove more scatter and therefore have a greater contrast improvement factor. This results in a higher-contrast image.

Image Receptor. With film/screen image receptor systems, the primary determinant of the shape of the D log E curve is the physical composition of the film emulsion. As the slope of the curve becomes steeper, contrast is increased. Intensifying screens create an inherently higher-contrast image. Contrast is always lower for a film exposed to x-rays only than it is for the same film exposed to light from intensifying screens. Increasing film developer time, temperature, or replenishment rate from the optimal range will increase the chemical fog on the film. These changes produce a decrease in the slope of the curve, which results in a decrease in contrast. Decreasing film development time, temperature, or replenishment rate from the optimal range will decrease the film's density, which in turn will decrease contrast.

With digital imaging systems, the primary determinant of the scale of contrast is the post-processing histogram and look-up table sequence that sets the range of information that will be supplied to the monitor, where it will be displayed in a range of brightness. These exposure differences are displayed through various bit-depth values along the z axis of the image. These can then be adjusted on the monitor through the manipulation of the window width. With digital image receptor systems, sufficient differences in exposure to the receptor are necessary for the individual pixels to exhibit different exposure values.

SUMMARY

Contrast is one of the two photographic properties that comprise visibility of detail. Visibility of detail refers to the fact that the radiographic image is visible to the human eye only because sufficient contrast (and density/IR exposure) exists to permit structural details to be perceived. Image contrast is the difference between adjacent densities. It can be mathematically evaluated as the percentage or ratio of the differences between densities. These differences can range from clear white through various shades of gray to black.

Dynamic range describes the range of contrast as it is displayed on a digital image. Window width describes the process that produces changes in the range of density/IR exposure. Sufficient differences in exposure to the receptor are necessary for the individual pixels to exhibit different exposure values. These exposure differences are displayed through various bit depth values along the z axis of the image.

When the differences between adjacent densities that comprise contrast are great, the image is described as high contrast. The result is fewer discernible shades of gray. Conversely, when the differences are minimal, the image is described as low contrast.

Short scale contrast is also called high contrast, or increased contrast, whereas long scale contrast is called low contrast, or decreased contrast. Physical contrast is the total range of density/IR exposure values recorded by the image receptor, whereas visible contrast is the total range of density/IR exposure values that can be perceived by the human eye in a single image.

Image contrast is the total amount of contrast acquired from both the anatomical part and the image receptor. These are described as image receptor contrast and subject contrast, respectively. Film contrast depends on four factors: the use of intensifying screens, film density, the D log E curve, and film processing. Digital receptor contrast primarily depends on post-processing operations, including histogram analysis and the application of the look-up table. Subject contrast is the range of differences in the intensity of the x-ray beam after it has been attenuated by the subject. It is dependent on kilovoltage and the amount and type of irradiated material.

The major consideration in evaluating visible contrast is verification that a proper range of densities is visible throughout the anatomical area of interest on the image. Proper density/IR exposure alone is not enough. The anatomical structures of interest can be visualized only when sufficient contrast between the densities exists. To perceive a contrast change, exposure should be maintained at a uniform level. The 15 percent rule is an acceptable method of achieving this.

A wide variety of factors can affect contrast. These factors are classified as either controlling or influencing factors. The controlling factor is kVp and it should be used as the principal method for altering the contrast. The influencing factors include milliamperage-seconds, focal spot size, anode heel effect, distance, filtration, beam restriction, anatomical part, grid construction, and image receptors.

When the controlling factor or any of the influencing factors is altered, some change in contrast will occur; however, with some of the factors the effect is often negligible. Table 27-3 illustrates the effect on contrast when the various factors are changed. For the purpose of this review, assume that compensation has been made for the changes in the density/IR exposure. Remember that if no compensation is made for the changes in density/IR exposure, and the resulting image is over- or underexposed, contrast will always decrease. ■

TABLE 27-3. Effects of Changing Factors on Contrast

+ = increases contrast
− = decreases contrast
∅ = negligible effect
Controlling Factor
− Increasing kilovoltage
+ Decreasing kilovoltage
− Increasing number of pulses in the generator waveform
+ Decreasing number of pulses in the generator waveform
Influencing Factors
∅ Increasing milliamperage-seconds*
∅ Decreasing milliamperage-seconds*
∅ Focal-spot size changes
∅ Anode heel effect
∅ Increasing SID
∅ Decreasing SID
+ Increasing OID
− Decreasing OID
− Increasing filtration
+ Decreasing filtration
+ Increasing beam restriction/collimation
− Decreasing beam restriction/collimation
− Increasing amount of irradiated tissue
+ Decreasing amount of irradiated tissue
+ Increasing the differences between the atomic number of the tissues
− Decreasing the differences between the atomic number of the tissues
− Increasing density of tissue
+ Decreasing density of tissue
+ Using contrast media (increasing or decreasing atomic number)
− Additive pathological conditions
+ Destructive pathological conditions
+ Increasing grid ratio
− Decreasing grid ratio
∅ Increasing film/screen relative speed
∅ Decreasing film/screen relative speed
+ Use of intensifying screens
− Increasing or decreasing film processing developer time and temperature beyond optimal

*For example, changing mAs while maintaining density/IR exposure by SID changes.

REVIEW QUESTIONS

1. Define contrast.
2. How do high-contrast images differ from low-contrast images?
3. What is the difference between physical and visible contrast?
4. What factors affect image receptor contrast and subject contrast?
5. How does density/IR exposure affect image receptor contrast?
6. What is the controlling factor of subject contrast and how does it affect it?
7. How do variations in the anatomical part affect contrast?
8. What is the effect of a grid on contrast?
9. How do the histogram and look-up table affect display contrast?

REFERENCES AND RECOMMENDED READING

Abildgaard, A., & Notthellen, J. A. (1992). Increasing contrast when viewing radiographic images. *Radiology, 185*(2), 475–478.

Bauer, R. G. (1970). High kilovoltage chest radiography with an air gap. *Radiologic Technology, 42*, 10–14.

Bierman, A., & Boldingh, W. H. (1951). The relation between tension and exposure times in radiography. *Acta Radiologica, 35*, 22–26.

Cahoon, J. B. (1961). Radiographic technique: Its origin, concept, practical application and evaluation of radiation dosage. *The X-Ray Technician, 32*, 354–364.

Carlton, R. R., & McKenna, A. (1989). Repeating radiographs: Setting imaging standards. In E. Frank (Ed.), *Postgraduate advances in radiologic technology.* Berryville, VA: Forum Medicum.

Carroll, Q. B. (1993). *Evaluating radiographs.* Springfield, IL: Charles C Thomas.

Carroll, Q. B. (2003). *Fuchs's radiographic exposure, processing, and quality control* (7th ed.). Springfield, IL: Charles C Thomas.

Chow, M. F. (1988). The effect of a film's sensitivity to its speed, contrast, and latitude. *The Canadian Journal of Medical Radiation Technology, 19*(4), 147.

Clark, K. C. (1953). An introduction to high-voltage technique. *Radiography, 19*, 21–33.

Cullinan, A., & Cullinan, J. (1994). *Producing quality radiographs* (2nd ed.). Philadelphia: J. B. Lippincott.

Distance—technique relationship of angulated projections. (1980). *Radiologic Technology, 52*(3), 301.

Eastman Kodak Company. Health Sciences Markets Division. (1980). *The fundamentals of radiography* (12th ed.) (Kodak Publication M1-18). Rochester, NY: Author.

Fauber, T. (2008). *Radiographic imaging and exposure.* St. Louis: Mosby.

Files, G. W. (1935). Maximum tissue differentiation. *The X-Ray Technician, 7*, 17–24+.

Files, G. W. (1952). *Medical radiographic technique.* Springfield, IL: Charles C Thomas.

Fuchs, A. W. (1940). Balance in the radiographic image. *The X-Ray Technician, 12*(3), 81–84, 118.

Fuchs, A. W. (1948). Relationship of tissue thickness to kilovoltage. *The X-Ray Technician, 19*, 287–293.

Fuchs, A. W. (1950). The rationale of radiographic exposure. *The X-Ray Technician, 22*, 62–68, 76.

Fuchs, A. W. (1958). *Principles of radiographic exposure and processing.* Springfield, IL: Charles C Thomas.

Funke, T. (1966). Pegged kilovoltage technic. *Radiologic Technology, 37*, 202–213.

Gratale, P., Turner, G. W., & Burns, C. B. (1986). Using the same exposure factors for wet and dry casts. *Radiologic Technology, 57*(4), 325–328.

Hiss, S. S. (2003). *Understanding radiography* (4th ed.). Springfield, IL: Charles C Thomas.

Jenkins, D. (1980). *Radiographic photography and imaging processes.* Lancaster, England: MTP Press Limited.

Jerman, E. C. (1928). *Modern x-ray technic.* St. Paul, MN: Bruce.

Kelsey, C. A. (1982). Comparison of nodule detection with 70 kVp and 120 kVp chest radiographs. *Radiology*, 609.

Kodera, Y., Schmidt, R. A., Chan, H., & Doi, K. (1984). Backscatter from metal surfaces in diagnostic radiology. *Radiology*, 231.

Koenig, G. F. (1957). Kilovoltage as a qualitative factor. *The X-Ray Technician, 29*, 1–4, 13.

Lauer, O. G., Mayes, J. B., & Thurston, R. P. (1990). *Evaluating radiographic quality: The variables and their effects.* Mankato, MN: The Burnell Company.

Mattsson, O. (1955). Practical photographic problems in radiography. *Acta Radiologica Supplementum*, 1201–1206.

McEnerney, P. (1960). Evaluation of radiographic contrast after uncompensated factor changes. *Radiologic Technology, 32*(1), 23.

Mitchell, F. (1991). Scattered radiation and the lateral lumbar spine part 1: Initial research. *Radiography Today, 57*(644), 18–20.

Mitchell, F., Leung, C., Ahuja, A., & Metreweli, C. (1991). Scattered radiation and the lateral lumbar spine part 2: Clinical research. *Radiography Today, 57*(645), 12–14.

Morgan, R. H. (1946a). An analysis of the physical factors controlling the diagnostic quality of roentgen images: Part III. Contrast and the intensity distribution function of a Roentgen image. *American Journal of Roentgenology and Radiation Therapy, 55*(1), 67–89.

Morgan, R. H. (1946b). An analysis of the physical factors controlling the diagnostic quality of roentgen images: Part IV. Contrast and the film contrast factor. *American Journal of Roentgenology and Radiation Therapy, 55*(5), 627–633.

Newman, H. (1933). Relation of kilovolts to thickness of part—x-ray technic. *The X-Ray Technician, 5*, 21–26.

Roderick, J. F. (1950). Photographic contrast in roentgenology. *The X-Ray Technician, 22*, 141–150, 163.

Schwarz, G. S. (1959). Kilovoltage and radiographic effect. *Radiology, 73*, 749–760.

Schwarz, G. S. (1960). Kilovoltage conversion in radiography. *The X-Ray Technician, 31*, 373–379, 436.

Schwarz, G. S. (1961). *Unit-step radiography.* Springfield, IL: Charles C Thomas.

Seeman, H. E. (1968). *Physical and photographic principles of medical radiography.* New York: Wiley & Sons.

Seeram, E. (2011). *Digital radiography: An introduction.* Clifton Park, NY: Delmar Cengage Learning.

Spiegler, G. (1950). The story of contrast and definition. *Radiography, 41*(189), 177–182.

Thompson, M. A., Hattaway, M. P., Hall, J. D., & Dowd, S. B. (1994). *Principles of imaging science and protection.* Philadelphia: W. B. Saunders.

Trout, E. D., Graves, D. E., & Slauson, D. B. (1949). High kilovoltage radiography. *Radiology, 52,* 669–683.

United States War Department. (1941, July 3). *Technical manual: Roentgenographic technicians* (TM 8–240). Washington, DC: Author.

Wallace, J. E. (1995). *Radiographic exposure: Principles & practice.* Philadelphia: F.A. Davis.

Wegelius, C. (1954). The diagnostic use of high voltage rays in relationship to the physical background of mass absorption. *Acta Radiologica Supplementum, 116,* 589–597.

Wilsey, R. B. (1921). The intensity of scattered x-rays in radiography. *American Journal of Roentgenology, 8,* 328–338.

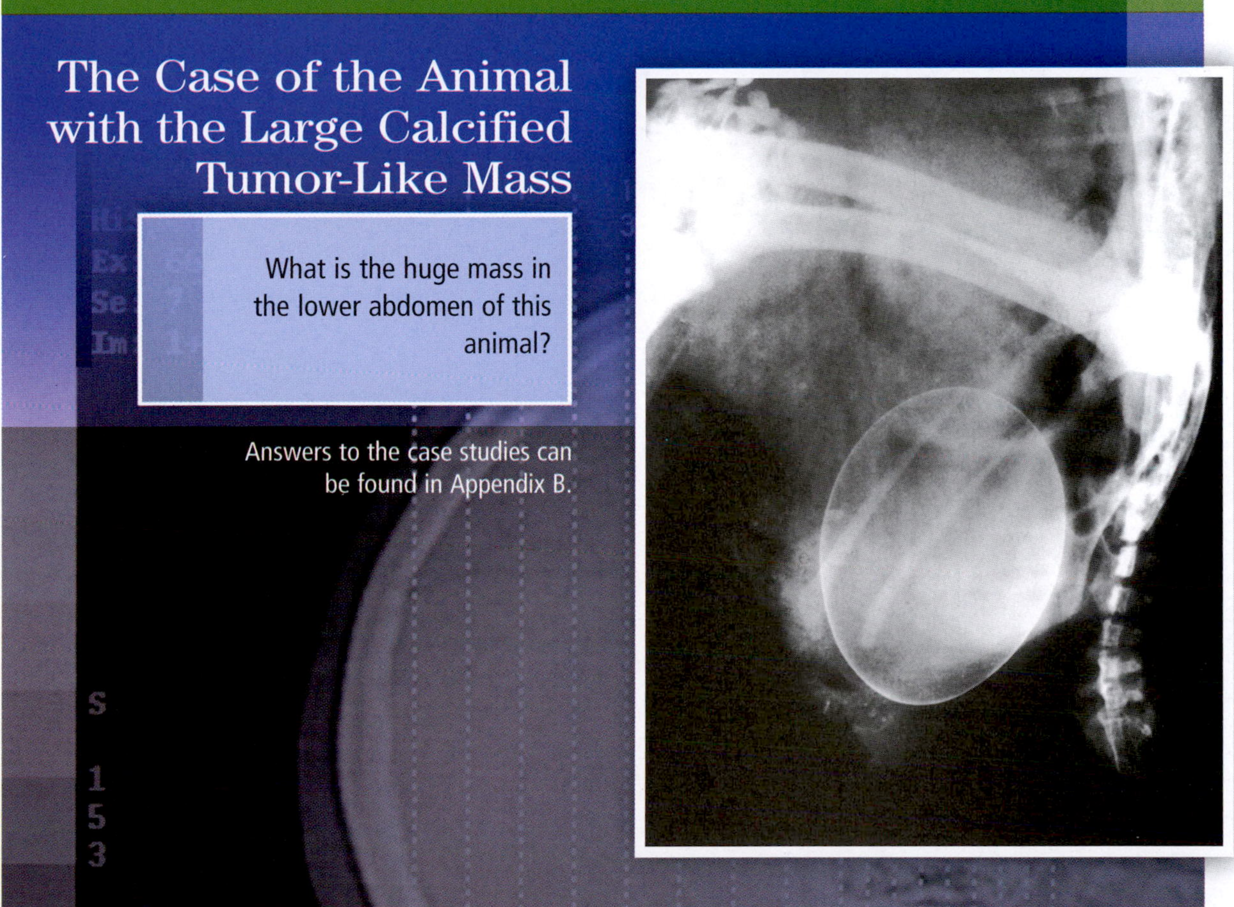

Courtesy of Dr. Marion Frank

CHAPTER 28

Recorded Detail

KEY TERMS

aliasing
definition
detail
edge spread function (ESF)
imaging noise
line spread function (LSF)
modulation transfer function (MTF)
Nyquist criterion
point spread function (PSF)
quantum mottle
quantum noise
recorded detail
sharpness
spatial resolution
unsharpness

One look is worth a thousand listens.

Merrill C. Sosman, "A Radiologist's Opinion of the Stethoscope"

OBJECTIVES

Upon completion of this chapter, the student should be able to:

- Define recorded detail, including synonymous terms and derived units.
- Explain the effect of various distances on recorded detail.
- Describe the factors that affect penumbra/point spread function size.
- Describe the effect of digital imaging systems and film/screen combinations on the resolution of recorded detail.
- Explain digital image receptor factors that control recorded detail.
- Describe appropriate techniques to prevent patient motion.
- Synthesize various geometrical factors into a clinical protocol for improving resolution.
- Recommend techniques for reducing motion, including immobilization devices.

ASSESSING RECORDED DETAIL

Recorded detail is one of the two geometric properties of image quality. Unlike the photographic properties of density/image receptor (IR) exposure and contrast, which control the visibility of detail, the geometric properties control detail itself. Recorded detail is the degree of geometric sharpness or accuracy of the structural lines actually recorded in the image. Good detail exists even when it cannot be seen due to poor visibility of detail or, in other words, when the density/IR exposure and/or contrast are poor. Recorded detail is one of the easiest of the prime technical factors to evaluate and adjust.

Recorded detail is also referred to as **definition**, **sharpness**, **spatial resolution**, or simply as **detail**. When the term *detail* is used by itself, it usually refers to the recorded detail of the radiographic image. Detail is easily quantified and even has a derived unit. The term *spatial resolution* is applied to quantified discussions of recorded detail.

The primary film/screen **unit of resolution** is line pairs per millimeter (lp/mm) or cycles per mm. A radiographic resolution tool is composed of pairs of lines a set distance from one another (Figure 28-1). The point at which the viewer can discern the closest pair of lines from each other represents the lp/mm reading. Most human visual acuity is limited to the range of 5 lp/mm. At this level each line is 0.1 mm wide, so a structure of this size could be discerned. Unfortunately, most radiographic imaging systems do not provide this level of resolution.

Digital imaging recorded detail (or spatial resolution, as it is more commonly called) is determined primarily by matrix size, pixel size, and grayscale bit depth. These correspond to the x, y, and z axes of the digital image. Digital imaging recorded detail is most commonly described in terms of spatial frequency. Spatial frequency is usually discussed as high or low. A shorter-wavelength signal (with higher frequency) represents pairs of lines that can be visualized very close together. This is high resolution. The opposite is true for low-frequency spatial resolution, as this signal has a longer wavelength (and lower frequency) representing pairs of lines that are further apart. This is low resolution. Spatial resolution is measured by several different units, including point spread function (PSF), line spread function (LSF), modulation transfer function (MTF), and system noise.

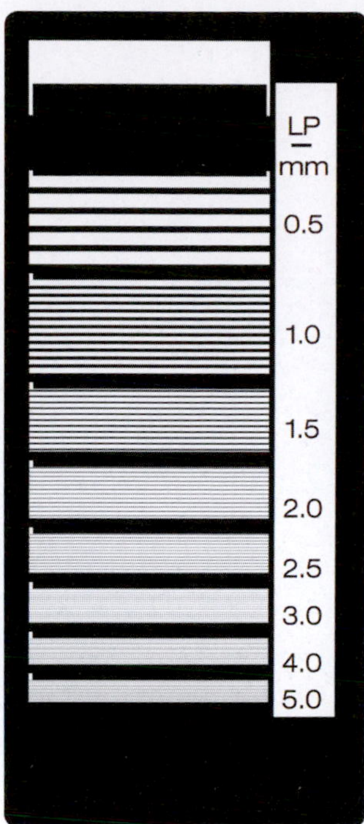

FIGURE 28-1. A resolution tool. The tool is read by discerning the point at which the finest lines are still visible as separated from one another. This point is then compared to the scale to determine the lp/mm reading. High spatial resolution represents a high-frequency signal that is capable of imaging smaller objects. Low spatial resolution represents a lower-frequency signal that can only image larger objects. *(Courtesy of Fluke Biomedical.)*

All radiographic images have less recorded detail than the object itself. In other words, the radiographic image exhibits some, but never all, of the detail of the anatomical part. The art of radiography involves controlling the degree of **unsharpness** so that it does not interfere with image diagnosis.

The effect of poor resolution on the image is seen as a lack of sharp definition of fine detail. This is caused by unacceptable levels of penumbra as compared to the umbral shadows that are expected from the part. Point spread function (PSF)

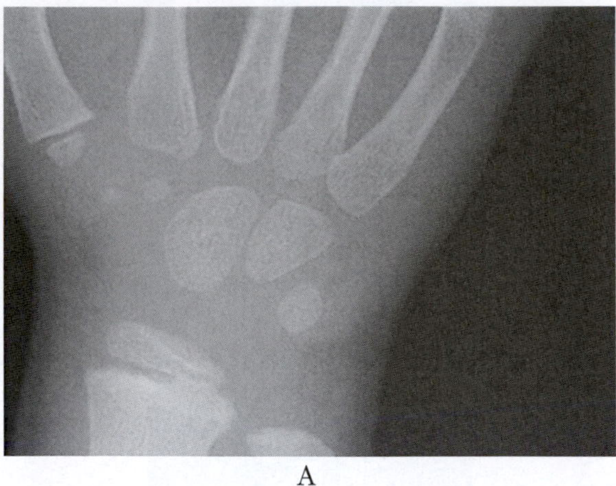

A

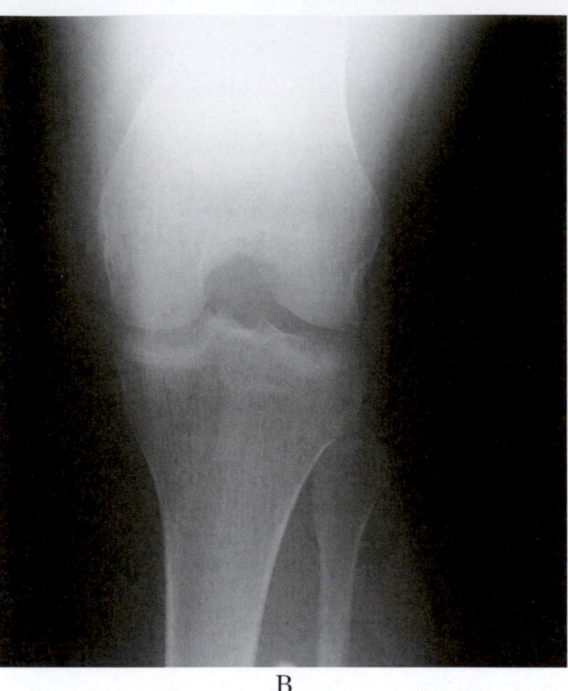

B

FIGURE 28-2. Assessing resolution. (A) A pediatric wrist exhibiting good resolution. (B) An adult knee exhibiting fair resolution in the tibia and poor resolution in the femur. *(Radiographs courtesy of Arlene Adler and Richard R. Carlton.)*

measures penumbra and is used to quantify digital system spatial resolution. Evaluation of resolution is best accomplished when an image has high contrast and a diagnostic-quality density/IR exposure.

Recorded detail is usually evaluated during quality control testing by imaging a resolution test tool. In a clinical situation, small structures are the easiest to examine to evaluate recorded detail. The trabeculae of bone is an excellent guidepost to image resolution. Much of the ability to assess when the resolution is too poor to be of diagnostic quality is a matter of clinical experience (Figure 28-2).

Spatial Resolution

Digital imaging requires a more specific term for resolution. *Spatial resolution* describes the ability of an imaging system to accurately display objects in two dimensions. Spatial resolution is higher when two objects can be demonstrated to be smaller or closer together.

Spatial resolution for digital images can be expressed in terms of three dimensions of the image. These are known as the x-axis, y-axis, and z-axis. Understanding how each of these dimensions is displayed can become extremely complex when different sources of data (such as CT and MRI) must be considered. However, there are common imaging parameters or measures that form the basis of all modalities, and these are fairly easy to understand. Although each measure must be considered separately, together they express the quality of the spatial resolution of the image. The spatial resolution quality measures are summed in Table 28-1.

To understand each measure, it is important to remember that most medical images use a two-dimensional format to illustrate a three-dimensional region of interest in the human body. However, these two-dimensional images contain three dimensions of information in that not only can structures be located according to height and width in an x-y grid matrix, but individual pixels

TABLE 28-1. Spatial Resolution Quality Measures

Spatial Resolution	Object Size	Object Distance	Unit(s) of Measurement	Modulation Transfer Function (MTF)	Point Spread Function (PSF)
High	Small	Close	High lp/cm or lp/mm	High (near 1.0)	Low
Low	Large	Distant	Low lp/cm or lp/mm	Low (0.0 to <1.0)	High

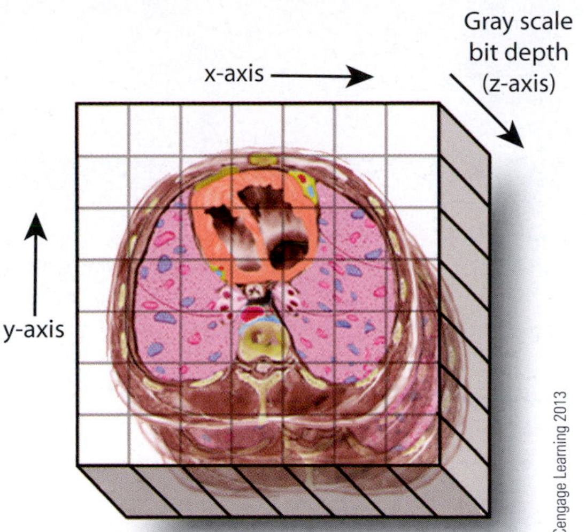

FIGURE 28-3. Spatial resolution and grayscale bit depth. Horizontal x-axis, vertical y-axis, and the z-axis that are represented by the value of the information collected in a single pixel (according to the grayscale shade displayed).

TABLE 28-2. Grayscale Bit Depth (Z-Axis)

Bits	Exponential Representation	# of Shades of Gray
1	2^{1}	2
6	2^{6}	64
8	2^{8}	256
10	2^{10}	1,024
12	2^{12}	4,096
16	2^{16}	65,536
24	2^{24}	16,777,216
32	2^{32}	4,294,967,296

A 1-bit pixel is capable of displaying two shades of gray (2^{1}).

are also represented by various shades of gray (the grayscale) (Figure 28-3).

The x-y grid matrix dimensions make up the spatial resolution because this information is represented through various points in space. The grayscale (sometimes called the z-axis) represents a depth to the information in the image. The grayscale is a summation of the information in the voxel that is represented by each pixel. Digital image quality is very much concerned with the grayscale bit depth, which is a measure of how many shades of gray can be displayed by each z-axis pixel in the x-y matrix. Grayscale bit depth (z-axis) values are shown in Table 28-2.

There are a number of different measures of spatial resolution. Those used most often to describe and compare imaging systems are point spread function, line spread function, spatial frequency, modulation transfer function, and noise. Although these sound intimidating, it is possible to understand why each is important as it relates to digital imaging without using a graduate degree in medical physics to calculate their values.

Point Spread Function (PSF). **Point spread function (PSF)**, **line spread function (LSF)**, and **edge spread function (ESF)** all express the boundaries of an image. In conventional radiography this aspect was called penumbra or blur. PSF is determined by complex mathematical measurement of the image produced from a single point. Figure 28-4 illustrates how a single point from a line extending through the imaging plane is isotropically imaged by an imaging system. The raw data for PSF measurements in imaging are usually in µm, but the PSF itself is valid only after application of an appropriate PSF, LSF, or ESF formula. For x-ray imaging (such as computed radiography), a point is made by drilling a tiny hole in a sheet of lead and then producing an x-ray image of the hole. Nuclear

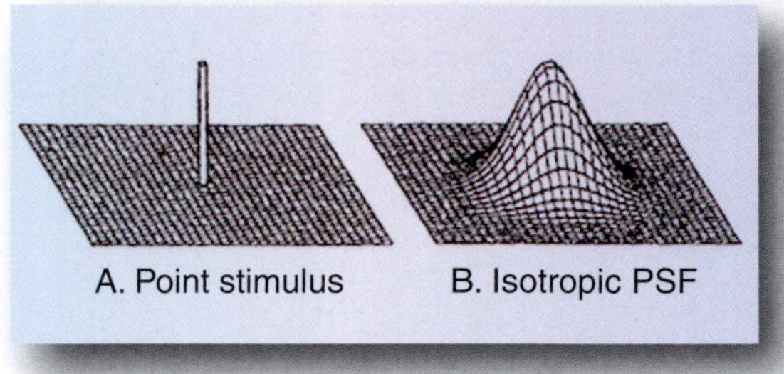

FIGURE 28-4. Point spread function. (A) A vertical line creates a point when it intersects the horizontal imaging plane. (B) 3D graphic representation of the imaging receptor response to the point is the point spread function (PSF). Note that the imaging receptor responds isotropically. *(Note: From The Essential Physics of Medical Imaging [2nd ed., p. 264], by J. Bushberg, J. Seibert, E. Leidholdt, and J. Boone, 2002, Philadelphia: Lippincott. Reprinted with permission.)*

medicine uses a point source of radioactivity; computed tomography, a thin metal wire; sonography, a monofilament; and MRI, a small water-filled hole in a tissue-equivalent phantom.

Spatial Frequency. High spatial resolution represents a high-frequency signal that is capable of imaging smaller objects. Low spatial resolution represents a lower-frequency signal that can only image larger objects. This parameter is determined by measuring the distance between pairs of lines that can be imaged as distinct from one another. The test tools are simply pairs of lines that are different distances from one another. The tool is imaged by the system, and the viewer determines the smallest pair of lines that can be visualized. The pairs of lines are then measured as line pairs per unit of length (usually mm or cm). Figure 28-5 illustrates how pairs of lines are transferred to the spatial frequency unit of cycles per unit of length. This is similar to the more common frequency measurements in cycles per unit of time, as with electrical power at 60 cycles per second. The higher the spatial frequency, the closer together the sine waves, and the closer together the line pairs.

Modulation Transfer Function (MTF). **Modulation transfer function (MTF)** measures the accuracy of an

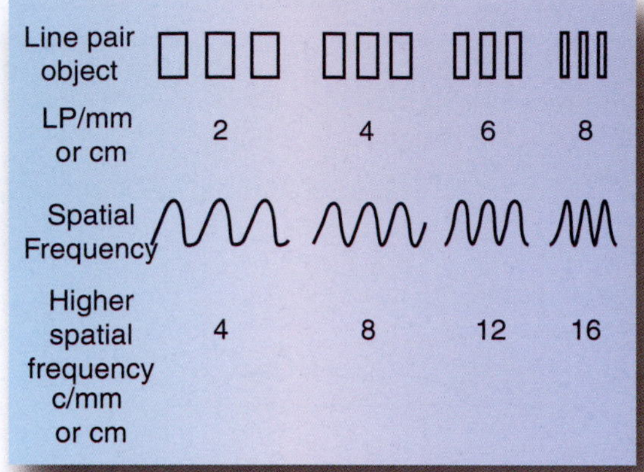

FIGURE 28-5. Spatial resolution can be measured by how close together pairs of lines can be displayed (top), by the units measuring the distance between the line pairs (lp/mm or cm), by a sine wave representing this distance (which is actually the spatial frequency), or by the spatial frequency in cycles per unit of length (c/mm or cm).

image compared to the original object on a scale of 0 to 1. This is sometimes called the fidelity (or trueness) of the image. Mathematically, MTF measures the percentage of object contrast that is recorded. Because this measurement varies according to the size of the object (a greater percentage of object contrast is recorded for larger objects), MTF is more useful when represented as a graph of MTF versus the size of the object (the spatial frequency), as shown in Figure 28-6.

An MTF of 0 represents no signal and therefore no image. An MTF of 1 represents a signal of such extremely high fidelity that it records the image perfectly. MTF values for imaging modalities can reach 1.0 for large objects such as those with a spatial frequency of 1.0 lp/cm for computed tomography or 1.0 lp/mm for computed radiography. As the spatial frequency of objects rises, the MTF decreases. For example, a CT system may demonstrate an MTF of 1.0 for a spatial frequency of 1.0 lp/cm but drop to an MTF of 0.4 for a spatial frequency of 2.0 lp/cm (see Figure 28-6).

Noise. **Imaging noise** is simply background information that the image receptor receives. As long

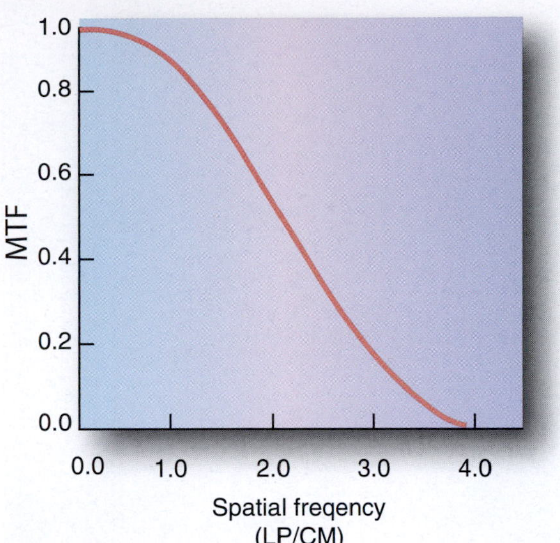

FIGURE 28-6. A typical modulation transfer function (MTF) curve measures the accuracy of an image compared to the original object on a scale of 0.0 to 1.0. Because this measurement varies according to the size of the object, MTF curves are plotted according to the size of the object (the spatial frequency). This graph demonstrates that when the spatial frequency is 1.0 lp/cm, the MTF is close to a perfect 1.0. However, when the spatial frequency rises to 3.0 lp/cm, MTF drops to around 0.10. The CT system represented by this graph produces relatively low imaging resolution for objects with a spatial frequency greater than 2.0 lp/cm.

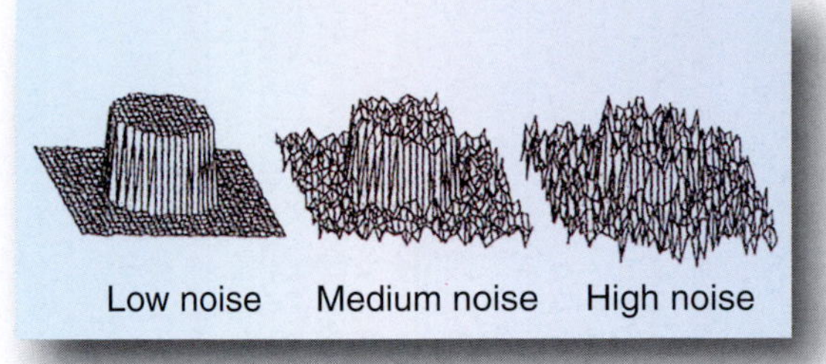

FIGURE 28-7. Noise. Imaging noise is represented as increasing from A through B to C. When the noise level rises, more complex computer processing algorithms may be necessary. When their limits are reached, degradation of the image occurs. *(Note: From The Essential Physics of Medical Imaging [2nd ed., p. 273], by J. Bushberg, J. Seibert, E. Leidholdt, and J. Boone, 2002, Philadelphia: Lippincott. Reprinted with permission.)*

as the background noise is significantly less than the amount of information that is coming from the image receptor, computer processing algorithms can easily filter out the noise. When the noise level rises, as shown in Figure 28-7, more complex algorithms may be necessary. When their limits are reached, degradation of the image occurs.

Quantum noise refers to a lack of sufficient incoming data for processing. The word *quantum* means "counted or measured," and the term has been used in radiography to indicate an insufficient number of incoming x-ray photons reaching the image receptor. This results in a blotchy or mottled image. For this reason, the phenomenon is also called **quantum mottle**. The solution to the problem remains the same—increase the number (or quanta) of incoming signals, whether it requires increasing the mAs of an x-ray beam (the most common solution), or a stronger signal from an ultrasound transducer, radioactive isotope, or RF coil in an MRI unit.

Digital Sampling (Nyquist Criterion) and Aliasing (Moiré Pattern)

Digital systems are susceptible to a few imaging problems that are unique to the way they collect information. Because all digital systems sample the incoming signal at discrete points, they do not collect as much information as an analog system. Digital imaging requires that the spatial resolution frequency signal be sampled twice from each cycle. This is known as the **Nyquist criterion** or limit because it is the processing algorithm that averages the incoming analog data by using the distance between the imaging detector elements (to ensure that data is not missed or double-sampled). This is sometimes stated as signal averaging over the detector aperture width.

Aliasing occurs when the Nyquist criterion is violated. This occurs when the spatial frequency exceeds the Nyquist frequency and the incoming data are sampled less than twice per cycle. Data collected under these conditions are said to be aliased

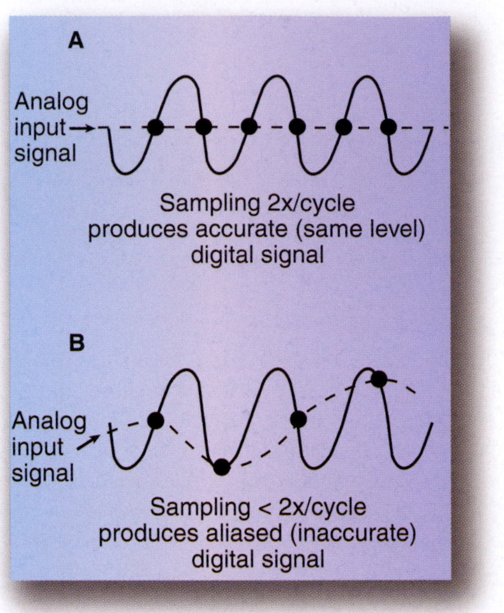

FIGURE 28-8. Aliasing. Improper sampling not in accordance with the Nyquist criterion produces aliasing (often visualized as a moiré pattern). (A) Nyquist criterion sampling 2x/cycle produces an accurate-level high-frequency digital signal. (B) Violation of the Nyquist criterion sampling 2x/cycle produces an inaccurate, fluctuating, low-frequency digital signal.

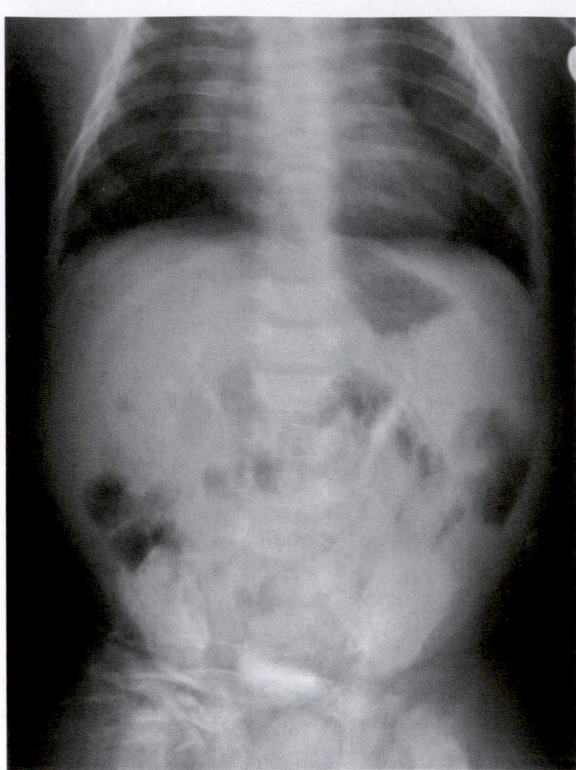

FIGURE 28-9. Motion unsharpness. The diaphragm, heart, and bowel are all unsharp due to motion of this pediatric patient. *(Radiograph courtesy of Arlene Adler and Richard R. Carlton.)*

(Figure 28-8). These images look like a moiré pattern. When a computed radiography image demonstrates this pattern, the first reaction of experienced radiographers is to troubleshoot the grid, especially a reciprocating grid mechanism, for malfunction. The image is more often the result of inadequate sampling of the incoming data. Essentially what occurs in the computer is that a low-frequency aliased image wraps around over the high-frequency image. This creates a visual impression of two slightly out-of-alignment images in a moiré pattern.

EFFECTS ON IMAGE APPEARANCE

Resolution affects the image appearance by demonstrating fine detail structures, often very close to the size limits of the naked eye. When fine detail is lacking, the image will often appear blurred.

Motion unsharpness is often not perceived by the beginning student, partially because students must learn to critically examine each image in a methodical manner. Another reason is that a thorough knowledge of how various anatomical structures should appear radiographically is necessary in order to recognize when motion causes them to appear unacceptable (Figure 28-9). The assessment of motion is a matter of obtaining sufficient clinical experience. Progress in professional competence has been achieved when the beginning radiographer easily discerns motion unsharpness.

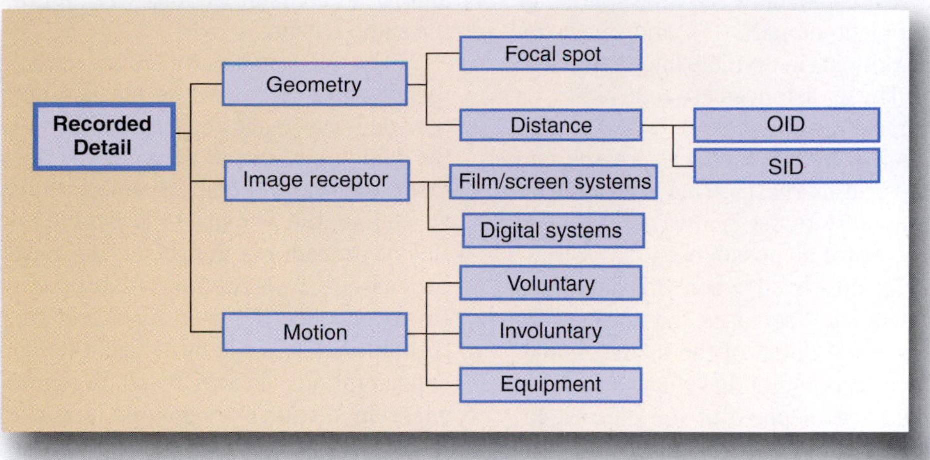

FIGURE 28-10. Image analysis: factors affecting recorded detail.

FACTORS AFFECTING RECORDED DETAIL

The factors that control recorded detail are shown in Figure 28-10. Close consideration of these factors will reveal that recorded detail is often improved through factors that increase the patient dose. This makes consideration of how much resolution is necessary for a particular study a patient radiation protection issue. Resolution problems should be approached in this order:

1. Eliminate motion;
2. Reduce OID;
3. Reduce focal spot size;
4. Reduce intensifying-screen phosphor size and concentration; and
5. Increase SID.

Geometry

The geometry of the beam is the most important factor in establishing the level of resolution desired for recorded detail. Because the x-ray beam emanates from a small point (the focal spot), the further the photons move from their source, the further they diverge. In Figure 28-11 note how much more tissue is imaged and exposed at the level of the spine than at the level of the collimator light beam. This is the basis of the inverse square law and it applies to the geometry of the beam as well.

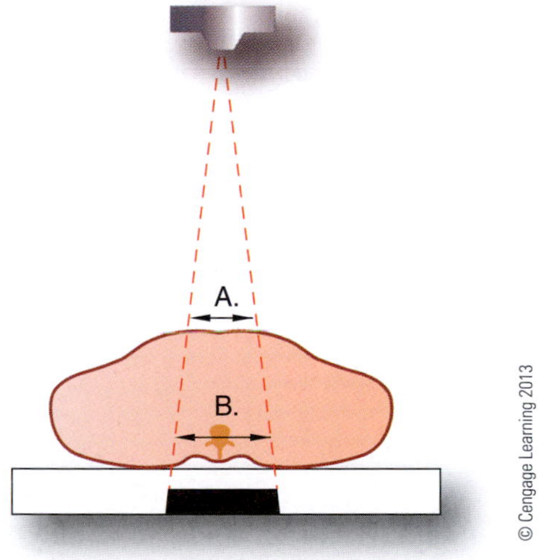

FIGURE 28-11. Divergence of the x-ray beam. More tissue is imaged and exposed at the level of the spine (point B) than at the level of the collimator light beam (point A).

Distance. The distances between the source or focal spot (S), object or part (O), and image receptor (I) are critical in establishing sufficient recorded detail. These distances are referred to, as shown in Figure 28-12, so that SOD × OID = SID. Resolution is improved when OID decreases and degraded whenever it increases. This is why the affected side or part of interest is always positioned as close to the receptor as possible.

Resolution is improved when SID increases and degraded when it decreases. Increasing SID improves the recorded detail of the image enough that it has been recommended that a routine 48″ (120-cm) distance in place of the current 40″ (100-cm) distance would be worthwhile.

When it is necessary to make adjustments in order to improve detail, OID should be evaluated first. The minimum OID should be used to improve detail. The details of the positioning and the equipment in use should be carefully considered. In many instances a change in positioning will accomplish a remarkable improvement in detail. In fact, most positioning routines were established with OID as a critical factor. For example, the PA chest projection is preferred because it places the heart closer to the image receptor than does the AP projection. The left lateral stomach, AP kidney, and AP lumbar projections were all developed for the same reason.

The OID can also be minimized by considering the distance between the surface supporting the part and the image receptor. Differences between the tabletop-to-image receptor or Bucky tray distance can have a considerable influence on OID. Of course, the minimal OID is obtained with non-Bucky procedures that place the part directly on the cassette, as is routine in extremity radiography. However, once the need for a grid supersedes the resolution that is lost by using a Bucky tray, careful consideration can still result in significant differences in detail. For example, some radiographic tables will permit an OID of 1–2 cm, whereas a floating-top table may permit a minimum OID of 10 cm. The differences in image quality are significant (Figure 28-13).

Once the OID has been minimized, resolution is improved when SID increases and degraded when it decreases. Again, positioning routines were established to take advantage of this relationship. For example, the lateral cervical is usually performed at 72″ (180 cm) instead of 40″ (100 cm) because the OID cannot be reduced due to the distance between the neck and shoulder. Increased SID is the only method that can produce a lateral

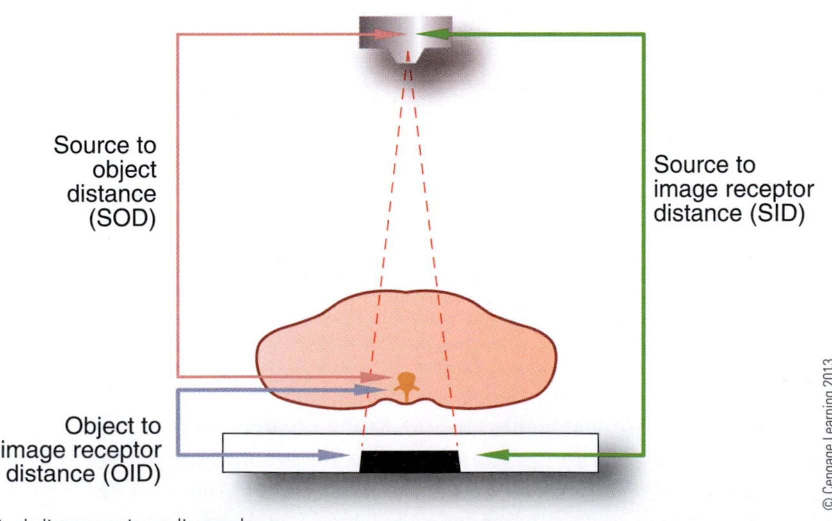

FIGURE 28-12. Critical distances in radiography.

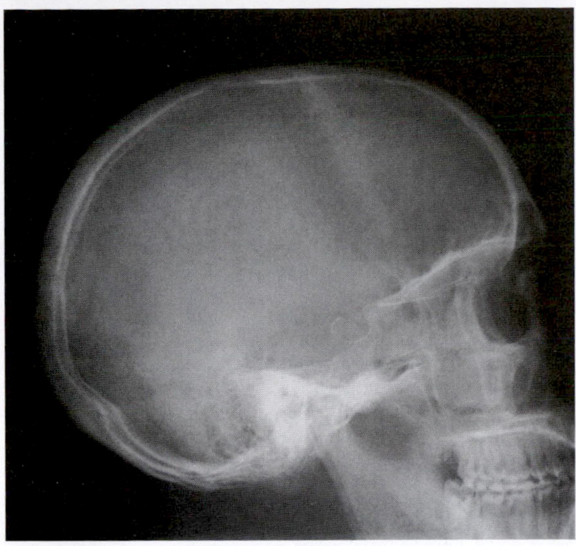

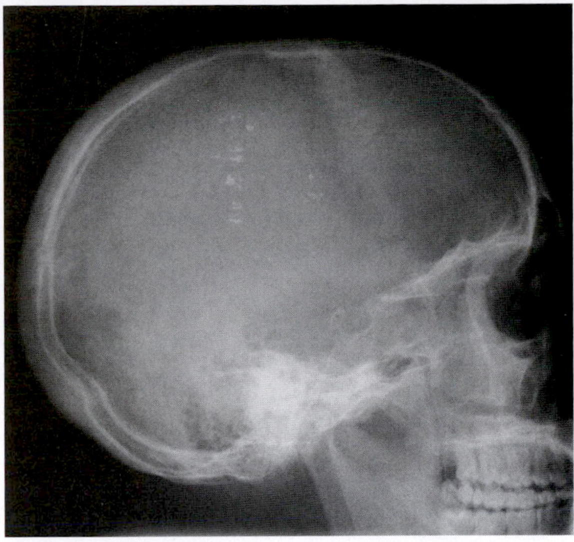

FIGURE 28-13. (A) 7 cm OID (OFD); (B) 14 cm OID (OFD). *(Radiographs courtesy of Arlene Adler and Richard R. Carlton.)*

image comparable to the AP and oblique projections, which have a much smaller OID.

Focal Spot Size. Focal spot size is controlled by the line focus principle (see Figure 6-13). A multitude of tube designs have been used over the years to minimize the effective focal spot while maximizing the actual focal spot to absorb the heat.

The umbra is the distinctly sharp area of a shadow or the region of complete shadow. The penumbra is the imperfect, unsharp shadow surrounding the umbra. With light, it is the region of partial illumination that surrounds the complete shadow. It is also referred to as the edge gradient. Digital systems are evaluated for this factor as part of spatial resolution by measuring their point spread function (PSF) and line spread function (LSF).

The focal spot size is a major controller of image resolution because it controls penumbra. The fact that the source of the x-ray photons is not a point source, although it is sometimes convenient to think of it as such, is what causes penumbra. Figures 28-14A and B illustrate the umbra and penumbra caused by the focal spot size and configuration. As the focal spot decreases in size, penumbra also decreases, thus increasing resolution. Focal spots are usually not capable of imaging structures smaller than the focal spots themselves.

The width of the penumbra (unsharpness) can be mathematically calculated using the following formula:

$$P = \frac{\text{Focal Spot Size} \times \text{OID}}{\text{SOD}}$$

EXAMPLE: Calculate the penumbra for an image taken with a 1.0-mm focal spot, at a 40″ distance and an OID of 3″.

Answer:

$$P = \frac{\text{Focal Spot Size} \times \text{OID}}{\text{SOD}}$$

If the SID is 40″ and the OID is 3″, then the SOD = 40″ –3″ = 37″.

$$P = \frac{1.0 \times 3''}{37} = \frac{3}{37} = 0.08 \text{ mm}$$

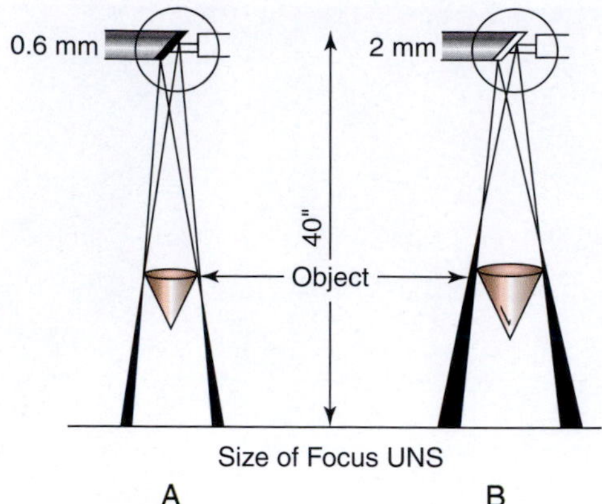

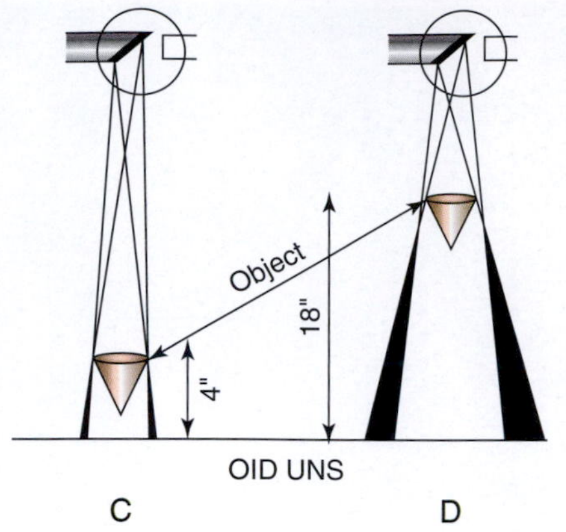

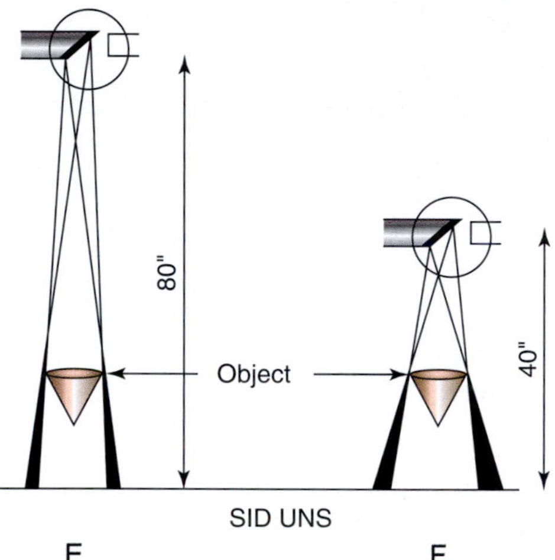

FIGURE 28-14. Umbra and penumbra. The umbral area receives essentially no photons. The penumbral area receives more photons at the outer edges with progressively fewer photons toward the umbral area, thus creating an imperfect, unsharp shadow around the umbra. (A and B) The effect of focal-spot size on resolution. The geometry of the beam reduces penumbra and increases resolution as focal-spot size decreases. (C and D) The effect of object-to-image receptor distance (OID) on resolution. As the OID decreases, penumbra is reduced and resolution increases. (E and F) The effect of source-to-image receptor distance (SID) on resolution. As SID increases, penumbra is reduced and resolution increases.

EXAMPLE: Calculate the penumbra for an image taken with a 2.0-mm focal spot, at a 40″ distance and an OID of 3″.

Answer:

$$P = \frac{\text{Focal Spot Size} \times \text{OID}}{\text{SOD}}$$

If the SID is 40″ and the OID is 3″, then the SOD = 40″ – 3″ = 37″.

$$P = \frac{2.0 \times 3''}{37} = \frac{6}{37} = 0.16 \text{ mm}$$

EXAMPLE: Calculate the penumbra for an image taken with a 1.0-mm focal spot, at a 40″ distance and an OID of 8″.

Answer:

$$P = \frac{\text{Focal Spot Size} \times \text{OID}}{\text{SOD}}$$

If the SID is 40″ and the OID is 8″, then the SOD = 40″ – 8″ = 32″.

$$P = \frac{1.0 \times 8''}{32} = \frac{8}{32} = 0.25 \text{ mm}$$

> ***EXAMPLE:*** Calculate the penumbra for an image taken with a 1.0-mm focal spot, at a 72″ distance and an OID of 3″.
>
> ***Answer:***
>
> $$P = \frac{\text{Focal Spot Size} \times \text{OID}}{\text{SOD}}$$
>
> If the SID is 72″ and the OID is 3″, then the SOD = 72″ − 3″ = 69″.
>
> $$P = \frac{1.0 \times 3''}{69} = \frac{3}{69} = 0.04 \text{ mm}$$

From these examples, it is evident that penumbra decreases when the focal spot decreases, when the OID decreases, and when the SID increases.

Figures 28-14C and D illustrate that as OID decreases, penumbra also decreases. Figures 28-14E and F illustrate that as SID increases, penumbra decreases. When penumbra decreases, resolution is increased.

Penumbra is increased by another phenomenon known as attenuation or absorption unsharpness. Because of the divergence of the incident x-ray beam, only an object that is trapezoidal would have a perfectly sharp edge (Figure 28-15A). A trapezoidal object would have a relatively equal object thickness that would attenuate the beam, causing an equal proportion of the beam to reach the image. A square object would project an edge with a gradually increasing attenuation (Figure 28-15B). Circular objects, which predominate in the human body, have an attenuation that varies throughout the entire object, reaching a maximum at a single point (Figure 28-15C). Consequently, the attenuation of the object itself causes a continuously varying projected density/IR exposure, which, when added to the penumbra, causes structures in the human body to have gradual instead of sharp, abrupt edges.

Image Receptor

Film/Screen Systems. Film/screen combinations are most commonly classified by speed. Within a single phosphor type, there is an inverse relationship

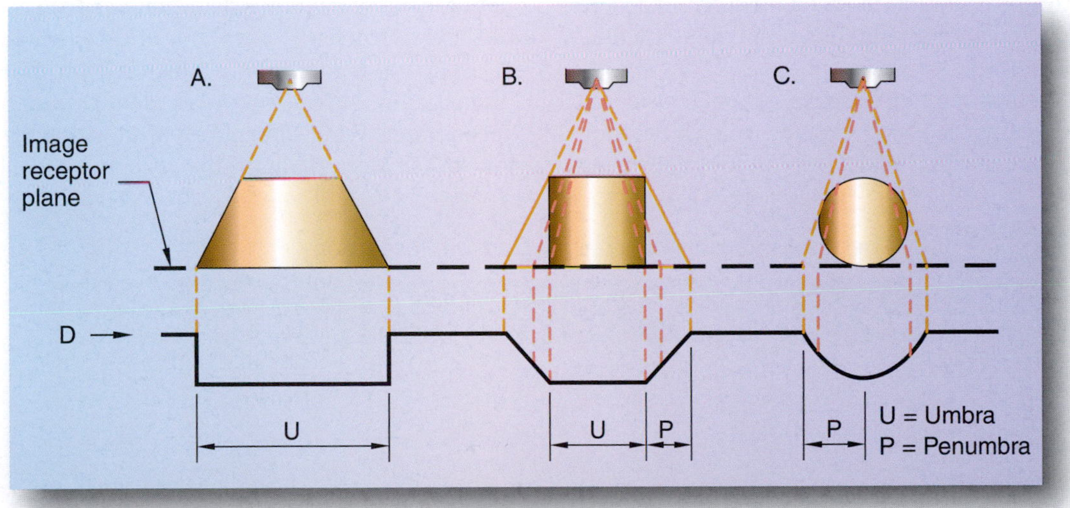

FIGURE 28-15. Attenuation unsharpness. The D line represents the amount of density that would occur in the image receptor under each object. (A) A trapezoidal object shaped congruent to the divergence of the beam. (B) A square object produces density shadings that form the penumbra. (C) A round object produces a penumbra that is incorporated into the continuously varying density of the shape itself.

between film/screen combination speed and resolution. In other words, a slow film/screen combination will demonstrate better resolution than a fast one. This is such a definite relationship that many slow film/screen combinations are labeled as detail combinations.

Once the geometrical considerations of recorded detail have been maximized, the most common source of better resolution is the film/screen combination. Most institutions utilize at least two different film/screen combinations in recognition of the better detail required by extremity examinations. This policy permits higher speed film/screens to be used to reduce patient dose for other examinations that do not require such high resolution.

Although various types of film have a wide variety of resolving capabilities, in radiography the intensifying screen always has poorer resolution than the film. Radiographic film usually has resolving capabilities in the range of 100 lp/mm, far beyond the ability of any screen or human eye. As long as the film is sensitive to the light emitted by the screens, film speed and resolution are not important issues in radiographic imaging.

Although obsolete due to excessive patient dose, nonscreen or direct exposure film possesses the highest resolution possible. Direct exposure film often required 20–100 times the mAs of a film/screen exposure.

Adjustment of film speed is seldom considered for resolution purposes. However, when a decision is made to use a higher-resolution intensifying screen, its slower speed may be somewhat compensated for by using a higher-speed film to help reduce patient dose.

The resolving power of an intensifying screen depends on three factors: **phosphor size, phosphor layer thickness,** and **phosphor concentration**. The relationship of these factors to recorded detail, patient dose, and density/IR exposure is shown in Table 28-3. As phosphor size and layer thickness decrease, resolution increases along with patient dose; however, increasing phosphor concentrations will result in an intensifying screen that is better able to record details while reducing patient dose. Overall, as intensifying-screen speed is decreased, there is a gain in resolution but patient dose must be increased. This creates a classical confrontation in radiography that pits recorded detail against patient dose. The decision is often left to the radiographer, who must consider all elements of both sides of the issue. Detail-speed screens can resolve about 15 lp/mm, regular-speed screens about 10 lp/mm, and high-speed screens about 7 lp/mm. These differences in recorded detail are easily visualized (see Figure 23-3).

Recall that because of their higher conversion efficiency, rare-earth phosphors have significantly better resolving abilities than similar speed calcium tungstate screens.

Quantum mottle is a phenomenon that may dramatically affect recorded detail when high-speed intensifying screens are used with extremely low mAs. Modern intensifying-screen technology

TABLE 28-3. Effects of Intensifying-Screen Factors on Resolution

Phosphor Change	Effect on Image Resolution	Effect on Patient Dose	Effect on Film Density/ IR Exposure
Phosphor size			
increases	decreases	decreases	increases
decreases	increases	increases	decreases
Layer thickness			
increases	decreases	decreases	increases
decreases	increases	increases	decreases
Phosphor concentration (packing density)			
increases	increases	decreases	increases
decreases	decreases	increases	decreases

is so advanced that it is now possible to obtain screens that are so sensitive that sufficient radiographic density/IR exposure can be achieved at extremely low mAs. If the total number of incident photons reaching the intensifying screen is insufficient to activate enough phosphors to emit light to cover the entire surface of the film, quantum mottle results (see Figure 22-6). When using diagnostic radiographic intensifying screens, quantum mottle is corrected **only** by increasing mAs.

When resolution is unsatisfactory and the geometric solutions have been exhausted, a higher-resolution film/screen combination should be used. It is important to remember that this decision includes a significant increase in patient dose. Conversely, if resolution is more than satisfactory for the examination, a lower-resolution film/screen combination should be considered to reduce patient dose.

The radiographic film and intensifying screens are sandwiched together in the cassette by pressure pads that keep them in immediate direct contact with one another. When the film/screen contact is broken, even over a small area of the cassette, the image detail is not as sharp because of increased penumbra (see Figure 22-5).

The only adjustment for poor film/screen contact is repairing or discarding the cassette. The procedures for testing cassettes for film/screen contact are part of a quality control program.

Digital Systems. The primary factors affecting the recorded detail of digital imaging systems are the detector geometric properties and the image processing system. Table 25-2 provides a comparison of the differences in the detector systems for each of the most common CR/DR systems.

Photostimulable phosphor systems, which are often called computed radiography (CR), have recorded detail limitations very similar to those of film/screen intensifying-screen phosphor systems. This is because they depend on a phosphor to acquire incoming x-ray photon data. The factors are phosphor size, layer thickness, and concentration. Additional limits on recorded detail may occur in CR systems during the scanning of the phosphor screen and during the processing phase. The major factors that limit photostimulable phosphor systems are the intensifying screen and scanning system.

Indirect digital radiography (flat panel) systems are of two types. One uses an intensifying screen with a CCD detector, and the other uses a silicon detector with a CsI scintillator. The screen/CCD system has the same limitations that affect recorded detail in film/screen intensifying-screen systems (phosphor size, layer thickness, and concentration). The silicon/scintillator/TFT system also has limitations due to the fill factor. The fill factor is the area of the detector that is light sensitive. A high fill factor produces higher resolution. Each interface between system elements reduces recorded detail, for example, CsI scintillator to silicon detector to TFT charge reader. The processing phase is also a factor. The major factor that limits indirect digital systems is the size of the detector element.

Direct digital radiography (flat panel) selenium detectors can be made much thicker because photons traveling through them maintain a much more vertical path than in silicon detectors. There is virtually no blurring during direct detection of photons. However, they cannot be made as small as silicon detectors. The major factor that limits direct digital systems is the size of the detector element.

The image processing system also sets a limit on recorded detail (spatial resolution) depending on the acquisition and display matrix size, pixel pitch, and grayscale bit depth. These correspond to the x-, y-, and z-axes of the digital image (see Figure 28-3).

Motion

Motion affects recorded detail because it fails to permit enough time for a well-defined image to form. Instead, the image is spread over a linear distance and appears as a blurred series of densities in which no fine detail can be perceived.

Voluntary Motion. Voluntary motion is that which is under the direct control of the patient. For the most part, this comprises the voluntary nervous system in cognizant adults (children and incognizant adults may be excepted in some cases). For all patients, including children and incognizant adults, **communication,** especially in a manner that establishes a professional and competent atmosphere, is the best method of controlling voluntary motion. There are a few examinations, such as most headwork, where immobilization greatly decreases the potential need for a repeated exposure.

For most examinations, when the radiographer effectively communicates positioning instructions, the patient is able to cooperate in reducing motion. Instructions must be given in a kindly and concerned manner. They must be in an understandable language, which includes avoiding medical terminology when appropriate; use proper pronunciation of foreign language instructions; and be at a proper volume and properly enunciated. Even infants and incognizant adults will respond to a kindly tone of voice and gentle handling. Never assume that your patient is unable to understand your instructions. Many young children can be amazingly cooperative when they wish to be and incognizant adults will often remember fragments of conversations when they regain full cognizance.

Involuntary Motion. Involuntary motion is not under the conscious control of the patient. For the most part, involuntary motion is controlled by the involuntary nervous system and is physiological in nature. Heartbeat and peristalsis are the most common examples. Involuntary motion can be best reduced by decreasing exposure time.

Equipment Motion. Although often overlooked, motion of equipment can also be an occasional problem. If the movement of the reciprocating grid mechanism is not dampened, it can cause vibration of the cassette in the Bucky tray. If the x-ray tube suspension system is not balanced and isolated from other moving devices, especially overhead suspended units, it can vibrate or drift. This type of motion is extremely difficult to detect. It is usually suspected only when various patients examined with the same x-ray unit appear to have motion problems.

Communication. The best method of reducing motion is patient communication. It is assumed that appropriate aids to positioning, such as foam pads, angle sponges, and sandbags, are already in use. The radiographer should consider the instructions that are given to be sure that they are clear, concise, and understandable.

Exposure Time Reduction. When the patient is unable to cooperate, the best method is a reduction in exposure time with a corresponding increase in mA to maintain sufficient mAs and film density/IR exposure. Involuntary motion can be best reduced by a reduction in exposure time. Other methods of decreasing exposure time while maintaining exposure include using higher-speed film and screens, decreasing SID, and increasing kVp. Increasing kVp is not a preferred method because of the accompanying contrast change. Table 28-4 summarizes the pros and cons of each method.

Immobilization. When communication and exposure time reduction are not sufficient to reduce motion, partial immobilization must be considered. Immobilization devices, such as foam pads, angle sponges, and sandbags, should be considered routine positioning aids. Patient motion can be expected when these aids are not provided. If students find it uncomfortable or difficult to hold radiographic positions during laboratory positioning practice, imagine how an ill patient who is in pain (most likely lying on the most acute area) must feel. The use of positioning aids is part of professionalism. Even when they are in short supply, the radiographer should try to locate the proper aids for the patient.

For some examinations, especially headwork, immobilization greatly reduces the potential need for

TABLE 28-4. Effects of Various Methods for Reducing Exposure Time to Avoid Motion

Method	Density/IR Exposure	Contrast	Resolution	Distortion
mA increase	maintains	maintains	maintains	maintains
kVp increase	maintains	decreases	maintains	maintains
Film/screen speed increase	maintains	maintains	decreases	maintains
SID decrease	maintains	maintains	decreases	increases

repeated exposures and should be used routinely. Widely ranging immobilization devices and techniques have been developed over the years; some are available commercially and others are homemade.

Experienced radiographers often say that tape is the radiographer's best friend. Tape should certainly be carried at all times by radiographers and used freely when warranted. A strip of tape across the forehead (folded sticky side out across skin surfaces) has avoided many repeated cranial exposures.

Some devices, especially in pediatrics, are designed to immobilize the entire body. Pediatric boards, mummy wrapping techniques, Pig-O-Stats™, and compression bands are common examples. Individual parts can usually be immobilized with combinations of tape, sandbags, long-handled paddles, compression bands, and sheet wrapping. As a last resort, human immobilizers may be used to hold the patient in position. Male relatives are the first choice, female relatives second, then nonradiology hospital personnel and nonprofessional radiology personnel. Radiographers are the last choice. Under no circumstances should anyone be expected to routinely hold patients.

SUMMARY

Recorded detail is one of the two geometric properties of radiographic image quality. Unlike the photographic properties of density/IR exposure and contrast, which control the visibility of detail, the geometric properties control detail itself. Recorded detail is the degree of geometric sharpness or accuracy of the structural lines actually recorded in the radiographic image. Good detail exists even when it cannot be seen due to poor visibility of detail or, in other words, when the density/IR exposure and/or contrast are poor.

Recorded detail is also referred to as definition, sharpness, resolution, or simply as detail. When the term *detail* is used by itself, it usually refers to the recorded detail of the radiographic image. Detail is easily quantified and even has a derived unit. The term *resolution* is applied to quantified discussions of recorded detail. The unit of resolution is line pairs per millimeter (lp/mm) or cycles per mm.

The factors that affect recorded detail are geometry, including SID, OID, and focal spot size; image receptor; and motion.

When the factors that affect recorded detail are altered, some change in the recorded detail will occur. No effect will occur unless one of these factors is altered. Table 28-5 illustrates the effect on recorded detail when the various factors are changed. ■

TABLE 28-5. Effect of Changing Factors on Recorded Detail

+ = increases recorded detail (resolution)
− = decreases recorded detail (resolution)
Geometry
+ Increasing SID
− Decreasing SID
− Increasing OID
+ Decreasing OID
− Increasing patient thickness
+ Decreasing patient thickness
− Increasing focal spot size
+ Decreasing focal spot size
Film/Screen Combination
− Increasing film/screen speed
+ Decreasing film/screen speed
+ Good film/screen contact
− Poor film/screen contact
Motion
− Increasing motion
+ Decreasing motion

REVIEW QUESTIONS

1. What is recorded detail?
2. How is resolution measured?
3. How do the SID and the OID affect recorded detail?
4. What is the relationship between focal spot size and recorded detail?
5. What is the difference between umbra and penumbra?
6. What three factors affect the resolving power of intensifying screens?
7. What is the difference between voluntary and involuntary motion?
8. What are the methods that can be used to reduce the possibility of motion?

REFERENCES AND RECOMMENDED READING

American Registry of Radiologic Technologists. (1987). Use of "penumbra" studied. *Radiologic Technology, 58*(1), 74.

Ball, J., & Price, T. (1995). *Chesneys' radiographic imaging* (6th ed.). Oxford: Blackwell Scientific.

Bushong, S. C. (2008). *Radiologic science for technologists: Physics, biology, and protection* (9th ed.). St. Louis, MO: C.V. Mosby.

Cahoon, J. B. (1961). Radiographic technique: Its origin, concept, practical application and evaluation of radiation dosage. *The X-Ray Technician, 32,* 354–364.

Carroll, Q. B. (2003). *Fuchs's radiographic exposure, processing, and quality control* (7th ed.). Springfield, IL: Charles C Thomas.

Crooks, H. E. (1973). Some aspects of radiographic quality with special reference to image sharpness. *Radiography, 39*(468), 317–327.

Cullinan, A., & Cullinan, J. (1994). *Producing quality radiographs* (2nd ed.). Philadelphia: J. B. Lippincott.

Eastman Kodak Company. (1977a). *Image insight 1: The quality image* (Publication M3-182). Rochester, NY: Author.

Eastman Kodak Company. (1977b). *Image insight 2: Geometry of image formation: Detail* (Publication M3-184). Rochester, NY: Author.

Engel, T. L. (1979). Effect of kilovoltage and milliamperage on focal spot size. *Radiologic Technology, 50*(5), 559–561.

Fauber T. (2008). *Radiographic imaging and exposure.* St. Louis, MO: Mosby.

Files, G. W. (1935). Maximum tissue differentiation. *The X-Ray Technician, 7,* 17–241.

Files, G. W. (1952). *Medical radiographic technique.* Springfield, IL: Charles C Thomas.

Fuchs, A. W. (1940). Balance in the radiographic image. *The X-Ray Technician, 12*(3), 81–84, 118.

Fuchs, A. W. (1950). The rationale of radiographic exposure. *The X-Ray Technician, 22,* 62–68, 76.

Fuchs, A. W. (1958). *Principles of radiographic exposure and processing.* Springfield, IL: Charles C Thomas.

Geometrical fallacies. (1983). *Radiologic Technology, 54*(4), 297.

Haus, A. G. (1980, October). Effects of geometric and screen-film unsharpness in conventional and 350 kVp chest radiography. *Radiology,* 197.

Haus, A. G. (1985). Evaluation of image blur (unsharpness) in medical imaging. *Medical Radiography and Photography, 61*(1–2), 42–53.

Hiss, S. S. (2003). *Understanding radiography* (4th ed.). Springfield, IL: Charles C Thomas.

Jenkins, D. (1980). *Radiographic photography and imaging processes.* Lancaster, England: MTP Press Limited.

Jerman, E. C. (1928). *Modern x-ray technic.* St. Paul, MN: Bruce.

Lauer, O. G., Mayes, J. B., & Thurston, R. P. (1990). *Evaluating radiographic quality: The variables and their effects.* Mankato, MN: The Burnell Company.

Morgan, R. H. (1945a). An analysis of the physical factors controlling the diagnostic quality of Roentgen images: Part I. Introduction. *American Journal of Roentgenology and Radiation Therapy, 54*(2), 128–135.

Morgan, R. H. (1945b). An analysis of the physical factors controlling the diagnostic quality of Roentgen images: Part II. Maximum resolving power and resolution coefficient. *American Journal of Roentgenology and Radiation Therapy, 54*(4), 395–402.

Morgan, R. H. (1949). An analysis of the physical factors controlling the diagnostic quality of Roentgen images: Part V. Unsharpness. *American Journal of Roentgenology and Radiation Therapy, 62*(6), 870–880.

Seeman, H. E. (1968). *Physical and photographic principles of medical radiography.* New York: Wiley & Sons.

Sparks, O. J. (1960). Possibilities and limitations of definition. *Radiologic Technology, 32*(2), 148.

Spiegler, G. (1950). The story of contrast and definition. *Radiography, 41*(189), 177–182.

Stears, J. G., Gray, J. E., & Frank, E. D. (1989). Radiologic exchange (resolution by focal spot size). *Radiologic Technology, 60*(5), 429–430.

Stockley, S. M. (1986). *A manual of radiographic equipment.* Edinburgh: Churchill Livingstone.

Sweeney, R. J. (1975). Some factors affecting image clarity and detail perception in the radiograph. *Radiologic Technology, 46*(6), 443.

Thompson, M. A., Hattaway, M. P., Hall, J. D., & Dowd, S. B. (1994). *Principles of imaging science and protection.* Philadelphia: W. B. Saunders.

United States War Department. (1941, July 3). *Technical manual: Roentgenographic technicians* (TM 8-240). Washington, DC: Author.

Wallace, J. E. (1995). *Radiographic exposure: Principles & practice.* Philadelphia: F.A. Davis.

Wilks, R. J. (1981). *Principles of radiological physics.* Edinburgh: Churchill Livingstone.

CHAPTER 29

Distortion

KEY TERMS

caudad
cephalad
distortion
elongation
foreshortening

Hans Castorp peered through the lighted window, peered into Joachim Ziemssen's empty skeleton. The breastbone and spine fell together in a single dark column. The frontal structure of the ribs was cut across by the paler structure of the back. Above, the collar-bones branched off on both sides, and the framework of the shoulder, with the joint and beginning of Joachim's arm, showed sharp and bare through the soft envelope of flesh. The thoracic cavity was light, but blood-vessels were to be seen, some dark spots, a blackish shadow.

Thomas Mann, Der Zauberberg (The Magic Mountain)

OBJECTIVES

Upon completion of this chapter, the student should be able to:

- Define size and shape distortion.
- Explain the effects of SID and OID on image distortion.
- Discuss various methods of minimizing distortion through variation of SID and OID.
- Explain why elongation and foreshortening are relational definitions.
- Describe the routine relationships between central ray, anatomical part, and image receptor.
- Explain the proper terms used to describe angulation direction and degree.
- Differentiate distorted images from routine projections.

OBJECTIVES (continued)

- Calculate the magnification factor when given SID and SOD.
- Calculate the actual size of an object when given the projected size, SID, and OID.
- Describe adjustments of SID and OID that will minimize magnification.
- Describe adjustments of central ray, anatomical part, and image receptor that will minimize shape distortion.

ASSESSING DISTORTION

Distortion is the second of the two geometric properties affecting radiographic image quality. Unlike the photographic properties of density/image receptor (IR) exposure and contrast, which control the visibility of detail, the geometric properties control detail itself. Distortion is a misrepresentation of the size or shape of the structures being examined. It creates a misrepresentation of the size and/or shape of the anatomical part being imaged. This misrepresentation can be classified as either size or shape distortion. Distortion, like detail, exists even when it cannot be seen due to poor visibility or, in other words, when the density/IR exposure and/or contrast are poor. The evaluation and adjustment of distortion require a thorough familiarity with normal radiographic anatomy. Unless the normal size and shape of a structure are known, comparison of the size and shape cannot be accomplished. Distortion can be difficult to determine even when normal sizes and shapes are known. Because the objective of radiography is to provide accurate images of structures, methods of minimizing distortion are important to diagnosis.

The factors that control distortion are shown in Figure 29-1. Careful examination of these factors will reveal that distortion is directly related to positioning. Only careful attention to the distances, direction, and angulation between the anatomical part, central ray, and image receptor can minimize distortion.

FACTORS AFFECTING SIZE DISTORTION

Magnification is the only possible size distortion in radiography. During acquisition of the image, minification is impossible, due to the divergent property of x-ray photons. Because it is not possible to reflect or refract x-ray photons by ordinary methods, they can only diverge from their point source. Thus, only magnification is possible and all size distortion

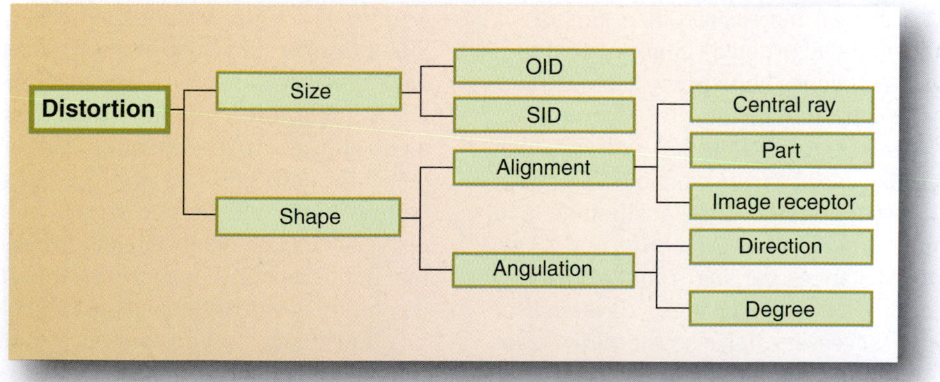

FIGURE 29-1. Image analysis: factors affecting distortion.

is controlled by the radiographic distances, SID and OID. In digital image receptor systems post-processing can resize the image.

In all instances, reduced magnification size distortion increases the resolution of recorded detail. Therefore, the objective in most radiography is to minimize magnification as much as possible. Magnification radiography is an exception to this rule. In this instance, the principles of magnification geometry are used to increase the size of structures that are too small to be easily visualized. Special conditions must be created to achieve diagnostically acceptable magnification images.

Magnification size distortion is controlled by positioning the body part and tube to maximize SID while minimizing OID. This can be accomplished by various procedures and by positioning. For example, an upright oblique cervical vertebra projection can be performed at 72″ (180 cm), whereas a supine projection is performed at 40″ (100 cm). An AP chest may place the heart 6″ (15 cm) from the image receptor, whereas a PA projection would place it 2″ (5 cm) away.

Source-to-Image-Receptor Distance

The SID has a major effect on magnification (Figure 29-2). The greater the SID, the smaller the magnification, because as SID increases, the percentage of the total distance that makes up OID decreases. The OID is the critical distance for magnification and resolution.

Although 40″ (100 cm) has developed as the current routine SID, this was not always so. The popular SID has been increasing since the advent of radiography and will probably continue to do so. The first x-ray techniques book in the United States is generally recognized to be the 1918 *Extract from the United States Army X-Ray Manual*, in which 20″ (50 cm) is discussed as a reasonable SID. When Ed Jerman developed the first positioning and technique book, *Modern X-Ray Technic*, in 1928, he recommended distances varying from 25″ (63 cm) to 36″ (90 cm). Of course, in those days shorter distances were necessary because the x-ray tubes were not capable of handling the load required to provide sufficient density/IR exposure with the film and screens of the time. As generator technology advanced, the SID increased.

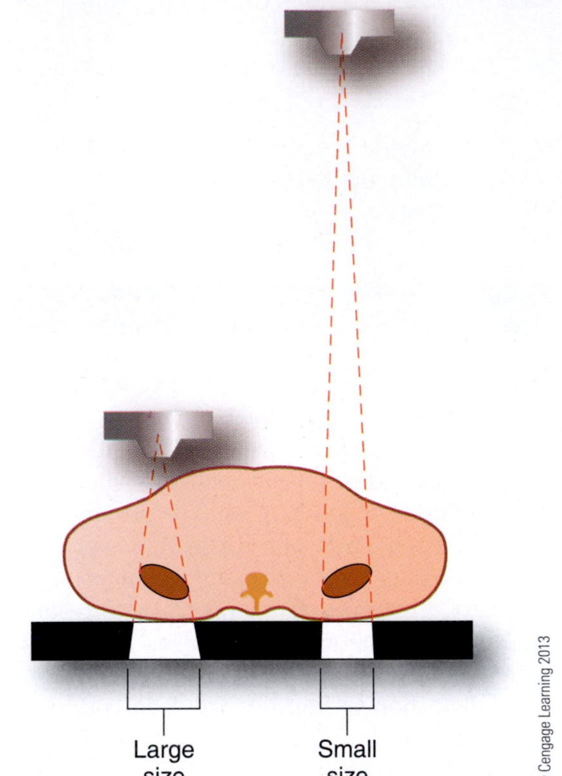

FIGURE 29-2. The effect of SID on image size magnification. Magnification size distortion is minimized by increasing SID.

Glenn Files's 1945 book, *Medical Radiographic Technic*, established the 40″ (100-cm) SID. For over 65 years this has remained the standard distance, but there are institutions that use 48″ (120 cm) as a routine distance, and the movement appears to be growing. Although a change demands new grids as well as careful consideration of x-ray unit design so that tube-to-tabletop distances can be achieved, and low table design so that radiographers can reach the tube, the increased resolution is worth the expense and trouble.

For many, many years chest radiography has routinely been performed at 72″ (180 cm) because the erect positioning arrangement permits a horizontal beam to be used and the increased SID effectively minimizes the magnification of the heart shadow. Any examination that permits a horizontal beam to be used can easily be established at an SID greater than 40″ (100 cm), and in many places the lateral cervical vertebral examination is performed at 72″ (180 cm) as well.

The source-to-object distance (SOD) is seldom discussed because it is included in descriptions of SID and OID, which are more critical. The SID is the distance that must be established by the radiographer when positioning.

The SID must be maximized to decrease magnification. Examinations of body parts with large inherent OID, such as the lateral cervical vertebra and the chest, use large SID whenever possible. In addition, the historical trend to increase the routine SID should be continued.

Object-to-Image-Receptor Distance

The OID is also a critical distance in both magnification and resolution. Figure 29-3 illustrates two major facets of OID. First, when objects within a structure are at different levels (Figure 29-3, objects A and B), they will be projected onto the image as different sizes. This is similar to the manner in which the eye processes information for depth perception; smaller objects are perceived as more distant and larger objects as closer.

The radiographer should develop a stereoscopic perception of the radiographic image, which is difficult because radiographic perceptions are in reverse of the normal information the eye is accustomed to processing. This is because objects that are further from the image receptor will be magnified. For example, in a chest radiograph the ribs are seen as wider as they become more posterior. This effect should make them appear closer, which is the opposite of the truth for the PA projection. Nevertheless, the perception of three-dimensionality can be developed and then used to determine object-to-image-receptor distance visually. When describing objects, it is important to remember that the size and distance relationship in

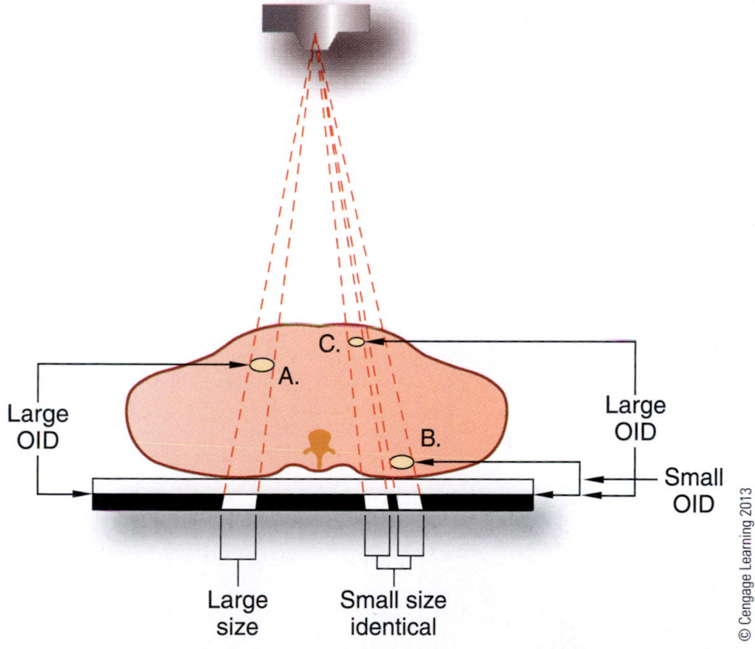

FIGURE 29-3. The effect of OID on image size magnification. Objects A and B are identical in size but their images as projected on the receptor are of significantly different sizes. Object C is significantly smaller than B, yet the image sizes are identical because of C's greater OID.

a radiographically projected image is the opposite of that perceived visually.

A more important size relationship that is controlled by OID is shown in Figure 29-3 between objects B and C, where object C appears identical in size to object B. This is an illusion because object C is much smaller but is magnified more because of its location in the part. This illustrates that a thorough knowledge of normal radiographic anatomy is a prerequisite to making judgments about size relationships. This is also one of the reasons radiographic examinations must include two projections, as close to 90° from one another as possible. When AP and lateral projections cannot be performed because of superimposing structures, as in an examination of the kidneys, it is important to include two oblique projections at 90° to one another. The two 90° opposing images can be used to verify the positional relationship of structures. This is also a shape distortion issue.

The OID is also important in dosimetry because it establishes the source-to-entrance skin distance that is the benchmark maximum exposure to the patient. Because OID varies with the part size and position of the patient, it accounts for the increased exposure that is part of many examinations. For example, there is a significant difference in the OID between an AP and a lateral projection (Figure 29-4). Note that the SOD changes dramatically in the figure as well. Obviously the entrance skin exposure would be greater with the lateral, even if the same exposure factors were used. Consequently, larger patients receive a greater exposure simply because their entrance skin surface is closer to the source, making their SOD much less. The increased mAs that is often used to provide sufficient image receptor exposure then increases the patient entrance skin exposure even more.

The OID must be minimized to decrease magnification. Examinations of body parts with large inherent OID, such as the kidneys and chest, use positioning techniques to achieve as small an OID as possible.

Calculating Size Distortion

Size distortion is present in any radiographic image and can be measured very accurately by using simple geometry. Magnification, or size distortion, can be assessed by calculation of the magnification factor. The magnification factor is the degree of magnification and is calculated by:

$$M = \frac{SID}{SOD}$$

where: M = magnification factor

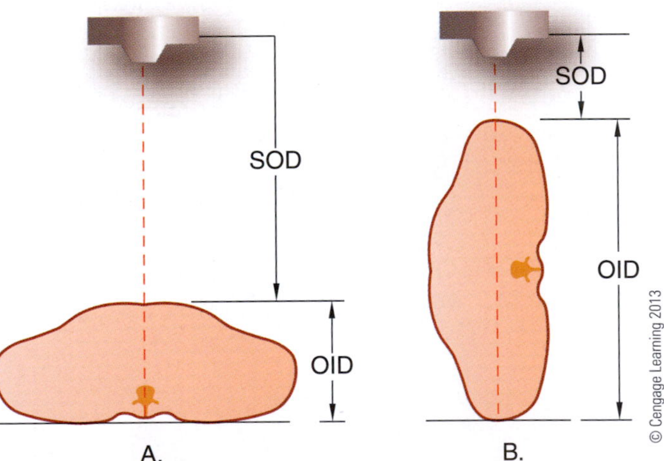

FIGURE 29-4. Variation in OID with size and projection. (A) Short OID, large SOD, low entrance skin exposure. (B) Large OID, short SOD, high entrance skin exposure.

The mnemonic device shown can be used by placing a fingertip over the variable for which you wish to solve and then viewing the mathematical relationship (see discussion of Ohm's law in Chapter 3).

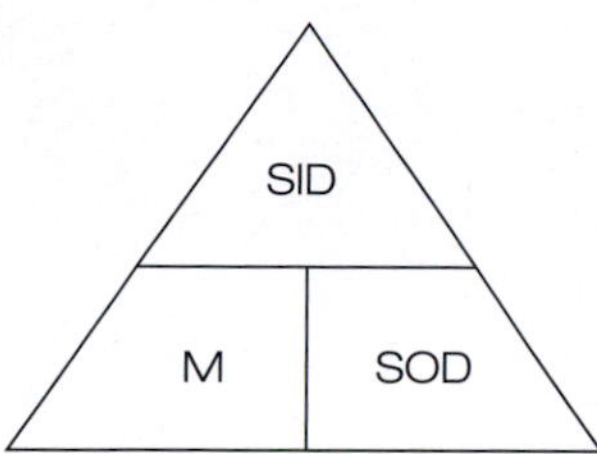

EXAMPLE: If the SID is 40″ (100 cm) and the SOD is 30″ (75 cm), what is the magnification factor?

Answer:

$$M = \frac{SID}{SOD}$$

$$M = \frac{40''}{30''} \text{ or } M = \frac{100\text{ cm}}{75\text{ cm}}$$

$$M = 1.33$$

The magnification will be 33 percent or the image will be 133 percent of the object size.

EXAMPLE: If the SID is 40″ and the OID is 2″, what is the magnification factor?

Answer: Because the SOD is not supplied, it must be found by using the formula:

$$SID = SOD + OID$$

$$40'' = SOD + 2''$$

$$SOD = 40'' - 2''$$

$$SOD = 38''$$

then

$$M = \frac{SID}{SOD}$$

$$M = \frac{40''}{38''}$$

$$M = 1.05$$

The magnification factor permits calculation of the actual size of an object that is projected as an image by using the formula:

$$O = \frac{I}{M}$$

where: O = object size
I = image size
M = magnification factor

The following mnemonic device can be used.

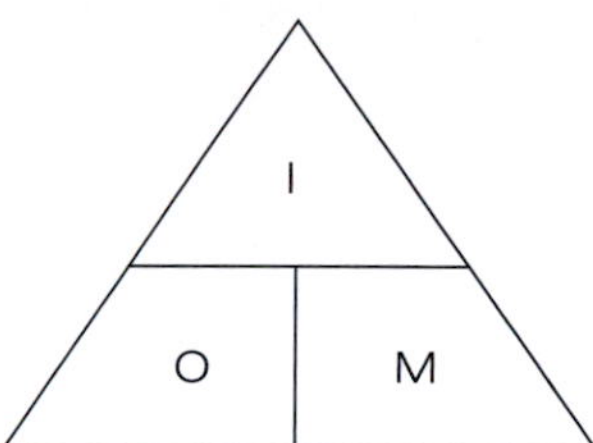

EXAMPLE: If a projected image measures 5″ and the magnification factor is 1.02, what is the size of the actual object?

Answer:

$$O = \frac{I}{M}$$

$$O = \frac{5''}{1.02}$$

$$O = 4.9''$$

EXAMPLE: If object B in Figure 29-3 is 2″ in diameter on the image and is measured to be 3″ from the image receptor (by using a lateral projection), what is its actual size if the SID is 40″?

Answer: Because the SOD is not supplied, it must be found by using the formula:

$$SID = SOD + OID$$

$$40'' = SOD + 3''$$

$$SOD = 40'' + 3''$$

$$SOD = 37''$$

(continues)

(continued)

then

$$M = \frac{SID}{SOD}$$

$$M = \frac{40''}{37''}$$

$$M = 1.08$$

then

$$O = \frac{I}{M}$$

$$O = \frac{2}{1.08}$$

$$O = 1.85''$$

If the image size and the object size are known, the percent of magnification can be determined using the following formula:

$$\frac{I - O}{O} \times 100 = \text{percent of magnification of the object}$$

EXAMPLE: If an object measures 5 cm and the image measures 6 cm, what would be the percent magnification of the object?

Answer:

$$\frac{I - O}{O} \times 100 = \text{percent of magnification of the object}$$

$$\frac{6 - 5}{5} \times 100 = \text{percent of magnification of the object}$$

$$\frac{1}{5} \times 100 = \text{percent of magnification of the object}$$

$$0.2 \times 100 = 20 \text{ percent of magnification of the object}$$

The magnification formula assumes that the focal spot is a point source. Because it is not, when the object size approaches the effective focal spot size or smaller, special problems develop from penumbral overlap (Figure 29-5). Therefore, objects smaller than the effective focal spot cannot be demonstrated and the magnification formula must be modified to consider the width of the focal spot.

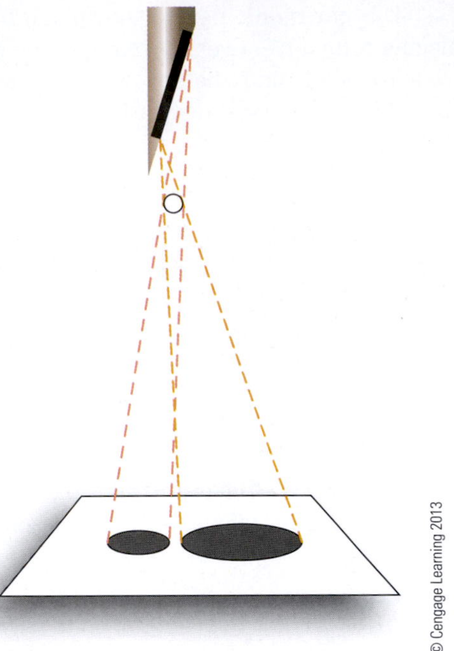

FIGURE 29-5. Objects smaller than the focal spot itself cannot be imaged due to penumbral overlap. The entire image is composed of overlapping penumbra with no umbra to define the edges.

FACTORS AFFECTING SHAPE DISTORTION

Shape distortion is the misrepresentation by unequal magnification of the actual shape of the structure being examined (Figure 29-6). Shape distortion displaces the projected image of an object from its actual position and can be described as either elongation or foreshortening. **Elongation** projects the object so it appears to be longer than it really is, whereas **foreshortening** projects it so it appears shorter than it really is. Elongation occurs when the tube or the image receptor is improperly aligned. Foreshortening occurs only when the part is improperly aligned. Changes in the tube angle cause elongation, never foreshortening.

Shape distortion often results because structures lie normally at different levels within the body. Shape distortion also occurs because of the divergence of the x-ray beam. The projected length

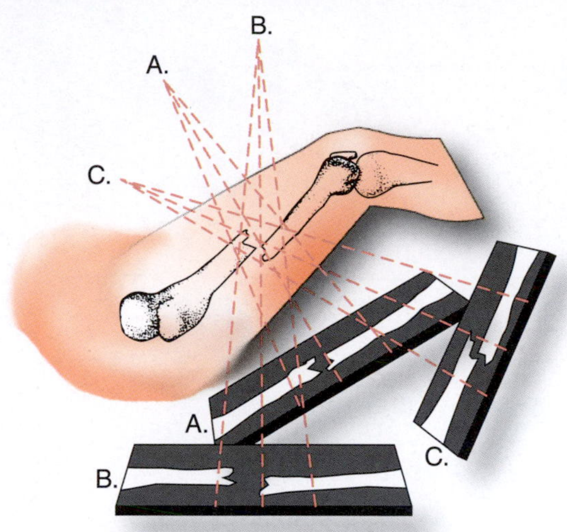

FIGURE 29-6. Shape distortion due to unequal magnification. Note how the alignment of the part appears different depending on the degree of distortion. *(Note: Adapted with permission from Producing Quality Radiographs, by A. M. Cullinan, copyright 1987, Philadelphia: J.B. Lippincott.)*

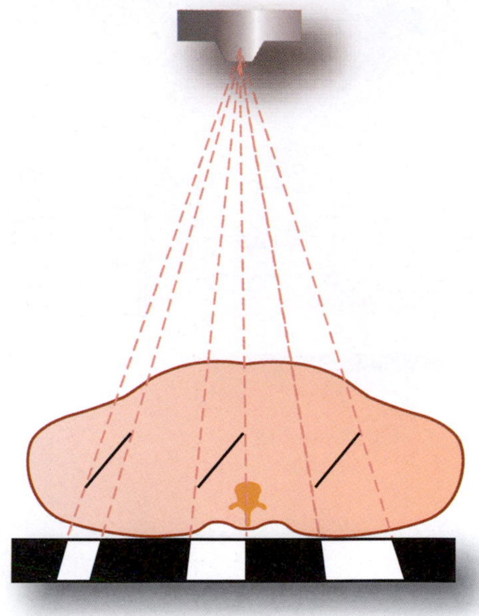

FIGURE 29-7. Shape distortion due to the angle between the object and the diverging beam. Although all three objects are at the same angle to the image receptor, the projected length varies according to the angle between the object and the diverging beam.

varies, depending on the angle between the object and the diverging beam (Figure 29-7).

Adjustment of shape distortion requires careful consideration of the beam-part-image-receptor geometry involved in the projection. This information must be combined with a knowledge of the normal projection of the structures to determine exactly how improvements can be achieved.

Alignment

Shape distortion can be caused or avoided by careful alignment of the central ray with the anatomical part and the image receptor. Proper positioning is achieved when the central ray is at right angles to the anatomical part and to the image receptor. This means the part and the image receptor must be parallel. When the position of the body part or object within the body does not permit this alignment, creative positioning must be utilized. The half-axial 30° angulation of the cranium to demonstrate the occipital bone, the 25° cephalad angulation of the pelvis to demonstrate the sigmoid colon, and the 10° caudad angulation of the coccyx are all examples of routine procedures that were developed to minimize distortion.

Alignment adjustments involve bringing the tube central ray, the part, and the image receptor back into their correct relationship—part and image receptor parallel to one another with the central ray perpendicular to both. Incorrect centering may occur from off-centering the tube (misalignment of the central ray), incorrectly positioning the part, or off-centering the image receptor (Figure 29-8).

Central Ray. The central ray is the theoretical photon that exits from the exact center of the focal spot. Ideally the central ray is intended to be projected perpendicular to both the anatomical part and the image receptor. Whenever the central ray is not perpendicular, some degree of shape distortion will result. This occurs in every image because only the central ray is truly perpendicular. Any structure that is not positioned at the central ray will be

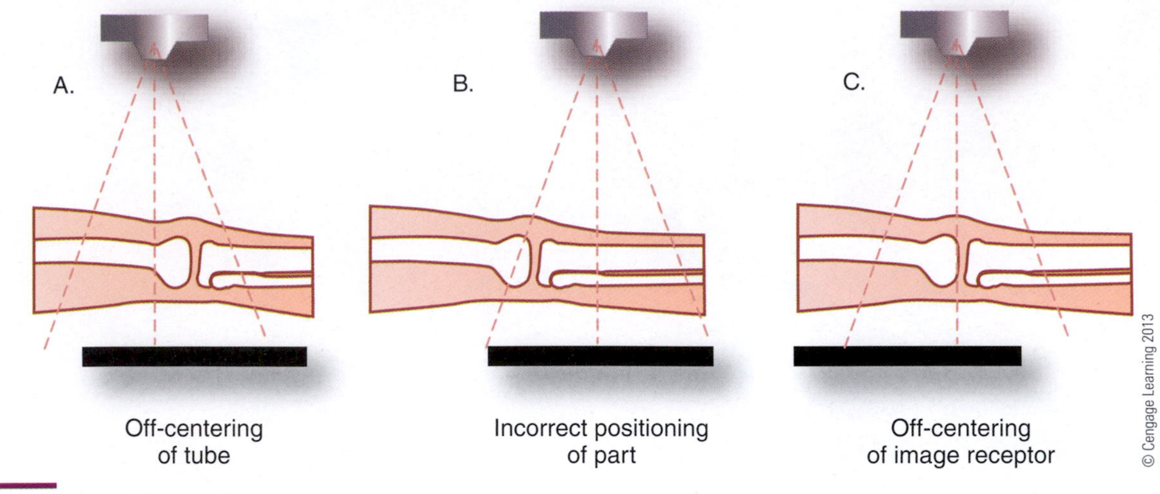

FIGURE 29-8. Incorrect centering.

distorted because of the divergence of the beam—the farther from the central ray, the greater the distortion. This applies as distance from the central ray increases transversely as well as longitudinally. For example, an AP pelvis will have more distortion of an object near the right greater trochanter than an object near the symphysis pubis. This is why it is so important to position according to standardized central ray locations.

Long bone length studies are an example of a procedure developed to ensure accurate central ray centering. The procedure shown in Figure 29-9 uses a radiopaque ruler, positioned from above the hip joint to below the ankle joint, as a measurement control. Spot exposures of the critical joints—hip, knee, and ankle—are then made with the central ray perpendicular to the joint space to ensure accurate measurement.

Centering away from the specified central ray entrance point is equivalent to angling the tube away from perpendicular because the entire perspective of the anatomical part is distorted. Some projections take advantage of this type of distortion. For example, a PA lumbar projection uses the divergence of the beam to open the lordotically curved intervertebral joints (Figure 29-10).

The central ray is normally positioned perpendicular to the anatomical part and to the image receptor. When the part is superimposed over other structures, central ray angulation can be a useful tool to provide a projection that would otherwise be impossible to differentiate from overlying structures. The use of the semiaxial AP projection of the skull to project the occipital region free of facial bone superimposition is an example. Failure to maintain the correct relationship between the part and the image receptor will produce a projected image that may not be comparable to norms and is therefore useless in the diagnostic process.

Anatomical Part. The long axis of the anatomical part, or object, is intended to be positioned perpendicular to the central ray and parallel to the image receptor. When these positions are incorrect, distortion may occur. Elongation occurs when there is poor alignment of the tube and/or image receptor. Foreshortening occurs only when there is poor alignment of the part (Figure 29-11). Figure 29-11A shows the intended relationships of central ray, part, and image receptor. In Figure 29-11B the entire object is foreshortened because of the improper part-to-image-receptor relationship. In addition to the entire object being foreshortened, one end is more magnified due to increased OID, which indicates that size distortion is also occurring.

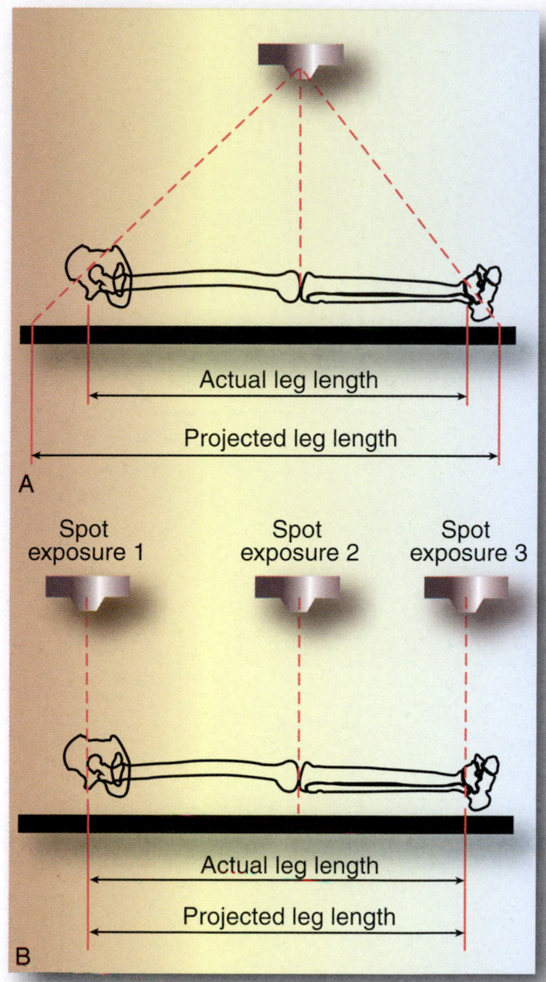

FIGURE 29-9. A long bone leg length study. Exact central ray location is critical to ensuring an accurate measurement of the bone lengths. (A) Inaccurate leg lengths due to beam divergence at the joints from a single exposure. (B) Accurate leg lengths with three spot exposures, each perpendicular to a joint.

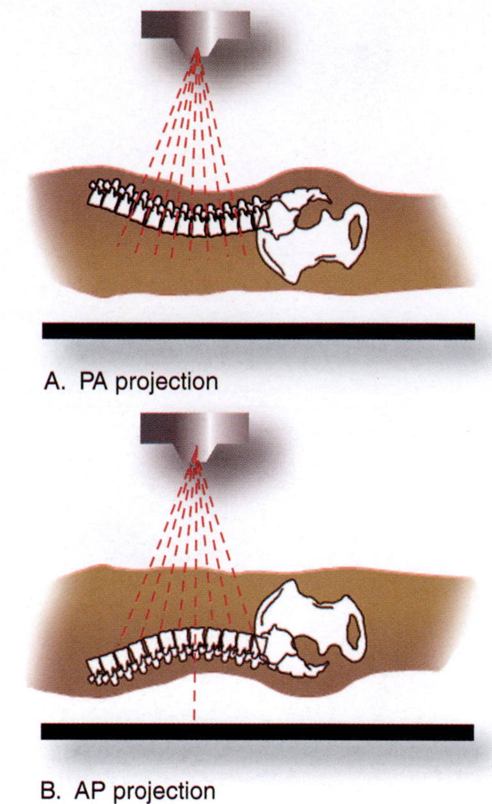

FIGURE 29-10. Divergence of the beam used to advantage. The lordotic curvature of the lumbar spine and the divergence of the beam can be used to open the intervertebral joints in a PA projection.

In Figure 29-11C the entire object is again foreshortened, with one end being more magnified due to increased OID. However, because of the differences in the actual size of the two ends, the increased size distortion of the smaller end makes both ends appear the same size.

Note especially the vast differences in the projected images of these anatomical part relationships. Figure 29-11A projects an accurate image. Figure 29-11B projects distortion of both size and shape so the entire object is foreshortened and the large end appears larger than it really is. Figure 29-11C also projects distortion of both size and shape but has distorted the relationship so both ends appear the same size.

The anatomical part is normally positioned with its long axis perpendicular to the central ray and parallel to the image receptor. As with the central ray, some routine projections are designed to vary from this standard to avoid superimposition. Failure to maintain the specified relationships between the central ray and the image receptor can result in an image that is not comparable to norms

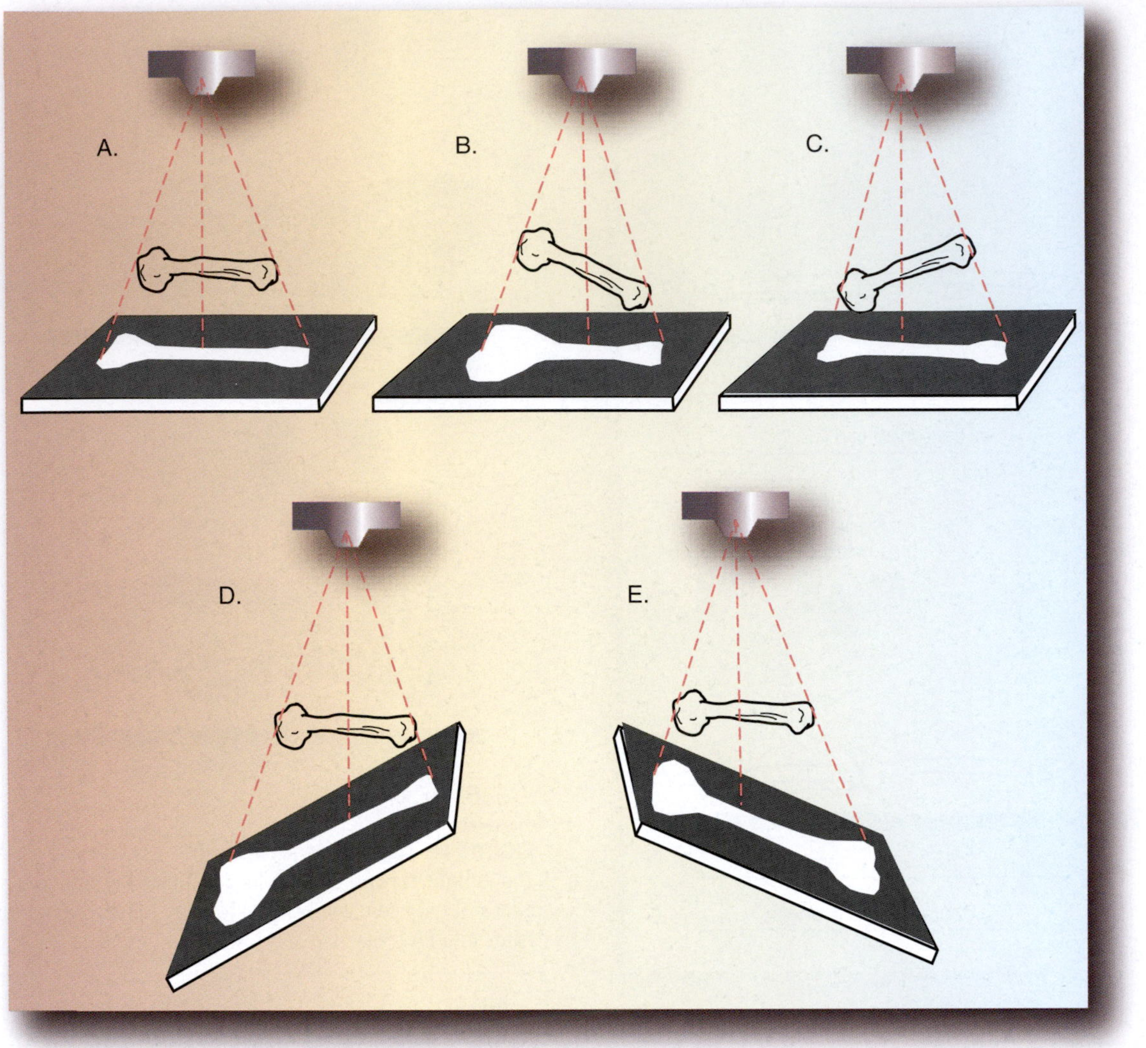

FIGURE 29-11. Foreshortening and magnification due to anatomical part and image receptor alignment. (A) Normal relationship between part and image receptor. (B and C) Foreshortening and magnification due to changes in anatomical part alignment. (D and E) Elongation and magnification due to changes in part/image receptor and central ray/image receptor alignment.

and therefore of limited value in the diagnostic process.

Image Receptor. The image receptor is intended to be positioned perpendicular to the central ray and parallel to the anatomical part. As long as the image receptor plane is parallel to the object, the only result of off-centering of the image receptor is the clipping of a portion of the area of interest. Although this will usually result in a repeated exposure, there is no distortion of image size or shape.

However, when the image receptor plane is not parallel to the object, or if the central ray is not centered to the part, serious shape distortion results exactly as if the object were not parallel. Figures 29-11D and E illustrate for the image receptor the same examples shown for the object in Figures 29-11B and C.

The image receptor plane is normally positioned perpendicular to the central ray and parallel to the anatomical part. Even in routine projections designed to vary from this standard, the specified relationships must be maintained to obtain a useful diagnostic image.

Angulation

Angulation refers to the direction and degree the tube is moved from its normal position perpendicular to the image receptor. Numerous radiographic projections utilize angulation to avoid superimposition of parts. The semiaxial AP projection of the cranium, tangential calcaneus, and axial clavicle are all examples.

The angulation of the tube is designed to cause a controlled or expected amount of shape distortion to avoid superimposition. As long as the specified angulation is applied, the image is comparable to norms and is of diagnostic quality. Angulation of the tube also changes the SID, which, unless compensated for by a new SID, will produce a decrease in image receptor exposure.

Direction

The most common direction of tube angle is longitudinal. Longitudinal angulations are usually termed **cephalad** when the tube is angled toward the head of the patient, and **caudad** when it is angled toward the patient's feet. Some radiographic tubes can also be angled transversely (sometimes referred to as "roll"). Transverse angulations are usually identified as right and left (in reference to the patient).

The direction of the tube angle is specified according to patient position and must be maintained as specified. When the patient position is reversed, the direction of tube angle must also be reversed to maintain the relationship. For example, 25° cephalad for an AP projection is identical to 25° caudad for a PA projection.

Degree. Degree is simply a method of describing the exact amount of angulation and is usually stated as the angle between the central ray and the image receptor plane from the standard reference point of perpendicularity. Because the standard reference point is 90° from the patient's head, radiographic angles must be added or subtracted from that point. For example, 5° cephalad is 5° from perpendicular, as is 5° caudad. It is important to maintain the correct degree of angle specified for a given procedure. Tube angulations also change SID, which will produce changes in magnification. Table 29-1 provides conversions for common tube angulations.

TABLE 29-1. SID Compensations for Common Tube Angulations

Tube Angulation	Overhead Scale	True SID
5°	39.8″	40″
10°	39.4″	40″
15°	38.6″	40″
20°	37.6″	40″
25°	36.2″	40″
30°	34.6″	40″
35°	32.8″	40″

From *Radiologic Technology, 52,* pp. 3, 304, by Robert J. English, 1980, by permission of the American Society of Radiologic Technologists.

Evaluating Shape Distortion

Shape distortion is a more subjective evaluation than size. It is much more difficult to assess because there is no effect that can be calculated, as in the magnification factor for size distortion. Instead, the entire assessment relies on the radiographer's knowledge of normal anatomy and the normal projected images for each position.

EFFECT ON IMAGE APPEARANCE

Size

Size distortion is generally a matter of magnification (Figure 29-12). All magnification involves a degree of loss of resolution, even when special systems are designed to minimize the loss.

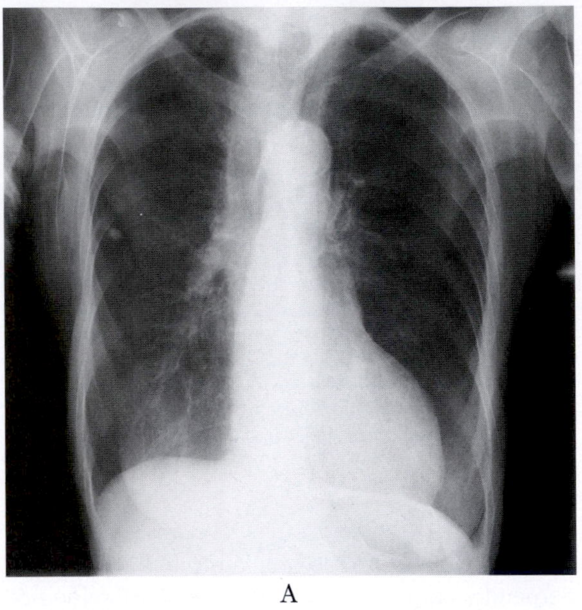

A

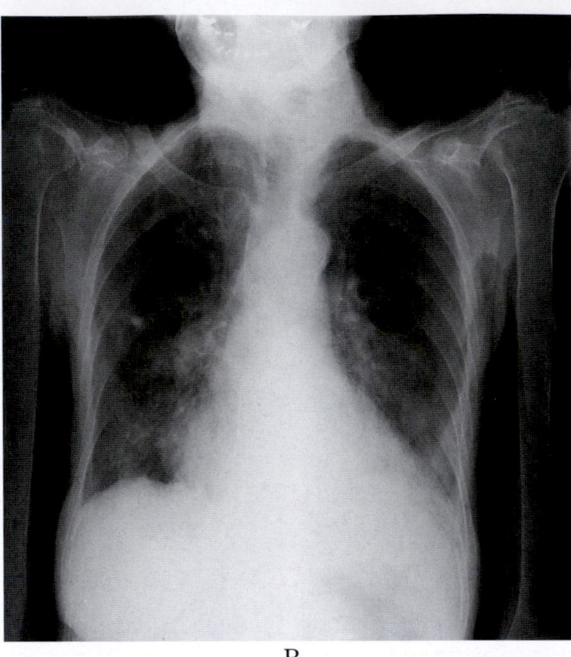

B

FIGURE 29-12. Magnification size distortion. (A) Minimal heart size magnification in PA chest. (B) An AP projection of the same patient demonstrating greater heart size magnification. *(Courtesy of Tracy Thegze, RT[R] Community Hospital, Munster, Indiana.)*

Shape

Shape distortion involves both elongation and foreshortening and is a serious alteration in the projected image (Figure 29-13). There are situations where shape distortion can be used to advantage, as in a tangential calcaneus.

60 kVp	15 mAs	72" SID
No grid	100 Rs	11.9 mR

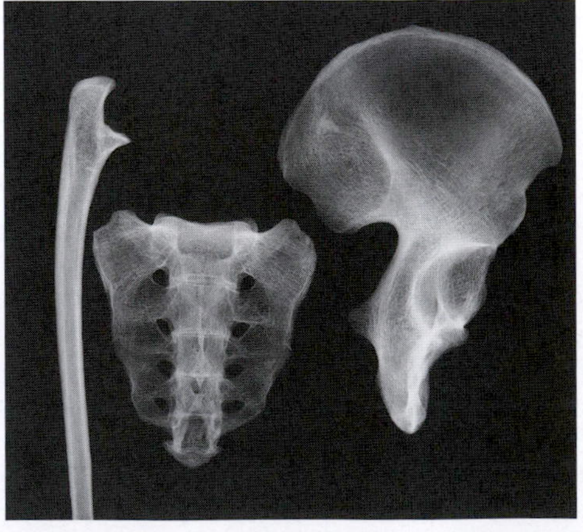

A

FIGURE 29-13. Shape distortion. (A) This radiograph was taken with the central ray perpendicular and centered to the center of the image receptor. (B) This radiograph was taken with the central ray perpendicular but off center to the left (away from the pelvis). The effect on distortion is not significant; however, changes in the image appearance are evident, particularly when studying the pelvis, which was furthest from the central ray angle of 25° and centered to the center of the image receptor. Notice the significant distortion created by angling the central ray. *(Radiographs courtesy of Arlene Adler and Richard R. Carlton.)*

60 kVp	15 mAs	72" SID
No grid	100 Rs	11.9 mR

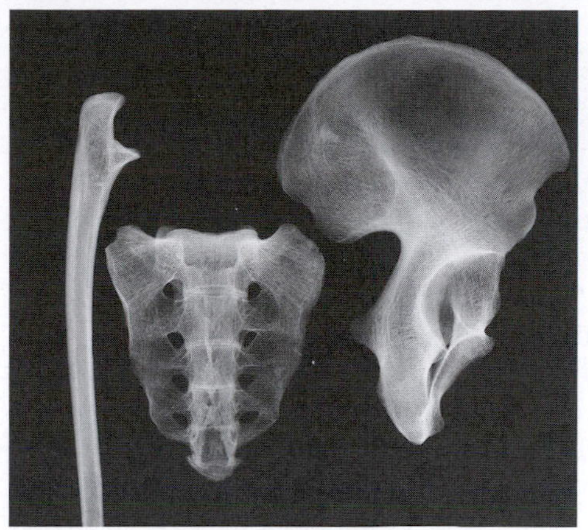

B

60 kVp	15 mAs	72" SID
No grid	100 Rs	11.9 mR

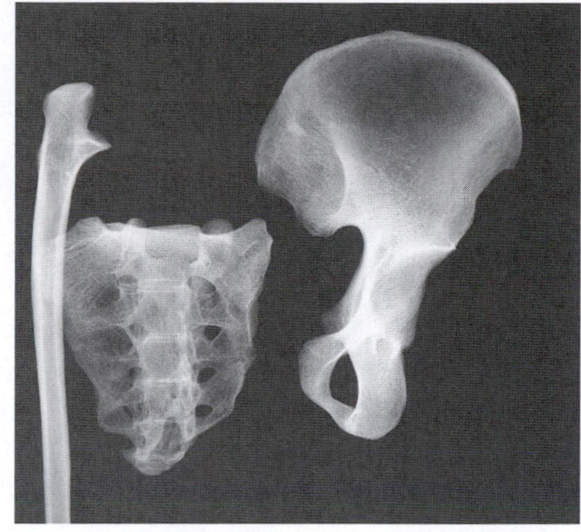

C

FIGURE 29-13. *(continued)*

SUMMARY

Distortion is the second of the two geometric properties affecting image quality. Unlike the photographic properties of density/IR exposure and contrast, which control the visibility of detail, the geometric properties control detail itself. Distortion is the difference between the structures being examined and the recorded image. It creates a misrepresentation of the size and/or shape of the anatomical part being imaged. This misrepresentation can be classified as either size or shape distortion. Distortion, like detail, exists even when it cannot be seen due to poor visibility or, in other words, when the density/IR exposure and/or contrast are poor. The evaluation and adjustment of distortion require a thorough familiarity with normal radiographic anatomy. Unless the normal size and shape of a structure are known, comparisons of size and shape cannot be accomplished.

When the factors that affect size and shape distortion are altered, some change in distortion will occur. No change will occur unless one of these factors is altered. Table 29-2 illustrates the effect on distortion when the various factors are changed. ■

TABLE 29-2. Effect of Changing Factors on Distortion

+ = increases distortion
− = decreases distortion
Size Distortion
− Increasing SID
+ Decreasing SID
+ Increasing OID
− Decreasing OID
+ Increasing patient thickness
− Decreasing patient thickness
Shape Distortion
+ Improper central ray alignment
+ Improper anatomical part alignment
+ Improper image receptor alignment
+ Improper direction of central ray angle
+ Improper degree of central ray angle

REVIEW QUESTIONS

1. What is distortion?
2. What is the difference between size and shape distortion?
3. How do the SID and the OID affect size distortion?
4. What is the magnification factor formula?
5. What is the difference between elongation and foreshortening?
6. How does the alignment of the anatomical part affect shape distortion?
7. How do the direction and degree of angulation affect shape distortion?
8. How can shape distortion be used to advantage?

REFERENCES AND RECOMMENDED READING

Ball, J., & Price, T. (1995). *Chesneys' radiographic imaging* (6th ed.). Oxford: Blackwell Scientific.

Bushong, S. C. (2008). *Radiologic science for technologists: Physics, biology, and protection* (9th ed.). St. Louis, MO: Elsevier.

Cahoon, J. B. (1961). Radiographic technique: Its origin, concept, practical application and evaluation of radiation dosage. *The X-Ray Technician, 32,* 354–364.

Carroll, Q. B. (2003). *Fuchs's radiographic exposure, processing, and quality control* (7th ed.). Springfield, IL: Charles C Thomas.

Cullinan, A., & Cullinan, J.(1994). *Producing quality radiographs* (2nd ed.). Philadelphia: J. B. Lippincott.

Distance—technique relationship of angulated projections. (1980). *Radiologic Technology, 52*(3), 301.

Distortion in imaging. (1989). *Radiography Today, 55*(628), 31.

Eastman Kodak Company. (1977). *Image insight 2: Geometry of image formation: Detail* (Publication M3-184). Rochester, NY: Author.

English, R. J. (1980). Distance-technique relationship of angulated projections. *Radiologic Technology, 52*(3), 301–304.

Fauber T. (2008). *Radiographic imaging and exposure.* St. Louis, MO: Mosby.

Files, G. W. (1952). *Medical radiographic technique.* Springfield, IL: Charles C Thomas.

Haus, A. G. (1980, October). Effects of geometric and screen-film unsharpness in conventional and 350 kVp chest radiography. *Radiology,* 197.

Haus, A. G. (1985). Evaluation of image blur (unsharpness) in medical imaging. *Medical Radiography and Photography, 61*(1–2), 42–53.

Hiss, S. S. (2003). *Understanding radiography* (4th ed.). Springfield, IL: Charles C Thomas.

Jenkins, D. (1980). *Radiographic photography and imaging processes.* Lancaster, England: MTP Press Limited.

Jerman, E. C. (1928). *Modern x-ray technic.* St. Paul, MN: Bruce.

Lauer, O. G., Mayes, J. B., & Thurston, R. P. (1990). *Evaluating radiographic quality: The variables and their effects.* Mankato, MN: The Burnell Company.

Morgan, J. A. (1977). *The art and science of medical radiography* (5th ed.). St. Louis, MO: Catholic Hospital Association.

Morgan, R. H. (1945). An analysis of the physical factors controlling the diagnostic quality of Roentgen images: Part I. Introduction. *American Journal of Roentgenology and Radiation Therapy, 54*(2), 128–135.

Morgan, R. H. (1945). An analysis of the physical factors controlling the diagnostic quality of Roentgen images: Part II. Maximum resolving power and resolution coefficient. *American Journal of Roentgenology and Radiation Therapy, 54*(4), 395–402.

Morgan, R. H. (1949). An analysis of the physical factors controlling the diagnostic quality of Roentgen images: Part V. Unsharpness. *American Journal of Roentgenology and Radiation Therapy, 62*(6), 870–880.

Pearson, G. R. (1951). Radiographic projection studies. *Radiologic Technology, 23*(1), 1.

Riles, G. W. (1943). *Medical Roentgenographic technique.* Springfield, IL: Charles C Thomas.

Seeman, H. E. (1968). *Physical and photographic principles of medical radiography.* New York: Wiley & Sons.

Stockley, S. M. (1986). *A manual of radiographic equipment.* Edinburgh: Churchill Livingstone.

Tarrant, R. M. (1952). Maintaining desired anode-film distance and alignment after angling the x-ray tube. *Radiologic Technology, 23*(5), 349.

Thompson, M. A., Hattaway, M. P., Hall, J. D., & Dowd, S. B. (1994). *Principles of imaging science and protection.* Philadelphia: W. B. Saunders.

United States War Department. (1941, July 3). *Technical manual: Roentgenographic technicians* (TM 8–240). Washington DC: Author.

Wallace, J. E. (1995). *Radiographic exposure: Principles & practice*. Philadelphia: F.A. Davis.

Wilks, R. J. (1981). *Principles of radiological physics.* Edinburgh: Churchill Livingstone.

Case of the Line in the Stomach

Although barium has been used to coat this stomach for the air contrast study, an odd line appears at its midpoint. What is causing the line?

Answers to the case studies can be found in Appendix B.

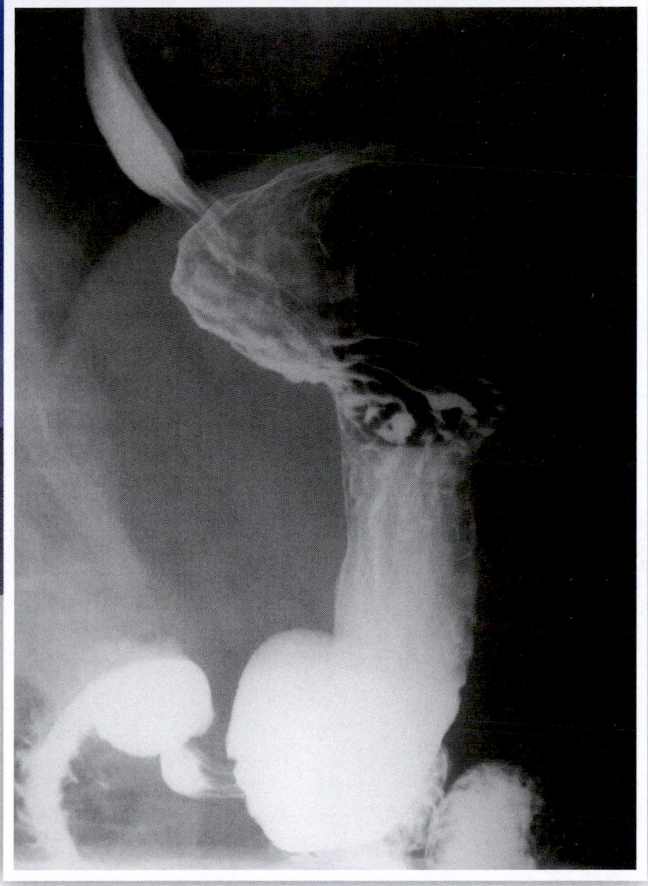

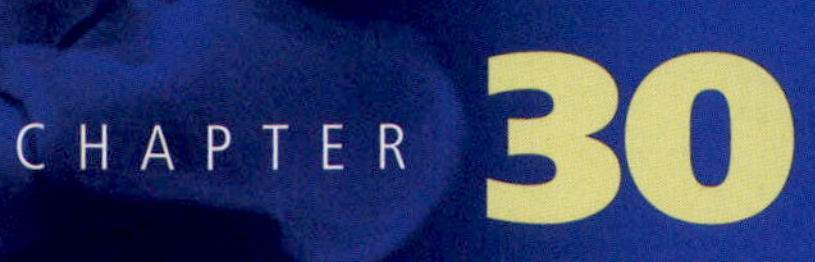

CHAPTER 30 The Art of Image Critique

> If all the factors involved in the making of a … radiograph are known, it then becomes a simple matter, by means of … (a) method of analysis, to decide what may be done to improve the quality of that radiograph.
>
> *Ed. C. Jerman, the "father of radiologic technology"*

OBJECTIVES

Upon completion of this chapter, the student should be able to:

- Discuss the elements of a diagnostic image as they relate to the art of image critique.
- Identify the steps of the decision-making process.
- Describe an effective image critique method, incorporating critical problem-solving skills.
- Use an effective image critique method.
- Explain the differences among technical factor problems, procedural factor problems, and equipment malfunctions.
- Apply an effective image critique method to a wide range of problems specific to clinical situations beyond those presented in this chapter.

IMPLEMENTING IMAGING STANDARDS

Radiographers are required to make critical decisions every day about the quality of their radiographic images. Critiquing an image is a very complex process that requires a thorough knowledge of all aspects of radiography. Deciding if an image is acceptable or unacceptable should be approached in a logical, organized manner. Image critique is an analytical process that involves many of the steps of diagnostic decision making, including critical problem solving. This process remains ever more critical in digital imaging systems even though it is possible to post-process the image to bring it into the human visual range.

The Diagnostic Image

The art of image critique revolves around the concept of deciding exactly where in the diagnostic-quality spectrum a particular radiographic image lies. A practical technical definition of a diagnostic-quality image has never been established because the artistic elements involved to produce the required medical information vary so much from one situation to another. The exponential number of variables involved makes radiography as much an art as a science.

The production of a diagnostic image involves an overwhelming number of variables, including such elements as patient anatomy, pathological conditions, radiographic positioning, patient preparation, radiation protection, x-ray equipment, prime technical factor selections, collimation, digital image acquisition, image receptors, processing, post-processing, density/image receptor (IR) exposure and contrast perceptions, detail, and distortion. In other words, nearly all of the elements of anatomy, positioning, physics, and principles of exposure are involved. The art of image critique is the application of scientific knowledge to an analysis of the image.

The Analytical Process

It is important to remember that not even radiologists are trained in the finer points of creating and analyzing the quality of a radiographic image. The radiographer is the expert and has the responsibility of proceeding with image analysis. Only with an acceptable image can a radiologist make an accurate diagnosis. It is the radiographer's professional responsibility to create the best possible image given each individual circumstance.

To determine whether an image is of diagnostic quality, the steps of an analytical decision-making process must be followed.

The process begins with a review of the entire image. This is essential to avoid premature narrowing. During the review the radiographer watches for anything that is different from a diagnostic-quality image. When differences are noticed, a pattern is sought, especially when there is more than one cue. Cues and patterns focus attention on a suspicious area, thus narrowing the search. Cues and patterns are then used to seek hypotheses. An effort is made to formulate a hypothesis that will explain all the cues. Cues that do not fit the hypothesis are held in reserve. The hypothesis is then tested by guided information seeking, with general questioning to produce more cue information. The last step is an evaluation of the final hypothesis. The hypothesis attempts to resolve the greatest number of cues and patterns.

There are myriad factors that can affect the quality of a radiographic image, and these factors can act upon each other to create an astronomical number of possible imaging problems. An image critique system uses the diagnostic problem-solving process to critically think through the problem and help resolve the situation.

IDENTIFYING AN IMAGING PROBLEM

The identification of an imaging problem requires the use of a full range of radiographic expertise. The radiographer must first recall that the purpose of the radiographic image is to provide information about the medical condition of the patient. The information needed may vary greatly, depending on the suspected medical problem and the anatomical region to be examined. For example, alignment of a nail during a hip-pinning operation requires a type of information different from that needed for detection of a small blood vessel constriction during cerebral angiography.

The meaning of the expression "diagnostic-quality image" is quite different in these two cases. The hip pinning requires two images at right angles to one another as fast as possible with a major consideration being patient dose. The cerebral angiograph requires maximum visibility of detail and resolution from a high-speed exposure with less consideration of patient dose. Any definition of a diagnostic-quality image must consider the clinical situation while providing a good balance between visibility of detail (density/IR exposure and contrast) and the geometry of the image (recorded detail or distortion).

The primary problem encountered by radiographers in successfully critiquing images is the tendency to glance at images instead of critically evaluating them for image quality. The professional approaches each image as a window in the diagnostic process.

In her introductory text for radiologists, *Fundamentals of Radiology*, Dr. Lucy Frank Squire emphasizes to aspiring radiologists that, "While the single-glance approach has its value, it is full of danger to the patient, because the presence of a very obvious abnormality tends to suppress psychologically your search for more subtle changes." She suggests that students utilize a systematic approach to evaluating images, primarily by looking at various structures in a deliberate order, concentrating on each structure while excluding the superimposed shadows of other structures. Radiographers should adopt an identical process by looking at each technical and procedural factor in a systematic fashion before jumping to any "glancing" conclusions.

AN EFFECTIVE IMAGE CRITIQUE METHOD

An effective image critique method is a three-step process involving:

1. the classification of the image,
2. the determination of the cause of the problem, and
3. the recommendation of corrective action (Figure 30-1).

This approach is designed to provide the radiographer with an organized and systematic protocol for critiquing an image. When consistently used, the system will be found to be a thorough and dependable method for establishing and maintaining professional skills at the very highest level of competence. The form in Figure 30-2 illustrates the application of this image critique method.

Classification of the Image

The first step in classifying the image is to evaluate it to determine if it is within the diagnostic acceptance limits. If the image is within the acceptance limits it should be critically examined to determine if it is of **optimal** diagnostic quality. If it is satisfactory in every respect, the pride of professional competence is the radiographer's reward. If the image is within acceptance limits but not of optimal diagnostic quality, the radiographer should continue the critique to refine his or her technical skills. Although the image may be submitted for diagnosis, a continued critique provides an opportunity to improve the quality of care for future patients.

If the image is outside the acceptance limits, a continued critique is mandatory prior to attempting to repeat the exposure. Failure to continue the critique is ethically unacceptable for a radiographer because it subjects the patient to additional radiation exposure without ascertaining how to produce an acceptable image.

Determination of the Cause of the Problem

The actual diagnostic problem solving begins with determination of the cause of the unacceptable or suboptimal image. In most instances there is more than one cause, and this can complicate the problem-solving process immensely. Searching for cues or patterns is primarily a matter of clinical experience. It is best to slowly narrow the search process by first trying to classify the problem into one of three major categories:

1. a technical factor problem,
2. a procedural factor problem, or
3. an equipment malfunction problem.

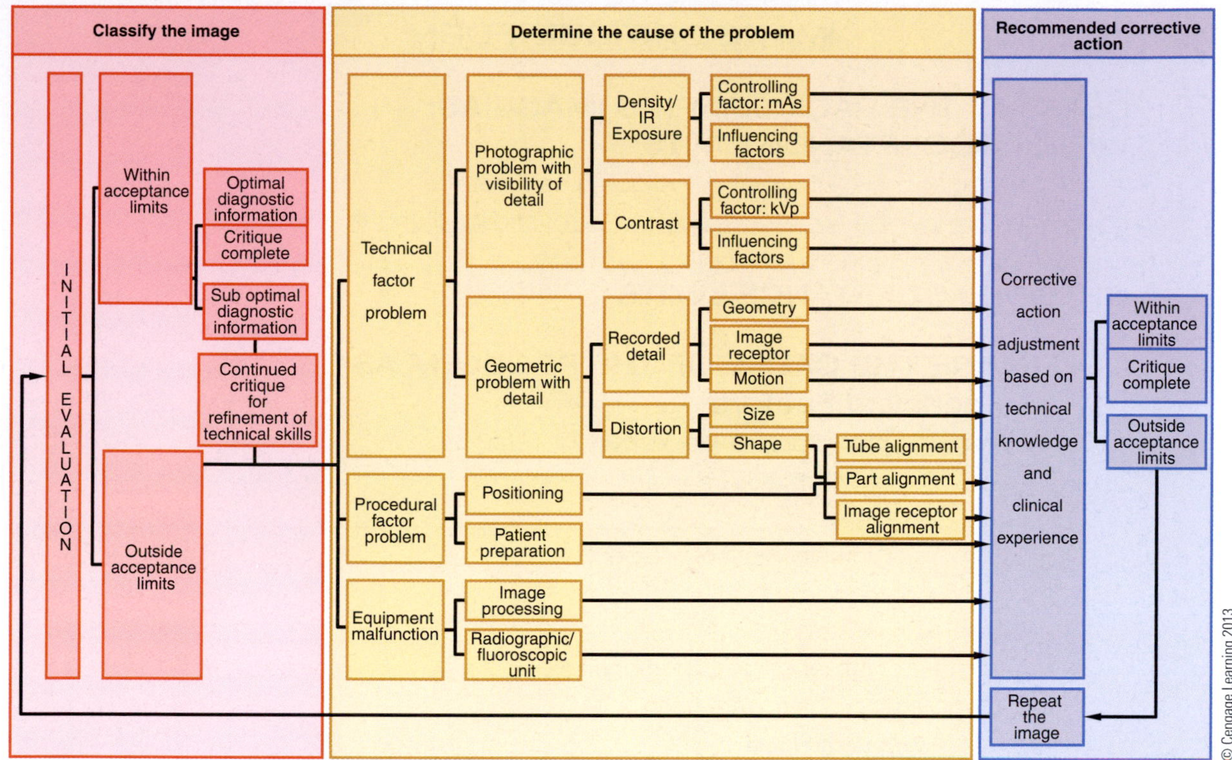

FIGURE 30-1. An effective image critique method.

All of these categories are then further subdivided in an effort to determine the exact cause of the problem.

Technical Factor Problems. Technical factor problems can be arranged into two categories: a problem with visibility of detail or a geometric problem with detail itself. (Of course, some images will have problems with both visibility of detail and detail.) Problems with visibility of detail concern maintaining sufficient density/IR exposure and contrast to make the detail of the image visible. Even with good detail present, anatomical structures cannot be visualized unless appropriate density/IR exposure and contrast are also present. An image that appears totally black may still possess good detail; it is simply beyond the ability of the human eye to discern it. Although digital systems can post-process such images and bring them into the human visual range, the fact that the image detectors received too little or too much radiation does not provide the optimal viewing data. Geometric problems directly concern the production of detail (also called definition, sharpness, and resolution). (See Figure 27-6, Image analysis phase.)

Problems with visibility of detail are further classified as density/IR exposure or contrast problems. Density/IR exposure problems may be the result of the mAs selection and/or a variety of other influencing factors, including the image receptor, the selected kVp level, distance, grid selection, beam restriction, a pathology problem, and so on. Contrast problems are the result of the kVp selection and/or a variety of influencing factors, including field size, patient thickness, grid selection, and so on.

IMAGE CRITIQUE FORM

I. CLASSIFY THE RADIOGRAPHIC IMAGE AS:

- [ ] **WITHIN ACCEPTANCE LIMITS**
  - [ ] Optimal diagnostic information (critique is complete)

(all checkmarks below this line require completion of section II and III)

  - [ ] Suboptimal diagnostic information
- [ ] **OUTSIDE ACCEPTANCE LIMITS**

II. DETERMINE THE CAUSE OF THE PROBLEM AS:

- [ ] **A: Technical Factors**
  - [ ] Photographic problem with visibility of detail
    - [ ] Density/IR Exposure
      - [ ] mAs ______________________
      - [ ] Influencing factor (specify) ______________________
    - [ ] Contrast
      - [ ] kVp ______________________
      - [ ] Influencing factor (specify) ______________________
  - [ ] Geometric problem with detail
    - [ ] Recorded detail
      - [ ] Geometry (specify) ______________________
      - [ ] Image Receptor ______________________
      - [ ] Motion ______________________
    - [ ] Distortion
      - [ ] Size (Magnification) (specify) ______________________
      - [ ] Shape (Part/Image Receptor/Tube Alignment) (specify) __________
- [ ] **B: Procedural Factors**
  - [ ] Patient Positioning
    - [ ] Tube Alignment ______________________
    - [ ] Part Alignment ______________________
    - [ ] Image Receptor Alignment ______________________
  - [ ] Patient Preparation (specify) ______________________
- [ ] **C: Equipment Malfunction**
  - [ ] Processing Equipment (specify) ______________________
  - [ ] Radiographic/Fluoroscopic Equipment (specify) ______________________

III. RECOMMENDED CORRECTIVE ACTION For each cause specified above:

____

____

____

FIGURE 30-2. Form used for image critique.

Geometric problems with detail are further classified as recorded detail or distortion problems. Recorded detail problems are the result of the geometry of the beam (focal spot size, SID, or OID), the image receptor, and/or patient motion. Distortion is further classified as size distortion (magnification) or shape distortion. Size distortion problems are the result of SID or OID. Shape distortion problems are the result of improper tube, part, and/or image receptor alignment.

Procedural Factor Problems. A procedural factor problem can be classified as one that involves patient positioning or patient preparation for the x-ray examination. Proper patient positioning results when the part, the image receptor, and the tube (central ray) are correctly aligned with one another. The result is an image that demonstrates the anatomical structures of interest from the proper perspective. Of course, a thorough knowledge of the anatomy being visualized for a given radiographic procedure is essential to determine if the positioning is accurate. When studying an image for accuracy in positioning, three alignment factors should be reviewed separately:

1. the tube alignment,
2. the part alignment, and
3. the image receptor alignment.

The second procedural factor problem involves preparation of the patient for the examination. Proper patient preparation includes removing radiopaque objects from the area of interest (e.g., jewelry, safety pins, etc.), proper bowel cleansing for a gastrointestinal study, recording a thorough history, communicating clear instructions to the patient, and so on.

Equipment Malfunction. The last major category in the classification of the causes of an imaging problem is equipment malfunction. Although the technical and procedural factors may have been correctly determined, a problem can still result when the equipment being used for the examination does not function properly. Problems normally occur with the processing equipment or with the radiographic/fluoroscopic equipment. These problems can be kept to a minimum through an effective quality control program.

Recommendation of Corrective Action

Each identified cause requires an appropriate corrective action that will resolve the problem. Corrective action adjustments are based on knowledge and clinical experience. Clinical experience is gained through careful attention to problems and successes. Remember that clinical knowledge is gained by critiquing acceptable but suboptimal images, analyzing repeated images, and recording successful results.

It is recommended that radiographers purchase or make a personal technique system booklet that can be easily carried while performing clinical examinations. This booklet should record appropriate technical factors, including the specific tube used (by room number or location), kVp, mAs, distance, grid, the relative speed of the image receptor, anatomical projection, part thickness, and any other variable factors (adjustable filtration, focal spot size, etc.). By using a personal technique system booklet, the radiographer has a quick reference for establishing the technical and procedural factors for a specific examination. Additionally, this guide can be useful for determining accurate adjustments in order to correct a problem.

APPLYING THE IMAGE CRITIQUE METHOD

Figure 30-3 illustrates how to use the image critique method that has been outlined. The radiograph in Figure 30-3A is classified as an image that is outside the acceptance limits of image quality. To determine the cause of this problem, the entire image should be studied for technical and procedural accuracy as well as for potential equipment malfunction problems.

From this review, it is determined that the image exhibits a technical factor problem and a procedural problem but no apparent equipment problem. Further searching narrows the technical factor problem to a photographic problem of visibility of detail and the procedural problem to patient positioning. This narrowing is based on

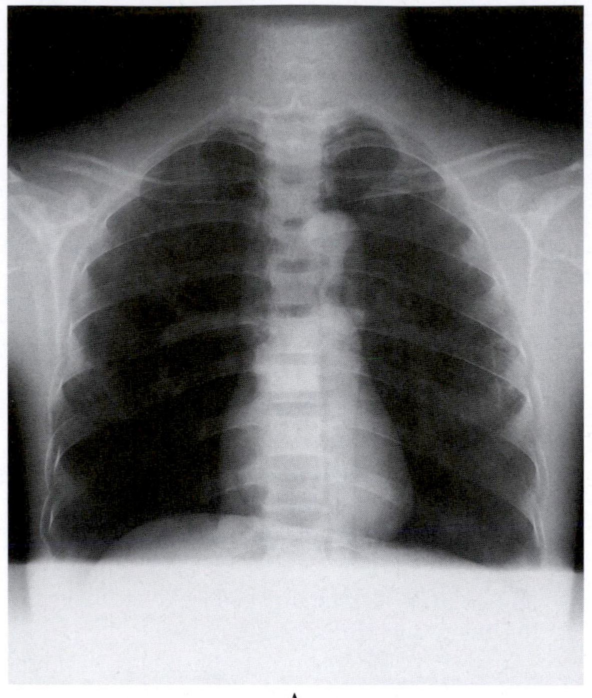

A

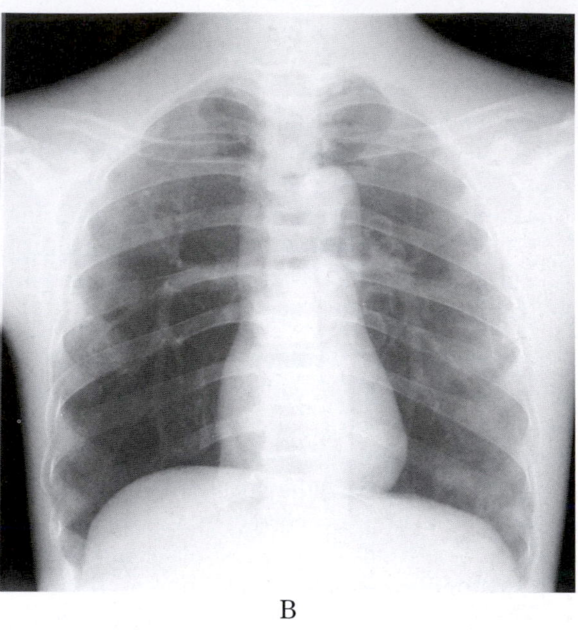

B

FIGURE 30-3. (A) Original radiograph. (B) Repeated radiograph. *(Radiographs courtesy of Arlene Adler and Richard R. Carlton.)*

observations that the image is overexposed and that not all of the anatomical structures of interest are demonstrated on the image. These two cues narrow the search by eliminating geometric problems of detail, patient preparation, and equipment malfunction as probable causes. Once suspected problem areas are defined, the cues and patterns should be used to form a hypothesis about the probable cause of the problem.

The photographic problem of visibility of detail can be further narrowed to an exposure problem. The possible causes of excessive exposure are then reviewed to determine the most likely cause. Although too much mAs is the most common cause, a number of secondary factors, such as the film/screen combination, the grid selection, and the kVp level, need to be considered and checked to test the hypothesis. This is a necessary part of evaluating the hypothesis.

Next, the procedural problem should be reviewed to determine the most likely cause. The problem is first narrowed to a patient positioning problem and then to an alignment problem.

The possible causes of alignment problems should then be reviewed to determine the most likely cause. Careful review of the image reveals that the central ray was not correctly aligned to the center of the image receptor. Because of this improper central ray alignment, some of the anatomical structures of interest (the lower lungs and costophrenic angles) are not visualized.

The final step is recommending corrective action. In the example, the corrective action involves changes in technical factor selection and patient positioning. The mAs is reduced by one-half the original amount to correct the density/IR exposure problem and the central ray is properly aligned to the midline of the image receptor. Figure 30-3B illustrates the result after these adjustments were made.

A thorough understanding of the concepts involved in producing an acceptable diagnostic-quality image is important. Because of the large number of variables in the imaging process, acceptable images will not always result from the initial exposure. Even the best of radiographers will be required to repeat images because of the vast number of variables. By applying a systematic image critique method, radiographers are practicing one of the most complex skills of the profession. This analytical and effective image critique method will help to ensure the best possible patient care by minimizing the need to repeat an exposure.

SUMMARY

Critiquing an image is a very complex process that requires a thorough knowledge of all aspects of radiography. Deciding if an image is acceptable or unacceptable should be approached in a logical, organized manner. Image critiquing is an analytical process that utilizes many of the steps involved in diagnostic decision making, including critical problem solving.

To determine whether an image is of diagnostic quality, the steps of an analytical decision-making process must be followed.

The process begins with a review of the entire image to avoid premature narrowing. When differences are noticed, a pattern is sought, especially when there is more than one cue. Cues and patterns focus attention on a suspicious area, thus narrowing the search. Cues and patterns are then used to seek hypotheses. An effort is made to formulate a hypothesis that will explain all the cues. The hypothesis is then tested by guided information seeking, with general questioning to produce more cue information. The last step is an evaluation of the final hypothesis. The hypothesis attempts to resolve the greatest number of cues and patterns.

An effective image critique method is a three-step process involving: (1) the classification of the image, (2) the determination of the cause of the problem, and (3) the recommendation of corrective action.

In the first step, the image is classified to determine if it is within the diagnostic acceptance limits. If the image is within acceptance limits but not of optimal diagnostic quality, the radiographer should continue the critique to refine his or her technical skills. If the image is outside the acceptance limits, a continued critique is mandatory prior to attempting to repeat the exposure.

The actual diagnostic problem solving begins with determination of the cause of the unacceptable or suboptimal image. Searching for cues or patterns is primarily a matter of clinical experience. It is best to slowly narrow the search process by first trying to classify the problem into one of three major categories: (1) a technical factor problem, (2) a procedural factor problem, or (3) an equipment malfunction problem.

Each identified cause requires an appropriate corrective action that will resolve the problem. Corrective action adjustments are based on knowledge and clinical experience. Clinical experience is gained through careful attention to problems and successes.

Even the best of radiographers will be required to repeat images. Using an effective image critique method will help to ensure the best possible patient care by minimizing the need to repeat an exposure. ■

REVIEW QUESTIONS

1. What is the purpose of image critique?
2. During the analytical process of critiquing a radiograph, how are cues and patterns used?
3. What are the three steps in an effective image critique method?
4. What are the three classifications of imaging problems?
5. What are the two categories of technical factor problems?
6. A necklace is seen on a chest radiograph. What type of imaging problem would this be?
7. A digital image is created using the wrong procedure definition (i.e., the digital system is programmed for a lateral cervical spine but a knee was radiographed). What type of imaging problem would this be?
8. How does a radiographer determine the appropriate corrective action for an imaging problem?

REFERENCES AND RECOMMENDED READING

Adler, A. M., & Carlton, R. R. (1989). Repeating radiographs: Critiquing the image. In E. Frank (ed.), *Postgraduate advances in radiologic technology.* Berryville, VA: Forum Medicum.

Adler, A. M., & Carlton, R. R. (1990). Perceiving the radiographic image. In E. Frank (Ed.), *Postgraduate advances in radiologic technology.* Berryville, VA: Forum Medicum.

Carlton, R. R., (1992). Another dimension of quality assurance in radiology. In L. T. Gurley & W. J. Callaway (Eds.), *Introduction to radiologic technology* (3rd ed., pp. 149–166). St. Louis, MO: C. V. Mosby.

Carlton, R. R., & McKenna, A. (1989). Repeating radiographs: Setting imaging standards. In E. Frank (Ed.), *Postgraduate advances in radiologic technology.* Berryville, VA: Forum Medicum.

Carnevali, D. L., & Thomas, M. D. (1993). *Diagnostic reasoning and treatment decision making in nursing.* Philadelphia: J. B. Lippincott.

Cullinan, A., & Cullinan, J. (1994). *Producing quality radiographs* (2nd ed.). Philadelphia: J. B. Lippincott.

Cullinan, J. E. (1981). A "perfect" chest radiograph—or a compromise? *Radiologic Technology, 53*(2), 121.

Doenges, M. E., & Moorhouse, M. F. (2008). *Application of nursing process and nursing diagnosis: An interactive text for diagnostic reasoning* (5th ed.). Philadelphia: F.A. Davis.

Goldman, L. W. (1977). Effects of film processing variability on patient dose and image quality. *Second Image Receptor Conference: Radiographic Film Processing: Proceedings of a Conference held in Washington, DC, March 31–April 2, 1977* (HEW Publication [FDA] 77-8036, 55–63). Rockville, MD: U.S. Department of Health, Education, and Welfare, Public Health Service, Food and Drug Administration, Bureau of Radiological Health.

Hiss, S. S. (2003). *Understanding radiography* (4th ed.). Springfield, IL: Charles C Thomas.

Jean Nagelkerk (2000). *Diagnostic Reasoning: Case Analysis in Primary Care Practice.* Philadelphia: Saunders.

Jerman, E. C. (1926). An analysis of the end-result: The radiograph. *Radiology, 6,* 59–62.

Lauer, O. G., Mayes, J. B., & Thurston, R. P. (1990). *Evaluating radiographic quality: The variables and their effects.* Mankato, MN: The Burnell Company.

McQuillen-Martensen, K. (1997). *Radiographic critique of the posteroanterior and lateral chest. Seminars in Radiologic Technology, 5*(2), 59–69, 89–95.

McQuillen-Martensen, K. (2010). *Radiographic image analysis* (3rd ed.). Philadelphia: Saunders.

Novelline, R. A. (2004). *Squire's fundamentals of radiology* (6th ed.). Cambridge: Harvard University Press.

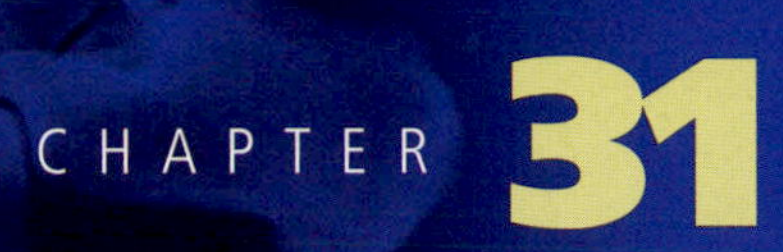

CHAPTER 31 Quality Management

KEY TERMS

detective quantum efficiency (DQE)
external beam evaluation
film processing system
quality assurance
quality control
total repeat rate

. . . a quality assurance program maximizes the likelihood that the images will consistently provide adequate diagnostic information for the least possible radiation exposure and cost to the patient.

William R. Hendee and Raymond P. Rossi, Quality Assurance for Radiographic X-Ray Units and Associated Equipment

OBJECTIVES

Upon completion of this chapter, the student should be able to:

- Define quality assurance and quality control and discuss their relationship to excellence in radiography.
- Describe the process of identifying imaging requirements, developing equipment specifications, selecting equipment, installing and testing equipment, and training the technical staff.
- Describe the objectives and responsibilities of monitoring equipment performance.
- Discuss primary quality control tests for external radiation beam monitoring of diagnostic radiographic systems, fluoroscopic systems, tomographic systems, and automatic exposure controls.
- Discuss appropriate monitoring factors for digital radiography detectors.
- List primary quality control tests for miscellaneous ancillary equipment, including cassettes and viewboxes.

(continues)

OBJECTIVES (continued)

- Explain the rationale behind the data collection process and the basic analysis of a radiographic repeat-rate study.
- Describe a basic troubleshooting procedure.

QUALITY ASSURANCE AND QUALITY CONTROL

Regulation and Accreditation

In the United States, the federal government initiated radiologic and imaging sciences quality management regulations after the Radiation Control and Safety Act of 1968. The 1981 Consumer-Patient Radiation Health and Safety Act added considerably to the scope of this effort, as did the 1990 Safe Medical Devices Act (SMDA) and the 1992 Mammography Quality Standards Act (MQSA). Today these acts and others relating to radiologic and imaging sciences are developed and enforced by the Center for Devices and Radiological Health (CDRH), which is part of the Food and Drug Administration (FDA) under the Department of Health and Human Services (HHS). In 1996 the Health Insurance Portability and Accountability Act (HIPAA) was enacted with the intention of simplifying standards by encouraging electronic transactions. This law also safeguards patient security and confidentiality (for which it is best known). Essentially, HIPAA established national standards for (1) electronic record security; (2) standardized electronic formats for record keeping; (3) standardized electronic identifiers and codes for institutions, personnel, diagnoses, and treatments; and (4) requirements for confidentiality and privacy rules. Failure to comply with this law can result in significant legal penalties (up to $250,000 and 10 years in prison).

Of the acts currently in place, the SMDA and MQSA have had the greatest impact on the practice of the radiologic and imaging sciences. SMDA mandates that any serious injury or death due to a medical device be reported. MQSA requires mammography facilities to be approved by the FDA.

There are also voluntary accreditation procedures available, and they are used by the vast majority of hospitals in the United States. The largest hospital accreditation agency is The Joint Commission (TJC) on the Accreditation of Healthcare Organizations (JCAHO). Its approval is linked to many medical activities, most importantly to reimbursement by the federal and state governments and many insurance companies. Accreditation agencies establish quality standards, assess them, and provide certification that individual institutions have met the agency's standards.

Although there are numerous quality measurement consultants, books, and process methods, one is worthy of remembering in all medical settings. The Hospital Corporation of America's FOCUS-PDCA method has gained great acceptance. It functions as shown in Table 33-1.

Quality management consists of a coherent system designed to monitor equipment performance through a variety of quality assurance and quality control standards or benchmarks.

Quality Assurance

Quality assurance consists of activities that provide adequate confidence that a radiology service will render consistently high-quality images and services. It is an evolutionary process that assesses everything that affects patient care. It may be medically, technically, or managerially oriented. Quality assurance includes evaluating activities such as interpretation of examinations, maintenance of equipment, performance of procedures, filing systems, staff development, scheduling of examinations, and supply lines.

The quality assurance process operates by identifying problems or potential problem areas,

TABLE 31-1. FOCUS-PDCA Method

Find and define a problem.
Organize a team to work on improvement.
Clarify the problem with current knowledge.
Understand the problem and its causes.
Select a method to improve the process.
Plan implementation.
Do the implementation and measure change.
Check the results.
Act to continue improvements.

monitoring the problem, and then resolving it. Monitoring problems involves several steps, including establishing criteria, performing monitoring, and collecting, analyzing, and evaluating data. It is these steps of the monitoring process that are of greatest concern to the quality assurance radiographer.

Quality Control

Quality control is the aspect of quality assurance that monitors technical equipment to maintain quality standards. The concept of **quality control** is rooted in the need to stabilize the various equipment components of the radiographic imaging chain. From incoming-line current through x-ray production to the processing of the radiograph, erratic equipment performance causes repeat radiographs and unnecessary patient exposure to radiation. The term *quality control* is sometimes used to describe the evaluation of individual radiographs according to acceptance limits standards. It is probably better to think of this image evaluation process as image critiquing or quality checking rather than quality control, although the quality control process is certainly a critical part of the critique evaluation.

Technical expertise will ensure success in radiography when quality assurance is used to ascertain that the equipment is reliable. Because radiographic equipment changes as it ages, there are often great differences between the results obtained on one unit and those obtained on another. The same unit cannot be counted on to produce exactly the same beam for the radiographer to control and analyze unless it is properly checked on a regular basis. The system of checks to accomplish a measure of consistency in beam output is the quality control.

Ensuring the quality of the radiographic image is a prime responsibility of the radiologic technologist. Every patient expects to receive the highest possible quality, or excellence, of service, from a medical facility. No one wants to be exposed to ionizing radiation by a radiographer incapable of producing excellent images.

It is important that quality control be seen as a method of controlling the radiographic image from start to finish. To do this requires a series of procedures (Figure 31-1). Unfortunately, some quality control begins with the last step instead of the first. An effective program cannot be achieved simply by monitoring equipment performance, although this is unquestionably the most involved step. The thought process preceding equipment purchase is critical.

PURCHASING EQUIPMENT

Identification of Imaging Requirements

It is not always apparent exactly what type of equipment is needed when new purchases are being considered. Historically, this decision was made by the chief radiologist or administrative technologist.

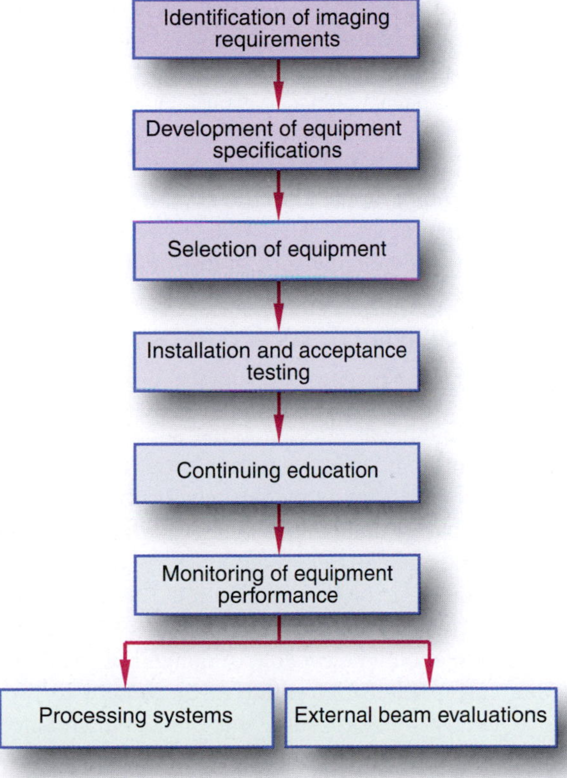

FIGURE 31-1. A total quality control system. *(Adapted from W. R. Hendee and R. P. Rossi,* Quality Assurance for Radiographic X-Ray Units and Associated Equipment *[HEW Publication FDA 79-8094], 1979, Rockville, MD: U.S. DHEW, PHS, FDA, Bureau of Radiological Health.)*

Rarely are the actual operators of the equipment, the radiographers, consulted. The result has been that nearly every x-ray department owns a radiological monstrosity that is avoided by radiographers and radiologists alike. These units are often inconvenient, overly sophisticated, or unable to produce quality images. Careful identification of imaging requirements can prevent these problems.

It is not necessary to be an expert in imaging physics and technology in order to be capable of contributing to the process of identifying the imaging requirements. Each member of the radiological team can contribute his or her expertise. The person who will make the final decision should interview the radiologists, administrators, supervisors, and staff technologists who will use the equipment. In many instances the needs of the radiologist will determine the basic parameters for the purchase. Administrators must often impose financial and space restraints, although they can also create new funds and space when necessary. Supervisors are often able to provide important information on patient flow and staffing needs. After the radiologists, the radiographers are the most important persons to have input because their experiences with equipment provide a wealth of information.

Development of Equipment Specifications

Generic equipment specifications should be developed from the interview information. It is important that the person formulating the specifications has the technical background to state exactly what is needed to meet the imaging requirements. An imaging physicist should be involved at this point. The best specifications include detailed statements of what the equipment should be capable of doing. For example, "Maintain mA linearity within ± 10 percent to produce a consistent exposure when mAs is maintained but mA is varied." This must include a change from highest to lowest setting. When the specifications are complete they are sent to vendors for bidding.

Selection of Equipment

The actual selection of equipment becomes simple if the investigation into the first two steps has been thorough. When the bids arrive they can be compared for meeting specifications, cost, and service. The actual decision is then academic. A pitfall in the process can occur when radiologists in the institution show a preference to a particular vendor, thus weakening the bargaining position of the department administrator. In many institutions this pitfall should be expanded to include interference by administrative officers unfamiliar with imaging equipment.

Installation and Acceptance Testing of Equipment

Installation and acceptance testing of equipment is the responsibility of the vendor and/or manufacturer. The quality control technologist must verify that the equipment specifications have been met. Normally this includes supervising the testing procedures and results. It is suggested that the exact methods for acceptance testing be included in the original specifications. The data from these tests will form the standard for all future quality control monitoring.

Continuing Education

It is normally the responsibility of the vendor to familiarize the users of the equipment with its proper operation. With simple equipment, such as ancillary devices, the equipment manual may be sufficient for use in in-service training. More complex equipment should be demonstrated and explained by the vendor **to at least two persons** as part of the purchase contract. Continuing education **must** be an ongoing procedure. It is advisable to include both the quality control and in-service education coordinators in the initial training demonstrations. A good in-service program will include an orientation procedure as well as periodic updates on all complex equipment.

MONITORING EQUIPMENT PERFORMANCE

The final procedure of a total program is commonly considered to be the whole of quality control. Monitoring equipment performance includes routine checks of all radiographic equipment. Although they are interdependent, monitoring can be divided into two parts: (1) **film processing systems** and (2) **external beam evaluation**. Objectives for a performance monitoring system are to:

1. monitor the quality of the image processing systems,
2. measure the quality of the external radiation beams, and
3. specify faults within these systems to allow corrective measures to be taken.

Evidence shows that a properly working quality control system will reduce equipment downtime and the number of repeated exposures. This will also reduce patient dose, patient waiting time, and supply costs, as well as increase confidence in diagnostic consultation and boost departmental morale.

Responsibility

Professional service personnel or medical physicists are not required to perform routine quality control procedures. Many procedures must be done daily, and to use these experts would be too costly. Radiographers, who are more available and knowledgeable about potential problems, should do the equipment monitoring. An initial cost outlay for testing equipment is required. To maintain a program, staff technologists must be given time to perform the procedures and to evaluate them.

Processor Monitoring

Processor monitoring is designed to permit an automatic film processor to fluctuate within set limits. These tests may be performed by anyone who has been oriented to the use of the equipment involved. Only a radiographer or processor maintenance person should perform the corrective actions.

Action must be taken to correct problems whenever the limits are exceeded. A quality control program that is not backed up by a commitment to shut down processors that are outside limits is of little value. Manufacturers' suggestions should be followed for the start-up and for the regular maintenance of the processor.

There are also several monitoring tests that should be done on a daily basis. These include a darkroom fog test, also known as a safelight test, and processor sensitometry to monitor speed, contrast, and base fog of film. See Chapters 19, 20, and 21 for details.

External Beam Evaluation

The second part of performance monitoring involves the evaluation of the external primary radiation beam. These tests must be performed by a radiographer who has knowledge of the physical operation of the equipment and all related accessories. Corrective action should be taken only by an authorized service person.

Some monitoring equipment can be made very inexpensively; other equipment must be purchased. A dosimeter is an essential piece of equipment, and reasonable quality control cannot be performed without one. Computerized dosimeters are available that permit readouts and printouts of many quality control parameters from a single exposure. The Duke University quality assurance tool is one such device. Figure 31-2 illustrates common quality control equipment. A room log should be kept to record test results, maintenance, and repairs performed on each x-ray tube and other system in each room.

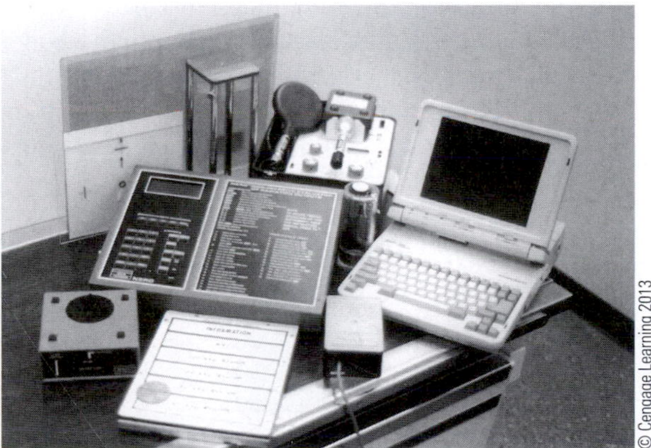

FIGURE 31-2. Radiographic quality control equipment. Clockwise from upper left: wire mesh film/screen contact tool, collimator accuracy tool, pinhole focal spot camera, digital dosimeter with computer, synchronous spinning top and penetrometer tool, and kVp test cassette with star pattern focal spot tool. In center: noninvasive beam evaluator (NERO™ computerized unit with ionization chamber) and resolution pattern focal spot test tool.

Diagnostic Radiographic Systems. The tests that should be performed on diagnostic radiographic systems should be done on a **semiannual** schedule. The tests for x-ray tubes should include the following.

Focal spot size estimation. An estimate of focal spot size is important so that it is kept within acceptable limits to ensure proper image detail. There are three types of focal spot test tools: line pair resolution tools, star test patterns, and pinhole cameras. Both line pair resolution tools and star test patterns function by imaging a resolution pattern on a film. The image can then be analyzed to estimate the focal spot size. A pinhole camera permits measurement of the focal spot by creating an image of the effective focal spot on a film (Figure 31-3).

The National Electrical Manufacturers Association (NEMA) specifies that focal spots of 0.3 mm and smaller may be measured with a star test pattern. Focal spots larger than 0.3 mm should be measured with a pinhole camera. In clinical quality control assurance testing, a pinhole camera is avoided because it is difficult to use accurately and requires massive tube loading. A star test pattern will satisfactorily monitor focal spot size growth in most instances. When the focal spot grows to an unacceptable size, the x-ray tube must be replaced. NEMA specifies that focal spots smaller than 0.8 mm may be 50 percent larger than the stated nominal size. Focal spots between 0.8 mm and 1.5 mm may be 40 percent larger than nominal, and focal spots larger than 1.5 mm may be 30 percent larger than nominal. For example, a 0.5-mm focal spot may actually be 0.75 mm and still be considered acceptable.

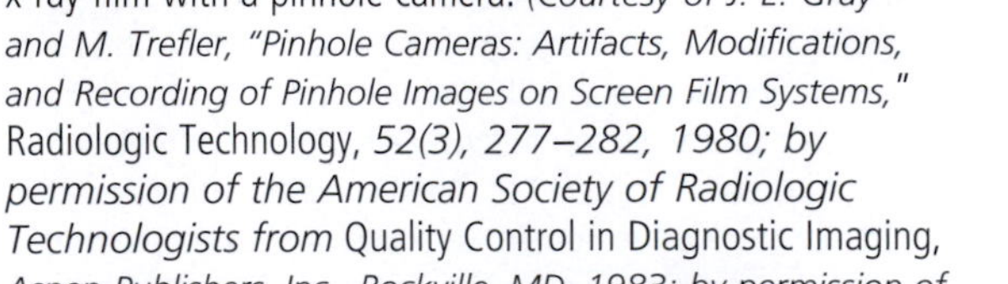

2.0mm 1.0mm 1.0mm

FIGURE 31-3. Focal spot images produced on dental x-ray film with a pinhole camera. *(Courtesy of J. E. Gray and M. Trefler, "Pinhole Cameras: Artifacts, Modifications, and Recording of Pinhole Images on Screen Film Systems,"* Radiologic Technology, *52(3), 277–282, 1980; by permission of the American Society of Radiologic Technologists from* Quality Control in Diagnostic Imaging, *Aspen Publishers, Inc., Rockville, MD, 1983; by permission of the Mayo Foundation for Medical Education and Research.)*

Half-value layer. The amount of total filtration in the primary beam is important for both radiation protection and image quality. Radiation protection is ensured by eliminating low-energy photons that are incapable of reaching the image receptor. Image quality is ensured by making appropriate contrast adjustments. Half-value layers are measured by using dosimetry equipment to detect the quality of aluminum filtration that will reduce the beam intensity to half the original value. Computerized quality control dosimeters provide a digital readout of the half-value layer. Half-value layer recommendations or requirements vary depending on the kVp. If insufficient filtration is present, the tube housing must be modified to supply additional aluminum filtration.

Collimator, central ray, and bucky tray accuracy. The congruence of the projected centering light field and the central ray with the actual collimated primary x-ray beam and bucky tray is of critical importance for radiation protection. Radiation protection is ensured by avoiding repeated images due to overcollimation errors and by avoiding irradiation of tissue unless it will be imaged. A collimator test tool is simply a lead marker for each corner of the light beam plus crosshairs or a lead marker, placed several centimeters above the cassette surface, for the central ray. A 2 percent SID error is allowed between the primary beam image and the light field size (this is a U.S. federal standard). The centering mark should be within 1 percent of the light field central ray. The positive beam limitation (PBL) mechanism should not permit the primary beam to be larger than the cassette in the bucky tray unless the override lock is activated. When these margins of error are exceeded, the collimator light or PBL mechanism must be adjusted.

Distance and centering indicators' accuracy. Many older x-ray units have inaccurate distance indicators located on tube support stands or overhead readouts. In addition, both distance and centering locks, stops, and detents may not be accurate. Assurance that distance and centering are accurate avoids the need for repeated exposures due to the inverse square law, misalignment of the central ray, and primary beam collimation. Distance indicators should be checked with a tape measure (point zero should be measured from the focal spot, which is approximately 1 cm from the bottom of the tube housing end cap). Centering indicators can be checked by visual inspection of the collimator light beam (assuming a collimator and central ray accuracy test has been done). Distance indicators should be ± 10 percent, and centering indicators should be ± 2 percent. If the indicators are not within these limits they should be adjusted.

Angulator or protractor accuracy. X-ray tables, bucky units, and tubes with angulators or protractors must provide accurate readings for positioning baselines. They can be evaluated by using a large protractor for angle measurements and a level to verify that locks, stops, and detents are set to establish horizontal and perpendicular surfaces. Angles should be ± 1 percent, with adjustments made when necessary.

The tests for x-ray generators should include the following.

Kilovoltage accuracy. Kilovoltage settings tend to drift over time, primarily as a result of tube aging. Their accuracy is essential in maintaining image quality. The scale of contrast and density cannot be predicted unless the kVp is accurate. Verification and calibration of the kVp ensure that technique exposure charts will produce diagnostic-quality images. Computerized dosimeters provide digital readouts or printouts of average and single-pulse kVp. If the settings drift beyond ± 5 kVp of the labeled setting, the generator must be recalibrated.

Timer accuracy. Exposure time settings also tend to drift over time. Their accuracy is essential in maintaining image quality because exposure cannot be predicted unless the time is accurate. Verification and calibration of the timer ensure that technique exposure charts will produce diagnostic-quality images. Computerized dosimeters provide digital readouts or printouts of the exposure time, or a spinning top may be used to measure 1φ generators and a motorized synchronous top may be used for 3φ units. The tops are less accurate, more time-consuming, and difficult to use. Exposure time settings should be maintained within ±5 percent of the label. If the settings drift beyond this limit, the timing circuit or mechanism must be recalibrated.

mR/mAs and milliamperage linearity. Milliamperage settings also tend to drift over time, primarily as a result of tube aging. Their accuracy is essential to maintaining image quality because exposure cannot be predicted unless the mA is accurate. Assurance is needed that technique exposure charts will accurately produce diagnostic-quality images. Milliamperage cannot be measured by noninvasive quality control methods. Consequently, mA station accuracy must be inferred by comparing mR/mAs measurements after both time and kVp accuracy have been verified. Comparative measurements are made for the same mAs at different mA and time settings to evaluate the linearity of the mA stations. Computerized dosimeters provide digital readouts or printouts of mR/mAs. Milliamperage stations should be maintained within ± 10 percent of each other, but some sources recommend maintaining the entire generator within ± 10 percent. If the settings drift beyond the established limit, the generator must be recalibrated.

Exposure reproducibility. Generators must be capable of repeating exposures accurately. This is ensured by measuring the mR/mAs of several different exposures with the same technical factors. Computerized dosimeters provide digital readouts or printouts of mR/mAs. Reproducibility should be maintained within ± 5 percent. If the readings are beyond this limit, the entire series of tube and generator tests should be analyzed to attempt to isolate the problem.

Specialized radiographic systems, such as fluoroscopy, tomography, and automatic exposure controls, require additional tests.

Fluoroscopic Systems. The tests for fluoroscopic systems should include the following.

Exposure reproducibility. Fluoroscopic spot film devices use automatic exposure controls (AECs), and they should be evaluated according to the AEC tests that follow.

Exposure rate. Fluoroscopic exposure rates are measured by a dosimeter exactly as diagnostic mR/mAs. The exposure rate should not exceed 5 R/min. If the rate exceeds this limit, the automatic brightness control or other systems may require calibration or repair.

Field size accuracy and beam alignment. As with collimation accuracy in diagnostic radiography, fluoroscopic units should not be capable of irradiating tissue outside the image receptor area. In addition to the evaluation performed for a diagnostic unit, fluoroscopic units should display everything within 1 cm of the edges of the image intensifier tube, and the primary beam should be aligned to the center of the image intensifier. Correction of the tube collimation, image intensification system, or video display system may be required (further testing by a service engineer is necessary).

Source-to-skin distance limits. Fluoroscopic units should not be capable of placing the tube target closer than 15″ (38 cm) (or 12″ [30 cm] for a mobile fluoroscopy unit) to the patient's skin surface (this is a U.S. federal requirement). Without making any exposure, the source-to-image-receptor distance should be verified. If it is not within limits, the unit should not be used until a mechanical device is fitted to set a minimum source-to-skin distance.

Intensifier viewing system resolution. Because fluoroscopic resolution is much poorer than radiographic resolution, periodic assurance that it has not deteriorated is critical in maintaining confidence in diagnosis. A fluoroscopic mesh test tool or a resolution pattern test tool can be imaged to permit visualization of the maximum resolving ability of the system. If the resolution appears to be deteriorating, a service engineer should be consulted.

Intensifier viewing system contrast. Because fluoroscopic contrast is much higher than radiographic contrast, it is important to periodically determine approximately how low contrast a structure may be imaged. Special low-contrast fluoroscopic test tools are available that consist of two plates of aluminum with holes of 1–7 mm drilled in one of the plates. When the plates are sandwiched together and imaged on a fluoroscopy system, low-contrast evaluation can be made based on the smallest visible hole.

Image display systems. Fluoroscopic systems use video systems for image display because of the reduction in patient dose. Although a video signal generator is the test tool of choice, its expense and limited application in radiography usually prohibit its use for routine testing. A fluoroscopic mesh test tool or a resolution test tool and a piece of wire mesh are more commonly used. The resolution test tool can be imaged on the fluoroscopy unit to permit visual measurement of the system resolution. The wire mesh can be imaged to permit visualization of distortion (Figure 31-4). When degradation in resolution or distortion is observed, a service engineer should be consulted.

Automatic brightness control. Although there are a number of types of automatic brightness controls, the term is used here in a generic sense. These controls are designed to function like an AEC in that variations in subject density are automatically compensated for, resulting in a relatively uniform image density. A computerized dosimeter can be used to measure exposure after the beam passes through a phantom. When the phantom thickness is decreased by half, the exposure should be similarly reduced. If there is a great discrepancy between phantom thickness and exposure reduction, a service engineer should be consulted.

Tomographic Systems. The tests for tomographic systems should include the following.

Uniformity and completeness of motion. Tomography relies on the motion of the tube during exposure to produce a sectional image of the subject. Assurance of the uniformity and completeness of tube motion are basic tests. The test tool is simply a lead mask with a pinhole

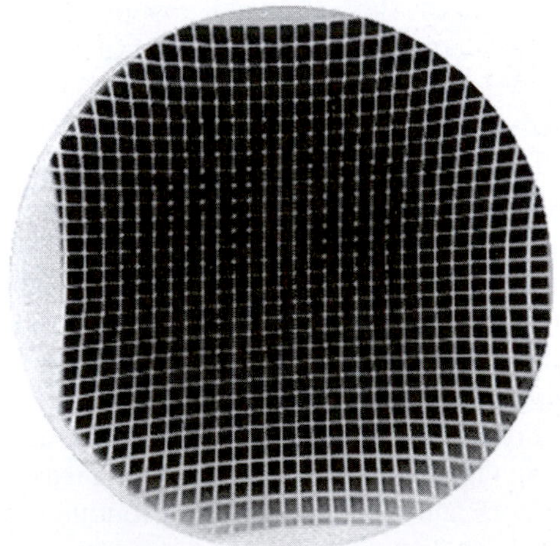

FIGURE 31-4. Normal distortion of a wire mesh test tool imaged with a conventional fluoroscopy system. *(By permission of Mayo Foundation for Medical Education and Research. All rights reserved.)*

that is positioned several centimeters above the tomographic fulcrum. If the pinhole is centered to the image receptor and then imaged with a full tomographic motion, images similar to Figure 31-5 may be obtained. Erratic tube motion is demonstrated by the uneven densities. If the motion were incomplete, there would not be a full length of the tracing. If the motion is erratic or incomplete, the mechanisms involved in the tomographic motion should be cleaned (rails, guidewheels, etc.) and the test repeated. If the problem continues, a service engineer should be consulted.

Section depth indicator accuracy. Tomographic units are designed to provide an image that is sharp (possessing good detail) only at the fulcrum level. Assurance that the fulcrum indicator is accurate is essential in diagnosing the location of structures within the subject. Commercial test tools are available or a penetrometer with lead numbered steps can be used. When a tomographic image is made of the test tool, the number that was at the level of the fulcrum should appear sharp. If it does not, the fulcrum indicator should be adjusted to the appropriate level. Additional testing may be required to ascertain the proper adjustment.

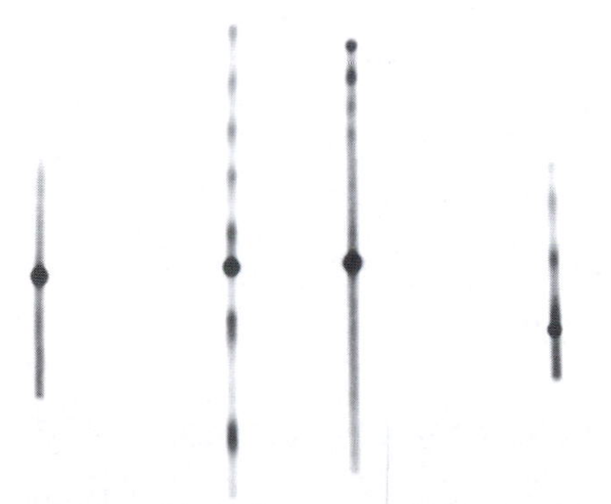

FIGURE 31-5. Tomographic uniformity and completeness of motion test with a pinhole trace image. Both exposures were erratic, as demonstrated by the uneven densities along the entire pinhole exposure. *(By permission of Mayo Foundation for Medical Education and Research. All rights reserved.)*

Section thickness accuracy. The sharp section of a tomograph should be of a known thickness, depending on the total arc of the tomographic motion (exact section thickness per arc is usually stated in the equipment manual). Commercial test tools are available or an angled wire mesh can be used. When the angled resolution mesh is imaged, the section thickness can be determined by measuring the region of sharpness on the image. If the section thickness is inaccurate, the pinhole trace should be consulted. If it appears unacceptable, a service engineer should be consulted.

Resolution. Tomographic resolution is determined by imaging a resolution test pattern at the fulcrum level. The resulting image can be visually inspected to determine the resolving capability of the system. When resolution deteriorates, standard diagnostic quality control measures should be consulted first, then a service engineer.

Automatic Exposure Controls. The tests for automatic exposure controls (AECs) should include the following.

Exposure reproducibility. The same reproducibility standards for diagnostic radiography systems are applied to AECs. Using the same procedure, with the addition of a subject phantom, densitometer readings of images produced with the AEC should be within OD ± 0.1 in the same areas. Reproducibility cannot be achieved on an AEC with dosimeter mR/mAs readings. Radiographs must be produced and measured with a densitometer. If the readings are not within limits, the generator AEC circuits must be calibrated.

Ion chamber sensitivity. Most AECs utilize three ion chambers and permit activation of various combinations during exposures. It is important to ensure that each ion chamber is equally sensitive by comparing the reproducibility of each chamber individually. Exact chamber locations should be verified by producing an image of the ion chambers by using the AEC without a subject at extremely low kVp. After this step is completed, the test is done by using a lead brick to block all chambers but the one to be tested. The AEC reproducibility test is then performed for the unblocked chamber. If all chambers do not respond within ± 10 percent, a service engineer should be consulted to recalibrate the generator AEC circuitry.

IR exposure variation control accuracy. Nearly all AEC units provide controls to decrease and increase image receptor (IR) exposure (density) by changing the sensitivity of the ion chamber. These controls vary tremendously from one unit to another. Consultation of equipment manuals will provide the percentage of change each control is designed to produce. A computerized dosimeter can then be employed to obtain mR/mAs measurements to verify the intensity differences for each control. If the controls are not accurate, the generator AEC circuits must be calibrated.

Response capability. Each AEC has a minimum response capability (which varies with manufacturer and model). If the AEC cannot respond at the minimum time, there is no assurance that diagnostic-quality images can be produced. Response capability is best evaluated by using a computerized dosimeter readout or printout to determine exposure time for AEC exposures made with a small lucite phantom. As the phantom thickness is reduced, the AEC should produce exposures within ±10 percent mR/mAs of one another until a time below the minimum exposure time is used. If the minimum response time is greater than specified, the AEC should not be used until the problem is corrected.

Backup timer verification. Occasionally, even the best radiographers will forget to activate the proper tube or AEC. When this occurs, patient radiation protection requires that AEC backup timers be functioning to terminate exposures and protect both patient and tube. When a lead plate is placed over the AEC ionization chamber and an exposure is made, the backup timer should terminate the exposure and a visual and an audible warning should occur. If the backup timer or signals fail, the AEC should not be used until the problem is corrected.

Digital radiography detectors. Most digital radiography vendors offer a quality control test tool for the periodic evaluation of their detector systems. The primary quality assurance parameter in these systems is known as **detective quantum efficiency (DQE)**. DQE measures the ratio of the transfer efficiency of the detector as the signal-to-noise ratio squared going into the system compared to that coming out. The formula is:

$$SNR^2_{output} / SNR^2_{input}$$

These values range from 0 to 1, with 1 representing a perfect system. Higher DQE values increase the ability to view small or low-contrast structures and are greatly valued in digital mammography systems.

Digital quality assurance tools may also measure other parameters given earlier in this chapter, such as system linearity, contrast evaluation, and so on.

ANCILLARY EQUIPMENT

Ancillary equipment must also be monitored on a regular basis. This includes cassette cleaning, film/screen contact tests, and viewboxes and display monitors.

Cassette Cleaning and Inspection

During normal use, radiographic intensifying screens are exposed to dust and other foreign particles as cassettes are opened during loading and unloading of film. Periodic cleaning of the screens with a specially formulated antistatic solution removes these artifacts and eliminates the potential for misdiagnosis. At the time they are cleaned, cassettes should also be inspected for wear at corners, edges, and especially at hinges. When excessive wear is observed, the cassette should be tested to see if it is lightproof. All cassettes should have a leaded identification number to assist in locating the source of artifacts during use.

Film/Screen Contact

Cassette backs and fronts may warp due to improper storage or traumatic handling. This can lead to loss of contact between the film and the intensifying screen. When poor film-to-screen contact exists, the diverging light photons from the screen cause loss of detail and contrast. A wire mesh test tool should be imaged and the radiograph examined for areas of poor detail. Although rescreening cassettes will replace the pressure pads and sometimes resolve the problem, many institutions prefer to replace the entire cassette.

Viewbox Uniformity

Viewboxes, or illuminators, should emit a uniform intensity of light. One of the greatest sources of misunderstanding between radiographers and radiologists is the difference in light intensity of different viewboxes because it directly affects the perceived radiographic density. When radiographs consistently exhibit different densities on different viewboxes, they become difficult to evaluate. Viewboxes should be monitored with a light meter periodically to alleviate this problem. Viewboxes are measured in NITs, the unit of luminance (1 NIT = 1 candela/m^2). Normal viewboxes emit around 1,700 NIT, whereas mammography viewboxes should be in the 3,500-NIT range. When inconsistencies are discovered, they should be brought to the attention of all professional staff.

Correction of the problem, when many viewboxes are involved, can be expensive because most institutions have collected viewboxes of different models and manufacturers over many years. The thickness and translucency of the plastic surface must be identical for all viewboxes. Differences in the plastic are the most common cause of illumination problems. Old viewboxes may require painting of their reflectors so the exact tone and reflecting ability of the paint matches newer models. Finally, the bulbs of all viewboxes must not only be of the same manufacture and model but should be from the same production run. Attempts to solve viewbox problems should be carried out in the order just described.

Digital Radiography Detector Systems

Digital radiography PSP systems require regular erasure of the plates as well as periodic inspection for cracks and surface markings. Erasure should be performed daily unless all PSPs are used every day. Visual inspection for cracks and surface markings should be performed semiannually (with any plates creating artifacts removed from use immediately in the interval). Semiannual performance of exposure tests is also recommended.

Display Monitors

Digital imaging display monitors require regular quality assurance to ascertain image quality and to monitor phosphor decay. These factors are sometimes referred to as monitor degradation. Both spatial resolution and optical density/brightness must be evaluated on a regular basis.

Spatial resolution is evaluated through the display of a standardized image, the SMPTE test pattern (as shown in Figure 26-1), and a grayscale tool. All three display axes must be evaluated (x, y, and z). The x- and y-axes are evaluated by imaging spatial resolution test tools to evaluate point spread function (PSF), line spread function (LSF), and modulation transfer function (MTF). This measures the matrix and pixel size accuracy. These factors are discussed in detail in Chapter 30. The z axis is evaluated through imaging a grayscale performance tool that is often generated form the storage memory of the monitor itself. This measures the grayscale bit depth. As with all quality assurance, the change in results over time is the critical test. Consequently it is important to maintain a log of the test results for each monitor and to use it to predict when calibration and replacement should be scheduled.

Optical density/brightness is evaluated through measurements of dynamic range with a luminance meter in unit of foot-Lamberts (fL) or candela per square meter (cd/m^2). Dynamic range is measured by setting the greatest visible black-and-white level by using the monitor contrast and brightness controls. Readings from both levels are obtained with a luminance meter. The dynamic range is calculated from the formula:

$$OD = \log (L_{max}/L_{min})$$

The SMPTE test pattern includes a 10-step grayscale that can be used to construct a D log E curve. This curve can be used to monitor grayscale performance over time. Brightness uniformity is the difference between luminance measurements at the center of the display compared to the corner edges. The brightness uniformity specification is 15 percent. When a workstation has more than one monitor, the recommendation is that the luminance measurements match within 5 percent.

PACS SYSTEMS

Because each imaging modality has developed quality assurance measures, the primary quality issue for a PACS system is the accuracy of the interface between the specific modality system and the electronic medical record (EMR) in the hospital information system (HIS) and radiology information system (RIS). Some experts in PACS management recommend that data from any system be held in a storage area (sometimes called the fix-queue or penalty box) until the data can be matched with the modality, HIS, and RIS data or until human intervention resolves the mismatched data. This avoids problems with incomplete patient information being dumped into the PACS, where it adds to unfinished work lists, skews data, and contributes to misfiled patient information. It is also important that a quality check is done on the interface between each element of the PACS system. This should include an item list that is developed with the manufacturer to assure the expectations of the clinical site are being met. One example that is often used is the proper setting for modality autosend switches. These features are designed to permit real-time transmission of images from a modality to the PACS system as the technologist or sonographer completes them. However, service technicians and modality operators may turn them off to increase the speed of the modality functions and may forget to reactivate them so physicians and radiologist assistants have immediate access to the images.

REPEAT-IMAGE STUDIES

The careful analysis of repeated images has proven a valuable aid in diagnosing the radiographic process. Repeated radiographs are also referred to as reject, retake, or double-dose studies. Even excellent repeat-image studies need take little time or effort to pinpoint conditions that may be easily corrected. Significant reductions in patient dose, radiographer time and effort, and supply costs can be achieved with properly executed repeat-image studies.

TABLE 31-2. Causes of Repeated Image

Total exposure		55 percent
Underexposure	34 percent	
Overexposure	21 percent	
Positioning		30 percent
Motion		3 percent

Obtaining Data

A repeat-image study involves retaining all repeated radiographs, regardless of cause, for analysis. Any image outside the acceptance limits and scrap film should be included. Boxes labeled as to cause of repeat should be provided near each processor and the room and tube used should be noted on each image before it is discarded. Typical causes of repeats are shown in Table 31-2.

The most important rule when analyzing repeated images is to not discipline radiographers based on the information obtained. The analysis must be used in a constructive manner to improve working conditions and to point out areas where further technical training may be helpful. Radiographers must be informed of the intent of the study and asked to cooperate in a positive manner to improve both patient care and working conditions. Most radiographers are aware of numerous items they believe contribute to repeat radiographs and welcome an opportunity to find justification for their change. Incompetent radiographers should be disciplined through normal administrative procedures based on actual performance, not as a finding of a repeat-image study. Failure by management to follow this suggestion may result in inaccurate repeat-study data when images are not submitted for analysis.

Analysis of Data

The analysis of collected data begins with the classification and counting of images by cause of repeat, room, tube, and radiographer. Data should also be separated according to time (weekly is most common). The compiled data should be examined for obvious problems. For example, a large number of images from a single room with an artifact in the same location might indicate a barium or iodine stain on a grid or table. Once obvious problems are addressed, the data should be examined for unequal distribution of repeats. Tables 31-3 and 31-4 illustrate how distributions can be diagnosed.

TABLE 31-3. Retake Percentage by Room

	Room #				
Reason	**1**	**2**	**3**	**4**	**5**
Overexposure	29	37	36	33	33
Underexposure	(45)	31	32	32	37
Positioning	20	18	18	19	17
Centering	10	11	(20)	9	9
Motion	6	7	6	5	5
Other	8	6	7	7	6
Total:	118	110	119	105	107

Technique exposure chart error? (Room 1, Underexposure)

Collimator misaligned? (Room 3, Centering)

TABLE 31-4. Retake Percentage by Technologist

	Technologxist #				
Reason	**1**	**2**	**3**	**4**	**5**
Overexposure	35	31	32	30	43
Underexposure	32	31	31	34	30
Positioning	20	18	18	(30)	17
Centering	13	12	11	12	11
Motion	5	(11)	4	4	4
Error	(10)	4	5	3	3
Other	5	7	6	6	7
Total:	120	112	107	119	115

Need to be more careful? (Technologist 1, Error)

Using long exposure times? (Technologist 2, Motion)

Has difficulty with some exams? (Technologist 4, Positioning)

(Tables 31-3 and 31-4 adapted from *Analysis of Retakes: Understanding, Managing and Using an Analysis of Retakes Program for Quality Assurance* [HEW Publication FDA 79-8097], 1979, Rockville, MD: U.S. DHEW, PHS, FDA, Bureau of Radiological Health.)

The **total repeat rate** is a valuable figure to monitor over long periods of time. It is calculated as a percentage of the total number of images produced during the period of the study. The total image figure can be extracted from institutional data in some cases or can be estimated by multiplying the number of examinations by the average number of images produced per examination. For example, a chest unit that produced 600 examinations in a week could be calculated to have produced 1,200 images (PA + lateral × 600). Repeat rates may suffer from a start-up effect where data may not be reliable for the first three weeks due to unfamiliarity with the requirements of the study or various psychological phenomena from stress to hypermotivation. Data indicate that radiographer repeat rates should be between 3 and 10 percent, with the average at 8 percent. One study demonstrated the student reject rates average to be slightly above 9 percent. Data also appear to indicate that when the rate drops below 3 percent there is a problem in data collection or an extremely wide acceptance limit in effect. It is important to realize that repeat rates are not only affected by processing equipment, x-ray equipment, patient condition, and radiographer competence, but also by the acceptance limits of the radiologists. In some instances a high repeat rate may indicate extremely high quality standards in the institution, whereas the same rate may also indicate poor-quality radiographers. Caution in interpretation is essential, and all aspects of the analysis should be carefully studied before conclusions are drawn.

TROUBLESHOOTING

Troubleshooting (locating problems when equipment malfunctions) is a diagnostic process. The same reasoning process that a physician uses to diagnose a disease can be applied to radiographic equipment. Beginning with the symptoms, the radiographer can work step by step through a problem-solving procedure to eliminate possible problems until the source of trouble is isolated.

Although radiographers are not qualified to perform invasive procedures on electronic equipment, they can often pinpoint the general source of the problem. For example, an increase in exposure could be caused by nearly all equipment in the radiographic imaging chain. However, a problem-solving approach may discover that all radiographs have increased exposure, not just the radiographs from a single unit. This might focus attention on the film processor. If the developer temperature is checked and found to be within normal limits, the radiographer might then check the replenishment tank only to discover that it is empty. To solve the problem, the radiographer might fill the tank, remove air locks from the replenishment lines, and restock the developer tank solution. A complete troubleshooting guide is provided in Appendix B.

SUMMARY

Quality assurance consists of activities that provide adequate confidence that a radiology service will render consistently high-quality images and services. Quality assurance includes evaluating activities such as interpretation of examinations, maintenance of equipment, performance of procedures, filing systems, staff development, scheduling of examinations, and supply lines. The quality assurance process operates by identifying problems or potential problem areas, monitoring the problem, and then resolving it.

Quality control is the aspect of quality assurance that monitors technical equipment to maintain quality standards. The concept of quality control is rooted in the need to stabilize the various equipment components of the radiographic imaging chain. From incoming-line current through x-ray production to the processing of the radiograph, erratic equipment performance causes repeat radiographs and unnecessary patient exposure to radiation.

Equipment purchasing decisions should involve each member of the radiological team. Specific imaging requirements should be identified and equipment specifications should be developed. Once the equipment is selected, it is then installed and tested.

Monitoring equipment performance is an integral part of quality assurance. It involves the processing systems as well as the external radiation beams. Ancillary equipment should also be checked.

Monitoring the quality of the processing systems includes routine processor sensitometry and darkroom safelight testing. External beam evaluations involve monitoring the diagnostic radiographic systems, fluoroscopic systems, tomographic systems, and automated exposure controls. Numerous tests on each of the systems are performed to ensure equipment accuracy. Ancillary equipment, such as cassettes viewboxes, and display monitors, are also evaluated. PAC system interface accuracy is also important.

A careful analysis of repeat radiographs is also a valuable aid in diagnosing the radiographic process. Significant reductions in patient dose, radiographer time and effort, and supply costs can be achieved with properly executed repeat-image studies. ■

REVIEW QUESTIONS

1. Why are quality assurance and quality control so important?
2. What factors should be considered when making equipment purchasing decisions?
3. How should film processing systems be monitored?
4. How often should tests be performed on diagnostic radiographic systems?
5. What tests should be performed routinely on the x-ray generator?

6. What tests should be performed routinely on automatic exposure controls?
7. What tests should be performed routinely on digital radiography detectors?
8. Why are repeat-image studies a valuable part of quality assurance?

REFERENCES AND RECOMMENDED READING

Adams, M. J., Barsotti, J. B., Kohler, T. D., & Reel, L. A. (1994). Film processor quality assurance: Increasing reliability while decreasing costs. *American Journal of Roentgenology, 163,* 709–710.

Adler, A. M., & Carlton, R. R. (1989). Repeating radiographs: Critiquing the image. In E. Frank (Ed.), *Postgraduate advances in radiologic technology.* Berryville, VA: Forum Medicum.

Adler, A. M., Carlton, R. R., & Wold, B. (1992a). An analysis of radiographic repeat rate data. *Radiologic Technology, 63*(5), 308–314.

Adler, A. M., Carlton, R. R., & Wold, B. (1992b). A comparison of student radiographic reject rates. *Radiologic Technology, 64*(1), 26–32.

American Association of Physicists in Medicine. (1978). *Diagnostic radiology committee task force on quality assurance protocol: Basic quality control in diagnostic radiology* (AAPM Report No. 4). Chicago: Author.

American College of Radiology. (1981). *Quality assurance in diagnostic radiology and nuclear medicine—the obvious decision* (HEW Publication [FDA] 81–8141). Rockville, MD: U.S. Department of Health, Education, and Welfare, Public Health Service, Food and Drug Administration, Bureau of Radiological Health.

Ardran, G. M., & Crooks, H. E. (1968). Checking diagnostic x-ray beam quality. *British Journal of Radiology, 41,* 193.

Ardran, G. M., Crooks, H. E., & James, V. (1969). Testing x-ray cassettes for film-intensifying screen contact. *Radiography, 35*(414), 143.

Barber, T. C., & Thomas, M. (1983). *Radiologic quality control manual.* Reston, VA: American College of Radiology.

Basart, J. A. (1974). Developer pH: Its significance in quality control. *Radiographic Technology, 45*(6), 413.

Berry, G. C., Starchman, D. E., & Howland, W. J. (1980). Objective equipment selection and performance evaluation. *Radiology Management, 2*(5), 14.

Bowers, J., Lin, P., & Rogers, L. (1978, May 12–13). Impact of equipment specifications on purchases. *Workshop in Purchase Specifications and Performance Evaluation of Radiologic Imaging Equipment Proceedings.* Chicago: Midwest Chapter American Association of Physicists in Medicine, Northwestern University Medical School and Northwestern Memorial Hospital.

Brookstein, J. J., & Steck, W. (1971). Effective focal spot size. *Radiology, 98,* 31–33.

Burkhart, R. L. (1983). *A basic quality assurance program for small diagnostic radiology facilities* (HHS Publication FDA 83–8218). Rockville, MD: U.S. Department of Health and Human Services, Public Health Service, Food and Drug Administration, National Center for Devices and Radiological Health.

Carlton, R. (1980). Establishing a total quality assurance program in diagnostic radiology. *Radiologic Technology, 52,* 23–38.

Carlton, R. R. (1992). Another dimension of quality assurance in radiology. In L. T. Gurley & W. J. Callaway (Eds.), *Introduction to radiologic technology* (3rd ed., pp. 149–166). St. Louis, MO: C. V. Mosby.

Carlton, R. R., & McKenna, A. (1989). Repeating radiographs: Setting imaging standards. In E. Frank (Ed.), *Postgraduate advances in radiologic technology.* Berryville, VA: Forum Medicum.

Carroll, Q. B. (1993). *Fuchs's radiographic exposure, processing, and quality control* (5th ed.). Springfield, IL: Charles C Thomas.

Chu, W. K., Ferguson, S., Wunder, B., Smith, R., & Vanhoutte, J. J. (1979). A two-year reject/retake profile analysis in pediatric radiology. *Health Physics, 42*(1), 53–59.

Corr, B. (1978). A basic quality control system—Part 1. *The Canadian Journal of Medical Radiation Technology, 9*(3), 129.

Corr, B. (1985). Quality control in radiology: An administrative overview. *The Canadian Journal of Medical Radiation Technology, 16*(1), 4.

Crooks, H. E. (1975). Control of image quality, voltage, and filtration. *Radiography, 41*(481), 3.

Crooks, H. E. (1980). A device for checking the speeds and quality of x-ray films and efficiency of film processors. *Radiography, 46*(545), 128.

Cullinan, A., & Cullinan, J. (1994). *Producing quality radiographs* (2nd ed.). Philadelphia: J. B. Lippincott.

Cullinan, J. E. (1981). A "perfect" chest radiograph—or a compromise? *Radiologic Technology, 53*(2), 121.

Dodd, B. C. (1983). Repeat analysis in radiology: A method of quality control. *The Canadian Journal of Medical Radiation Technology, 14*(2), 37.

Dreyer, K., Mehta, A., & Thrall, J. (2002) PACS: A guide to the digital revolution. New York: Springer Verlag.

Eastman, T. R. (1993). Technique charts are vital to quality. *Radiologic Technology, 65*(1), 19.

Eisenberg, R. L., Akin, J. R., & Hedgcock, M. W. (1980, March). Optimal use of portable and stat examination. *American Journal of Roentgenology,* 523–524.

Engel, T. L. (1979). Effect of kilovoltage and milliamperage on focal spot size. *Radiologic Technology, 50*(5), 559.

Everson, J. D., & Gray, J. E. (1987). Focal-spot measurement: Comparison of slit, pinhole, and star resolution pattern techniques. *Radiology, 165*(1), 261–264.

Fairbanks, R., & Doust, C. (1979). Methods for studying the focal spot size and resolution of diagnostic x-ray tubes. *Radiography, 45*(533), 89.

Finney, W. (1999). Introduction to radiographic quality assurance. In P. W. Ballinger (Ed.), *Merrill's atlas of radiographic positions and radiologic procedures* (7th ed., pp. 305–320). St. Louis, MO: C. V. Mosby.

Gilbert, M., & Carlton, W. (1978). Performance evaluations for diagnostic x-ray equipment. *Radiologic Technology, 50,* 243–248.

Gildenhorn, H. L., Rehman, I., Pape, L., & Baker, S. (1960). Standardization of physical factors in radiographic exposures. *Radiology, 75,* 262–267.

Goldman, L. W., & Beech, S. (1979). *Analysis of retakes: Understanding, managing, and using an analysis of retakes program for quality assurance* (HEW Publication [FDA] 79–8097). Rockville, MD: U.S. Department of Health, Education, and Welfare, Public Health Service, Food and Drug Administration, Bureau of Radiological Health.

Gray, J. E., & Trefler, M. (1980). Pinhole cameras: Artifacts, modifications, and recording of pinhole images on screen film systems. *Radiologic Technology, 52*(3), 277.

Gray, J. E., Winkler, N. T., Stears, J. G., & Frank, E. D. (1983). *Quality control in diagnostic imaging: A quality control cookbook.* Rockville, MD: Aspen.

Guglielmo, J. (1980). Processor quality control science. *Radiology Management, 2*(4), 2.

Hall, C. L. (1977). Economic analysis from a quality control program. *Proceedings of the Society of Photo-optical Instrumentation Engineers, 127,* 271–275.

Hangiandreou, N. J., Fetterly, K. A., & Felmlee, J. P. (1999). Optimization of a contrast-detail-based method for electronic image display quality evaluation. *Journal of Digital Imaging, 12*(2), 60–67.

Haus, A. G. (1993). *Film processing in medical imaging.* Madison, WI: Medical Physics.

Hendee, W. R., & Ritenour, R. (1993). *Medical imaging physics* (3rd ed.). St. Louis, MO: C. V. Mosby.

Hendee, W. R., & Rossi, R. P. (1979). *Quality assurance for radiographic x-ray units and associated equipment* (HEW Publication [FDA] 79–8094). Rockville, MD: U.S. Department of Health, Education, and Welfare, Public Health Service, Food and Drug Administration, Bureau of Radiological Health.

Hendee, W. R., & Rossi, R. P. (1980). *Quality assurance for conventional tomographic x-ray units* (HEW Publication [FDA] 80–8096). Rockville, MD: U.S. Department of Health, Education, and Welfare, Public Health Service, Food and Drug Administration, Bureau of Radiological Health.

High and normal speed rotors: Effect on focal spot size, resolution and density. (1981). *Radiologic Technology, 53*(1).

Irfan, A. Y., Pugh, V. I., & Jeffery, C. D. (1985). Some practical aspects of peak kilovoltage measurements. *Radiography, 51*(599), 251–254.

Joint Commission on Accreditation of Healthcare Organizations Diagnostic Radiology Services. (1994). *Accreditation manual for hospitals.* Chicago: Author.

Kalivoda, F. J. (1979, Fall). Ancillary audits in the radiology services: Improving patient care. *Radiology Management,* 2–10.

Kebart, R. C., & James, C. D. (1991). Benefits of increasing focal film distance. *Radiologic Technology, 62*(6), 434–441.

Lam, R. W., & Price, S. C. (1989). The influence of film-screen color sensitivity and type of measurement device on kVp measurements. *Radiologic Technology, 60*(4), 319–321.

Langston, P., Crawley, M. T., & Whiting, G. (2001). Management of an equipment quality control programme in diagnostic radiology. *Radiography, 7*(3), 171–179.

Lowthian, J., & McFadden, B. (1989). Quality control for chest radiography. *Canadian Journal of Medical Radiation Technology, 18*(2), 93–97.

MacLean, B. (1984). Quality Control Report 1981–82: 9 months of operations. *The Canadian Journal of Medical Radiation Technology, 15*(1), 4.

Martell, B., & Gale, J. (2002). Quality assurance on imaging monitors: Design and implementation. *Canadian Journal of Medical Radiation Technology, 33*(4), 3–12.

McEntee, M. F., Brennan, P. C., & Connor, G. O. (2004). The effect of X-ray tube potential on the image quality of PA chest radiographs when using digital image acquisition devices. *Radiography, 10*(4), 287–292.

McFadden, B. (1989). Half value layer calibration. *Canadian Journal of Medical Radiation Technology, 20*(2), 67–74.

McKinney, W. (1988). *Radiographic processing and quality control.* Philadelphia: J. B. Lippincott.

McKinney, W. E. J. (1993). Another look at film processor quality. *Radiologic Technology, 64*(4), 211–212.

McLemore, J. M. (1981). *Quality assurance in diagnostic radiology.* Chicago: Yearbook Medical.

Moores, B. M., Henshaw, E. T., Watkinson, S. A. A., & Pearcy, B. J. (1987). *Practical guide to quality assurance in medical imaging.* New York: Wiley.

National Electrical Manufacturers Association. (1985). *Measurements of dimensions and properties of focal spots of diagnostic x-ray tubes* (NEMA Standards Publication No. XR-5-1984). Rosslyn, VA: Author.

Nelson, M. T. (1994). Continuous quality improvement (CQI) in radiology: An overview. *Applied Radiology, 23*(7), 11–16.

Nelson, R. E., Barnes, G. T., & Witten, D. M. (1977). Economic analysis of a comprehensive quality assurance program. *Radiologic Technology, 49,* 129–134.

Paleen, R., Skundberg, P. A., & Schwartz, H. (1989). How much is quality assurance costing your department? *Radiology Management, 11*(1), 24.

Papp, J. (2006). *Quality management in the imaging sciences* (3rd ed.). St. Louis. MO: Mosby Elsevier.

Pirtle, O. L. (1994). X-ray machine calibration: A study of failure rates. *Radiologic Technology, 65*(5), 291–298.

Potsaid, M. S., Rhea, J. T., & Llewellyn, H. J. (1978, June). Quality assessment and assurance in diagnostic imaging. *Radiology,* 583–588.

Price, R. (1981). The continuous assessment of x-ray tubes and generators. *Radiography, 47*(553), 2.

Pugin, M. (1986). Teaching quality control in radiological imaging. *The Canadian Journal of Medical Radiation Technology, 17*(4), 14.

Rhatigan, L., & Montague, E. (1987). Computerized quality assurance. *Radiologic Technology, 58*(6), 523.

Roehrig, H. (1999a). Image quality assurance for CRT display systems. *Journal of Digital Imaging, 12*(1), 1–2.

Roehrig, H. (1999b). Image quality assurance for CRT display systems—Part II. *Journal of Digital Imaging, 12*(2), 49.

Rogers, K. D., Matthews, I. P., & Roberts, C. J. (1987). Variation in repeat rates between 18 radiology departments. *The British Journal of Radiology, 60,* 463–468.

Rouse, S., & Cowen, A. R. (1983). Quality assurance of fluorographic camera systems. *Radiography, 49*(587), 251.

Rozenfeld, M., & Jette, D. (1984, January). Quality assurance of radiation dosage: Usefulness of redundancy. *Radiology,* 241.

Siegel, E., & Kolodner, R. (2001). *Filmless radiology.* New York: Springer.

Stears, J. G., Gray, J. E., Webbles, W. E., & Frank, E. D. (1985). X-ray waveform monitoring for radiographic quality control. *Radiologic Technology, 57*(1), 9–15.

Stears, J. G., Gray, J. E., Webbles, W. E., & Frank, E. D. (1989). Radiologic exchange (kVp measurements). *Radiologic Technology, 60*(3), 233–236.

Stein, K. M. (2000). Quality assurance in CT. *Radiologic Technology, 72*(1), 67.

Sweeney, R. J. (1983). *Radiographic artifacts: Their cause and control.* Philadelphia: J. B. Lippincott.

Thompson, M. A., Hattaway, M. P., Hall, J. D., & Dowd, S. B. (1994). *Principles of imaging science and protection.* Philadelphia: W. B. Saunders.

Thornhill, P. J. (1987). Quality assurance in diagnostic radiography: Are we using it correctly and what is its future? *Radiography, 53*(610), 161–163.

Watkinson, S., & Moores, B. M. (1984). Reject analysis: Its role in quality assurance. *Radiography, 50*(593), 189–194.

Watkinson, S., Shaw, M., Moores, B. M., & Eddleston, E. (1983). Quality assurance: A practical programme. *Radiography, 49*(578), 27.

Watkinson, S. A. (1985). Economic aspects of quality assurance. *Radiography, 51*(597), 133.

Wheeler, W. N. (1980). Equipment specifications and performance standards for equipment pertaining to the nuclear medicine department. *Radiology Management, 2*(5), 43.

World Health Organization. (1982). *Quality assurance in diagnostic radiology.* Geneva: Author.

Zimmer, E. A. (1960). *Artifacts and handling and processing faults on x-ray films.* New York: Grune & Stratton.

The Case of the Deep Sea Rodeo

This creature was radiographed after a sojourn in the deep. What is it?

Answers to the case studies can be found in Appendix B. (Reprinted by permission of the International Society of Radiographers and Radiological Technicians from K. C. Clark Archives, Middlesex Hospital, London, England, Courtesy of Dr. Marion Frank)

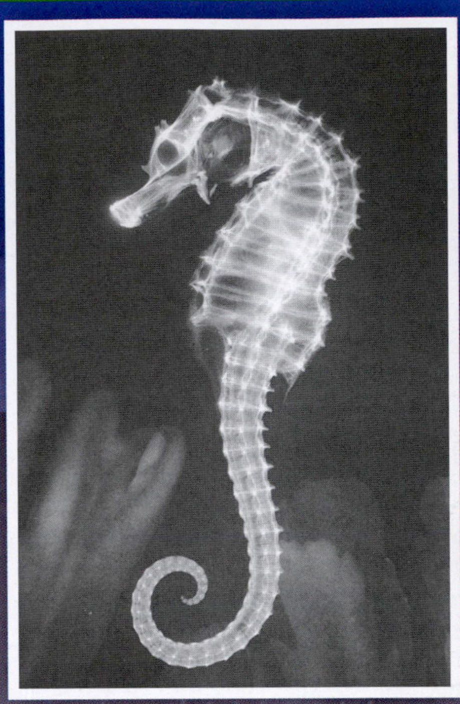

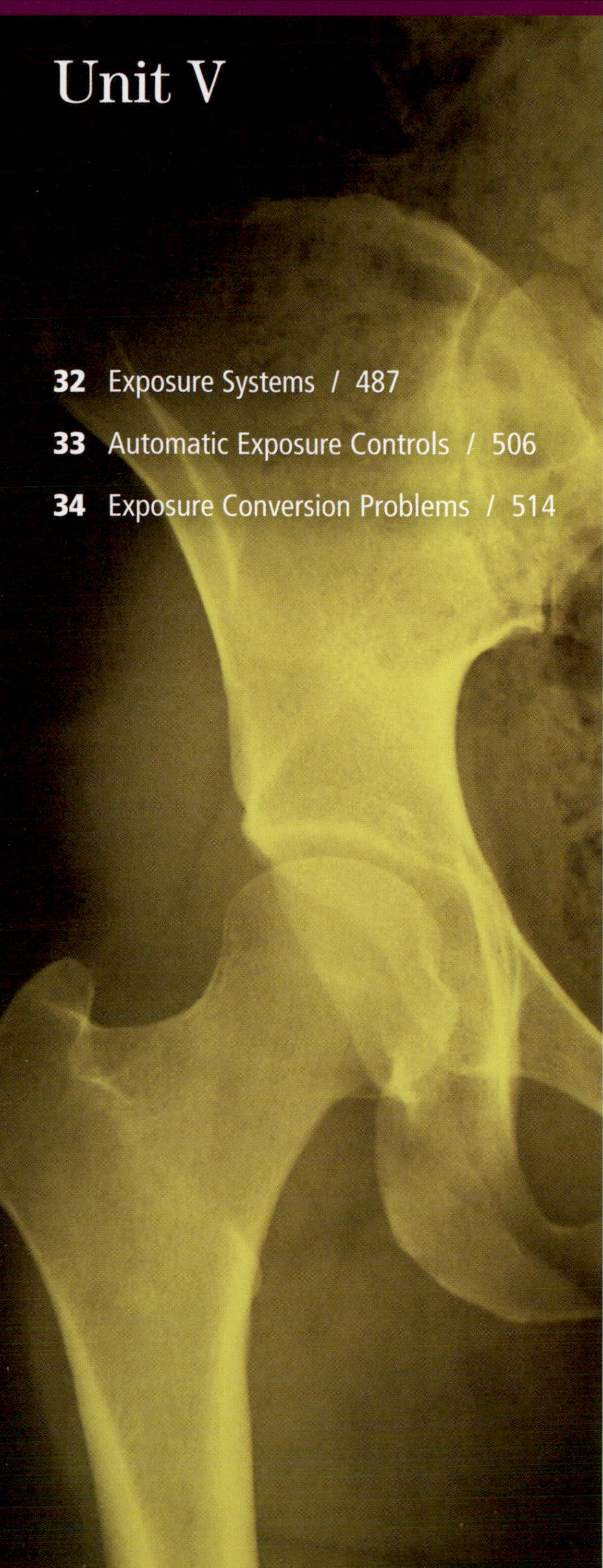

Unit V

Comparing Exposure Systems

32 Exposure Systems / 487

33 Automatic Exposure Controls / 506

34 Exposure Conversion Problems / 514

Once thorough background knowledge has been acquired, the radiographer must then analyze the clinical conditions and synthesize the information into a workable exposure system. The objective is to provide a method of producing consistent image quality. Consistency facilitates the diagnostic process by permitting more valid comparisons between examinations and confidence in the amount of information presented in the image. A balance must exist between image quality, patient situation, and dose.

This unit presents various exposure systems that have been developed and assists in evaluating which system is most appropriate for particular clinical situations. This process is especially important in digital radiography. All radiographers must have a thorough understanding of how an exposure system functions if it is to be used successfully. The practice of radiography involves so many nonroutine situations, unusual conditions, and unique patients that simply following guidelines established by someone else does not permit the radiographer with the necessary skills to provide the patient with the best quality of care.

It is even more important to establish appropriate exposure factors when using computed or digital radiography systems and automatic exposure control (AEC) devices (phototimers). These automated systems cannot function unless the incoming photons are at the correct intensity and proper attenuation ranges to permit the computer or mechanical system to provide an appropriate range of input data for the processing of the image.

Because of the tremendous number of variables in the radiographic imaging chain, the most successful exposure systems maintain them all except a single variable for a given range of conditions. For example, a variable kVp system maintains all factors except kVp, which is varied to obtain appropriate exposures for different subject densities and contrasts. This unit begins with a technical discussion on **exposure systems** and charts as a guide to establishing functional systems for clinical practice. This includes specific details in the development of fixed kVp systems and variable kVp systems, the most popular exposure systems. **Automatic exposure controls** follows and is used for more exposures than any other system. A full chapter of **exposure conversion problems** provides methods for solving complex problems similar to the nonroutine situations that arise in practice.

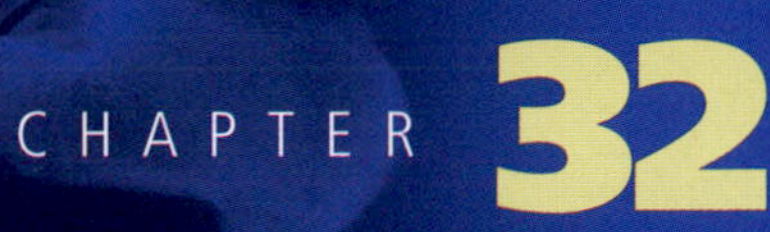

CHAPTER 32

Exposure Systems

KEY TERMS

anatomically programmed radiography
caliper
optimal kVp
patient equivalent phantom

> [The radiograph] is not an anatomical snapshot taken at random.
>
> *Arthur W. Fuchs, Preface to the first edition of Principles of Radiographic Exposure and Processing*

OBJECTIVES

Upon completion of this chapter, the student should be able to:

- Compare various exposure systems.
- Describe the advantages and disadvantages of fixed and variable kVp systems.
- Discuss other exposure systems that have influenced radiographic technique.
- Explain why measurement of part thickness is critical to the accurate use of technique systems.
- Describe the function of the radiographer when using automatic exposure control systems.
- Describe how programmed exposure control systems function.
- State the steps necessary to establish a technique system.
- Explain a basic phantom testing procedure.
- Describe the process of selecting an optimal image range.
- Extrapolate a technique system from a limited number of phantom test images.
- Describe the clinical trial and fine-tuning processes.

OBJECTIVES (continued)

- Describe the principles of fixed kVp technique theory.
- Define optimal kilovoltage.
- Explain how to establish fixed kVp for various subject parts.
- Describe the steps in establishing a fixed kVp technique system.
- Synthesize a fixed kVp technique system from control radiographs.
- Describe a variable kilovoltage technique system.
- State the 2-kVp/cm rule.
- Explain why more than a single kilovoltage scale is required.
- Calculate new exposure factors from a single satisfactory exposure when mAs ratios are provided.

EXPOSURE SYSTEM SELECTION

The foundations of the principles of radiographic exposure technique were laid in the 1920s by Ed. C. Jerman, known as the father of radiologic technology in the United States, and were developed into a scientific system in the 1940s by Arthur W. Fuchs.

Because radiographic exposure is such a complex process, technique systems function best when the large number of variables can be held constant while a single factor is permitted to vary. The goal of any radiographic exposure system is to provide a method of consistency in the quality of image production. These systems are often incorporated into preprogrammed control consoles through exposure factors. It is important to remember that they are suggested starting points that should be revised by the radiographer as necessary. Failure to follow this practice results in a higher personal repeat rate and excessive patient dose.

A radiography department can expect to produce consistent results only when technique systems are used for all x-ray units. Monitoring and revising these systems are part of the quality control function. Utilizing an accurate technique system is equally important with digital imaging systems.

Each exposure system has its advantages and disadvantages, and professionals quickly develop a rationale for their favorite system. The student must study each system in detail to learn its advantages and disadvantages before forming a personal professional judgment. It is important to recognize that any exposure system is designed to provide consistency in image quality and requires that all users of equipment in a single institution adhere to the same technique systems. Nearly all variables in exposure systems are changed according to the thickness of the anatomical part being radiographed. No exposure system can be expected to function accurately unless the radiographer measures part thickness. Part thicknesses for various regions in the average adult were detailed by Arthur Fuchs (Table 32-1).

It remains important to use calipers to determine body part size, and in fact this is probably the single most important quality control measure when not utilizing automatic exposure controls (AECs) (commonly called phototimers).

The device used to measure a part thickness is a **caliper**. Improper use of a caliper will result in improper technical factors and a repeated exposure. Caliper measurements are made either by central ray entrance and exit or by thickest part. It is critical that all radiographers using a particular technique chart measure by the same method and in exactly the same manner.

Central ray measurements should be made from the point of central ray entrance to exit. For example, in Figure 32-1, the chest should be measured at point B, not point A or C. Thickest part measurements should be made at the thickest part of the area of interest. If another special measurement point or method has been established, it must be followed by all users of the chart.

Although personal philosophy may differ from institutional procedures and policies, the professional must let personal preference become secondary to the primary goal of widespread consistency

TABLE 32-1. Average Adult Part Thickness by Region

Region		Average Thickness Adult—CMS AP	PA	Lat	Percent Frequency
Thumb, Fingers		1.5–4			99
Hand		3–5			99
				7–10	93
Wrist		3–6			99
				5–8	98
Forearm		6–8			94
				7–9	92
Elbow		6–8			96
				7–9	87
Arm		7–10			95
				7–10	94
Shoulder		12–16			79
Clavicle			13–17		82
Foot		6–8			
				7–9	
Ankle		8–10			
				6–9	
Leg		10–12			
				9–11	92
Knee		10–13			91
				9–12	86
Thigh		14–17			96
				13–16	85
Hip		17–21			76
Cervical	C1–3	12–14			77
Vertebrae	C4–7	11–14			98
	C1–7			10–13	90
Thoracic Vertebrae		20–24			76
				28–32	81
Lumbar Vertebrae		18–22			69
				27–32	77
Pelvis		19–23			78
Skull			18–21		96
				14–17	88
	Frontal		08-31		97
Sinuses	Max.		18–22		88
				13–17	96
Mandible				10–12	82
Chest			20–25		82
				27–32	84

Reprinted with permission of the American Society of Radiologic Technologists from Arthur W. Fuchs's "Relationship of Tissue Thickness to Kilovoltage." *The X-ray Technician* [now *Radiologic Technology*] *19*(6), 287–293, 1948.

in image quality. The following information outlines three exposure systems: fixed kVp, variable kVp, and anatomically programmed radiography systems.

Fixed Kilovoltage Systems

Fixed kVp systems were developed by Fuchs in 1943 during World War II. They have strong theoretical support in the literature and among many radiographers because they tend to decrease patient dose, provide more information on the image, increase the

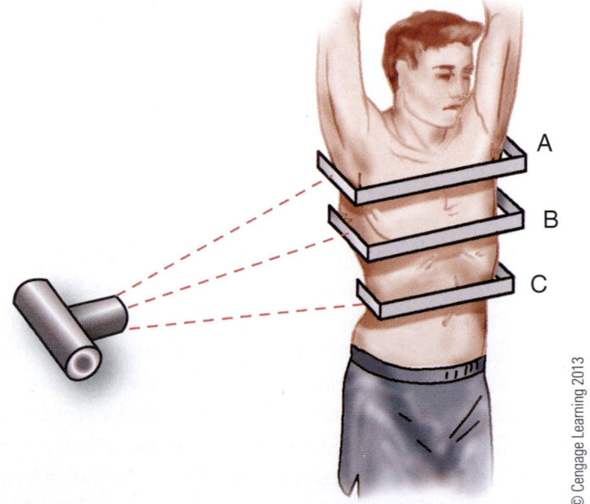

FIGURE 32-1. Proper caliper measurement of part thickness by using the central ray entrance-to-exit method as shown in B.

consistency of image receptor exposure, lengthen exposure latitude, reduce x-ray tube wear, decrease time settings and therefore patient motion, and are easier to remember. However, these systems produce more scatter radiation, which tends to provide a lower contrast than a variable kilovoltage system. Low contrast is usually perceived as less pleasing to the eye and for this reason many institutions have not adopted the fixed kVp system.

Variable Kilovoltage Systems

Variable kVp systems were the first methodical approach to radiographic technique. They were proposed by Jerman in 1925 and predominated until x-ray generators became powerful enough to support fixed kVp techniques in the 1940s. They permit small incremental changes in exposure to compensate for variation in body part thickness. Most x-ray generators permit finer adjustment of kVp stations than of time or mA settings. Variable kVp systems produce higher-contrast images, which enhance the visibility of fine detail and increase the perception of resolution. Institutions that have not adopted a variable kVp system cite the overwhelming advantages of fixed kVp to patient dose, image information, tube wear, and so on.

Anatomically Programmed Radiography Systems

Anatomically programmed radiography (APR) systems are commonly utilized computerized exposure control units that combine an automatic exposure control (AEC) system with exposure factors to correspond to specific anatomical procedures (Figure 32-2). The control console provides choice of an anatomical region along with suggested exposure factors. For example, when the radiographer selects a lumbar spine, a screen may provide a choice of projections. When the lateral projection is indicated, a suggested series of exposure factors may be set on the x-ray console. However, if the radiographer determines that nonroutine conditions exist, the exposure factors can be modified prior to exposure. The computerized control can be programmed to display any desired exposure system and then be fine-tuned to meet existing needs.

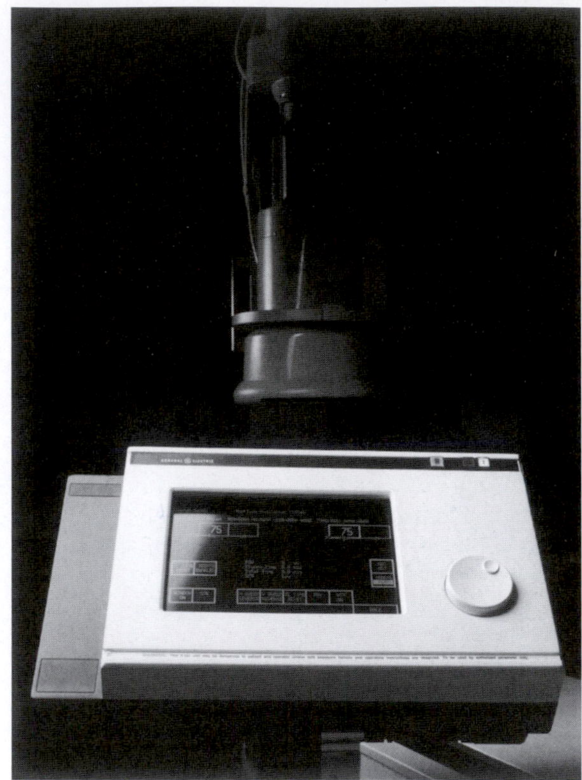

FIGURE 32-2. A programmed, computerized exposure control console. *(Courtesy of GE Healthcare.)*

When APR systems are used, they incorporate AEC devices in their programmed exposure factors. When AEC systems are used, the selection of exposure time factors, and thereby mAs selection, is eliminated. The radiographer must still exercise professional judgment to determine all other factors, including mA (which can be used to influence the time), kVp, distance, and so on. Part of the art of phototiming is learning when to use AECs and when to avoid them.

ESTABLISHING AN EXPOSURE SYSTEM

The process of establishing an exposure system begins with collecting exposure data. The first step is to make a single exposure that produces an optimal diagnostic-quality image. This original image must be at the optimal center of the acceptance limits curve. Although any projection can be used as a starting point in collecting data, it is preferred that the first data be from a subject part size and kVp in the middle of the diagnostic range. Ideal part sizes are 10–25 cm and ideal kilovoltage is in the 60–80 range. Figure 32-3 illustrates the steps in establishing an exposure system.

Initial Phantom Images

Initially, a series of test exposures is made to determine the optimal-quality image. This is accomplished by using an appropriate phantom to produce images at a variety of technical factor combinations both above and below the average level. It is essential that the exposure remain the same at a control point to avoid misperception of the contrast range. It is preferred that the images be produced using an AEC to control the exposure. If an AEC is not available, or cannot be used due to other circumstances, an exposure or density reference control point must be established and measured with a densitometer. For example, the exact center of the body of L4 could be measured on each image. It would be necessary to adjust milliampere-second values until all images exhibit the same exposure index numbers. An anatomical phantom can be used to achieve this. With film screen systems the recommendation was to set control point densities within OD 0.3 of one another.

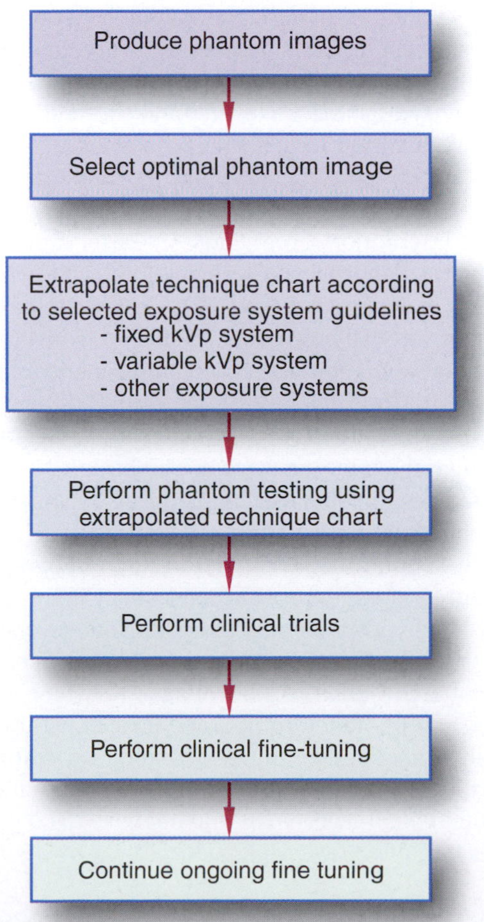

FIGURE 32-3. A systematic approach to establishing a technique chart.

Select Optimal Phantom Image

Once the series of phantom test images has been produced, it should be shown to radiologists and supervisory radiographers. These professionals should not be asked to select the best image but to select those images they believe to be outside acceptance limits, because when any group of professionals is asked to select the best image there will be differences of opinion, leaving no consensus as to which is the best image. Conversely, elimination of those images that are not acceptable will often result in a series of images that are acceptable to all, although "perfect" to only a few.

Extrapolate Technique Chart

Next, a series of preliminary clinical trials should be performed by preparing an exposure system that adjusts current technical factors to those that are newly established as optimal. Particular attention should be given to projections that have a narrow range of part thicknesses or few choices of technical factors. For example, the variations in a wrist or PA chest chart both require careful calculation, the wrist because the normal thickness range encompasses only about 3 cm and the PA chest because the extremely high kVp with a normal thickness range of only about 5 cm amplifies minute changes in mAs.

Phantom Testing

The new chart is then tested with a phantom to verify its effectiveness. Minimum phantom testing should include a median, small, and large part thickness. At this point the system is completed for all part thicknesses for each projection.

Clinical Trials

Finally, a limited series of clinical trial examinations should be performed using the new system. Each examination should be recorded and all repeated images should be saved for analysis. The series of clinical examinations should then be shown to each person who participated in the determination of the original standards. If the new image quality is accepted, a new exposure system should be designed and implemented. If the new image quality experiences limited acceptance, adjustments should be made to satisfy deficiencies and all of the phantom testing and clinical trial steps should be repeated. Under no circumstance should clinical trials be performed until phantom testing and the other preliminary steps have been properly completed. Whenever new equipment is added to the imaging chain, especially a new x-ray tube or a new image receptor system, the phantom testing and/or clinical trial steps should be repeated until confidence is reestablished.

Clinical Fine-Tuning

Clinical fine-tuning requires that the technical factors for each exposure be recorded, regardless of whether the image is within acceptance limits. Each image is then used to fine-tune the system. Excellent-quality images permit technical factors for the part thicknesses to be verified, whereas all other images permit adjustments of the technical factors for their respective part sizes.

Ongoing Fine-Tuning

It is important that a system of ongoing fine-tuning be established as a quality control monitoring method. The quality control radiographer should be consulted whenever a technique chart produces an unacceptable exposure and the cause is not evident. A series of unexplained rejected images may signify a change in one of the system's components that can be determined by quality control testing. The problem can often be fixed by a service engineer, although aging processes (such as filament wear, focal spot deterioration, and tube gas) may require adjustments of the exposure system.

ESTABLISHING FIXED KILOVOLTAGE EXPOSURE SYSTEMS

Because radiographic exposure is such a complex process, technique systems function best when the large number of variables can be held constant while a single factor is permitted to vary. In a fixed kilovoltage system, the kVp is held constant for a given range of subject densities and contrasts while the mAs is varied to achieve an appropriate image receptor exposure. The kVp has a profound effect on many radiographic factors, such as contrast, type of interaction, production of scatter radiation, and average photon energy. In addition, it varies depending on generator phase, filtration, machine calibration, intensifying-screen phosphor conversion efficiency, subject inner-shell binding energy range, and so on. Consequently, an exposure system that makes kVp a constant eliminates the effects of these variables on the system. The basis of a fixed kilovoltage exposure system therefore becomes the concept of the optimal kilovoltage peak.

In keeping with the goal of any radiographic exposure system to provide consistency in the quality of image production, a fixed kilovoltage system provides a relatively uniform contrast and an easily remembered series of kilovoltages to which mAs values can be added to produce images within established acceptance limits. The uniform contrast contributes to radiologists' confidence in the information in the image, as they do not have to contend with a variable grayscale.

Advantages and Disadvantages

There are a number of advantages to the fixed kilovoltage exposure systems. These systems tend to decrease patient dose, because the kilovoltage is always at the maximum possible level, and this permits decreased mAs in compensation. The decreased mAs contributes to decreased patient exposure. In addition, the consistency in kVp levels results in uniform contrast, permitting the radiologist to compare images of a given projection or patient, and provides more confidence in the diagnostic process. The higher average kVp that the optimal kVp concept produces lengthens exposure latitude. It also decreases mAs, thereby decreasing the average mA, which lowers x-ray tube heating and extends tube life, and/or decreasing time, which reduces the possibility of patient motion.

There are also disadvantages to a fixed kilovoltage exposure system. These systems tend to provide a lower overall contrast than do variable kilovoltage systems, and this is usually perceived by radiologists as less pleasing to the eye. Without question, the lower contrast produces much more scattered radiation and images that are less artistically beautiful. Additionally, small incremental changes in exposure for variations in body part thickness may not be possible with systems that fix kVp and vary mAs, due to less variety in mA stations and exposure times as compared to the kVp settings.

Optimal Kilovoltage Peak

The **optimal kVp** is the maximum kVp level that will produce images with appropriate contrast that are consistently within acceptance limits. This kVp level must ensure sufficient penetration of the subject as well as provide acceptable image contrast. Insufficient penetration of the area of interest, especially in contrast media studies, limits the diagnostic region to the edges of the contrast media. Sufficient penetration permits visualization through the contrast media and increases the diagnostic information available.

The use of the maximum kVp as optimal causes a corresponding decrease in the mAs required to produce acceptable density/image receptor (IR) exposure. The mAs reduction contributes to both reduced mA and time. Reduced mA decreases x-ray tube heating and prolongs filament and anode life. Reduced time minimizes the possibility of patient motion. The optimal kVp produces lower contrast and the minimum patient exposure. The fixed kVp system takes advantage of the only situation in radiography where image quality can be increased (low contrast and therefore more diagnostic shades of gray) and patient exposure decreased (less mAs and therefore less mR/mAs).

Establishing Optimal Kilovoltage Peak

Numerous optimal kVps are established for a fixed kVp system; each is specific for a range of subject densities and contrasts. In other words, the so-called fixed kVp is fixed only for a specific range of part thicknesses for a particular procedure. For example, where 80 kVp may be selected as the optimal kVp for noncontrast media abdominal examinations, 50 kVp may be determined to be the maximum for contrast that is acceptable for imaging the trabeculae of the smaller extremities. The optimal kVp should not be changed unless the conditions under which it was set have changed, or the acceptance limits are changed.

Initial Phantom Images

Setting up a fixed kVp system requires that a series of test exposures be obtained to determine the optimal kVp. This is accomplished by using an abdomen or pelvis phantom to produce images at a variety of kVps above and below the average level. It is essential that the exposure remain the same at a control point to avoid misperception of the contrast range (Figure 32-4). It is preferred that the images be exposed using an AEC, although an exposure or density reference control point can be used.

Select Optimal Phantom Image

Once the series of phantom test images has been produced, the optimal phantom image must be selected. The objective of optimal kVp is to determine the highest kVp and lowest contrast that is within acceptance limits, not the best image. The optimal kVp is the highest of the acceptable images. Remember that this process is one of elimination, not of selection. In other words, radiologists and quality control radiographers should be asked to eliminate unacceptable images, not to choose the single best-quality image.

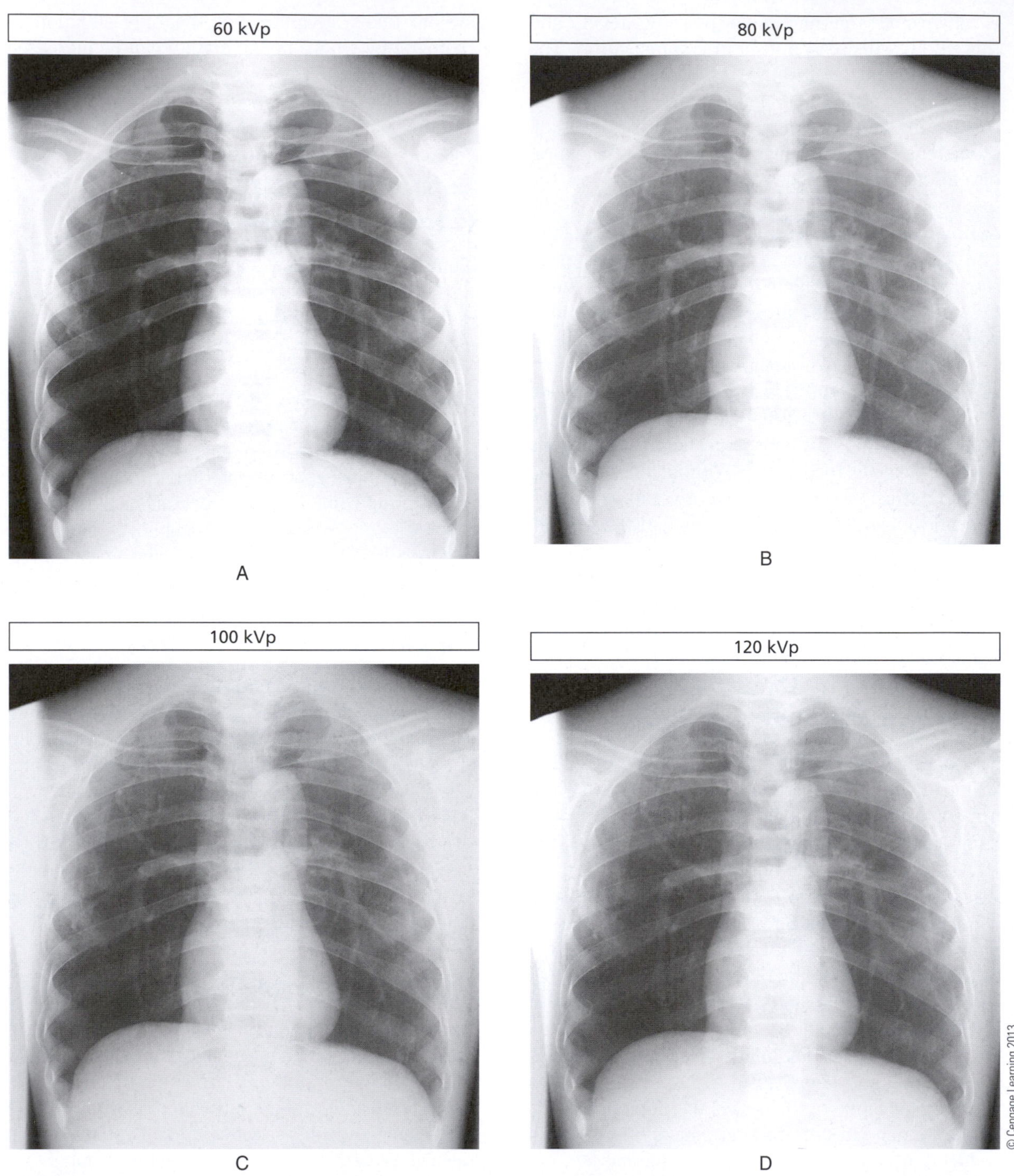

FIGURE 32-4. A series of chest images produced at 60, 80, 100, and 120 kVp to determine the optimal kVp. Whereas 60 kVp may be selected as optimal for ribs, 12 kVp may be determined to be optimal for the chest.

TABLE 32-2. Common Optimal kVp Ranges for the Major Body Regions

Region	Optimal kVp Range
Small extremities	50–60
Iodine-based contrast media studies	68
Large extremities	70
Skull	80
Abdomen and ribs	80
AP vertebral column	80
Lateral vertebral column	90
Chest	120
Barium-based contrast media studies	120

Careful consideration must be given to the variety of subject densities and contrasts in the human body before establishing the optimal kVps for other procedures. Table 32-2 illustrates common optimal kVp ranges for the major body regions, but individual requirements often vary.

Extrapolate Technique Chart

Once the optimal kVp has been determined, an extrapolated exposure chart should be obtained by adjusting current technical factors to the newly established optimal kVp.

Milliampere-seconds is designed to be the primary variable for a fixed kVp exposure system. The mAs values for the technique chart must be set at minimum increments of 30 percent because values less than 30 percent are not significant.

Because there is no linearity with some of the exposure variables, no accurate formula can be given for extrapolating mAs values. However, most systems have been found to operate in the range of doubling or halving the mAs for every 5 cm of subject thickness. For example, if 80 mAs produces a diagnostic-quality image of a 20-cm part, a 15-cm part will require about 40 mAs, whereas a 25-cm part will require about 160 mAs. This is often applied to variable kVp technique systems as a "2-kVp/cm rule," which is fairly consistent with the 15 percent rule and ensures sufficient penetration.

Phantom Testing

Phantom testing is recommended prior to performing patient examinations. As a minimum, phantom testing should be done for a medium, small, and large part size. Because of the nonlinearity of the exposure systems and the inadequacy of the 15 percent rule, phantom testing should always be employed when the part size is less than 10 cm or the kVp is outside the median diagnostic range of 60–80.

Phantom testing also serves as a fine-tuning mechanism for the extrapolated chart prior to clinical use. Once several mAs values have been set, extrapolation of the mAs for subject thickness can be done accurately. For example, if 68 kVp is set as the optimal fixed kVp for iodine-based contrast media abdominal work, a technique chart might be established from a base diagnostic-quality 20-cm phantom image at 50 mAs (Table 32-3). Step 1 illustrates a blank chart with the phantom technique. Using the 15 percent rule, several additional mAs values can be extrapolated for phantom testing, as shown in Step 2. Upon phantom testing, the extrapolated mAs values may require fine-tuning, as shown in Step 3. Once phantom fine-tuning is accomplished, the extrapolation of the final mAs values can be completed, as shown in Step 4. At this point the chart has been proven within acceptance limits by phantom testing and is ready for clinical trials.

Clinical Trials

Limited clinical trials are permissible with the new chart. All images should be recorded, with repeated images saved for analysis. When clinical trials are proceeding without excess repeated exposures, the new technique chart can move into the clinical fine-tuning stage.

Clinical Fine-Tuning

The clinical fine-tuning process will adjust and finally validate the entire chart. At this point the new technique chart can be adopted. However, ongoing fine-tuning then begins as a permanent process.

TABLE 32-3. Fixed kVp Technique Chart

Blank Chart with Phantom Technique			Extrapolation of Additional mAs Values	Fine-Tuning of Extrapolated mAs Values	Extrapolation of Final mAs Values
cm	kVp	Step 1 mAs	Step 2	Step 3	Step 4
16	68				30
17	68				35
18	68				40
19	68				45
20	68	50	50	50	50
21	68				60
22	68				70
23	68				80
24	68				90
25	68		100	100	100
26	68				115
27	68				130
28	68				145
29	68				160
30	68		200	180	180
31	68				215
32	68				250
33	68				285
34	68				320
35	68		400	360	360

Ongoing Fine-Tuning

Ongoing fine-tuning is the process that maintains the accuracy of the entire exposure system and gives radiographers and radiologists confidence in the exposure and diagnostic processes.

ESTABLISHING A VARIABLE KILOVOLTAGE PEAK EXPOSURE SYSTEM

A variable kilovoltage x-ray exposure technique system is one in which the kilovoltage to be used for a particular projection is varied depending on measured body part thickness. The thicker the body part, the higher the value of kilovoltage assigned. A milliampere-second value is specified for each body part to be examined. Its value depends on image receptor exposure and other parameters.

In use, the radiographer sets the mAs specified for the part and measured part thickness. The value of kVp corresponding to that thickness is found on the chart. For example, in Table 32-1, a 12-cm-thick part will require 54 kVp (e.g., an average shoulder).

Advantages and Disadvantages

Technique systems that use variable kilovoltage offer the advantage of permitting small incremental changes in exposure to compensate for variation in body part thickness. These changes in exposure may not be possible with systems that fix kilovoltage and vary milliampere-seconds because of an insufficient number of settings on the exposure timers of many x-ray generators.

A potential disadvantage of the variable kilovoltage technique arises when one considers the complexity of the effect of changing kilovoltage on the way the subject is imaged. Increasing kilovoltage reduces image contrast. Reducing contrast may be helpful if the initial kilovoltage is too low to provide adequate penetration of the part (Figure 32-5A). The reduction in contrast that occurs when kilovoltage is too high can reduce the radiologist's ability to see fine detail in the image (Figure 32-5C). A useful variable kilovoltage system must use values of kilovoltage that provide adequate penetration of the part and result in a level of contrast that is acceptable to the radiologist (Figure 32-5B). This is shown in Table 32-4.

The radiation exposure to the patient is strongly dependent on the kilovoltage used for the projection. In general, the higher the kilovoltage, the lower the patient dose. When kilovoltage is at an appropriate level for the body part examined, patient dose considerations are less of a factor when deciding whether to establish an exposure system using fixed or variable kVp.

Historical Development

In the early days of radiography it was common practice to use a change of 2 kVp for every 1 cm of tissue thickness. A kilovoltage progression could be readily computed by taking two times the centimeter measurement. To this value a constant, such as 30 kVp, was added to achieve a kVp value high enough to penetrate the part. This produces a basic variable kVp formula:

$$(2 \text{ kVp} \times \text{part cm}) + 30 \text{ kVp} = \text{new kVp}$$

It was found that multiple kilovoltage scales were needed because the values selected from the progression could be too low to provide adequate penetration of body parts, such as the shoulder or cervical spine, which contain dense bone with little soft tissue (Table 32-5A). Higher kilovoltage scales were created by increasing the base kilovoltage added. For example, if kilovoltage were computed using 40 kVp instead of 30 kVp, the formula would be:

$$(2 \text{ kVp} \times \text{part cm}) + 40 \text{ kVp} = \text{new kVp}$$

All values would be correspondingly higher with the new formula. For example, the values of shoulder and cervical spine views measuring 12 cm would be 64 kVp instead of the 54 kVp previously obtained. By increasing or decreasing the value of kVp added as a constant, it is possible to create an array of kilovoltage scales. The scales shown in Table 32-5A–C were computed using 30, 40, and 50 kVp as the constant:

$$(2 \text{ kVp} \times \text{part cm}) + 30 \text{ kVp} = \text{new kVp}$$
$$(2 \text{ kVp} \times \text{part cm}) + 40 \text{ kVp} = \text{new kVp}$$
$$(2 \text{ kVp} \times \text{part cm}) + 50 \text{ kVp} = \text{new kVp}$$

Note that the kilovoltage values for a 20-cm-thick body part are shown as 70 kVp, 80 kVp, and 90 kVp, depending on the scale selected.

Changes of 10 kVp in the base number added were used in the belief that a change of ±10 kVp would compensate for doubling and halving mAs. In practice 30, 40, or 50 can be easily added to centimeters, doubled by the radiographer mentally, and the assigned value of kVp can thus be readily determined when systems are not available. Milliampere-second values were found by trial and error but, once determined, were listed for a particular body part and kilovoltage selected by measuring the part. A useful technique chart was thus created.

It was found in practice that 80 kVp for a 20-cm abdomen using equipment and image receptors of the time was nearly ideal. In 1948, Fuchs suggested that kVp be fixed at 80 for the abdomen, with mAs varied to compensate for the size difference of patients. Fixed kilovoltage techniques, sometimes called optimum techniques, are described earlier in this chapter. They are mentioned here to point out that similar results may be obtained regardless of the system employed in order to handle the variables of kVp, mA, and time.

Although the kilovoltage scales shown in Table 32-5A–C were useful in practical patient radiography, and in fact would still be useful, two assumptions used in their computation were found

52 kVp	1200 mAs	42″ SID
16:1 grid	300 RS	1550 mR

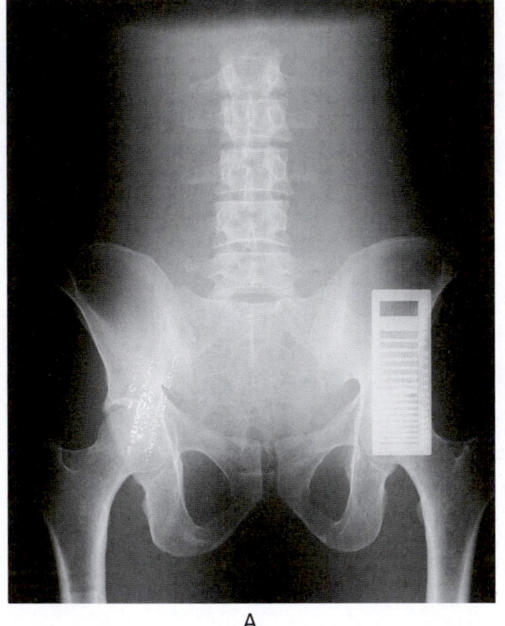

A

70 kVp	160 mAs	42″ SID
16:1 grid	300 RS	1550 mR

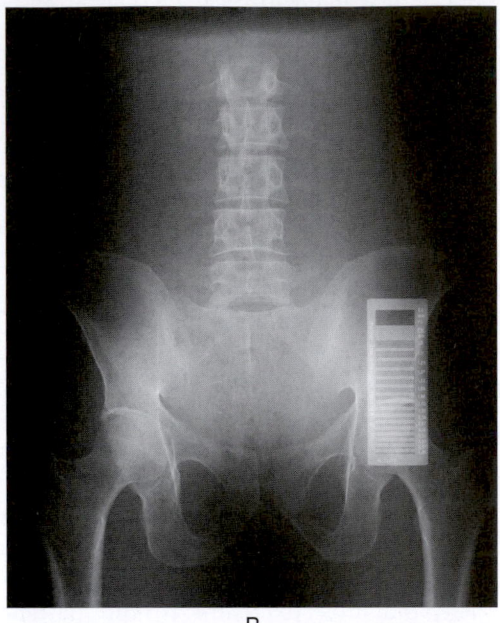

B

115 kVp	10 mAs	42″ SID
16:1 grid	400 RS	106 mR

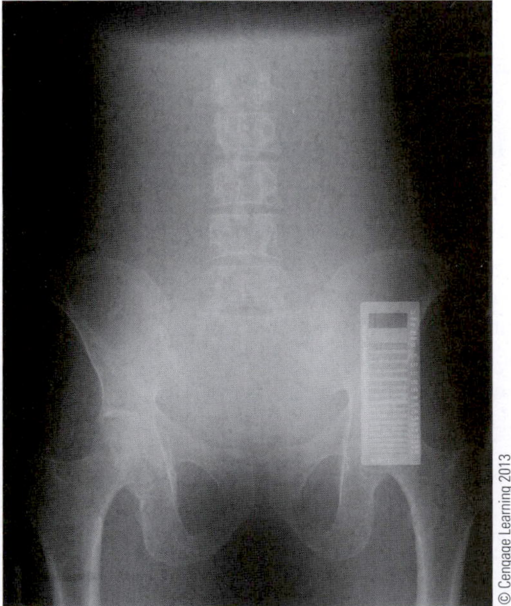

C

FIGURE 32-5. Comparison of contrast produced at three kilovoltage ranges: (A) high contrast at low (52) kilovoltage; (B) ideal contrast produced at approximate (70) kilovoltage; and (C) low contrast produced at high (115) kilovoltage.

TABLE 32-4. 2-kVp/cm Chart

cm	10	11	12	13	14
kVp	50	52	54	56	58

to be false. The notion that a ±10-kVp change will balance a change of double or half mAs has largely given way to the so-called 15 percent rule. This rule suggests decreasing kVp by 15 percent to reduce exposure by half and increasing kVp by 15 percent to double exposure. Although the 15 percent rule better reflects the exponentially nonlinear changes that occur when kilovoltage is altered, it is not totally accurate either. These relationships are among the most complex in radiography and remain difficult to quantify.

When the 15 percent rule is applied, it can be readily seen that a 7.5-kVp change is required at 50 kVp (15 percent × 50 kVp) to balance a 50 percent reduction in mAs, while at 100 kVp, a 15-kVp change (15 percent × 100 kVp) is required. This reflects the fact that at low kilovoltage a small change in kVp can have a large effect on exposure, whereas at higher kilovoltage a larger change will be required to produce the same effect. A uniform change of 2 kVp per centimeter in tissue thickness will not function satisfactorily over a wide range of tissue thicknesses. At a fixed value of mAs and proper exposure of an average patient, images of thicker patients will become increasingly underexposed as patient size increases.

Early users of variable kilovoltage techniques computed kVp scales using 2 kVp per centimeter plus a constant and ±10 kVp between the scales. They were able to use such systems successfully chiefly because the range of variation in adult body part thicknesses is small (see Table 34-1). Thus, kilovoltage values used for a particular body part are within a relatively narrow range. Because mAs values were found by trial and error using kilovoltage from the scales according to patient measurement, problems due to the use of the ±10-kVp change between the scales were minimized, if not entirely eliminated. In addition, a patient whose body habitus varies from the norm is easily recognized by an experienced radiographer, and it was common practice then,

TABLE 32-5. Variable Kilovoltage Scales

A 2 kVp/cm + 30		B 2 kVp/cm + 40		C 2 kVp/cm + 50	
cm	kVp	cm	kVp	cm	kVp
2	34	2	44	2	54
3	36	3	46	3	56
4	38	4	48	4	58
5	40	5	50	5	60
6	42	6	52	6	62
7	44	7	54	7	64
8	46	8	56	8	66
9	48	9	58	9	68
10	50	10	60	10	70
11	52	11	62	11	72
12	54	12	64	12	74
13	56	13	66	13	76
14	58	14	68	14	78
15	60	15	70	15	80
16	62	16	72	16	82
17	64	17	74	17	84
18	66	18	76	18	86
19	68	19	78	19	88
20	70	20	80	20	90
21	72	21	82	21	92
22	74	22	84	22	94
23	76	23	86	23	96
24	78	24	88	24	98
25	80	25	90	25	100
26	82	26	92	26	102
27	84	27	94	27	104
28	86	28	96	28	106
29	88	29	98	29	108
30	90	30	100	30	110
31	92	31	102	31	112
32	94	32	104	32	114
33	96	33	106	33	116
34	98	34	108	34	118
35	100	35	110	35	120
36	102	36	112	36	122

as now, to increase or decrease the mAs according to the radiographer's professional judgment in compensation for body habitus and known pathological conditions.

The kVp Scale

This problem is remedied by establishing a limited variable kilovoltage scale that meets three criteria:

1. All contrast is acceptable to the radiologists.
2. Small-part-size kVp recommendations provide adequate penetration.
3. Large-part-size kVp recommendations avoid excessive scatter fog.

Initial Phantom Images

The limited variable kilovoltage scale is determined by producing a series of radiographs according to straight variable kilovoltage charts such as those shown in Table 32-5A–C. A phantom in a variable depth water bath is used to simulate the various part thicknesses. A variable depth water bath is made by placing a radiographic phantom in a watertight Plexiglas box and then filling it with water to the desired centimeter thickness. A much less complicated, although suboptimal, simulation of this procedure is to simply image a phantom at various kVp levels without changing the part thickness (Figure 32-5). Both procedures will produce a series of phantom images ranging from very high (or even inadequate penetration) contrast to very low contrast with excessive scatter fog.

Select Optimal Phantom Image

If the resulting image is over- or underexposed, a repeat image with an appropriate mAs adjustment is made. This process is continued on subsequent patients until ideal diagnostic-quality images are obtained. The kVp should not be altered from the value shown for part thickness in Table 32-6.

The use of a **patient equivalent phantom** can reduce or eliminate the need for patient exposures. The American National Standards Institute (ANSI) patient equivalent phantom (PEP) is recommended for this purpose. Technical factors required to produce a density of OD 1.4 with the PEP are suited for use on a 21-cm AP lumbar spine patient. Use the kVp for a 21-cm patient from the chart and find the mAs required by trial exposures. If an ANSI phantom is not available, a smooth-bottom plastic wastebasket filled with tap water to a depth of 17 cm has been used successfully for technique development. Use kVp from the chart for a 21-cm AP lumbar spine, and by trial exposure find the mAs required to produce OD 1.4.

The series of images that is produced will demonstrate a wide range of contrast. The images are evaluated by all radiologists and those other physicians deemed critical to the image quality process. Each physician indicates those images he or she is not willing to accept for diagnosis. When this evaluation is complete, the variable kilovoltage scale is reduced to only those kVp levels that are within the acceptable diagnostic range for the physicians who will be diagnosing from the images. This reduction will eliminate some of the part sizes from the chart (see Table 32-6, Step 1).

Extrapolate Exposure System

Once the range of acceptable diagnostic images has been established, a complete exposure system can be computed. The elimination of suboptimal images leaves only the kVp ranges acceptable to the physicians and forms a limited "step" of acceptable kilovoltage. Steps should be formed in groups of 4- to 5-cm increments as this makes mAs adjustments much simpler.

The mAs Scale

Establishing the kVp steps in increments of 4–5 cm permits simple doubling or halving of mAs to maintain image density. Changes of 4–5 cm in tissue thickness require doubling or halving of mAs to maintain approximately the same image receptor exposure. The system is revised to eliminate the rejected kVp ranges by establishing extrapolated kVp steps for the entire system (see Table 32-6, Step 2). At this point in the development of the system it should be obvious that there are a number of inappropriate kVp ranges. For example, a 14-cm part should not be radiographed at 84 kVp, nor should a 31-cm part be radiographed

TABLE 32-6. Stepped Variable kVp Technique Chart

2 kVp/cm + 40							
Establishing a Limited Variable kVp Scale Step 1				Extrapolating kVp Steps Step 2		Fine-Tuning of Extrapolated kVp Values Step 3	
cm	kVp	mAs	evaluation	kVp	mAs	kVp	mAs
4	54	20	reject	70	5	70	5
6	56	20	reject	72	5	72	5
8	58	20	reject	74	5	74	5
10	60	20	reject	76	5	76	5
11	62	20	reject	78	5	70	10
12	64	20	reject	80	5	72	10
13	66	20	reject	82	5	74	10
14	68	20	reject	84	5	76	10
15	70	20	acceptable	70	20	70	20
16	72	20	acceptable	72	20	72	20
17	74	20	acceptable	74	20	74	20
18	76	20	acceptable	76	20	76	20
19	78	20	acceptable	78	20	78	20
20	80	20	acceptable	80	20	80	20
21	82	20	acceptable	82	20	82	20
22	84	20	acceptable	84	20	84	20
23	86	20	reject	70	80	78	40
24	88	20	reject	72	80	80	40
25	90	20	reject	74	80	82	40
26	92	20	reject	76	80	84	40
27	94	20	reject	78	80	78	80
28	96	20	reject	80	80	80	80
29	98	20	reject	82	80	82	80
30	100	20	reject	84	80	84	80
31	102	20	reject	70	320	78	160
32	104	20	reject	72	320	80	160
33	106	20	reject	74	320	82	160
34	108	20	reject	76	320	84	160
35	110	20	reject	78	320	78	320
36	112	20	reject	80	320	80	320
37	114	20	reject	82	320	82	320
38	118	20	reject	84	320	84	320

at 70 kVp. Therefore, it is necessary to fine-tune the extrapolated kVp steps to bring these kVp values within appropriate ranges for penetration and scatter control (see Table 32-6, Step 3). This is accomplished by applying the 4–5-cm rule and/or the 15 percent rule to modify the kVp to an appropriate value while maintaining an acceptable exposure. Note that in Table 32-6, Step 3, the kVp steps follow an even 4-cm doubling or halving of mAs pattern, with only the 20-mAs values utilizing the entire accepted range of 70–84 kVp. This is because the fine-tuning process determined that the upper kVp range (78–84 kVp) produced overpenetration of the small part sizes while the lower kVp range (70–78 kVp) did not adequately penetrate the larger part sizes.

Phantom Testing

Phantom testing is recommended prior to performing patient examinations. At the minimum, phantom testing should be done for a median, small, and large part size as a fine-tuning mechanism for the extrapolated chart prior to clinical use.

Clinical Trials

Limited clinical trials are then permissible with the new chart. All images should be recorded with repeated images saved for analysis. When clinical trials are proceeding without excess repeated exposures, the new technique chart can move into the clinical fine-tuning stage.

Clinical Fine-Tuning

The clinical fine-tuning process is designed to adjust and validate the entire chart. At this point the new technique chart can be adapted. However, ongoing fine-tuning then begins as a permanent process.

Ongoing Fine-Tuning

Ongoing fine-tuning is the process that maintains the accuracy of the entire exposure system and is crucial to both radiographers and radiologists developing a confidence in the exposure and diagnostic processes. It is performed by maintaining an accurate record of modifications to existing techniques for review by the person responsible for quality control.

SUMMARY

The goal of any radiographic exposure system is to provide a method of consistency in the quality of image production. Each type of exposure system functions in a different way to accomplish this goal, but all require the routine use of exposure systems.

Each exposure system has its advantages and disadvantages. It is important to recognize that any exposure system is designed to provide consistency in image quality, and this requires that all users of equipment in a single institution adhere to the same technique charts. Three popular exposure systems are the fixed kVp system, the variable kVp system, and the anatomically programmed system.

A systematic process for establishing a technique chart involves producing initial phantom images, selecting the optimal phantom image, extrapolating a technique chart for a given exposure system, performing phantom testing using the extrapolated technique chart data, performing clinical trials, clinical fine-tuning, and, finally, establishing a system of ongoing fine-tuning.

Fixed kilovoltage technique systems tend to decrease patient exposure because the kilovoltage is always at the maximum possible level. These systems tend to provide a lower overall contrast than do variable kilovoltage systems, and this is usually perceived by radiologists as less pleasing to the eye. The optimal kVp is the maximum kVp level that will produce images with appropriate contrast that are consistently within acceptance limits. Establishing a fixed kVp technique

SUMMARY (continued)

chart involves producing phantom images, selecting the optimal phantom image, extrapolating a technique chart, and performing phantom testing, clinical trials, clinical fine-tuning, and ongoing fine-tuning.

A variable kilovoltage x-ray exposure system is one in which the kilovoltage to be used for a particular projection is varied depending on measured body part thickness. A milliampere-second value is specified for each body part to be examined. Technique systems that use variable kilovoltage offer the advantage of permitting small incremental changes in exposure to compensate for variation in body part thickness. Increasing kilovoltage reduces image contrast. A useful variable kilovoltage system must use values of kilovoltage that provide adequate penetration of the part and result in a level of contrast that is acceptable to the radiologist. Initially, variable kVp systems were established using a 2-kVp change for each centimeter of tissue thickness. A constant was added to this value, such as 30, 40, or 50 kVp, to get the kVp level up to a value that would provide adequate penetration. ■

REVIEW QUESTIONS

1. What is the principal goal of an exposure system?
2. What are some of the advantages of the three exposure systems?
3. What are the steps involved in establishing an exposure system?
4. What is the basic principle of a fixed kVp exposure system?
5. How is the optimal kVp established?
6. Which exposure factor(s) become constant(s) in a variable kilovoltage technique system?
7. What is the 2-kVp/cm rule?

REFERENCES AND RECOMMENDED READING

Bryan, G. J. (1970). *Diagnostic radiography: A manual for radiologic technologists.* Baltimore: Williams & Wilkins.

Cahoon, J. B. (1961). Radiographic technique: Its origin, concept, practical application and evaluation of radiation dosage. *The X-Ray Technician, 32,* 354–364.

Carlstein, C. J. (1971). Radiography of compressed air workers using optimum kilovoltage. *Radiologic Technology, 43*(1), 10–14.

Carroll, Q. B. (1993). *Fuchs's radiographic exposure, processing, and quality control* (5th ed.). Springfield, IL: Charles C Thomas.

Clark, K. C. (1953). An introduction to high-voltage technique. *Radiography, 19,* 21–33.

Cullinan, A. & Cullinan, J. (1994). *Producing quality radiographs* (2nd ed.). Philadelphia: J. B. Lippincott.

Du Pont, E. I. de Nemours & Co. Medical Products Department, Customer Technology Center. *Bit system of technique conversion.* Wilmington, DE: Author.

Dyke, W. P. (1975). Depth resolution: A mechanism by which high kilovoltage improves visibility in chest films. *Radiology, 117,* 159–164.

Eastman, T. R. (1979). *Radiographic fundamentals and technique guide.* St. Louis, MO: C. V. Mosby.

Eastman Kodak Company Health Sciences Markets Division. (1980). *The fundamentals of radiography* (12th ed.) (Kodak Publication M1–18). Rochester, NY: Author.

Files, G. W. (1952). *Medical radiographic technique.* Springfield, IL: Charles C Thomas.

Fodor, J., & Malott, J. C. (1993). *The art and science of medical radiography* (7th ed.). St. Louis, MO: C. V. Mosby.

Fodor, J., Malott, J. C., Ross, J. A., & Porter, M. (1985). Indications for the use of high kVp in the plain film examination of the abdomen. *Radiologic Technology, 57*(2), 159–161.

Fuchs, A. W. (1934). Radiography of entire body employing one film and a single exposure. *Radiography and Clinical Photography, 10,* 9–14.

Fuchs, A. W. (1938). Higher kilovoltage technic with high-definition screens. *Radiography and Clinical Photography, 14*(3), 2–8.

Fuchs, A. W. (1943). The optimum kilovoltage technique in military Roentgenography. *American Journal of Roentgenology, 50,* 358–365.

Fuchs, A. W. (1945). Military photoroentgen technique employing optimum kilovolt (peak) principles.*The American Journal of Roentgenology, 53,* 587–596.

Fuchs, A. W. (1948). Relationship of tissue thickness to kilovoltage. *The X-Ray Technician, 19,* 287–293.

Fuchs, A. W. (1949). Control of radiographic density. *The X-Ray Technician, 20,* 271–273, 291.

Fuchs, A. W. (1950). The rationale of radiographic exposure. *The X-Ray Technician, 22,* 62–68, 76.

Fuchs, A. W. (1958). *Principles of radiographic exposure and processing* (2nd ed.). Springfield, IL: Charles C Thomas.

Funke, T. (1966). Pegged kilovoltage technic. *Radiologic Technology, 37,* 202–213.

Gratale, P., Turner, G. W., & Burns, C. B. (1986). Using the same exposure factors for wet and dry casts. *Radiologic Technology, 57*(4), 325–328.

Gyss, E. E. (1957). A medical radiographic technique chart based on constants. *Radiologic Technology, 29*(2), 76.

Hiss, S. S. (1975). Technique management. *Radiologic Technology, 46*(5), 369.

Hiss, S. S. (2003). *Understanding radiography* (4th ed.). Springfield, IL: Charles C Thomas.

Hopper, B. S. (1957). Radiography above 100 peak kilovolts. *The X-Ray Technician, 29*(1), 9.

Jenkins, D. (1980). *Radiographic photography and imaging processes.* Lancaster, England: MTP Press Limited.

Jerman, E. C. (1926a). Extremity technic. *Radiology, 6,* 252–254.

Jerman, E. C. (1926b). Potter-Bucky diaphragm technic. *Radiology, 6,* 336–338.

Jerman, E. C. (1928). *Modern x-ray technic.* St. Paul, MN: Bruce.

Koenig, G. F. (1957). Kilovoltage as a qualitative factor. *The X-Ray Technician, 29,* 1–4, 13.

Koenig, G. F. (1966). Potential. *Radiologic Technology, 37*(4), 184–198.

Lauer, O. G., Mayes, J. B., & Thurston, R. P. (1990). *Evaluating radiographic quality: The variables and their effects.* Mankato, MN: The Burnell Company.

Lex, J. K. (1957). The x-ray exposure chart. *The X-Ray Technician, 28*(4), 250.

Lyon, N. J. (1962). Optimum kilovoltage techniques. *The X-Ray Technician, 33,* 398–401.

Mahoney, G. J. (1959). A slide rule for kVp-mAs adjustments facilitating the use of high kilovoltage. *The X-Ray Technician, 31,* 35–38.

Mattsson, O. (1955). Practical photographic problems in radiography. *Acta Radiologica Supplementum, 120,* 1–206.

McDaniel, C. T. (1965). Tissue absorption theory applied to formulation of radiographic technique resulting in time as the variable factor. *Radiologic Technology, 37*(2), 51–55.

McFadden, B. (1985). Principles of radiographic exposure: A new approach. *The Canadian Journal of Radiography, Radiotherapy, and Nuclear Medicine, 16*(2), 45–54.

Merrill, H. F. (1960). High kilovoltage radiography. *The X-Ray Technician, 32*(3), 259.

Morgan, J. A. (1977). *The art and science of medical radiography* (5th ed.). St. Louis: Catholic Hospital Association.

Morgan, R. H. (1949). An analysis of the physical factors controlling the diagnostic quality of roentgen images. *American Journal of Roentgenology and Radiation Therapy, 54,* 128; *54,* 395; *55,* 67; *55,* 627.

Morgan, R. H. (1961). Physics of diagnostic radiology. *Physical foundations of radiology* (3rd ed.). New York: Paul Hoeber/Harper & Row.

Nemet, A., Cox, W. F., & Hills, T. H. (1953). The contrast problem in high kilovoltage radiography. *British Journal of Radiology, 26,* 185–192.

Ott, T. T. (1963). Extending the range of medical radiography to 150 kilovolts. *The X-Ray Technician, 34*(6), 335–343.

Revesz, G., Shea, F. J., & Kundel, H. L. (1982). The effects of kilovoltage on diagnostic accuracy in chest radiography. *Radiology, 142,* 615–618.

Roderick, J. F. (1950). Photographic contrast in Roentgenology. *The X-Ray Technician, 22,* 141–150, 163.

Roderick, J. F. (1952). Latitude in Roentgenology. *The X-Ray Technician, 24,* 187–196, 220.

Sante, L. R. (1942). *Manual of Roentgenological technique* (9th ed.). Ann Arbor, MI: Edwards Brothers.

Schwarz G. S. (1958). A simple universal unit system of radiographic exposures suited to departmental, national, and international standardization. *Radiology, 71,* 573–574.

Schwarz, G. S. (1959a). Extended range radiography. *Radiology, 69,* 419–423, 1957.

Schwarz, G. S. (1959b). Kilovoltage and radiographic effect. *Radiology, 73,* 749–760.

Schwarz, G. S. (1960). Kilovoltage conversion in radiography. *The X-Ray Technician, 31,* 373–379, 436.

Schwarz, G. S. (1961). *Unit-step radiography.* Springfield, IL: Charles C Thomas.

Seeman, H. E. (1968). *Physical and photographic principles of medical radiography.* New York: Wiley & Sons.

Thomas, J. B. (1959). High kilovoltage equipment and technique. *The X-Ray Technician, 30*(6), 500.

Thompson, M. A., Hattaway, M. P., Hall, J. D., & Dowd, S. B. (1994). *Principles of imaging science and protection.* Philadelphia: W. B. Saunders.

Trout, E. D., Graves, D. E., & Slauson, D. B. (1949). High kilovoltage radiography. *Radiology, 52,* 669–683.

Tuddenham, W. J., Hale, J., & Pendergrass, E. P. (1953). Supervoltage diagnostic Roentgenography. *American Journal of Roentgenology, 70*(5), 759–765.

United States Army. (1955, March). *Principles of radiographic exposure* (TM 8–282). Washington, DC: Author.

United States War Department. (1941, July 3). *Technical manual: Roentgenographic technicians* (TM 8-240). Washington, DC: Author.

van Dijk, D. (1955). Some factors influencing the results in radiography. *Medicamundi, 1,* 27–32.

Williams, W. A. (1960). Standardization of x-ray technique. *The X-Ray Technician, 32*(2), 137.

Wilsey, R. B. (1921). The intensity of scatter x-rays in radiography. *American Journal of Roentgenology, 8,* 328–338.

Wynroe, R. F. (1955). Some observations on kilovoltage variations. *Radiography, 21*(251), 242–243.

Yurcessen, E. H. (1954). Trend for higher kilovoltage for adequate penetration. *The X-Ray Technician, 26*(2), 96.

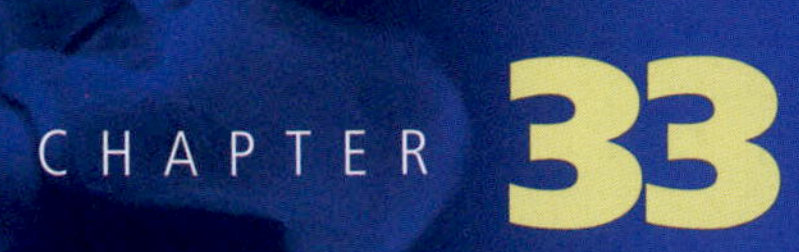

Automatic Exposure Controls

KEY TERMS

backup time
minimum response time

> The art of using AECs is the art of positioning.
>
> —*Richard Carlton*

OBJECTIVES

Upon completion of this chapter, the student should be able to:

- Explain why the art of automatic exposure control is the art of positioning.
- Accurately identify configuration size, shape, and position for various brands of ionization chambers.
- Describe how to modify image receptor exposure when using an automatic exposure control.
- Describe various common problems with subject density and subject contrast when using AECs.
- Explain the effect of collimation on AEC image quality.
- Provide solutions to problems with minimum response time and backup time.
- Explain how to modify the suggested technical factors on an anatomically programmed control unit.
- Discuss the advisability of the creative use of AECs.

The operation of ionization chamber automatic exposure controls (AECs) is discussed in Chapter 5, X-Ray Equipment. It is important to remember that although the term *phototiming* may be used in clinical practice, the generic terms *automatic exposure control* (AEC) and *automatic exposure device* (AED) refer to both antique phototiming devices and the ionization chambers currently in use. The term phototiming actually refers to the use of ionization chambers. Ionization chambers serve to measure the exposure to the receptor. In nearly all instances the principles are applicable to phototimers as well as ionization chambers.

AECs have been popular since their introduction by Russell H. Morgan in 1942. He designed the first phototimer for use with mass chest screening photofluorographic units.

The ionization chamber is designed for a single purpose, best illustrated by the proper term for the device—automatic exposure control. The single function of an AEC is to eliminate the need for the radiographer to set an exposure time. The radiographer loses control over time, and as a result mAs, when using an AEC. All other factors, especially mA and kVp, must still be set manually or may be preprogrammed as in an anatomically programmed radiography system.

Radiographers can fall into the habit of depending on AECs to produce diagnostic images in situations for which they were never designed. When using an AEC it is critical that the location of the ionization chamber be determined and the precise positioning of tissue over that location be achieved. These factors can be remembered by thinking of the use of AECs as another of the radiographic arts based on professional expertise and a sound technical understanding.

IONIZATION CHAMBERS

The most critical element in using AECs is the exact position of the ionization chambers because positions differ for various brands and models of equipment (Figure 33-1). Automatic exposure devices provide diagnostic-quality exposures only for structures positioned directly above the ionization chambers. Therefore, the most important fact to remember when using automatic exposure devices is that the art of using AECs is the art of positioning. Experienced radiographers become extremely adept, often to the point of being artistic, in carefully positioning exactly the right amount of tissue over the chambers.

Ionization chamber AECs are usually used in a three-chamber configuration. The most common relationship of the three chambers is with the center chamber at the center of the image receptor with right and left chambers slightly higher. This configuration places the center chamber below the duodenum and transverse colon for most abdominal examinations, thus eliminating problems with gastric and bowel gas being placed over the chamber. This configuration also places the right and left chambers away from the mediastinum and completely within the lobes of the lungs during chest radiography. As long as the exact chamber locations are known, this configuration will not affect phototiming ability during other examinations.

Determining Configurations

Determining the location of the AEC chambers can be a difficult task. Some manufacturers provide plastic inserts for collimators that project an image of the chamber location, size, and shape with the positioning light beam (Figure 33-2). These inserts are accurate for only the specified SID (usually printed in a corner of the insert). When projection inserts are not provided, the radiographer must be capable of determining the location, size, and shape. This can be accomplished by producing an image without a body part as the subject, exposed at very low kVp for maximum contrast (see Figure 33-1).

Controlling Configurations

AEC consoles permit various combinations of the ionization chambers to be activated in order to control the exposure. Most units permit any single cell or all three cells to be activated. Some units permit other combinations to be utilized, for example, right and left chambers together or all three at once. These options provide the radiographer with seven

52 kVp	4 mAs	72″ SID
16:1 grid	200 RS	3.12 mR

A

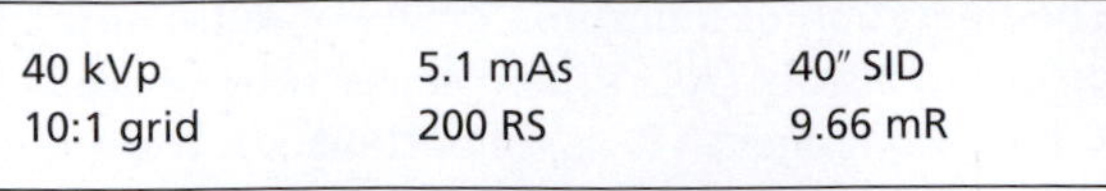

40 kVp	5.1 mAs	40″ SID
10:1 grid	200 RS	9.66 mR

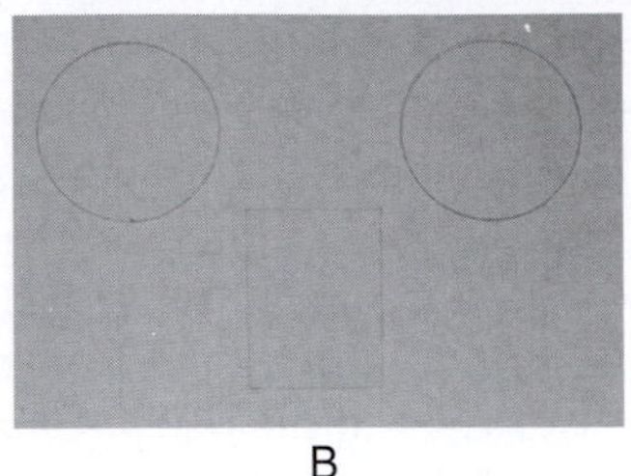

B

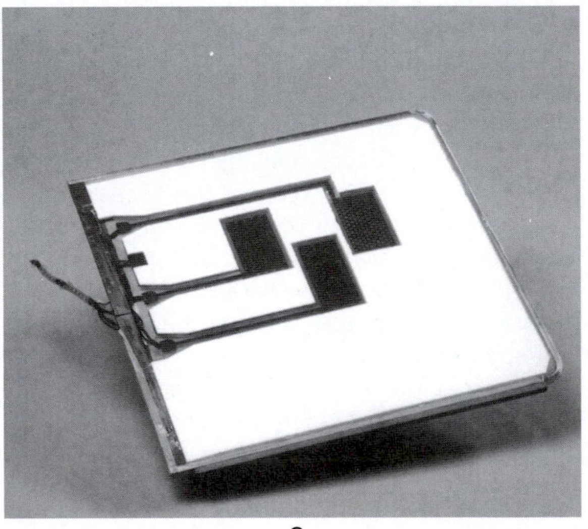

C

FIGURE 33-1. Automatic exposure control ionization chamber configurations. (A) An image of a configuration with square ionization chambers. The middle cell is centered to the image receptor while the outside cells are placed high. (B) An image of a configuration with both square and circular chambers (outlined in pencil). The middle cell is square and centered to the image receptor while the outside cells are round and high. (C) Actual square ionization chamber configuration. The middle cell is centered to the image receptor while the outside cells are high. Note the wire leads to each ionization chamber. *(By permission of Mayo Foundation for Medical Education and Research. All rights reserved.)*

different combinations of the three chambers. In these situations, often termed *averaging*, the signals from the cells are sent to a special operational amplifier, which sums the voltages received from each cell and divides by the number of cells that have been activated. When the appropriate voltage for a diagnostic-quality exposure is reached, the exposure is terminated by the operational amplifier. When more than one cell is activated, the cell receiving the most radiation will contribute the greatest electrical signal and therefore have the most influence on overall exposure. For example, if three cells are activated and an abdomen is positioned so that barium is over one cell and normal tissue over the other two cells, the resultant image will be slightly overexposed because the operational amplifier was dividing the incoming voltage by all three cells but only two cells were contributing to the signal. If the cell under the barium was the only one activated, the image would be greatly overexposed, probably to the backup time limit, because insufficient radiation was received to terminate the exposure. Cell selection is therefore determined by the radiographer based on knowledge of anatomy and positioning.

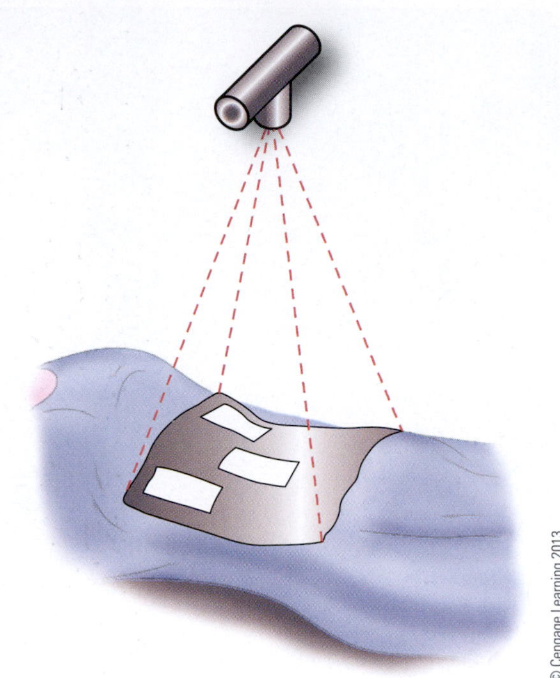

FIGURE 33-2. Projection of AEC locations from collimator positioning light.

Density Controls

All AEC systems permit the adjustment of the amount of radiation necessary to send the exposure termination signal. These controls regulate the image receptor exposure but often have different labels, depending on the manufacturer. Typical AEC density control labels are −3, −2, −1, 0, 1, 2, 3, or ¼, ½, N, 1¼, 1½. Most labels use the center control as the normal density (0 and N in the two examples) and permit both increases and decreases. Some units use a single density control, whereas others use a major and a minor control. Major controls operate large exposure changes, whereas minor controls operate fine adjustment.

The density controls should not be used to compensate for patient part thickness or kVp changes. The AEC system is designed to calculate this compensation automatically. Proper use of the density controls is accomplished when the configuration of the ionization chamber cells cannot be adapted to the necessary positioning, for example, when an image is produced that is slightly overexposed for the lung fields and a decrease in exposure is desired even though the patient and ionization chambers are properly positioned.

Exposure Technique Charts

Automatic exposure controls require the use of exposure technique charts that specify the technical parameters to be used. The only difference from non-AEC charts is that cell locations are given but time settings are eliminated, as the AEC fulfills that function automatically.

POSITIONING SKILLS

The AEC will produce a diagnostic exposure for whatever tissue is placed directly over the chamber. When the radiographer possesses good positioning skills, the vast majority of AEC exposures will produce diagnostic-quality results. Poor positioning skills result in an increased repeat rate when using AECs. There are numerous instances when variables in tissue density and contrast may complicate the precise location of the tissue of interest over the ionization chamber. Knowledge of when these instances are likely to occur and the experience to adequately compensate for them are important. When not enough of the structure of interest is positioned over the activated ionization chamber, the AEC cell will attempt to produce a diagnostic-quality exposure for whatever is over it (Figures 33-3 and 33-4).

The skilled radiographer detects the majority of these conditions through careful observation of the patient and consideration of the patient's history. A proper clinical history can reduce the number of repeated images and produce excellent images.

Subject Density and Contrast Problems

AEC problems with subject density and contrast occur whenever an unexpected density is present or when an expected density is lacking. For example, fluid in the lungs causes increased subject density and contrast, for which the AEC would remain on longer, making an aerated lung overexposed for

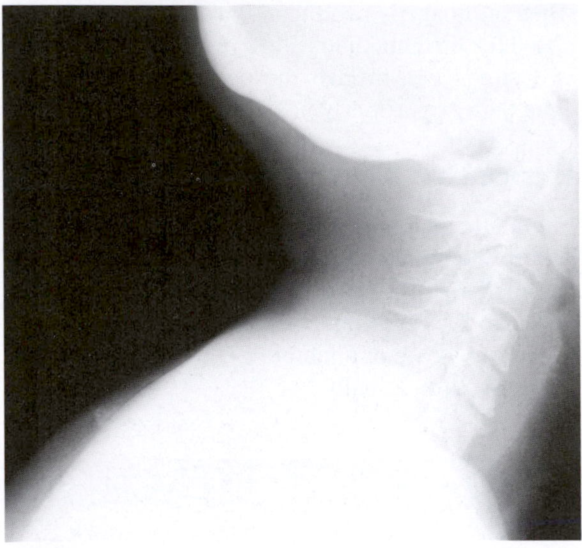

FIGURE 33-3. Improper positioning over AEC cell. Although this lateral cervical spine is underexposed, note that the region at the center of the image receptor, where the AEC cell was activated, is a nearly perfect exposure. *(Radiographs courtesy of Arlene Adler and Richard R. Carlton.)*

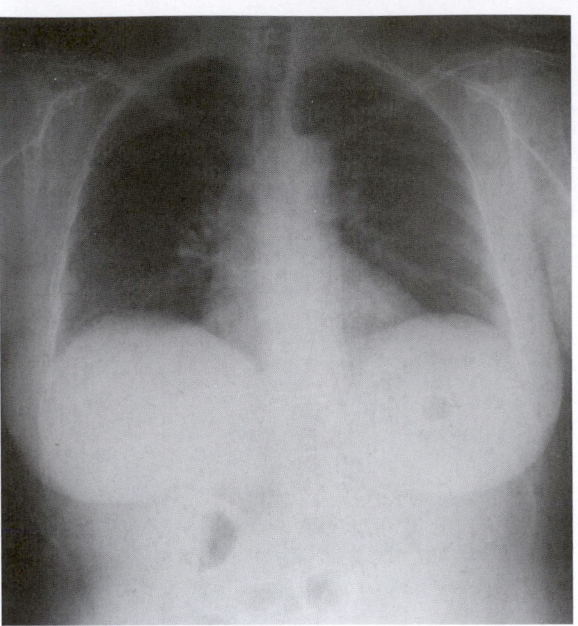

FIGURE 33-4. Improper AEC cell selection. Although this PA chest is overexposed, note that the region at the center of the image receptor, where the AEC cell was activated, is a proper exposure for the thoracic spine. *(Radiographs courtesy of Arlene Adler and Richard R. Carlton.)*

diagnosis. A case of emphysema would produce the opposite result.

Collimation

Collimation of the primary beam is another important consideration when using AECs. Attempts to tightly collimate should be avoided near ionization chamber locations. If the primary beam is collimated from an activated chamber, the chamber operates as if the tissue is extremely dense. The resulting long exposure will create an overexposed image.

The use of wider collimation can also create problems because the full primary beam will produce scatter radiation that may undercut the patient (Figure 33-5). This undercutting scatter will cause the AEC to terminate the exposure while some areas of the image are still underexposed.

Timing Problems

Minimum response time and the proper use of a **backup time** are important considerations when using AECs. The **minimum response time** is the length of time necessary for the AEC to respond to the ionization and send a signal to terminate the exposure. Modern AECs have a minimum response time in the region of 0.001 second. However, the use of extremely high-speed systems for smaller part sizes can cause problems when AECs need less than 0.001 second to produce a diagnostic-quality exposure. In these instances, mA should be decreased to permit longer AEC time.

The backup time establishes the maximum exposure time for the system in order to prevent overexposure. It should be set at 150 percent of the anticipated manual exposure time, although U.S. public law requires that generators automatically terminate AEC exposures at 600 mAs or 60 kilowatt seconds (kWs) (kVp × mA × time) above 50 kVp, and 2,000 mAs below 50 kVp. When the backup time is too short, it will terminate the exposure before the AEC signal, thus producing an underexposed image. In these instances, the backup time should be increased to a level where the AEC is terminating the exposure at the proper time.

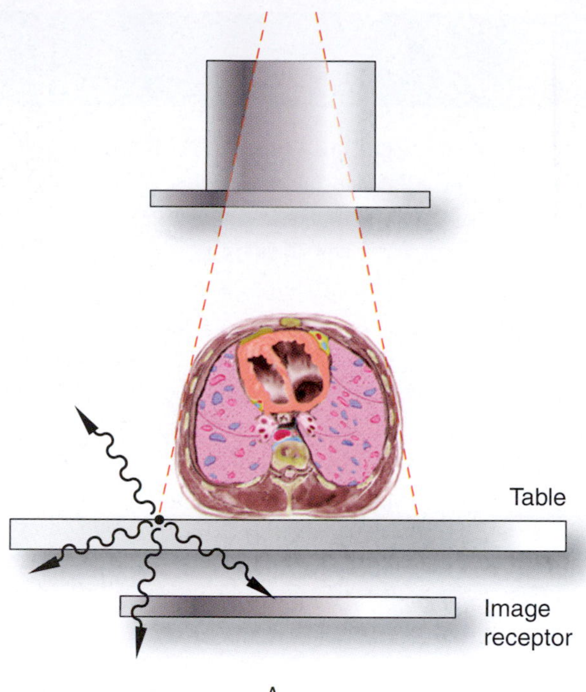

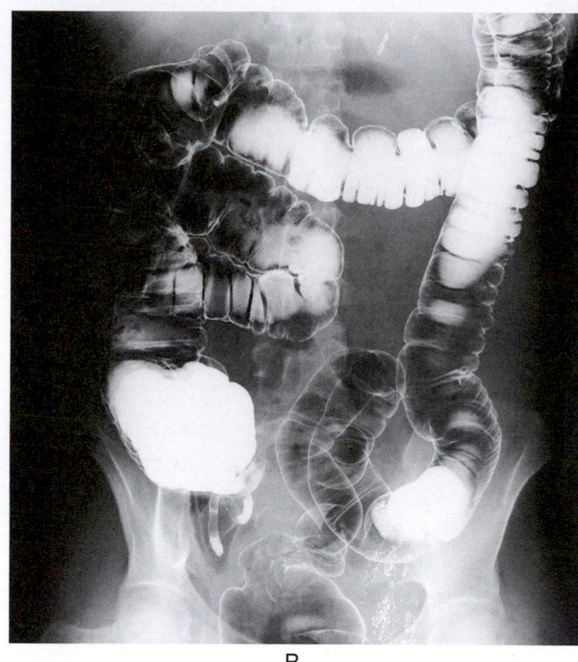

FIGURE 33-5. Undercutting scatter. (A) The uncollimated primary beam produces scatter that undercuts the patient and causes the AEC to prematurely terminate the exposure. (B) An image that is overexposed in the upper right quadrant due to undercutting. *(Reprinted with permission from the American Society of Radiologic Technologists from "Automatic Exposure Control: A Primer,"* Radiologic Technology, 59*(5), 1988, p. 425; radiograph courtesy of Seymour Sterling.)*

Anatomically Programmed Radiography

Anatomically programmed radiography (APR) units combine an AEC system with an exposure system that is computerized to correspond to anatomical procedures. The control console permits the choice of an anatomical region (for example, the chest) and the projection (for example, PA). This choice results in the computer entering the suggested average technique (for example, 120 kVp, 600 mA, with the right and left ionization chambers activated). The radiographer may override the suggested technique when patient condition, pathology, or other factors make it desirable to do so.

Creative Positioning

The experienced radiographer often becomes extremely adept at positioning exactly the right amount of tissue over the chambers. Experienced radiographers should remember that a manual technique will always provide a precisely repeatable exposure, whereas an AEC exposure leaves the radiographer guessing. More important, digital radiography systems rely on consistent use of the programmed parameters for image processing. Attempting to subvert this process only leads to additional difficulties, poor-quality images, and overexposure of patients.

Care must be taken when AEC cells are not completely covered by tissue. The most common compensation in this circumstance is to deactivate the uncovered cell. However, if no cell is covered by normal tissue for the area of interest, deactivation is not the answer. In these instances, creative techniques must be used. For example, if a cell is covered by an appropriate percentage of tissue, it may react with an appropriate exposure. These techniques require much experience and should not be attempted by inexperienced radiographers.

SUMMARY

The ionization chamber is designed for a single purpose, best illustrated by the proper term for the device—automatic exposure control. The single function of an AEC is to eliminate the need for the radiographer to set an exposure time. The radiographer loses control over time, and as a result mAs, when using an AEC. All other factors, especially mA and kVp, must still be set manually.

When using an AEC, it is critical that the location of the ionization chamber be determined and that the precise positioning of tissue over that location be achieved. AEC locations differ for various brands and models of equipment. Automatic exposure devices provide a diagnostic-quality exposure only for structures positioned directly above the ionization chambers. AECs are usually used in a three-chamber configuration. The most common relationship of the three chambers is with the center chamber at the center of the image receptor with right and left chambers slightly higher.

AEC consoles permit various combinations of the ionization chambers to be activated in order to control the exposure. When more than one cell is used, the signals from the cells are sent to a special operational amplifier that sums the voltages received from each cell, divides by the number of cells that have been activated, and then terminates the exposure.

All AEC systems permit the adjustment of the amount of radiation necessary to send the exposure termination signal. These controls regulate the density but often have different labels, depending on the manufacturer. Typical AEC density control labels are −3, −2, −1, 0, 1, 2, 3, or ¼, ½, N, 1¼, 1½. Some units use a single density control, whereas others use a major and a minor control.

Problems can result with the use of AEC devices when variations occur in subject density or contrast. Collimation must also be used consistently to ensure proper results. The AEC's minimum response time can also cause exposure problems when very fast systems are used. Backup times should be set at 150 percent of the expected manual technique time. ■

REVIEW QUESTIONS

1. What is the principal function of the automatic exposure control?
2. What are the typical number and configuration of the ionization chambers?
3. What is the purpose of an operational amplifier?
4. When should the density controls be used?
5. How can changes in subject density result in AEC problems?
6. How can collimation affect AEC image quality?
7. Define minimum response time.

REFERENCES AND RECOMMENDED READING

Bruce, G. (1976). Automatic exposure control: A few notes. *Radiography, 42*(503), 235.

Bushberg, J. T., Seibert, J. A., Leidholdt, E. M., & Boone, J. M. (2003). *The essential physics of medical imaging* (2nd ed.). Philadelphia: Lippincott Williams & Wilkins.

Bushong, S. C. (2008). *Radiologic science for technologists: Physics, biology, and protection* (9th ed.). St. Louis, MO: Elsevier/C. V. Mosby.

Croft, M. J. (1986). Filtration, the answer to the automatic exposure control response problem. *Radiologic Technology, 57*(5), 447.

Cullinan, A., & Cullinan, J. (1994). *Producing quality radiographs* (2nd ed.). Philadelphia: J. B. Lippincott.

Curry, T. S., Dowdey, J. E., & Murry, R. C. (1990). *Christensen's introduction to the physics of diagnostic radiology* (4th ed.). Philadelphia: Lea and Febiger.

Eastman, T. R. (1971). Automated exposures in contemporary radiography. *Radiologic Technology, 43*(2), 80–83.

Fodor, J., & Malott, J. C. (1993). *The art and science of medical radiography* (7th ed.). St. Louis, MO: C. V. Mosby.

Hiss, S. S. (2003). *Understanding radiography* (4th ed.). Springfield, IL: Charles C Thomas.

Jenkins, D. (1980). *Radiographic photography and imaging processes.* Lancaster, England: MTP Press Limited.

Karila, K. T. K. (1989). Manual or automatic exposure controller imaging in mammography. *Radiography Today, 54*(618), 35.

Morel, J. M. (1957). Phototiming. *Radiologic Technology, 29*(3), 165.

Morgan, R. H. (1942). A photoelectric timing mechanism for the automatic control of Roentgenographic exposure. *American Journal of Roentgenography and Radium Therapy, 48,* 220–228.

Morgan, R. H. (1943a). The automatic control of exposure in photofluorography. *Public Health Reports, 58,* 1533–1541.

Morgan, R. H. (1943b). The control of diagnostic quality in Roentgenograms of the chest. *American Journal of Roentgenography and Radium Therapy, 50,* 149–161.

Olson, A., & High, M. (1981). Performance of automatic exposure controls when used with rare-earth intensifying screens. *Radiology,* p. 491.

Seeram, E. (1985). *X-ray imaging equipment: An introduction.* Springfield, IL: Charles C Thomas.

Sprawls, P. (1987). *Physical principles of medical imaging.* Rockville, MD: Aspen.

Sprawls, P. (1990). *Principles of radiography for technologists.* Rockville, MD: Aspen.

Stears, J. G., Gray, J. E., & Frank, E. D. (1988). Radiologic exchange (automatic exposure control function). *Radiologic Technology, 59*(6), 521–522.

Sterling, S. (1988). Automatic exposure control: A primer. *Radiologic Technology, 59*(5), 421–427.

Thompson, T. T. (1985). *A practical approach to modern imaging equipment* (2nd ed.). Boston: Little, Brown.

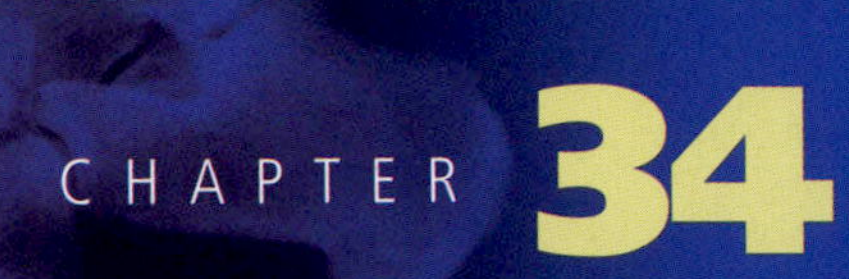

Exposure Conversion Problems

KEY TERMS

proportionally

> Never lose your courage.
>
> *Professor Wilhelm Röntgen*

OBJECTIVES

Upon completion of this chapter, the student should be able to:

- Discuss the limitations of standard conversion tables.
- Explain the concept of direct and inverse relationships versus proportions.
- Calculate appropriate new exposure factors for multiple changes in exposure factor variables.

STANDARD CONVERSION RELATIONSHIPS AND TABLES

A primary concern when using conversion tables is their tendency to oversimplify complex exposure problems. It is safer to think of radiographic exposure factors as relationships to one another rather than as direct conversions. The radiographer uses conversion tables as guidelines, with the realization that the great number of variables in any imaging system makes all conversion factors variables, not constants. Conversion tables are designed to assist in producing an image within acceptance limits. Production of an image of optimal diagnostic quality usually requires fine-tuning. Conversion tables, like all other factors, require fine-tuning before being integrated into an exposure system.

Most conversion tables are designed to provide a method of maintaining image receptor (IR) exposure. It is important to understand the interrelationship between variables and their effects on the four image quality factors: density/IR exposure, contrast, recorded detail, and distortion.

The effect of a particular variable is best described as either a direct relationship, in which an increase in the variable causes an increase in the effect, or an inverse relationship, in which an increase in the variable causes a decrease in the effect, and vice versa. The description of a relationship as direct or inverse does not necessarily indicate that the relationship is **proportionally** direct or inverse. In other words, a proportionally direct relationship would indicate that a linear relationship exists between the variable and the effect, whereas a direct relationship would simply indicate that as the variable changes, the effect changes in the same direction, not necessarily in a linear manner.

Table 34-1 is a master table indicating the relationship of most radiographic image variables to density/IR exposure, contrast, recorded detail, and distortion. Conversion tables are provided for the factors that are commonly considered when converting from one exposure factor or system to another, especially regarding maintaining image receptor exposure (Tables 34-2 through 34-10).

TABLE 34-1. Effects of Radiographic Exposure Variables on the Primary Factors

D = direct relationship (when the variable changes, the effect changes in the same direction).
I = inverse relationship (when the variable changes, the effect changes in the opposite direction).
X = decreases if variable is greater or less than optimal.
O = no effect
NOTE: Many effects are not linearly proportional.

Variable	Effect on Density/IR Exposure	Contrast	Recorded Detail	Distortion
EQUIPMENT				
Generator Phase	D	X	O	O
Kilovoltage	D	X	O	O
Millamperage-Seconds	D	O	O	O
SID	I	O	D	I
OID	I	X	I	D
TUBE				
Focal Spot Size	O	O	I	O
Filtration	I	I	O	O
Beam Restriction	I	D	O	O
SUBJECT				
Part Thickness	I	X	I	D
Tissue Type	I	X	O	O
Additive Pathology	I	X	O	O
Destructive Pathology	D	X	O	O
IMAGE RECEPTOR				
Grid Ratio	I	D	O	O
Film/Screen Relative Speed	D	O	I	O
Film Processing				
Developer Time	D	I	O	O
Developer Temperature	D	I	O	O
Developer Replenishment	D	I	O	O

TABLE 34-2. **Exposure Maintenance Rules**

All of these rules help maintain the same exposure

• 2-KVP/CM RULE

Variable kVp Theory

Maintains exposure by changing kVp for different part sizes.

Changes by 2 kVp for every cm of part size.

EXAMPLE: 60 kVp for 10 cm = 64 kVp for 12 cm

• 4–5-CM RULE

Fixed kVp Theory

Maintains exposure by changing mAs for different part sizes.

Double or halve mAs for every 4–5-cm part size.

EXAMPLE: 10 mAs for 20 cm = 20 mAs for 24 cm

• 15% RULE

Variable and Fixed kVp Theory

Maintains exposure when kVp is changed.

Increase kVp 15% AND decrease mAs to half

EXAMPLE: 60 kVp and 10 mAs = 69 kVp and 5 mAs

Decrease kVp 15% AND increase mAs double

EXAMPLE: 60 kVp and 10 mAs = 51 kVp and 20 mAs

Disclaimer: The above rules are not "Laws of Exposure" by any means. They are simply rules of thumb that have proven useful for generations of radiographers. The actual physical processes that determine exact exposure rates and image quality factors are extremely complex and vary not only from one radiographic unit to another, but over time with the same unit. These rules may be considered useful with a range of 1–2 densities for part sizes from 10–20 cm and kVp ranges of 60–80. However, they are often close enough to produce diagnostically useful images throughout the diagnostic radiography range of body part sizes and kVp levels.

TABLE 34-3. **Conversion Factors: Effect of Generator Phase on Exposure**

When Converting Generator Phase		To Maintain Exposure, Multiply mAs by a
From:	**To:**	**Conversion Factor of:**
1ϕ2p	**3ϕ/HF**	**0.5**
3ϕ/HF	**1ϕ2p**	**2.0**

TABLE 34-4. **The 15 Percent Rule**

To maintain exposure when increasing kVp: increase kVp 15% and reduce mAs to half.

To maintain exposure when decreasing kVp: decrease kVp 15% and double mAs.

TABLE 34-5. **The mAs Formula**

mA × seconds = mAs

TABLE 34-6. **The Exposure Maintenance Formula**

$$\frac{mAs_1}{mAs_2} = \frac{D_1^2}{D_2^2}$$

where: mAs_1 = original mAs

mAs_2 = new mAs

D_1 = original distance

D_2 = new distance

The same formula can be expressed as:

$$mAs_2 = \frac{mAs_1 \times D_2^2}{D_1^2}$$

TABLE 34-7. **Recommended Compensation for Subject Part Thickness**

mAs = 2X or 0.5X mAs per 5 cm

= 15%–20% mAs per cm

kVp = 2 kVp per cm

NOTE: Because scatter production varies with total part thickness, these figures are based on 60–80 kVp for a 20-cm part. The recommendations for changes are less accurate further from this average range.

TABLE 34-8. **Grid Conversion Formula**

$$\frac{mAs_1}{mAs_2} = \frac{GCF_1}{GCF_2}$$

TABLE 34-9. Grid Conversion Factors

(Approximate values based on clinical tests of pelvis and skull.)

Grid	60 kVp	85 kVp	110 kVp
No grid	1	1	1
5:1	3	3	3
8:1	3.75	4	4.25
12:1	4.75	5.5	6.25
16:1	5.75	6.75	8

Adapted with permission from *Characteristics and Applications of X-Ray Grids*, Liebel-Flarsheim division of Sybron Corporation, Cincinnati, Ohio.

TABLE 34-10. Relative Speed Formula

$$\frac{mAs_1}{mAs_2} = \frac{RS_2}{RS_1}$$

SOLVING COMPLEX EXPOSURE PROBLEMS

The most difficult part of developing technique exposure factor skills is learning how to use the information in actual clinical situations. The difficulty lies in the fact that clinical problems usually present complex situations with more than one variable. Now that each variable has been explored in detail, it is necessary to learn how to solve complex exposure problems with many variables.

Methodology

A very simple method can be used to assess a complex exposure problem. Although the analytical decision-making process can be used, it is simpler to work through the variables. If the same variables are considered for each problem, it is less likely that a factor will be missed.

Radiographic variables that should be considered when solving a clinical exposure problem can be classified into four major areas: equipment, tube, patient, and image receptor. Each of these four areas has its variables, as shown in Table 34-1. The variables are easier to remember than it first appears. Equipment is composed of phase plus the four primary factors (kVp, mA, time, and distance). The tube is focal spot, filtration, and field size. The subject consists of part density/IR exposure density and contrast. The image receptor includes grid and film/screen variables.

Mistakes in solving complex exposure problems are invariably caused by failure to consider one of these variables. Even when the solution to a problem appears self-evident, a moment taken to consider all the variables may reveal a hidden factor that would have been missed otherwise.

The following problems demonstrate this methodology.

EXAMPLE: A satisfactory image is produced as follows:

1ϕ2p, 80 kVp, 40 mAs, 40″ SID, 8:1 grid, 250 RS

If a new image is to be produced with the following changes—3ϕ/HF, 12:1 grid, 400 RS—what changes should be made to maintain the original exposure?

Answer: The following variables must be considered:

Equipment: generator phase from 1ϕ2p to 3ϕ/HF

Image receptor: grid from 8:1 to 12:1
Image receptor: film/screen combination from 250 RS to 400 RS

Each variable must be converted for the new exposure:

Equipment: generator phase from 1ϕ2p to 3ϕ/HF

The conversion factor for 1ϕ2p to 3ϕ/HF = mAs × 0.5

40 mAs × 0.5 = 20 mAs

Image receptor: grid from 8:1 to 12:1

The conversion factor formula for grid changes is

$$\frac{mAs_1}{mAs_2} = \frac{GCF_1}{GCF_2}$$

The conversion factor for an 8:1 grid = 4

The conversion factor for a 12:1 grid = 5.5, so

(continues)

(continued)

$$\frac{20 \text{ mAs}}{\text{mAs}_2} = \frac{4}{5.5}$$

$\text{mAs}_2 \times 4 = 20 \text{ mAs} \times 5.5$

$\text{mAs}_2 \times 4 = 110 \text{ mAs}$

$$\text{mAs}_2 = \frac{110 \text{ mAs}}{4}$$

$\text{mAs}_2 = 27.5 \text{ mAs}$

Image receptor: film/screen combination from 250 RS to 400 RS

The conversion formula for RS changes is

$$\frac{\text{mAs}_1}{\text{mAs}_2} = \frac{\text{RS}_2}{\text{RS}_1}$$

The RS change is from 250 RS to 400 RS, so

$$\frac{27.5 \text{ mAs}}{\text{mAs}_2} = \frac{400}{250}$$

$\text{mAs}_2 \times 400 = 27.5 \text{ mAs} \times 250$

$\text{mAs}_2 \times 400 = 6{,}875 \text{ mAs}$

$$\text{mAs}_2 = \frac{6{,}875 \text{ mAs}}{400}$$

$\text{mAs}_2 = 17.2 \text{ mAs}$

So the new exposure factor conditions require a change to 17.2 mAs to duplicate the original exposure factors.

EXAMPLE: A satisfactory image is produced as follows:

3ϕ/HF, 80 kVp, 20 mAs, 72″ SID, 12:1 grid, 400 RS

If a new image is to be produced with the following changes—1ϕ2p, 68 kVp, 100 mA, 8:1 grid, 200 RS—what changes should be made to maintain the original exposure?

Answer: The following variables must be considered:

Equipment: generator phase from 3ϕ/HF to 1ϕ2p

(continues)

(continued)

Equipment: kVp from 80 to 68

Equipment: mAs = time × 100 mA

Image receptor: grid from 12:1 to 8:1

Image receptor: film/screen combination from 400 RS to 200 RS

Each variable must be converted for the new exposure:

Equipment: generator phase from 3ϕ/HF to 1ϕ2p

The conversion factor for 3ϕ/HF to 1ϕ2p = mAs × 2.0

$20 \text{ mAs} \times 2.0 = 40 \text{ mAs}$

Equipment: kVp from 80 to 68

The conversion when decreasing kVp by 15 percent is doubling the mAs.

$80 \text{ kVp} \times 15\% = 12 \text{ kVp}$

$80 \text{ kVp} - 12 \text{ kVp} = 68 \text{ kVp}$

so, $40 \text{ mAs} \times 2 = 80 \text{ mAs}$

Image receptor: grid from 12:1 to 8:1

The conversion factor formula for grid changes is

$$\frac{\text{mAs}_1}{\text{mAs}_2} = \frac{\text{GCF}_1}{\text{GCF}_2}$$

The conversion factor for an 8:1 grid = 3.75

The conversion factor for a 12:1 grid = 4.75, so

$$\frac{80 \text{ mAs}}{\text{mAs}_2} = \frac{4.75}{3.75}$$

$\text{mAs}_2 \times 4.75 = 80 \text{ mAs} \times 3.75$

$\text{mAs}_2 \times 4.75 = 300 \text{ mAs}$

$$\text{mAs}_2 = \frac{300 \text{ mAs}}{4.75}$$

$\text{mAs}_2 = 63.2 \text{ mAs}$

Image receptor: film/screen combination from 400 RS to 200 RS

The conversion formula for RS changes is

$$\frac{\text{mAs}_1}{\text{mAs}_2} = \frac{\text{RS}_2}{\text{RS}_1}$$

The RS change is from 400 RS to 200 RS, so

(continues)

(continued)

$$\frac{63.2 \text{ mAs}}{\text{mAs}_2} = \frac{200}{400}$$

$$\text{mAs}_2 \times 200 = 63.2 \text{ mAs} \times 400$$

$$\text{mAs}_2 \times 200 = 25{,}280 \text{ mAs}$$

$$\text{mAs}_2 = \frac{25{,}280 \text{ mAs}}{200}$$

$$\text{mAs}_2 = 126.4 \text{ mAs}$$

(continues)

(continued)

Equipment: mAs = time × 100 mA

$$\frac{126.4 \text{ mAs}}{100 \text{ mA}} = \text{time}$$

$$1.26 = \text{time}$$

So the new exposure factor conditions require a change to 126.4 mAs to duplicate the original exposure factors. Using 100 mA, the exposure time would be set at 1.26 second.

SUMMARY

A primary concern when using conversion tables is their tendency to oversimplify complex exposure problems. It is safer to think of radiographic exposure factors as relationships to one another rather than as direct conversions. Conversion tables are designed to assist in producing an image within acceptance limits. Most conversion tables are designed to provide a method of maintaining image receptor exposure. It is important to understand the interrelationships between variables and their effects on the four image quality factors: density/IR exposure, contrast, recorded detail, and distortion.

The effect of a particular variable is best described as either a direct relationship, in which an increase in the variable causes an increase in the effect, or an inverse relationship, in which an increase in the variable causes a decrease in the effect, and vice versa. A proportionally direct relationship would indicate that a linear relationship exists between the variables.

The most difficult part of developing technique exposure factor skills is learning how to use the information in actual clinical situations. It is necessary to learn how to solve complex exposure problems with many variables. A very simple method can be used to assess a complex exposure problem. If the same variables are considered for each problem, it is less likely that a factor will be missed.

Radiographic variables that should be considered when solving a clinical exposure problem can be classified into four major areas: equipment, tube, patient, and image receptor. Mistakes in solving complex exposure problems are invariably caused by failure to consider one of the variables. Even when the solution to a problem appears self-evident, a moment taken to consider all of the variables may reveal a hidden factor that would otherwise have been missed. ■

REVIEW QUESTIONS

1. What is the primary purpose of conversion tables?
2. When making exposure factor conversions, it is important to consider the effect on which of the image quality factors?
3. What is the meaning of a direct relationship?
4. What is the difference between a relationship and a proportion?
5. When solving complex exposure problems, the variables can be classified into what four major areas?

REFERENCES AND RECOMMENDED READING

Cullinan, A., & Cullinan, J. (1994). *Producing quality radiographs* (2nd ed.). Philadelphia: J. B. Lippincott.

Du Pont, E. I. de Nemours & Co. Medical Products Department, Customer Technology Center. *Bit system of technique conversion.* Wilmington, DE: Author.

Eastman, T. R. (1979). *Radiographic fundamentals and technique guide*. St. Louis, MO: C. V. Mosby.

Eastman Kodak Company Health Sciences Markets Division. (1980). *The fundamentals of radiography* (12th ed.) (Kodak Publication M1-18). Rochester, NY: Author.

Files, G. W. (1952). *Medical radiographic technique.* Springfield, IL: Charles C Thomas.

Fodor, J., & Malott, J. C. (1993). *The art and science of medical radiography* (7th ed.). St. Louis, MO: C. V. Mosby.

Gratale, P., Turner, G. W., & Burns, C. B. (1986). Using the same exposure factors for wet and dry casts. *Radiologic Technology, 57*(4), 325–328.

Hiss, S. S. (2003). *Understanding radiography* (4th ed.). Springfield, IL: Charles C Thomas.

Jenkins, D. (1980). *Radiographic photography and imaging processes.* Lancaster, England: MTP Press Limited.

Jerman, E. C. (1928). *Modern x-ray technic.* St. Paul, MN: Bruce.

Kratzer, B. (1973). A technique computer: Scientific approach to radiologic technology. *Radiologic Technology, 42*(4), 142–150.

Lauer, O. G., Mayes, J. B., & Thurston, R. P. (1990). *Evaluating radiographic quality: The variables and their effects*. Mankato, MN: The Burnell Company.

Morgan, J. A. (1977). *The art and science of medical radiography* (5th ed.). St. Louis, MO: Catholic Hospital Association.

Sante, L. R. (1942). *Manual of Roentgenological technique* (9th ed.). Ann Arbor, MI: Edwards Brothers.

Schwarz, G. S. (1961). *Unit-step radiography.* Springfield, IL: Charles C Thomas.

The Case of the Dripping Film

What caused the horizontal lines and dripping marks on this radiograph?

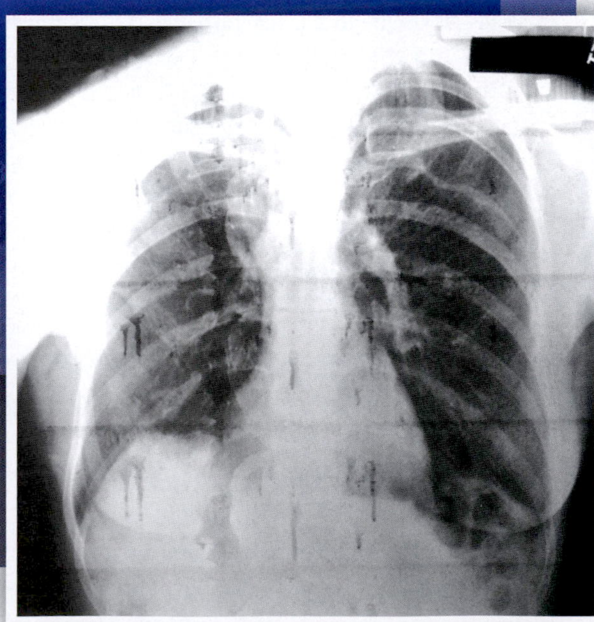

Answers to the case studies can be found in Appendix B

(By permission of Mayo Foundation for Medical Education and Research.

Unit VI

Special Imaging Systems and Modalities

35 Mobile Radiography / 523

36 Fluoroscopy / 533

37 Tomography and Digital Tomosynthesis / 548

38 Mammography / 561

39 Bone Densitometry / 589
Lisa King,RT(R)(M)(BD) CBDT

40 Vascular Imaging Equipment / 604

41 Computed Tomography / 617

42 Magnetic Resonance Imaging / 648
William Faulkner, BS, RT(R)(MR)(CT)FSMRT
Candi Roth, RT(R)(MR)(CT)(M)(CV)FSMRT

43 Nuclear Medicine and PET Scanning / 671
Christina Truluck, PhD, CNMT, RT(N)

44 Radiation Therapy / 703
Julie Hollenbeck, BS, RT(T)

45 Diagnostic Medical Sonography / 724
Sharon Lakia, MS, RT(R), RDMS, RVT

Several special imaging systems deserve consideration to complete a basic foundation in the principles of radiographic imaging. These include the use of specialized diagnostic equipment for **mobile radiography; fluoroscopy,** the oldest and most common dynamic radiographic modality; and **tomography and digital tomosynthesis** (which is now used in digital mammography).

The specialized systems utilized in **mammography, bone densitometry,** and **vascular imaging equipment** are explored as well as the unique design requirements of these fields of radiologic science. Most modern imaging modalities utilize computers to accomplish digital image processing. Those that rely completely on digital processing include **computed tomography (CT)** and **magnetic resonance imaging (MRI),** which, although recognized as specialty areas within radiologic technology, continue to serve as extensions of the radiographer's knowledge.

Also within the scope of departments of radiology, the specialty modalities of **nuclear medicine and PET scanning**, **radiation therapy** (oncology), and **diagnostic medical sonography** (ultrasound) are addressed in this text although they are recognized as separate established professional disciplines with their own accreditation and certification processes. Proper study of these professions generally requires a recognized educational program of one or more years in length encompassing the study of entire subjects beyond the realm of this text.

A thorough study of the six units of this text—**Creating the Beam, Protecting Patients and Personnel, Creating the Image, Analyzing the Image, Comparing Exposure Systems, and Special Imaging Systems and Modalities**—provides the thorough physical basis required of the radiologic or imaging sciences professional. Basic physical knowledge must be combined with an equally thorough and correlated knowledge in the anatomical sciences of anatomy, positioning, physiology, and pathology to form the complete basis of radiography knowledge. Only when this basis is added to an elementary understanding of human interactions and combined with clinical experience does the true professional radiographer emerge.

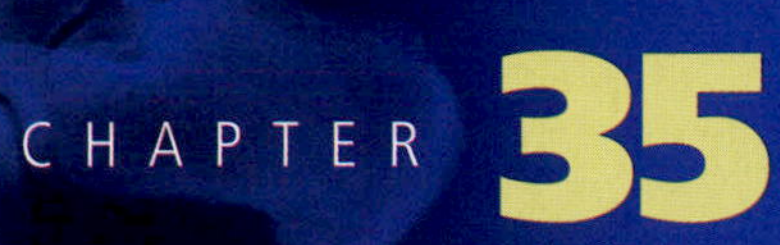

CHAPTER 35 Mobile Radiography

Come, come, and sit you down.

You shall not budge!

You go not till I set you up a glass

Where you may see the inmost part of you.

Shakespeare, Hamlet, III, iv, 18

OBJECTIVES

Upon completion of this chapter, the student should be able to:

- Determine factors that contribute to the difficulty of mobile radiography.
- Explain appropriate communication methods for mobile examinations.
- Describe items that must be considered when arranging a patient room for a mobile examination.
- Recommend methods for accomplishing acceptable variations of standard radiographic projections, especially chest examinations, for air-fluid levels.
- Assess the radiation protection rules for mobile radiography.
- Differentiate light-duty portable x-ray units from full-power mobile units.
- Evaluate the advantages of capacitor-discharge and battery-powered mobile units.

OBJECTIVES (continued)

- Explain why technical factor selection is more difficult during mobile radiography.
- Describe the effect of various generator waveforms on kVp.
- Identify advantages of standardizing mobile SID to one of 40″ (100 cm), 56″ (140 cm), or 72″ (180 cm).
- Determine appropriate grids for mobile examinations.
- Appraise various image receptor systems for mobile applications.

The mobile radiographic examination is often the ultimate test of the radiographer's competence and skill. Accomplishing an optimal-quality image without stationary equipment on the most difficult patients is a prime achievement. An understanding of the special considerations involved in mobile examinations is important for the radiographer.

SPECIAL PATIENT CONSIDERATIONS

Mobile examinations are more difficult to accomplish because there are so many additional variables—variables that would be constants with a stationary unit—when manipulating and positioning both patient and equipment. In many instances the reason an examination is requested at the bedside is to avoid transporting the patient because of his or her physical condition. Special adaptations of routine projections, imaginative equipment manipulation, and innovative technical factor considerations are often required.

In surgery or the emergency unit, the stress of performing in a high-tension environment may be added to the patient problems. These situations often include limitations due to aseptic conditions and the presence of additional critical equipment (e.g., ventilators, multiple intravenous solutions, cardiac lines, etc.).

Communication

Although good communication with the patient is not a special consideration during mobile examinations, it is advisable for the radiographer to park the mobile unit outside a patient's room before entering to establish the proper rapport. The patient's permission must be obtained before proceeding with the examination, an explanation of the procedure should be given, and some rearrangement of equipment and room furnishings must usually be accomplished before bringing the mobile unit into the room.

The unconscious or incognizant patient requires the same explanation that a cognizant patient would receive. In many instances conscious but incognizant patients will be more cooperative if they hear a kindly voice of explanation prior to being touched. In surgery, the attending physician or operating room nurse must be consulted before entering, and this procedure should be followed even in an emergency suite.

Manipulating Equipment

Extreme care must be taken when manipulating equipment in a high-technology environment such as intensive care, surgery, or the emergency unit. The importance of other equipment must be considered, especially when it must be moved to make room for the x-ray unit. Care must be exercised to ensure that power supplies, oxygen tubes, catheters, intravenous lines, and so forth have enough slack to permit movement. Finally, the radiographer must take care not to bump the bed or other equipment when moving the mobile unit out of the way or when driving it into position. Although this seems to be an obvious consideration, it is easily overlooked when one's mind is on the examination. Wall-suspended television units are especially hazardous to both the x-ray tube and the radiographer's head. Neither the radiographer nor the patient can afford to be in a hurry when preparing for a mobile examination. It is the radiographer's duty to return all items to their original locations prior to leaving the area.

Positioning and Pathology

Patients requiring examinations with mobile equipment are often unable to assume standardized positions. Clinical experience and a thorough knowledge of acceptable positioning variants are required for this problem. For example, the inability of the patient to sit on the side of a bed requires an AP projection of the chest instead of the preferred PA projection. A patient in orthopedic traction may not be able to straighten the knee. Thus, a distal knee joint and mid-shaft and proximal hip exposure will be required to avoid gross distortion and to satisfactorily demonstrate the entire femur from a single projection. However, routine positioning practices should still be carried out to the extent possible. For example, during chest radiography most cognizant patients are capable of moving the scapula from the lung fields by rolling their shoulders forward, as they would if the examination were performed on stationary equipment.

Even with difficult or uncooperative patients, chest radiography should be performed with the patient in a semi-erect position in the vast majority of instances. Patients who have been confined to a bed, especially when pathology is present, are prone to disease processes that cause collections of fluid. Even elevating the thorax to the level of a pillow (perhaps only 10° from supine) may provide an opportunity to demonstrate a fluid level. Ideally, air-fluid level demonstration is best accomplished with the patient in a completely erect position, utilizing a horizontal beam (Figure 35-1). Demonstration of

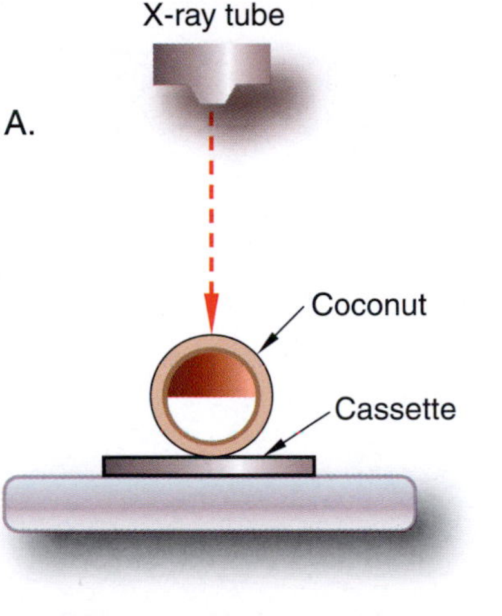

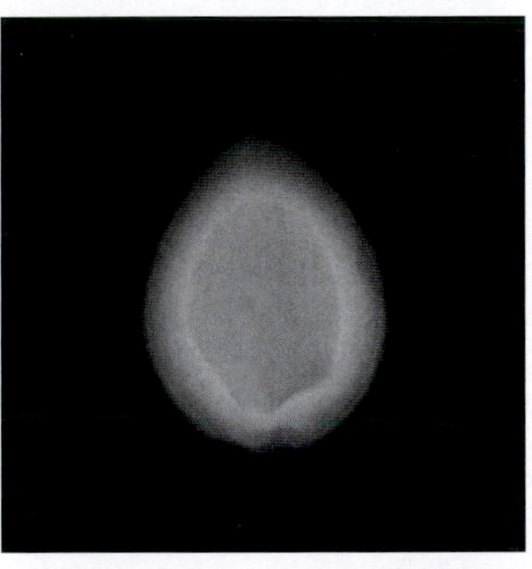

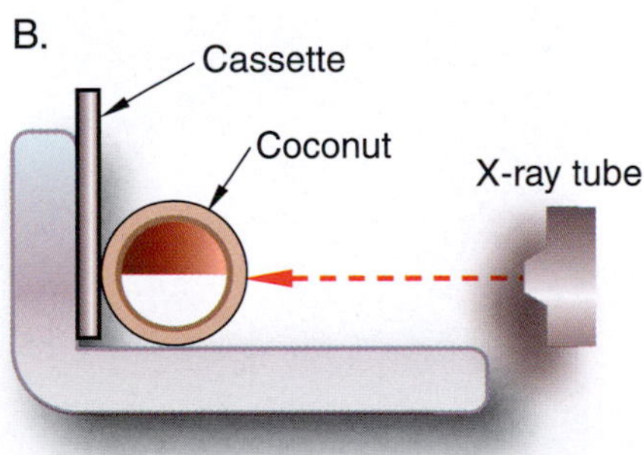

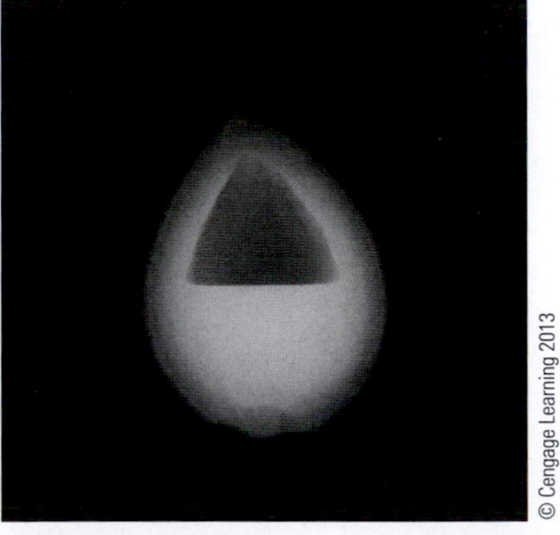

FIGURE 35-1. Demonstration of air-fluid levels. A coconut was used to demonstrate the effect of various positions and tube angles on air-fluid levels. (A) Recumbent AP projection with beam perpendicular to the air-fluid level. (B) Upright AP projection with beam parallel to the air-fluid level. (continues)

air-fluid levels when a patient is unable to assume an erect position causes gross distortion of anatomical structures (Figure 35-2). This distortion may be great enough to render the image useless for normal chest diagnosis. When it is determined that air-fluid demonstration is a priority, two projections may be necessary: one for air-fluid levels and the other for a normal projection of the chest.

The radiographer must not assume that an apparently well patient is able to be transported to stationary equipment. For example, an ambulatory patient on whom a mobile chest examination is requested may in fact be under observation for myocardial infarct and may be susceptible to the sudden onset of potentially serious symptoms.

The radiographer must also not assume that every mobile examination will result in a poorer image quality than examinations performed in the radiology department. The same myocardial infarct patient may be capable of providing a detailed history that makes delineation of the heart shadow the primary image quality goal, of assuming an erect position on the edge of a bed, and of holding a cassette to permit a 72″ (180-cm) PA projection essentially identical in quality to an image produced with a stationary unit.

Because the mobile examination is performed at the patient's bedside, there is an increased possibility of artifacts, such as personal items (e.g., dropped hair pins, jewelry, etc.), layers of coverings (e.g., insulated blankets, several sheets, etc.), and medical equipment (e.g., nasogastric tubes, intravenous lines, catheters, electrocardiographic leads, clamps, etc.). A careful and tactful examination of the area of interest should be performed prior to

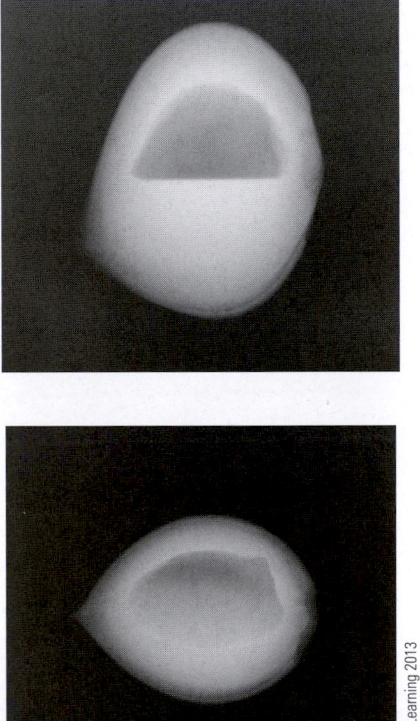

FIGURE 35-1. (continued) (C) The image receptor was at a 45° angle to the plane of the floor, with the beam parallel to the air-fluid level and therefore parallel to the floor. (D) The image receptor was at a 45° angle to the air-fluid level, with the beam perpendicular to the image receptor. Note that the central ray must be parallel to the floor to demonstrate distinct air-fluid levels.

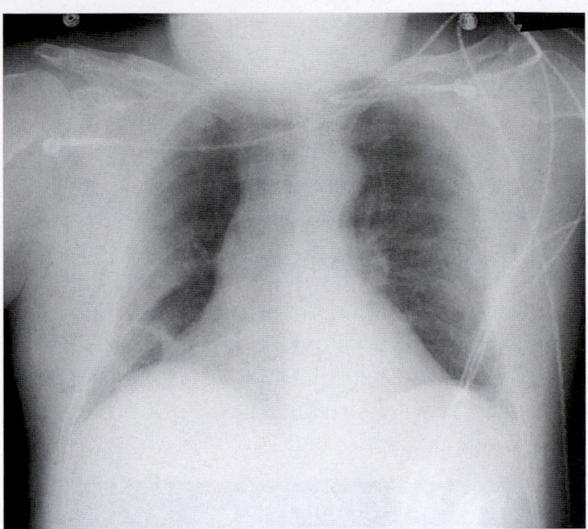

FIGURE 35-2. A chest radiograph demonstrating distortion due to improper source-to-image-receptor alignment during a mobile examination. The central ray and image receptor were not perpendicular to one another. *(Radiographs courtesy of Arlene Adler and Richard R. Carlton.)*

exposure to locate and remove as many of these artifacts as possible. It is usually possible to carry out this examination during positioning, which also presents an opportunity to check for a necklace, bra, brace, and so on. Clamps holding various tubes and lines should be moved as far from the area of interest as possible. For example, intensive care unit chest radiography often requires movement of intravenous, respiratory, and cardiac lines from over the lung fields. A nursing staff member or physician should be consulted before moving any lines, especially venous and arterial. It is desirable to limit coverings to a single smoothed layer of gown or sheet.

SPECIAL RADIATION PROTECTION CONSIDERATIONS

During a mobile examination the radiographer is bringing a radiation hazard into an area not designed for radiation protection. Professional responsibility for ensuring radiation protection becomes a fundamental operating procedure during all mobile radiography. This is a prime opportunity for radiographers to educate the public, health professionals, physicians, and other patients concerning proper radiation protection practices. A duty exists to protect the patient, health workers, the public, and oneself. The rules shown in Table 35-1 should never be violated. The mobile unit should not be used as a portable shield. When standing behind a mobile unit, a lead apron is required to ensure sufficient protection. Radiographers should also move to a maximum distance from the mobile unit by extending the exposure control cord prior to making the exposure. It is not unreasonable to ask others, especially patients sharing a room, if they would prefer to leave the area for a few moments while the exposure is made.

TABLE 35-1. Radiation Protection Rules for Mobile Radiography

1. Recognize a duty to protect your patient, health professionals, physicians, the public, and yourself.
2. Request the public, health professionals, physicians, and other patients to leave the immediate area prior to exposure. (Always inform these persons that you will be finished in a moment, request them to remain nearby, and inform them promptly when you are finished.)
3. Announce in a loud voice your intent to make each exposure and permit sufficient time for others to leave.
4. Carry at least two lead aprons: one for yourself, the other for your patient. If you have an assistant, he or she, too, must have an apron.
5. Never place your hand or any other body part within the primary beam.
6. Provide gonadal protection for your patient.
7. Achieve maximum distance from the patient (not the tube) immediately prior to exposure, in accordance with rules requiring the use of a 6′ cord on mobile units.
8. Label and handle each cassette carefully to avoid repeats.

TYPES OF EQUIPMENT

X-ray units are available in a wide array of sizes and capabilities, many of which can be classified as mobile. Although often described as portable units (the truly portable unit can be hand carried), the proper description is mobile. The need for mobile x-ray equipment has been apparent from the earliest days of radiography; one unit was designed to fit in a suitcase. During World War I, the Picker Corporation developed a mobile unit that became popular for bedside radiography in hospitals and was emulated by other vendors.

Today mobile equipment operates on rechargeable batteries. In addition, mobile units come with built-in monitors and flat panel detector systems for immediate display of the image. Detectors may be tethered to the unit or more commonly use wireless technology to send the exposure data to the unit for processing and display. This allows the radiographer to view the image at the bedside and to be sent to a PACS system for physician review (Figure 35-3).

Mobile units use batteries for a power supply and are recharged through 110- to 120-V wall outlets. There is circuitry that monitors battery strength, and normal maintenance procedures include periodic replacement of old batteries.

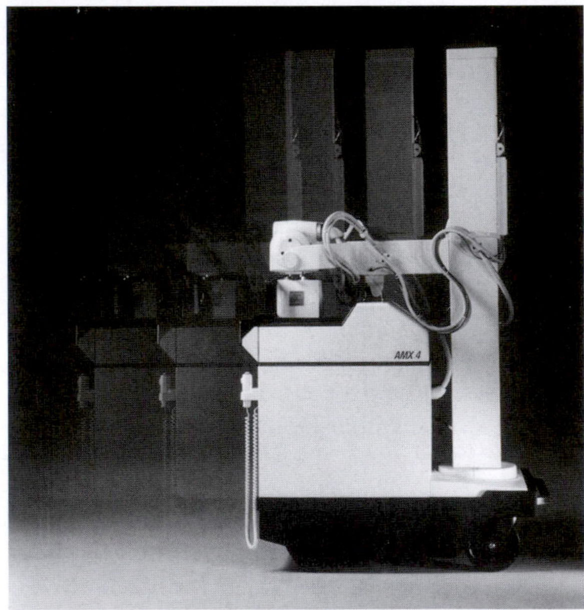

FIGURE 35-3. A typical full-powered mobile radiographic unit. *(Courtesy of GE Healthcare.)*

Generators in these units produce output that is essentially high frequency (Figure 35-4).

One advantage of a battery-powered unit is that power is available to drive the unit itself. The drive switch on a mobile unit should be of the deadman type so that its release immediately disengages the power drive. The size and weight of a battery-powered mobile x-ray unit are considerable, and extreme care must be observed when piloting it. Patients and staff could be seriously injured by careless driving. Radiographers must be cautious in looking ahead, especially at corners and intersections, just as when driving a car.

SPECIAL TECHNICAL FACTOR SELECTION CONSIDERATIONS

Kilovoltage

Mobile units produce an x-ray beam with an average photon energy that is fairly similar to that of stationary equipment. Full-power high-frequency units that are battery powered produce a waveform, as shown in Figure 35-4. Because this waveform has very little ripple, it is as efficient as a stationary unit.

Capacitor discharge units made exposures through the use of large capacitors, which allowed the proper kVp range when sufficient power was not available, before high-frequency mobile units were developed. As a result, capacitor discharge units often had serious kVp limitations.

Milliampere-Seconds

In the past it was common to make adjustments when setting mobile exposure factors due to the low power of the units. It is no longer necessary to make changes such as using higher kVp to substitute for lack of mAs to obtain sufficient image receptor exposure.

Distance

A primary cause of repeated mobile exposures is failure to measure distance. Every mobile procedure must have SID measured. Radiographers who

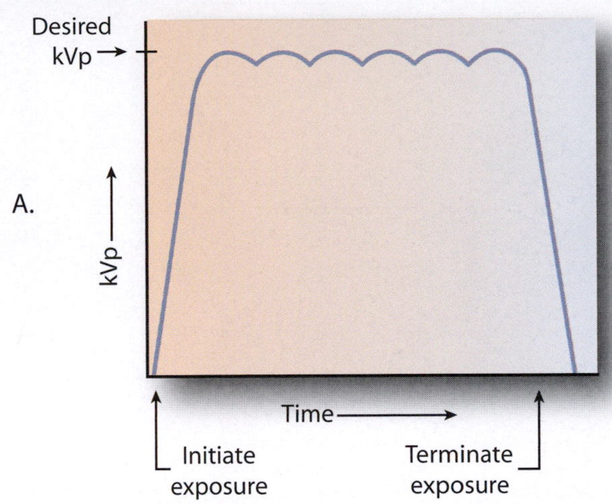

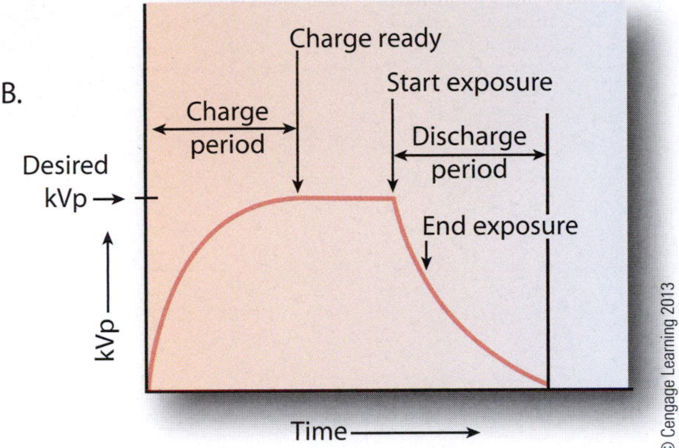

FIGURE 35-4. Mobile unit generator waveforms. (A) A battery-powered unit. (B) A capacitor discharge unit.

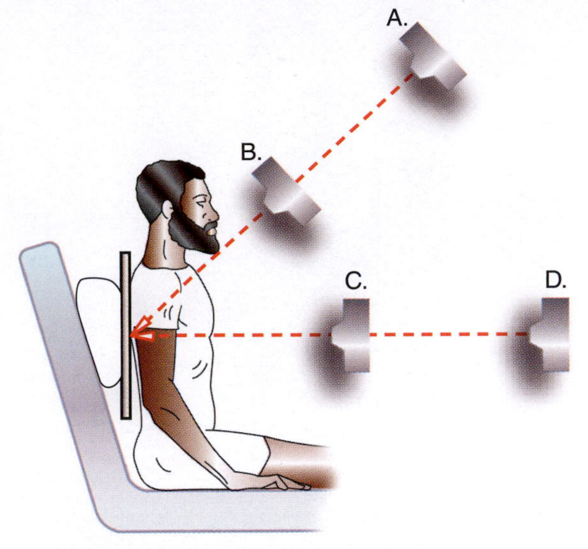

FIGURE 35-5. Common distance problems during mobile chest radiography.

estimate SID must be within 15 percent to avoid producing a significant exposure difference. A 72″ (180-cm) chest image must be exposed between 61″ (153 cm) and 83″ (208 cm) to produce an optimal exposure using 72″ (180-cm) factors.

Figure 35-5 illustrates common problems encountered in mobile chest radiography. The size of the room and the location of the bed and ancillary equipment may not permit a mobile unit to be manipulated into a position from which a standard 40″ (100-cm) or 72″ (180-cm) projection can be obtained. Position A may be unobtainable because of tube height limitations. Position B is usually obtainable but does not optimize information because at an SID of 40″ (100 cm) it magnifies the heart and, when the patient cannot sit erect, does not provide the geometry to demonstrate air-fluid levels. Positions C and D may be obtainable when air-fluid levels are required, but position C causes magnification.

The most reliable method of eliminating exposure fluctuations due to distance is to use only the two standardized distances, 40″ (100 cm) and 72″ (180 cm), with the addition of 56″ (140 cm) for mobile radiography. The 56″ (140-cm) distance should be employed only when 40″ (100 cm) is undesirable because of magnification, yet 72″ (180 cm) is not possible due to room and/or equipment limitations. As seen earlier in Table 26-3, mAs conversions are provided to maintain exposure at these distances according to the rule of doubling or halving mAs with each distance change (i.e., 40″ [100 cm] to 56″ [140 cm] to 72″ [180 cm]).

Grids

Proper alignment to a grid is difficult when the patient is supine but the grid is on a soft bedding surface, which easily permits the grid to

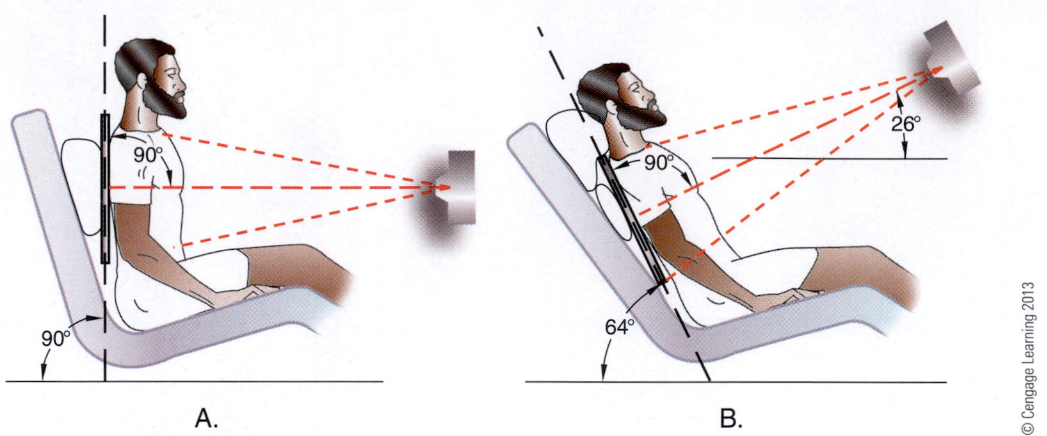

FIGURE 35-6. Alignment problems during mobile chest radiography. (A) A simple alignment problem correctly resolved. (B) A difficult alignment problem correctly resolved.

tilt, unless the patient's weight is almost exactly distributed around the center of the grid. Proper alignment is even more difficult when the image receptor is at an angle other than parallel or perpendicular.

Figure 35-6 illustrates the problems created by this common situation. The radiographer must attempt to align the central ray and the image receptor perpendicular to one another. Although this is a relatively simple task when the relationships are as shown in Figure 35-6A, it becomes very difficult when the reference points are not parallel or perpendicular.

Most people can draw a simple angle, such as 45°, quite accurately, but accuracy becomes more difficult when the baseline is at an angle. Figure 35-7 demonstrates this difficulty. Angling off-center to a focused grid by as little as 5° can result in sufficient grid cutoff to visibly reduce image receptor exposure.

Grids that permit wide exposure and centering latitude assist in these problems. Lower ratio (6:1 to 8:1), higher frequency (178–200 lpi), short dimension, and wide focal range grids (40″–72″) are preferred for mobile radiography.

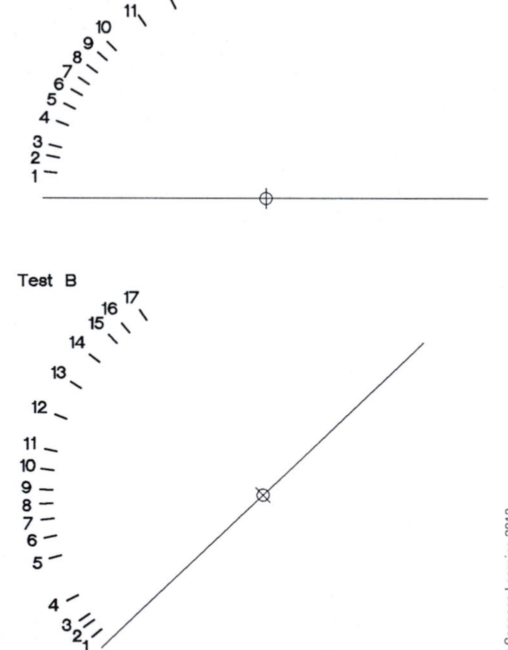

FIGURE 35-7: Difficulty of angle estimation with an angled baseline. If a line is drawn from one of the numbers to the dot, which number would create a 90° angle? A 15° angle? A 37° angle? Record your answers for both tests A and B, and then look on page 12 for the correct answers. Do not tilt your head or the book when completing Test B.

SUMMARY

Mobile examinations are more difficult because there are so many additional variables—variables that would be constants with a stationary unit—when manipulating and positioning both patient and equipment. In many instances the reason an examination is requested at the bedside is to avoid transporting the patient because of his or her physical condition. Special adaptations of routine projections, imaginative equipment manipulation, and innovative technical factor considerations are often required. Good communication with the patient is a necessary part of all radiographic procedures. The unconscious or incognizant patient requires the same explanation that a cognizant patient would receive.

Extreme care must be taken when manipulating equipment in a high-technology environment such as intensive care, surgery, or the emergency unit. Care must be exercised to ensure that power supplies, oxygen tubes, catheters, intravenous lines, and so forth have enough slack to permit movement.

Patients requiring examinations with mobile equipment are often unable to assume standardized positions. Clinical experience and a thorough knowledge of acceptable positioning variants are required for this problem. Because the mobile examination is performed at the patient's bedside, there is an increased possibility of artifacts, such as personal items, layers of coverings, and medical equipment.

During a mobile examination the radiographer is bringing a radiation hazard into an area not designed for radiation protection. A duty exists to protect the patient, health workers, the public, and oneself.

Mobile units operate on rechargeable batteries, and many units come with built-in monitors and flat panel detector systems for immediate display of the image. A number of factors should be considered when establishing exposure systems, including kilovoltage, milliamperage, distance, grids, and image receptor systems. ■

REVIEW QUESTIONS

1. Why are mobile procedures often more difficult than those performed using stationary units?
2. What should the radiographer do before bringing mobile equipment into a patient's room?
3. What must be considered when manipulating mobile equipment in a high-technology environment?
4. What must a radiographer do to adequately visualize air-fluid levels on a chest radiograph?
5. What type of generator waveform is produced with a full-power battery-operated mobile unit?
6. Why is it important to measure distance (SID) for all mobile procedures?
7. What type of grid is preferred for mobile procedures?

REFERENCES AND RECOMMENDED READING

Adler, A., & Carlton, R. R. (2010). *Introduction to radiography and patient care* (5th ed.) Philadelphia: Elsevier/Saunders.

Ball, J., & Price, T. (1989). *Chesneys' radiographic imaging.* Oxford: Blackwell Scientific.

Barnhard, H. J. (1978). The bedside examination: A time for analysis and appropriate action. *Radiology, 129*, 539–540.

Benbow, M. (1994). The selection of kVp during mobile radiography on the special care baby unit. *Radiography Today, 60*(686), 19–20.

Bushberg, J. T., Seibert, J. A., Leidholdt, E. M., & Boone, J. M. (2003). *The essential physics of medical imaging* (2nd ed.). Philadelphia: Lippincott Williams & Wilkins.

Bushong, S. C. (2008). *Radiologic science for technologists: Physics, biology, and protection* (9th ed.). St. Louis, MO: Elsevier/C. V. Mosby.

Cantwell, K. G., Press, H. C., & Anderson, J. E. (1978). Bedside radiographic examinations: Indications and contraindications.*Radiology, 129*, 383–384.

Cullinan, A., & Cullinan, J. (1994). *Producing quality radiographs* (2nd ed.). Philadelphia: J. B. Lippincott.

A device for improving the quality of bedside decubitus exams. (1979). *Radiologic Technology, 51*(1), 88.

Eisenberg, R. L., Akin, J. R., & Hedgcock, M. W. (1980). Optimal use of portable and stat examination.*The American Journal of Roentgenology, 134*, 523–524.

Evans, S. A., Harris, L., Lawinski, C. P., & Hendra, I. R. F. (1985). Mobile x-ray generators: A review. *Radiography, 51*(595), 89–107.

Floyd, C., Baker, A., Lo, J., & Ravin, C. (1992). Measurement of scatter fractions in clinical bedside radiography. *Radiology, 183*(3), 857–861.

Fry, O. E., & Gianturco, C. (1960). Bedside radiography reduction of patient exposure and orientation of grid cassettes. *Radiologic Technology, 31*(4), 387.

Hasse, R. A. (1991). New trends in portable x-ray batteries and technology. *Radiology Management, 13*(3), 42–44.

MacMahon, H., Yasillo, N., & Carlin, M. (1992). Laser alignment system for high-quality portable radiography. *RadioGraphics, 12*, 111–120.

Marlowe, J. E. (1983). *Surgical radiography.* Baltimore: University Park Press.

O'Donovan, P., Skipper, G., Litchney, J., Salupo, A., & Bortnick, J. (1992). Device for facilitating precise alignment in bedside radiography. *Radiology, 184*(1), 284.

Osborn, R. R. (1960). Improved portable radiographs of the trunk without the use of grids or Bucky. *Radiologic Technology, 32*(2), 145.

Rossi, R., Harnisch, B. D., & Hendee, W. R. (1982, December). Evaluation of an automatic exposure control device for mobile radiography. *Radiology*, 823.

Schaefer, C. (1989, December). Improved control of image optical density with low-dose digital and conventional radiography in bedside imaging. *Radiology*, 713.

Seeram, E. (1985). *X-ray imaging equipment: An introduction.* Springfield, IL: Charles C Thomas.

Thompson, M. A., Hattaway, M. P., Hall, J. D., & Dowd, S. B. (1994). *Principles of imaging science and protection.* Philadelphia: W. B. Saunders.

Trew, D. J. (1970). The "cordless" mobile x-ray machine. *Radiography, 36*(427), 159–164.

Weaver, K. E., Barone, G. J., & Fewell, T. R. (1978). Selection of technique factors for mobile capacitor energy storage x-ray equipment. *Radiology, 128*, 223–228.

Wolbarst, A. B. (1993). *Physics of radiology.* Norwalk, CT: Appleton & Lange.

Answers to Figure 35-7

Test A	Test B
90° = 15	90° = 15
15° = 3	15° = 4
37° = 8	37° = 7

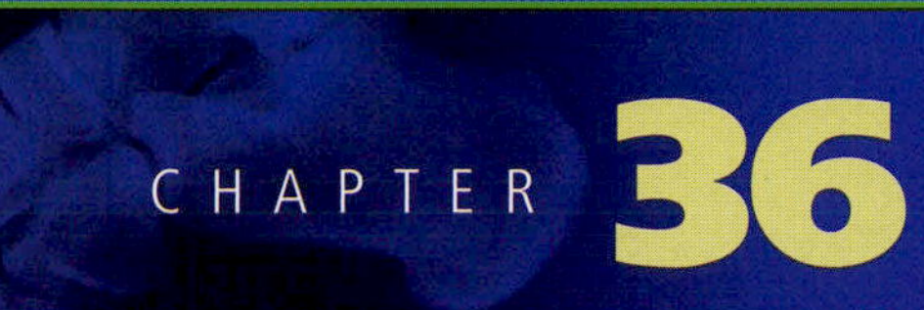

CHAPTER 36 Fluoroscopy

KEY TERMS

carriage
fluoroscopic screen
fluoroscopy
flux gain
image intensification tube
minification gain
total brightness gain

. . . in February, 1896, fantastic, vague, and startling reports emanated from the foreign press regarding a wonderful device "invented" by Professor Salvioni of Perugia, Italy, called the cryptoscope, that permitted instantaneous visualization of human, living, and moving bones. . . . At about the same time Professor McGie of Princeton University also developed a . . . skiascope. Edison also constructed a similar device about which extensive publicity soon developed. He named it the fluoroscope.

Arthur W. Fuchs, "Edison and Roentgenology," reprinted with permission from the American Journal of Roentgenology.

OBJECTIVES

Upon completion of this chapter, the student should be able to:

- Differentiate fluoroscopic examinations from static diagnostic radiographic examinations.
- Describe a typical basic fluoroscopic image chain.
- Explain the difference between the operation of a fluoroscopic and a diagnostic x-ray tube.
- Explain the functions and operation of the image intensification tube input screen, photocathode, electrostatic focusing lenses, and anode and output screen.
- Explain the basic function of a fluoroscopic automatic brightness control.
- Discuss the factors that affect fluoroscopic image contrast, resolution, distortion, and quantum mottle.

OBJECTIVES (continued)

- Explain the uses of dynamic and static fluoroscopic recording systems.
- Explain digital fluoroscopic image acquisition.
- Relate problems with mobile radiographic equipment to mobile fluoroscopic equipment.
- Discuss various methods of reducing dose to the patient, the radiographer, and the radiologist during a fluoroscopic examination.

HISTORICAL DEVELOPMENT

Fluoroscopy (fluoro) is a dynamic radiographic examination, compared to diagnostic radiography, which is static in character. Fluoroscopy involves active diagnosis during an examination. For this reason, fluoroscopy is primarily the domain of the radiologist. The radiographer's role becomes that of an assistant during the examination, although routine post-fluoroscopic radiography is the responsibility of the radiographer. Radiographers should perform fluoroscopy only for static examinations where diagnosis is not involved, such as spot imaging the terminal ilium.

The invention of the fluoroscope is credited to Thomas A. Edison in 1896, the year after Röntgen's discovery of x-rays. However, technically speaking, Röntgen discovered x-rays fluoroscopically when he noticed their ability to demonstrate skeletal anatomy as he brought a lead disc into the beam and observed the dynamic movement of his own fingers projected onto a fluorescent screen. Thus, fluoroscopic procedures have been a part of diagnostic radiography since its inception.

A fluoroscopic imaging chain consists of a specialized x-ray tube with an image receptor, called the **fluoroscopic screen,** that can be viewed during an x-ray exposure. The first fluoroscopes were held by hand in front of the patient and x-ray tube and included a viewing hood to eliminate extraneous light. Later units attached the fluoro screen to the x-ray table. In both systems, the radiologist's face and eyes received the full primary beam. A great number of the pioneers in radiology became martyrs of the science because of the design of early fluoro units. Once the biological hazards of radiation became apparent, the design of the fluoroscope was changed to permit viewing by an arrangement of mirrors. This arrangement shielded the primary beam in a leaded enclosure while the mirrors transmitted the optical image to the viewer. **Image intensification tubes** were developed in 1948, and they resulted in video camera and monitor systems (see Figure 5-1) that began to replace mirror viewers. By 2005 digital fluoroscopic systems began to predominate, with TFT matrices and post-processing capabilities.

FLUOROSCOPIC USES

Although the fluoroscopic image was preferred originally, the need to document findings, coupled with immense improvements in the resolution capabilities of diagnostic radiography, not to mention reductions in the dose to the patient, caused fluoroscopy to become less popular.

Fluoroscopic Positioning Previewing

Fluoroscopy is not intended to be used as a preview to positioning. Radiographers spend 2 years or more learning how to position the patient properly. There should be no reason for a radiographer to use fluoroscopy as a positioning guide. This procedure would cause unnecessary patient exposure to ionizing radiation. Radiographers should obtain a satisfactory image 95 percent of the time, and this degree of expertise entails not just positioning but technical factors and equipment variations as well.

TYPES OF EQUIPMENT

The fluoroscopic x-ray tube and image receptor are mounted on a C-arm to maintain their alignment at all times (Figure 36-1). In the United States, federal

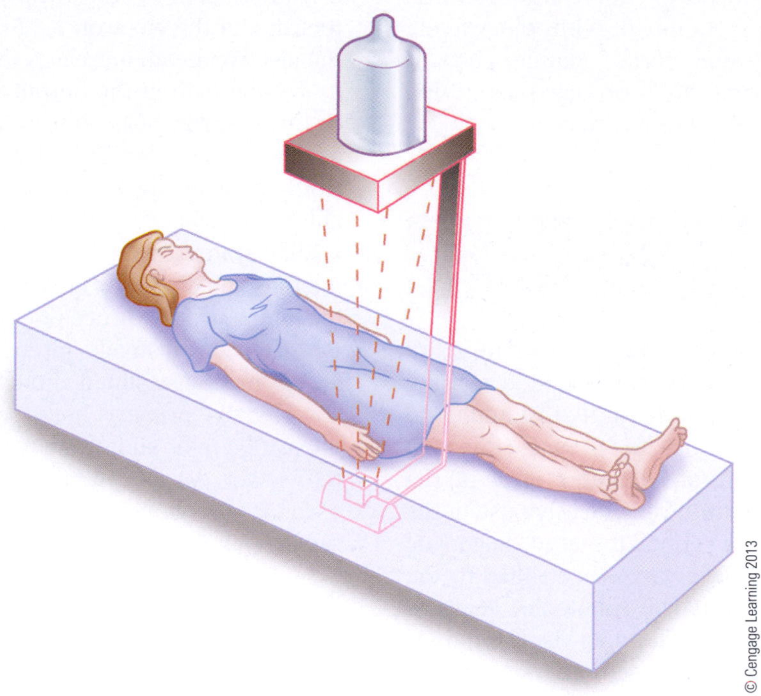

FIGURE 36-1. C-arm alignment of fluoroscopic x-ray tube and image receptor.

regulations prohibit the use of a fluoroscopic x-ray tube when the entire primary beam is not resulting in an image. The C-arm permits the image receptor to be raised and lowered to vary the beam geometry for maximum resolution while the x-ray tube remains in position. It also permits scanning the length and width of the x-ray table. There are two types of C-arm arrangements, both described by the location of the x-ray tube. Under-table units have the x-ray tube under the table, whereas over-table units suspend the tube over the patient.

The arm that supports the equipment suspended over the table is called the **carriage.** It typically includes an image intensification tube (on an under-table unit) or the x-ray tube (on an over-table unit), controls for power drive to the carriage, brightness (which regulates the tube mA), spot image selection, tube shutters, spot imaging and/or cine camera, video input tube, and other controls. Although it can be disengaged and pushed away from the table to gain access to the patient, exposure cannot commence until the carriage is returned to a full beam intercept position.

FLUOROSCOPIC X-RAY TUBES

Fluoroscopic x-ray tubes are very similar to diagnostic tubes except that they are designed to operate for longer periods of time at much lower mA. Where a typical diagnostic tube operates at 50–1,200 mA, the fluoroscopic mA range is 0.5–5.0 mA. The tube target must be fixed to prevent an SOD of less than 15" (38 cm). The fluoroscopic tube is operated by a foot switch, which permits the fluoroscopist to have both hands free to operate the carriage and position and palpate the patient. Care must be taken to not accidentally activate the foot switch when the unit is in operating mode before or after examinations. Fluoroscopic tubes are equipped with electrically controlled shutters that permit maintenance of close collimation from the fluoro carriage during both fluoroscopy and spot imaging.

IMAGE INTENSIFICATION TUBES

Early fluoroscopic screens were very dim. Dark adaptation, a procedure in which light levels are reduced for a period of at least 10–15 minutes to permit the rods of the eye to become activated, was a time-consuming and irritating part of the radiologist's work routine. The exclusive use of the rod cells constituted a serious threat to diagnostic accuracy because visual acuity is controlled by the cones, which require daylight (photopic) levels of light in order to function. Photopic visual acuity is about 10 times greater than scotopic acuity. The brightness of the fluoro image was not raised to daylight levels until image intensification technology was developed in 1948.

An image intensification tube was designed to electronically amplify the brightness of an image. Image intensifiers were capable of increasing image brightness 500–8,000 times.

A typical image intensifier is shown in Figure 36-2. The primary x-ray beam exits the patient and strikes the input screen of the image intensifier tube, which is a vacuum tube with a cathode and an anode. The fluorescent screen is built into the image intensifier as its input screen. The fluorescent screen absorbs the x-ray photons and emits light photons, which immediately encounter the photocathode (the cathode of the tube) that is in contact with the input screen to prevent divergence of the light beam. The photocathode absorbs the light photons and emits electrons. The electrons are then accelerated from the cathode toward the anode and the output screen by the potential difference that exists between the cathode and anode. At the same time the electron beam is focused onto the output screen, which is much smaller than the input screen. Electrostatic lenses are used to accelerate and focus the electrons. The primary brightness gain occurs from the acceleration and focusing of the electron beam. The acceleration of the electron beam increases its energy and its ability to emit light at the output screen. The focusing of the electron beam intensifies the image into a smaller area. The output screen absorbs the electrons and emits light photons, which are then available for viewing or further electronic processing by a video system. Note the changes in the quantity of photons and electrons in the image at each stage of the intensification process.

The entire image intensification tube is encased in a lead-lined housing that effectively absorbs the primary beam while permitting the intensified light photon image to be transmitted to the viewer. An ion pump device called a getter is used to remove ions produced during operation and to maintain the vacuum within the tube.

Input Screen and Photocathode

The input fluorescent screen consists of a 0.1- to 0.2-mm layer of sodium-activated cesium iodide (CsI) phosphors coated onto the concave surface of the image intensification tube. This surface may be made of glass, titanium, steel, or aluminum and ranges from 6" (15 cm) to 23"3 (58 cm) in diameter, depending on the manufacturer and use. The screen is concave to maintain the same distance between each point on the input screen and its corresponding location on the output screen. Failure to maintain this distance would result in distortion of the image because points farther from the center would be more magnified. The CsI phosphors are packed together very tightly so they absorb about 66 percent of the incident beam, producing a good conversion efficiency, or quantum yield. The phosphors then emit light photons vertically, in proportion to the absorption, thus reducing the lateral spread of light photons that would reduce the image detail. As an example, a single 25-keV incident photon would typically produce over 1,500 light photons. This conversion efficiency permits the fluoro system to function with minimal activation of the phosphors.

An extremely thin protective coating is applied to the input screen to prevent a chemical interaction with the photocathode. The

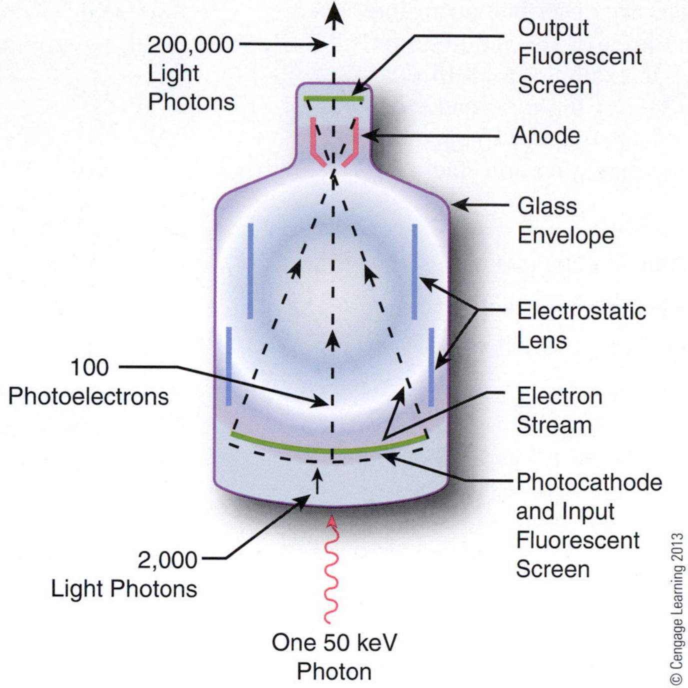

FIGURE 36-2. An image intensification tube. The quantity of photons and electrons in the image changes at each stage of the intensification process, with the output significantly greater than the input.

photocathode material is composed of photoemissive metals, usually cesium and antimony compounds, which are applied to the protective coating. The two materials appear to be a single coating when examined. The photoemissive materials absorb the light photons and emit electrons in a process called photoemission. The process is similar to thermionic emission except that the stimulation is light instead of heat.

Electrostatic Lenses

The electrostatic lenses are a series of charged electrodes located inside the glass envelope of the tube. Because the electrons are negative, the charge of the lenses accelerates and focuses the electron stream, which carries the fluoroscopic image. As with an optically focused image, the focal point reverses the image so the output screen image is reversed from the input screen image (right becomes left and superior becomes inferior). The concave input screen reduces distortion by maintaining the same distance between all points on the input screen and their corresponding locations on the output screen, regardless of the position of the focal point.

Magnification Tubes. The greater the voltage supplied to the electrostatic lenses, the greater the acceleration and the closer the focal point moves toward the input screen. Image intensification tubes can be designed to magnify the image electronically by changing the voltage on the electrostatic lenses. They are often called multifield, dual-field, triple-field, or quad-field intensifiers.

Increased voltage focuses the electrons at a point closer to the input screen, and this causes the image to be magnified when it reaches the output screen (Figure 36-3). Magnification image intensifiers are capable of 1.5–4 magnification, which is usually controlled at the fluoro carriage. Some tubes are capable of up to four different magnifications. Resolution can be increased from ≈4 lp/mm to ≈6 lp/mm when the magnification mode is used. The tubes are described according to the diameter of the area of the input screen that will be imaged. For example, a 23/15 dual-focus tube has a 9" (23-cm) input screen when operating normally and uses a 6" (15-cm) area when magnifying. The magnification factor is calculated as:

$$\text{magnification} = \frac{\text{input screen diameter}}{\text{diameter of input screen used during magnification}}$$

EXAMPLE: What is the magnification for an image viewed with an image intensification tube with an input screen diameter of 9″ (23 cm) that is using a 5″ (13-cm) diameter area during magnification?

Answer:

$$\text{magnification} = \frac{\text{input screen diameter}}{\text{diameter of input screen used during magnification}}$$

$$\text{magnification} = \frac{9''}{5''}$$

magnification = 1.8

The excess edges of the image are not transmitted by the output screen; therefore, the primary beam field should be collimated to the viewing field when these tubes are operated in magnification mode. Minimal magnification is used for most studies because it reduces contrast problems due to minification and flux gain and permits viewing of the entire primary beam field.

Anode and Output Screen

The anode is positively charged and is normally supplied with about 25 kV. This charge causes a tremendous attraction of the negative electrons from the photocathode. The anode is positioned inside the glass envelope, immediately in front of the output screen. It has a hole in its center that permits

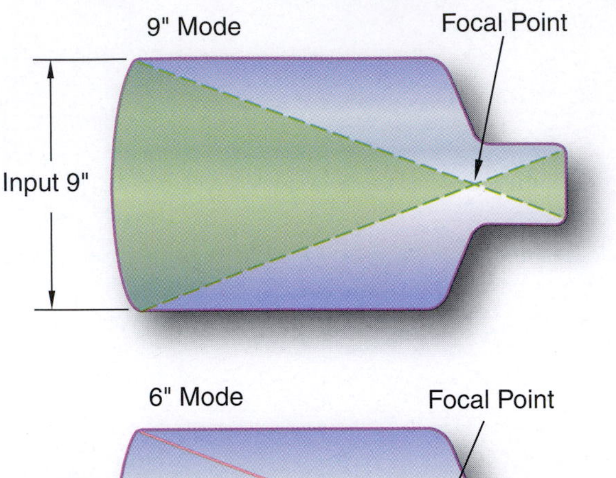

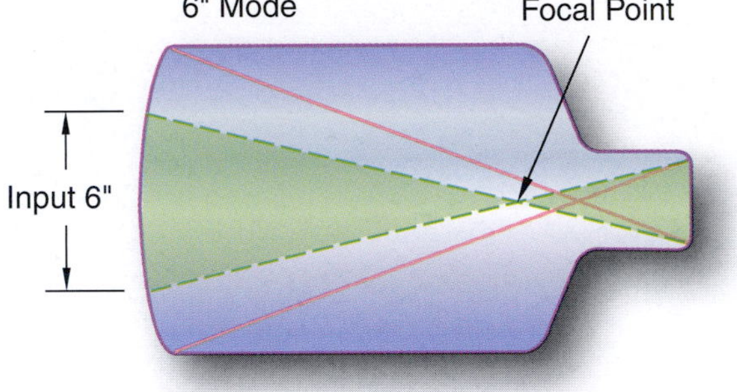

FIGURE 36-3. A magnification image intensification tube. Changes in the focal point produce the magnification.

the accelerated electrons to pass through the anode field and onto the output screen.

The output screen is also a glass fluorescent screen. It is a silver-activated zinc-cadmium sulfide phosphor (ZnS-CdS:Ag) that was also used as the input phosphor in early tubes. The phosphor is extremely small (1–2 mm), and the output anode screen is very thin (4–8 mm) to produce high resolution (≈70 lp/mm). The electrons that strike the screen are converted into green light photons that exit the tube. Because all phosphors emit light isotropically, an opaque filter is used under the output phosphor layer to prevent most of the light emitted in that direction from returning to the input screen, where it would degrade the image. Some newer intensifiers use a fiber-optic disc in place of the glass output screen. Fiber optics eliminate the isotropic emission problem and are capable of transmitting the image some distance without loss of resolution.

Total Brightness Gain

Total brightness gain is a measurement of the increase in image intensity achieved by an image intensification tube. It is determined by two factors: minification gain and flux gain.

Minification Gain. Minification gain occurs as a result of the same number of electrons that were produced at the large input screen being compressed into the area of the small output screen. Most image intensification tubes have input screens of 6" (15 cm) or 9" (23 cm), although 12" (30-cm) and larger tubes have been available for special applications. The typical output screen has a diameter of 1" (2.5 cm). The minification gain is calculated as the ratio between the area of the input and output screens.

$$\text{minification gain} = \frac{\text{input screen diameter}^2}{\text{output screen diameter}^2}$$

EXAMPLE: What is the minification gain for an image intensification tube with an input screen diameter of 6" (15 cm) and an output diameter of 1" (2.5 cm)?

Answer:

$$\text{minification gain} = \frac{\text{input screen diameter}^2}{\text{output screen diameter}^2}$$

$$\text{minification gain} = \frac{6^2}{1^2}$$

$$\text{minification gain} = \frac{36}{1}$$

$$\text{minification gain} = 36$$

Minification gain is simply an increase in brightness or intensity, not an improvement in the quality or number of photons making up the image.

Flux Gain. Flux gain is a measurement of the increase in light photons due to the conversion efficiency of the output screen. For example, if the output phosphor produces 50 light photons for each electron that strikes it, the flux gain would be 50. Flux gain does not take into account the conversion efficiency of the input screen. It deals only with the gain accomplished by the electron-to-light conversion at the output screen. Flux gain causes a decrease in image quality exactly as intensifying screens decrease resolution in diagnostic images as a result of the penumbral effect of individual phosphor crystals.

Total Brightness Gain. Total brightness gain can be calculated by several methods. As a function of minification and flux gain, the formula is:

$$\text{brightness gain} = \text{minification gain} \times \text{flux gain}$$

EXAMPLE: What is the total brightness gain for an image intensification tube with a minification gain of 36 and a flux gain of 60?

Answer:

$$\text{brightness gain} = \text{minification gain} \times \text{flux gain}$$

$$\text{brightness gain} = 36 \times 60$$

$$\text{brightness gain} = 2{,}160$$

However, the original formula was:

$$\text{brightness gain} = \frac{\text{intensity of output phosphor}}{\text{intensity of Patterson B-2 fluoroscopic screen}}$$

A Patterson B–2 fluoro screen was chosen as the reference point because it was in common use at the time. This formula has lost acceptance because the Patterson B–2 screens would vary from one batch to another and their deterioration was not linear.

Because the Patterson B–2 screen is no longer available, this standard is now obsolete. Although it appears that the term *brightness gain* will continue in use, its measure is a conversion factor that is the ratio of the intensity of the output phosphor to the input exposure rate.

$$\text{conversion factor} = \frac{\text{intensity of output phosphor}}{\text{mR/sec}}$$

Output phosphor intensity is measured in candelas (cd), the unit of luminous intensity.

$$\text{conversion factor} = \frac{\text{cd/m}^2}{\text{mR/sec}}$$

Typical values for modern image intensifier systems are

$$80 - 250\frac{\text{cd/m}^2}{\text{mR/sec}}$$

This represents a gain of 8,000–25,000 times.

Brightness gain deteriorates as much as 10 percent per year because, just as with intensifying-screen phosphors, the input and output screen phosphors age. Although difficult to measure, brightness gain can be evaluated by monitoring the radiation dose required to obtain a diagnostic image from a standard phantom, such as an abdomen or pelvis.

Various systems with different names are used to automatically maintain satisfactory fluoroscopic image density and contrast. Automatic brightness control (ABC) is the most common term, although automatic dose control (ADC) and automatic brightness stabilization (ABS) accomplish the same result. They maintain the brightness of the image by automatically adjusting the exposure factors as necessary according to subject density and contrast. Most ABC systems monitor the current flowing between the cathode and anode of the image intensification tube or the intensity of the output screen. In all systems, the primary beam is changed when current and intensity fall below established levels. Regulation of the primary beam can be accomplished by varying kVp, mA, and pulse time. Most ABCs use combinations of these methods in a manner similar to a stepped variable kVp technique system. For example, kVp is gradually increased to the maximum acceptable contrast level, then mA is doubled while kVp is stepped down to the lowest acceptable contrast level and the procedure is started over again. All ABCs have a relatively slow response time, which is noticeable during routine fluoroscopic scanning because the image density adjustment lags a moment behind rapid changes in tissue density. Automatic gain control (AGC) is part of the video camera control system. It responds very quickly to input information but does not change the x-ray exposure factors.

IMAGE QUALITY

Because the imaging chain of a fluoroscopic system is so complex, there are more factors that affect each of the quality elements of the image than in static radiography. In addition to contrast, resolution, and distortion, quantum mottle must also be considered.

Contrast

Contrast is controlled by increasing the amplitude of the video signal, although it is affected by other factors. Digital fluoroscopic system can also use post-processing functions, especially window width and various filtering algorithms, to improve image contrast. Image intensified fluoroscopic contrast is not only affected by scattered ionizing radiation but is also affected by penumbral light scatter in the input and output screens, and light scatter within the image intensification tube itself. By raising the lowest density value, it decreases the total visible contrast. The overall effect is of reduced contrast. There is also a decrease in image contrast near the edges of the images.

Resolution

The ability to resolve recorded detail in a fluoroscopic system will vary depending on the geometrical factors, just as in static radiography. However, the geometrical factors are different, including minification gain. CsI image intensifiers are capable of ≈2 lp/mm, whereas digital fluoroscopic systems often achieve 2 lp/mm (Table 36-1).

TABLE 36-1. Typical Limiting Spatial Resolution in Fluoroscopy

Field of View: cm (inches)	1,023-Line Video: Line Pairs/mm	525-Line Video: Line Pairs/mm
14 (5.5)	2.7	1.4
20 (7.9)	2.0	1.0
27 (10.6)	1.6	0.7
40 (15.7)	1.3	0.5

From *The Essential Physics of Medical Imaging* (2nd ed.), by J. Bushberg, J. Seibert, E. Leidholdt, and J. Boone, 2002, Philadelphia: Lippincott Williams & Wilkins. Reprinted with permission.

Distortion

Size distortion is caused by the same factors that affect static radiographic magnification, primarily OID. Although a magnified image often appears to have more distortion, the distortion is also present in the minified image. It is simply easier to detect when enlarged.

Shape distortion is caused primarily by geometric problems in the shape of the image intensification tube. Although the image intensifier input screen is concave, it does not completely eliminate edge distortion at the output screen. Electrons at the outer edges of the image tend to flare outward as they are electrostatically focused. Part of this problem is caused by the repulsion of electrons from one another due to their like charges. Figure 31-4 illustrates the edge distortion problem in image intensification tubes. This effect is called vignetting or pincushion distortion and may comprise 8–10 percent of the image area. Some of the vignetting effect is also caused by the effect of the divergence of the primary beam from the x-ray tube focal spot. Vignetting also causes image intensity to be greater at the center of the image and less at the edges. Consequently, distortion is minimized and contrast is improved at the center of the fluoro image. This problem has been completely overcome with the use of TFT matrices, as they have uniform resolution across the entire surface of the detector array.

Quantum Mottle

Quantum mottle is a blotchy or grainy appearance caused by insufficient radiation to create a uniform image. Because the quantity of photons is controlled by the mA and time settings, with static radiography any mA and time combination can be used to accumulate sufficient radiation to create a uniform image. With fluoroscopy, the time factor is controlled by the length of time the eye can integrate, or accumulate, light photons from the fluoro imaging chain. Because this period is 0.2 second, fluoroscopy must provide sufficient photons, through mA, to avoid mottle. Quantum mottle is also a large part of video noise and is a special problem during fluoroscopy because the units operate with the minimum number of photons possible to activate the fluoro screen. The factors that influence mottle are those that affect the total number of photons arriving at the retina of the eye. This includes radiation output, beam attenuation by the subject, the conversion efficiency of the input screen, minification gain, flux gain, total brightness gain, viewing system, and the distance of the eye from the viewing system. Increasing the efficiency of any of these factors can assist in reducing quantum mottle, but the most common solution is to increase the fluoro tube mA.

VIDEO VIEWING SYSTEMS

The most commonly used fluoroscopic viewing system is video. A system includes a video camera attached to the image intensification tube output phosphor and a display monitor for viewing. Fluoroscopic video cameras use charge-coupled devices (CCDs).

Video Camera Charge-Coupled Devices (CCDs)

A CCD is a semiconducting device capable of storing a charge from light photons striking a photosensitive surface. When light strikes the photoelectric cathode of the CCD, electrons are released proportionally to the intensity of the incident light. As with all semiconductors, the CCD has the ability to store the freed electrons in a series of P and N holes, thus storing the image in a latent form (see Chapter 4). The video signal is emitted in a raster scanning pattern by moving the stored charges along the P and N holes to the edge of the CCD, where they are discharged as pulses into a conductor. The primary advantage of CCDs is the extremely fast discharge time, which eliminates image lag. This is extremely useful in high-speed imaging applications such as cardiac catheterization. Other advantages are that CCDs are more sensitive than video tubes, they operate at much lower voltages, which prolongs their life, they have acceptable resolution, and they are not as susceptible to damage from rough handling.

Video Monitor

A video monitor is a high-resolution output screen that receives the final processed signal from the fluoroscopic processor. Flat screen monitors require regular calibration and quality assurance testing.

DIGITAL FLUOROSCOPY

Digital fluoroscopy is achieved through the use of a high-power generator operating in a pulse progressive fluoroscopy mode. Essentially this technology pulses the x-ray production from the fluoroscopic x-ray tube in synchronization with the detector signal, so that pulses of signals are received by the image processing unit. The length of time required for the generator to come on and achieve the necessary kVp and mAs levels is called the interrogation time. The extinction time is that required to shut the generator down in preparation for the next pulse.

This technology is combined with a detector comprised of a thin film transistor (TFT) in contact with the image intensifier (II) output anode screen. The TFT replaces the image intensifier in nondigital fluoro systems. A TFT is a pixelated unit with a photodiode connected to each pixel element.. A unique feature of TFTs is that they are relatively insensitive to x-ray photons. In fact, some manufacturers add a CsI scintillator element to the image receptor to increase sensitivity by adding back the x-ray photon energy. CsI phosphors absorb x-ray photons and emit light that can be recorded by the TFT. TFT limitations are primarily concerned with the electronic noise limits for flat panel amplification. The gain at fluoro levels is around 1–5 μR/frame, which adds a significant signal-to-noise ratio (s/n). Most digital fluoro manufacturers utilize a process called pixel binning by combining pixels 2×2 or 3×3. This results in lower noise, which in turn provides a more accurate diagnostic image. Details on the function of TFTs are part of Chapter 23, Digital Radiography.

Digital fluoroscopy resolution cannot be as high as in radiography because the clinical value is outweighed by patient exposure concerns. Consequently, digital fluoro pixels are between 200 μm and 300 μm (which translates to approximately 1–2 lp/mm), as compared to radiography pixels, which are 100–150 μm (which translates to approximately 10–12 lp/mm). Most digital fluoroscopic systems are capable of 8-bit processing (which provides up to 256 shades of gray per pixel). Some manufacturers combine up to four radiography pixels into a single image processing pixel for fluoroscopic functions.

Digital fluoroscopic systems are capable of very good separation of acquisition and display, which produces much higher contrast. When combined with the post-processing capabilities of the fluoro units, this provides significantly improved imaging ability.

Last image hold is a common function on most digital fluoroscopic units (including mobile C-arm equipment). This function simply maintains the last real-time fluoroscopic image until it is replaced by the unit being activated again. This allows physicians to continue to work from the most recent image without exposing the patient to additional radiation.

Numerous post-exposure image processing functions are also available with digital fluoroscopy. These include window level and width, filtering techniques (edge enhancement, temporal filtering, etc.), and digital subtraction technology (which can digitally remove background structures when a previous image is superimposed). See Chapter 40, Vascular Imaging Equipment, for more details on digital subtraction fluoroscopy.

Digital fluoroscopy reduces patient exposure considerably with both dynamic and static images recorded at reduced doses. This reduction can be on the order of elimination of up to 90 percent of the patient exposure.

RECORDING THE FLUOROSCOPIC IMAGE

Dynamic recording of fluoroscopic images can be achieved through the use of any recording media with adequate memory (e.g., DVDs). It is also possible to record static images from fluoroscopy with any digital recording device.

Digital Fluoroscopy

Digital fluoroscopy units process the image coming from the charge coupled device (CCD) by sending an analog signal through an analog-to-digital converter (ADC) microchip. See Chapter 23, Digital Radiography, for a complete discussion of this process.

Once the fluoroscopic image has been converted to a digital signal, it can be manipulated as desired and transferred repeatedly without loss of quality. Display on a monitor permits changes in density (digital window level), contrast (digital window width), magnification, filtration enhancements, and other techniques to be applied to the image.

Digitization also permits storage on computer disk, and transfer via electronic means such as teleradiology systems or the Internet.

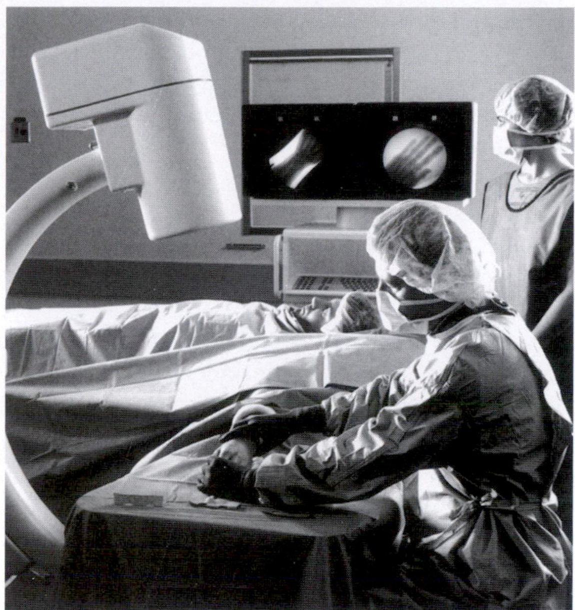

FIGURE 36-4. A mobile C-arm fluoroscopic unit. *(Courtesy of GE Healthcare.)*

MOBILE FLUOROSCOPIC EQUIPMENT

Mobile C-arm fluoroscopic units are extremely popular for surgical procedures (Figure 36-4). When coupled to a videodisc unit, both static and dynamic imaging can be instantly available. The units operate exactly as do stationary fluoroscopic units, although controls may have different labeling. All the cautions and adaptations for mobile radiography are applicable to mobile fluoroscopy.

RADIATION PROTECTION DURING FLUOROSCOPY

The Patient

Fluoroscopic units operate with the minimum radiation output possible for the efficiency of the imaging system. There is no appreciable difference in the patient dose between an optical mirror viewing system and a video system. The entrance skin exposure for the patient is the surface closest to the source. With an under-table unit the ESE is measured from the surface next to the tabletop. With an over-table unit it is measured from the surface toward the fluoro carriage. The tabletop exposure rate should not exceed 10 R/min and for most units should range from 1 to 3 R/min. The minimum source-to-skin distance is 12" (30 cm) for mobile fluoroscopic equipment and 15" (38 cm) for stationary equipment.

In the United States, federal law requires an audible 5-minute timer. Although it can be reset as many times as necessary to complete a procedure, it is intended to serve as a reminder to the radiologist of how much total exposure time is being used. Fluoroscopy is interrupted when the 5 minutes have elapsed and the radiographer must reset the timer to continue the procedure.

Magnification image intensifiers cause increased patient dose because the automatic brightness control (ABC) will increase the tube output to compensate for the loss of electrons within the image intensification tube during magnification. The x-ray tube should have the collimation shutters closed to the viewing image size when in the magnification mode. When magnifying, the output screen of the image intensification tube does not receive the entire image from the input screen, so it is possible to irradiate tissue that cannot be viewed. Although these image intensifiers may have interlocks that automatically collimate when magnifying, attention to this detail decreases patient dose.

The Radiographer and Radiologist

A lead apron of at least 0.5 mm Pb/eq must be worn by all persons (other than the patient) who are present in the fluoroscopic room during exposure. An apron designed to cover the front and sides of the body is usually sufficient, although a wraparound apron for both front and back should be considered if the radiographer is required to turn his or her back to the patient and x-ray tube during the procedure. Radiographers assisting during fluoroscopy must develop the ability to back and sidle around the room during exposures, always keeping the front of the body with its lead apron facing the patient and tube. If the hands must be placed within the primary beam, lead gloves of at least 0.5 mm Pb/q must be worn.

The primary source of exposure to the radiographer and radiologist is the patient. It is worth noting that the highest energy scatter occurs at a greater than 90° angle to the incident beam (skewed toward the tube) and is greatest at the entrance surface more than at deeper depths because of the lower attenuation of the beam at the surface. It is also worth remembering that according to the inverse square law, a single step back from the patient will decrease the dose exponentially (Figure 36-5). The slot immediately under the tabletop where the bucky tray is positioned for diagnostic radiography is also at the gonadal level. Fluoroscopic units must have a 0.25 mm/Pb eq. lead shield to cover this slot. However, it must be brought into position by moving the bucky tray to the head or foot of the table prior to beginning fluoro. Strips of lead rubber, forming a drape (which should be 0.25 Pb), are positioned between the fluoroscopist and patient to absorb the majority of the patient scatter. The radiographer has one advantage during fluoroscopy in that he or she may position himself or herself behind the radiologist. This not only adds an additional lead apron, but the entire body of the fluoroscopist is there to protect the radiographer.

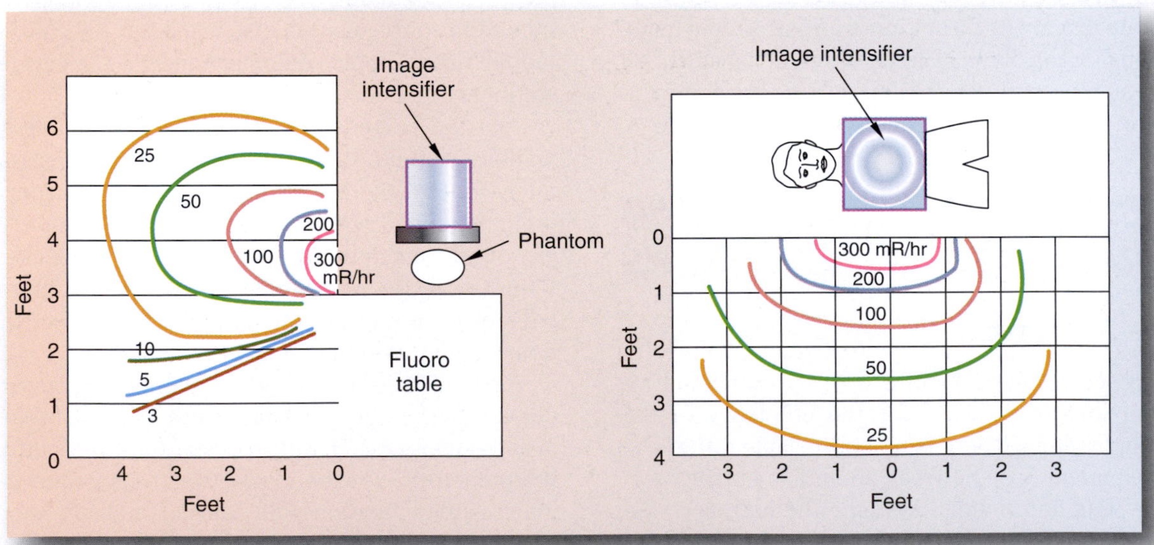

FIGURE 36-5. An isodose curve for a typical fluoroscopic unit. The shape of the curve illustrates areas of lesser dose during fluoroscopic procedures. *(Adapted with permission from Wold, G. J., Scheele, R. V., and Agarwal, S. K., April 1971, "Evaluation of Physician Exposure During Cardiac Catheterization,"* Fig. 3 and 4, p. 189, Radiology 99: 1, 188-190.*)*

Others

The radiographer has a duty to require that anyone present in the fluoroscopy room during an examination wear a lead apron. All persons, regardless of rank or authority, should be informed of this requirement. Fluoroscopy should not be initiated until everyone complies.

SUMMARY

Fluoroscopy (fluoro) is a dynamic radiographic examination that involves active diagnosis during the examination. For this reason fluoroscopy is primarily the domain of the radiologist, the radiologist assistant, and the physician assistant. The radiographer's role becomes that of an assistant during an examination. Fluoroscopy is currently used for studies that require observation of dynamic physiological functions, for example, the flow of barium through the gastrointestinal tract, swallowing, the injection of a contrast medium into the heart, and so on.

The fluoroscopic imaging chain consists of a specialized x-ray tube with an image receptor, called the fluoroscopic screen, that can be viewed during an x-ray exposure. The fluoroscopic x-ray tube and image receptor are mounted on a C-arm to maintain their alignment at all times. Fluoroscopic x-ray tubes are very similar to diagnostic tubes except that they are designed to operate for longer periods of time at much lower mA. During fluoroscopy, the primary x-ray beam exits the patient and strikes the input screen of the image intensifier tube. The fluorescent screen is built into the image intensifier as its input screen. The fluorescent screen absorbs the x-ray photons and emits light photons, which immediately encounter the photocathode (the cathode of the tube) that is in contact with the input screen to prevent divergence of the light beam. The photocathode absorbs the light photons and emits electrons. The electrons are then accelerated from the cathode toward the anode and the output screen by the potential difference that exists between the cathode and anode. At the same time, the electron beam is focused onto the output screen, which is much smaller than the input screen. Electrostatic lenses are used to accelerate and focus the electrons. The primary brightness gain occurs from the acceleration and focusing of the electron beam. Brightness gain is a measurement of the increase in image intensity and is determined by minification gain and flux gain. The acceleration of the electron beam increases its energy and its ability to emit light at the output screen. The focusing of the electron beam intensifies the image into a smaller area. The output screen absorbs the electrons and emits light photons, which are then available for viewing or further electronic processing by a video system. The primary factors that affect the quality of the fluoroscopic image include contrast, resolution, distortion, and quantum mottle.

During fluoroscopy, it is possible to record either a dynamic or a static image. Fluoroscopic units operate with the minimum radiation output possible for the efficiency of the imaging system. The entrance skin exposure for the patient is the surface closest to the source. The tabletop dose rate should not exceed 10 R/min and for most units should range from 1 to 3 R/min.

A lead apron of at least 0.5 mm Pb/eq must be worn by all persons (other than the patient) who are present in the fluoroscopic room during exposure. The primary source of exposure to the radiographer and radiologist is the patient, with the highest energy scatter occurring at a 90° angle to the incident beam. The radiographer has a duty to require that anyone present in the fluoroscopy room during an examination wear a lead apron. ■

REVIEW QUESTIONS

1. Why is fluoroscopy the domain of the radiologist, radiologist assistant, and physician assistant?
2. What is the typical basic fluoroscopic imaging chain?
3. How does a fluoroscopic x-ray tube differ from a diagnostic x-ray tube?
4. What is the basic function of the fluorescent screen, the photocathode, the electrostatic lenses, and the output screen?
5. What is the formula used for determining brightness gain?
6. What is the purpose of the automatic brightness control?
7. What is the primary limitation of resolution of the fluoroscopic image?
8. What radiation protection practices should be adhered to by the radiographer during fluoroscopy?

REFERENCES AND RECOMMENDED READING

American Association of Physicists in Medicine. (1998). *Managing the use of fluoroscopy in medical institutions (Report of Task Group 6, AAPM Report 58)*. College Park, MD: Medical Physics.

Barnes, G. T., & Tishler, J. M. (1981). Fluoroscopic image quality and its implications regarding equipment selection and use. In C. M. Coulam, J. J. Erickson, F. D. Rollo, & A. E. James. (Eds.), *The physical basis of medical imaging*. New York: Appleton-Century-Crofts.

Beekmans, A. G. (1982). Image quality aspects of x-ray image intensifiers. *Medicamundi, 27*, 25.

Birken, H., & Bejczy, C. I. (1978). A new generation of x-ray image intensifiers. *Medicamundi, 18*(3), 120.

Brink, G. S. (1973). Fundamentals of image intensification: Design and application. *Radiologic Technology, 44*(5), 317.

Bushberg, J., Seibert, J., Leidholdt, E., & Boone, J. (2002). *The essential physics of medical imaging* (2nd ed.). Philadelphia: Lippincott Williams & Wilkins.

Bushong, S. C. (2008). *Radiologic science for technologists: Physics, biology, and protection* (9th ed.). St. Louis, MO: Elsevier Mosby.

Curry, T. S., Dowdey, J. E., & Murry, R. C. (1990). *Christensen's introduction to the physics of diagnostic radiology* (4th ed.). Philadelphia: Lea and Febiger.

De Voss, D. (1985). *Basic principles of radiographic exposure* (2nd ed.). Baltimore: Williams & Wilkins.

Fuchs, A. W. (1947). Edison and Roentgenology. *The American Journal of Roentgenology, 57*(2), 145–156.

Gough, L. (1987). Remote-controlled fluoroscopy in a pediatric hospital. *The Canadian Journal of Medical Radiation Technology, 18*(3), 93.

Gray, J. E., Stears, J. G., Lopez, F., & Wondraw, M. A. (1984, February). Fluoroscopic imaging: Quantitation of image lag or smearing. *Radiology*, 563.

Gray, J. E., Winkler, N. T., Stears, J. G., & Frank, E. D. (1983). *Quality control in diagnostic imaging: A quality control cookbook*. Baltimore: University Park Press.

Hynes, D. M., Edmonds, E. W., & Baranoski, D. (1981). Reducing fluoroscopic dosage and cause. *Diagnostic Imaging, 3*, 32–37.

Image intensification systems. (1974).*Radiologic Technology, 46*(3), 196.

Morgan, D. (1990). Applying 100 millimetre and digital technology to general radiography. *Radiography Today, 56*(642), 11–13.

Pooley, R., McKinney, J., & Miller, D. (2001).The AAPM/RSNA physics tutorial for residents: Digital fluoroscopy. *RadioGraphics, 21*, 521–534.

Rich, J. E. (1970). *The theory and clinical application of intensified fluoroscopy in the radiology department*. Milwaukee, WI: General Electric Company Medical Systems Division.

Seeram, E. (1978). Some characteristics of the cesium iodide x-ray image intensifier. *The Canadian Journal of Radiography, Radiotherapy, and Nuclear Medicine, 9*(1), 42–43.

Seeram, E. (1985). *X-ray imaging equipment: An introduction*. Springfield, IL: Charles C Thomas.

Seeram, E. (2011). *Digital radiography, an introduction*. Clifton Park, NY: Delmar Cengage Learning.

Siedband, M. P. (1981). Fluoroscopic imaging. In C. M. Coulam, J. J. Erickson, F. D. Rollo, & A. E. James, (Eds.), *The physical basis of medical imaging*. New York: Appleton-Century-Crofts.

Skucas, J., & Gorski, J. W. (1976). Comparison of image quality of 105 mm film with conventional film. *Radiology, 118*, 433–437.

Stears, J., Gray, J. E., & Frank, E. D. (1989). Radiologic exchange (dose reduction with 105 mm spot films). *Radiologic Technology, 60*(6), 515–516.

Thompson, M. A., Hattaway, M. P., Hall, J. D., & Dowd, S. B. (1994). *Principles of imaging science and protection.* Philadelphia: W. B. Saunders.

Wesenberg, R. L., & Amundson, G. M. (1984). Fluoroscopy in children: Low exposure technology. *Radiology, 153*(1), 243–247.

Wolbarst, A. B. (1993). *Physics of radiology.* Norwalk, CT: Appleton & Lange.

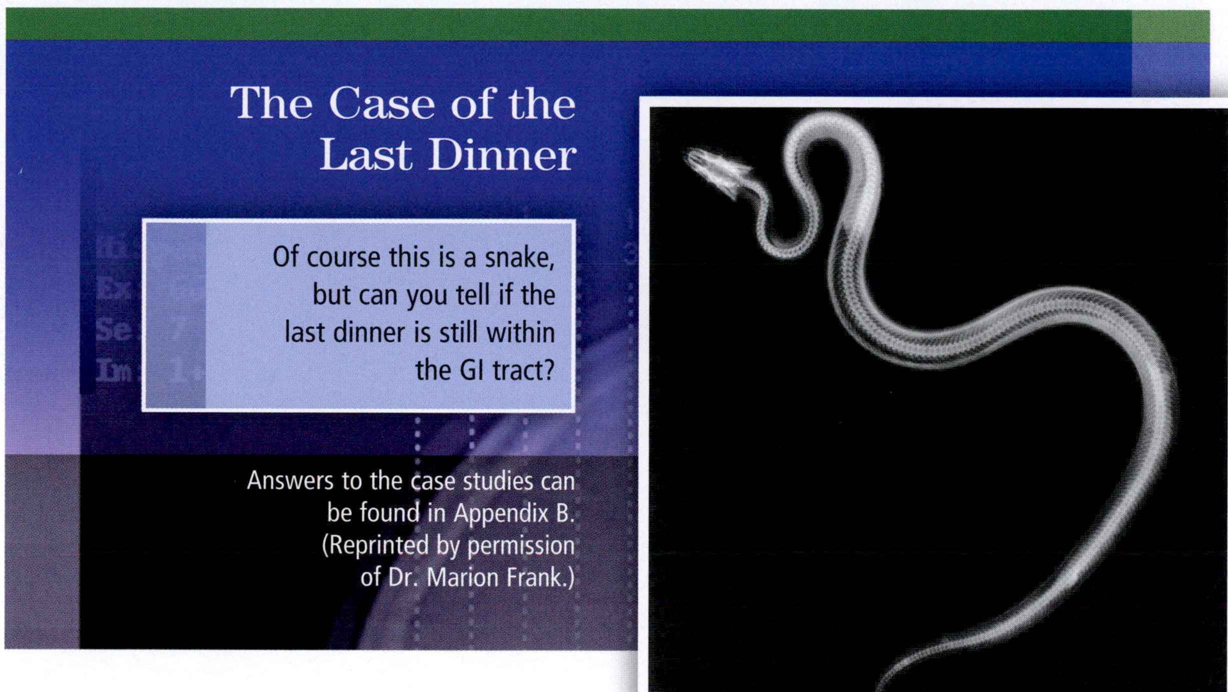

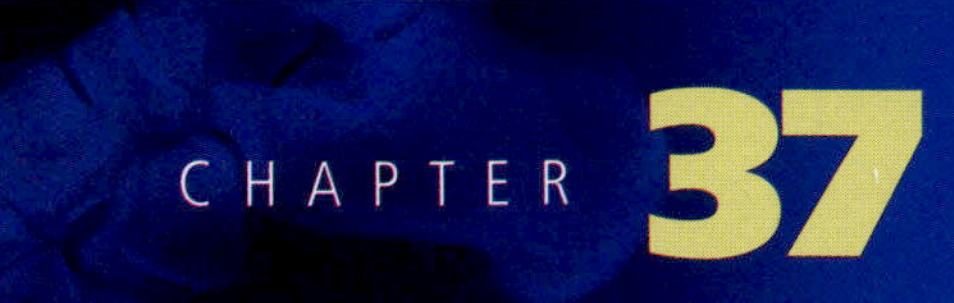

Tomography and Digital Tomosynthesis

KEY TERMS

blur
digital tomosynthesis
exposure amplitude
focal plane
fulcrum
pantomography
section interval
section thickness
tomographic amplitude
tomography

. . . there exists between (tube and plate), in space, a single fixed plane, in which each point always has a corresponding image point on the plate; hence, only the organs contained in this plane are in focus.

André-Edmund-Marie-Bocage, from "Method of, and apparatus for, radiography on a moving plate"

OBJECTIVES

Upon completion of this chapter, the student should be able to:

- Define tomography.
- Explain the tomographic principle.
- Explain the relationship of tomographic amplitude to exposure amplitude.
- Describe the effects of tomographic amplitude, distance from the fulcrum, distance from the image receptor, and the orientation of tube motion on image blur.
- Explain the causes of tomographic phantom images.
- Explain the function of the fulcrum.
- Describe the dimensions of the focal plane.
- Correlate changes in exposure amplitude with their effect on section thickness.
- Describe a section interval.
- Evaluate linear tomographic quality parameters.

OBJECTIVES (continued)

- Establish a tomographic procedure, including section thickness and interval, for a clinical problem.
- Describe the specialized tomographic techniques.
- Select appropriate exposure factors for a tomographic examination after a satisfactory preliminary scout radiograph has been produced.
- Explain the process of acquiring a digital tomosynthesis image.

Tomography is a radiographic technique that employs motion to show anatomical structures lying in a plane of tissue while blurring or eliminating the detail in images of structures above and below the plane of interest. It primarily demonstrates coronal sections, although sagittal sections of most body parts and transverse sections of the head may be accomplished through positioning.

First developed in 1921, and long the premier investigative procedure for removing superimposing structures, tomography is now used in only a few limited areas. Since the advent of modern computerized sectional imaging techniques (i.e., computed tomography and magnetic resonance imaging), its use has declined rapidly, although it is still considered of value for routine examination of the kidneys during intravenous pyelography. Tomography has also been found useful when computerized modalities are too costly or unavailable, and digital tomosynthesis is establishing its value as a routine diagnostic modality.

Although many have claimed credit for the development of tomography, only nine investigators actually had a part in its development, beginning with André Edmund Bocage (French dermatologist 1892–1953) and including the American radiographer Jean Kieffer. Tomography has been called planigraphy, stratigraphy, and laminography over the years, and it is still sometimes called body section radiography.

THE TOMOGRAPHIC PRINCIPLE

The principle of tomography is based on synchronous movement of two of the three elements in a tomographic system: the x-ray tube, the object, and the image receptor. Most tomographic units synchronize the movements of the x-ray tube and the image receptor in opposite directions around a stationary **fulcrum** (pivot point) during the exposure. Their alignment is maintained by a rigid attachment, such as a metal rod. The object to be examined is placed at the fulcrum (Figure 37-1). The result is a tomographic image in which the area located at the fulcrum is sharp because it has not moved in its relationship to the tube and the image receptor during the exposure (Figure 37-2). However, structures above and below, which would have been superimposed, are now blurred due to the motion.

Although tomography is a dynamic process, it can be understood by careful consideration of the tomographic concept. Oblique projections or tube angle

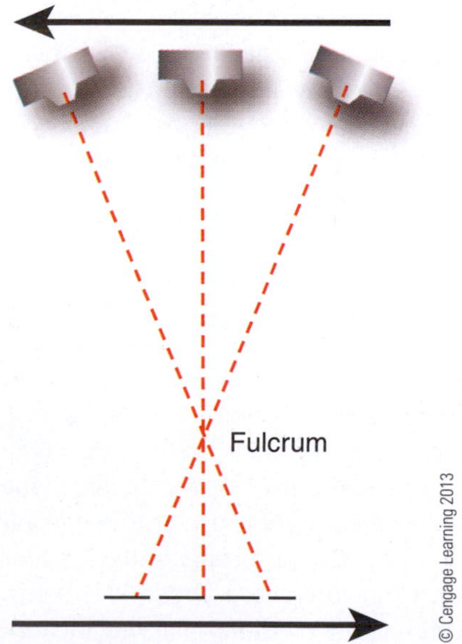

FIGURE 37-1. The tomographic principle—the interrelationships. The x-ray tube and image receptor are attached so they move in opposite directions while maintaining their alignment. The fulcrum, as the point around which the movement occurs, remains the single unmoving point. Objects placed at the fulcrum are imaged sharply, while all other objects are blurred.

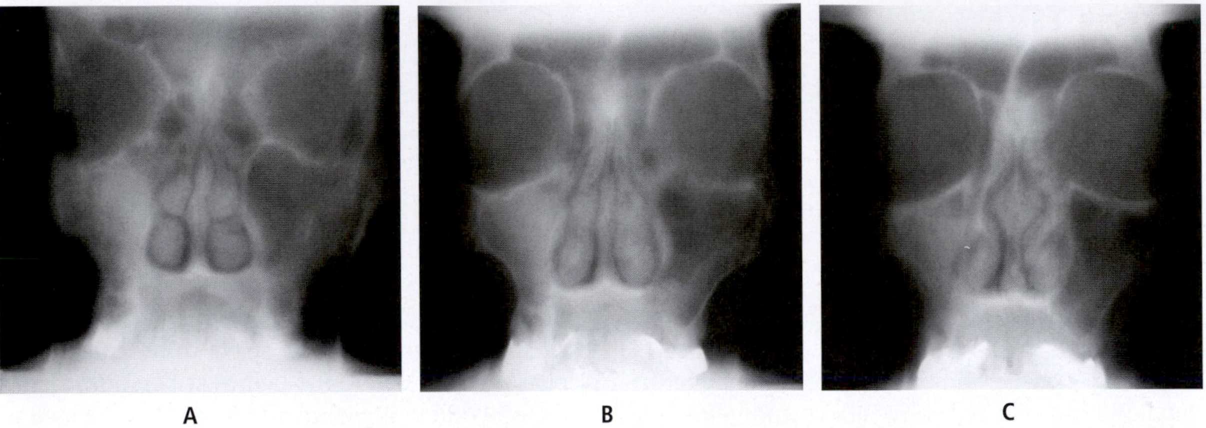

FIGURE 37-2. A tomogram of the maxillary sinuses in an AP projection with the fulcrum (A) 19 cm from the table; (B) 20 cm; and (C) 21 cm. The structures that are sharp are located within the fulcrum focal plane. Structures above and below the focal plane are blurred. Note the opacification of the right maxillary sinus and the thickening of the mucosal wall in the inferior left sinus. *(Radiographs courtesy of Arlene Adler and Richard R. Carlton.)*

projections are used to project objects away from one another. Tomography builds on this geometry in a dynamic manner (Figure 37-3). As the tube proceeds through the tomographic motion, the projected images are first at a severe tube angle, which gradually decreases to a perpendicular beam, which then increases to a severe tube angle in the opposite direction. The resulting projection of superimposed objects first to one side, then to the other, causes their projected image to be streaked, or blurred, across the length of the image receptor. The longer the blurring, the less opportunity to create a sharp image. The shorter the blurring, the sharper the image. Therefore, there is a direct relationship between distance from the fulcrum and blurring. The greater the distance from the fulcrum, the greater the blurring, and vice versa.

Those images that lie in the plane of the fulcrum will be projected onto exactly the same location on the image receptor because the image receptor is moving at exactly the proper rate to maintain their location. Objects located above and below the fulcrum will be projected onto varying locations on the image receptor as it moves, thus blurring their images. The farther the object is from the fulcrum, the greater the difference between its projected motion and the motion of the image receptor. This causes its image to be projected at various locations. The more its image is blurred, the easier it is to visualize sharp, unblurred structures through the blurring.

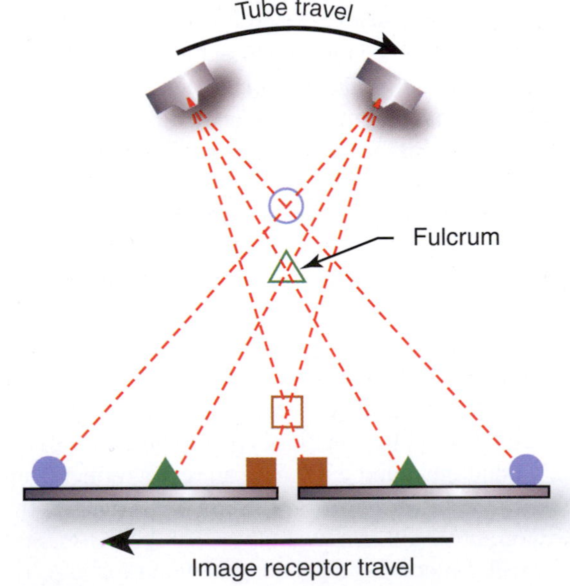

FIGURE 37-3. The tomographic concept. The ball is projected to the right of the triangle as the exposure begins but is blurred completely across the triangle to appear at the left by the end of the exposure. Also note that the box goes through the same blurring, but in the opposite direction.

Because the creation of a section of sharply defined tissue is similar to cutting slices out of the body for examination, terms such as *cuts* and *slices* have evolved. Because these phrases can easily cause immense distress when overheard by patients, the radiographer should strive to adhere to the term *section*, avoiding *cut* and *slice*.

TOMOGRAPHIC QUALITY

Tomographic Amplitude

The **tomographic amplitude,** arc, or angle is the total distance the tube travels (Figure 37-4). The x-ray tube does not have to be engaged in an exposure for the entire tomographic angle. However, the tomographic amplitude is always greater than or equal to the exposure amplitude. There is an inverse relationship between the tomographic amplitude and the section thickness, as discussed later.

Exposure Amplitude

The **exposure amplitude,** arc, or angle is the total distance the tube travels during the exposure (see Figure 37-4). The x-ray tube is engaged in an exposure for the entire exposure angle. The exposure amplitude is always equal to or less than the tomographic amplitude.

Blur

Blur is the streaking or smearing that results in the loss of nearly all recorded detail of objects outside the focal plane. There is an inverse relationship between blurring and the image receptor exposure of objects. Increased blurring causes decreased exposure, thus making an object more transparent. This permits objects within the focal plane to be seen through the blurring. Blur is affected by the exposure amplitude, distance from the fulcrum, distance from the image receptor, and orientation of tube motion.

Exposure Amplitude. The exposure amplitude has a direct linear relationship to blur width. As the exposure amplitude increases, blur increases in direct proportion. For example, doubling the exposure amplitude will double image blur.

Distance from the Fulcrum. The distance from the fulcrum has a direct relationship to blur width. As the distance of an object from the fulcrum increases, blur increases.

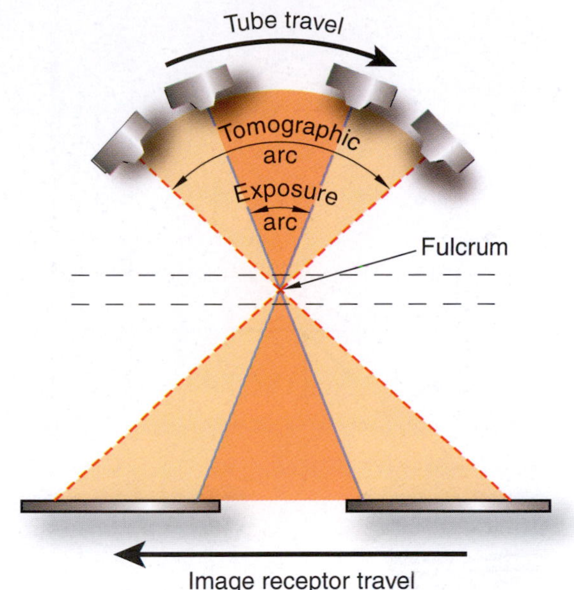

FIGURE 37-4. Tomographic and exposure amplitude, arc, or angle.

Distance from the Image Receptor. The distance from the image receptor has a direct relationship to blur width. As the distance of an object from the image receptor increases, blur increases. For example, blurring of superimposed structures around a pulmonary lesion is greater when the affected side is positioned down for lateral decubitus tomograms because this positions the unaffected lung farther from the image receptor.

Orientation of Tube Motion. The orientation of tube travel has a direct relationship to blur width. As the orientation of tube travel approaches perpendicularity, blur increases. Figure 37-5 shows the difference between an image of a structure that is perpendicular to a linear tomographic motion and one that is parallel.

Phantoms

Phantoms are sometimes called blur edges or blur margins. They are images that do not correspond to existing structures. They are false images and, as such, are dangerous to the diagnostic process. Phantoms are produced during complex tomographic motions, especially circular, when the tube motion is parallel to the long axis of the structure (Figure 37-6). They are also caused

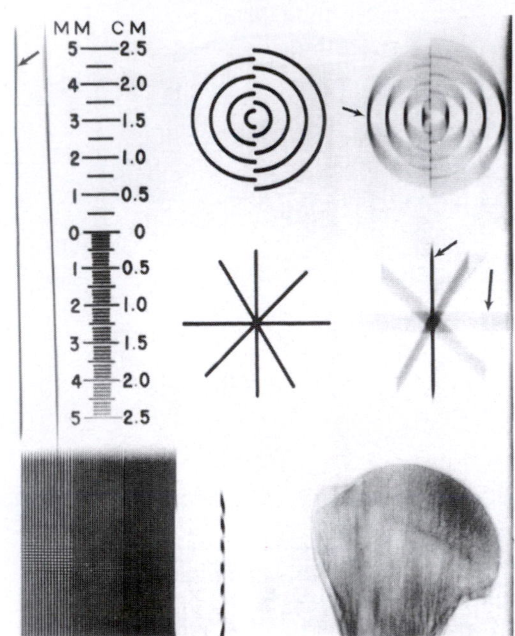

FIGURE 37-5. The effect of the orientation of tube motion on the long axis of the object. The tomographic phantom has a star pattern of wires. When the fulcrum is 1cm below the wires, blurring occurs. The image was produced with a linear motion from the top to the bottom of the radiographic image. Arrows illustrate where the wire perpendicular to the direction of motion is projected with maximum blurring. The wire parallel to the direction of motion is projected with no lateral blurring. (The linear motion causes blurring only as elongation at the ends of the wire.) The wires at 45° are projected with intermediate amounts of blurring. *(Courtesy of Philips Medical Systems, N.A.)*

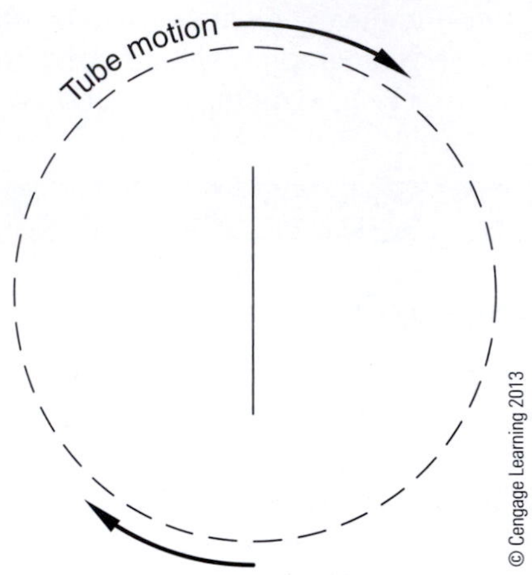

FIGURE 37-6. Phantoms caused by circular tomographic motion. Although the top and bottom of the circle produce motion that is perpendicular to the long axis of the object, the sides produce parallel motion. During the time the parallel motion occurs, the image blurring is decreased, thus producing a sharper and more dense image. This sharper and more dense image is the phantom, blur edge, or blur margin.

by blur overlap (Figure 37-7) and displacement of blur margins due to the tomographic motion. For example, a dense bony structure may have its blur margin projected into a soft tissue area. Especially in cranial and chest tomography, the decreased blur density may simulate a pathological soft tissue condition. Reduced section thickness and increased exposure amplitude decrease phantom images.

Fulcrum

The fulcrum is the pivot point around which the motions of the tube and the image receptor are centered. It determines the focal plane and thereby controls the section level. The fulcrum may be fixed so that the patient is moved up and down to change the section level (the Grossman principle). More commonly, the fulcrum is adjustable so that it moves up and down while the patient remains stationary.

Focal Plane

The **focal plane** is often referred to as the section, although the terms *section level*, *layer height*, *object plane*, and *depth of focus* have also been used. It is the region within which the image exhibits satisfactory recorded detail and is controlled by the level of the fulcrum. The focal plane is not an exactly defined region. Objects located near the fulcrum are less blurred, whereas objects located farther from the fulcrum are more blurred. Consequently, gradually increasing recorded detail eventually reaches a point where it is considered of diagnostic sharpness. This point defines the margins of the focal plane.

Section Thickness

Section thickness is the width of the focal plane and is controlled by the exposure angle (Figure 37-8). Exposure angle is inversely proportional to section thickness. As the exposure angle increases, section thickness decreases. Conversely,

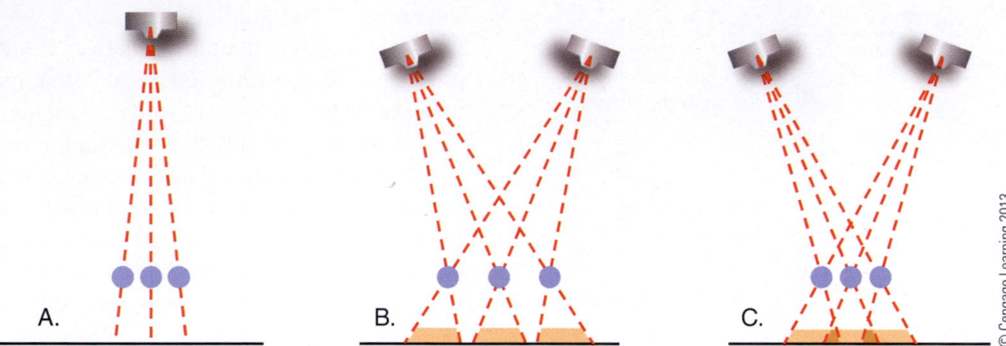

FIGURE 37-7. Tomographic blur overlap phantoms. (A) The sharp image of three wires produced by a static radiograph. (B) The blurred image of three wires produced by a small exposure amplitude. (C) The blur overlap that produces two phantom images from three wires imaged with a large exposure amplitude.

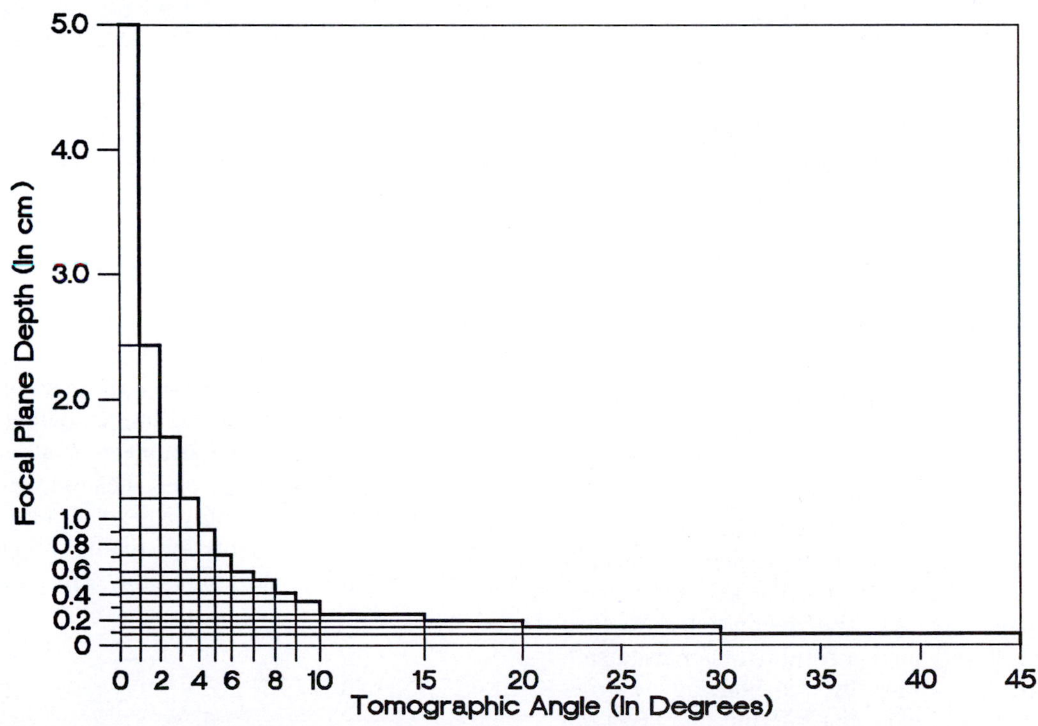

FIGURE 37-8. The effect of exposure angle on section thickness. *(Courtesy of Railfare Enterprises Limited.)*

as the exposure angle decreases, section thickness increases.

Section thickness occurs in a plane parallel to the image receptor (Figure 37-9). Although there is an increase in magnification due to the increased OID of object C in Figure 37-9 as the x-ray tube moves to the left, there is also a corresponding increase in the SOD and SID. The ratio of SID to SOD, the magnification ratio, remains the same, as do the ratios for objects A and B. Therefore, although

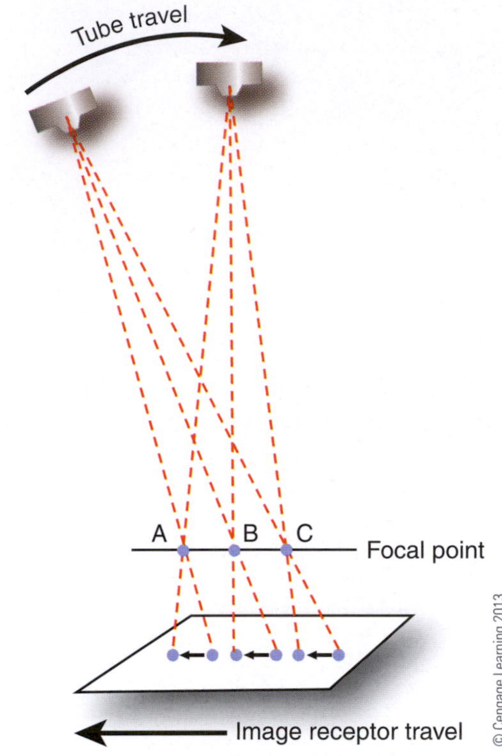

FIGURE 37-9. The effect of tomographic movement on magnification of objects in the focal plane.

magnification has an effect on the detail and sharpness of tomographed objects, tomographic motion does not change the total effect from that seen in a static radiograph of the same area.

Most tomographic images exhibit less contrast than static images of the same regions because of the decreased tissue density that is being imaged with a single section. The decreased difference in subject density also constitutes decreased subject contrast. Additionally, the blurring of structures above and below the fulcrum increases the base density of the image. Increased base density decreases contrast because fewer densities remain within the diagnostically visible range of densities.

Section Interval

The distance between fulcrum levels is the **section interval.** During tomographic procedures, the section interval should not exceed the section thickness. Tomographing an object with section intervals greater than the section thickness creates gaps of unexamined tissue that may permit misdiagnosis.

A procedure must be planned to establish appropriate section intervals. At least one full section above and below the area of interest is required to prove completion of the sectioning. Careful consideration of section thickness permits the use of section intervals that create a slight overlapping of sections. For example, an exposure amplitude that produces a 0.5-mm section thickness should be used with fulcrum changes of 0.4 mm to permit a 0.1-mm overlap (0.05 mm at the top and bottom of each section).

TYPES OF MOTION

Tomography was first achieved with a linear motion. Although numerous motions to minimize section thickness were developed, only the linear motions remain in common use.

Linear tomography occurs when the movement of the tube and image receptor is along a straight line (Figure 37-10A). Linear motion has a major quality problem because the SID and OID change as the tube moves. Both SID and OID are greater at the extreme left and right positions than at the center position. During the tomographic motion the distances are in constant fluctuation.

Linear tomography also has a significant decrease in image quality because blurring is dependent on the orientation of the structure to the linear motion. Structures that are parallel to

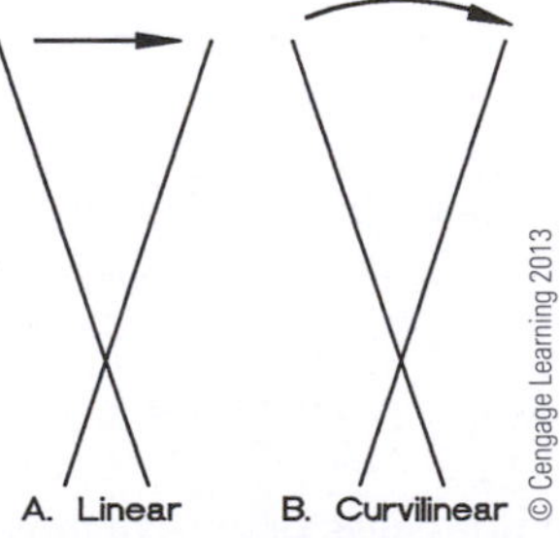

FIGURE 37-10. The two most common tomographic motions.

the motion are not so much blurred as they are streaked. Figure 37-5 illustrates the blurring of lines perpendicular to linear motion and the streaking (elongating) of parallel lines. Linear streaking causes sharp images from structures as much as several centimeters away from the fulcrum. Elongated linear streaking is not a phantom image; it is the image of structural margins that were not blurred.

Linear motion places severe limitations on the total tomographic amplitude. Because the angle of the tube to the object and the image receptor has limits beyond which shape distortion is objectionable, the thinness of the tomographic section is also limited (Figure 37-11). Total tomographic arc is limited to 48°. The only method of decreasing section thickness is to develop complex tomographic motions that permit greater amplitude.

Linear tomography remains popular because it is an inexpensive addition to a diagnostic x-ray unit. It requires a rod to attach the x-ray tube and the bucky tray, an adjustable fulcrum through which the rod may pivot, and a motor to drive the x-ray tube stand. All other tomographic motions require specialized units designed to provide the desired motion through complicated tracks, gears, pivots, and so forth.

Because the motion of the tomographic unit creates the tomographic sectional image, it is critical to maximize the motion. This is accomplished by aligning the long axis of the part of interest to the direction of the tube motion. Inability to accomplish this type of positioning for numerous areas of the body is a disadvantage of linear tomography.

Curvilinear tomography improves on the linear motion by maintaining SID and OID and reducing magnification differences (see Figure 37-10B). It is still of limited value due to the single, linear direction of the motion.

DIGITAL TOMOSYNTHESIS

Digital radiographic tomography is called **digital tomosynthesis** because the computed radiographic images are manipulated by a post-acquisition algorithm to simulate tomographic exposures instead of actually producing additional images.

Digital tomosynthesis combines digital image capture and processing with simple tube/detector motion as used in conventional radiographic tomography. Although it is similar to computed tomography (CT), it is a separate process. Tomosynthetic processing requires about 10 exposures to establish an adequate image base from which reprocessing can be done. Higher-resolution detectors are used, thus allowing very high in-plane resolution, even if the z-axis resolution is poor. The primary interest in tomosynthesis is in breast imaging, as an extension to mammography, where

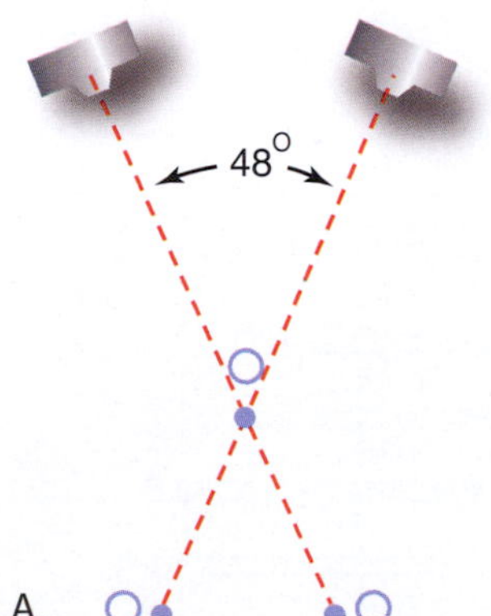

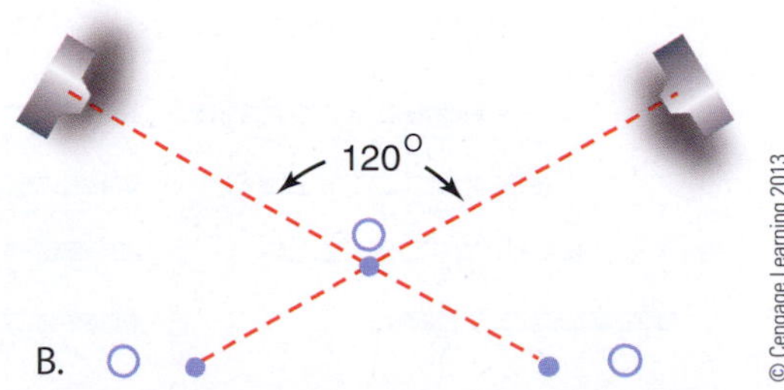

FIGURE 37-11. Limitations to total linear tube amplitude due to excessive distortion produced at the extreme edges of large angles such as 120°.

it may offer better detection rates with little extra increase in radiation exposure. The primary advantage over traditional film/screen tomography is that the resulting images can be manipulated as well as re-created in various planes without re-exposing the patient. Reconstruction algorithms for tomosynthesis are significantly different from those of conventional CT. Figure 37-12 explains the tomosynthetic process in detail.

Flat panel image receptors (as used in direct computed radiography) are best for tomosynthetic systems because they provide rapid readout. The image dataset is acquired by making about 10 static exposures at slightly different central ray angles through the region of interest (ROI). Post-acquisition image processing permits reconstruction of any desired plane through the exposed area. In addition, post-acquisition algorithms for modifying blur, density/brightness, contrast, and other quality factors can be used as necessary.

TOMOGRAPHIC PROCEDURES

Tomography is most often used to localize objects that are difficult to see due to superimposed structures. Because the section thickness determines how much tissue is visualized for each section, each examination must be evaluated to determine an appropriate series of tomographic sections. Routine procedures often begin with a preliminary scout exposure for diagnostic comparisons. This image is also useful in establishing exact structural locations and verifying exposure factors.

Exposure Factors

Choosing proper technique exposure factors for tomography requires special attention to compensate for the time needed for the exposure amplitude.

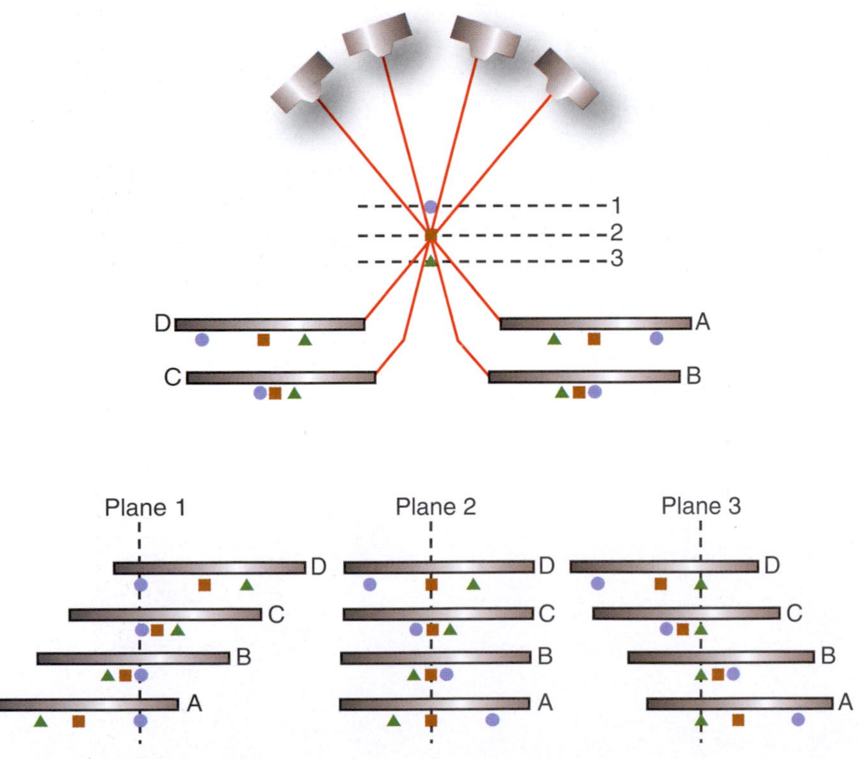

FIGURE 37-12. Digital tomosynthesis. *(Note: From* The Essential Physics of Medical Imaging *[2nd ed.], by J. Bushberg, J. Seibert, E. Leidholdt, and J. Boone, 2003, Philadelphia: Lippincott Williams & Wilkins. Reprinted with permission.)*

Time. It is critical that the time be set first. The exposure time must match the length of time required for the x-ray tube to complete the exposure amplitude. An exposure time that is less than the amplitude will not permit full blurring and will project erratic phantoms. An exposure time that is greater than the amplitude will increase the density of the image at the final tube position, thus increasing the recorded detail while decreasing the blurring of structures outside the focal plane. Complex tomographic motions often require 3- or 6-second exposures.

Milliamperage. Dedicated tomography unit generators provide special stations below 100 mA to permit appropriate mAs to be set with the long times required for complex tomographic motions. Stations of 10, 15, 20, 25, 30, 40, and 50 mA are extremely helpful in these situations. Approximately 30 percent more mAs is required for a wide-angle tomogram due to the loss of scatter density caused by the air gap at the extremes of the tomographic motion. Zonographic tomograms usually require the same mAs as static images.

Kilovoltage. All fine exposure adjustments must be accomplished by variations of kVp because of the limitations imposed by the fixed time settings. The 15 percent rule is a critical tool in determining these adjustments. It is also useful to recall that a 5 percent change in kVp is required to produce a visible exposure difference in most images. Because these adjustments tend to increase kVp to the point where contrast may become a problem, every possible device that will eliminate scatter radiation should be employed. These include maximum collimation (to the exact area of interest), lead masks at the tabletop, high ratio grids, and compression bands.

Specialized Techniques

Narrow-Angle Tomography (Zonography). Narrow-angle tomography (exposure amplitudes of less than 10°) is used when localization is necessary because the exact location of a structure is unknown or when a survey is being performed, for example, on a lesion of the lung or on the kidneys. A small exposure amplitude is used to produce a thick section (Figure 37-13A). Narrow-angle tomography has reasonable contrast but poor recorded detail because of the thick section.

Wide-Angle Tomography. Wide-angle tomography is used when a lesion has been localized or a specific structure has been determined to require a more detailed examination. A series of thinner sections may then be used (see Figure 37-13B). Wide-angle tomography has inherently low contrast but a reasonable amount of recorded detail because of the thin section. It is useful in the examination of small bone structures, such as the inner ear, although computed tomography now has much to offer in this area of diagnosis.

Panoramic Tomography. Specialized equipment has been developed to permit slit scan radiography of the curved surfaces of the face and head, especially of the mandible (Figure 37-14). The terms **pantomography**, *orthopantomography*, and *panoramic tomography* have been used to describe

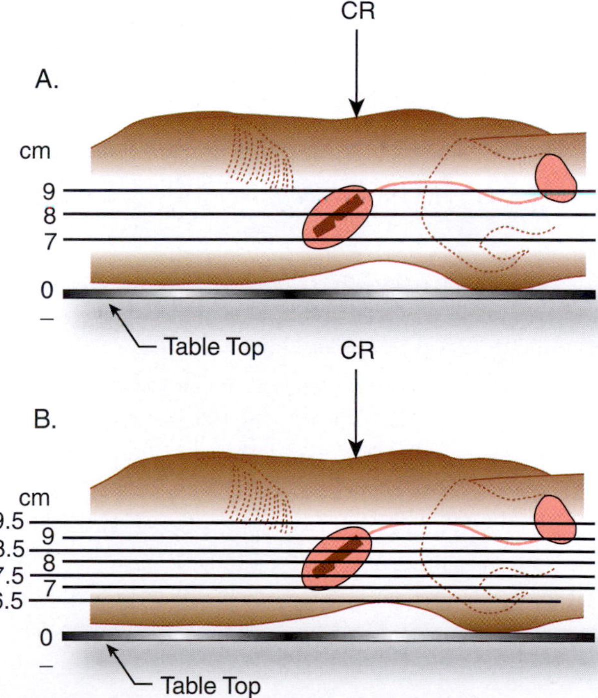

FIGURE 37-13. The effect of exposure amplitude on section thickness. (A) A small exposure amplitude to produce a thick section for localization or as a survey examination. (B) A larger exposure amplitude to produce thin sections for detailed examination. *(Reprinted with permission from Littleton, J. T. [1976]. Tomography: Physical Principles and Clinical Aplications. Baltimore, MD: The Williams & Wilkins Co.)*

this type of x-ray unit. Slit scan radiography uses only the perpendicular photons of the primary beam by using a lead mask to collimate the beam to a narrow slit. Both the x-ray tube and the image receptor rotate past the slit during the exposure to lay out the structure of interest, much like rolling paint from a roller onto a wall (Figure 37-15).

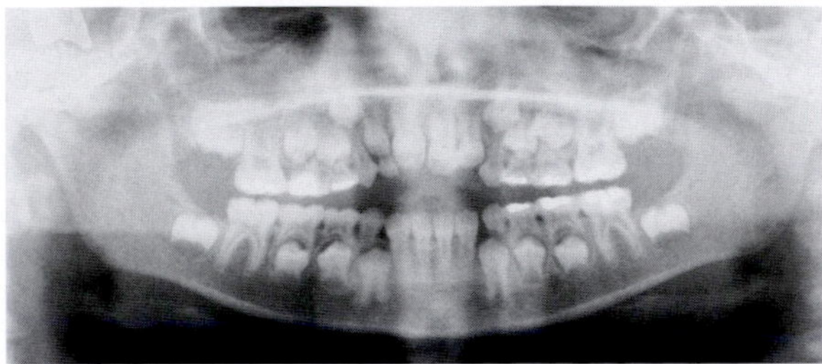

FIGURE 37-14. A panoramic projection of the mandible. *(Radiograph courtesy of Arlene Adler and Richard R. Carlton.)*

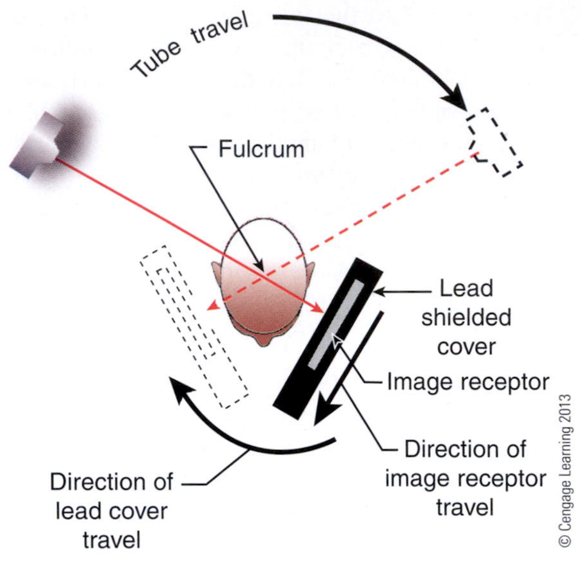

FIGURE 37-15. Panoramic tomographic equipment.

SUMMARY

Tomography is a radiographic technique employing motion to show structures lying in a plane of tissue while blurring or eliminating the detail in images of structures in other planes. It primarily demonstrates coronal sections, although sagittal sections of most body parts and transverse sections of the head may be accomplished through positioning.

The principle of tomography is based on synchronous movement of two of the three elements in a tomographic system: the x-ray tube, the object, and the image receptor. Most tomographic units synchronize the movements of the x-ray tube and the image receptor in opposite directions around a stationary fulcrum during the exposure. Those images that lie in the plane of the fulcrum will be projected onto exactly the same location on the image receptor because the image receptor is moving at exactly the proper rate to maintain their location. Objects located above and below the fulcrum will be projected onto varying locations on the image receptor as it moves, thus blurring their images.

The tomographic amplitude, arc, or angle is the total distance the tube travels. The exposure amplitude, arc, or angle is the total distance the tube travels during the exposure. The exposure amplitude is always equal to or less than the tomographic amplitude. Blur is the streaking or smearing that results in the loss of nearly all recorded detail of objects outside the focal plane and is affected by the tomographic amplitude, distance from the fulcrum, distance from the image receptor, and orientation of tube motion. Blur edges and blur margins are called phantoms.

The focal plane is often referred to as the section, although the terms *section level, layer height, object plane*, and *depth of focus* have also been used. It is

SUMMARY (continued)

the region within which the image exhibits satisfactory recorded detail and is controlled by the level of the fulcrum. Section thickness is the width of the focal plane and is controlled by the exposure angle. The distance between fulcrum levels is the section interval. During tomographic procedures, the section interval should not exceed the section thickness.

Choosing proper exposure factors for tomography requires consideration of exposure time, milliamperage, and kilovoltage. Specialized tomographic techniques include narrow-angle, wide-angle, and panoramic tomography. ■

REVIEW QUESTIONS

1. Define tomography.
2. How does a basic tomographic system operate?
3. What is the difference between tomographic amplitude and exposure amplitude?
4. What factors affect tomographic blur?
5. What is the function of the fulcrum?
6. How is section thickness controlled?
7. Which of the tomographic motions alters distance during the exposure arc?
8. What are the advantages of complex tomographic motions?
9. Why is it important to establish the exposure time prior to setting the other exposure factors for a tomogram?
10. Differentiate between the uses of narrow-angle and wide-angle tomography.

REFERENCES AND RECOMMENDED READING

Ball, J., & Price, T. (1989). *Chesneys' radiographic imaging.* Oxford: Blackwell Scientific.

Barnes, G. T., & Moreland, R. F. (1981, October). A linear tomographic alignment test object. *Radiology*, 247.

Bushberg, J. T., Seibert, J. A., Leidholdt, E. M., & Boone, J. M. (2003). *The essential physics of medical imaging* (2nd ed.). Philadelphia: Lippincott Williams & Wilkins.

Bushong, S. C. (2008). *Radiologic science for technologists: Physics, biology, and protection* (9th ed.). St. Louis, MO: Elsevier/C. V. Mosby.

Coulam, C. M., Erickson, J. J., & Gibbs, S. J. (1981). Image and equipment considerations in conventional tomography. In C. M. Coulam, J. J. Erickson, F. D. Rollo, & A. E. James (Eds.), *The physical basis of medical imaging.* New York: Appleton-Century-Crofts.

Cullinan, A., & Cullinan, J. (1994). *Producing quality radiographs* (2nd ed.). Philadelphia: J. B. Lippincott.

Curry, T. S., Dowdey, J. E., & Murry, R. C. (1990). *Christensen's introduction to the physics of diagnostic radiology* (4th ed.). Philadelphia: Lea and Febiger.

Dowdell, L. C. (1984). *The joy of sectioning.* Toronto: Railfare.

Durzich, M. L. (1978). *Technical aspects of tomography.* Baltimore: Williams & Wilkins.

Forster, E. (1985). *Equipment for diagnostic radiography.* Lancaster: MTP Press.

Littleton, J. T. (1976). *Tomography: Physical principles and clinical applications.* Baltimore: Williams & Wilkins.

Littleton, J. T., & Durizch, M. L. (1983). *Sectional imaging methods: A comparison.* Baltimore: University Park Press.

Lockery, R. M. (1971). Principles of body-section radiography. *Radiologic Technology, 42*(5), 335.

Marlowe, N. A. (1983). The application of blurred under-subtraction in polytomography. *Radiologic Technology, 54*(6), 455.

Milner, S. C., & Case, J. (1984). Tomographic exposure angle: A comparison of two tests. *Radiography, 50*(592), 177.

Moore, C. J., Hopewell, R., Moores, B. M., & Eddleston, B. (1979). Test procedures for conventional tomographic x-ray equipment. *Radiography, 45*(540), 284.

Niklason, L., Christian, B., Niklason, L., Kopans, D., et al. (2005). Digital tomosynthesis in breast imaging. *Radiology*, 399–406.

Ramthun, B. (1988). Tomography of the posterior cervical spine fusion: A new concept. *Radiologic Technology, 60*(1), 27–31.

Smith, W. V. J. (1971). A review of tomography and zonography. *Radiography, 37*(433), 5.

Soni, V. P. (1977). A review of tomography. *Canadian Journal of Radiography, Radiotherapy, and Nuclear Medicine, 8*(4), 172–189.

Tomographic exposure angle. (1984). *Radiography, 50*(594), 291.

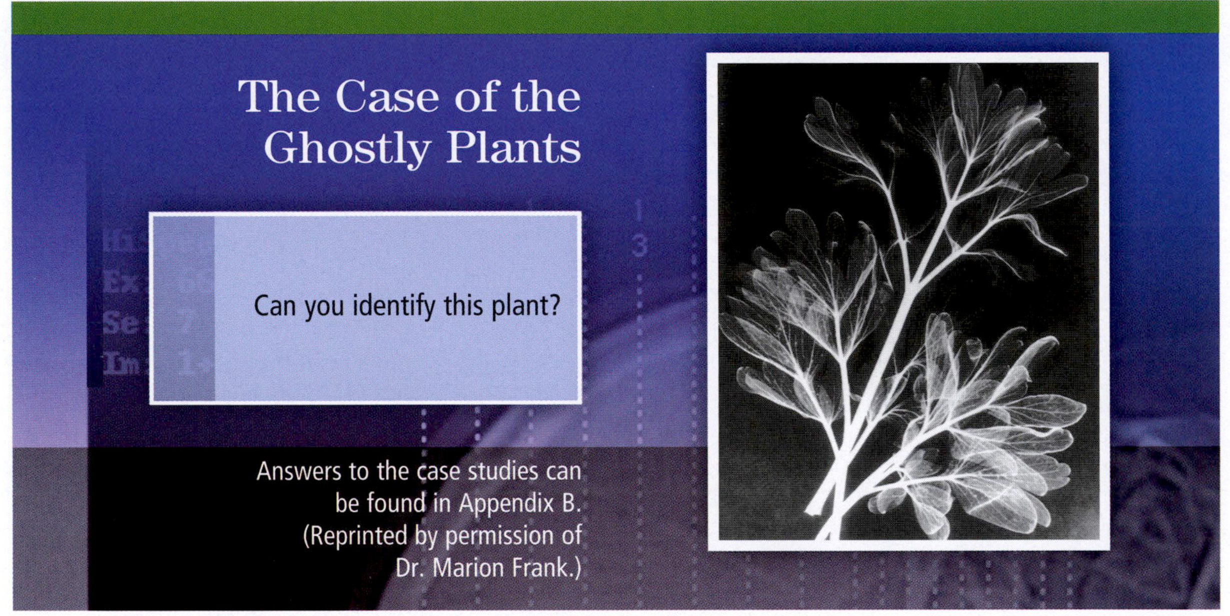

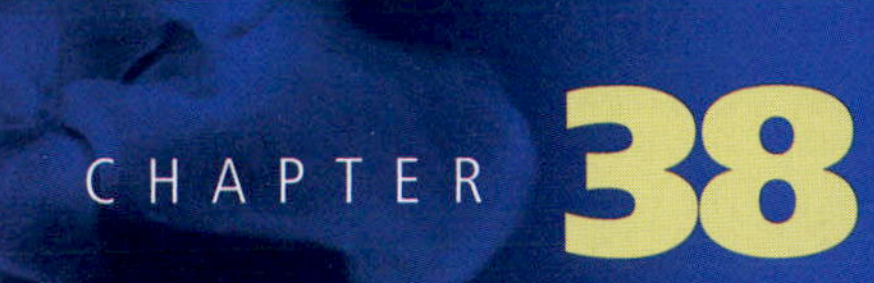

Mammography

KEY TERMS

bias focusing
digital mammography unit
effective target angle
molybdenum
reciprocity law failure
reference axis
reference axis target angle
rhodium

> Whenever the art of medicine is loved, there is also love for humanity.
>
> *Hippocrates*

OBJECTIVES

Upon completion of this chapter, the student should be able to:

- Explain the development of the regulations and guidelines underlying the performance of mammography.
- Describe the unique aspects of the mammography x-ray generator.
- Describe the distinctive design and application of the mammography x-ray tube and its associated components.
- Specify the accessory components of the mammography machine, detailing their unique design and function in producing quality images.
- Assess the critical importance of specialized equipment in producing breast images.
- Explain the basic elements of digital mammography.

HISTORICAL DEVELOPMENT

Mammography, today, has evolved into one of the most critical and demanding x-ray examinations performed. Every aspect of the examination has to be carried out with the utmost precision. The current technical and clinical aspects of the procedure are guided by strict regulations and specific guidelines. Mammography is presently the only radiography examination fully regulated by the federal government. Mammography requires a team approach. Several professionals are involved, including the radiologist, medical physicist, and, most important, an ARRT-registered radiographer, preferably with credentials in mammography.

There is much attention and regulation placed on the technical and clinical aspects of mammography due to the following: The American Cancer Society estimates that 209,000 women will be diagnosed with breast cancer annually and that 40,000 women will die of this disease (about 1,900 men will be diagnosed also). Approximately one out of eight women will develop breast cancer over a lifetime. Until recently, breast cancer was the leading cause of death from cancer among women. Lung cancer has now become the leader. Breast cancer is the leading cause of cancer deaths in females between the ages of 15 and 54. Most notably, the incidence of breast cancer, as a result of participation in screening, has increased 3 to 4 percent annually since 1982. The overall age-adjusted incidence rates are higher in white women compared with African American women. However, for African American women under age 50, the incidence is nearly three times higher. The size of the population at risk for developing breast cancer is also growing every year.

It is well known that mortality from breast cancer can be reduced significantly through widespread participation in breast screening. For women whose cancers are detected when they are small and confined to the breast, the vast majority are alive and well 10 years later. The diagnosis of breast cancer is not easily made. The highest resolution and contrast attainable has to be brought out in the breast image—more than any other x-ray examination. Remember, from previous chapter readings, that very high resolution and contrast cannot occur in the x-ray image without a corresponding increase in radiation exposure. The risk from ionizing radiation, therefore, is always of concern in mammography.

Although radiation exposures in mammography are relatively safe today as a result of improvements in technology, and certainly due to stringent regulations, one has to recognize that patient exposure is still an important consideration, and the exposure is relatively high in comparison to x-ray examinations of other body parts. The entrance skin exposure (ESE) for a 5-cm compressed breast is approximately 1,000 mR, and the ESE for a 21-cm lumbar spine AP projection is 220 mR.

1900s

Mammography has been performed since the early 1900s. In those early years, it was not a technologically well-developed examination. The results were unpredictable, and the technical quality of the images was very poor. Dr. Raul Leborgne of Uruguay was one of the first physicians to perform extended research on mammography, and he published the first textbook on the topic in 1953.

1960

Research into mammography continued at a very low level until about 1960, when Dr. Robert Eagan, then at M. D. Anderson Hospital in Houston, first described the use of a high-mA, low-kVp exposure technique with direct exposure industrial x-ray film. He introduced the technique of removing the aluminum filter from the port of the x-ray tube so the low-energy x-rays could exit. He also introduced the use of a cylindrical extension cone to reduce scatter radiation. Mammography in the 1960s was performed using a conventional x-ray machine. The x-ray tube at that time had a tungsten anode, and a large 2-mm focal spot was common. Typical exposure techniques utilized 28 kVp and 300 mA, with exposure times up to 6 seconds (1,800 mAs). Direct exposure x-ray film was used without a grid. Unfortunately, the exposure to the patient was extremely high. Exposures during this era were between **50 to 100 times higher** than exposures applied today. Early mammographers reported exposures greater than **50 R** per projection. If repeat radiographs were performed, erythema of the skin would often occur. Eagan's development of a special technique to optimize the x-ray equipment to image the breast prompted the beginning of widespread research into the use of mammography.

1967

In 1967, CGR (France) introduced the first **dedicated** mammography machine (Figure 38-1). The production model of this machine featured a molybdenum anode, 0.7-mm focal spot, and a beryllium window port. In addition, the unit had a built-in device to compress the breast. As a result of these technical improvements, contrast and resolution in the breast image were greatly enhanced. However, exposure to the patient increased compared to Eagan's technique because of the continued use of direct exposures on industrial x-ray film and because a higher mAs was required due to the reduced x-ray output of the molybdenum anode.

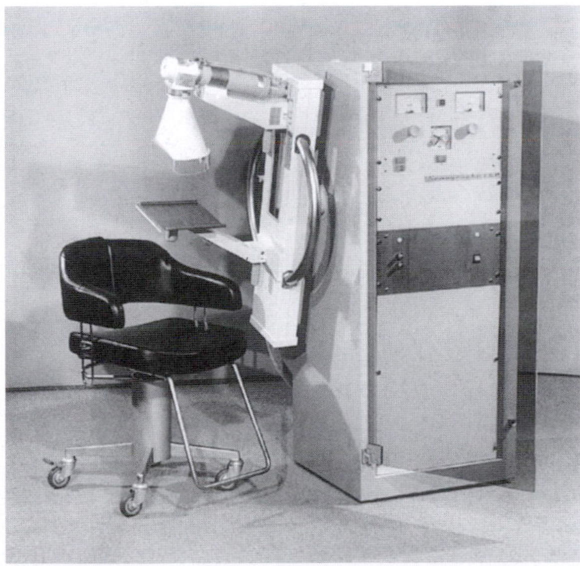

FIGURE 38-1. A 1967 Senograph, produced by CGR (France), became the first commercially available dedicated mammography machine. The unit contained the first molybdenum anode, 0.7-mm focal spot, beryllium window port, and compression device. *(Courtesy of GE Healthcare.)*

The radiography community during this time was discovering an uncomfortable tradeoff. High-resolution and high-contrast breast images could not be produced without introducing high exposure to the patient. It was during this time that the **benefit-versus-risk debates** about mammography practice ensued.

Research continued, and in the early 1970s, Siemens (Germany), Philips (Netherlands), and Picker and General Electric (USA) also introduced dedicated mammography machines. During the early 1970s, nearly every large radiology department in the world was performing mammography.

1971

In 1971, Xerox (USA) introduced a commercially available system of imaging the breast known as xeromammography. The Xerox **dry process** system utilized a conventional overhead x-ray tube with a tungsten anode. However, the filter had to be removed from the port and a low kVp of 40–50 set on the generator. The x-ray exposure was made on an electrically charged imaging plate instead of using screen and film. The imaging plate was then placed in a special development unit and the breast image came out on heavy paper in shades of blue. No film processors or viewboxes were needed. Although a dedicated x-ray machine did not have to be purchased, a special processing machine was needed. Xeromammography was extensively used until the mid-1980s because it produced high-contrast and high-resolution images (Figure 38-2). Radiation exposures to the patient were lower than in Eagan's technique. However, the exposure, which ranged from 2 R to 4 R per projection, was still relatively high. Continued research led to significant improvements in screen/film mammography and lower exposures. Major changes in the design and use of the dedicated mammography machine prompted a large decline in the use of xeromammography for breast imaging by the late 1980s.

1972

In 1972, during the intensive growth and research period in mammography, Du Pont (USA) introduced the first dedicated screen/film system for

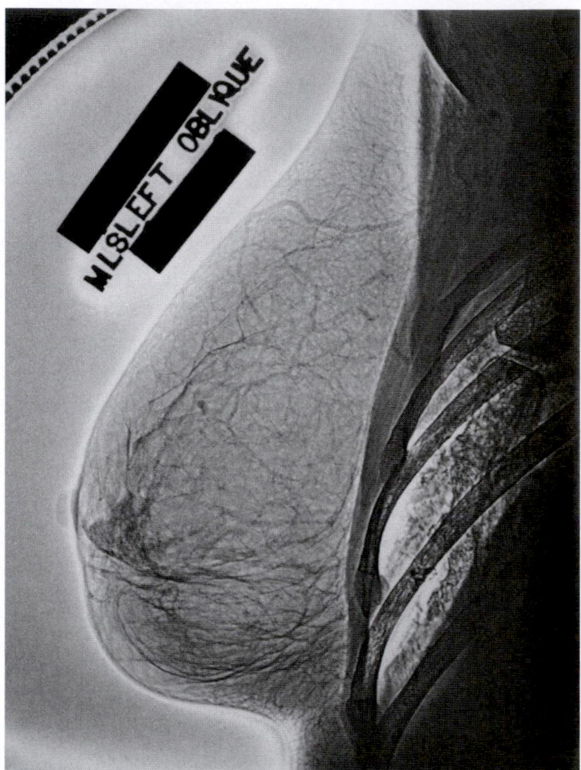

FIGURE 38-2. A 1978 xeroradiographic breast image. Xeromammography produced high contrast and high resolution at doses lower than direct x-ray film exposure. Images were obtained with conventional radiographic equipment, tungsten target, aluminum filter, and 45 kVp. *(Xerogram courtesy Richard R. Calrton.)*

mammography, **Lo Dose I.** The system utilized a single-emulsion film and a single-emulsion calcium tungstate screen that was placed in a light-safe polyethylene bag and vacuum sealed. Utilizing a screen for the first time in mammography prompted a major reduction in exposure time and a corresponding reduction in radiation exposure to the patient of nearly **20×**. Use of a screen increased the very low inherent subject contrast of the breast in the image. Unfortunately, there was also a corresponding reduction in resolution when compared to direct x-ray exposure and xeromammography. However, the combined effects of a dramatic increase in contrast, reduced motion unsharpness, and corresponding exposure reduction was so significant that screen/film mammography gradually became commonplace. During the 1970s, radiologists debated whether to use the Xerox process or screen/film imaging, and many departments chose to use both.

1975

In 1975, a significant event occurred when Kodak (USA) introduced its specially designed for mammography **Min-R** screen, film, and cassette system. The Min-R single-emulsion screen, which used the new green emitting rare-earth phosphor, gadolinium oxysulfide, was paired with an orthochromatic (green- and blue-sensitive) single-emulsion film also called Min-R. The increased screen speed prompted an exposure reduction and there was very negligible loss of resolution. The screen was mounted in a specially designed low-absorption cassette and the screen and film placed so they were as close to the breast as possible (Figure 38-3). Using the cassette saved darkroom time and problems associated with the polyethylene bags. Also during this time, Du Pont introduced an increased-speed version of its screen/film—**Lo Dose II.**

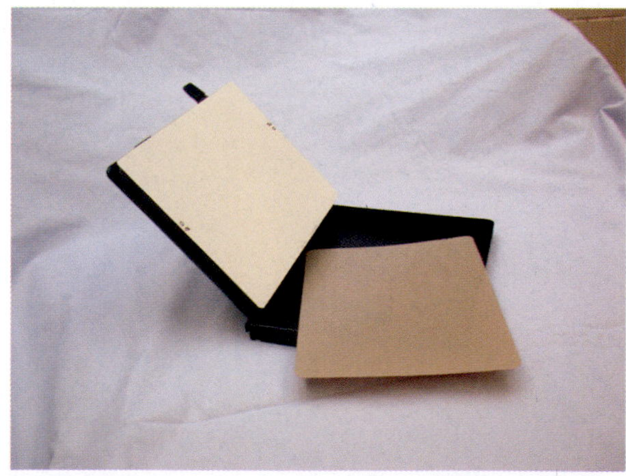

FIGURE 38-3. A 1975 Kodak mammography cassette, the first cassette developed especially for mammography. It contained a Min-R rare-earth phosphor single-emulsion screen (black arrow) and green-sensitive Min-R single-emulsion (white arrow) film. Design of the cassette allowed the screen and film to be placed close to the breast. Top of cassette is indicated by double arrows. *(Xerogram courtesy Richard R. Carlton.)*

1978

The most recent and technologically significant event in mammography occurred in 1978 when Philips (Netherlands) introduced a new generation of dedicated mammography machines (Figure 38-4). This new machine contained the first reciprocating grid. It was also equipped with a foot-pedal; power-driven breast-compression device; aluminum and molybdenum filter selection; automatic exposure control (AEC); a microfocus focal spot; magnification capability; and a high-output generator. Although the introduction of the grid increased the radiation exposure by a factor of **2 to 3×,** the high-contrast image that resulted from the reduction in scattered x-rays, in particular for large and dense breasts, was a dramatic improvement in image quality. Fortunately, at this very same time, Kodak introduced an increased-speed version of its Min-R film, Ortho-M, which reduced the radiation exposure by 50 percent, entirely offsetting the increase in exposure from the use of the grid. The modern era of mammography had begun.

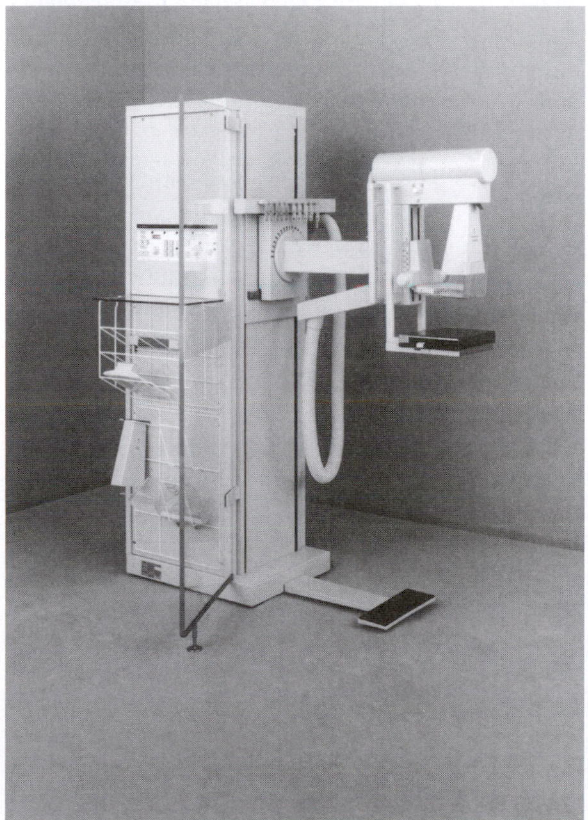

FIGURE 38-4. A 1978 Philips (Netherlands) dedicated mammography machine containing the first reciprocating grid. Introduction of this generation of mammography machines ushered in the modern era of utilizing dedicated machines for mammography. *(Courtesy of Philips Medical Systems.)*

1985–1990

In 1985, a Nationwide Evaluation of X-ray Trends (NEXT) study discovered a wide variation in mammographic image quality and in radiation exposures to the patient. Independent studies done later supported the NEXT data and found similar and additional unacceptable variations in image quality. Citations found in the studies included poor processor performance, inexperienced operators of the equipment, improper physician interpretation, poor exposure techniques, and a general inability to perform the examination in a consistent manner.

Concern about the quality of mammography led to the development of the American College of Radiology (ACR) accreditation program in 1987. This voluntary program required mammography sites to meet quality standards to ensure that optimally exposed breast images were being produced at low radiation exposures to the patient. Components of the ACR program included an assessment of both mammographic phantom and actual clinical images for optimal resolution and contrast, measurement of the average glandular dose to the breast, and processor performance. In 1990, additional standards were set forth, which included specific aspects of the equipment and accessory devices, personnel, and the documentation of an effective quality control program. By June 1994, 66 percent of the mammography machines in the United States had passed the ACR voluntary accreditation. Of those that failed, the three most common reasons for failure, in descending order, were poor clinical images, failure of the phantom image to demonstrate appropriate contrast and resolution, and poor processor performance.

1991

In 1991, the American Registry of Radiologic Technologists (ARRT) implemented its first **advanced-level** examination specifically for mammography. The examination was designed to ensure that the radiographers who perform mammography have appropriate comprehension of exact positioning techniques, have knowledge of the broad spectrum of mammography projections, understand technical factor selection, and know other specific technical, clinical, and affective aspects related to the performance of the examination. Radiographers who pass the advanced-level mammography examination are formally recognized to perform mammography and use the initial (M) after their radiography credential RT(R).

1992–1994

In 1992, as a result of the American Cancer Society's high-visibility public relations campaign that all women over 40 undergo screening mammography, and also because of federal legislation that provided reimbursement for screening mammography in women eligible for Medicare, the federal government enacted the Mammography Quality Standards Act (MQSA). The act was written because of lobbying from the ACR due to the great concern about the poor-quality mammography being performed. The act went into effect on October 1, 1994, and requires all sites (except VA facilities) that provide mammography service to meet quality standards and become certified for operation by the secretary of the Department of Health and Human Services (DHHS). Enactment of the MQSA marks the first time the use of an x-ray machine and a specific x-ray examination were regulated by the federal government.

1999

On April 28, 1999, the Final Rule of the MQSA went into effect after several years of public comments. MQSA is now officially known as Public Law 105-248. Today, dedicated mammography machines are produced by a variety of manufacturers. These machines are mechanically and electronically designed to meet the stringent radiographic and positioning requirements of breast imaging, and they are used with specially designed screens, film, and cassettes. There are no xeromammography systems in use today. Mammography equipment is presently capable of producing extremely high-contrast images with very high resolution, and the radiation exposures to the patient are reasonably low. However, researchers continue to seek higher contrast and resolution for breast images and methods for lowering the exposure.

2000

In February 2000, the first **digital mammography unit** was approved for sale in the United States. The machine was the General Electric Senographe 2000 D. The U.S. Congress passed legislation authorizing increased Medicare reimbursement for this technology, and digital mammography has become the new gold standard.

2011

Digital tomosynthesis is a specialized tomographic unit used primarily for mammography. Development began in 1997, but it was not until 2008 that the equipment and procedures began being used in clinical practice in Europe. The U.S. Food and Drug Administration approved digital tomosynthesis for clinical use in 2011. The process combines digital image capture and processing with simple tube/detector motion as used in conventional radiographic tomography (Figure 38-5). Although there are some similarities to computed tomography (CT), it is a separate technique.

CT uses a source and detector combination that makes a complete 360° rotation about the subject. This obtains a complete set of data from which images may be reconstructed. By comparison, digital tomosynthesis acquires a small rotation angle (e.g., 40°) with a small number of discrete exposures (e.g., 10). These data are processed to yield images similar to those of conventional tomography but with a limited depth of field. Because the image is acquired digitally, a series of sections at different depths and thicknesses can be reconstructed from the same acquisition. Tomosynthesis cannot produce narrow sections, but higher-resolution

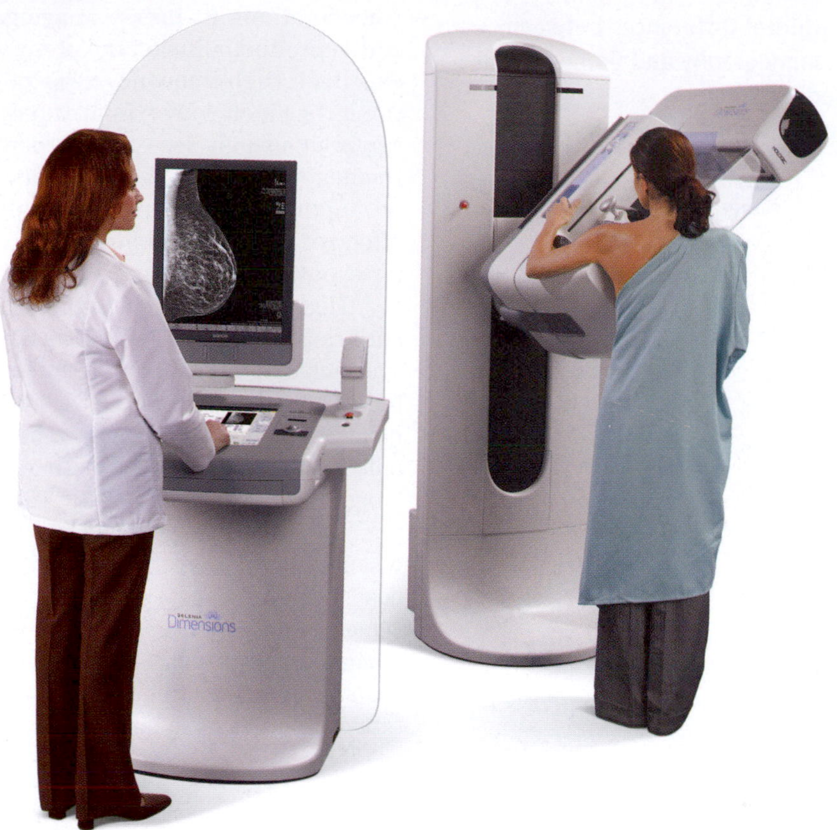

FIGURE 38-5. Reconstructed tomosynthesis slices reduce or eliminate the problems caused by tissue overlap and structure noise in mammography imaging offering improved diagnostic confidence and enhanced patient care. *(Image courtesy of Hologic, the women's health company.)*

detectors can be used, allowing high in-plane resolution, even when z-axis resolution is poor.

This chapter maintains a discussion of the technical aspects of both screen/film and digital mammography, although digital mammography now predominates. The reader should note that every component in the mammography system is modified from conventional radiology. Each component is designed specifically to maximize contrast and resolution while at the same time engineered to keep the radiation exposure to the patient at minimal levels. Table 38-1 illustrates the primary technical differences between mammography and conventional x-ray machines. The light-weight (some weigh only 500 lbs.) entirely self-contained mammography unit, which can easily be pushed around a room and simply plugged in, is a relatively sophisticated x-ray machine. Its sole design and purpose is to image the human breast.

GENERATOR CHARACTERISTICS

Manufacturers of dedicated mammography machines use the new high-frequency generators (see Chapter 5) that were introduced by Siemens (Germany) in 1987. There are several reasons for using high-frequency generators in mammography. These generators virtually eliminate voltage regulation problems and allow very precise control of kVp, mA, and exposure time—important

TABLE 38-1. Technical Differences between Mammography and Conventional Radiography

	Mammography	Conventional
Generator*	1φ high frequency	1φ, 3φ, Capacitor discharge, Falling load
Voltage frequency*	> 10,000 Hz	60 Hz
Voltage ripple	< 4%	4–100%
kVp†	25–28	50–130
mA†	20–160	100–1000
Exposure time (s)†	0.4–4.0	0.01–2.0
Power rating	3–10 kW	50–200 kW
AEC	1 detector	3 detectors
Film density (OD)††	> 1.30	1.10
Backup timer (mAs)	600 grid,	600 300 non-grid
Focal spot size (mm)	0.1 or 0.3	0.6 or 1.2
SID (cm)	60–65	102–122
X-ray beam utilized	Anode side only	Anode and cathode side equally
Effective target angle‡	22°–24°	7°–17°
Reference target angle**	7.5°–12°	7°–17°
Anode	Molybdenum or Rhodium	Tungsten
Tube port	Beryllium	Glass
Filter	Molybdenum or Rhodium	Aluminum
HVL (mm AL)	0.3 (30 kVp)	2.3 (80 kVp)
Grid	4:1 or 5:1	6:1–16:1
Screen–film speeds‡‡	100–320	100–1,200
Resolution (lp/mm)	12–20	5–10

* Some high-frequency generators are being introduced in conventional radiology.

† Range used in clinical practice.

†† Mammography density measured on the ACR Plexiglas™ phantom. Conventional density measured on 21-cm Plexiglas™ phantom.

‡ Measured from the vertical central ray.

** Measured from the reference axis/center of image receptor.

‡‡ Relative speeds of mammography screens are slower than those of conventional screens with same number.

considerations in breast imaging. The linearity and reproducibility of the x-ray exposures are excellent. High-frequency x-ray output waveform ripple is much lower than three-phase, 6-pulse ripple at usually less than 4 percent. The high frequency (100 kHz) allows more efficient x-ray production, and therefore produces a higher effective energy x-ray beam. The result is higher x-ray output for a given kVp and mA setting.

High-frequency generators do not require an autotransformer, line compensation circuit, or space-charge compensation circuit. This greatly reduces equipment bulk, cost, and space requirements. The high-frequency generator system is uniquely housed within the single-standing mammography unit (Figure 38-6). These new generators operate on single-phase incoming-line power, which simplifies installation and greatly reduces cost. High-frequency generators can also be designed to operate from batteries for use in mobile mammography vans. Several manufacturers have designed the high-frequency generator and x-ray tube within the same housing.

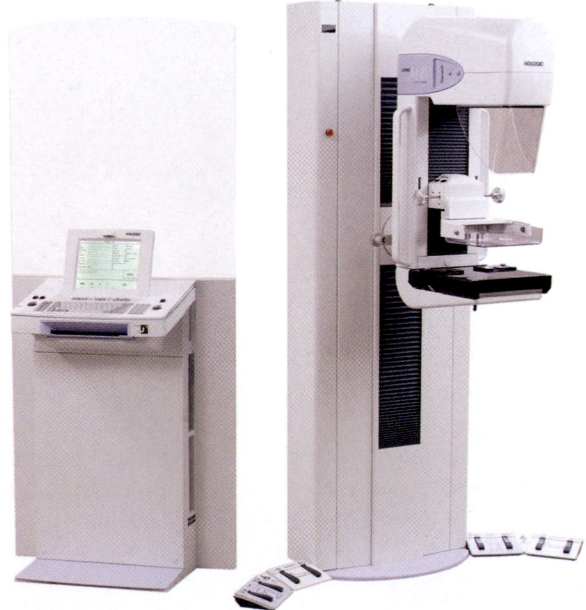

FIGURE 38-6. The Hologic M-IV screen-film mammography system. *(Image courtesy of Hologic, the women's health company.)*

kVp

A significant difference between mammography and conventional x-ray machines is the low kVp utilized. The kVp selections on the generator will range from 22 to 40 kVp. The kVp commonly used in clinical practice varies between **25 and 28 kVp.** The advantage of using low kVp is its ability to produce a very low-energy (soft) x-ray beam that produces high radiographic contrast. High contrast is desirable in breast images because the radiologist must be able to delineate clearly the normal and diseased structures of the breast tissue. Breast tissue is considered soft tissue and it is entirely made up of glands, fibers, and fat, which have very low inherent subject contrast (Figure 38-7). The radiologist must have sufficient contrast available in the image to visualize microcalcifications as small as 0.1 to 0.3 mm, and other subtle parenchymal structures. The major disadvantage of using kVp in the 20s range is that there is a high absorption of the low-energy x-rays in the breast, which contributes significantly to patient dose.

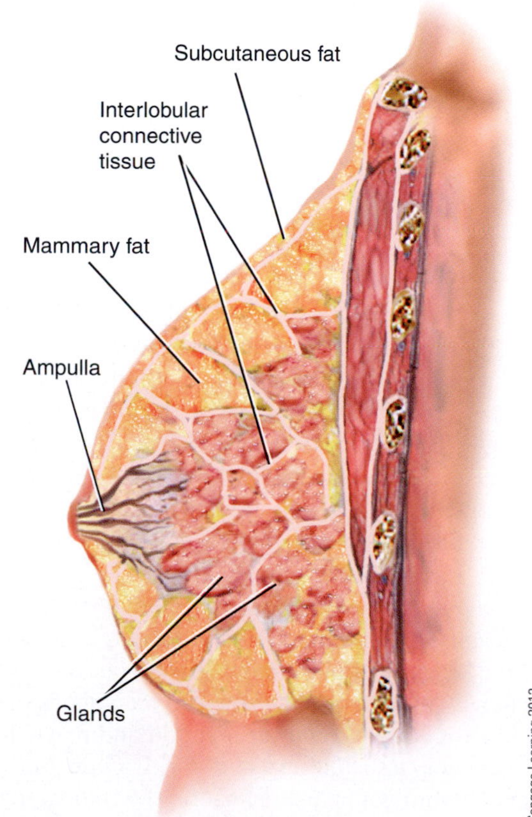

FIGURE 38-7. Female breast made up entirely of glands, fibrous tissues, and fat. This creates low inherent subject contrast in the mammographic image.

Exposure Time, mA, mAs

Mammography generators also utilize low mA settings. Depending on the manufacturer, the mA can vary from about 2 to as high as 180. Generators typically will have a variable mA selection from **20 to 100,** and many manufacturers design a single mA setting for the small focal spot (e.g., 20 mA) and one for the large focal spot (e.g., 80 mA). Low mA settings are necessary because of the power rating limitations placed on the smaller sized anode and the small focal spot sizes. The power ratings of mammography generators vary between 3 and 10 kilowatts (kW) compared to 50 to 1,200 kW on conventional x-ray generators.

In clinical practice, the specific mA selected is determined based on the principle of keeping exposure times short enough to decrease patient motion. However, the time should not be extremely short, which would cause grid artifacts (textured or structured patterns) to appear in the image. Because the mammography system produces a high-resolution image, grid lines have the potential of being prominently shown and will degrade image quality. Conversely, exposure times that exceed 1 second will result in **reciprocity law failure.** Typical exposure times in clinical practice will vary from **0.4 to over 1 second** for standard projections. Exposure times for projections using the magnification technique are much longer, varying from **2 to 4 seconds** due to the low mA used with the 0.1-mm focal spot. When performing magnification studies, mammographers must be very cautious, and explicit instructions must be given to the patient so motion is kept to a minimum during these longer exposures. Unfortunately, the screen response to the long exposure times that occur during magnification studies prompts reciprocity law failure, for which the radiographer must compensate. Additional exposure times from **10 to 30 percent** are required to maintain optimal density at these long exposure times. Fortunately, high-quality mammography machines have sophisticated built-in circuitry that will automatically compensate for reciprocity law failure so that repeat radiographs are kept to a minimum.

Automatic Exposure Control

Automatic exposure control (AEC) is an integral component on every dedicated mammography generator. Like the AEC circuitry used on conventional radiography equipment, its design and purpose is to provide consistent image receptor exposure for the various thickness and density compositions of breast tissues and for the range of kVp used. Because of the high-contrast imaging environment in mammography, there is minimal exposure latitude in terms of film density. Small variations in film density will affect the contrast required to visualize the subtle breast tissue and to diagnose cancer.

Automatic control of exposure techniques is crucial in breast imaging because of the wide range of breast thicknesses and density compositions. A 4-cm compressed breast on a number of similarly aged women can cause a range of x-ray exposure times from **0.05 ms to over 1 second**! It is virtually impossible for the radiographer to determine the exact density composition of breast tissues; therefore, it is difficult to determine the exact exposure time required if AEC is not used. The introduction of AEC on dedicated mammography machines, in particular the current generation of machines, prompted a significant reduction in repeat rates for mammography.

The AEC system on most mammography machines utilizes a single radiation-sensitive detector located **behind** the cassette. The detector is capable of moving toward the nipple, from its primary position at the chest wall, to allow for maximum variations in breast size and for critical magnification work (Figure 38-8). Most detectors will have 10 stops between the chest wall and the nipple. The AEC system should be capable of being calibrated for two different screen/film systems and also for non-grid, grid, and magnification options.

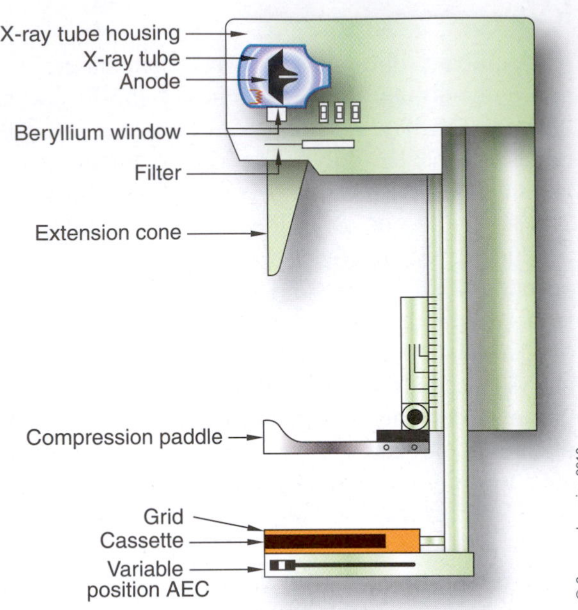

FIGURE 38-8. General design of a mammography machine and its accessory components. Note vertical alignment of the chest wall edge of cassette and compression paddle, straight portion of extension cone, and angle of the anode.

The optical density (OD) of the ACR Plexiglas™ mammographic phantom image should not be less than **1.20** and preferably about **1.30 OD.** The film density, as measured using the ACR standardized exposure technique, should be within ± 0.15 OD for the range of kVps used and for phantom Plexiglas™ thicknesses from 2 to 6 cm. The generator must contain a **density compensation circuit** that contains at least two + and two − settings. Each setting, or step, should result in a 12 to 15 percent change in mAs, or approximately a 0.15 change in optical film density, to allow maximum flexibility for all imaging requirements. Mammography generators have a **backup timer** similar to conventional AEC systems. The backup timer for grid techniques must be set at **600 mAs,** and for non-grid and magnification techniques, **300 mAs.** If the backup time is reached during a breast exposure, the radiographer should select a **higher kVp** setting for the repeat radiograph. The density compensation circuit should not be increased as is typically done in conventional AEC imaging. The primary reason backup time is reached in breast imaging is because of the inability of the low-energy photons to penetrate the breast. (This will usually occur on large or dense breasts.) A density compensation circuit increase will only prompt the backup timer to be reached again because the energy of the x-ray beam did not change; therefore, penetration of the breast will not occur. If the AEC system is left on during imaging of a breast with an implant in place, the backup time will also be reached. (Only **manual** exposure techniques should be used for implant imaging.)

Quality mammography generators have highly sophisticated microprocessor controlled circuits that provide accurate and reproducible film densities over the entire range of kVp settings required and for the different thicknesses and densities of breast tissue. Well-designed AEC circuitry can automatically compensate for reciprocity law failure during long exposures. Current machines may also contain circuits that can automatically adjust the kVp to a higher level during the actual exposure. This allows the film to be properly exposed and the backup time will not be reached if the breast is large or dense. The circuit adjusts the kVp by sensing the radiation intensity during the first 100 milliseconds of the exposure. If the current is too low, the kVp is automatically increased. When purchasing a new mammography machine, the AEC nomenclature should be carefully checked and tested to ensure that it has accurate density tracking, and therefore will reproduce film densities for all requirements within ± 0.10 OD.

X-RAY TUBE

Design

The most distinctive aspect of the mammography machine is the design and application of its x-ray tube and peripheral components. Each component described in this section has a very novel design compared to its counterpart in conventional radiology. The specific design or use of some components will increase contrast, resolution, or radiation exposure. Other components counteract this and cause a decrease in contrast, resolution, or exposure. The production of a high-quality breast image involves many tradeoffs. Taken altogether, however, the x-ray tube design and the components are capable of achieving high resolution and high contrast at moderate radiation exposure levels. First and foremost, the mammography equipment must be engineered to provide the high contrast and resolution required to visualize microcalcifications and the subtle parenchymal structures of the breast. Achieving the right balance of contrast, resolution, and low radiation exposures is a formidable challenge in breast imaging.

Heel Effect

The anode configuration in a mammography x-ray tube produces a prominent heel effect due to the short source-to-image-receptor distance (SID) and the use of a narrow target angle. Because the x-ray tube is aligned with the cathode placed directly over the chest wall area and the anode outward toward the nipple end, the heel effect fortunately can be used to maximum advantage (Figure 38-9).

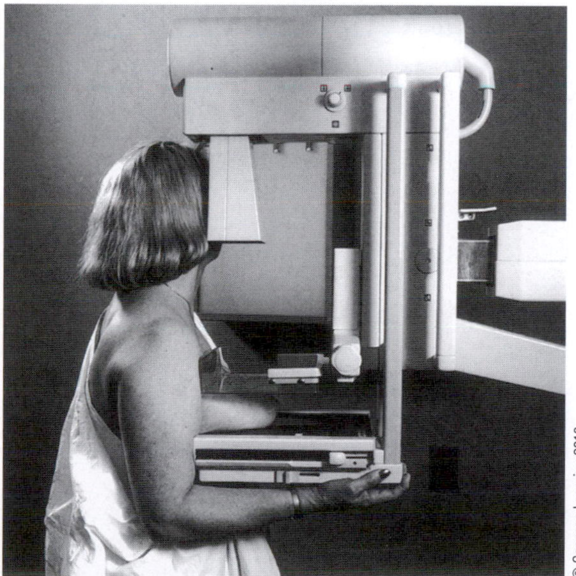

FIGURE 38-9. Patient positioned on a mammography machine. Note the short SID of 60 cm, which produces a prominent heel effect. The cathode side of the x-ray tube is placed over the patient's head and the anode side outward toward the nipple. This orientation allows the bulk of the x-ray tube housing to be placed away from the patient's head for ease of positioning.

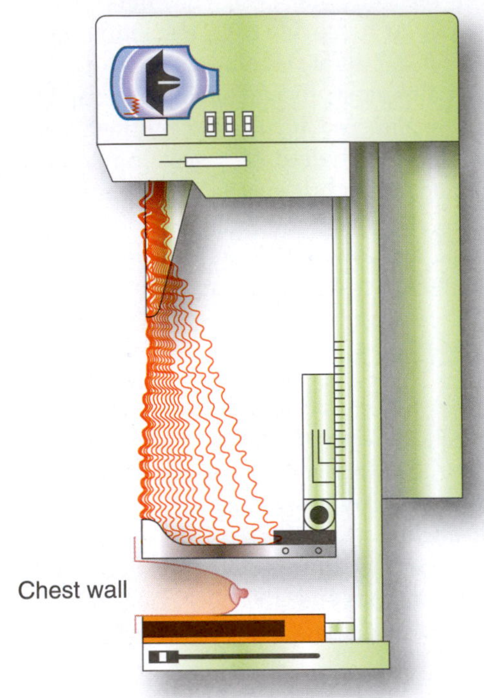

FIGURE 38-10. Mammography x-ray tube oriented with the cathode side placed over the chest wall area and the anode side placed outward toward the nipple end. Heel effect is used to maximum advantage with this orientation. Greater-intensity x-rays are placed over the chest wall area where the breast is thicker, producing a more uniform-density image.

Recall that the cathode side of the x-ray beam has a significantly greater intensity of x-rays compared to the anode side. A more uniform-density breast image can be produced because the more intense x-rays are at the chest wall where there is greater tissue thickness (Figure 38-10). The primary reason the cathode end of the x-ray tube is placed directly over the chest wall edge of the image is to take advantage of the prominent heel effect of the anode.

Cathode

The cathode in a mammography x-ray tube consists of standard helical-shaped tungsten filaments in a focusing cup. Mammography tubes typically utilize a single filament wire for both the large and small focal spots. When the small focal spot is engaged, a negative voltage is applied to the focusing cup, which acts to reduce the size of the electron stream creating the smaller focal spot. This is called **bias focusing** (see Chapter 6). Some machines utilize two separate filaments for the small and large focal spots.

The high resolution needed in mammography requires substantially smaller effective focal spot sizes than those used in conventional radiography. In addition, the majority of mammography machines utilize a relatively short SID of only **60 to 76 cm** (24 to 30 inches), which necessitates the use of microsized focal spots to diminish the increased geometric unsharpness. A nominal **0.3-mm large** focal spot is used for the routine contact images and a nominal **0.1-mm small** focal spot is used for magnification images.

In all x-ray tubes, the effective focal spot size varies in length along the cathode-anode axis at the plane of the film due to the line-focus principle. As a result, a larger focal spot size is always projected on the cathode side (Figure 38-11A). Because mammography tubes are oriented with the cathode side placed over the chest wall, the focal spot shape and size phenomenon creates a serious dilemma: resolution is substantially decreased at the chest wall where many lesions are found. The phenomenon is more pronounced for magnification techniques. Another phenomenon that can complicate breast imaging occurs if the actual focal spot and central ray are positioned over the center of the image as in conventional radiology. Due to the short SID, several millimeters of posterosuperior breast tissue will not be imaged (Figure 38-11B). These two negative geometric properties associated with the focal spot in mammography are diminished via the **off-center placement** of the glass x-ray tube unit within the tube housing. The glass tube is moved maximally toward the chest wall so the focal spot on the anode and vertical central ray are positioned **directly over the chest wall** (Figure 38-12A and B). The geometric dilemma is diminished by **eliminating** the entire cathode side of the x-ray beam. Although the effective focal spot size remains larger at the chest wall, utilizing the anode half of the beam provides slightly greater resolution because the projected focal spot sizes at the image plane are smaller on this side. Therefore, a smaller

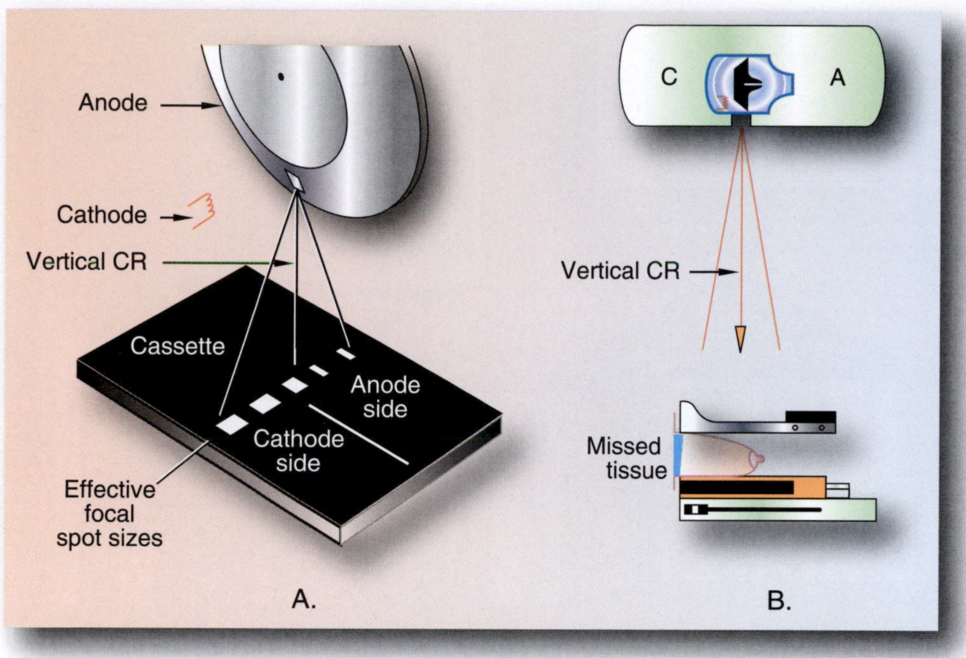

FIGURE 38-11. (A) Conventional radiography x-ray tube with focal spot and vertical central ray positioned over center of the cassette. Note that the focal spot length is projected larger in size toward the cathode end due to the line-focus principle. (B) Conventional focal spot and vertical central ray positioned over center of cassette prompting posterosuperior breast tissue to be missed on the image.

effective focal spot is projected at the important chest wall area (see Figure 38-12A). Placing the x-ray tube off center also enables the vertical central ray to enter **straight in** at the chest wall, eliminating the possibility of missing the posterosuperior breast tissue in the image (see Figure 38-12B). The heel effect continues to be advantageous because there remains greater intensity at the vertical central ray point than at the anode end. Recall that the x-ray intensity decreases gradually from the cathode toward the anode.

This unique design prompts a change in the orientation of the mammography x-ray beam. Because the vertical central ray is positioned at the chest wall (edge of the film), the x-ray directed to the center of the cassette is actually the midportion of the anode half of the x-ray beam. This new **angled** central ray is termed the **reference axis** in mammography (see Figure 38-12B).

The physical size of the focal spot in mammography is determined and measured by the manufacturers at the reference axis point on the image receptor plane, not at the vertical central ray point as in conventional radiography. The target angle will measure smaller from the reference axis perspective, and therefore the focal spot will also measure smaller. The nominal 0.30-mm large and nominal 0.10-mm small focal spots measure this size in the center of the film at the reference axis point. Therefore, the projected **length** and overall size of the effective focal spot at the vertical central ray point and chest wall will be at least **2 × larger.** This geometric phenomenon results from the line-focus principle and cannot be overcome. The high resolution in the image is maintained, in part, via the use of very small focal spot sizes. This may appear to not be an ideal engineering design; however, a tradeoff must be made. Overall, it is more advantageous to

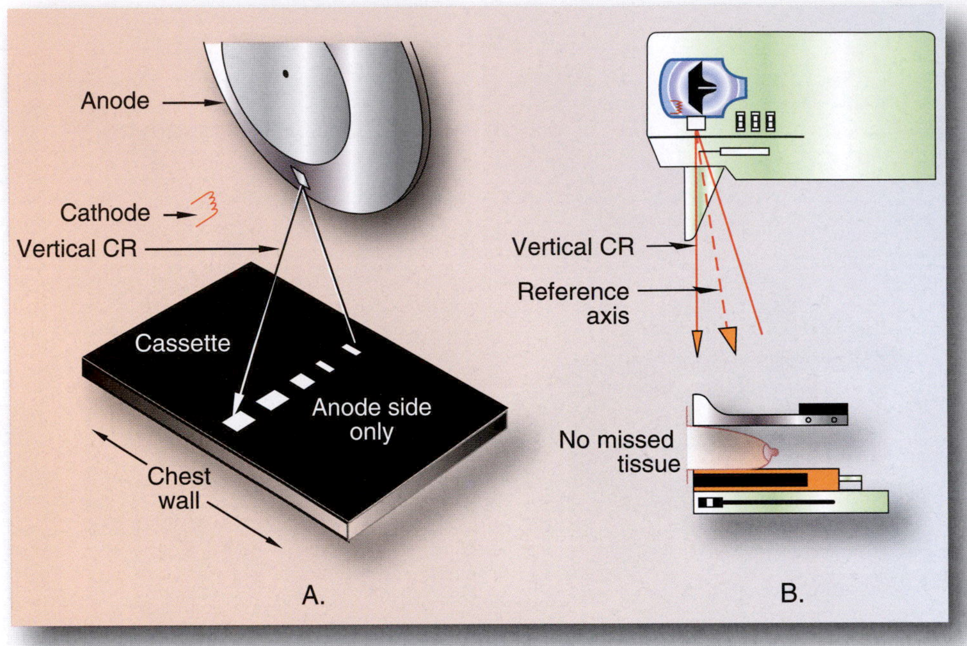

FIGURE 38-12. Off-center placement of the x-ray tube within the tube housing. The cathode side of the x-ray beam is eliminated. (A) Focal spot and vertical central ray placed directly over the chest wall. (B) Vertical central ray placed directly over chest wall structure, allowing the posterosuperior breast tissue to be imaged. Note that the new central ray is termed the reference axis. The nominal focal spot size is measured at the reference axis point on the image receptor.

have the cathode end over the more dense chest wall structures to take advantage of the **heel effect.** In addition, this orientation allows the bulk of the x-ray tube housing to be placed away from the patient's head for ease of positioning (see Figure 38-9).

Anode Configuration

Mammography tubes use rotating anodes to take advantage of the increased tube loading. This is particularly important because it enables the use of a higher mA and allows exposure times to be maintained under 1 second.

The **effective target angle** (measured from the vertical central ray point) is **greater** in a mammography tube, varying from **22° to 24°.** The larger effective angle is necessary so the x-ray beam will cover a 24-cm × 30-cm cassette at the 60- to 65-cm SID (Figure 38-13A and B). However, the **reference axis target angle** (measured from the center of the x-ray beam as in conventional radiography) is **smaller,** varying from **7.5° to 12°.** The reference axis target angle is specified in mammography tubes because it defines the size of the focal spot as measured in the center of the image.

Most manufacturers prefer to use a narrow target angle, as measured from the vertical filament, because it allows greater anode heat capacity for a given effective focal spot size. However, to utilize a narrower angle and maintain x-ray coverage on the cassette, the x-ray tube must be **tilted** (see Figure 38-13B). One manufacturer utilizes a unique design in which the anode is oriented with the stem placed in a vertical position and the x-ray tube steeply tilted. This allows the **edge** of the anode disk to be used as the actual target rather than the face of the anode (Figure 38-14A and B). The anode edge is designed with two distinct surfaces, one for

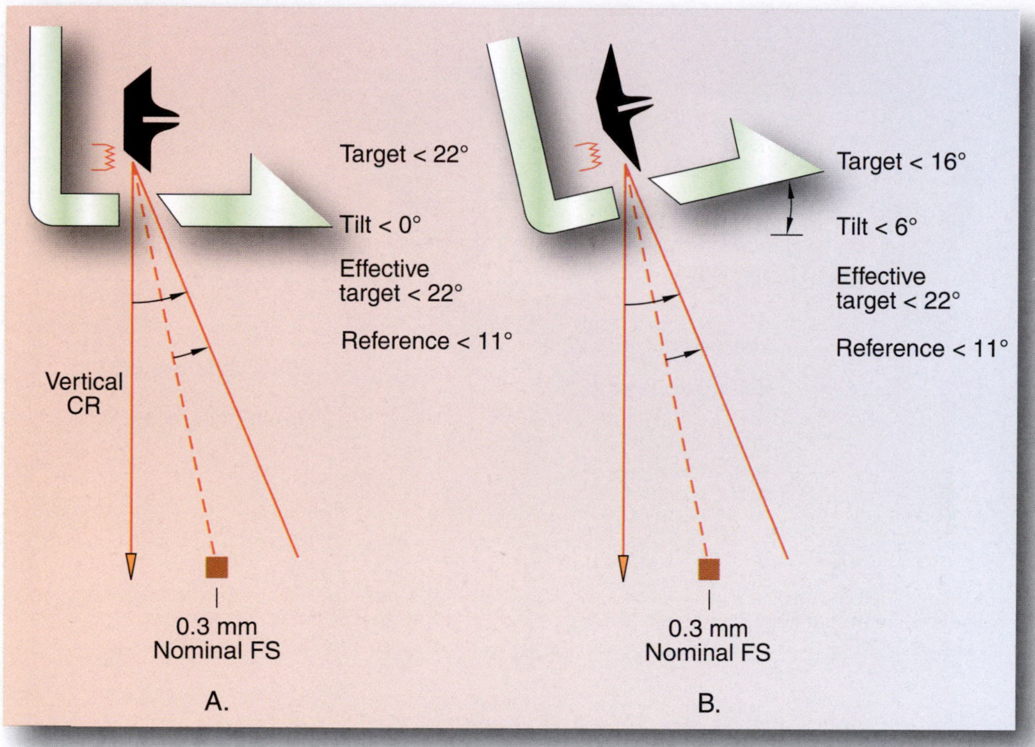

FIGURE 38-13. Mammography x-ray tube configurations. (A) Horizontal tube placement and 22° target angle. The large effective target angle of 22° allows x-ray coverage of the cassette at a short SID. The reference axis target angle of 11° creates a 0.3-mm focal spot size in the center of the image. (B) Tilting the tube 6° allows use of a smaller target angle of 16° and prompts the same effective angle of 22° and reference axis of 11° as the horizontal tube. Tilting allows greater anode heat capacity due to the smaller target angle.

each focal spot. This design allows radiation coverage of the film with the large focal spot, achievement of maximum anode heat capacity, capability of producing a small effective focal spot, and placement of the effective small focal spot closer to the chest wall, allowing greater resolution. Designing the anode configuration to achieve a small effective focal spot size, allowing maximum x-ray coverage of the cassette, and producing optimal resolution at a short SID are engineering challenges.

Anode Material

The anode in mammography x-ray tubes is made of **molybdenum.** Some manufacturers use a solid molybdenum disk and others design the molybdenum anode with graphite backing similar to conventional radiography. In order to prevent anode surface roughness and pitting, which could ultimately decrease x-ray output, the molybdenum may be doped with about 3 percent vanadium. Like tungsten, molybdenum has a high melting point, and conducts heat well.

Molybdenum is used as the anode material of choice over tungsten for several reasons. Studies indicate that x-ray energies ranging between 17 keV and 25 keV are required to differentiate the inherent low-contrast structures of all types of breasts. Specifically, x-ray energies between the narrow range of **17–20** are preferred. These specific x-ray energies must be present in the mammography x-ray beam to maximize subject contrast and visualize

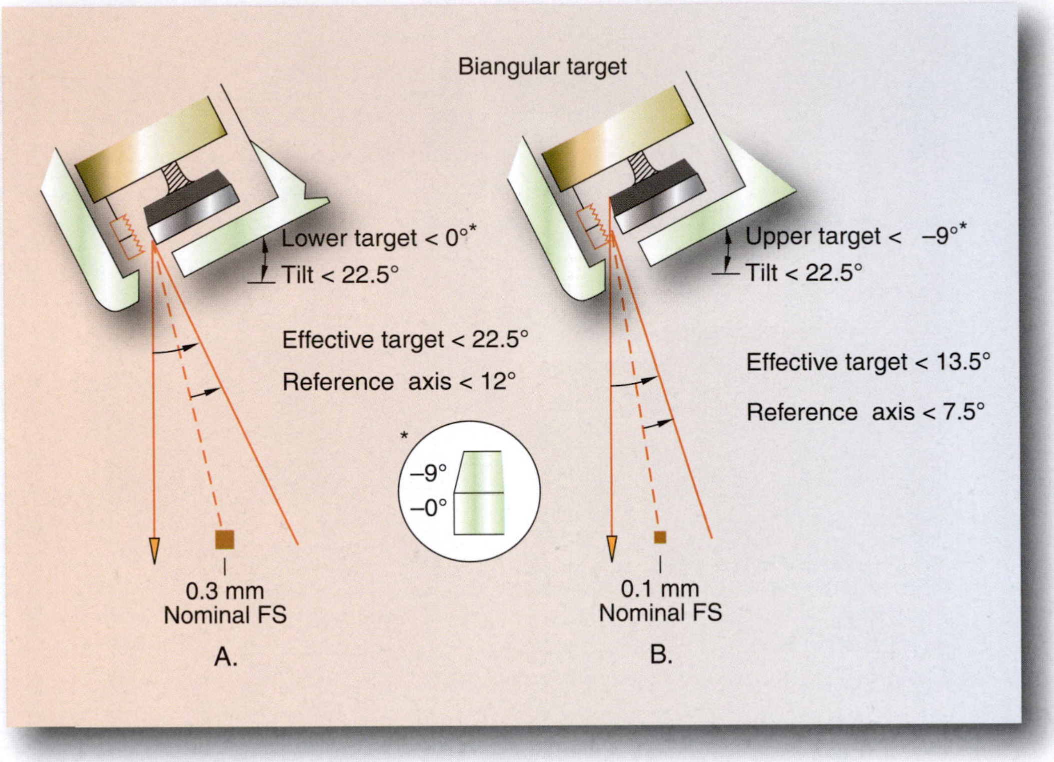

FIGURE 38-14. Anode oriented with stem placed in a vertical position, a biangular anode disk end used as the target, and the tube steeply tilted. Circular inset shows anode end in true vertical position with a 0° lower edge and −9° upper edge. (A) Lower edge of anode disk used for large focal spot. Steep 22.5° tube tilt produces a 22.5° effective target angle to allow x-ray coverage of the cassette and a 12° reference axis angle creates a 0.30 nominal focal spot. (B) Upper edge of anode disk used for small focal spot and magnification studies. The 22.5° tilt produces a 13.5° effective target angle, which allows adequate coverage for magnification images. The 7.5° reference axis angle creates a 0.10 nominal small focal spot. The small focal spot is projected closer to the chest wall structure, allowing greater resolution.

microcalcifications. If the x-ray beam contains energies higher than this narrow range, the x-rays will overpenetrate, scatter, and decrease radiographic contrast. A relatively large number of **photoelectric absorption** interactions is needed to produce the high radiographic contrast that will improve the visibility of detail in the image. Low kVp is necessary to produce the 17–20 keV range of x-ray photons that will create the photoelectric interactions. Unfortunately, this will introduce a higher radiation exposure to the patient. As in all areas of mammography, a tradeoff must be made. Without low-kVp x-rays and high photoelectric absorption, radiographic detail of the breast structures cannot occur.

The three primary breast tissues—adipose, fibrous, and glandular—have very low atomic numbers ranging from 6 to 8. Approximately 40 percent of cancers in the breast contain microcalcifications that have an atomic number of 20. Therefore, kVp settings around 25 are necessary. One must set the generator kVp slightly higher than the atomic number of the tissues being imaged so there is adequate penetration. Figures 38-15A and 38–15B illustrate an x-ray emission spectrum for a conventional tungsten anode x-ray tube and a molybdenum anode mammography tube operating at 26 kVp. Note that the tungsten anode will produce x-ray photons with energies in the preferred 17- to 20-keV range.

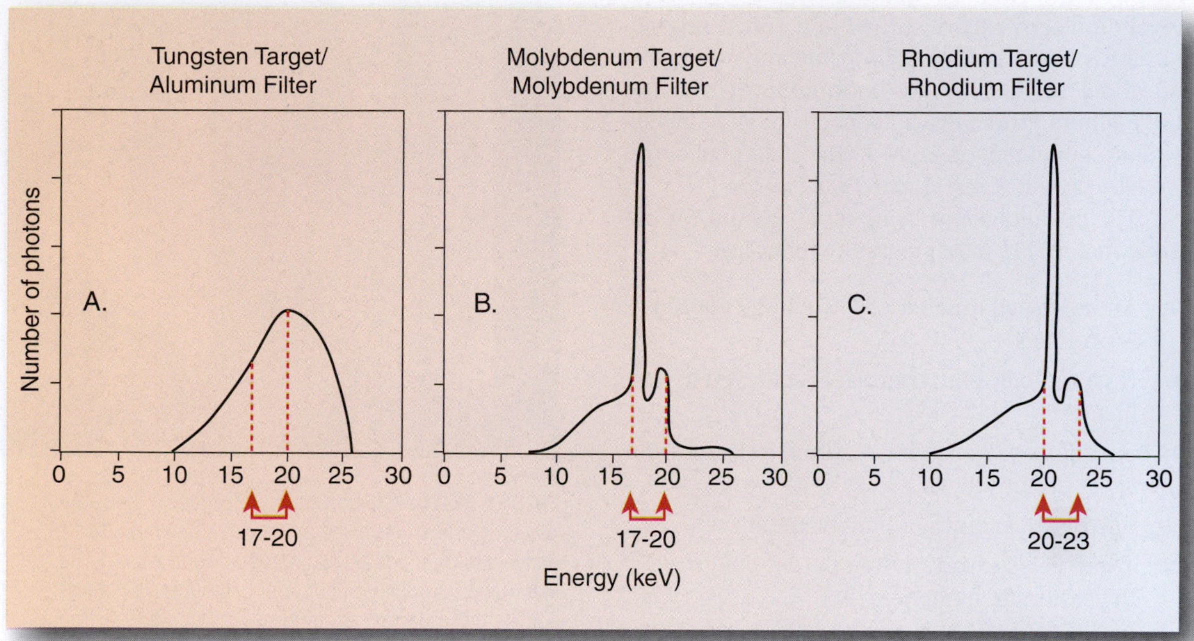

FIGURE 38-15. X-ray emission spectrums produced at 26 kVp. (A) Conventional tungsten target with aluminum filter. A high volume of photons is produced above the preferred mammography range of 17 to 20 keV and a high volume is produced below this range. Note that the entire x-ray beam is bremsstrahlung photons. (B) Mammography molybdenum target and molybdenum filter producing prominent characteristic photons at 17 and 20 keV in the preferred energy range. Very few photons are produced above this range. (C) Mammography rhodium target and rhodium filter. The spectrum shape is identical to B but produces a higher-average-energy x-ray beam than molybdenum. Note the prominent characteristic photons at 20 and 23 keV, which provide better penetration for larger or more dense breasts at a lower dose to the patient.

It also produces a high volume of photons above this range and a relatively large number below the range. The x-ray photons above the preferred mammography range will produce Compton interactions that decrease contrast, and the x-ray photons below this range all will be virtually absorbed via the photoelectric process and only contribute to patient dose. The entire tungsten-produced x-ray beam consists of bremsstrahlung x-rays.

The x-ray emission spectrum produced from the molybdenum anode has a drastically different shape. Note that the most prominent x-ray photons are **characteristic.** The characteristic x-rays are created from displacement of the K-shell binding electrons in the molybdenum atom (Table 38-2). Characteristic x-rays will account for approximately 30 percent of the total x-rays in the molybdenum beam at 30 kVp. Most important, there is an increased volume of characteristic x-ray photons produced at exactly 17 and 20 keV in the preferred range, which creates a nearly perfect x-ray beam for breast imaging. When properly filtered, the molybdenum anode produces very few x-ray photons above the preferred mammographic

TABLE 38-2. Characteristic X-Rays from Mammography X-Ray Targets

Electron Shells	Molybdenum (Z-42)	Rhodium (Z-45)
	keV*	
L to K	17	20
M to K	20	23

energy range. The x-ray photons below this range are photoelectrically absorbed and aid in producing high subject contrast. Unfortunately, they also contribute to dose. Many textbooks refer to the molybdenum x-ray emission spectrum as being essentially homogeneous due to the high concentration of x-rays in a very narrow range.

The advantages of using molybdenum for the anode material in mammography tubes are:

- An increased number of low-energy photons is produced.
- High radiographic contrast is achieved in the image.
- Specific x-ray energies required for breast imaging are produced.

The disadvantages of molybdenum are:

- There is less x-ray photon output due to a lower atomic number—42.
- Increased mAs is required to maintain image receptor exposure.
- Increased dose to the patient results.

The higher-contrast image produced by the molybdenum target is illustrated in Figure 38-16.

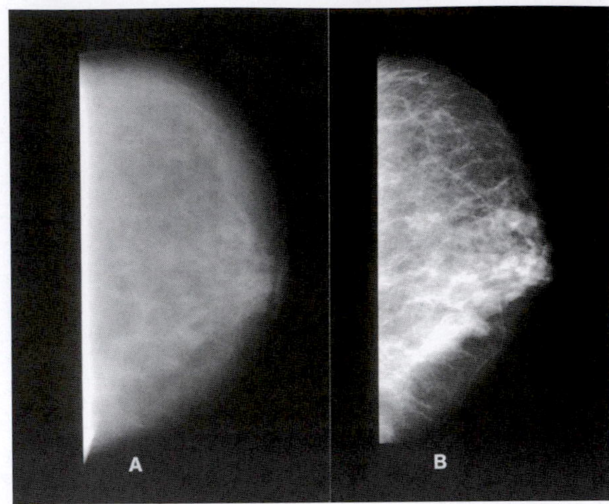

FIGURE 38-16. Craniocaudal projection of the same patient's breast produced at 30 kVp, showing effect of molybdenum anode on radiographic contrast. (A) The tungsten anode produces suboptimal radiographic contrast. (B) The molybdenum anode produces significantly higher contrast and greater visibility of detail. *(Images courtesy of C. Vyborny, MD, PhD.)*

Recently, a new anode material, **rhodium,** was introduced for use in mammography. The slightly higher atomic number of rhodium, 45, creates higher-energy x-ray photons (see Table 38-2). The primary advantage of using rhodium is that the characteristic x-rays it produces have energies that are **2–3 keV higher** than those of molybdenum. In the rhodium x-ray emission spectrum, the x-ray photon energies shift slightly to the right and the characteristic x-rays are prominent at **20 and 23 keV** (Figure 38–15C). This provides better penetration of large breasts or those breasts that are very dense. Of significance also is that rhodium's higher average energy x-ray beam prompts a reduction in exposure time of approximately 25 percent. When used with the appropriate filter, use of a rhodium anode can decrease x-ray exposure by 50 percent or more. The primary disadvantage of rhodium as an anode material is that its higher energy beam is not appropriate for use on small to regular-sized breasts, or those breasts that are not dense. Therefore, it cannot be the sole anode material. To take advantage of the inherent properties of rhodium, one manufacturer has designed a **biangular** anode, similar to Figure 38-14, in which the same disk contains a track for molybdenum and a separate track for rhodium, selectable by the operator. The x-ray tube can be moved in one of two positions, one for each of the two focal spots. This allows both focal spot sizes to be available for each track. Interestingly, another manufacturer has recently introduced a dual-track anode that contains molybdenum and **tungsten,** selectable by the operator also. The tungsten anode is used with a rhodium filter and, like the rhodium anode, is designed to be used on the larger or more dense breasts at a significantly reduced exposure. Altohugh molybdenum is the primary anode material used, all machines will have either rhodium or tungsten as an alternate choice.

Filtration

The port of the x-ray tube in mammography is specially designed. **Beryllium,** with an atomic number of 4, is used in the port of all mammography x-ray tubes to allow the low-energy x-rays to exit. Glass cannot be used because it would attenuate most of the low-energy x-rays needed to produce the breast image.

Filtration must be used at the tube port on all mammography machines. As in conventional radiography, the primary purpose of filtration is to attenuate the very low-energy x-rays that are not needed to produce the breast image. Without filtration, a relatively large number of 5- to 10-keV x-rays would exit the tube. In addition, a larger number of 20- to 30-keV x-rays at the higher-energy end of the spectrum would also exit. The 5- to 10-keV x-rays would all be absorbed in the breast and drastically increase the dose. The 20- to 30-keV x-rays would degrade image quality by decreasing radiographic contrast. A specific function of the filter in mammography, therefore, is to decrease most of the low- and some high-energy bremsstrahlung x-rays to maximize subject contrast. To accomplish this, mammography filters are made of the **same element** as the anode material. For a molybdenum anode the filter is **0.03-mm molybdenum,** and for the rhodium target, **0.025 mm rhodium.** The x-ray emission spectrums for molybdenum and rhodium in Figure 38-15 show the effect of this filtration. Eliminating much of the high 20- to 30-keV photons provides a nearly perfect x-ray beam for breast imaging.

Many mammography machines provide a selectable molybdenum or rhodium filter that can be used with the molybdenum anode. Selection of the rhodium filter with the molybdenum anode will produce an emission spectrum that lies halfway between the molybdenum and the rhodium configurations. The rhodium filter used with the molybdenum anode will produce a higher-energy x-ray beam that is more desirable for larger or dense breasts. Use of the rhodium filter will also reduce radiation exposure by about 38 percent. Caution must be exercised to ensure that the rhodium filter is not used with small and regular-sized breasts or non-dense breasts, because it will produce a lower-contrast image that would not provide the appropriate visibility of detail.

The half-value-layer (HVL) is an indirect measurement of the total filtration in the path of the x-ray beam. It is expressed in millimeters of aluminum (mm Al). In a mammography machine, the HVL will include the attenuation properties of the beryllium window, molybdenum filter, mirror, and the plastic compression paddle. The minimum HVL is specified by government regulations and should not measure less than **0.30 mm Al** at 30 kVp or **0.25 mm Al** at 25 kVp. This will ensure that adequate filtration is present in the x-ray beam, and the patient will not receive excessive radiation exposure. If the HVL is too high, image quality can be degraded. Excessive filtration, although it would reduce exposure, will decrease overall radiographic image contrast. Therefore, the HVL should not exceed **0.40 mm Al** at 30 kVp. It is recommended that the HVL be maintained as close as possible to the minimal level to ensure that image contrast is maintained at a high level.

Magnification

Magnified projections of the breast are additionally requested when the visibility of detail in very small breast structures and when microcalcifications need to be enhanced. They are also requested when breast structures that lie close together and overlap have to be separated. As many as 10 percent of patients require additional projections using the magnification technique.

The magnification factor on the mammography machine varies slightly among manufacturers and is standardized between 1.5 × and 1.8 ×. Some manufacturers design their equipment with two magnification selections—the second may be as high as 2.0 ×. To magnify the breast, a raised platform is placed on the cassette holder unit and the breast is placed on top of the platform for the exposure (Figure 38-17).

Magnified projections of the breast provide the following enhancements:

- **Increased resolution** due to the small focal spot and reduced quantum mottle
- **Reduction in scatter radiation** reaching the film due to the air gap
- **Improved visibility of detail** due to the larger field of view.

Magnifying the breast will technically reduce resolution in the image due to an increase in

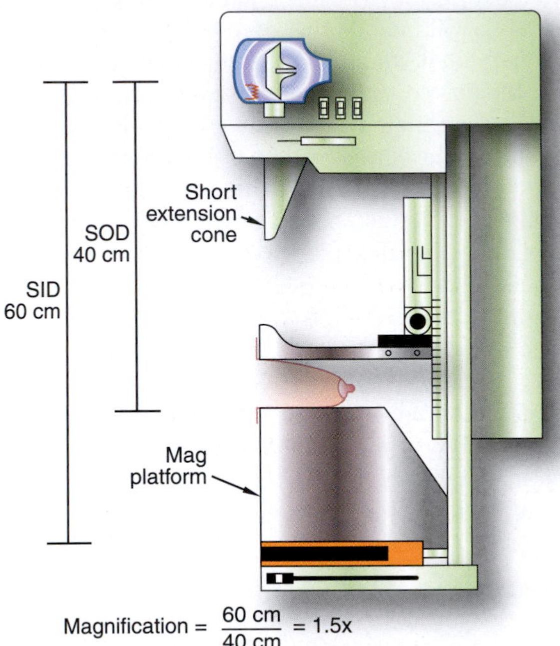

FIGURE 38-17. Breast in position on a raised platform to produce a 1.5× magnification image. There is greater intensity of radiation at the breast when placed closer to the x-ray tube. Magnification technique requires the use of a 0.10 focal spot to maintain resolution. *(Image courtesy of Eugene Frank.)*

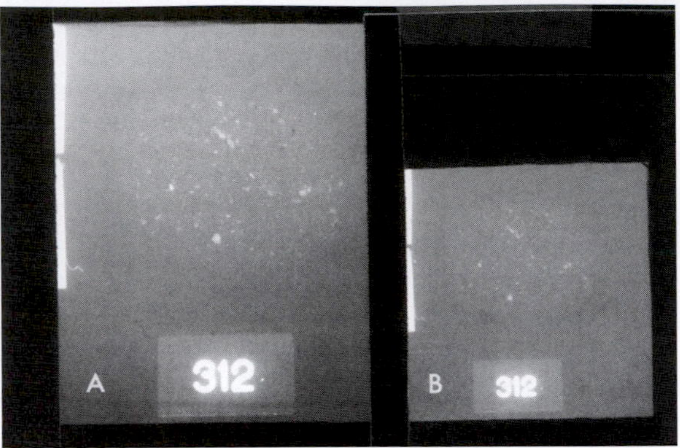

FIGURE 38-18. (A) Magnification image of calcifications in a Plexiglas™ breast phantom at 1.5× and 26 kVp. (B) Nonmagnified image of same phantom as A. *(Image courtesy Lynn Carlton.)*

geometric unsharpness. A magnification of 1.5 × will reduce resolution by at least 50 percent from about 20 lp/mm to 10 lp/mm. To regain the lost resolution, a very small 0.10-mm focal spot is utilized, which returns the resolution to the 20-lp/mm level. This is the smallest focal spot size employed anywhere in radiology. Effective resolution may even be improved in magnified images due to a **reduction in noise.** Recall that noise is primarily a product of the screen/film combination (quantum mottle). The screen/film combination typically is not changed for magnification techniques. Noise is therefore reduced by about 30 percent for 1.5 × magnification because significantly more x-ray photons are used per unit volume of tissue to produce the image. This is due to the breast being placed closer to the x-ray tube where there is a higher volume of x-rays available to form the image. For 1.5 × magnification, a given square of tissue covers approximately 2.25 × more area on the film compared to the contact image, and many more screen phosphors are utilized to form the image.

Scattered radiation is reduced somewhat as a result of the air gap between the cassette and breast. The reduced scatter increases radiographic contrast and, fortunately, a grid does not have to be used. The breast structures are seen much better when the magnification technique is used due to a combination of the microsized focal spot, the reduction in noise, and the reduction in scatter radiation. When the breast structures are magnified, they are spread apart and the anatomical field of view is enhanced (Figure 38-18A and B).

Radiation exposure to the patient is a major concern in magnification radiography of the breast. Radiation to the breast can increase **2–3** × during a single exposure, even without the use of a grid. This results from the breast being placed much closer to the x-ray source where the radiation intensity is greater. The exact exposure increase will vary among different manufacturers' units depending upon their specific design and magnification factor. The increase in radiation is due also to the additional exposure required because of reciprocity law failure. Use of the 0.10 focal spot requires that the mA be reduced considerably (e.g., 100 mA to 25 mA) due to tube loading. The reduction in mA will prompt exposure times to be increased to **2–4 seconds.** The long exposure time will require the mammographer to explain the procedure carefully and to watch the patient during the exposure so motion does not degrade image quality.

ACCESSORIES

Grids

Scatter control plays an important role in the production of a high-quality mammographic image. Scatter radiation is produced from the breast during the exposure, which contributes to the overall image receptor exposure, and the effect is a reduction in radiographic contrast. Scatter increases significantly for larger and more dense breasts and with higher kVp settings. With the introduction of the grid on dedicated mammography machines in 1978, scatter and secondary radiation reaching the image receptor has been reduced and high contrast maintained in the image. The grid will remove about 80–90 percent of the scatter. Use of a grid in mammography greatly improves radiographic quality, and today grids are used for all mammographic images. The use of a grid will, however, increase radiation exposure to the patient by a factor of **2–3 ×**.

Mammography grids are the linear type with a very low ratio of 4:1 or 5:1. The grid frequency will range from 30 to 50 lines/cm. The grid strips are made of lead as in conventional radiography. However, wood or carbon-fiber is used as the inner space material instead of aluminum in order to keep the Bucky factor as low as possible. All mammography grids in use today are a moving type—moving in one direction only. They do not reciprocate. A separate grid device is used for each of the two image receptor sizes used.

Grids are capable of producing artifacts in the image. Typically this occurs with the use of ultrashort exposure times that can be controlled by using an appropriate mA setting that will prevent short exposure times. Grids can also contain inherent artifacts. Upon purchase, mammography grids should be carefully checked before use to ensure they are free of artifacts. A basic quality control check can be performed by making a lighter-density film exposure with the grid stationary and another lighter-density exposure with the grid moving. If artifacts appear on the image made with the moving grid, the grid should probably be replaced.

Compression Device

All mammography machines contain a compression device that is used to compress the breast (see Figures 38-8 and 38-9). Improvements in breast compression technology in recent years have greatly improved the visibility of detail in breast images. Appropriately applied compression is one of the critical components in the production of a high-quality mammogram. The overall function of compression is to decrease the thickness of the breast, bring the breast structures as close to the image receptor as possible, and increase radiographic contrast (Figure 38-19). The specific advantages of this technique are:

- **Reduced magnification** lessens geometric unsharpness and increases resolution.
- **Reduced tissue thickness** requires less kVp, prompting a reduction in scattered radiation and an increase in radiographic contrast.
- **Reduced radiation exposure** occurs because less exposure time is required due to the decreased tissue thickness.
- **Reduced motion unsharpness** occurs because the breast is completely immobilized.
- **Improved visualization** of breast structures occurs because the structures are spread out over a larger area. There is also less superimposition of overlying structures.
- **More uniform image receptor exposure** occurs due to the flattening effect of compression permitting optimal exposure of the entire breast.

The effect of scatter and contrast is dramatic. A 6-cm-thick breast measuring 9 cm in diameter will have a scatter-to-primary ratio of about 0.8, or 80 percent of the exposure results from scatter. If the breast thickness is reduced to 3 cm with the breast area increased to 12 cm due to vigorous compression, the scatter-to-primary ratio is

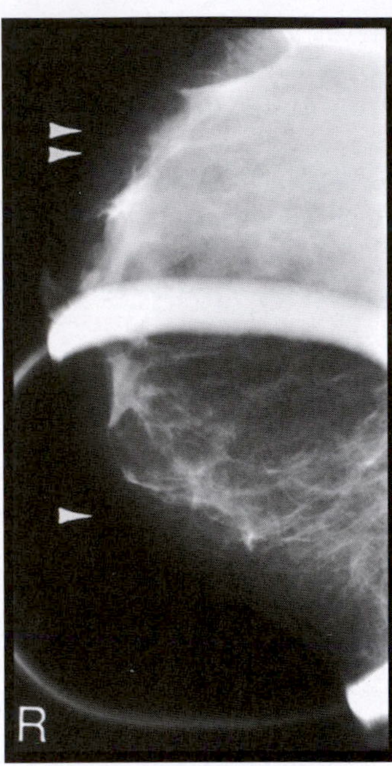

FIGURE 38-19. Effect of compression on the breast image. The spot compression on half of the breast (arrow) shows excellent contrast and resolution. The noncompressed side (double arrows) shows decreased density due to a thicker breast when no compression is applied. Significantly increased technical factors would be required to penetrate and achieve appropriate image receptor exposure if compression were not applied, and dose would be considerably higher. *(Image courtesy of Lynn Carlton.)*

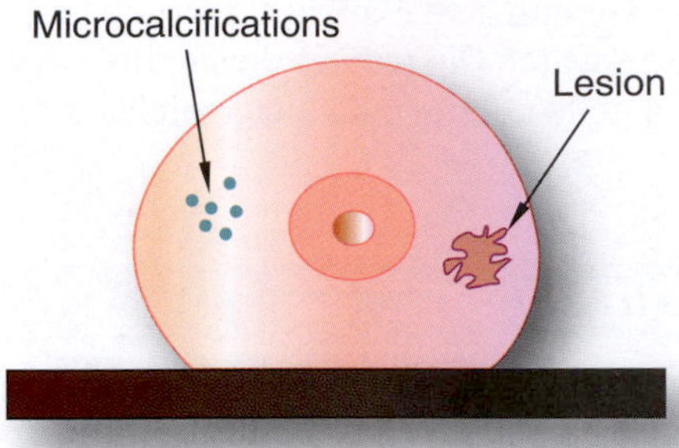

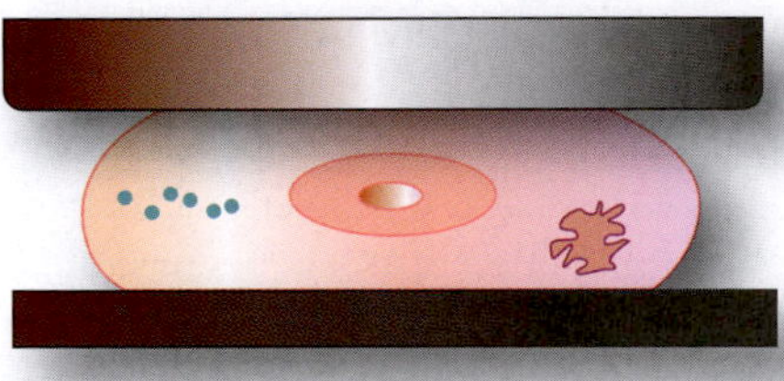

FIGURE 38-20. Breast compression. (A) No compression and scatter to primary ratio of 0.8. Note location of microcalcifications and lesion. (B) Compression decreases scatter to primary ration to 0.4; breast structures are brought closer to the film and spread out. Decreased tissue thickness and reduction in scatter radiation prompts greater radiographic contrast. Decreased magnification of structures creates greater resolution.

reduced to 0.4, or only 40 percent of the image receptor exposure results from scatter. Radiographic contrast would increase two-fold (Figures 38-20A and B).

The compression device is made of a plastic that allows transmission of the low energy x-rays. The device should have a straight chest wall edge to allow the compression to grasp the breast tissues close to the chest wall edge. Compression is controlled by the radiographer and must be capable of being applied at 25–45 lb. of force. In addition to the standard compression device, a smaller "spot" device is used to compress localized areas. The device should be checked regularly to ensure that it is working properly and applying the correct amount of pressure.

Film/Screen Systems

Like many of the previously described components of the mammography unit, the cassettes and screen/film combination used are also designed specifically to image the breast. Specially designed cassettes containing a single-emulsion screen are used with a single-emulsion film.

Mammography cassettes are manufactured of plastic or low attenuation carbon-fiber. Carbon-fiber enables the maximum number of x-rays to reach the intensifying screen, thereby keeping exposures at minimum levels. The screen is mounted on a foam pressure pad, and when closed, is placed at the extreme top of the cassette as close to the breast as possible (see Figure 38-3). The single screen is placed behind the film so there is high x-ray absorption of the screen phosphors closest to the film emulsion, thereby reducing the diffusion of light emitted from the screen (line-spread function). This arrangement prompts less image noise and greater resolution (Figure 38-21). The x-ray photons that exit the breast enter the top of the cassette and go through the film before reaching the screen phosphor.

Mammography screens are manufactured by a variety of companies and they are all very similar in design. Each company offers at least two different screen speeds—typically one screen will be twice as fast as the other. The majority of manufacturers use green emitting gadolinium oxysulfide as the screen phosphor material. Mammography screens are much slower than those used in conventional radiography. A slow screen offers reduced noise and increased resolution. The disadvantage of using a screen is the decrease in resolution and increased image noise. However, a tradeoff must once again be made due to the unacceptably high radiation exposure from the direct exposure technique. Uniformity of the speed of all the screens used is important. The difference between the minimum and maximum optical densities in all the screens shall not exceed 0.30 OD.

Mammography film is designed to be very high in contrast and resolution. Because the breast structures contain very low inherent subject contrast, a high-contrast film is needed to enhance the anatomical structures. Mammography film, like the screen, is single emulsion and designed to be slow in speed. The slow speed prompts low image noise and high resolution. Mammography film is green sensitive to match the spectral characteristics of the green emitting screen. Manufacturers offer at least two different film speeds and two films with different contrast levels. An antihalation coating is placed on the nonemulsion side of the film. The coating prevents screen light from going through the film and scattering back to the film, which would decrease resolution. Caution

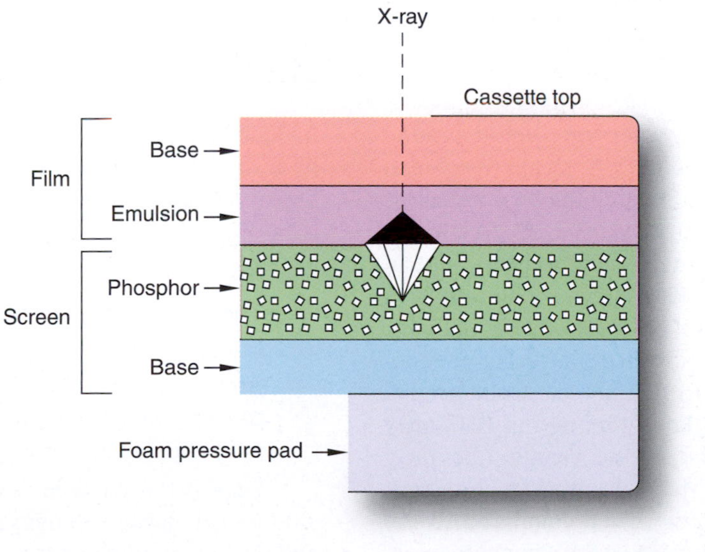

FIGURE 38-21. Cross-section of mammography screen and film in cassette. A single screen is placed behind the film as a back screen. Single-emulsion film is placed in contact with the single-emulsion screen. This design allows high absorption of x-rays in the screen phosphors closest to the film emulsion, which reduces diffusion of light emitted from the screen.

must be exercised so the nonemulsion side of the film (shiny side) is not placed in contact with the screen. The screen and film emulsions must always be in direct contact with each other.

The relative speed of a mammography screen/film combination should not be associated directly with a conventional screen/film system. A 100-speed mammography system will typically be 50 to 75 percent slower than a 100-speed conventional system. The stated speed will depend primarily upon the specific speed of the screen, the type and specific speed of film, and processing.

RESOLUTION

Dedicated mammography systems are capable of producing high-image resolution. Digital mammography systems provide spatial resolution of at least 10 lp/mm. This results in a pixel pitch of 50 microns or less. Many components, used together, play a role in achieving high resolution, most notably the microsized focal spots, compression, and low kVp. Cancer and other pathology can be identified although magnification is often required to view the small structures in the images and to actually see the high resolution.

Mammography images provide very high spatial resolution (Figure 38-22). Federal government regulation has mandated that consistent high-quality images be produced wherever mammography machines have met the MQSA standards. Mean glandular dose (MGD) provides the best indicator of risk to the patient instead of ESE. According to the federal government's MQSA program, in 1997 the average MGD for a single screen/film/grid study was 160 mRads (1.6 mGy). Dose data for digital mammography indicates a lowering of exposure when compared to film screen. Comparative MGD's per view have been reported at 2.37 mGy for screen/film mammography versus 1.86 mGy for digital systems. The risk from mammography at these levels is low when compared to the decreased deaths that result through screening. The lifetime risk of death from mammography is 5 in 1 million. With doses at their current levels, image noise and resolution are greater considerations than dose.

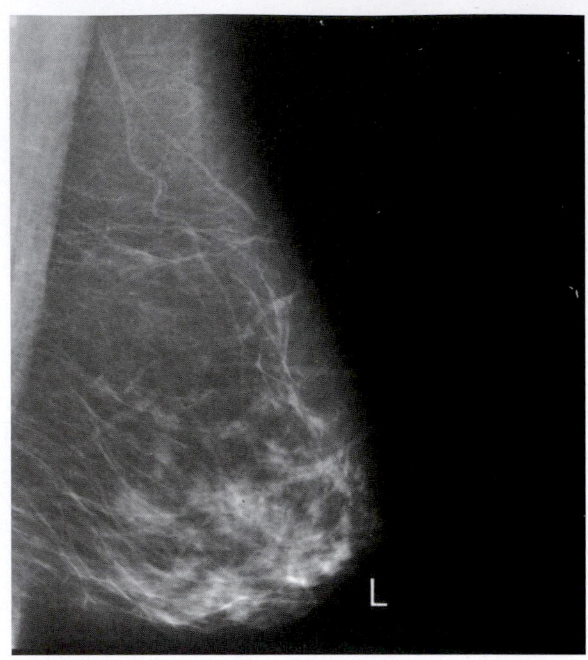

FIGURE 38-22. Mediolateral oblique projection of the breast produced on a current-generation mammography machine. High-quality image demonstrates optimal resolution and contrast. Radiation dose is low. *(Mammogram courtesy of Lynn Carlton.)*

DIGITAL MAMMOGRAPHY

In digital mammography, the film screen is replaced by a digital detector. The principal advantages of digital mammography include the following:

- The capacity to manipulate the image's contrast and density
- The capacity to transmit images for consultation, teaching, and so forth
- Archiving [picture and archiving communication system (PACS)] for simplified storage and ready access of images

One of the goals in mammography is to provide a high level of contrast between the lesion and the surrounding tissue. Unfortunately, because the breast tissue has similar densities, the attenuation differences between normal breast tissue and cancer are small. In digital mammography, the screen/film system is replaced by a detector, which produces an electric signal that is digitized and stored. Additional information about digital systems can be found in Chapter 23.

Various types of detectors are currently used by the current manufacturers of digital equipment. A phosphor flat panel system consists of a large-area plate that contains phosphors of thallium-activated cesium iodide (CsI) deposited onto photodiodes. In this system, the photodiodes detect the light emitted by the phosphor and create an electrical signal that is sent to the computer. A phosphor charge-coupled device (CCD) system is a second type of detector that also uses the CsI phosphor. Rather than using a large-area plate, the detector is a narrow 1 cm × 24 cm in size. The x-ray beam is collimated to match this detector and both are then scanned over the breast. With this design, the light of the phosphor is sent to a CCD, which converts the light into an electric signal. A third system is the selenium flat panel. This system does not use a phosphor; instead, the x-ray absorber is amorphous selenium. X-rays absorbed by this material are converted into an electrical charge by a system of electrode pads (Figure 38-23). With these digital detector systems, except in computed radiography (CR), it is no longer necessary to have AEC sensors under the plate. The digital detector device acts as a multielement sensor. The traditional CR system is also used in digital mammography as a fourth type of digital system. With CR, removable imaging plates are used with the Bucky tray. After exposure, the plates have to be transported to a reader device where the photostimulable phosphor in the plate is read by a laser light and converted into an electrical signal.

Images produced with digital mammography can be printed out in hard copy; however, one of the advantages of digital systems is that the images can be stored in a PACS. For maximum efficiency and cost reduction, digital images should be read on the computer monitor in a specially designed viewing station. Storage of digital images continues to be a challenge. A four-view exam will require as much as 240 megabytes of space. A major advantage of using digital mammography is that the images can easily be sent electronically to other physicians for interpretation, to other health-care institutions the patient may go to, and to efficiently call back for comparison purposes.

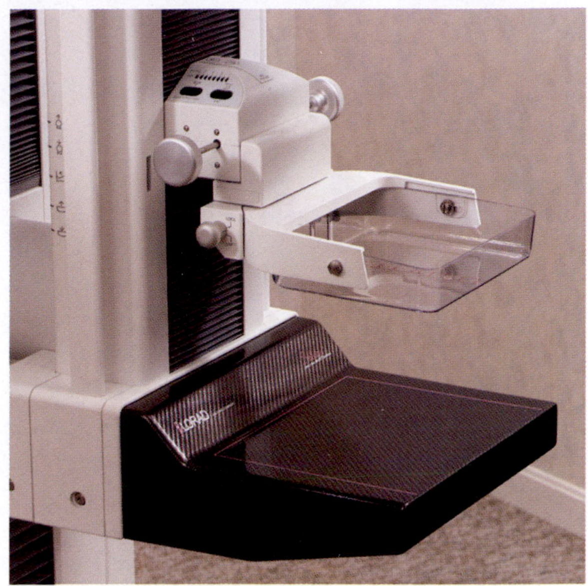

FIGURE 38-23. A digital direct conversion detector replaces the Bucky and film device. This digital detector is 24 cm × 29 cm and contains an amorphous selenium detector. Note the absence of the Bucky/IR opening. *(Courtesy of Hologic.)*

QUALITY CONTROL

The production of an optimal-quality breast image may be the most technically challenging of all radiographic examinations. Quality control tests are required under the rules of the MQSA to ensure that high standards of image quality are achieved daily. Some states may require additional tests. The ACR provides a quality control manual for medical physicists that contains a section for radiographers. The manual describes the quality control tests that should be carried out along with their frequency. The tests must be carried out accurately and at the minimum frequency stated. If problems occur in the production of images, the tests may need to be done more frequently. Regular quality control testing is the only means of ensuring that high image quality is always maintained. Slight changes in equipment performance, in particular the film processor and the accessory devices, can affect the contrast, resolution, or radiation exposure.

SUMMARY

Early detection of breast cancer depends on consistently reliable high-quality images. Image quality standards have been set forth by the American College of Radiology and the federal government's Mammography Quality Standards Act. The imaging requirements needed for mammography are more demanding than for other x-ray examinations. Mammography requires very high radiographic contrast and resolution so microcalcifications as small as 0.1 mm or less can be visualized along with the inherently low-contrast breast tissues. It is essential to use an imaging system that produces low noise. The radiation exposures associated with the examination must be sufficiently low to ensure that there is minimal risk to the patient.

The high subject contrast needed for effective mammography requires the use of low-kVp techniques along with a molybdenum anode and a molybdenum filter. The low x-ray energy range will enhance the breast structures and improve the visibility of detail. Two new options for imaging large and dense breasts have recently been introduced. These include the use of rhodium anodes with rhodium filtration and tungsten anodes with rhodium filtration.

Geometric unsharpness is minimized and resolution increased during mammography by using micro-focus focal spots, uniquely designed x-ray tube configurations, the heel effect to advantage, low magnification, and firm breast compression. Although the breast structure is small and low energy is utilized, there is still a significant component of scatter radiation that can obscure contrast. Therefore, low-ratio grids are required, along with breast compression, to reduce scattered radiation.

Dedicated mammography systems produce high-spatial-resolution images of 10 lp/mm or better. Digital mammography uses various types of detectors, including flat panel systems, CCD systems, and CR systems. Quality control tests are required under the rules of the MSQA. ■

REVIEW QUESTIONS

1. Discuss the advantages digital tomosynthesis has for mammographic applications.
2. List two reasons why high-frequency generators are used in mammography.
3. What is the kVp range for mammography?
4. What is the AEC backup time for a grid technique?
5. Which end of the mammography tube is placed over the chest wall area?
6. What are two focal spot sizes used in mammography tubes?
7. Which half of the x-ray beam, anode or cathode, is eliminated in mammography?
8. What is the most common anode material used in mammography?
9. List two reasons why x-ray tubes are tilted.
10. What material is the port of the x-ray tube in mammography made of?
11. List two advantages of producing magnified images of the breast.
12. State the two common grid ratios used in mammography.
13. List three advantages of using breast compression in mammography.
14. List three advantages of using digital mammographic systems.

REFERENCES AND RECOMMENDED READING

American Cancer Society. (2003). *Cancer facts and figures—2003.* Atlanta: Author.

American College of Radiology. (1999a). *Mammography quality control for medical physicists.* Reston, VA: Author.

American College of Radiology. (1999b). *Mammography quality control for technologists.* Reston, VA: Author.

Andolina V, Lillé S. (2010). *Mammographic imaging: A Practical guide.* Philadelphia: Lippinoctt Williams & Wilkins.

Barnes, G. T., & Brezovich, I. A. (1978). The intensity of scattered radiation in mammography. *Radiology, 126,* 243–247.

Barnes, G. T., Wu, X., Wagner, A. J., & Rubin, E. (1989). Scatter control in mammography: Past, present and future [abstract]. *Radiology, 173,* 472.

Buchanan, R. A., Finkelstein, S. I., & Wickersheim, K. A. (1976). X-ray exposure reduction using rare earth oxysulfide intensifying screens. *Radiology, 118,* 183–188.

Bushberg, J. T., Seibert, J. A., Leidholdt, E. M., & Boone, J. M. (2002). *The essential physics of medical imaging* (2nd ed.). Philadelphia: Lippincott Williams & Wilkins.

Chan, H., Wei, J., Sahiner, B., Rafferty, E., Wu, T., et.al. (2005). Computer-aided detection system for breast masses on Digital tomosynthesis mammograms: Preliminary experience. *Radiology.* 237(3):1075–80.

Egan, R. L. (1964). *Mammography.* Springfield, IL: Charles C Thomas.

Egan, R. L., McSweeney, M. B., & Sprawls, P. (1983). Grids in mammography. *Radiology, 146,* 359–362.

Elmore, J. G., Barton, M. B., Mocert, V. M., et al. (1998). Ten-year risk of false-positive screening mammograms and clinical breast examinations. *New England Journal of Medicine, 338,* 1089–1096.

Feig, S. D., & Ehrlich, S. M. (1990). Estimation of radiation risk from screening mammography: Recent trends and comparison with expected benefits. *Radiology, 174,* 638–647.

Gray, J. E., Winkler, N. T., Stears, J. G., & Frank, E. D. (1983). *Quality control in diagnostic imaging: A quality control cookbook.* Baltimore: University Park Press.

Haus, A. G., Metz, C. E., Chiles, J. T., & Rossmann, K. (1976). The effect of x-ray spectra from molybdenum and tungsten target tubes on image quality in mammography. *Radiology, 118,* 705–709.

Haus, A. G., Paulus, D. D., Dodd, G. D., Cowart, R. W., & Bencomo, J. (1979). Magnification mammography: Evaluation of screen film and xeroradiographic techniques. *Radiology, 133,* 223–226.

Hendrick, R. E. (1990). Standardization of image quality and radiation dose in mammography. *Radiology, 174,* 648–656.

Hendrick, R. E. (1992). Quality assurance in mammography: Accreditation, legislation, and compliance with quality assurance standards. *Radiological Clinics of North America, 3,* 243–255.

Hendrick, R. E., Pisano, E. D.,Averbukh, A.,Moran, et al. (2010, February). Comparison of acquisition parameters and breast dose in digital mammography and screen-film mammography in the American College of Radiology Imaging Network Digital Mammographic Imaging Screening Trial. *American Journal of Roentgenology, 194(2),* 362–369.

Kimme-Smith, C., Bassett, L. W., Gold, R. H., Roe, D., & Orr, J. (1987). Mammographic dual screen, dual emulsion film combination: Visibility of simulated microcalcifications and effect on image contrast. *Radiology, 165,* 313–318.

Kimme-Smith, C., Rothchild, P. A., Bassett, L. W., Gold, R. H., & Moler, C. (1989). Mammographic film processor temperature, development time, and chemistry: Effect on dose, contrast and noise. *American Journal of Roentgenology, 173,* 65–69.

Kimme-Smith, C., Wang, J., Debruhl, N., Basic, M., & Bassett, L. W. (1994). Mammograms obtained with rhodium vs molybdenum anodes: Contrast and dose differences. *American Journal of Roentology, 162,* 1313–1317.

Logan, W. W., & Norlund, A. W. (1979). Screen-film mammography technique: Compression and other factors. In W. W. Logan & E. P. Muntz, (Eds.), *Reduced dose mammography* (pp. 415–431). New York: Masson.

National Council of Radiation Protection and Measurements. (1988). *Quality assurance for diagnostic imaging* (NCRP Report No. 99). Bethesda, MD: Author.

Niklason, T., Christian, B., Niklason, L., Kopans, D., et. al. (1997). Digital tomosynthesis in breast imaging. *Radiology.* 205(2):399–406.

Pisano, E. D. (2000). Current status of full-field digital mammography. *Radiology,* 214, 26–28.

Sickles, E. A., & Feig, S. A. (1993). American College of Radiology statement on screening mammography for women 40–49.*ACR Bulletin, 49,* 5.

Tabar, L., & Haus, A. G. (1989). Processing mammographic films: Technical and clinical considerations. *Radiology*, *173*, 65–69.

Vyborny, C. J., & Schmidt, R. A. (1992). Technical image quality and the visibility of mammographic detail. In A. G. Haus & M. J. Yagge (Eds.), *Syllabus: A categorical course in physics: Technical aspects of breast imaging* (pp. 85–93). Oak Brook, IL: Radiological Society of North America.

Yaffee, M. F., & Rowlands, J. A. (1997). X-ray detectors for digital radiography. *Physics in Medicine and Biology*, *42*, 1–39.

Yaffe, M. J. (1990). Physics of mammography: Image recording process. *RadioGraphics*, *10*, 341–363.

CHAPTER 39

Bone Densitometry

Lisa J. King, RT(R)(M)(BD) CBDT

KEY TERMS

bone mineral density (BMD)
dual photon absorptiometry (DPA)
dual x-ray absorptiometry (DXA)
energy-switching system
K-edge filter
osteoporosis
peripheral quantitative computed tomography (pQCT)
quantitative computed tomography (QCT)
quantitative ultrasound (QUS)
remodeling cycle
single photon absorptiometry (SPA)
single x-ray absorptiometry (SXA)
T-score
Z-score

Break the bone and suck out the very substance.

—*François Rabelais*

OBJECTIVES

Upon completion of this chapter, the student should be able to:

- Describe x-ray, computed tomography, and ultrasound methods of obtaining bone densitometry data.
- Describe the process of bone remodeling.
- Explain risk factors associated with osteoporosis.
- Explain WHO diagnostic criteria.
- Discuss the difference between K-edge filtered and energy switching measurement systems.
- Describe the positioning details of three different bone compartments for BMD measurements.
- List factors that adhere to ALARA concepts for BMD.

Bone densitometry is a noninvasive procedure for the measurement of **bone mineral density (BMD)** and plays an important role in the early diagnosis of osteoporosis, monitoring therapy, and predicting fracture risk. Although its development began over 100 years ago, it has just been in the last 20 years that we have seen significant advancements in the use of this technology.

HISTORY AND OVERVIEW

Early developments of this technology began in the field of dentistry with the use of plain radiographs of the mandible over 100 years ago. Plain radiographs have a limited ability in determining bone density because a bone loss of at least 40 percent must occur before it can be visualized by the unaided eye.

In the 1930s, pioneers reported their efforts of better defining bone loss by the introduction of radiographic absorptiometry (RA). In this technique, a step wedge of known densities was imaged simultaneously with the extremity to more accurately quantify bone mass.

Researchers also began studying changes in actual cortical thickness to develop various grading and indexing techniques. The qualitative spinal morphometric technique utilized a unique grading system that was dependant on the study of plain spinal radiographs, which were examined for a loss of trabecular pattern and the appearance of the cortical shell. Another technique, known as the Singh Index, was developed for the proximal femur.

In the 1960s, radiogrammetry was introduced, which was applied to plain radiographs of the appendicular skeleton. In this method, the diameter of cortical thickness at the bone's mid-diaphysis was compared to the total bone width to determine bone loss. The metacarpals were most often studied utilizing this technique, but other sites included the phalanx, distal radius, and femur.

Since that time, various other techniques have been developed utilizing both photon and x-ray absorptiometry and ultrasound, as follows:

- **Single photon absorptiometry (SPA)** was the first bone densitometer to be used clinically. This device offered a single energy measurement and utilized a sealed radionuclide source (^{125}I). Imaging was limited to the forearm only, which took about 15 minutes to perform.
- **Single X-ray absorptiometry (SXA)** was a modification of the SPA forearm scanner, but instead of a radioactive source it used x-rays.
- **Dual photon absorptiometry (DPA)** was the first dual energy bone densitometer that made possible the measurement of the hip and spine. It used a radioactive source (Gd^{153}) that naturally emitted photons of two different energies (40 and 100 keV).
- **Dual energy X-ray absorptiometry (DXA)** uses two **x-ray** beams of different **energy levels.** Soft tissue absorption is subtracted out and a bone mineral density (BMD) value is acquired from this data.
- **Quantitative computed tomography (QCT)** (Figure 39-1) is a special software applied to an existing CT scan to determine a true three-dimensional (3D) or volumetric (unit of measure g/cm^3) measurement of bone density as opposed to the two-dimensional (2D) or areal (unit of measure g/cm^2) provided by DXA. This allows for the separation of the values for cortical and trabecular bone compartments within the lumbar spine vertebral body. For this procedure, the patient lies on top of a phantom that contains known body composition values (bone/muscle/fat), and both the patient and phantom are scanned simultaneously. Some researchers use a smaller, dedicated CT unit for extremities only, in which case it is referred to as **peripheral quantitative computed tomography (pQCT)**.
- **Quantitative ultrasound (QUS)** of the bone is a technique used in more recent years for determining the interrogation of bone. It is most commonly used at the heel, which is rich in trabecular bone. The bone density in QUS is based on values of the broad-band ultrasound attenuation (BUA) and speed

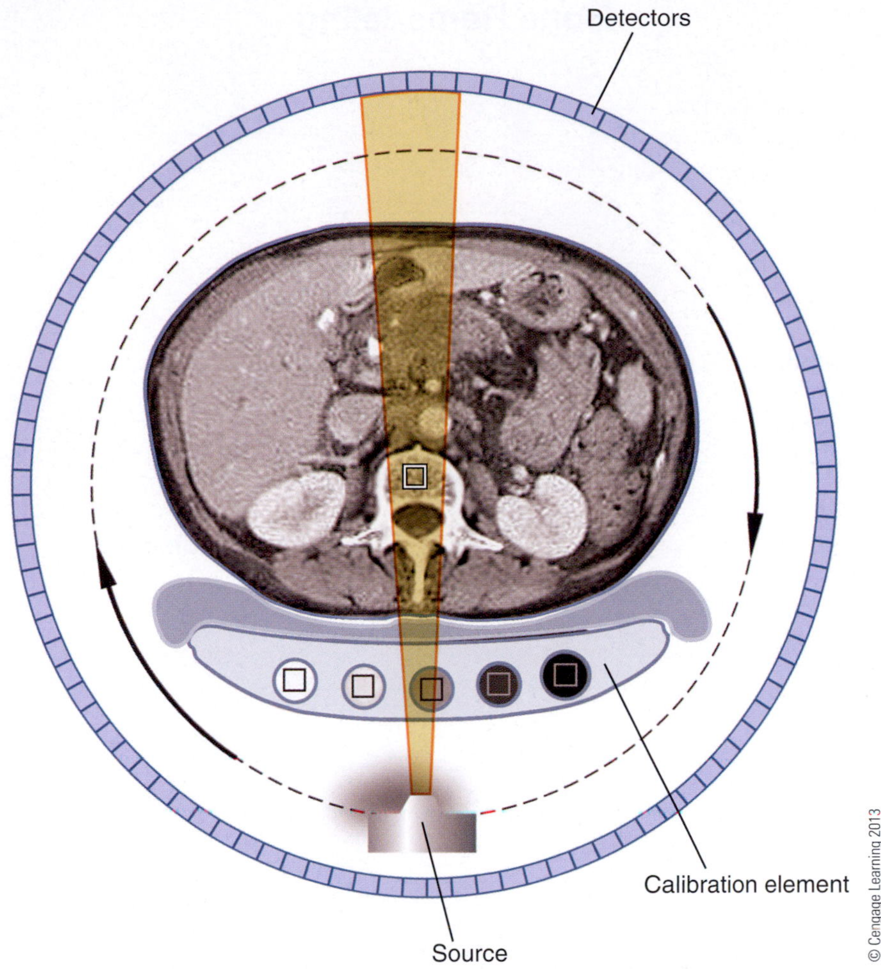

FIGURE 39-1. Quantitative computed tomography.

of sound [(SOS) – US]. The advantages of QUS over DXA is that it is less expensive, is more portable, and does not use x-ray. Even though QUS has proven to correlate with DXA results in predicting fracture risk in elderly women, studies have not proven it to be a reliable tool in the diagnosis of **osteoporosis**.

Of these technologies, the primary technologies still in use today include DXA, QUS, and QCT. However, DXA is the most widely used and validated for clinical use in the diagnosis and treatment of osteoporosis.

BONE SCIENCE

Cortical, or compact, bone is the extremely dense and protective outer portion of the bone. It is located along the exterior aspect shaft of bone, and makes up 80 percent of the skeletal mass. The sites with the highest concentration of cortical bone are the forearm (100 percent at the 1/3 portion) and hip (75 percent). Trabecular, or cancellous, bone, metabolically very active, provides the supportive inner aspect of bone, exhibits a spongy, lattice-work appearance, and contributes 20 percent of the body's skeletal mass. The skeletal sites

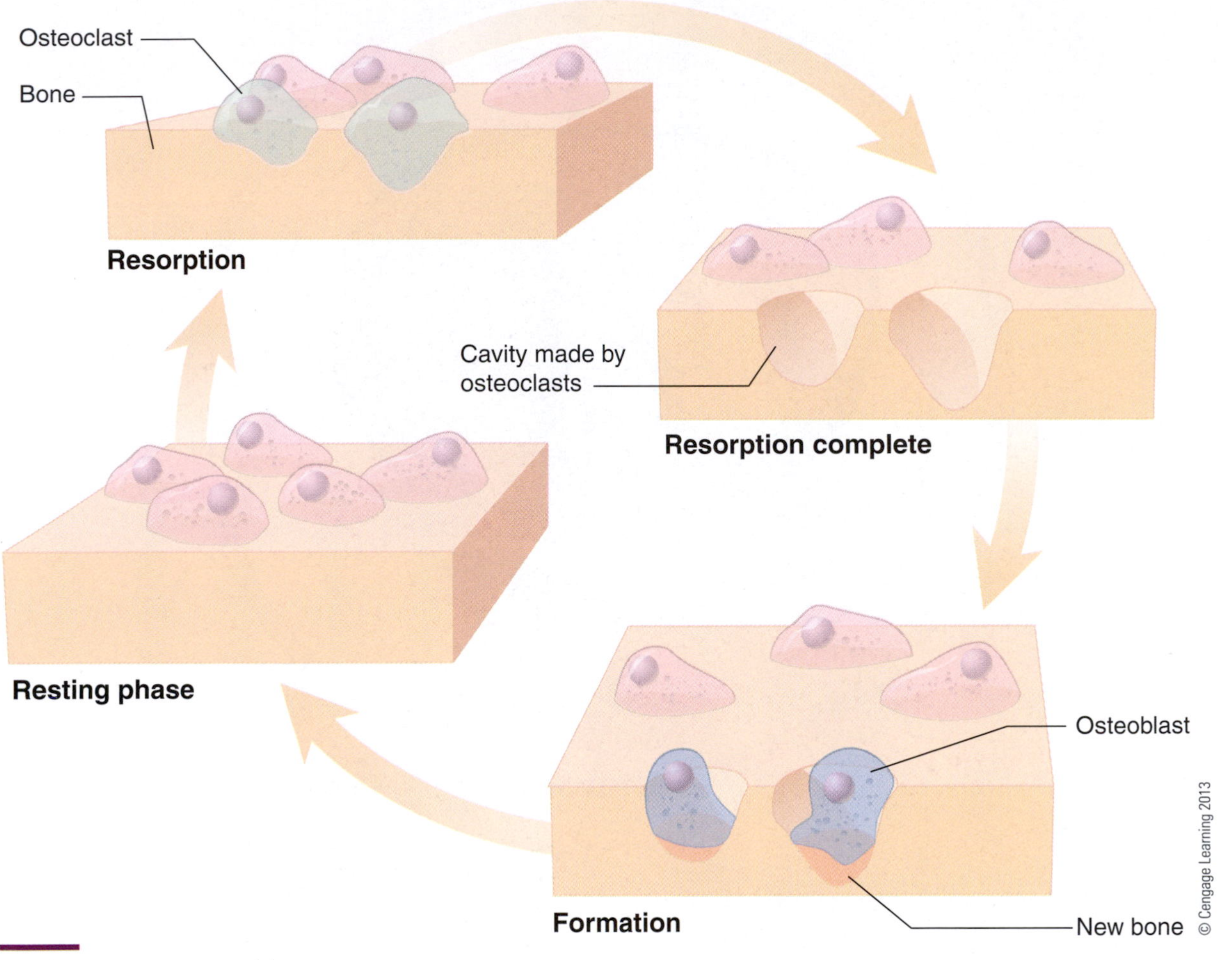

FIGURE 39-2. Bone remodeling.

richest in trabecular bone are the spine (66 percent), greater trochanter (50 percent), ultradistal (UD) radius (66 percent), and the calcaneus (95 percent).

At the cellular level, osteoclasts and osteoblasts work together in maintaining a balance between bone growth and breakdown in what is called the **remodeling cycle**. Osteoclasts are responsible for the break down of bone, or resorption. The formation, or building, of bone is provided by osteoblast cells. A decrease in bone density occurs when the removal of bone (resorption) occurs too quickly or when the deposit (formation) of new bone occurs too slowly. Such imbalances in the remodeling cycle lead to osteoporosis and increased fracture risk (Figure 39-2).

OSTEOPOROSIS

Osteoporosis, as defined by the World Health Organization (WHO), "is a systemic skeletal disease characterized by low bone mass and microarchitectural deterioration of bone tissue, with a

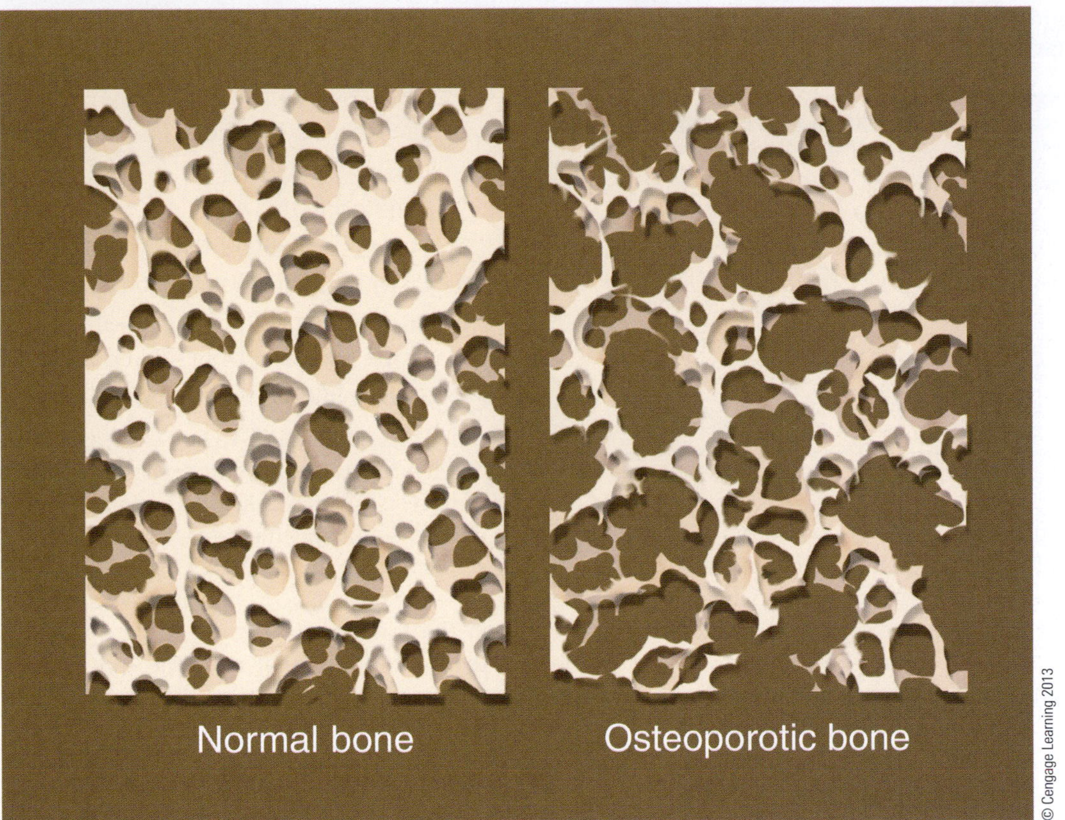

FIGURE 39-3. Osteoporosis.

consequent increase in bone fragility and susceptibility to fracture" (Figure 39-3).

Osteoporosis is categorized into two basic types, primary and secondary. With primary osteoporosis, the loss of bone occurs within the bone itself, and no other recognizable causes are present. This is usually the result of an imbalance of the bone remodeling cycle.

Within the primary category, the condition is further defined as type I and type II. Type I osteoporosis is the title used for post-menopausal osteoporosis, which is associated with the decrease in estrogen levels. Type II is another name for senile osteoporosis, where the only known cause is the process of aging.

Secondary osteoporosis occurs secondary to (or as a result of) a medical condition or a medication. Some examples of secondary causes are osteomalacia, hyperparathyroidism, hyperthyroidism, multiple myeloma, metastatic disease, or gluticocorticoid excess.

A patient's likelihood of developing osteoporosis may be linked to a number of risk factors, though some patients may present with osteoporosis and have no risk factors at all (Table 39-1). Some risk factors can be changed, whereas others cannot.

Even though having a thorough understanding of these risk factors is important, clinical assessment does not accurately predict fracture risk. Osteoporosis often presents as a "silent disease" until a fracture occurs, most commonly in the spine, hip, or wrist. Fractures of the hip are the most severe and contribute the most to morbidity, mortality, and the cost burden in health care. Of patients who survive a hip fracture, as many as 20 percent die within the first year following the fracture, and 50 percent experience a reduced ability to function in their daily tasks.

However, bone fragility can best be assessed by measuring the bone mineral density (BMD). Dual x-ray

TABLE 39-1. Risk Factors Associated with Osteoporosis

CANNOT change	CAN change
Female gender	Sex hormone deficiency
Increased age	Poor diet: Anorexia nervosa and/or poor calcium and vitamin D intake
Small body frame	Medications: Long-term use of glucocorticoids, some anticonvulsants, and certain other medications
Caucasian and Asian ethnicity	Sedentary lifestyle or immobilization
Family history	Cigarette smoking Alcohol abuse

absorptiometry (DXA) is considered the "gold standard" of noninvasive methods in the role of diagnosing osteoporosis, predicting fracture risk, and monitoring therapy. DXA uses two x-ray beams of different energy levels. After soft tissue absorption is subtracted out, the BMD can be calculated. Some of the advantages DXA offers over other methods are as follows:

- Noninvasive
- Short scan times
- Measures critical "central" or "axial" skeletal sites where early bone loss and fractures occur: hip and spine
- Offers high precision
- Low patient and operator dose
- Provides high-resolution imaging at low cost
- Primary test used to monitor therapy approved by the Food and Drug Administration (FDA)
- Stable calibration of equipment

DXA quantifies BMD by expressing the amount of mineralized tissue of the area scanned (g/cm^2). The BMD results for an individual patient are related to databases containing the values of young, healthy adults at peak bone mass (20–29 years), ideally matched in terms of sex and ethnicity and applied clinically in the form of a "**T-score**" (Figure 39-4). Basically, the T-score, as defined by the WHO's international reference standards, is applied in the diagnosis and treatment of osteoporosis (see Figures 39-5 and 39-6).

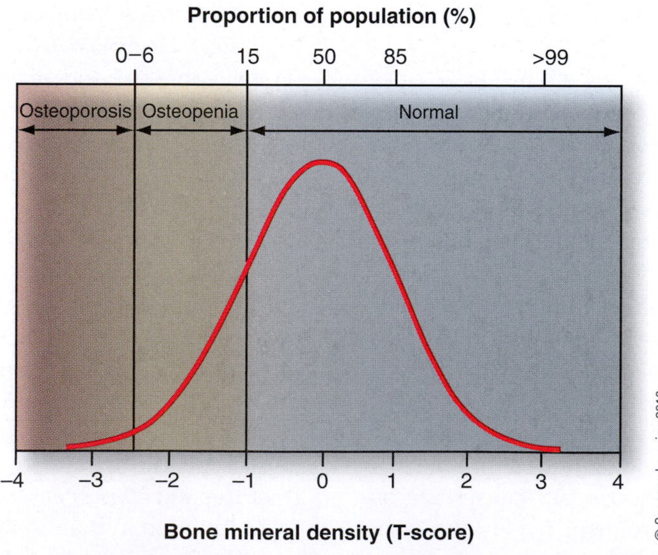

FIGURE 39-4. T-score distribution of bone mineral density in healthy women aged 30–40 years.

WHO DIAGNOSTIC CRITERIA

This T-score is related to the WHO international reference standards in the diagnosis and treatment of osteoporosis (Figure 39-5) and is a "widely used parameter to assist in the interpretation of BMD results." The T-score marks how far a patient's BMD is deviated from the mean of a sex-matched young adult population (ages 20–35) of individuals who have reached their peak bone mass. The WHO defines peak bone mass as "the amount of bony tissue present at the end of the skeletal maturation."

A **Z-score** is conceptually similar to a T-score, except the reference population is matched by the patient's age. The Z-score is recommended for use when reporting in pre-menopausal females and males of ages less than 50.

The WHO references any T-score of −1 or greater as "normal" bone mass. T-score values from −1.1 to −2.4 are defined as low bone mass or osteopenia. Once a T-score is −2.5 or less, the diagnosis of osteoporosis can be made, and if the patient has incurred a fragility fracture (fracture involving little to no trauma) also, then he or she is considered to possess "severe osteoporosis" (Figure 39-6).

Once a diagnosis of osteoporosis is made, DXA results can aid in the monitoring of efficacy of therapy. When performing serial measurements in these patients, good precision becomes vitally important. Precision relates to the ability of the system to reproduce the same results in repeated measurements of the same object. Accuracy describes the ability of the system to truly measure an object"s value (Figure 39-7).

Diagnostic Classification

Classification	T-score
Normal	–1 or greater
Osteopenia	Between –1 and –2.5
Osteoporosis	–2.5 or less
Severe Osteoporosis	–2.5 or less and fragility fracture

FIGURE 39-5. Diagnostic classification of T-scores.

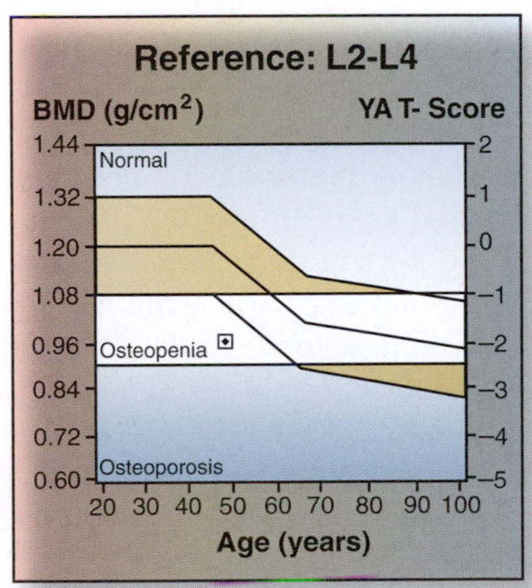

FIGURE 39-6. BMD measured in grams/cm squared.

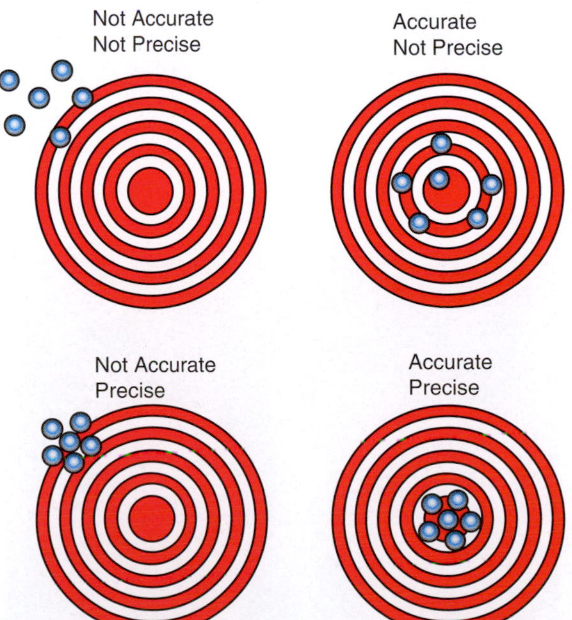

FIGURE 39-7. Target images.

DXA PRINCIPLES AND INSTRUMENTATION

Machine Components

A *workstation unit* includes a computer, display monitor, printer, keyboard, and power module.

Quality Control Phantom and Positioning Aids: Each DXA unit requires various quality control (QC) phantoms and positioning aids, both of which are manufacturer specific.

Exam Table and C-Arm (Figure 39-8): Included with the exam table is a radiolucent table mattress for added comfort as the patient lies supine for the exam. Table movement controls and a crosshair laser indicator light are useful when positioning the patient at the proper start point. The C-arm houses the x-ray source (below) and detector array (above), maintaining their alignment to one another. The x-ray beam passes through the patient before reaching the detector system and finally is processed by the computer system.

The principle behind the DXA technology is dependent on the "attenuation coefficient on atomic number and photon energy." To differentiate soft tissue from bone, two different energy x-ray spectrums are required. Of the three primary DXA equipment manufacturers (Lunar, Norland, and Hologic), two different methods are used to obtain this.

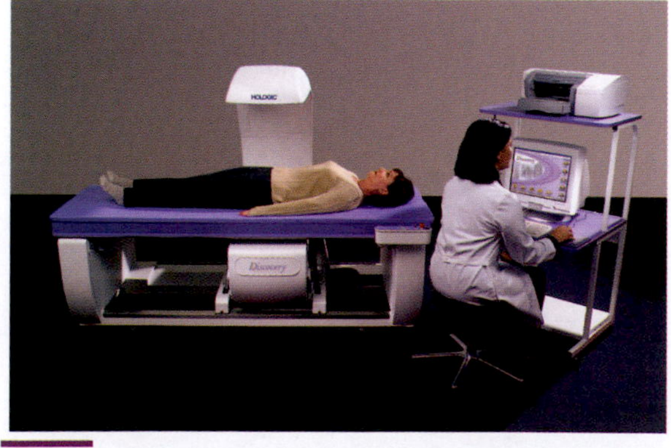

FIGURE 39-8. DXA system. *(Courtesy of Hologic, Inc.)*

K-edge Filtered

A rare-earth or **K-edge filtered** x-ray source is used by Lunar and Norland. In this instance, a primary beam with a peak energy of near 50 keV passes through the rare-earth filters, which causes the spectrum to then contain two different energy peaks (near 40 and 70 keV). This system also utilizes a special pulse counting detector system and must be calibrated regularly with the use of an external phantom.

Energy-Switching System

Hologic uses a synchronous **energy-switching system** that switches the kVp between 100 and 140 (Figure 39-9). The result is a primary beam with two different energy peaks (near 40 and 80 keV). Calibration with this system occurs internally and continuously. As scanning occurs, the beam passes through a calibration wheel that contains three sectors: air gap, soft tissue equivalent, and bone equivalent. This technique allows for a simpler detector system that doesn't have to separate photons.

SCAN ACQUISION AND ANALYSIS

DXA equipment is very versatile in that it allows for the scanning of peripheral and central sites. This is achieved through the selection of the appropriate collimator/detector (Table 39-2). The most commonly measured areas are the hip and spine. The forearm is the next most common site measured and should be measured when the hip and spine areas cannot be measured, when the patient has hyperparathyroidism, or when the patient is very obese (over the weight limit for DXA table).

There are three principal sites of osteoporotic fractures. These are called bone compartments or sites (Figure 39-10).

FEMUR

The most dependable method in predicting hip fractures lies in the measurement of the hip BMD (Figure 39-11). Most commonly, the left hip or

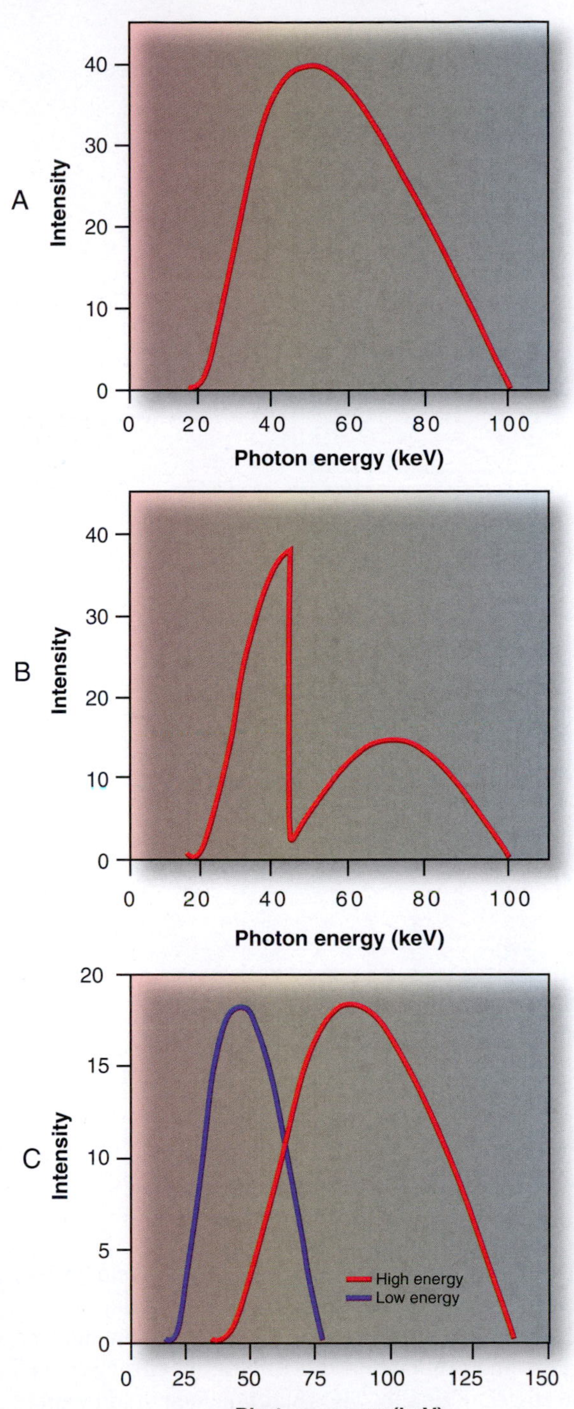

FIGURE 39-9. Energy spectra (keV) for x-ray sources used in bone densitometry.

TABLE 39-2. DXA Collimator/Detector Types

Pencil Beam	Fan (Array) Beam
Circular pinhole collimator	Narrow "slit" collimator
Single detector	Multi-element detector
X-ray beam moves in a serpentine (rectilinear) direction	X-ray beam moves in only one direction (length of patient)
Scan times 5–7 min	Faster scan times < 1 min
Good resolution and reproducibility	Less resolution and reproducibility than pencil beam C-arm permits for lateral lumbar spine to be performed Careful centering of pt necessary to avoid parallax (geometric distortion at outer edges)

bilateral hips are selected, but this may be affected by the patient's fractures and/or surgical history. Once this determination is made, scan parameters are selected according to manufacturer recommendations. To aid in precise patient positioning, most manufacturers provide a foot positioning guide. This helps to ensure a proper internal rotation of 15–25 degrees of the femoral neck. The following criteria will help in determining proper patient positioning:

- The lesser trochanter is rotated to the posterior portion of the femur and will have limited to no visibility.
- The greater trochanter's profile will be fully visible.
- The femoral neck will be fully visible, resulting in separation between the femoral head and greater trochanter.
- The femoral neck should be positioned parallel to the long axis of the table and appear straight on the reference image.
- Adequate separation between the ischium and femoral neck should be demonstrated.

The regions of the hip that are analyzed for BMD values include the femoral neck, trochanteric, inter-trochanteric, Ward's triangle (considered unreliable by some sources), and/or total hip.

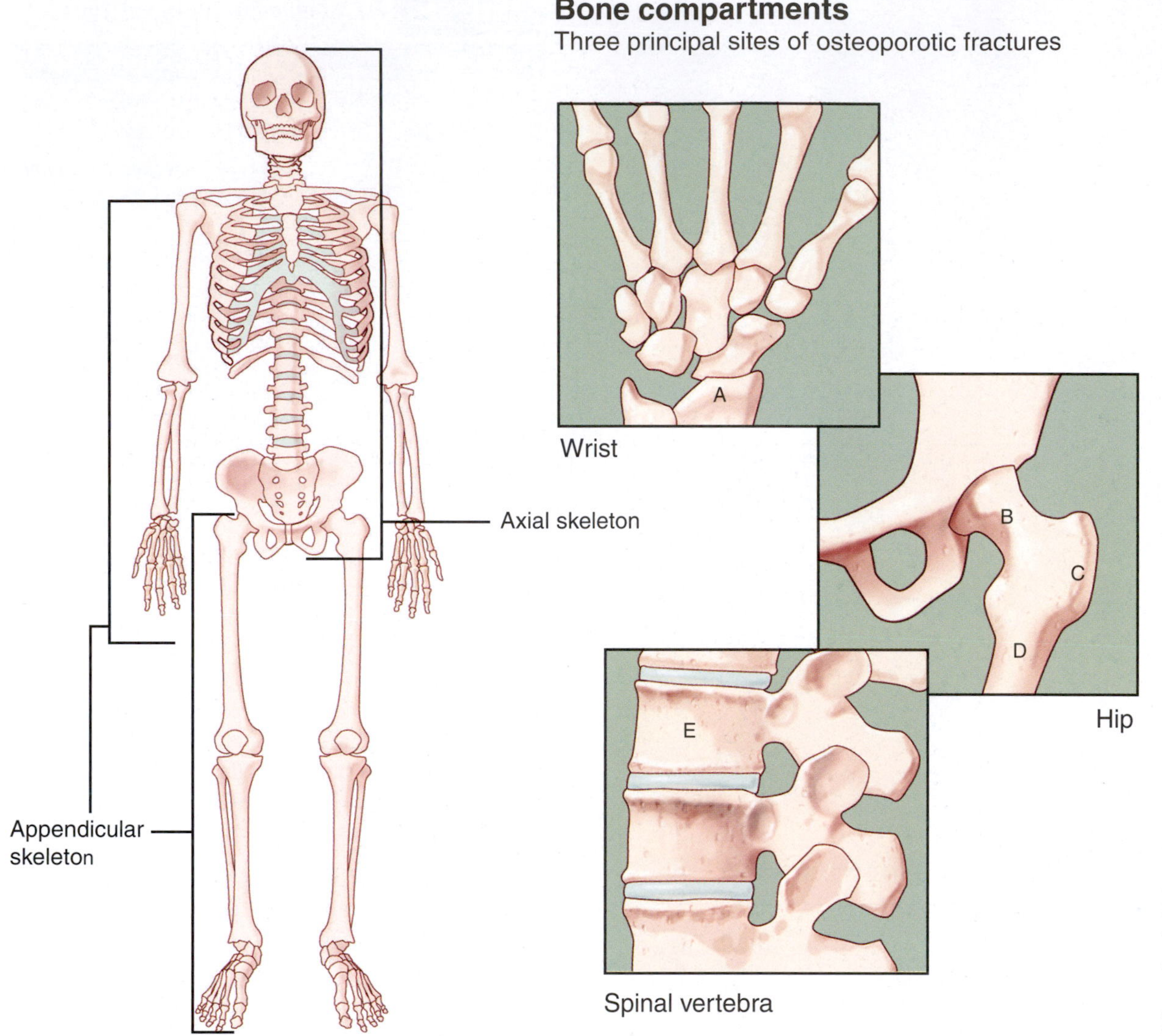

FIGURE 39-10. Bone compartments used in bone densitometry.

SPINE

The L1-L4 spine is used in measuring the spine's BMD and is considered the optimum site in monitoring therapy due to its rich content of highly metabolic trabecular bone (Figure 39-12).

For the PA projection of the spine, the patient is placed on the table in a supine position, aligned straight and in the center of the table. The patient's lower legs are elevated and placed on a large block provided by the equipment manufacturer. Scanning begins at 1" to 2" below the iliac crest and ends when the 12th set of ribs is viewed in the scan image. The final image should begin at about the middle of L5 at the bottom and extend up through the middle of T12, where the 12th ribs are attached. The spine should be centered and straight on the image, indicated by an even amount of soft tissue visualized on each side of spine.

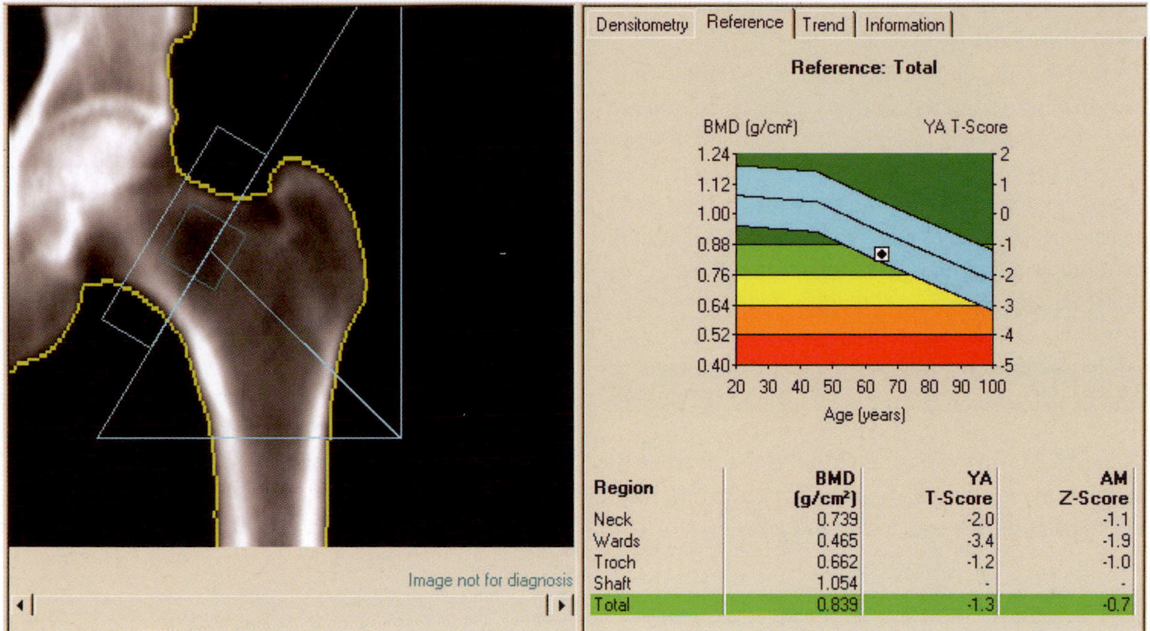

FIGURE 39-11. DXA scan of proximal femur. *(From Bonnick, Sydney, 2004, Bone Densitometry in Clinical Practice, New York: Springer. With kind permission of Springer Science + Business Media.)*

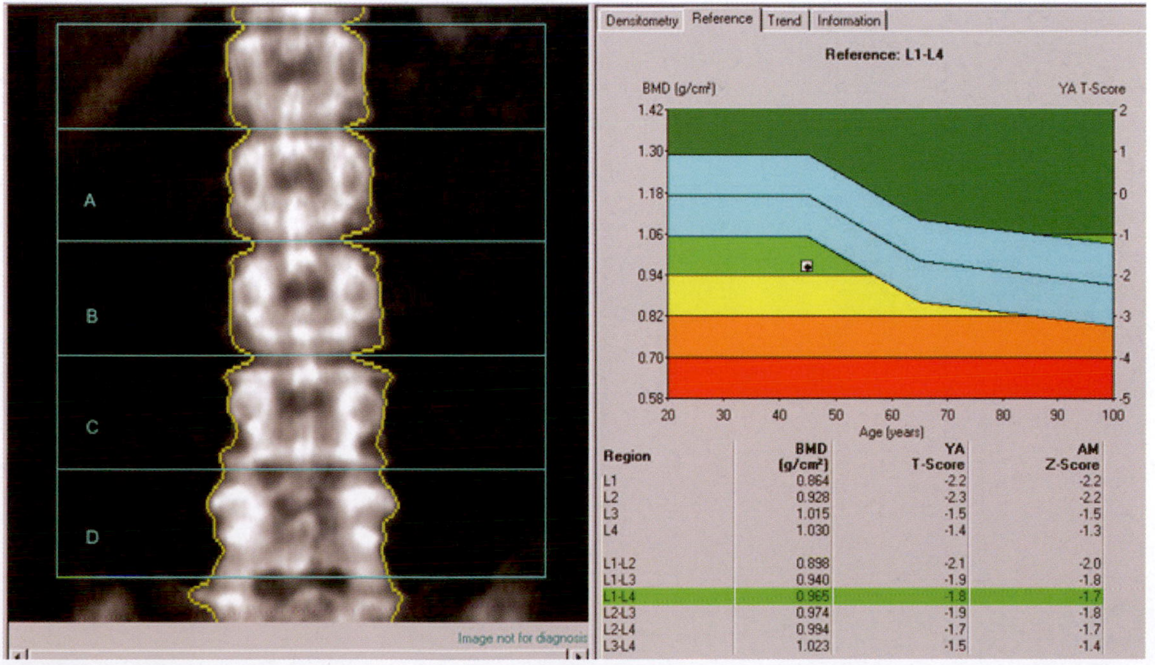

FIGURE 39-12. DXA scan of spine. *(From Bonnick, Sydney, 2004, Bone Densitometry in Clinical Practice, New York: Springer. With kind permission of Springer Science + Business Media.)*

The iliac crest is displayed in the lower, lateral aspects of the image.

Occasionally it is necessary to exclude individual vertebrae from the analysis if the vertebrae are clearly abnormal or if there is more than 1.0 T-score difference between the vertebra in question and the adjacent vertebrae. Sometimes a lateral or vertebral fracture assessment (VFA) can aid in determining some causes of spinal BMD differences, such as spinal fractures, spurs, and calcified aorta.

FOREARM

The distal forearm (radius and ulna) is the first site of choice involving the diagnosis of hyperparathyroidism because this disease is characterized by cortical bone loss and the 1/3 radius (33 percent) region is 99 percent rich in cortical bone (Figure 39-13). The other area of interest of the forearm is the ultradistal (UD) region of the radius and ulna (measured from a distance of 4 or 5 percent of the overall ulnar length, as measured from the tip of the styloid process). This area is predominantly trabecular bone and is the site for pathological Colle's fractures. Generally, the patient's non-dominant forearm is selected for scanning. Studies have proven the non-dominant arm to have the lowest BMD values (by 2–3 percent) and the databases used clinically to diagnose and predict fracture risk were developed using population studies where the non-dominant forearm was the standard.

For the forearm, the patient is seated in a chair with a back but no arms or wheels at a 90-degree

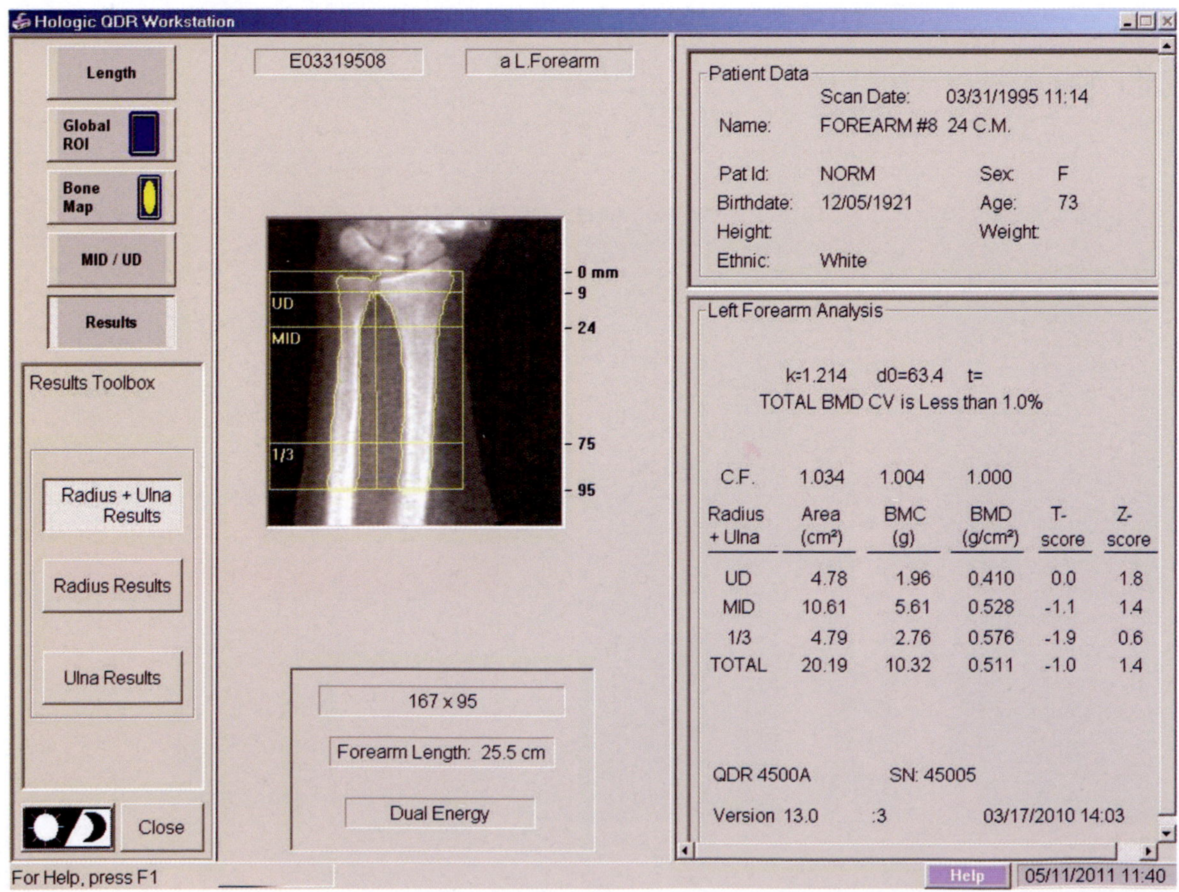

FIGURE 39-13. DXA of forearm. *(Courtesy of Hologic, Inc.)*

angle to the long axis of the table. The patient's arm is abducted and the forearm is extended across the table to allow the elbow to form a 90-degree angle.

The resultant image should display the forearm centered (with adequate soft tissue and air on both sides of the forearm) and straight vertically. At the top of the image, the first row of carpal bones should be visible to ensure the inclusion of the entire shaft of the distal radius and ulna. The image should also be free of all artifacts, including motion, jewelry, surgical hardware, and old fractures.

QUALITY CONTROL

It is important to implement and maintain strict quality control (QC) procedures in bone densitometry in order to ensure the generation of accurate and precise patient results. These practices greatly influence efficacy and integrity in managing patient bone health.

With DXA, a daily QC procedure is conducted to ensure that the system and software components are operational prior to scanning the first patient.

Upon installation, a spine phantom is scanned to establish bone and soft tissue baseline values, which then becomes the calibrated standard by which daily phantom scan data are compared (usually automatically by the software). This phantom is usually constructed of hydroxyapatite and an epoxy resin, which possess attenuation properties similar to bone mineral and soft tissue, respectively. The BMD values for a phantom never change, but the BMD values in humans change slowly over time. A daily phantom ensures the machine's scanning stability and thus the reproducibility of measurements; the phantom must be scanned daily prior to the scanning of patients.

RADIATION SAFETY AND PROTECTION

Compared to conventional radiography, the effective radiation dose for DXA is relatively low (Table 39-3).

The operator dose involved in DXA is approximately <0.1 mrem/hr for pencil beam, and <0.3 mrem/hr for fan beam.

In view of the low doses involved with DXA, the application of the ALARA (as low as reasonably achievable) principle is not that difficult to obtain. The ALARA protective methods for DXA are time, distance, and shielding.

Time limitations can be achieved through proper training of technologists to prevent unnecessary poor positioning and repeated scans, thus reducing scan times.

Distance limitations can be achieved through positioning the computer workstation at least 1 meter (3 feet) from the side of the scan table. Some facilities prefer to extend that distance to 3 meters (9 feet) when using fan beam or using a portable shield between the scanner and the workstation. Additional room shielding or operator protection is not needed to comply with ALARA regulatory requirements.

TABLE 39-3. Radiation Safety and Patient Dose

Annual Natural Background Exposure	240 mrem
Lateral Lumbar Spine X-Ray	70 mrem
Mammogram	45 mrem
Dental X-ray	10 mrem
Transcontinental Flight, Round Trip	6 mrem
Chest X-ray	5 mrem
One Week Ski Vacation	1.5 mrem
GE Lunar Prodigy AP Spine	3.7 mrem

SUMMARY

Bone densitometry is a noninvasive procedure for the measurement of bone mineral density (BMD) that plays an important role in the early diagnosis of osteoporosis. This disease affects more than 25 million people in the United States, and over 1.3 million fractures annually are associated with this disease. Osteoporosis is categorized into two types: primary and secondary. Primary osteoporosis is the loss of bone within the bone itself when no other recognizable causes are present. Secondary osteoporosis occurs secondary to a medical condition or a medication. Dual energy absorbtiometry (DXA) is the primary method for diagnosing osteoporosis. It utilizes two x-ray beams of different energy levels. Soft tissue absorption is subtracted out and a bone mineral density (BMD) value is acquired from these data. It is likely that over the next several years, more emphasis will be placed on applying the use of DXA in the prevention, detection, and treatment of osteoporosis. ■

REVIEW QUESTIONS

1. Which type of cell is chiefly responsible for bone reabsorption in the remodeling cycle?
2. How much bone loss must occur before it can be seen on a plain radiograph?
3. Identify the risk factors associated with osteoporosis.
4. List the two methods used to obtain the two energy X-ray spectra required in DXA.
5. Describe how osteoporosis is defined by the WHO.
6. Explain the types of collimation used in DXA instrumentation.
7. What are the two most commonly used sites in DXA when measuring a patient's BMD?
8. What regions are analyzed for BMD values when scanning the hip?
9. Which site is considered the optimum site when clinically monitoring therapy?
10. Which region is the first site of choice when scanning a patient with hyperparathyroidism?

REFERENCES AND RECOMMENDED READING

AAPM. (1977). *Report no. 4, basic quality control in diagnostic radiology*. Reston, VA: AAPM.

American Medical Association. (2004). *Module 2: Osteoporosis management: Recommendations for BMD measurement and technique for testing. Dec. 2004–Dec. 2006*. Chicago: American Medical Association.

Blake, G., Wahner, H., & Fogleman, I. (1998). *The evaluation of osteoporosis: Dual energy x-ray absorptiometry and ultrasound in clinical practice*. London: Martin Dunitz.

Bonjour, J. P., Theintz, G., Law, F., Slosman, D., & Rissoli, R. (1994). World Health Organization Collaborating Center for Osteoporosis and Bone Disease. Department of Medicine, University Hospital, Geneva, Switzerland. *Osteoporosis International*, *4*(Suppl. 1), 7–13.

Bonnick, S. L., & Lewis, L. A. (2002). *Bone densitometry for technologists*. Totowa, NJ: Humana Press.

Borg, J., et al. (1995). Single x-ray absorptiometry: performance characteristics and comparison with single photon absorptiometry. *Osteoporosis International*, *5*, 377–381.

Cooper, C., Atkinson, E. J., Jacobsen, S. J., O'Fallon, W. M., & Melton, L. (1993). Population-based study of survival after osteoporotic fractures. *American Journal of Epidemiology, 137*(9), 1001–1005.

Fogleman, I., & Blake, G. M. (2000). Different approaches to bone densitometry. *Journal of Nuclear Medicine, 41*, 2015–2025.

Hologic Inc. (2000–2006). *QDR for Windows XP reference manual.* Bedford, MA: Author.

Lentle, B. C., & Prior, J. C. (2003). Osteoporosis: What a clinician expects to learn from a patient's bone density examination. *Radiology, 228*, 620–628.

National Institutes of Health (NIH). (2009). Osteoporosis overview. Retrieved from http://www.niams.nih.gov/bone.

Orwoll, E., & Bliziotes, M. (2003). *Osteoporosis—pathophysiology and clinical management.* Totowa, NJ: Humana Press, Inc.

Périard, M. *X-ray and gamma photon bone densitometry in clinical diagnosis—a review by Consumer and Clinical Radiation Protection Bureau*, Health Canada. Ottawa. Consumer and Clinical Radiation Protection Bureau.

Rogene Tesar, R., Avery, G., Caudill, J., Colquhoun, A., et al. (2008). *ISCD International Society for Bone Densitometry Technologist Course Syllabus*, Version 8. Middletown, CT: ISCD.

Theodorou, D., Stavroula, T., & Sartoris, D. (2002). Dual-energy x-ray absorptiometry in diagnosis of osteoporosis: Basic principles, indications, and scan interpretation. *Comprehensive Therapy, 28*(3), 190–200.

World Health Organization. (1993, June). Consensus Development Conference: Diagnosis, prophylaxis, and treatment of osteoporosis. *Journal of the American Medical Association 94*, 646–650.

World Health Organization. (2003). *Prevention and management of osteoporosis.* WHO Technical Report Series #921. Report of a WHO Scientific Group. Geneva: Author.

World Health Organization. (2007, May). WHO Scientific Group on the Assessment of Osteoporosis at Primary Health Care Level. Summary Meeting Report, May 5–7, 2004, Brussels, Belgium.

The Case of the Mysterious Mammal

This computed tomography is of an animal found on the roadside near Jolly Beach, South Carolina. Look carefully at the bone structure to determine what it is.

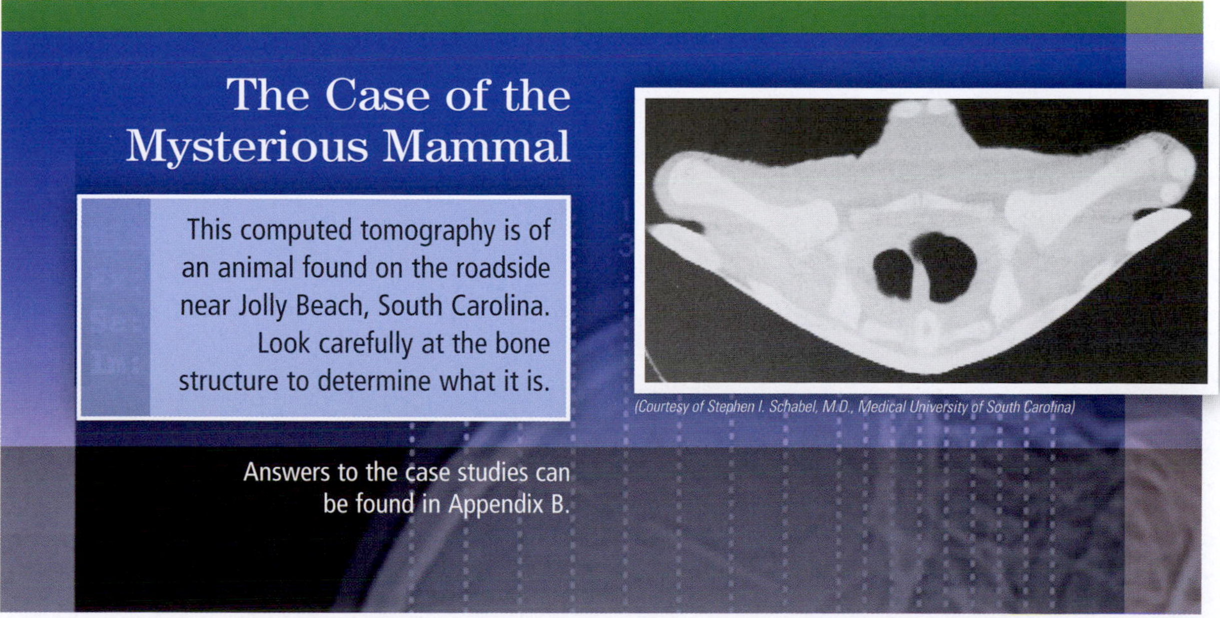

(Courtesy of Stephen I. Schabel, M.D., Medical University of South Carolina)

Answers to the case studies can be found in Appendix B.

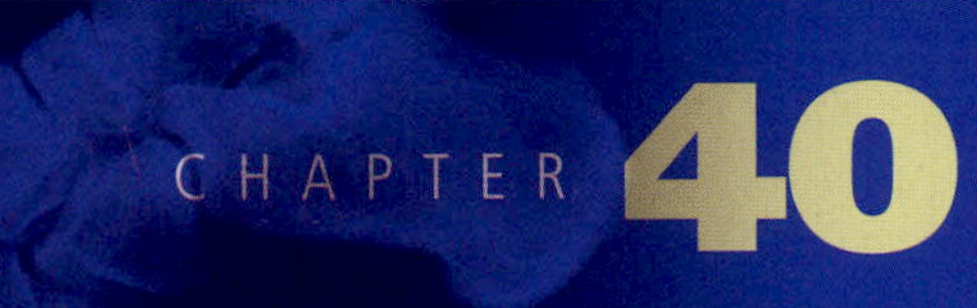

Vascular Imaging Equipment

KEY TERMS

contrast medium injection device
digital angiography
digital cineradiography
digital subtraction angiography

During World War I the demand for x-ray technicians in military hospitals was so great that a shortage of technical workers became acute at home. The value of the well-trained technician was emphasized, and the radiologist was no longer satisfied with someone who knew only how to throw the switch and develop films.

Margaret Hoing (the "first lady of radiologic technology")
From A History of the American Society of X-Ray Technicians, 1952

OBJECTIVES

Upon completion of this chapter, the student should be able to:

- Differentiate among the different types of historic image recording devices.
- Describe the components of digital image acquisition.
- Differentiate among the modes of digital image acquisition.
- Identify various image post-processing functions.
- Describe the structure and function of the C-arm assembly.
- Describe the structure and function of the angiographic table.
- Describe the structure and operation of contrast medium injection devices.
- Explain the various quality control measures taken with vascular imaging equipment.

The equipment in the vascular imaging laboratory is unique in nature. The imaging equipment must accommodate for rapid image acquisition while withstanding high amounts of heat. In order for this to occur, special generators and x-ray tubes are required. The generators should offer high-performance capabilities to produce optimal images while reducing patient exposure. The x-ray tubes must work with the fluoroscopic and computer system to produce quality digital images for each particular exam. The x-rays tubes must accommodate different modes of digital image acquisition. Once the images are acquired, they are manipulated using a computer system. Additional equipment, such as a contrast medium injector, is required to assist in the diagnostic process. A quality control program is implemented and maintained in order for high-quality image production to continue. This chapter highlights these key points as they pertain to vascular imaging equipment and vascular imaging procedures.

HISTORY OF VASCULAR IMAGING

Image recording in the vascular imaging laboratory has changed quite drastically over the years. Historically, images were recorded on radiographic film using various devices that allowed for rapid-sequence filming. Today, however, radiographic film is almost obsolete with the use of digital imaging.

There were three main types of rapid-sequence filming devices used: the roll film changer, the cut film changer, and the cineangiographic camera. The roll film changer consisted of a 60-foot continuous roll of radiographic film that allowed for approximately 60 exposures. This rapid film changer consisted of a grid, upper and lower intensifying screens, pressure plate, film cutter, and supply and receiving bins (Figure 40-1). The grid, which was located between the upper intensifying screen and the patient, was used to absorb scatter radiation generated in the patient before it reached the film and degraded image quality. The upper and lower intensifying screens enhanced the ability of the x-ray beam to produce a diagnostic image on the film. The pressure plate helped in this process by compressing the upper and lower intensifying screens against the film, ensuring uniform film/screen contact. Unexposed film was contained in the supply bin until it was exposed. After exposure, the film was housed in the receiving bin until it could be developed. A film cutter near the receiving bin was used to manually cut the exposed images away from the rest of the unexposed roll of radiographic film.

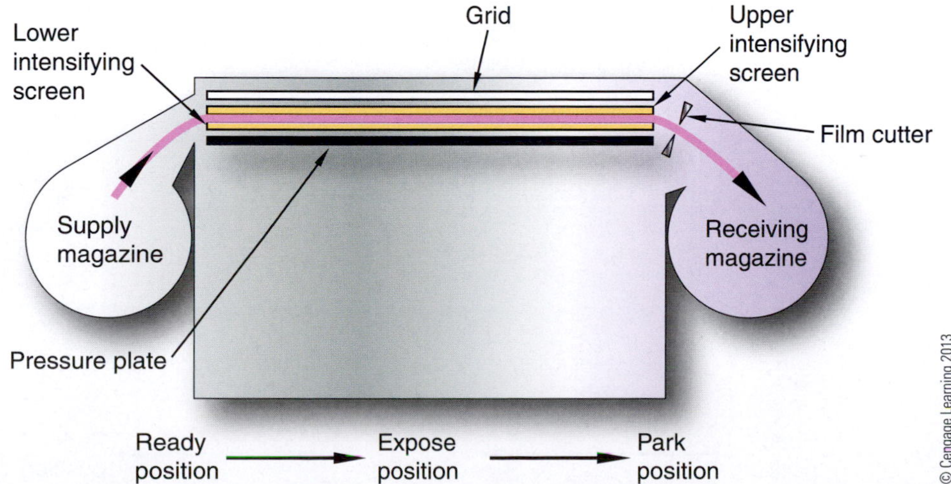

FIGURE 40-1. The roll film changer. This diagram demonstrates how film travels from the supply magazine (ready position) between the intensifying screens (expose position) into the receiving magazine (park position).

The cut film changer assembly resembles the roll film changer, except the radiographic film was precut to a size, usually 14″ × 14″. In addition, the supply magazine only allowed for a maximum of 30 unexposed films to be held (Figure 40-2).

Cineangiographic cameras, which resembled movie cameras, replaced the television camera tube to record images on film for later playback. These cameras were generally used during cardiac catheterizations where detailed images of fast-moving anatomic structures were needed. Cine cameras provided better spatial image detail than electronically acquired images but with an increased radiation dose to the patient.

Cineangiographic systems consisted of a camera and x-ray tube that were synchronized. This means that the x-ray tube was energized only during the cineangiographic film exposure and not during film advancement. This synchronization, which prevents any unnecessary exposure to the patient, was accomplished through the work of the synchronous motors.

The cineangiographic imaging system consisted of three very important components: automatic brightness control, beam-splitting mirror, and cine camera. The automatic brightness control, or ABC, was used to compensate the beam quality and/or quantity for differences in anatomic thickness or density by adjusting the kVp, mA, or both. The beam-splitting mirror permitted simultaneous filming and viewing of the images during the procedure. This mirror would direct 10 percent of the image to the television monitor and the other 90 percent to the cine camera. The cine camera, which resembles a movie camera, was a complex device that allowed for the filming of the cineangiographic images.

The cine camera consisted of a lens, iris diaphragm, shutter, aperture, pressure plate, transport mechanism, film supply, and take-up reels (Figure 40-3). The optical lens would focus light from the output phosphor of the image intensifier tube onto the cine film. The iris diaphragm, which was located between the lens and the shutter, restricted the divergence of the light from the lens. The shutter was a rotating half-disk situated in front of the aperture that interrupted the flow of light to the film as it rotated. The shutter opening was approximately 160° to 180°. The aperture was a rectangular opening that further restricted the amount of light entering the camera. The pressure plate, which was located behind the aperture in the cine camera, functioned in maintaining a firm contact between the film and the aperture. The transport mechanism transported the unexposed film from the supply reel to the aperture for exposure and finally to the take-up reel until it could be developed.

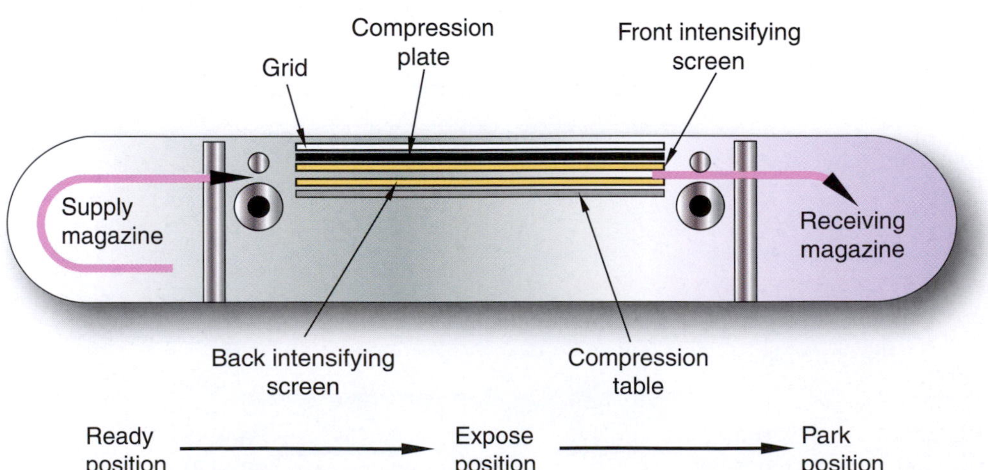

FIGURE 40-2. The cut film changer. This diagram demonstrates how film travels from the supply magazine (ready position) between the intensifying screens (expose position) into the receiving magazine (park position).

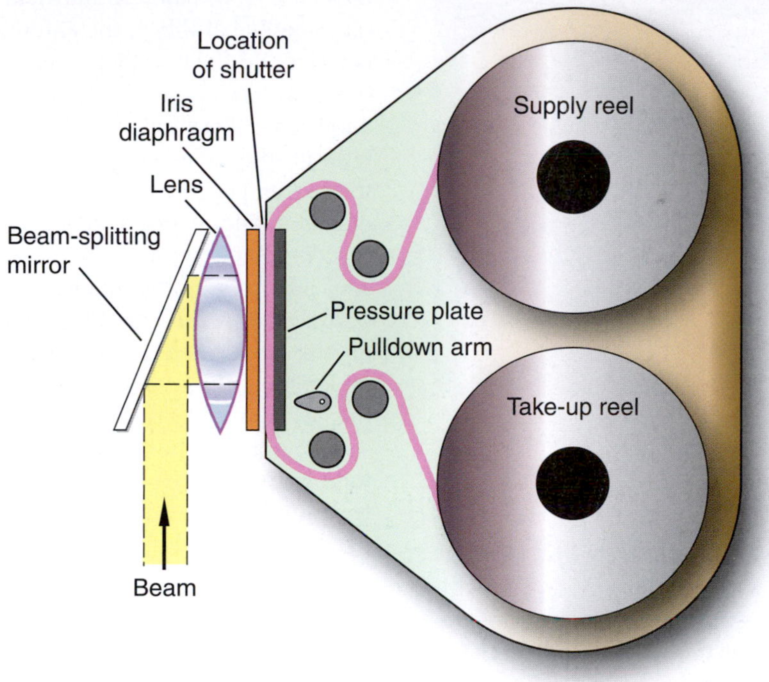

FIGURE 40-3. The cine camera.

Exposures in a cine camera could be made by either the action of the shutter or the action of the x-ray beam. In shutter exposure, the shutter opens for exposure to the film and closes for advancement of the cineangiographic film. In x-ray beam exposure, constant potential generators allowed for the pulsating of the x-ray beam. The pulsating beam not only allowed for the advancement of the film after the exposure but also eliminated the need for the shutter.

DIGITAL IMAGE ACQUISITION

The invention of digital image acquisition has improved the imaging ability of the angiographic suite. Digital image acquisition involves using computers in conjunction with the imaging equipment to produce quality diagnostic digital images. These computers have increased the resolution of the image while reducing radiation dose to the patient. In addition, there is a reduction in cost to the patient and institution. Digital images can be manipulated after acquisition, therefore decreasing the need for repeat exposures. For example, the contrast can be adjusted on an image that is too light. Digital images are easier to store than conventional images because they take up less space and are easier to obtain when they are needed. These images can be stored in an archive system that can be accessed at any time. Digital image acquisition requires the use of specialized equipment in order to produce a digital image. This specialized equipment includes a high-frequency generator, an x-ray tube, an image intensifier, and an image processor (Figure 40-4).

Generator

High-frequency generators, usually in the multiphasic or three-phase format while offering 12 pulses per second, are selected for vascular imaging laboratories because of their high-performance capabilities. These generators allow for high mA stations,

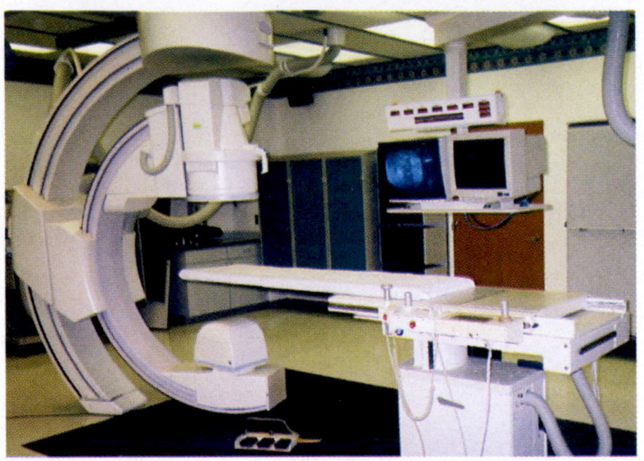

FIGURE 40-4. A vascular imaging laboratory. *(Image courtesy of Arlene Adler.)*

usually 800–1,000 mA, with relatively low kVp settings, usually 50–100 kVp. A high mA station with a low kVp setting will improve the visibility of the contrast medium against the surrounding soft tissue structures. In addition, using high mA stations allows for short exposure times.

The x-ray tube in the vascular imaging laboratory operates in the radiographic mode even during digital fluoroscopy. To prevent the x-ray tube from overheating, the high-frequency generator is switched off and on very rapidly, causing pulsing of the x-ray beam. This pulsing is known as pulse-progressive fluoroscopy. Interrogation time is the time required to prepare the x-ray tube for exposure—in other words, the time needed for the x-ray tube to be switched on and reach the selected kVp and mA stations. Extinction time is the time required to stop the exposure or shut off the x-ray tube. Vascular imaging requires high-frequency generators that allow for interrogation and extinction times of less than 1 ms.

X-Ray Tube

Vascular imaging x-ray tubes vary slightly from general imaging x-ray tubes in their ability to withstand high amounts of heat while providing optimal images. High heat amounts are produced by extended periods of fluoroscopy and rapid sequences of exposures made over a short period of time. Because heat production occurs at the anode, this will determine heat tolerance. Short-term loading ability is the amount of heat an anode can tolerate for a sequence of exposures. Continuous heat-loading ability is the amount of heat the anode can tolerate during a fluoroscopic exposure. Overall, the heat-loading ability is determined by the size and construction of the anode disk. Larger-diameter anode disks, usually 15 cm or greater, are combined with a large target angle or focal spot size to accommodate for the increased heat production. A thicker anode disk, usually 5 cm or greater, constructed of molybdenum with a graphite backing, improves the heat-loading capacity of the vascular x-ray tube.

The heat capacity ability of the vascular x-ray tube is measured by the calculation of heat units generated at the anode. Heat units are calculated by multiplying the peak kilovoltage, milliamperage, time in seconds, rectification constant, and number of consecutive exposures together. The rectification constant is determined by the type of generator being used. A single-phase generator has a rectification constant of 1, while the three-phase and multiphasic generators have a rectification constant of 1.35 and 1.40, respectively. Vascular imaging requires an x-ray tube with a 1-MHU (mega heat unit) heat capacity in order to keep up with the daily imaging requirements.

Image Intensifier

The image intensifier can either be analog or digital in nature. An analog image intensifier requires the use of charge-coupled devices (CCDs) and an analog-to-digital converter to produce a digital image (see Chapter 36). The CCD replaces the television camera in the vascular imaging system. The CCD consists of crystalline silicon that is located on the output phosphor of the image intensifier. Digital images are obtained when the silicon is illuminated, causing generation of an electrical charge. This electrical charge is then sent as a signal to the analog-to-digital converter. The analog-to-digital converter digitizes the signal from the CCD by converting the signal into pixels or picture elements. On the other hand, a digital image intensifier acquires the images digitally so no special conversion equipment is needed. Digital image intensifiers are composed of silicon pixel detectors and are known as flat panel or digital detectors.

Image Processor

The last part of the digital image acquisition system is the image processor. The image processor consists of image-processing hardware and a computer. The image-processing hardware controls the speed of the imaging equipment. This hardware allows for real-time viewing of the images, meaning images are seen as they are acquired. The computer controls the various components of the imaging system, including the generator, x-ray tube, image-processing hardware, and image storage device. This computer allows for the different modes of digital image acquisition. In addition, the computer allows for manipulation of the digital images. Once manipulated, these images are stored as part of a picture archiving and communication system (PACS) or network system. These images can also be printed using a laser printer or transferred to a compact disc or videotape.

MODES OF DIGITAL IMAGE ACQUISITION

Digital image acquisition can occur in three different modes: **digital angiography** (DA), **digital subtraction angiography** (DSA), and **digital cineradiography** (cine). Once images are acquired, the image processor can manipulate, export, or store these images (Table 40-1).

Digital Angiography

Digital angiography, also known as spot filming, replaced traditional spot-film devices in the vascular imaging laboratory. Digital angiography involves the production of one image, similar to the last fluoroscopy hold image. This mode of acquisition is generally used when only a few images are needed for a procedure. For example, a spot film is taken post-insertion of a peripherally inserted central catheter (PICC) to check tip placement and as a record of the procedure.

Digital Subtraction Angiography

Digital subtraction angiography involves eliminating bone and soft tissue structures from an image so that only the contrast-filled vessels remain. In order for DSA acquisition to occur, three steps must be accomplished. First, a scout or mask image must be obtained. The scout image contains all of the anatomy of interest prior to the injection. Next, the injection process must occur. The resulting image, known as the native image, displays all of the anatomy, including the contrast-filled vessels. Finally, the mask image is laid over the native image. The computer then subtracts all of the like structures, leaving only the contrast-filled vessels in the image (Figure 40-5). However, if patient motion (voluntary or involuntary) occurs between the scout image and the injection, an artifact will appear on the resulting image. DSA is normally used when imaging vessels of the head, chest, and extremities.

Digital Cineradiography

The last mode of digital image acquisition, digital cineradiography, is used primarily for cardiac catheterization. This type of acquisition involves taking numerous exposures, known as frames, in a second of time. Typically, cardiac catheterization involves exposure rates of 15, 30, or 60 frames per second.

TABLE 40-1. Modes of Digital Image Acquisition

Mode	Number of Images	Use
Digital Angiography	Single image	When only a few images are needed for the procedure (e.g., interventional radiology procedures)
Digital Subtraction Angiography	Numerous frames per second	Carotid and cerebral angiography Abdominal and peripheral angiography
Digital Cineradiography	Numerous frames per second	Cardiac catheterization

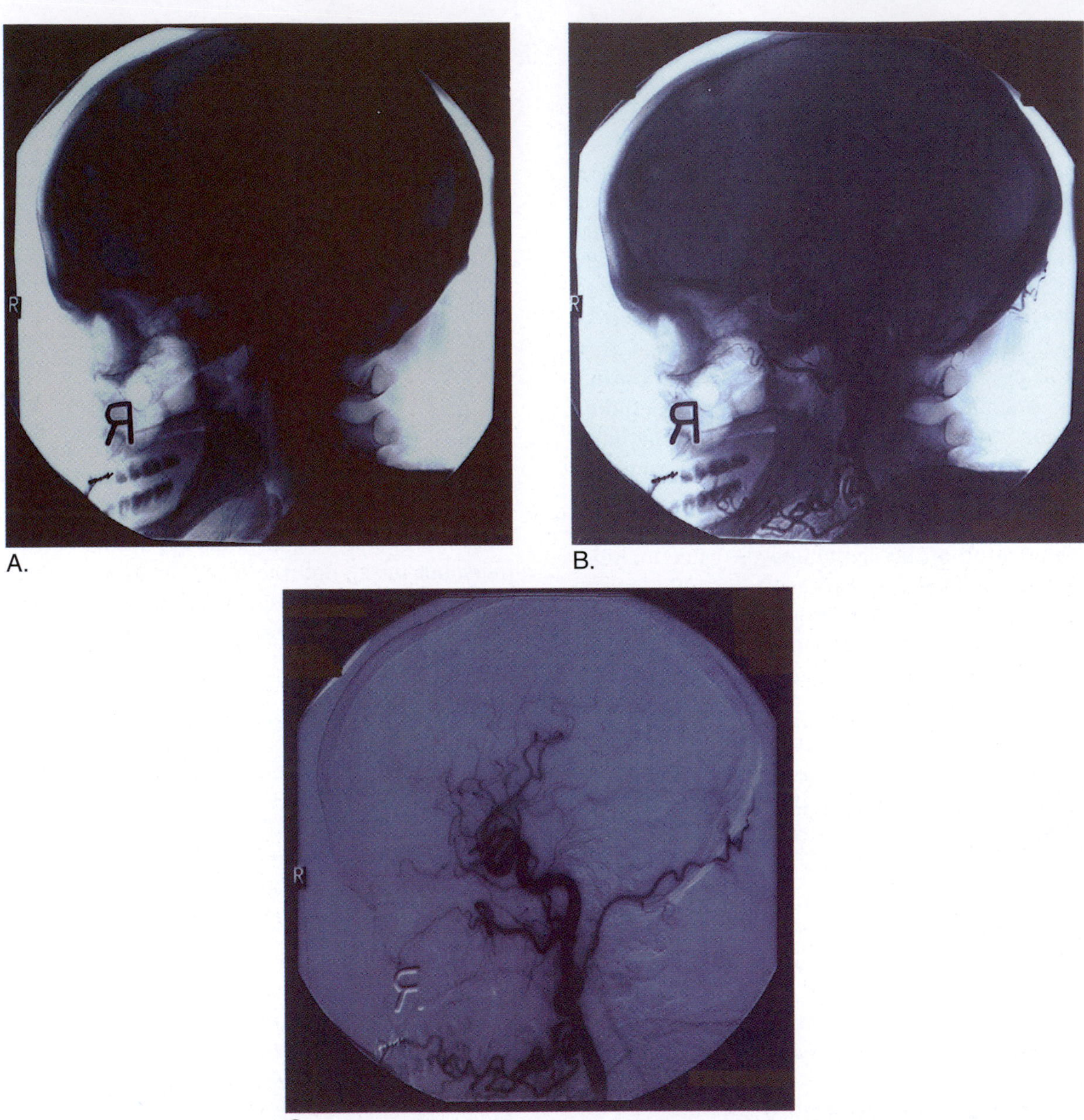

FIGURE 40-5. Digital subtraction angiography. This figure depicts the stages involved in digital subtraction angiography: (A) scout image; (B) injection image; and (C) resulting subtracted image. *(Images courtesy of Arlene Adler.)*

These high frame rates provide higher-resolution images as compared to general fluoroscopy. In fact, cineradiography can demonstrate events that are normally too fast or cannot be seen by general fluoroscopy. However, as the number of frames per second increases, the patient dose also increases.

IMAGE POST-PROCESSING

After image acquisition occurs, digital images are manipulated or post-processed before they are permanently stored. Manipulating the images before they are stored helps eliminate the need for repeat exposures. The type of post-processing depends on the mode of digital image acquisition.

Windowing, annotation, zoom, and analytic functions can be used on any type of digital image acquisition. Window level involves adjusting the density, while window width adjusts the contrast or brightness of an image. Images that are too light or too dark can be adjusted to make them diagnostic quality, providing the image has had adequate but not excessive exposure. The annotation function allows the user to dictate on the image itself. This allows the user to identify right or left sides for future viewers. In addition, the user can add comments to the image, such as the size and type of a particular catheter. Zoom allows the user to zone in on and magnify a particular area of interest. This function is useful when locating smaller structures such as aneurysms. The final function, analytic tools, involves using various methods to quantify distances, calculate degree of stenosis, and measure blood flow. These tools can be extremely helpful to vascular imaging personnel during and after the procedure.

The post-processing functions—remasking, pixel shifting, view tracing, and edge enhancement—pertain only to digital subtraction angiography. Remasking involves selecting another mask image in order to obtain the best subtracted image of the anatomy of interest. This function is used when there is a significant amount of patient motion after the initial mask image. Another post-processing function that compensates for patient motion is called pixel shifting. This function is used when the patient moves slightly from the mask image to the injection image. Pixel shifting allows the user to move the mask image to correspond to the patient movement. The next function, view tracing, involves combining numerous frames into one image to demonstrate a completely filled contrast structure. For example, this function may be used to demonstrate a contrast-filled abdominal aorta from the celiac axis to the iliac bifurcation. The final function, edge enhancement, is used to accentuate the edges of vessels or small structures so they can be seen (Figure 40-6). However, too much edge enhancement can cause distortion of the image.

C-ARM ASSEMBLY

The design of equipment in the vascular imaging laboratory is similar to the design of the portable radiographic equipment used during surgical procedures known as the C-arm assembly. Vascular imaging equipment, however, is much larger in size and is not portable.

A typical C-arm assembly consists of four parts: the x-ray tube, the image intensifier, the

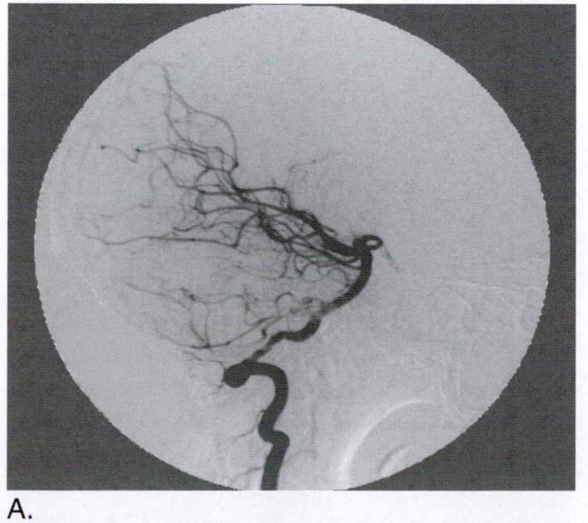
A.

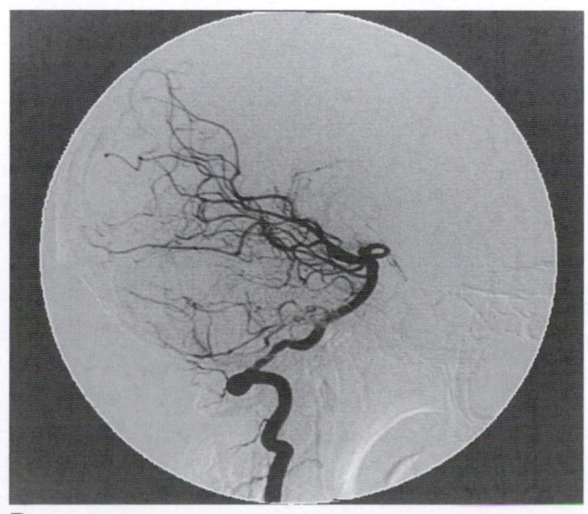
B.

FIGURE 40-6. Demonstration of edge enhancement (A) normal image and (B) edge enhanced image. *(Images courtesy of Arlene Adler.)*

gantry, and the point of attachment (Figures 40-7 and 40-8). The x-ray tube is similar in construction to that of a tube found in a digital fluoroscopy room. The x-ray tube is mounted on the bottom of the C-arm assembly.

The image intensifier can be either analog or digital in nature. An analog image intensifier requires the use of a CCD and an analog-to-digital converter to digitize the image. A digital intensifier acquires the image digitally so no special conversion equipment is needed. The image intensifier is mounted on the top of the C-arm assembly.

The final two parts of the C-arm work together to allow manipulation of the assembly. The gantry mounts the C-arm assembly to the floor or ceiling of the vascular imaging laboratory. The point of attachment connects the C-arm assembly to the gantry. The point of attachment allows for 180° rotation of the C-arm assembly. This attachment also allows for craniocaudal and oblique angulations needed to image the required anatomy for cardiac or vascular imaging procedures. Therefore, the patient never has to be moved during the procedure.

The most important feature of the C-arm assembly is the relationship of the x-ray tube and image intensifier. In this design, the central ray of the x-ray tube is always perpendicular to the image intensifier and therefore at right angles to the body part.

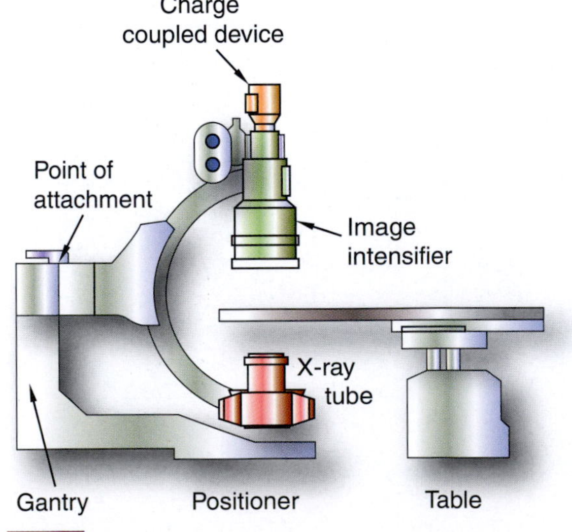

FIGURE 40-7. C-arm assembly.

ANGIOGRAPHIC TABLES

Tables used in vascular imaging laboratories must meet three requirements. First, angiographic tables must be easy to use and convenient for the vascular imaging laboratory personnel. The table must be able to provide support and comfort for the patient. Finally, the angiographic table must not degrade the diagnostic quality of the image.

A typical design of an angiographic table involves a table base and a table plate (Figures 40-9 and 40-10). The table base attaches to the floor while the table plate rests on the top of the table base. This design allows for the capability of free floating of the table plate in all directions. In addition, table plate has the potential to be raised or lowered as needed. Sometimes the table plates can be interchanged

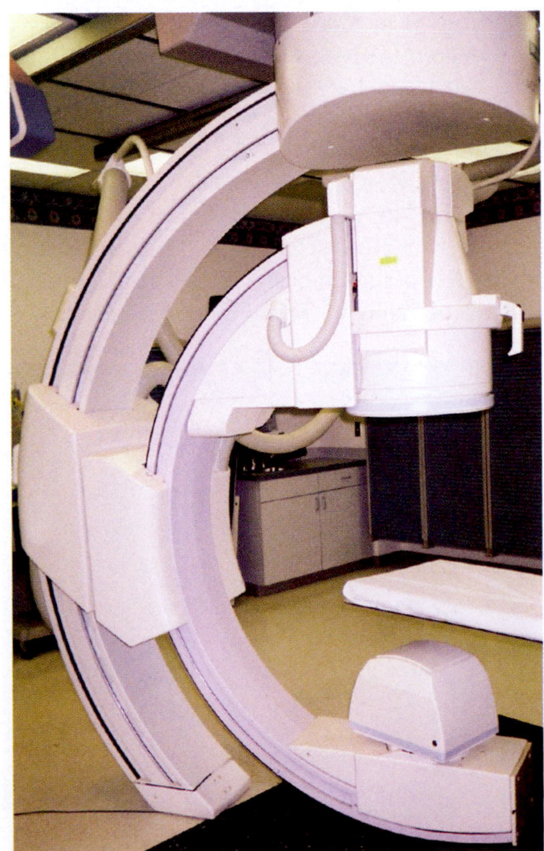

FIGURE 40-8. C-arm assembly. *(Image courtesy of Arlene Adler.)*

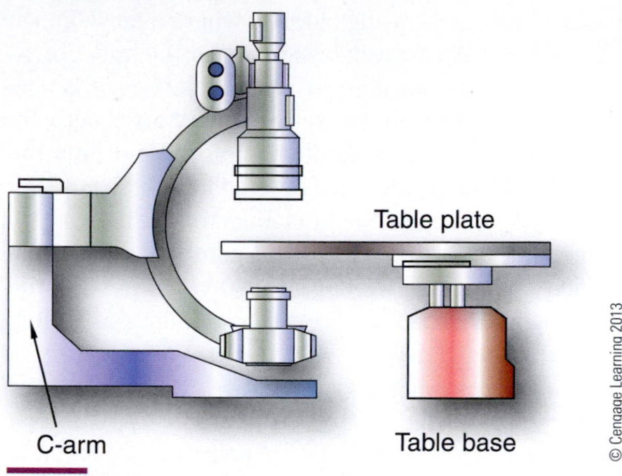

FIGURE 40-9. Table assembly.

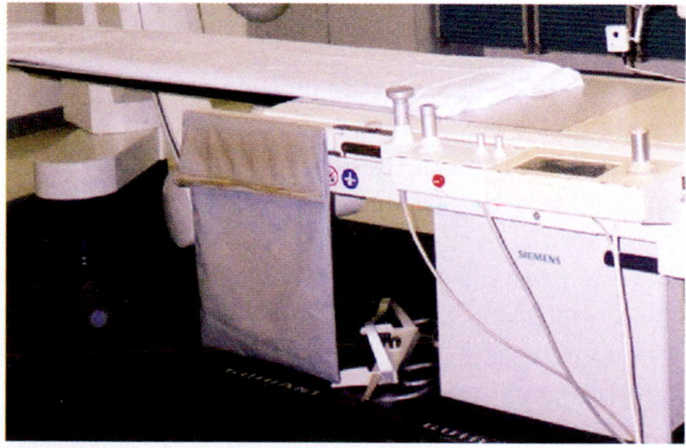

FIGURE 40-10. Table assembly. *(Image courtesy of Arlene Adler.)*

according to the procedure being performed. For example, a cerebral angiogram may require a table plate that is narrower at the head end to accommodate for lateral projections. The table plate allows for the attachment of various equipment needed for the procedure, such as manual controls, IV poles, restraining devices, contrast medium injection devices, lead shields, and hemodynamic monitoring devices.

Angiographic tables are equipped with a foam pad for patient comfort. This foam pad should be thin enough so image quality is not degraded but thick enough for patient comfort. In addition to the foam pad, arm boards are attached to the angiographic table to support the patient's extremities during the angiographic procedure.

The design material for the angiographic table should not degrade image quality. A low radiation-absorbing plastic and carbon fiber material is the preferred material of composition. A low attenuation table prevents degradation of the image quality, and it also lowers radiation levels to the patient and the vascular imaging laboratory personnel.

CONTRAST MEDIUM INJECTION DEVICES

Contrast medium injection devices allow for the safe delivery of a preset amount of contrast. These devices allow for large bolus injections that are too difficult to be performed by hand. Newer devices even allow for smaller bolus injections that previously could only be performed manually.

A typical contrast medium injection device consists of the control panel, syringe, warming device, and pressure mechanism (Figure 40-11). The control panel displays the injection parameters, which are manipulated by the cardiovascular interventional technologist. The injection parameters include flow rate, rise, total volume, pressure, and delay. The flow rate is the rate at which the contrast medium is going to be injected. It is measured in cubic centimeters per second (cc/sec) and is dependent on factors such as catheter length, inner catheter diameter, number of catheter side holes, injection pressure, and viscosity of the contrast medium (Table 40-2). The rise, also known as linear rise, is the time it takes to reach the desired flow rate. Rise is measured in seconds. The total volume is the desired amount of contrast to be delivered. Total volume can be calculated by multiplying the flow rate by the injection duration ($V = cc^2/sec \times seconds$). Total volume is measured in cubic centimeters. The injection pressure is the force needed for a specific dose of contrast medium. Injection pressure is dependent on the size of the vascular structure and the type of catheter used for the injection. Typically, smaller vessels require lower injection pressures. Manufacturer insert information should be consulted for determining safe pressure limits for each specific catheter. Injection pressure is measured in pounds per square inch (psi). The range for injection

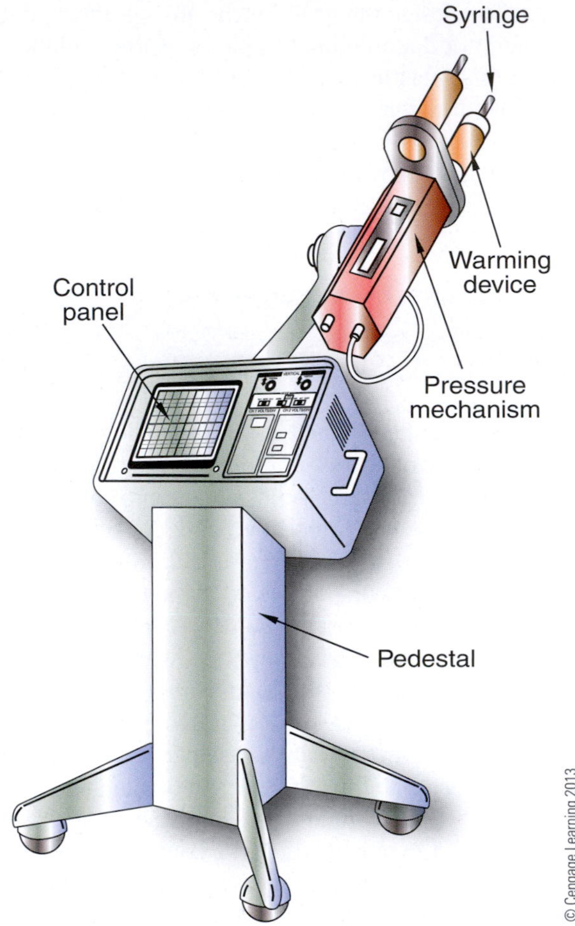

FIGURE 40-11. Contrast medium injection.

TABLE 40-2. Factors Affecting Flow Rate

Viscosity	Lower viscosity permits higher flow rates.
Catheter Length	Shorter catheters permit higher flow rates.
Catheter Internal Diameter	Larger internal diameters permit higher flow rates.
Injection Pressure	Higher psi permits higher flow rates.
Catheter Sideholes	The presence of sideholes in the catheter permits higher flow rates.

pressures is 100 to 1,200 psi. The last injection parameter, delay, can be either injection or x-ray in nature. An injection delay allows for image acquisition to begin before the injection occurs. This is useful in digital subtraction angiography where a mask image is required. An x-ray delay allows for the injection to occur before image acquisition occurs. This is useful when performing lower extremity arteriography via a catheter in the abdominal aorta and only the vessels distal to the knee need to be visualized.

The contrast medium injector syringe is removable and disposable. The contrast syringe capacity can range from 40 to 260 cc. A new sterile syringe is loaded in the syringe-loading assembly prior to each case.

The warming device is a thermal sleeve placed over a preloaded syringe to maintain the contrast medium temperature at or near body temperature (37°C; 98.6°F). The warming device maintains temperature but does not increase it from room temperature to body temperature. Therefore, the contrast medium should be warmed prior to the syringe being filled.

The pressure mechanism is an electromechanical motor attached to a jackscrew that drives the piston into or out of the syringe. This piston movement causes the syringe plunger to move forward or backward as needed.

Contrast medium injectors are equipped with numerous safety mechanisms to prevent damage to the catheter and danger to the patient (Table 40-3). Function-monitoring devices, such as a flashing light,

TABLE 40-3. Safety Mechanisms for Contrast Medium Injectors

Function-Monitoring Device	A flashing light, audible tone, or written message used to notify personnel of any problems
Volume-Limiting Device	Prevents excessive amounts of contrast from being delivered to the patient
Pressure-Limiting Device	Prevents the injection pressure from exceeding a maximum pressure set prior to the injection
Acceleration Regulators	Allow the electromechanical drive motor to accelerate over an exact duration of time to prevent whiplash of the catheter
Rate-Rise Control	Prevents an instant surge of injection pressure by gradually increasing the psi to the preset limit

audible tone, or written message, are used to notify the cardiovascular interventional technologist of any problems. The problem may be an injector malfunction or operational error such as an omission of an injection parameter. A volume-limiting device prevents excessive amounts of contrast from being delivered to the patient. A pressure-limiting device prevents the injection pressure from exceeding a maximum pressure set prior to the injection. Acceleration regulators allow the electromechanical drive motor to accelerate over an exact duration of time to prevent whiplash of the catheter. Finally, the rate-rise control prevents an instant surge of injection pressure by gradually increasing the psi to the preset limit.

QUALITY CONTROL

Quality control programs in the vascular imaging laboratory are established by the organization to ensure that the angiographic equipment is operating properly and safely. In addition, they are established to ensure that the highest-quality image is produced while limiting the radiation exposure to the patient and ultimately lowering the cost to both the patient and the organization.

Components of the quality control program should include periodic monitoring of the x-ray viewing and image storage stations, evaluation of the x-ray beam, and assessment of the ancillary equipment. X-ray viewing and image storage systems should be tested regularly for their effectiveness. X-ray equipment should be monitored to maintain high-quality images and prevent equipment malfunction. Ancillary equipment, such as the contrast medium injectors and cardiac monitoring device, should be inspected regularly to prevent malfunctions during a procedure. In order for this to occur, scheduled maintenance should be established between the equipment manufacturer and the organization.

In addition to contracts for preventative maintenance and service with the manufacturer, the organization should have members of the biomedical instrumentation department trained to monitor or correct faulty equipment in case of an emergency. By utilizing the biomedical instrumentation department, the vascular imaging laboratory can produce high-quality images while reducing patient dose and lowering cost.

SUMMARY

The vascular imaging laboratory contains specialized radiographic equipment that produces high-quality images of contrast-filled structures within the body. Special high-frequency generators permit the use of high mA settings, short exposure times, and relatively low kVp settings. The high mA stations allow for short exposure times, thus reducing patient exposure. In addition to the high-frequency generators, specialized x-ray tubes are required for high-quality digital images. These x-ray tubes must work in conjunction with the image intensifier and computer system for image acquisition. Image acquisition can be either analog or digital in nature. The x-ray tubes should allow for the different modes of digital image acquisition. Once the images have been acquired, the computer system allows the images to be manipulated as needed.

The vascular imaging laboratory also contains specialized ancillary equipment needed to produce high-quality images of contrast-filled structures within the body. The most commonly used device is the contrast medium pressure injector. This equipment allows for large bolus injections that are too difficult to be performed by hand. Newer devices also allow for smaller bolus injections that were previously performed by hand.

For a vascular imaging laboratory to run successfully, it is very important that a quality control program be established and implemented. This program should include scheduled maintenance of the x-ray tube and image acquisition system, image manipulation and viewing systems, and ancillary equipment. The quality control program should be used to maintain safe and successful operation of the equipment, produce the highest image quality, and reduce exposure to the patient and imaging staff. ■

REVIEW QUESTIONS

1. What determines the heat-loading ability of a vascular x-ray tube?
2. What are the total heat units generated by a vascular x-ray tube for a series of 12 exposures using 600 mA, 0.5 second, 89 kVp on a multiphasic unit?
3. When using an analog image intensifier, what two devices are required to produce a digital image?
4. What is the purpose of the image processor in a digital image acquisition system?
5. Describe the process of digital subtraction angiography.
6. Which image post-processing function is used when there is a significant amount of motion in a digital subtraction angiography acquisition?
7. What is the most important design feature in the C-arm assembly?
8. What are the three requirements that an angiography table must meet in order to be used in a vascular imaging laboratory?
9. What is the total volume for an injection that has a flow rate of 15 cc/sec and injection duration of 2 seconds?
10. List the safety mechanisms that contrast medium injection devices are equipped with.
11. List the components of a vascular imaging laboratory quality control program.

REFERENCES AND RECOMMENDED READING

Bushong, S. C. (2008 and 9th ed.). *Radiologic science for technologists: Physics, biology, and protection* (8th ed.) St. Louis, MO: Elsevier/C. V. Mosby.

Cullinan, A., & Cullinan, J. (1994). *Producing quality radiographs* (2nd ed.). Philadelphia: J. B. Lippincott.

Curry, T. S., Dowdey, J. E., & Murry, R. C. (1990). *Christensen's introduction to the physics of diagnostic radiology* (4th ed.). Philadelphia: Lea & Febiger.

Laudicina, P., & Wean, D. (1994). *Applied angiography for radiographers.* Philadelphia: W. B. Saunders.

Snopek, A. M. (2006 and 5th ed.). *Fundamentals of special radiographic procedures* (4th ed.). Philadelphia: W. B. Saunders.

Tortorici, M. R., & Apfel, P. J. (1995). *Advanced radiographic and angiographic procedures: With an introduction to specialized imaging.* Philadelphia: F. A. Davis.

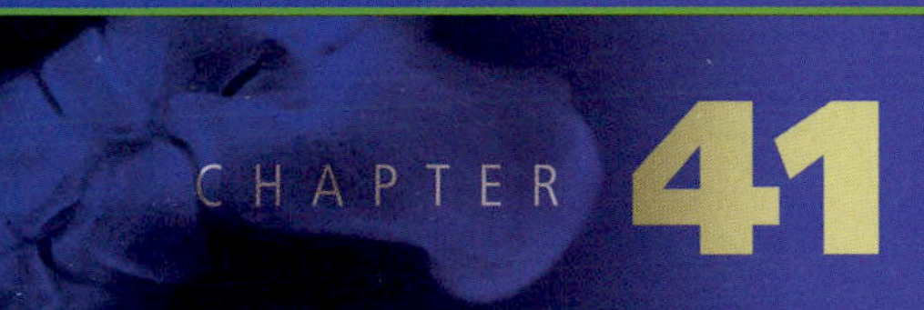

CHAPTER 41 Computed Tomography

KEY TERMS

collimator pitch
convolution
deconvolution
gantry
mask
pitch
targeting

The physicians seem to be quite keen on it.

Allan Cormack upon being informed that he and Godfrey Hounsfield were to share the 1979 Nobel Prize for Medicine for the invention of computed tomography

OBJECTIVES

Upon completion of this chapter, the student should be able to:

- Explain the invention of computed tomography.
- Describe typical gantry components.
- Explain the basic features of each generation of CT scanners, especially multidetector (MDCT) units.
- Explain why CT tabletops have patient weight limits.
- Compare the requirements for a CT x-ray tube with those of a routine diagnostic tube.
- Explain the operation of a scintillation crystal and photomultiplier tube CT detector.
- Explain the operation of a xenon-gas–filled ionization chamber CT detector.
- Discuss the importance of detector alignment and calibration.
- Discuss the use of a CT computer menu or index.
- Describe the major display features possible with advanced software.

OBJECTIVES (continued)

- Describe the calculation and use of Hounsfield units.
- Explain reformatting image reconstruction.
- Explain how CT display image density and contrast are controlled.
- Describe the factors affecting resolution, including voxel, pixel, and matrix size.
- Discuss methods of reducing CT image noise and motion.
- Illustrate section shape, partial volume effect, and scan arc in relation to scanning procedures.
- Explain a variety of common CT artifacts.
- Discuss radiation protection of the patient and others during CT examinations.

Computed tomography (CT) produces a digital tomographic image from diagnostic x-rays. The basic principle of CT involves digitizing an image received from a slit scan projection of the patient's body and then back-projecting the image through mathematical algorithms.

Although CT scanning is usually performed transversely, digital processing of information can produce sagittal and coronal sections (Figure 41-1). Because the CT x-ray beam is confined to a slit, much scatter radiation is eliminated from the image. The combination of the transverse sectioning procedure with slit scanning produces an image of significantly better quality than that available with other imaging methods. Primarily the image differentiates various types of soft tissues (e.g., gray matter, white matter, blood, tumor, cerebrospinal fluid, etc.). When digital image data manipulation is added, CT provides more diagnostic information than any other ionizing radiation imaging modality.

As with other tomographic modalities, the terms *cut* and *slice* are used in clinical practice. Because these phrases can easily cause distress when overheard by a patient, the radiographer should strive to adhere to the term *section*, avoiding *cut* and *slice*.

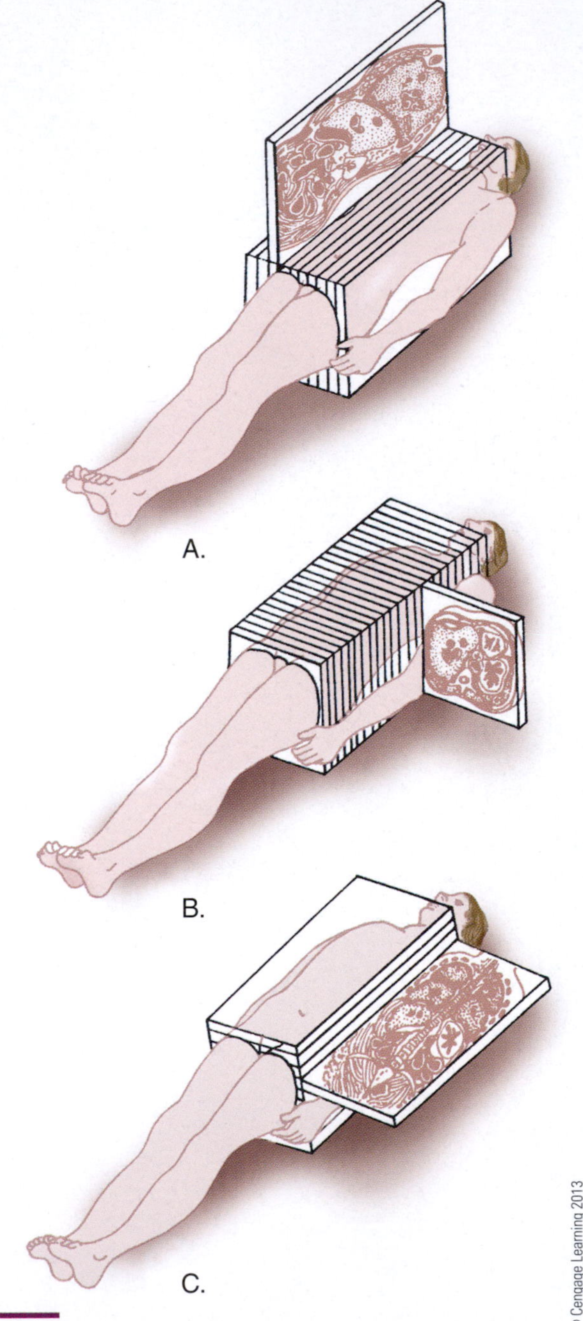

FIGURE 41-1. Computed tomography sections: (A) sagittal; (B) transverse; (C) coronal.

THE INVENTION OF COMPUTED TOMOGRAPHY

The invention of CT has been credited to Godfrey N. Hounsfield for his work in 1970–1971, although preliminary work was done by Oldendorf in 1961 and Cormack in 1963, and all three based their work on the investigations of the Austrian mathematician J. Radon, who proved in 1917 that an image of a three-dimensional object could be produced from its mathematical projections. Hounsfield was a research engineer with Electro-Musical Instruments Ltd. (EMI), the English firm that gained international renown as the Beatles' music publishers during the 1960s. His original scanner was built on a lathe bed and required 9 days to produce a single section image. Although the company sold its CT business, it continues to operate American and British EMI. Hounsfield and Cormack were awarded the 1979 Nobel Prize for Medicine. Hounsfield's invention parallels Röntgen's discovery of x-rays as the two most outstanding contributions to medical imaging.

Early CT units were capable of only axial tomography, and the term *computerized axial tomography* (CAT) scanning became popular. Modern CT units are capable of diverse modes much more complex than simple axial scanning. However, the term *CAT scanning* may endure, as have other antiquated radiologic terms (e.g., flat plate and wet reading). A modern CT unit includes a gantry, table, x-ray tube, detectors, computer, display console, and image storage units (Figure 41-2).

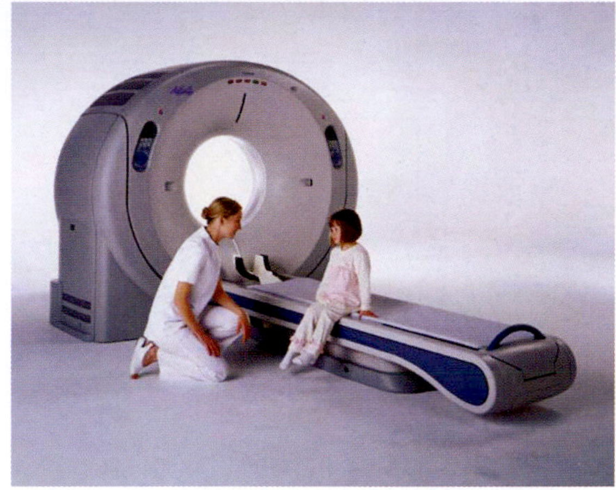

FIGURE 41-2. A computed tomography unit. *(Courtesy of GE Healthcare.)*

SCANNER GENERATIONS

Computed tomography technology advanced very rapidly after Hounsfield's discovery. Scanners are sometimes described by their generation, with the original EMI head scanner considered to be the first. Descriptions of various computed tomography equipment refer to both rays and projections (also called views). A **ray** is a pencil-thin beam of radiation that strikes a single detector. A **projection** (or **view**) is composed of a set of rays striking a detector array (a group of detectors). Although there are no distinct lines between the generations, Table 41-1 illustrates the major characteristics of each.

First Generation

First-generation CT scanners were single-ray systems designed for examination of the head only (Figure 41-3). The head was surrounded by a water bag to eliminate air interfaces. A single x-ray tube and a pair of detectors were aligned on a fixed C-arm. The detectors were sodium iodide scintillation crystals with photomultiplier tubes. A pencil-thin slit field, 3 mm × 26 mm, scanned a 180° arc around the patient's head. Each detector was exposed to a 3 mm × 13 mm field. First-generation units used a rotating scan and index system that scanned the head linearly (from one side to the other), indexed 1°, repeated the scanning process, indexed another 1°, and so on, for the entire 180° (Figure 41-4). This is also called a translate (scan) and rotate (index) system. The x-ray tube was on during scanning and off during indexing. Although the pair of detectors did not decrease the 180° scanning time, they permitted two anatomical sections to be scanned simultaneously, thus reducing the total examination time by half.

The detectors measured the attenuation coefficient of the exit radiation beam at overlapping 1.7-mm intervals 240 times during each scan.

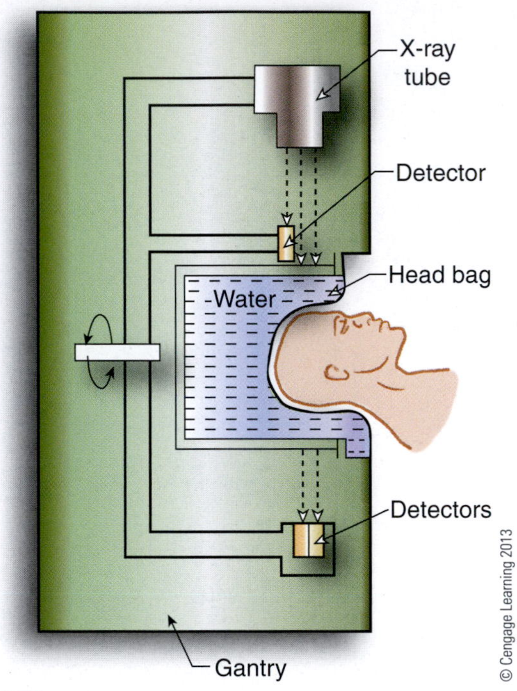

FIGURE 41-3. A first-generation CT head scanner.

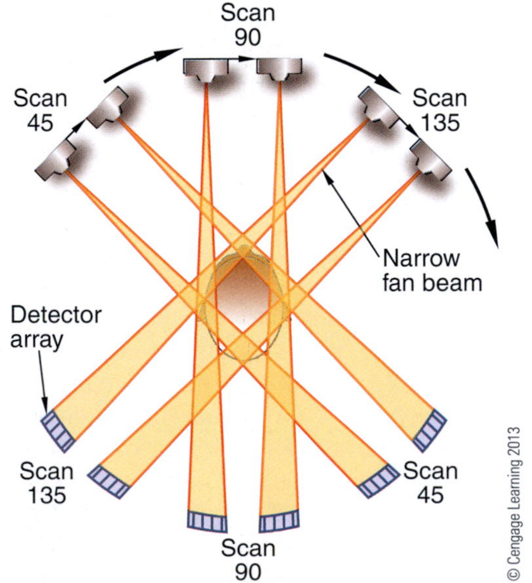

FIGURE 41-4. First-generation CT scan and rotate system. Only three scans (the 45th, 90th, and 135th) are shown to simplify the illustration. A single scan and rotate required 180 scans, each 1° apart.

TABLE 41-1. Major Characteristics of CT Unit Generations

First generation	head only linear scan and rotate (180 scans, 1° rotations) paired detectors (160 measurements per scan) 4.5- to 5-minute scan time single-ray pencil beam single detector
Second generation	single-projection, fan-shaped beam (permitting whole-body scanning) up to 30 detectors 10- to 90-second scan time linear scan and rotate (6 scans, 30° rotations)
Third generation	single-projection, fan-shaped beam up to 300 detectors 2- to 10-second scan time 360° rotation of x-ray tube and detectors crude dynamic capabilities
Fourth generation	single-projection, fan-shaped beam 360° ring of stationary detectors 2- to 10-second scan time 360° rotation of x-ray tube dynamic capabilities
Fifth generation	electron beam scanners stationary tube annular targets cardiac imaging 50 msec imaging
Sixth generation helical/spiral	multiple-projection, fan-shaped beam 360° ring of stationary detectors 360° rotation of x-ray tube computer-controlled table movement through gantry bore continuous scanning throughout entire examination
Seventh generation	Multidetector CT (MDCT) $>$ 10K detector elements 0.5-mm section thickness $>$ 20 simultaneous contiguous detectors $\approx$ 12- to 15-sec procedure time (body region scan time)

The unit required 4.5 minutes to complete a pair of full 180° scans and 5 minutes to reconstruct the images. Each section was derived from 43,200 measurements (180° × 240) and was displayed on an 80 × 80 matrix. Each display pixel represented a voxel of tissue 3 mm × 3 mm × 13 mm, although a 1.5-mm pixel display became available. A common examination routine for the head consisted of 10–12 sections, which required 25–35 minutes to obtain.

Second Generation

Second-generation CT units used a single-projection, fan-shaped beam instead of a pencil slit and a linear array of as many as 30 detectors (Figure 41-5). They too are no longer available. The fan-shaped beam and increased number of detectors permitted scanning and rotation with fewer linear movements. For example, a 30-detector unit could complete the 180° linear movement in only six rotations of 30° each. However, the loss of collimation increased the amount of scatter radiation detected. This is a major disadvantage of all fan beam scanners. A lead mask was added to the detectors to assist in reducing the scatter reaching the detectors. Scan time was reduced to between 10 and 90 seconds, a reasonable respiratory suspension time, thus permitting examination of the whole body.

Third Generation

Third-generation CT units used a wider fan-shaped beam and a curved array of 250–750 detectors to achieve a single projection (Figure 41-6). The fan-shaped beam was wide enough to include the entire body in a single exposure and rotated 360° within the gantry, thus eliminating the linear scan and rotate system. A typical third-generation scanner might produce 700,000 measurements per section. Various scanning arcs were usually possible, for example 220° or 360°. Scan time was reduced to between 1 and 12 seconds, permitting sequential images to crudely approximate dynamic functions. Third-generation units that featured dynamic scanning usually performed at about four scans per minute, which equals the routine scanning time of a fourth-generation unit. Because they had only a single detector array, third-generation scanners were prone to ring artifacts (see Figure 41-34c).

Fourth Generation

Fourth-generation CT units were developed as a result of a competitive contract awarded to the American Science and Engineering Company (AS&E) by the U.S. National Institutes of Health (NIH). They use a single-projection, fan-shaped beam with 600–2,000 stationary detectors arrayed in a 360° ring (Figure 41-7). The ring of detectors eliminates movement of the detectors, thereby decreasing calibration requirements. As many as

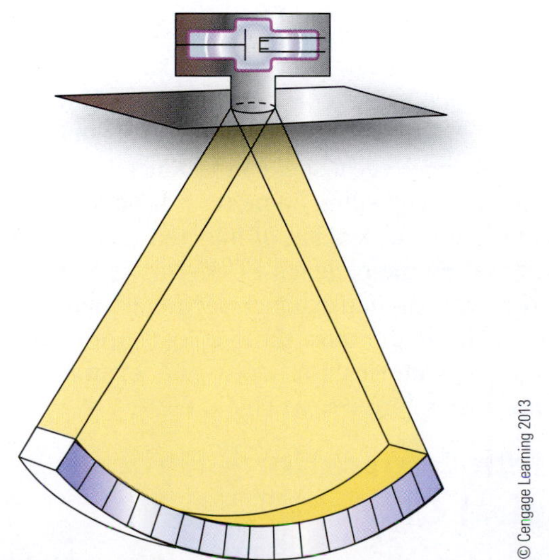

FIGURE 41-5. A fan-shaped beam.

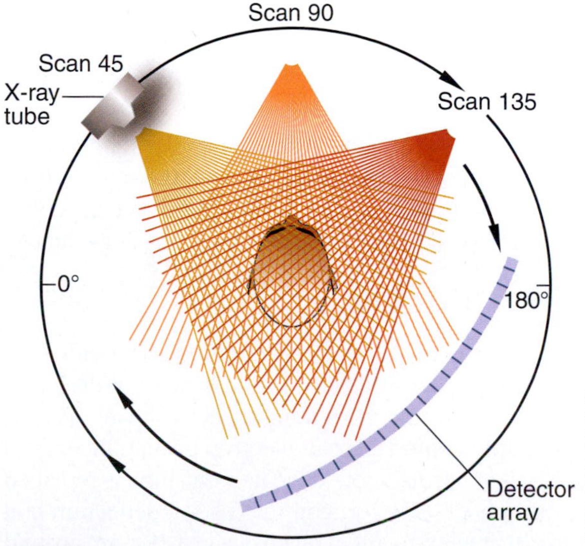

FIGURE 41-6. A third-generation CT scanner.

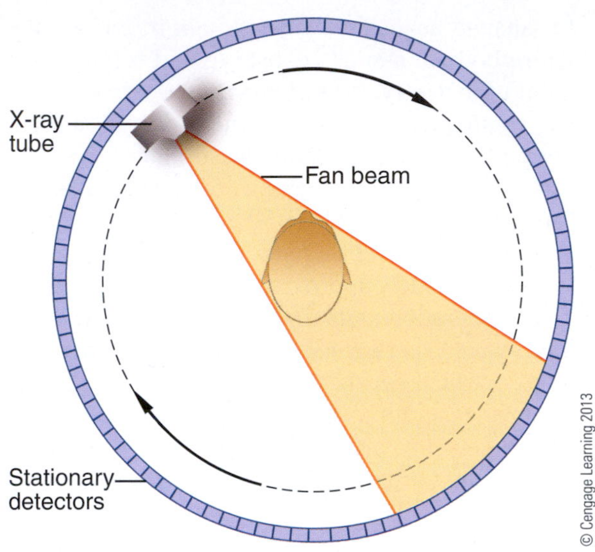

FIGURE 41-7. A fourth-generation CT scanner.

1,200,000 measurements may be processed per section. A wider range of scan arcs, including arcs over 360°, is usually possible, with scan times ranging from 0.5 to 10 seconds.

Some fourth-generation scanners are capable of dynamic scanning rates in the range of 15 scans per minute. The limiting factor is the interscan time and the computer processing time, not the actual scanning time. Dynamic scanning is usually achieved by reducing the interscan time to 1–2 seconds and not indexing the gantry. Scanning occurs first in a clockwise direction, then counterclockwise, and so forth. Another technique, called overscan, may also be available. Overscanning uses a scan of more than 360°. The overscan may be displayed as segmented data from two, three, or four scans as a single image.

Fifth Generation

The fifth generation of scanners is represented by the technology utilized in a dedicated cardiac unit designed around a rotating electron beam. This is sometimes referred to as electron beam tomography (EBT) or cardiac cine CT. The x-ray tube is replaced with a huge electron gun that uses a deflection coil to direct a 30° beam of electrons in a 210° arc around a 360° anode ring (Figure 41-8). The fan beam that is produced is intercepted by a 360° detector array.

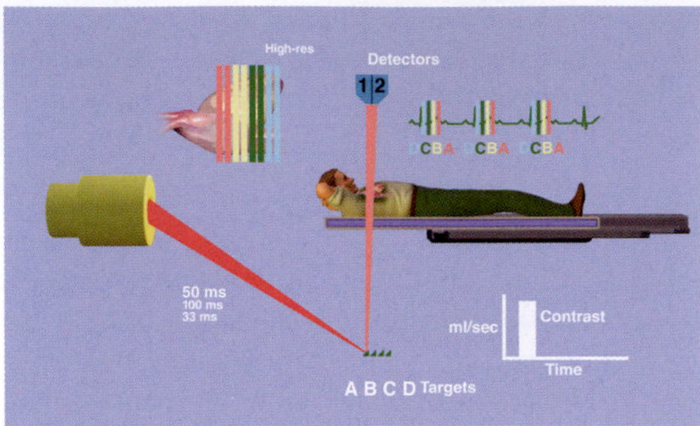

A.

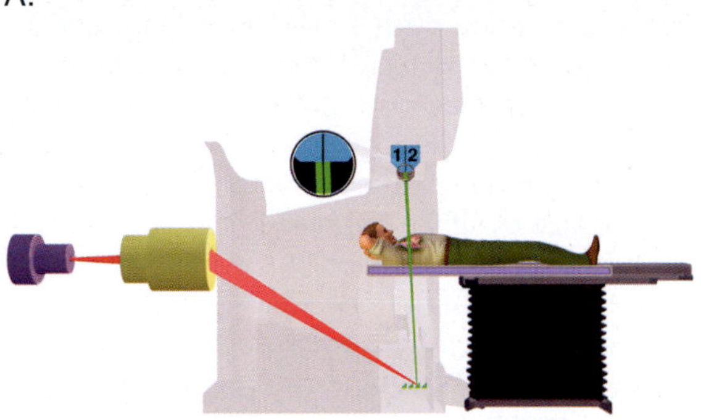

B.

FIGURE 41-8. Fifth-generation electron beam tomography (EBT) or cardiac cine CT. (A) Scanner components. (B) Multidetector operation with contrast media injection triggered by patient ECG. *(Courtesy of GE Healthcare.)*

Because the electron beam rotates around the anode ring, there is no moving gantry in this design. The patient is placed within the anode ring, somewhat akin to being inside the x-ray tube itself. This unit is a dynamic scanner because it can produce four sections simultaneously within 50 msec. It is also capable of multisection sequencing of injected contrast media triggered by the patient's ECG. This is fast enough to provide real-time dynamic sectional images of the beating heart. Because these images are essentially anatomical movies (or cine), the examination is sometimes referred to as cine CT.

Sixth Generation—Helical/ Spiral CT

Helical (spiral) scanners were made possible by advances in slip ring connection technology. Slip rings consist of brushes that fit into grooves to permit the

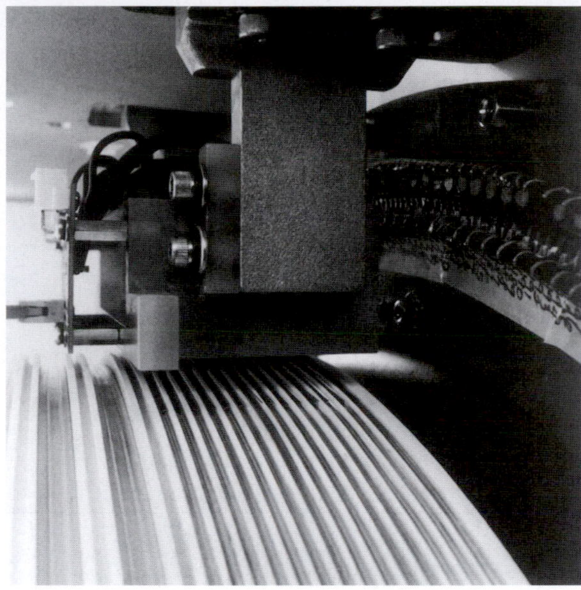

FIGURE 41-9. A helical computed tomography scanner slip ring. The brushes are contained in the large unit at the center of the photograph. They fit into grooves in the ring underneath. As the x-ray tube rotates, the necessary electrical connections are maintained without interruption. *(Courtesy of Philips Medical System, Inc. All rights reserved.)*

current and voltage to the x-ray tube to be supplied while the tube is in continuous rotation around the gantry (Figure 41-9). This permits scanning of the entire body in a helical pattern without stopping the tube. When the patient table is moved slowly during the x-ray exposure while the tube is in continuous rotation, data comprising a continuous helical scan of the patient is acquired. Both low- and high-voltage slip rings have been developed by different manufacturers.

The term *spiral* is a misnomer. A spiral is a circular motion with a decreasing or increasing diameter. The actual scanning motion has a set circular diameter, which is a helix. The data are acquired in a helical, not a spiral, motion (Figure 41-10).

The primary advantage of helical scanning is a much shorter total scan time (30–40 seconds for the entire abdomen). This in turn permits the use of less contrast media. Not only are patients at less risk of contrast media reaction, but the throughput of patients is greatly increased. Another advantage is that for many patients the entire examination

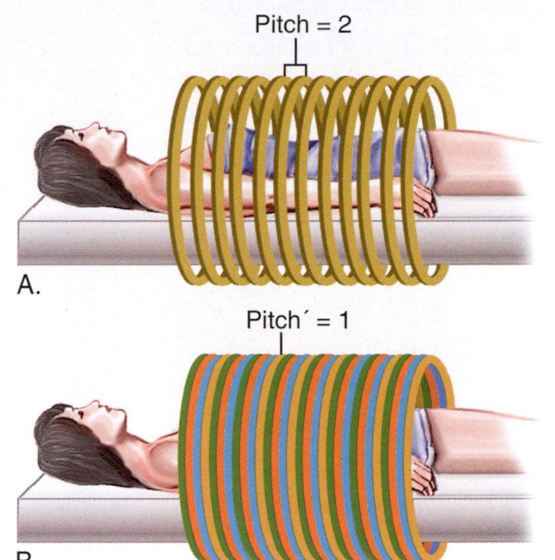

FIGURE 41-10. Helical and MSCT/MDCT scan and pitch. (A) A single helical scan motion with a pitch of 2. (B) MSCT/MDCT collimator pitch of 1.

can be completed in one breath hold, eliminating overlaps and missed areas due to variations in the amount of air in the lungs between scan sections. This also reduces the possibility of motion artifacts.

The primary disadvantage is that a full 360° set of data is not acquired for each section because the patient is continuously advancing through the gantry bore during the exposure. The sectional image is created from computer reconstructions of planar sections that approximate the acquisition of planar reconstruction data. Both the advantages and disadvantages are detailed in Table 41-2.

Pitch. Because the patient table moves during the exposure, a method to measure and reproduce this motion must be established. **Pitch** is the term that is used to define this extension or contraction of the helix. Pitch is simply the ratio of the distance the table moves (feed) during one 360° tube rotation to the total beam collimation (Figure 41-10). The formula for pitch is:

$$P = \frac{I}{B}$$

where: P = pitch
I = table increment per 360°
B = beam width in mm

EXAMPLE: If the table is moving at 15 mm/sec and a section thickness of 10 mm is being acquired, what is the pitch?

Answer:

$$P = \frac{I}{S}$$

$$P = \frac{15}{10} = 1.5$$

EXAMPLE: If a pitch of 0.8 is being used and a section thickness of 8 mm is being acquired, what is the proper table speed?

Answer:

$$P = \frac{I}{S} \text{ or } I = PB$$

$$I = 0.8 \times 8$$

$$I = 6.4 \text{ mm/sec}$$

EXAMPLE: If the table is moving at 5 mm/sec. and a pitch of 1.0 is being used, what is the section thickness?

Answer:

$$P = \frac{I}{B} \text{ or } B = \frac{I}{P}$$

$$B = \frac{5}{1.0}$$

$$B = 5 \text{ mm}$$

TABLE 41-2. Advantages and Disadvantages of Helical (Spiral) Computed Tomography

Advantages
Requires less contrast media, resulting in decreased patient risk of contrast media reactions.
Eliminates overlap and missed areas due to variations in breathing for some patients and examinations where the entire scan can be completed in one breath hold.
Motion artifacts are reduced.
Faster scan time increases patient throughput.
Pitch settings can be set to oversample sections of interest.
Reconstruction section thickness can be smaller than the acquisition section thickness.
Disadvantages
Full 360° projection data are not acquired for each section.
Sections are reconstructed to represent approximate acquisition of planar data.

Collimator Pitch. Multidetector CT changes the way pitch is calculated because the beam is intercepted and acquired by multiple detectors instead of a single detector receiving the entire beam. The term **collimator pitch′** ("pitch prime") refers to the pitch of a single detector within an MDCT array of image receptors, not the total beam collimation. Table 41-3 includes both pitch formulas.

Increasing the pitch value permits a greater field of view (FOV) to be imaged in a shorter time. However, it is important to understand that pitch values less than 1.0 imply data oversampling. Pitch

TABLE 41-3. CT Pitch Formulas

Single Section Pitch or Multiple Section Pitch (Beam Width)	P = I/B,	where: P = pitch I = table increment per 360° B = beam width in mm
Multiple Section Pitch (Section Width)	CP = I/S,	where: CP = collimator pitch I = table increment per 360° S = section width in mm

values greater than 1.0 imply that some data are being missed. The ability to set the pitch less than 1.0 and produce oversampling of areas of interest is also an advantage of helical scanning. Another major advantage is that image reconstruction can be set for smaller section thicknesses than those that were acquired.

Resolution. Image resolution in helical scanners (which includes multisection scanners as well) is vastly improved over older models. Resolution issues must be considered from two perspectives: the image matrix pixel size in both the x and y planes and the helical pitch (which forms the z-axis), as shown in Figure 41-11.

Increased resolution in the x and y planes is accomplished by technologies that decrease the size of the detectors. Both computer processing and display resolution far exceeds current detector acquisition technology.

Increased resolution in the z plane is accomplished by using the smallest detector size combined with a pitch ≤ 1.

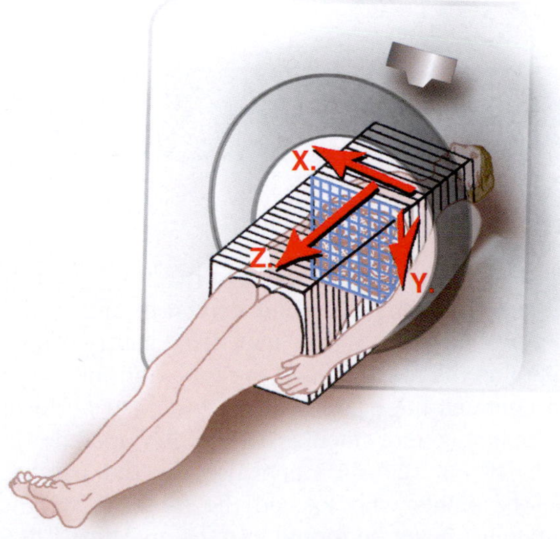

FIGURE 41-11. Image resolution in helical and MSCT/MDCT scanner is improved in all three planes. Resolution is increased in the x and y planes by decreasing detector size. Resolution is increased in the z plane by using the smallest detector size and pitch ≤ 1.

Seventh Generation—MSCT

Computed tomography units with multiple detectors are known by several terms. **Multisection or multislice computed tomography** (MSCT), **multidetector computed tomography** (MDCT), and **multiple detector array scanners** (MDA) have all appeared in the literature to date. The most appropriate term to use is **multisection computed tomography** (MSCT) because the term *slice* is professional slang and just because a scanner has multiple detectors does not necessarily indicate that multiple sections of data are being collected simultaneously.

Multisection CT units represent a major change in CT technology because multiple detectors are exposed simultaneously (Figure 41-12). At the turn of the century there were major advancements in detector technology that permitted an array of thousands of parallel bands of detectors to operate simultaneously instead of the single bands of detectors that had been in use up until then. This permitted a single beam exposure to produce multiple sets of image receptor data. When this technology is combined with helical scanning, total examination time is reduced dramatically, with an entire chest or abdomen procedure completed in 15–20 sec.

Because section thickness can be reduced with MSCT, resolution can be increased remarkably. Section thickness with single-section CT scanners is determined by the collimator size, not the width of the detector. Because MSCT scanners are exposing multiple detectors simultaneously, section thickness is determined by the width of the detector, even though the collimation of the beam is wide enough to expose several other bands of detectors (see Figure 41-12). For this reason, resolution in MSCT scanners is determined by the width of the detector, not the width of the collimator.

The MSCT design is more efficient, reduces patient exposure, increases image resolution, and allows post-acquisition reconstruction at new levels as well. For example, a 20-mm collimated beam width can be used to simultaneously expose an array of four 5-mm detector bands (as shown in Figure 41-12). The dataset that is acquired from this exposure can be displayed as four 5-mm sections, two 10-mm sections, or one 20-mm section. Nearly unlimited choices in section thickness become available to the interpreting physician or radiologist assistant.

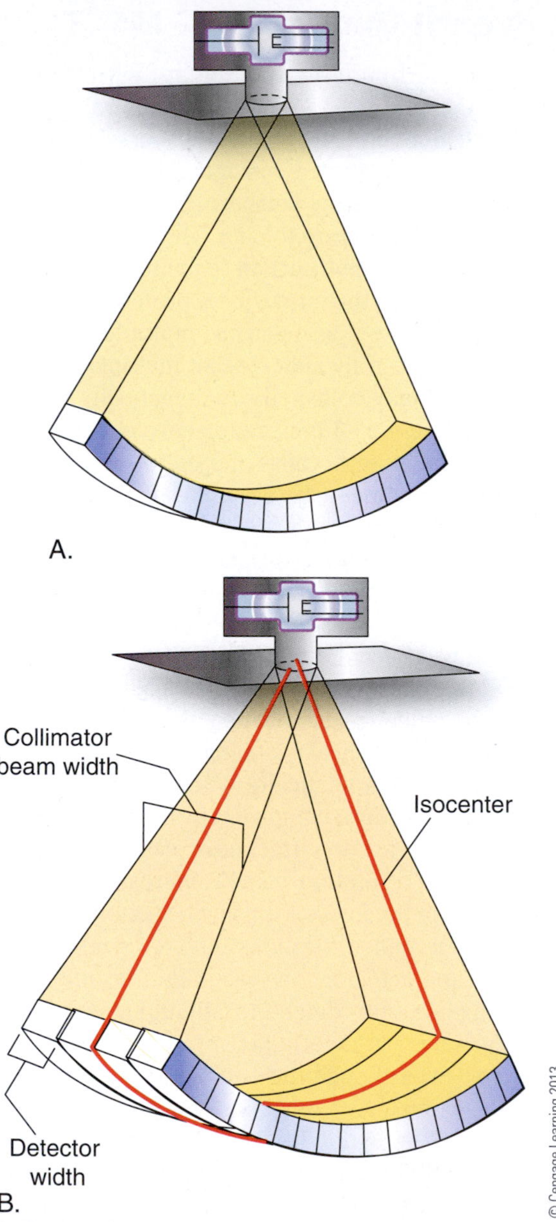

FIGURE 41-12. Multisection computed tomography (MSCT) resolution. (A) Single section CT resolution is determined by the width of the collimator beam. (B) Multisection CT resolution is determined by the width of the detector.

Some MSCT scanners allow users to set the pitch < 1 in order to increase the mAs/section available. This increases the quantity of data to each detector without overloading the x-ray tube. Some manufacturers only allow preset pitch.

All MSCT units use a helical scan system that produces extremely rapid scanning time while maintaining the advantages of higher resolution and reconstruction flexibility. Figure 41-12 illustrates how a four-detector-row, single-beam helical scan sequence would appear. MSCT units are rated according to the number of detector rows that can be exposed from a single beam collimation. The figure illustrates only four rows to demonstrate the concept. Current CT units offer multiple section capabilities, up to 320 sections. These scanners produce thousands of images for each procedure and have created considerable concern over radiologist liability because questions have not yet been answered regarding reasonable standards for how many of these images should be viewed to provide an adequate diagnosis. Three-dimensional reformation also helps with the viewing of so many images. In the United Kingdom, graduate degree programs for radiographers have been developed to assist in screening huge quantities of images in collaboration with radiologists, and there is now development of radiologist assistant programs in the United States that may provide some relief for this responsibility as well as additional career opportunities for highly qualified and motivated radiographers.

THE COMPONENTS OF A CT UNIT

The Gantry

The **gantry** is the movable frame of the CT unit. It contains the x-ray tube and detectors and is the most visible part of the unit. The gantry frame maintains the alignment of the tube and detectors and contains the equipment necessary to perform the scanning movements. The gantry includes a 50- to 85-cm (20″–34″) aperture for the patient. Obese patients who exceed the tabletop weight limits must never be forced into the aperture. They may become stuck.

Most gantrys can be angled up to 30° to permit positioning for partial coronal images. This is especially desirable in obtaining transverse scans perpendicular to the vertebral column. Table angulation can sometimes be used in place of gantry angulation. Scanners with the x-ray beam placed near the table side of the aperture permit more comfortable positioning of the patient and may permit coronal or sagittal scanning of some body parts, especially of the head. Both magnetic resonance imaging and CT reconfiguration software may be used in place of positions designed to achieve coronal or sagittal sections.

Positioning lights are usually mounted on the gantry as well. Intense white halogen lights and low-power red laser lights are used for positioning. The body part of interest must be properly centered to the aperture because the extreme edge of the scanning field produces a severely degraded image. There are often three positioning lights for accurate sagittal, coronal, and transverse centering.

Table

The CT table may be either flat or curved. It is usually made of carbon graphite fiber to decrease beam attenuation. Because the top must extend beyond the table to move the patient into the gantry aperture, it must be capable of supporting the entire weight of the patient without sagging when fully extended. Tabletops are rated for maximum weight, and it is critical that the radiographer make sure that this weight is not exceeded. Extensive damage to the table may result when attempts are made to examine very large patients who exceed the tabletop weight limit. Physicians must be informed if the CT unit cannot move obese patients into the aperture for examination. Examinations of patients over the weight limit may remove the CT unit from clinical use for all patients for a considerable time while the top is replaced. The top is motor-driven to permit the patient to be moved the exact desired distance between sections. Section intervals may be controlled automatically by a program initiated at the control console. The table must also be capable of vertical movement, both for positioning within the aperture and for ease of patient transfer.

X-Ray Tubes

The rapid sequential exposures required to produce CT images produce massive amounts of heat in the x-ray tube. Most CT x-ray tube difficulties have revolved around attempts to solve this problem. The early scanners used a stationary anode with a 2 mm × 16 mm focal spot operating at 120 kVp and 30 mA. This reduced image resolution significantly. However, since first-generation images were usually displayed on an 80 × 80 matrix, the x-ray tube was not the problem in this system.

As matrix size increased to 512 × 512, rotating anode tubes with focal spots as small as 0.6 mm × 1.2 mm came into use. Small-focal-spot scanners use a pulsed beam to reduce the heat load. Modern pulsed scanner tubes operate at 120 kVp, 1- to 5-msec pulses, and up to 1,000 mA. Some units permit 80 and 140 kVp to be selected, sometimes in alternate pulses, for dual energy scanning in which comparisons can be made between images at different kVp values. In addition, 0.5–5.0 million heat unit anodes of layered alloys, cylindrical anodes, and liquid-cooled and air-cooled tube housing designs have been developed. A CT tube may produce 30 exposures per examination. Because most CT units are scheduled for 10–20 examinations per day, a tube may accumulate 10,000 exposures in a single month. It is not unusual for a CT tube to fail after several months. Only a few last a full year.

The radiation beam is double collimated, once at the tube exit and again at the detector entrance. This assists in eliminating scatter information. Collimation controls the voxel length. Collimation is variable from 1 mm to 13 mm and is usually controlled by the software program. The dimension of the collimation width determines the voxel length, or section thickness.

Detectors

Detectors must be capable of responding with extreme speed to a signal, without lag, must quickly discard the signal, and then prepare for the next. They must also respond consistently and be small in size. They are usually placed with a source-to-image-receptor distance of 44″ (110 cm).

CT detectors should have high **capture efficiency,** high **absorption efficiency,** and high **conversion efficiency.** These three parameters are called the **detector dose efficiency.**

capture efficiency
absorption efficiency
+ conversion efficiency
dose efficiency

The capture efficiency is how well the detectors receive photons from the patient. It is controlled primarily by detector size and the distance between detectors. Absorption efficiency is how well the detectors convert incoming x-ray photons. It is determined primarily by the materials used (for example, the scintillation crystal or the gas) as well as the size and thickness of the detector. Conversion efficiency is determined by how well the detector converts the absorbed photon information to a digital signal for the computer.

CT detectors should also have high **stability,** fast **response time,** and a wide **dynamic range.** Stability is controlled by how often the detectors must be recalibrated to meet quality control standards. Response time is the speed with which the detector can react to recognize an incoming photon and recover for the next input. The dynamic range is the ratio of the largest signal that can be measured to the smallest. Typical modern scanners are capable of dynamic ranges of 1,000,000 to 1.

Scintillation Crystals and Photomultiplier Tubes. Early detectors consisted of a scintillation crystal in contact with a photomultiplier tube (Figure 41-13). This system was used in nuclear medicine for many years prior to the advent of CT. A sodium iodide (NaI) crystal absorbs an x-ray photon and produces light flashes (scintillations) in proportion to the energy of the photon and at the exact location where the photon struck within the crystal. This light (photo) is then amplified (multiplied) by the photomultiplier (PM) tube. The light photon strikes the cathode of the PM tube, where it is converted into electrons. The electrons are then amplified by a series of dynodes as they move through the tube. Each dynode has a higher voltage, thereby increasing the number and voltage of the electrons as they move toward the anode. Upon striking the anode, the electrons are converted into a digital signal that can be processed by the computer.

Although sodium iodide scintillation crystals are nearly 100 percent efficient within the diagnostic x-ray range, they exhibit phosphorescent afterglow, or lag. This makes them useless with the rapid sequential exposures in the later-generation scanners. Some units were produced using calcium fluoride (CaF_2), bismuth germinate ($Bi_4Ge_3O_{12}$), cesium

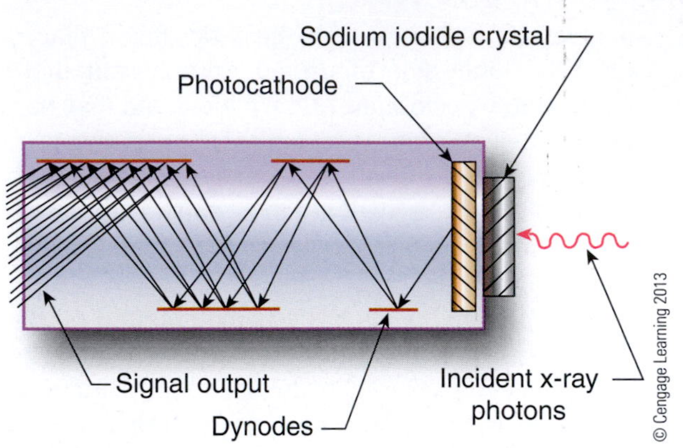

FIGURE 41-13. A scintillation crystal and photomultiplier tube detector.

iodide (CsI), gadolinium ceramics, and cadmium tungstate ($CdWO_4$) scintillation crystals, which, although less efficient (90 percent), have minimal afterglow. These materials are often bonded directly to the photocathode. A major disadvantage of scintillation-PM detectors was their size and interspace material, which prohibited packing them closer in the detector array. This reduced their total detection efficiency to less than 50 percent.

Xenon Ionization Chambers. Inexpensive CT scanners may use xenon-gas–filled ionization chamber detectors (Figure 41-14). They operate on the same principle as an ionization chamber. Essentially, they measure ionization in air by attracting to an electrode the ions created by x-ray photons in the air. The electrodes are usually thin tungsten plates spaced 1.5 mm apart. This spacing determines the maximum detector (and therefore display pixel size) resolution. The electrodes are alternately charged with positive and negative voltages. The quantity of ionic charge at the electrode is proportional to the energy of the photons detected between the electrodes. The detected energy comprises a digital signal that is sent to the computer.

Gas detectors range in efficiency from 60 to 90 percent but exhibit no lag. Ion chamber detectors were not used in the original EMI scanner because they were not sensitive enough. This disadvantage was overcome by using a long ion chamber and filling it with krypton or xenon, the heaviest inert gas, at high compression (20–30 atmospheres).

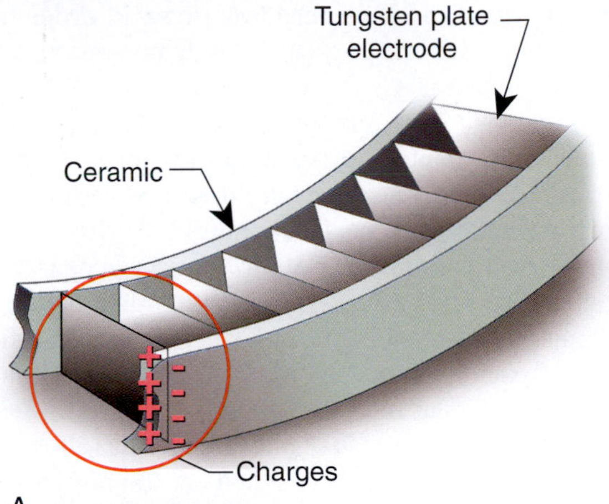

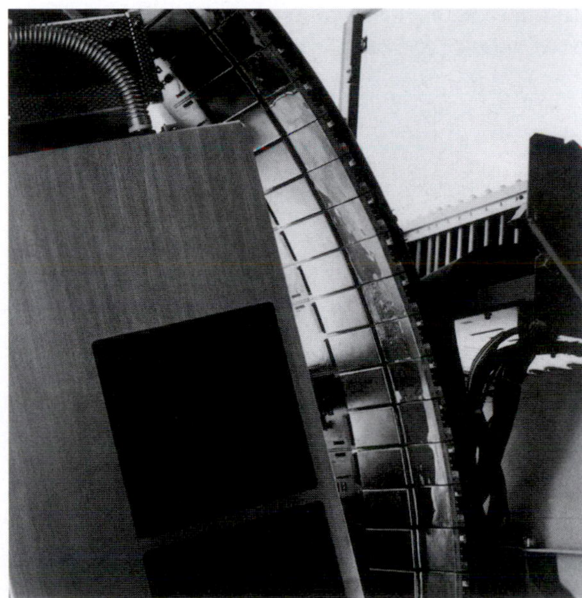

FIGURE 41-14. (A) A xenon-gas-filled ionization chamber CT detector. The tungsten plate electrodes are alternately charged with positive and negative voltages. (B) A detector ring in a helical CT unit. *(Courtesy of Philips Medical Systems, Inc. All rights reserved.)*

Although gas-ion detector efficiency may be only 60 percent, these detectors can be packed extremely close in the detector array, permitting a detection efficiency of slightly less than 50 percent, which is similar to that of scintillation-PM detectors.

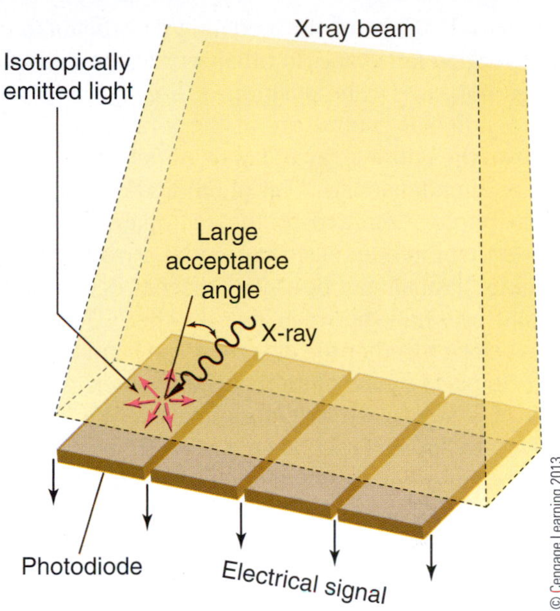

FIGURE 41-15. Solid-state detector. A scintillator is bonded to the top of the photodiode. When the incoming x-ray beam activates the scintillator, light photons are emitted, which are detected by the photodiode and converted into an electrical signal. Note the large acceptance angle of the scintillator. This accounts for the vastly increased sensitivity of solid-state detectors and permits the incoming x-ray beam to be a diverging fan shape.

Xenon detectors are highly directional. In other words, they must be set in a fixed position oriented to the x-ray source. This is why helical scanners do not use xenon detectors.

Solid State. Solid-state detectors are used in all helical and MSCT scanners. They are similar to the detectors used in digital radiography systems but with different performance requirements.

Solid-state detectors combine a calcium tungstate ($CdWO_4$), yttrium, or gadolinium ceramic scintillator with a photodetector (Figure 41-15). The scintillator is bonded to the top of the photodiode to assure accurate pickup of the emitted photons. When the incoming x-ray beam photon activates the scintillator, light photons are emitted isotropically in proportion to the intensity of the incoming light. A major advantage of the scintillator is that it has a large acceptance angle for incoming x-ray photons. This greatly increases the sensitivity of the detector by allowing the incoming x-ray beam to be a diverging fan shape. In other words, the detector does not have to be positioned directly under the perpendicular central ray of the x-ray beam. This allows the entire array of bands of detectors to operate simultaneously. The photodiode detects the light photons emitted by the scintillator and converts them into an electrical signal. However, they require a small gap between adjacent detectors to avoid crosstalk between one another. This limits how close together the detectors can be placed and this impacts the resolution of the scanner.

CT solid-state detectors used in MSCT scanners are typically 1.0 mm × 1.5–15 mm. Digital radiography systems use detectors that are much smaller (typically 0.1–0.2 mm on each side). One reason CT detectors are so much larger is because the CT signal must be very low noise in order to achieve the 20-bit grayscale depth necessary for effective diagnosis.

Because the crosstalk between adjacent detectors is related to the angle of the incoming x-ray beam, some scanners are designed with more narrow detectors at the isocenter of the x-ray beam where the incoming x-ray photons arrive at near 90° angles (Figure 41-16). A typical setup might include 1.0-mm wide detectors at the isocenter with gradually increasing widths of 1.5-, 2.0-, or 2.5- to 5.0-mm wide detectors at the outer edges of the collimated beam. Back illumination of photodiodes has allowed closer placement of detector cells at the isocenter. Together these innovations have allowed manufacturers to achieve submillimeter detection widths at the center of the beam. It must be remembered that

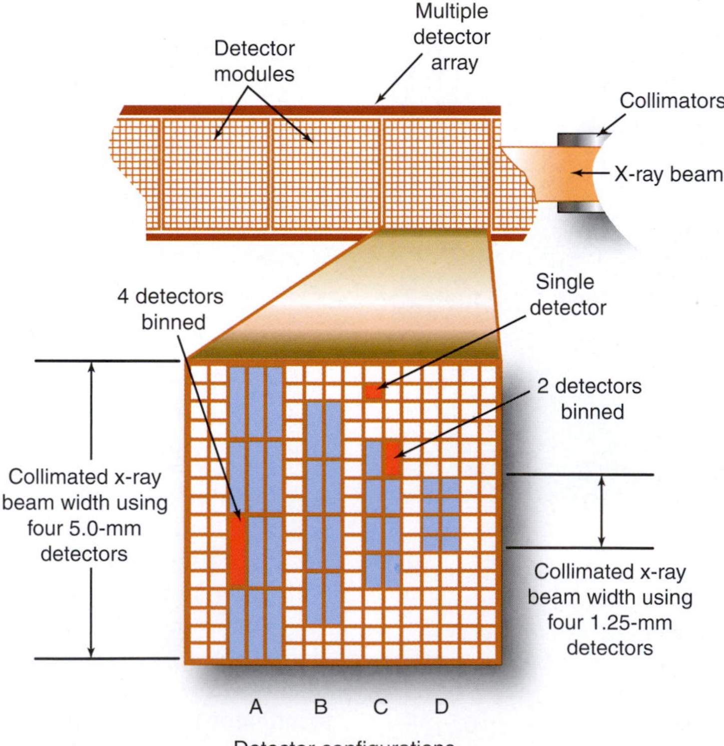

FIGURE 41-16. Multiple-array solid-state detector. When multiple detectors are arrayed in bands, a wide variety of image acquisition modes is possible. For example, although the collimated beam covers 20 mm and includes four 5.0-mm detectors, there are many options for binning detectors. A single detector can be used or combinations of two or four detectors can be binned together. *(Note: From* The Essential Physics of Medical Imaging *[2nd ed.], by J. Bushberg, J. Seibert, E. Leidholdt, and J. Boone, 2002, Philadelphia: Lippincott, Wilkins & Wilkins. Reprinted with permission.)*

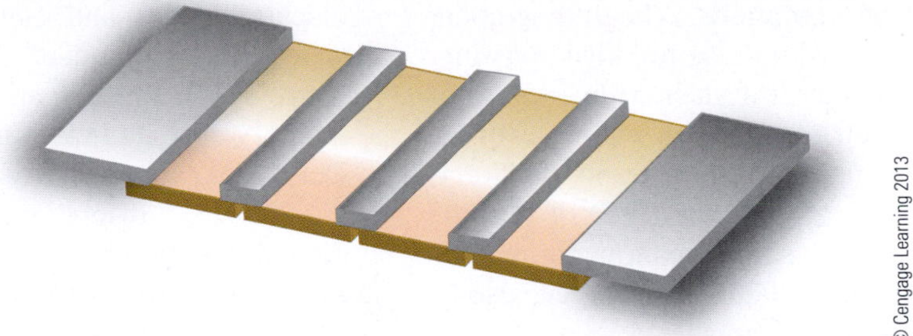

FIGURE 41-17. Solid-state detector septal and post-patient collimators. A single row of detectors makes up an array as shown. The gray plates on each side represent the post-patient collimator. The gray strips down the length of the detector row represent the thin septal collimators that divide each row of detectors in order to reduce crosstalk and increase resolution.

submillimeter resolution is not available across the entire MSCT helically scanned beam. It is possible only at the isocenter.

Additional techniques for decreasing detector crosstalk include both pre- and post-patient collimation. The post-patient collimator is a set of lead shields immediately in front of the detectors. Septal collimators are also being used as high-resolution collimators between detector rows in multiarray MSCT scanners (Figure 41-17).

There are also innovative post-acquisition algorithms that show promise of additional increases in resolution by correlating information from overlapping sets of binned detectors.

Detector Calibration. Tube and detector alignment is critical in CT because of the tight collimation of the tube and the collimator mask at the detector. The slightest misalignment may produce a concentric ring artifact image that completely overrides clinical information.

The calibration field of view (also called the scan field of view, or SFOV) is the area within the gantry from which the raw data for calibration will be acquired. Most CT units offer a number of fields and vectors for calibration. It is important to choose an appropriate field and vector (i.e., 25 mm for head calibration). Once the SFOV has been selected, the detector calibration program can be run. It is also important to realize that the field of view (FOV) (also called the display field of view [DFOV], target, or zoom region) comprises the maximum data compilation area. The calibration performed on the SFOV is only valid for smaller DFOVs.

Rotating anode tubes are aligned with their long axis perpendicular to the scanning plane. This prevents the anode heel effect within the useful beam while eliminating the gyroscopic effect on the rotating anode.

Detectors must remain in close calibration at all times. Scanner software does this automatically during scanning operations. Detectors that are out of calibration may cause artifacts that destroy image quality.

Computer

The CT computer is designed to control data acquisition, processing, display, and storage. The CT console provides the radiographer with access to the software program that controls data acquisition, processing, and display. Remote consoles may also be linked to the system to permit display and storage functions. Control of data storage may be available at the control console, remote workstations, or at the storage units themselves.

A systems program is used to start up the CT unit. This program turns on and performs quality assurance checks on numerous components in both the x-ray equipment and computer hardware systems, warms up the x-ray tube, and so forth. It also permits the radiographer to record various problems that need the attention of the service engineer. One of its main functions is to perform calibration checks on the detectors, although this may be an ongoing process during scanning. A diagnostics program with specific quality assurance tests is used by service engineers to troubleshoot the systems.

The CT console operates from a menu or index directory of operations. The radiographer simply uses a keyboard, mouse trackball, or other input device to indicate the desired operation. At the beginning of each examination, patient information, such as identification, history, and the like, is entered or input via a radiology (RIS) or hospital (HIS) data system. This information permits retrieval of the images at a later date and will also be displayed adjacent to each image.

The data acquisition program controls a variety of operations, including tube and detector collimation (pixel size), matrix size, gantry angle, tabletop entrance into the gantry aperture, section increment movements of the tabletop, x-ray tube voltage and amperage, scan speed, pitch, detector/resolution, and the direction of detector signals to the digital image processing section of the computer.

Display Console

The processing and display program controls the digital image production process, including the series of mathematical formulas (algorithms) that compile the image and the display parameters, such as window level and width, reconstructions, and enhancements.

The display console is often part of the main console and appears as a separate flat screen with controls (Figure 41-18). Also available are separate reporting workstations that permit radiologists to display images and electronically report the results, and independent consoles that contain their own CPU to retrieve and display images from the memory storage units and to receive images from examinations in progress.

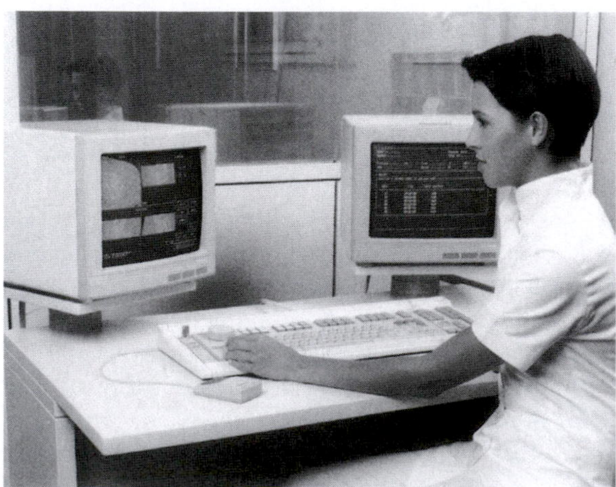

FIGURE 41-18. CT main console. *(Courtesy of Siemens Medical Systems, Inc.)*

Most CT display units permit a wide range of display features to enhance diagnosis. These vary by manufacturer but often include the following.

Scanogram/Sinogram. A localization image scanogram or sinogram is often displayed as the first image of an examination. It is displayed prior to the examination by slit scanning as the tabletop moves the patient through the tightly collimated primary beam. The resolution of the image is affected by the speed of the scan and the exposure output of the tube. The poorer the scan, the less the patient dose. Because these images are used primarily for localization, image quality is seldom important. The radiographer should advocate the highest-speed scan and the lowest-exposure output possible. The addition to the slit scan of dotted lines corresponding to the section intervals provides a convenient reference guide when viewing the sectional images. The scanogram can serve as a diagnostic tool in radiation therapy treatment planning by using a cursor to delineate the margins of a tumor on a series of transverse sections. The scanogram can then compile the cursor delineations to provide a coronal and sagittal outline of the tumor. The scanogram is sometimes called by one of a number of trademark names.

Grid Application. A grid pattern may be added to any image. Radiographers use the grid to confirm exact centering of the patient; radiologists use the grid pattern to describe precise structural locations.

Cursor. A cursor can be used to outline an area of interest. The area can be recorded on film and the Hounsfield unit mean or standard deviation can be displayed for the tissue within the marked area. Hounsfield units (HUs) are discussed in the later section titled "CT Numbers (Hounsfield Units)." A line can be drawn between any two cursor locations, displaying the area's measurement within the patient. A cursor can also be used by itself to mark an area of interest. Mapping and volume estimates are achieved through cursor guidance as well.

Density contouring software is available that permits selection of a single point by a cursor, with the program highlighting all pixels of matching HU. This feature can be used to outline a tumor or other object to compile volume estimates.

Special software is also available to facilitate **radiation therapy treatment planning** through the use of cursors and integration with dosimetric data from a dosimetry computer.

Reverse Display. Reverse display is available to reverse the image from left to right and/or reverse the density display so that blacks appear white and whites appear black.

Magnification. Although nearly unlimited magnification may be accomplished, distortion usually becomes objectionable beyond 3×.

Suppression. Originally designed to suppress the information from surgical clips, this feature permits a problem area, such as a surgical clip, to be outlined and then deleted from the reconstruction data.

Annotation. Text may be added to images for descriptions or anatomical labeling.

Histograms. A histogram is a bar graph that may provide useful diagnostic data in some instances. Software is available to produce these graphs by Hounsfield units and by time versus motion. Volumetric analysis is possible with some histographic data.

A histogram of the Hounsfield units along a line drawn between two cursor points may be useful in some diagnoses. Histograms of various motions versus time may also be displayed for diagnosis of vascular flow or heart motion. These histograms are of limited value in CT because other modalities, especially ultrasonography and nuclear medicine, produce more accurate information.

Three-Dimensional Imaging. Software is available that will reconstruct CT data into three-dimensional images (Figure 41-19) that can be manipulated in all three dimensions. The image can be rotated, tumbled, or tilted to demonstrate structures that would otherwise be hidden. Images can be adjusted to various degrees of translucency and can be divided. For example, an image of the head may have soft tissue density reduced to 25 percent, bone density reduced to 50 percent, and the right half of the image removed to permit viewing of the left side of the sella turcica.

CT NUMBERS (HOUNSFIELD UNITS)

The true linear attenuation coefficients of the tissue voxels are not exactly represented by the data received by the CT computer. Therefore, a series of tissue density values has evolved for CT measurements. Originally named *computed tomography numbers*, they were renamed Hounsfield units (HUs) after the Nobel Prize was awarded to Godfrey Hounsfield in 1979. These numbers are calculated by comparing the linear attenuation coefficient of each pixel to the linear attenuation coefficient of water, according to the following formula:

$$\text{CT Number} = 1.000\,\frac{\mu_p - \mu_w}{\mu_w}$$

where: μ_p = linear attenuation coefficient of measured pixel, and
μ_w = linear attenuation coefficient of water.

Therefore, the HU of water is always 0, average bone +1,000, and air −1,000. Table 41-4 illustrates the HU of other tissues. The CT unit can display the HU of any given volume of tissue. Most units use a cursor to delineate the pixels to be measured and then display the HU on the screen next to the image. Radiologists may use HUs occasionally to assist in diagnosis even though the original hope of defining HUs for specific pathologies has not been realized. The attenuation data received by CT detectors is accurate ±0.2 percent; therefore, HUs are accurate ±2.

IMAGE RECONSTRUCTION

The detectors send information proportional to the attenuation coefficient of the voxel of tissue lying between the detector and the x-ray tube. The CT image is then reconstructed using a mathematical algorithm (usually based on Fourier transformation or a

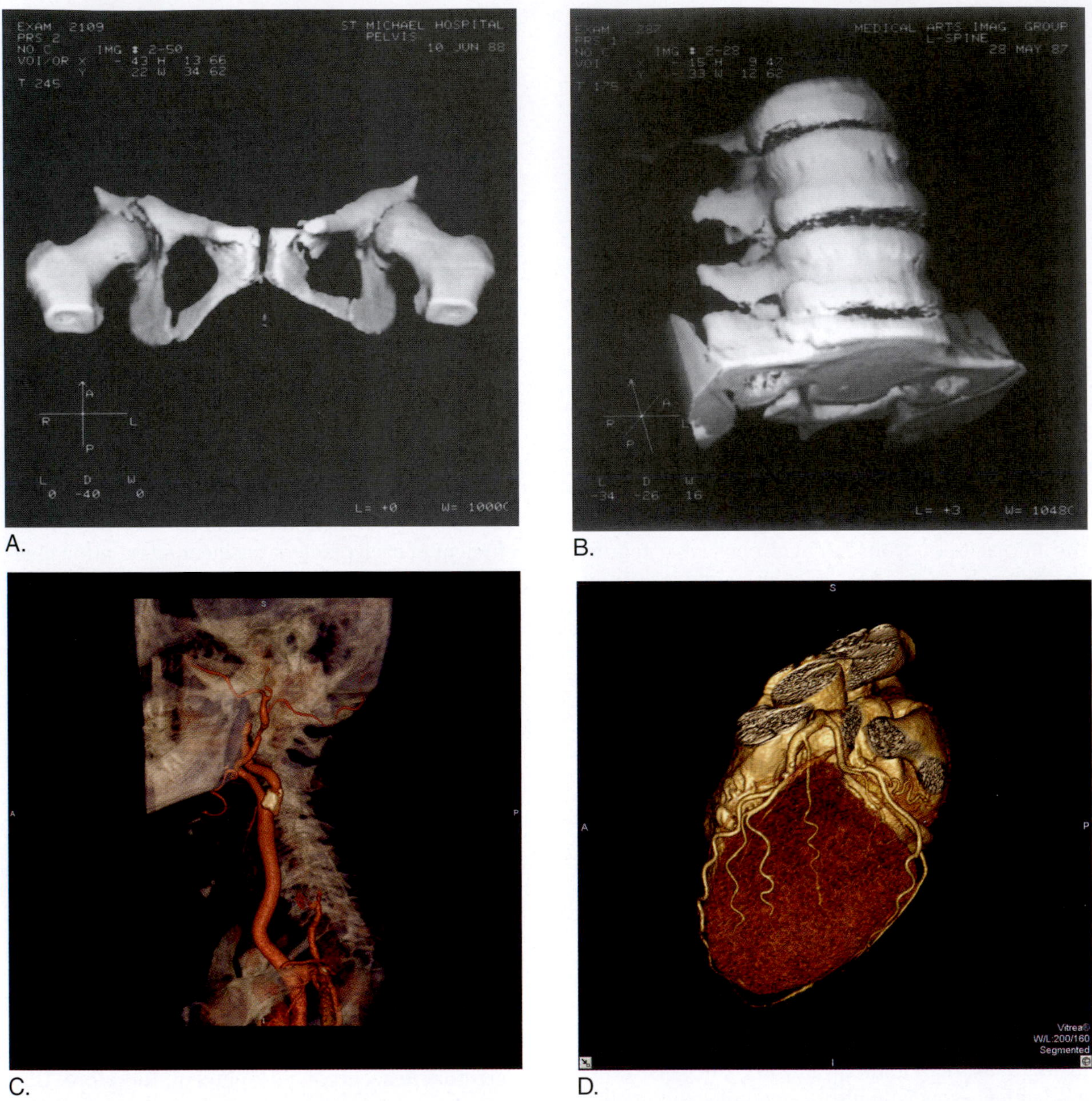

FIGURE 41-19. Three-dimensional CT reconstructions. (A) Pelvis, (B) spine, (C) carotid arteries, and (D) coronary arteries. *(Courtesy of Toshiba America Medical Systems, Inc.)*

combination of convolution and back-projection) of the digitized information received by the computer.

The programs used by CT scanners compensate for numerous intrinsic and extrinsic factors, including the emission spectrum of the beam, and weighting factors for the geometrical aberrations caused by beam divergence and semicircular detector arrangement. Reconstruction often requires up to 30 seconds. However, when an array processor is used, reconstruction time can be decreased to less than 1 second, which is desirable for dynamic studies.

TABLE 41-4. Hounsfield Units (HUs) (CT Numbers) of Various Tissues

Tissue	HU
Bone, petrous	+ 3,000
Bone, average	+ 1,000
Bone, cortical	+ 800
Blood, clotted	+ 55–75
Spleen	+ 50–70
Liver	+ 40–70
Pancreas	+ 40–60
Kidney	+ 40–60
Aorta	+ 35–50
Muscle	+ 35–50
Brain, white matter	+ 36–46
Cerebellum	+ 30
Brain, gray matter	+ 20–40
Blood	+ 13–18
Cerebrospinal fluid	+ 15
Tumors	+ 5–35
Gallbladder	+ 5–30
Water	0
Orbits	− 25
Fat	− 100
Lungs	− 150–400
Air	− 1,000

Fourier Transformation and Back-Projection

The primary mathematical method used in the creation of computerized medical images is the Fourier transformation. Transformations are simply conversions of data to more useful forms, as when radiation doses are changed from rems to mSv. Visual transformations can also be useful, as when a decubitus abdomen radiograph is viewed horizontally to facilitate detection of air-fluid levels.

Fourier's mathematics accomplishes transformations of extremely complex functions into separate but simpler functions. For example, a Fourier transform can be applied to separate music into functions of varying amplitudes, frequencies, and timing phases. This data can then be recorded for use in a magnetic tape player or CD-ROM. The Fourier transform permits the reconstruction of portions of the data when the other portions and their relationships are known. It is also possible to use the inverse Fourier transform to change back to the original data.

In digital imaging, the Fourier transform is used on data representing image intensities at specific locations. For example, Figure 41-20 demonstrates different attenuation coefficients at specific image receptor locations.

The information received by the image receptors can be processed through a variety of mathematical formulas (often referred to as algorithms or kernels). The Fourier algorithm is a fundamental formula used in image reconstruction.

It is based on algebraically adding several sets of incoming data from the image receptor. For example, in Figure 41-21, the top two waveforms have been combined to produce the bottom wave. Figure 41-22 illustrates how several different additions would change to combined waveforms. Finally, Figure 41-23 shows how numerous additions would produce a square waveform. Various mathematical algorithms can change or transform the amplitude

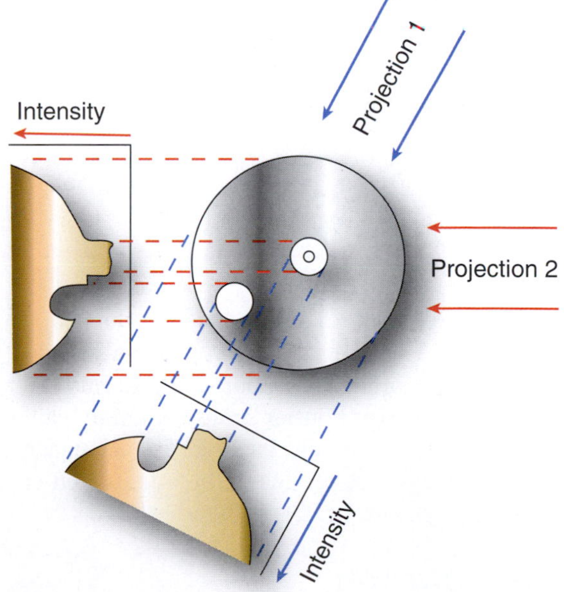

FIGURE 41-20. Image receptor data correlated to specific spatial locations. *(Reprinted from* Computers in Radiology, *Greenfield, G. B. & Hubbard, L. [1984] with permission from Elsevier.)*

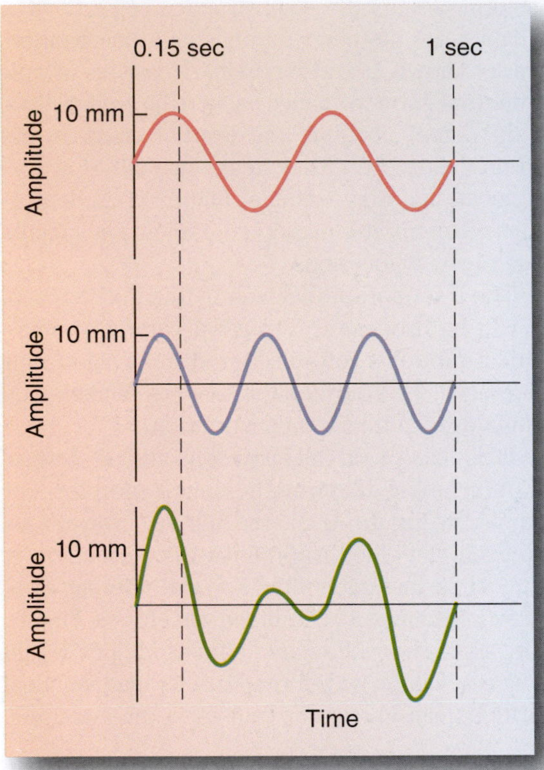

FIGURE 41-21. Basic Fourier algorithm. The top two waveforms have been combined to produce the bottom wave. *(Used by permission from Hedrick, W. R., & Hykes, D. L. [1992]. "A Simplified Explanation of Fourier Analysis,"* Journal of Diagnostic Medical Sonography, *J.B. Lippincott, Philadelphia, PA, 8[6], 302–303.)*

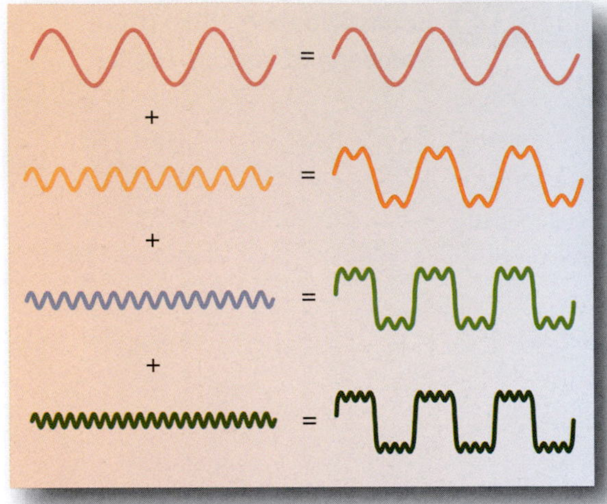

FIGURE 41-22. Basic Fourier algorithm. Several different additions changed to a combined waveform. *(Used by permission from Hedrick, W. R. ,& Hykes, D. L. [1992]. "A Simplified Explanation of Fourier Analysis,"* Journal of Diagnostic Medical Sonography, *J.B. Lippincott, Philadelphia, PA, 8[6], 302–303.)*

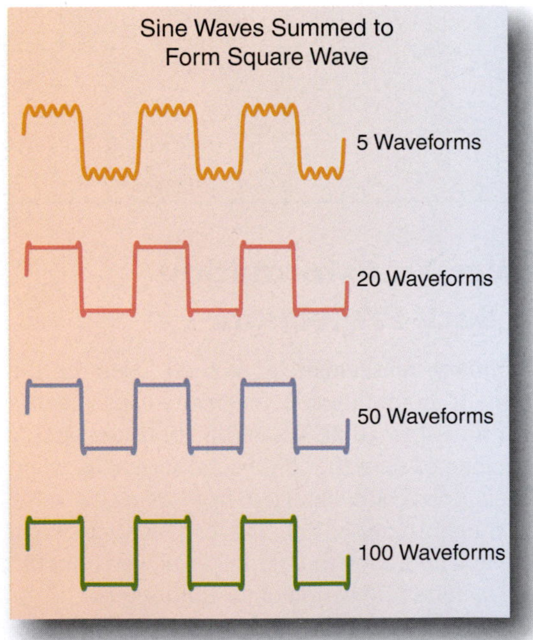

FIGURE 41-23. Basic Fourier algorithm. Numerous additions producing a square waveform. *(Used by permission from Hedrick, W. R., & Hykes, D. L. [1992]. "A Simplified Explanation of Fourier Analysis,"* Journal of Diagnostic Medical Sonography, *J.B. Lippincott, Philadelphia, PA, 8[6], 302–303.)*

and time domain to the frequency domain, and vice versa. This transformation process is called a Fourier transform or fast Fourier transform (FFT).

The inverse Fourier transformation can be used to mathematically back-project an image of the structures that produced the attenuation coefficients, as demonstrated in Figure 41-24.

Convolution and Deconvolution

It is sometimes useful to modify the value of each pixel to enhance or suppress a visual characteristic of the image. This process is actually mathematical filtering. **Convolution** is the process of modifying

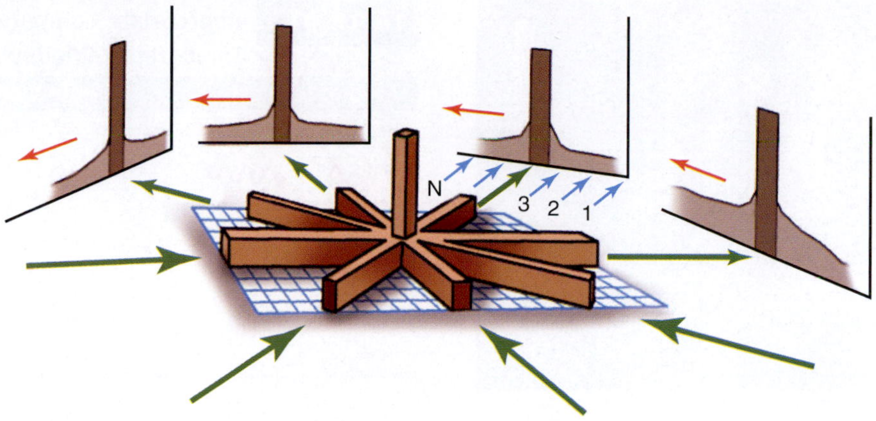

FIGURE 41-24. Image receptor data correlated to specific spatial locations. *(Reprinted from* Computers in Radiology, *Greenfield, G. B. & Hubbard, L. [1984] with permission from Elsevier.)*

pixel values by a mathematical formula. It is sometimes called a **mask** because a set of mathematical operations is placed over each pixel, the pixel value is changed, the mask is then applied to the next pixel, and so on. The total process is one of sliding the mask over all the pixel data and then displaying the modified image. **Deconvolution** is the process of returning the pixel values to their original level by a reverse process.

Helical Interpolation

Helical scanning occurs in a pattern that is at an angle to the perpendicular plane that is desired for imaging. To "straighten up" the sectional image, it is necessary to apply post-acquisition algorithms to the dataset. This process is called interpolation. Figure 41-25 shows how these algorithms function. Essentially, the raw dataset is projected, or interpolated, forward or backward into a theoretical perpendicular section. It is possible to use these algorithms to create a wide variety of sections that are reconstructions of data, not additional radiation exposure to the patient.

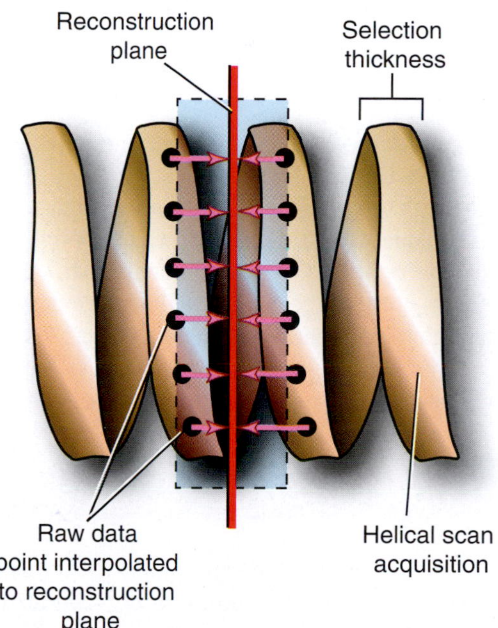

FIGURE 41-25. Helical scanning interpolation. The red line represents the theoretical perpendicular section into which the true helical raw data set is projected (whether forward or backward). This theoretical perpendicular section forms the image that is displayed. The section thickness is controlled by the pitch of the raw helical scan acquisition.

Reformatting

Reconstruction software is available that permits reformatting the information from a series of sectional images to produce an image of a section not actually scanned. For example, the extracted coronal image could be formed by reconstruction of only the appropriate voxels from each of the transverse sections. A typical reformatted CT image is shown in Figure 41-26. It is also possible to reconstruct images through an interactive process

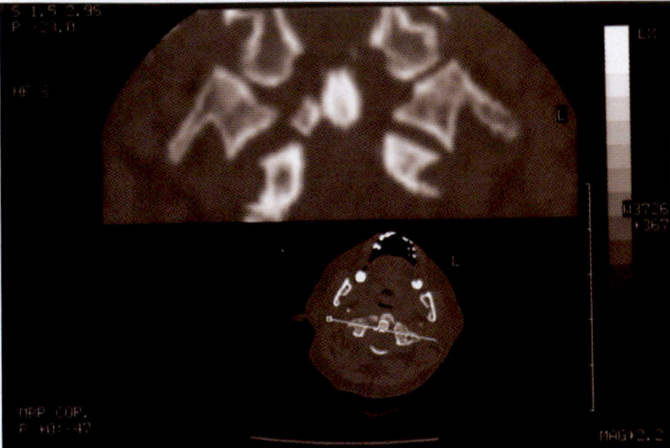

FIGURE 41-26. A reformatted CT image. The upper image is a coronal reconstruction from data acquired during axial transverse scanning of the cervical spine. Note the square bone fragment from the fracture. It is against the left side of the circular dense of C-2 at the center of the image. *(Courtesy of Barbara Imber and St. Rita's Medical Center, Lima, Ohio.)*

that accesses the raw data set to re-create other perspectives of the information.

Reformatting may also be used for a magnification technique called **targeting,** which permits an area of interest to be selected for reformatting. The reformatting process reconstructs the image data in a smaller pixel size to permit magnification with less distortion. This technique is used for regions in which extremely fine detail is necessary, such as the inner ear.

IMAGE QUALITY

Computed tomography image quality is primarily controlled by resolution and noise considerations. Density and contrast, as with any digitized image, can be manipulated by the computer. The prime consideration of the radiographer when making decisions regarding how to perform a particular CT examination must involve obtaining the necessary resolution while limiting noise.

Density and Contrast

Display density and contrast differences are varied with window level and width controls. Most CT images can demonstrate contrast differences of as little

TABLE 41-5. Appropriate Computed Tomography Window Widths

Area of Interest	Window Width (HU)
Head	70–200
Spine	350–750
Orbits	350–700
Heart	250–350
Abdomen	250–450
Thorax for lungs	1,200–1,400
Inner ear	2,000–4,000

as 0.4 percent (4 HUs), as compared to a minimum of 10 percent for a diagnostic radiograph. Appropriate CT window widths are shown in Table 41-5.

Resolution

The resolution of the CT image depends on pixel, voxel, and matrix size. High-contrast objects 1.5 times the pixel size or larger can be imaged reliably. For example, a pixel size of 0.5 mm can resolve an object 0.75 mm in size. Low-contrast objects may require a larger pixel size to permit the detectors to provide sufficient data to reach a visible difference between the attenuation coefficients. Therefore, low-contrast objects may actually be seen better with a larger pixel size, although the total resolution is reduced. The current spatial resolution possible is about 0.35 mm, as compared to 0.25 mm and better with diagnostic radiography. However, this resolution is not possible under routine scanning conditions.

Voxel, Pixel, and Matrix Size. Discussion of CT imaging detail must consider voxel, pixel, and matrix size. It is possible to have pixels and matrix size equal yet the voxel width may have a considerable effect on image quality. Matrix sizes offered on CT units have included 256 × 256, 320 × 320, 360 × 360, and 512 × 512. Because most CT images are processed and displayed with a circular field, the actual number of image pixels is less than if the matrix were square. For example, a 512 × 512 circular field matrix has slightly over 200,000 pixels.

Voxel width may be varied between 8 mm and 13 mm. A common voxel size might be 1 mm × 1 mm × 10 mm, with 10 mm representing the voxel width. The 20 percent additional tissue volume of a 13-mm voxel requires 60 percent more radiation exposure to produce an image of comparable quality. Therefore, patient dose considerations in CT are similar to those in diagnostic radiography.

Interface Artifacts. Depending on the mathematical algorithm used, imaging aberrations displayed as density differences may occur when two objects have more than a 60 percent difference in attenuation coefficients. These artifacts are called undershoot and overshoot. Any object of greatly different contrast, such as metallic surgical clips, bullets, an old contrast medium, and air, is likely to cause a star pattern artifact. The effect can be somewhat modified by using a larger matrix. However, different reconstruction algorithms that mathematically filter or compensate for the effect have been designed for various body parts. For example, a soft tissue algorithm is useless during examination of the inner ear. A special bone algorithm is required to produce useful information when numerous small bony structures are in close proximity to one another.

Magnification. The display or reconstruction **field of view** (FOV) is different from the scan field of view (SFOV). True CT magnification is achieved by choosing a smaller display field of view. This produces an image with less tissue per voxel, which in turn provides higher resolution and a larger image of a smaller area of interest. Magnification of the matrix field size has no effect on image resolution. When a CT image matrix is magnified it may be possible to perceive individual pixels. This causes the image to appear less sharp. Therefore, most radiologists prefer to diagnose from images of a smaller size that are sharp.

Noise. All digital images have noise problems. **Noise** on a CT image is directly related to the amount of data collected by the detector. It appears as quantum mottle (best seen in an image of a water phantom) and normally comprises 3–5 percent of the image. Most CT image noise is a result of statistical fluctuation in the information recorded by the detector, not a result of computer reconstruction mathematics. The amount of noise controls the low-contrast resolving ability of the CT unit. A standard CT quality assurance measurement is a daily noise evaluation that is done by imaging a phantom and using a cursor to read the HUs for control areas. Each reading should average at least 100 pixels (10 × 10 matrix).

Motion. Motion on a CT image is a function of exposure time, just as in diagnostic radiography. The exposure time in CT is controlled by the quantity of data detected. Because insufficient data results in a poor-quality image, motion during a CT scan is displayed as a series of very-poor-quality images. For example, a rib that moves is recorded in a series of locations due to the movement instead of in a stationary location as would result if respiration had been suspended. Each of the movement images is of poor quality because the detector received too little data to permit reconstruction of a normal-quality image (Figure 41-27). Helical and MSCT scanners can perform interrupted or skip-scanning to compensate for patient breathing motion.

SCANNING PROCEDURES

Section Interval and Thickness

The section interval is the distance between scan sections. The section thickness is the width of the volume of tissue being examined (the voxel). Section thickness is usually slightly less than voxel width because of the divergence of the beam. Both the section interval and the thickness are affected by the section shape.

Although section thickness is equivalent to voxel width, or slightly less, a section does not have parallel sides due to the divergence of the x-ray beam. Figure 41-28 illustrates the section shape problem that either overlaps or excludes tissue between sections. One author has described the total scan volume as more like a stack of frisbees than a stack of coins (Figure 41-29). The scanning procedure must take this geometry into account. Overlapping, which occurs with section intervals equal to voxel width, is desirable. For example, a voxel width of 13 mm should use section intervals of 13 mm. In most procedures it is important that no sections of tissue miss examination. Overlap and exclusions must be considered when designing the section interval sequence for the scanning

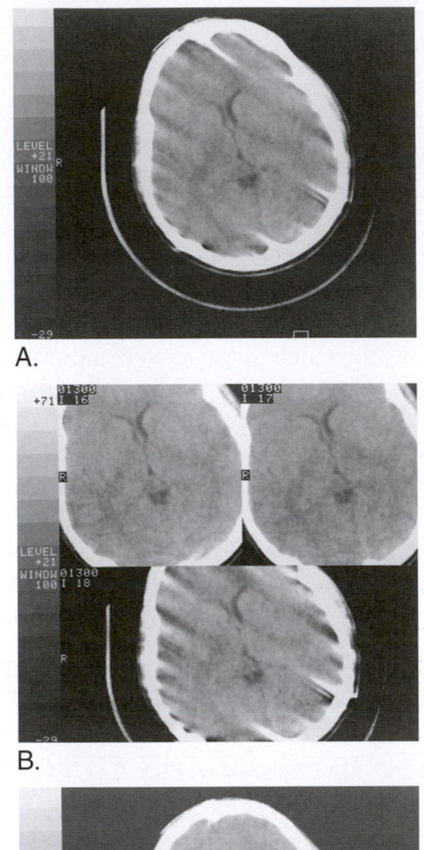

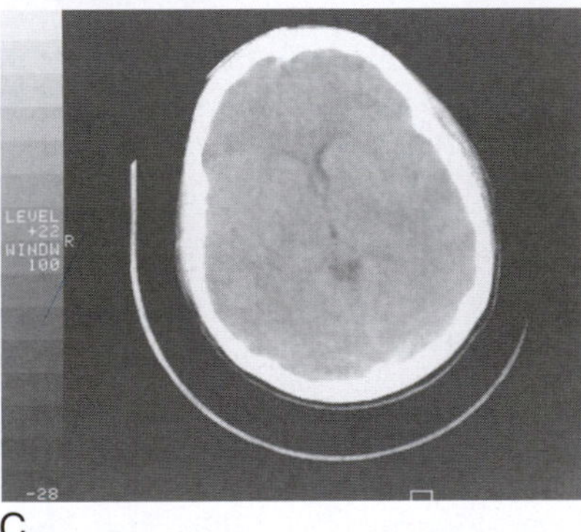

FIGURE 41-27. Computer correction of motion: (A) motion artifacts obscuring information; (B) separate images for each third of the scan time reveal all the motion that occurred during the final third of the scan; and (C) reconstruction using only the first two-thirds of the scan time produces a diagnostic-quality image. *(Images courtesy of Richard R. Carlton.)*

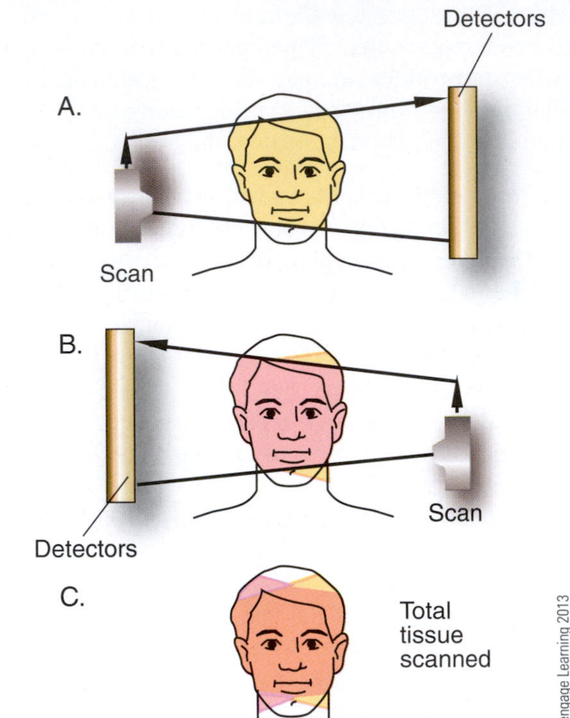

FIGURE 41-28. Section shape due to divergent beam geometry. (A and B) The first scan produces a wedge-shaped volume of scanned tissue. (C) The final scan produces a concave volume of double-scanned tissue with a convex volume of single-scanned tissue at the edges.

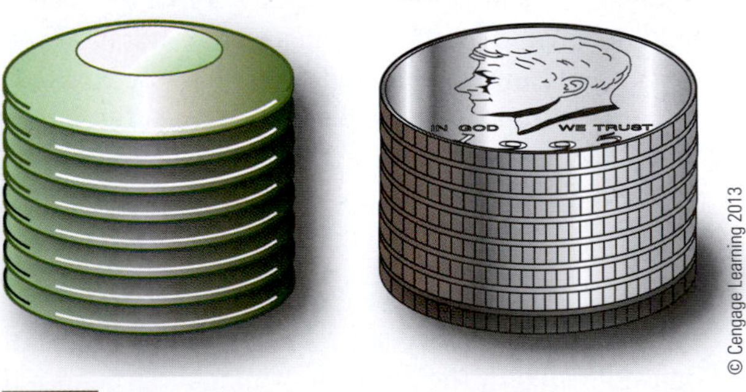

FIGURE 41-29. The total scan volume is more like a stack of Frisbees than a stack of coins.

procedure. Most CT unit programs have standardized scanning procedures for the various examinations, although they can be modified to fit specific circumstances and institutional requirements.

Exposure Factors

Most CT scanning is performed at a set kVp. Time is not a factor, as it must be controlled by the scanning program to provide sufficient exposure to the detectors. The CT radiographer can vary the mA to control the primary beam. However, dual energy scanning units require scanning with different kVp values, usually 80 kVp or 140 kVp.

Algorithms

As discussed earlier under image reconstruction techniques, the proper reconstruction algorithm must be used to mathematically filter unwanted artifacts. The CT console often combines the proper algorithm with the scanning procedure. High-pass and low-pass filters and other mathematical manipulations can also be performed to improve image quality.

Scan Field of View (SFOV) Size

The SFOV is set to accommodate the size of the part under examination. The smaller the scan field size, the better the image resolution and the faster the scan time. Common field sizes are 25 cm for the head and magnification of the spine, 35 cm for small bodies, and 48 cm for large bodies.

ARTIFACTS

Motion

Motion is a problem in CT because it produces streak artifacts through the image (Figure 41-30). The algorithm faults when it receives the changes in attenuation that occur at the edges of the moving part. This produces blank pixels, which appear as streaks in these regions.

Metal or Star

The presence of metallic materials in the patient also cause streak artifacts but may also produce star artifacts (Figure 41-31). The metal objects attenuate nearly 100 percent of the primary beam, which produces an incomplete projection. This may produce a star artifact if the reconstruction algorithm has been unable to create a full set of surrounding projections to smooth the edges of the object. Some CT units have software algorithms designed to reduce and partially correct for these artifacts.

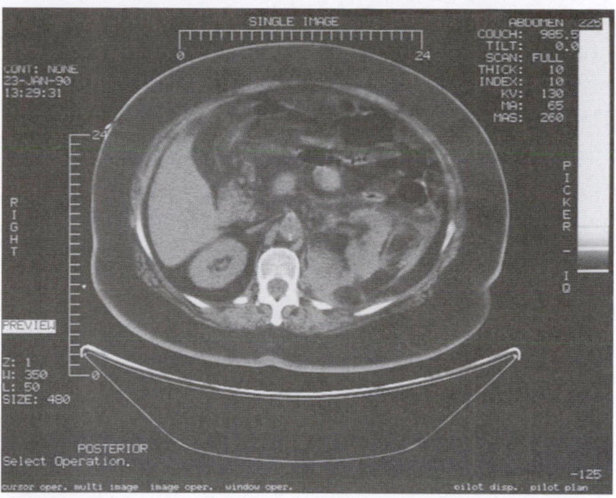

FIGURE 41-30. A typical computed tomography motion artifact. *(Courtesy of Wil Reddinger, Lima Technical College, Lima, Ohio.)*

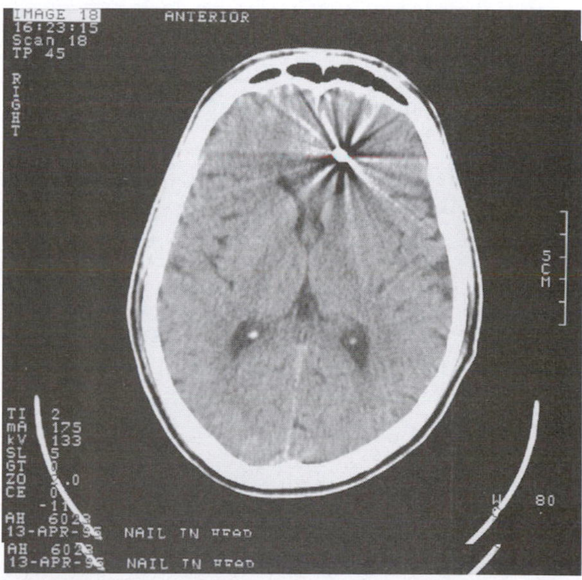

FIGURE 41-31. A typical computed tomography metal or star artifact. *(Courtesy of Wil Reddinger, Lima Technical College, Lima, Ohio.)*

Beam Hardening

Beam hardening artifacts are a result of the attenuation of the beam as it passes through the patient. The CT number of a posterior structure may be much different from that of a similar anterior structure because the beam reaching the posterior structure has already been significantly attenuated. Beam hardening artifacts are often described as broad dark bands or streaks known as cupping artifacts (Figure 41-32). A capping artifact occurs when the algorithm overcompensates for the beam hardening artifact. Cupping artifacts have lower CT numbers than expected, whereas capping artifacts have higher CT numbers than expected. Software algorithms are available to reduce or partially correct for their effect on the image.

Partial Volume Effect

Because the data from an entire section thickness is averaged together to form the image, the exact location of a section may cause small structures or portions of large structures to be hidden when they comprise only a small percentage of the total section. This is a common concern during CT of the vertebral column when a section interval happens to produce a section where an intervertebral disc comprises a small percentage of the total section volume (Figure 41-33). This is called the partial volume effect. It may obscure any object that is smaller than the voxel width (section thickness) when that object is scanned by two sections. Compensation for the partial volume effect may be overcome in some instances by slightly overlapping sections.

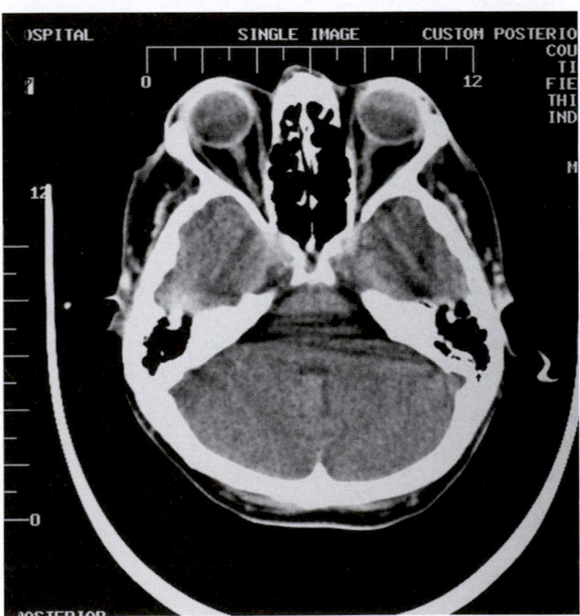

FIGURE 41-32. A typical computed tomography cupping or beam hardening artifact. *(Courtesy of Wil Reddinger, Lima Technical College, Lima, Ohio.)*

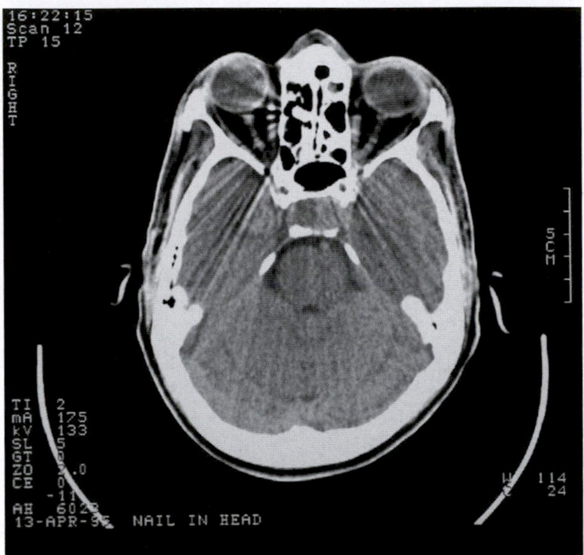

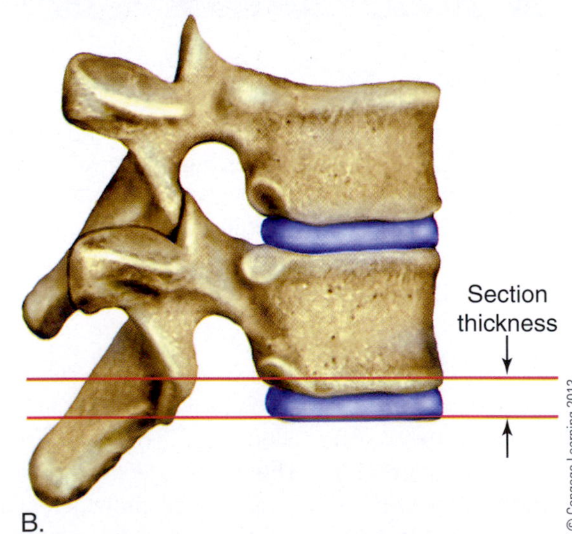

FIGURE 41-33. (A) A typical computed tomography out-of-field artifact demonstrating a severe partial volume averaging effect. *(Courtesy of Wil Reddinger, Lima Technical College, Lima, Ohio).* (B) A graphic illustration of the partial volume effect.

Ring Artifacts

When a single detector goes out of calibration and does not properly record incoming attenuation data, the projection (or view) includes a detector error, as shown in Figure 41-34A. When this error is multiplied during the scan, an annular or ring artifact, such as that illustrated in Figures 41-34B and C, is produced.

Numerous artifacts are unique to computed tomography. The more common include motion, metal, beam hardening, partial volume effect, and ring artifacts.

RADIATION PROTECTION

Patient Dose

Lowering Dose. The Alliance for Radiation Safety in Pediatric Imaging recommends the following practices for reducing doses to children:

- Significantly reduce, or child-size, the amount of radiation used
- Do not overscan:
  - Scan only when necessary
  - Scan only the indicated region
  - Scan once; multiphase scanning (pre- and post-contrast, delayed exams) is rarely helpful
- Be a team player:
  - Involve medical physicists to monitor pediatric CT techniques
  - Involve technologists to optimize scanning

Patient dose during computed tomography was originally measured according to the concepts of diagnostic radiology. Because the CT scan irradiates tissue via a tightly collimated beam that is moved over the patient, it became necessary to find a new method to measure patient dose during CT examinations. In 1981 the U.S. Food and Drug Administration (FDA) Bureau of Radiological Health (BRH), now known as the Center for Devices and Radiological Health (CDRH), developed the computed tomography dose index (CTDI) and the multiple scan average dose (MSAD). The CTDI measures the radiation dose to the patient as measured within the primary beam of the CT scanner. The MSAD represents the average dose a patient receives during

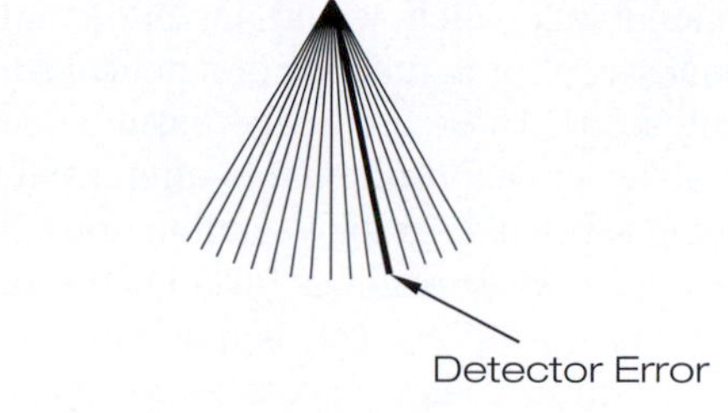

Ring Artifact

B.

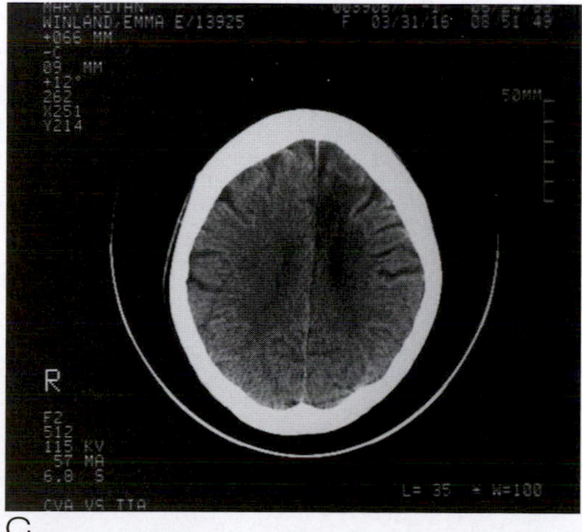

FIGURE 41-34. A typical tomography ring artifact. (A) The effect of a defective detector cell on a single projection. (B) The sum effect of the multiple projections that comprise the entire image. (C) An example scan with a ring artifact. *(Courtesy of Wil Reddinger, Lima Technical College, Lima, Ohio.)*

an examination, which would include numerous individual scans (or in the case of a helical scanner, a moving scan). These are actual tissue doses, not the entrance skin exposure that is often used to describe diagnostic radiography examinations.

Example MSAD readings for a head scan vary from 4–8 rads (4–8 cGy). This is much greater than the typical entrance skin exposure for a single skull radiograph, which may range from 0.105 to 0.24 rad (0.105–0.24 cGy). Of course, the comparisons are somewhat absurd as the CT examination provides vastly more information than a single radiograph, or even the entire series of exposures that would comprise a full skull examination.

Filtration is used in CT in a manner similar to that in diagnostic radiography, although CT uses much greater amounts of filter. A special "bow tie" filter has been developed for CT that matches the beam divergence and shape of the patient's body in transverse section (Figure 41-35).

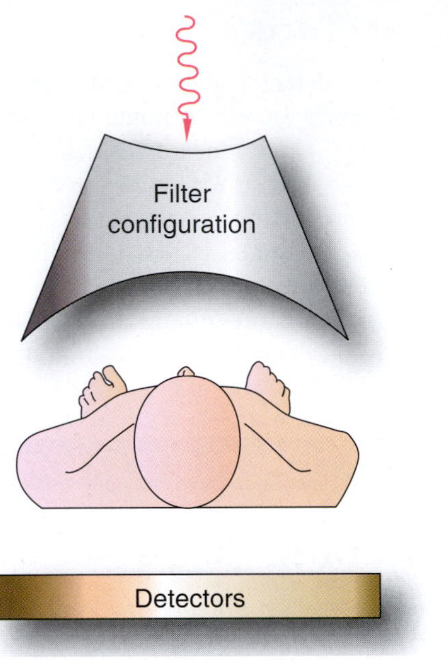

FIGURE 41-35. A CT bow tie filter.

Dose to Others

Dose to other persons in the scanning room results primarily from scatter from the patient, as during fluoroscopy. Lead aprons and other appropriate protective equipment should be used by anyone in the scanning room during examinations. A routine scan might produce a scatter dose of 2 to 5 mrads per section at 1 meter from the patient. Unless absolutely necessary, no one should be present in the scanning room while the unit is in operation. When someone must be present, he or she should remain as far from the patient as possible to take best advantage of the inverse square law. Standard radiation protection procedures should be followed. The most desirable person to stay with a patient is a relative, then a nonradiology staff member. A radiology department member is the last to be considered. Although use of a remotely controlled power injector is preferred, persons who must manually inject a contrast medium during scanning procedures should stand behind a lead shield, as far from the gantry as possible.

SUMMARY

Computed tomography (CT) produces a digital tomographic image from diagnostic x-rays. The basic principle of CT involves digitizing an image received from a slit scan projection of the patient's body and then back-projecting it through mathematical algorithms.

A modern CT unit includes a gantry, table, x-ray tube, detectors, computer, display console, and image storage units. The gantry is the movable frame of the CT unit. It contains the x-ray tube and detectors and is the most visible part of the unit. The gantry frame maintains the alignment of the tube and detectors and contains the equipment necessary to perform the scanning movements. CT tables are usually made of carbon graphite fiber to decrease beam attenuation and must support the entire weight of the patient without sagging when fully extended. They are rated

SUMMARY (continued)

for maximum weight. Modern pulsed scanner x-ray tubes operate at 120 kVp, 1- to 5-msec pulses, and up to 1,000 mA. CT detectors include xenon-gas-filled ionization chambers, which measure ionization in air by attracting to an electrode the ions created by x-ray photons in the air, and solid-state detectors.

The CT computer is designed to control data acquisition, process and display, and storage. The CT console operates from a "menu" or index directory of operations. The radiographer uses a keyboard, light pen, or other input device to indicate the desired operation. The data acquisition program controls a variety of operations, including tube and detector collimation (pixel size), matrix size, gantry angle, tabletop entrance into the gantry aperture, section increment movements of the tabletop, x-ray tube voltage and amperage, scan speed, and direction of detector signals to the digital image processing section of the computer. The processing and display program controls the digital image production process. The display console permits a wide range of display features, including the scanogram, grid pattern, cursor, density contouring, radiation therapy planning, reverse display, magnification, suppression, annotation, histograms, and three-dimewwnsional imaging. Hounsfield units (HUs), or CT numbers, represent the tissue density values for each pixel.

Computed tomography image quality is primarily controlled by resolution and noise considerations. Density and contrast, as with any digitized image, can be manipulated by the computer and are varied with window level and width controls. The resolution of the CT image depends on pixel, voxel, and matrix size. Imaging aberrations (artifacts) displayed as density differences may occur when two objects have more than a 60 percent difference in attenuation coefficients. Noise on a CT image is directly related to the amount of data collected by the detector. Motion on a CT image is a function of exposure time, just as in diagnostic radiography.

The section interval is the distance between scan sections. Its determination is effected by the section shape and the partial volume effect. Section thickness is equivalent to voxel width, or slightly less. Because the data from an entire section thickness is averaged together to form the image, the exact location of a section may cause small structures or portions of large structures to be hidden when they comprise only a small percentage of the total section. This is called the partial volume effect.

Numerous artifacts are unique to computed tomography. The more common include motion, metal, beam hardening, partial volume effect, and ring artifacts.

Because of the strictly collimated primary beam, most CT examinations have a patient dose much greater than that of the same part in diagnostic radiography examinations. Filtration is used in CT in a manner similar to that in diagnostic radiography. Dose to other persons in the scanning room results primarily from scatter from the patient, as during fluoroscopy. Lead aprons and other appropriate protective equipment should be used by anyone in the scanning room during examinations. ■

REVIEW QUESTIONS

1. What are the major components of a modern MSCT unit?
2. What is the gantry?
3. Why are tabletops rated for maximum weight?
4. What is the purpose of the detectors in a CT unit?
5. What operations are controlled by the data acquisition program?
6. What is a scanogram?
7. How are Hounsfield units (HUs) (CT numbers) calculated?

8. What controls the density, contrast, and resolution of the CT image?
9. Explain the partial volume effect.
10. Explain how a ring artifact is produced.
11. How does patient dose in CT compare to the doses for routine radiography?

REFERENCES AND RECOMMENDED READING

AAPM. (2011). Definition of a qualified medical physicist. Retrieved from http://www.aapm.org/medical_physicist/fields.asp.

ACR. (2011). Technical standard for diagnostic medical physics performance monitoring of computed tomography (CT) equipment. Retrieved from http://www.acr.org/SecondaryMainMenuCategories/quality_safety/guidelines/med_phys/ct_equipment.aspx.

Ambrose, J., & Hounsfield, G. (1973). Computerized transverse axial tomography. *British Journal of Radiology, 46*(148), 1023–1047.

Berland, L. L. (1987). *Practical CT technology and techniques.* New York: Raven Press.

Brenner, D. J., Elliston, C. D., Hall, E. J., Berdon, W. E. (2001). Estimated risks of radiation induced fatal cancer from pediatric CT. *American Journal of Radiology, 176*, 289–296.

Brooker, M. J. (1986). *Computed tomography for radiographers.* Lancaster, UK: MTP Press Limited.

Brooks, R. A., & DiChiro, G. (1975). Theory of image reconstruction in computed tomography. *Radiology, 117*, 561.

Brooks, R. A., & DiChiro, G. (1977). Slice geometry in computer assisted tomography. *Journal of Computer Assisted Tomography, 1*(2), 191–199.

Bushberg, J. T., Seibert, J. A., Leidholdt, E. M., & Boone, J. M. (2002). *The essential physics of medical imaging* (2nd ed.). Philadelphia: Lippincott Williams & Wilkins.

Bushong, S. C. (2009 9th ed.). *Radiologic science for technologists: Physics, biology, and protection* (8th ed.). St. Louis, MO: Elsevier/C. V. Mosby.

Chiu, L. C., Lipcamon, J. D., & Yiu-Chiu, V. S. (1995). *Clinical computed tomography for the technologist* (2nd ed.). New York: Raven.

Coulam, C. M., Erickson, J. J., Rollo, F. D., & James, A. E. (1981). *The physical basis of medical imaging.* New York: Appleton-Century-Crofts.

Crawley, M. T., Booth, A., & Wainwright, A. (2001). A practical approach to the first iteration in the optimization of radiation dose and image quality in CT. *British Journal of Radiology, 74*, 607–614.

Curry, T. S., Dowdey, J. E., & Murry, R. C. (1990). *Christensen's introduction to the physics of diagnostic radiology* (4th ed.). Philadelphia: Lea and Febiger.

Forster, E. (1985). *Equipment for diagnostic radiography.* Lancaster, UK: MTP Press.

Fox, S. H., & Toth, T. (2002). Dose reduction on GE CT scanners. *Pediatric Radiology, 32*(10), 718–723.

Frush, D. (2002). Pediatric CT: Practical approach to diminish the radiation dose. *Pediatric Radiology, 32*(10), 714–717.

Frush, D. P. (2002). Strategies of dose reduction. *Pediatric Radiology, 32*(4), 293–297.

Frush, D. P., Slack, C. C., Hollingsworth, C. L., Bisset, G. S., et al. (2002). Computer-simulated radiation dose reduction for abdominal multidetector CT of pediatric patients. *American Journal of Roentgenology, 179* (5), 1107–1113.

General Electric. (1976). *Introduction to computed tomography* (Publication 4691). Milwaukee, WI: General Electric Company, Medical Systems Division.

Harper, C. (1979). CT scanners: The industry behind the science. *Radiologic Technology, 51* (2), 199–202.

Hendee, W. R. (1983). *The physical principles of computed tomography.* Boston: Little, Brown and Co.

Hounsfield, G. N. (1973). Computerized transverse axial scanning (tomography): Part I. Description of system. *British Journal of Radiology, 46*, 1016–1022.

Hounsfield, G. N. (1979). Computed tomography: Past, present, and future. In L. Kreel & R. E. Steiner (Eds.), *Medical imaging.* Chicago: Year Book.

Huda, W. (2002). Dose and image quality in CT. *Pediatric Radiology, 32*, 709–713.

Huda, W., Chamberlain, C. C., Rosenbaum, A. E., et al. (2001). Radiation doses to infants and adults undergoing head CT examinations. *Medical Physics, 28*, 393–399.

Huda, W., Scalzetti, E. M., & Levin, G. (2000). Technique factors and image quality as functions of patient weight at abdominal CT. *Radiology, 217*, 430–435.

Instruction manual for testing the ACR CT phantom. (2011). Retrieved from http://www.acr.org/accreditation/computed/qc_forms/Phantom_Testing_Instruction_Final.aspx.

Kalender, W. A., Arkadiusz, P., & Christoph, S. (1994). A comparison of conventional and spiral CT: An experimental study on the detection of spherical lesions. *Journal of Computer Assisted Tomography, 18* (2), 167–176.

Knapp, R. H., Vannier, M. W., & Marsh, J. L. (1985). Generation of 3-D images from CT scans: Technological perspective. *Radiologic Technology, 56* (6), 391–398.

Kreel, L., & Steiner, R. E. (Eds.). (1979). *Medical imaging.* Chicago: Year Book.

Kuni, C. C. (1988). *Introduction to computers and digital processing in medical imaging.* Chicago: Year Book.

Lee, J. K., Sagel, S. S., & Stanley, R. J. (1990). *Computed body tomography* (2nd ed.). New York: Raven Press.

Lucaya, J., Piqueras, J., Garcia-Pena, P., et al. (2000). Low-dose high resolution CT of the chest in children and young adults: Dose, cooperation, artifact incidence, and image quality. *American Journal of Roentgenology, 175*, 985–992.

McCollough, C., Branham, T., Herlihy, V., et al. (2006). Radiation doses from the ACR CT accreditation program: Review of data since program inception and proposals for new reference values and pass/fail limits. Presented at the RSNA 92nd Scientific Assembly and Annual Meeting, 2006.

McCullough, E. C., & Payne, J. T. (1977). X-ray transmission computed tomography. *Medical Physics, 4*, 85.

Morgan, C. L. (1983). *Basic principles of computed tomography.* Baltimore: University Park Press.

Morgan, H. T. (2002). Dose reduction for CT pediatric imaging. *Pediatric Radiology, 32* (10), 724–728.

Moss, A. A., Gamsu, G., & Genant, H. K. (1984). *Computed tomography of the body.* Philadelphia: W. B. Saunders.

Nagel, H. (2005). Multislice CT technology. Retrieved from http://www.multislice-ct.com/www/page.php?guide=en_introduction_36 retrieved 7-29-05.

New CT accreditation dose requirements effective January 1, 2008. (2008). Retrieved from http://www.acr.org/accreditation/FeaturedCategories/ArticlesAnnouncements/NewDoseReq.aspx.

Parker, J. A. (1990). *Image reconstruction in radiology.* Boca Raton, FL: CRC Press.

Parkinson, L. (1991). Assessment of dose in computerized tomography. *Radiography Today, 57* (650), 23–28.

Paterson, A., & Frush, D. P. (2007). Dose reduction in paediatric MDCT: General principles. *Clinical Radiology, 62* (6), 507–517.

Reiser, M., Taskahashi, M., Modic, M., & Becker, C. (2004). *Multislice CT* (2nd ed.). New York: Springer.

Ritman, E. L., Kinsey, J. H., Robb, R. A., Harris, L. D., & Gilbert, B. K. (1980). Physical and technical considerations in the design of the DSR: A high temporal resolution volume scanner. *American Journal of Roentgenology, 134*, 369–374.

Romans, L. E. (2011). *Computed tomography for technologists: A comprehensive text.* Philadelphia: Kluwer Lippincott Williams & Wilkins.

Seeram, E. (1978). Computed tomography: An overview. *Radiologic Technology, 49* (4), 491–496.

Seeram, E. (1983). A course on CT for radiologic technologists: A conceptual framework. *The Canadian Journal of Medical Radiation Technology, 14* (1), 11.

Seeram, E. (1989). *Computers in diagnostic radiology.* Springfield, IL: Charles C Thomas.

Seeram, E. (2008). *Computed tomography: Physical principles, clinical applications, and quality control* (3rd ed.). St. Louis: Elsevier Saunders.

Shope, T. B., Gagne, R. M., & Johnson, G. C. (1981). A method for describing the doses delivered by transmission x-ray computed tomography. *Medical Physics, 8*, 488–495

Short, A. J. (1981). Reconstructions in computerized transverse axial radiography. *Radiography, 47* (557), 119.

Shrimpton, P. (1994). Patient dose in CT and recommendations for reduction. *Radiography Today, 60* (683), 9–11.

Ter-Pogossian, M. M. (1983). Physical principles and instrumentation. In J. K. T. Lee, S. S. Sagel, & R. J. Stanley (Eds.), *Computed body tomography.* New York: Raven.

Varchena, V. (2002). Pediatric phantoms. *Pediatric Radiology, 32*, 280–284.

Westerman, B. R. (2002). Radiation dose from Toshiba CT scanners. *Pediatric Radiology, 32* (10), 735–737.

Whitmore, R. C., Bushong, S., Archer, B., & Glaze, S. A. (1979). Radiation dose in neurological computed tomography scanning. *Radiologic Technology, 51* (1), 21–26.

Wolbarst, A. B. (1993). *Physics of radiology.* Norwalk, CT: Appleton & Lange.

Wong, E. T., Yu, S. K., Lai, M., Wong, Y. C., & Lau, P. C. (2001). MAPD—an objective way to select mAs for paediatric brain CT. *British Journal of Radiology, 74*, 932–937.

Yaffe, M., Fenster, A., & Johns, H. E. (1977). Xenon ionization detectors for fan beam computed tomography scanners. *Journal of Computer Assisted Tomography, 1* (2), 419–428.

Yoshizumi, T. T., Suneja, S. K., & Teal, J. S. (1989). Practical CT dosimetry. *Radiologic Technology, 60* (6), 505.

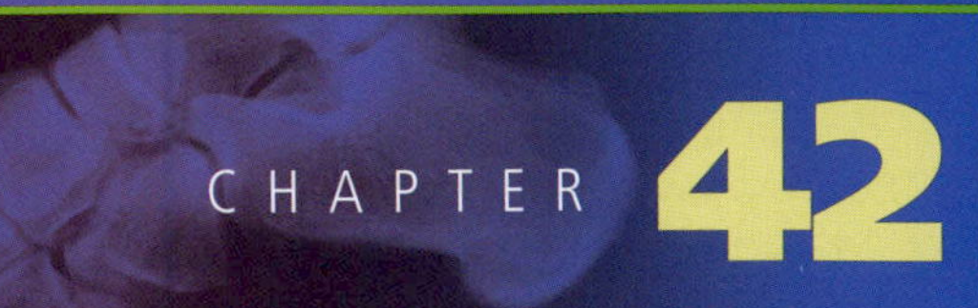

CHAPTER 42

Magnetic Resonance Imaging

William Faulkner, BS, RT(R)(MR)(CT), FSMRT,
and Carolyn Kaut-Roth, RT(R)(MR)(CT)(M)(CV), FSMRT

KEY TERMS

cryogen
gyromagnetic ratio
Larmor frequency
precession
radiofrequency (RF)
specific absorption rate (SAR)
surface coil
time of inversion (TI)
T_1
T_2
tesla

We are dealing not merely with a new tool but with a new subject, a subject I have called simply nuclear magnetism . . . the history of ordinary magnetism . . . has been rich in difficult and provocative problems, and full of surprises. Nuclear Magnetism . . . is like that too.

Edward M. Purcell, from his Nobel Lecture, December 11, 1952
Reprinted from Edelman, 1990, Clinical Magnetic Resonance Imaging, with permission from Elsevier.

OBJECTIVES

Upon completion of this chapter, the student should be able to:

- Describe the source of the magnetic fields within the body that are used during MRI.
- Describe the properties of proton precession as used in MRI.
- Define T_1, T_2, p, TR, TE, and TI.
- Explain the functions of x, y, and z gradient coils in selecting an image section by the use of the Larmor equation and a gradient magnetic field.
- Describe the use of RF pulses in the various MRI pulse sequences.
- Describe the components of an MRI unit, including the stationary magnet, gradient and RF coils, table, and computer consoles.
- Explain how MR image contrast is controlled.
- Describe the use of paramagnetic contrast agents.
- Discuss methods of reducing MRI image noise.
- Discuss safety measures for protection of all persons who approach the MRI unit magnetic field.

HISTORY

Magnetic resonance imaging (MRI) had its beginning as nuclear magnetic resonance (NMR). Primarily used by chemists, its basic principles date back to the days of Nikola Tesla, who discovered the rotating magnetic field in 1892 in Budapest, Hungary. Sir Joseph Larmor (1857–1942) developed an equation (now known as the Larmor Equation) that shows the relationship between the resonant (**precessional**) frequency of nuclei and an externally applied magnetic field. In 1937, Professor Isidor I. Rabi discovered the phenomena dubbed "nuclear magnetic resonance" based on the interaction of magnetically active nuclei in a strong magnetic field. Felix Bock (Stanford University) and Edward Purcell (Harvard University) received the Nobel Prize for Physics for their work in developing the instruments to measure the magnetic resonance in materials such as liquids and solids. This represented the birth of NMR spectroscopy. Beginning in the 1970s, Dr. Raymond Damadian (Downstate Medical Center, New York) demonstrated relaxation time differences between normal and abnormal tissues. In 1973, Paul Lauterbur (University of Illinois) described a technique he termed as zeugmatography, which utilized gradient magnetic fields to produce two-dimensional images using back-projection. In 1975, Richard Ernst described two-dimensional NMR using phase and frequency encoding along with Fourier transform for image reconstruction (as opposed to back-projection). In 1977, Dr. Damadian published an image through the human chest acquired using a technique he termed FONAR.

Beginning with the first commercial scanners installed during the 1980s, magnetic resonance imaging (as it is now known) has become a major method for imaging not only anatomic structures but also physiologic functions of the human body.

MRI uses the magnetic properties of hydrogen (^{1}H) to produce images of the body. It requires the patient to be placed within a large externally applied magnetic field in order to magnetize the tissue. **Radiofrequency (RF)** coils produce a pulsed magnetic field (radio waves) to rotate the magnetic field of the tissues through a receiving coil (antenna), inducing an MR signal. Additional coils within the MRI system produce gradient magnetic fields (magnetic fields that vary in intensity), which are utilized to spatially encode the detected signals. Currently, the most widely used technique for MR image reconstruction is the fast Fourier transform (FFT).

The contrast of the resultant MR images is a function of the particular type of technique or sequence used to acquire the data and the type and timing of the RF pulses. Contrast agents based on materials with magnetic properties can be utilized to enhance visualization of structures and/or lesions.

It is not the purpose of this chapter to teach in detail the concepts and clinical applications of MRI but rather to provide the reader with an overview of this marvelous and useful tool for imaging the human body.

INSTRUMENTATION

Given that MRI does not utilize ionizing radiation to produce images of the body, as with CT, very different hardware and electronics are required. The main components of an MRI unit include: the main magnet, the radiofrequency subsystem, and the gradient coil subsystem (Figure 42-1). As with most digital imaging modalities, there is a patient couch (or table), an operator console, and the computer subsystem (Figure 42-2).

Magnet

The magnet produces the externally applied static magnetic field referred to as the B_0 field. The purpose of the B_1 field is to magnetize the tissue. The strength of field produced by the system magnet (field strength) is expressed in units of **tesla** and is measured at isocenter (the precise center of the magnet where the patient lies). One (1) tesla (1 T) equals 10,000 Gauss. Current MR systems used for clinical imaging range in field strengths from 0.2 T to 3.0 T. As a point of reference, the earth's magnetic field is approximately 0.5 G. A 3.0-T system (30,000 G) is therefore approximately 60,000 times stronger than the earth's magnetic field. The higher

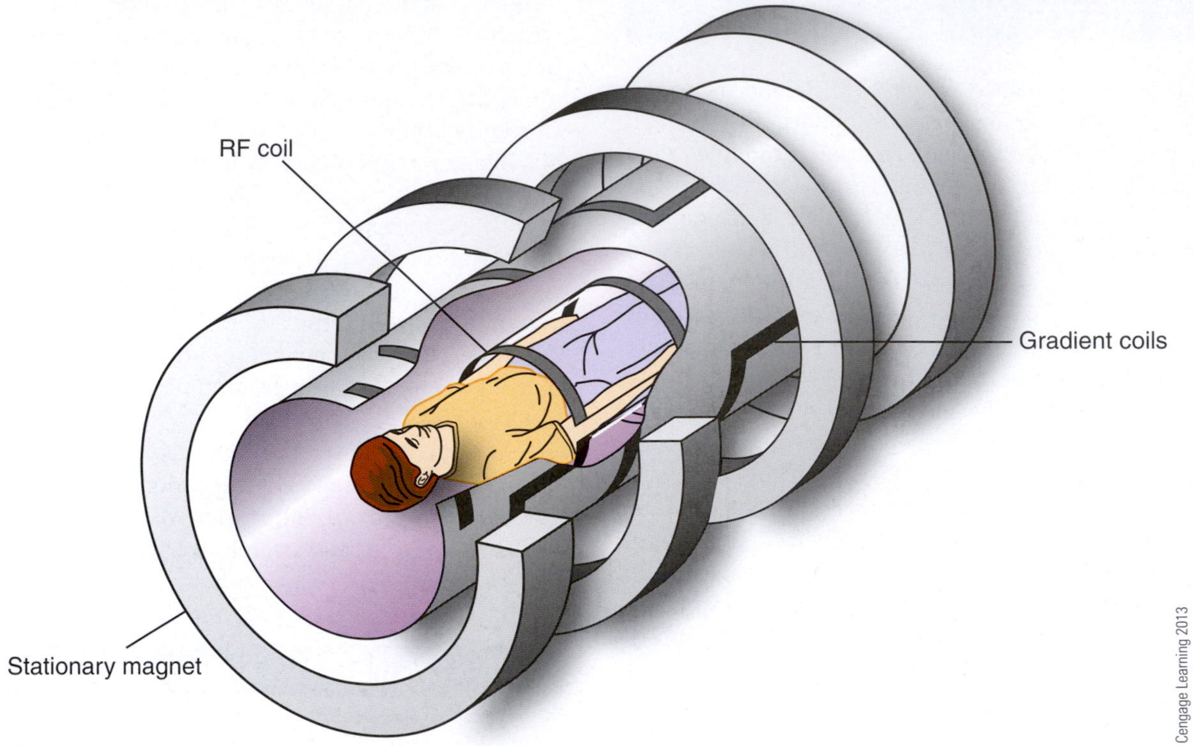

RF coil

Gradient coils

Stationary magnet

FIGURE 42-1. A typical magnetic resonance imaging unit.

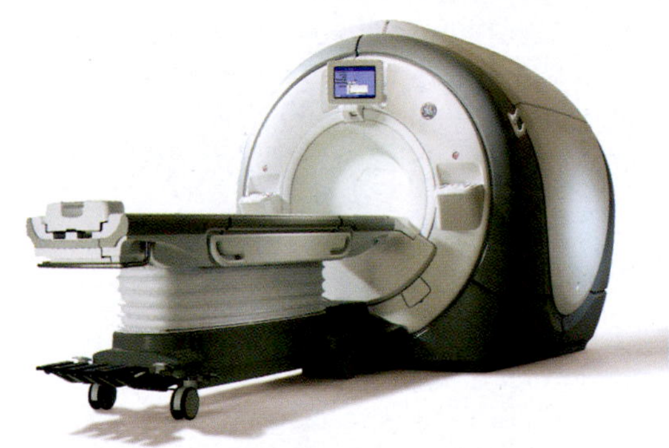

FIGURE 42-2. An MRI system. *(Courtesy of GE Healthcare.)*

the field strength of an MR system, the greater the tissue is magnetized and therefore the greater the available signal from the tissues being imaged. Increasing the available signal from the tissue is important, as this provides greater flexibility in acquisition techniques—primarily either by allowing for shorter acquisition times or higher spatial resolution.

There are primarily three types of magnet designs used for MR systems: permanent, resistive, and superconducting, as discussed next

Permanent Magnets. Permanent magnets, as the name implies, are constructed of "bricks" of material that are naturally magnetic. They are arranged such that the systems have a magnet above and below the patient table. The magnets are supported by aniIron frame that also serves to return the field. Given the design, the magnetic field direction is oriented along the y axis of the patient, resulting in a vertical field. Many have referred to these types of systems as *open MRI*. This term, however, is a marketing-derived term and should not be applied only to these types of magnets, as, in truth, all magnets are open in some respects. The field strength typical of various permanent MRI systems ranges from approximately 0.2 T up to approximately 0.35 T.

Resistive Magnets. Another method for the creation of the magnetic field is with electricity. These types of magnets are known as electromagnets. When direct current is passed through a wire, a static magnetic field is created around the wire. If these wires are configured in the shape of a coil or a "Slinky"™, this is known as a solenoid electromagnet. Solenoid electromagnets are lighter than permanent magnets, are low in field strength, and require a power supply. These types of electromagnets are known as resistive systems. Although they are low in field strength, these resistive systems can be "turned off" when not in use (unlike other MR imaging systems). The field strength typical of various resistive MR systems ranges from approximately 0.2 T up to approximately 0.7 T.

Superconducting Magnets. Permanent and resistive MR systems are limited with respect to how strong a magnetic field can be produced using those technologies. In order to obtain a higher field strength, superconducting technology is utilized. Because the property of resistance is temperature dependent, reducing temperature will reduce resistance. Therefore, to create a system without resistance, the solenoid electromagnet can be "submerged" into a cryogenic liquid. The **cryogen** most commonly used in superconducting MRI systems is liquid helium (He). The temperature of liquid He is 4 Kelvin (K), or – 452° Fahrenheit (F). This resistance-free system is known as a superconducting system. Currently, most MR systems in clinical use are superconducting systems.

The main magnetic field is located within the imager, but also extends out and around the imager. This field (outside the imager) is known as the fringe field or stray field. In order to confine the fringe field, magnetic field shielding is used. Magnetic field shielding can be applied either passively or actively. Passive shielding is similar to the shielding used in radiography, whereby the imaging room walls are lined with metal. In x-ray this metal shielding is lead; in MRI the passive shielding (for the static field B_0) is iron. (Bear in mind that MR systems are also shielded for RF. RF shielding will be discussed in the radiofrequency (B_1) section.) Another method for shielding in MRI is known as active shielding. The term *active* implies activity or current. For MRI, active shielding uses additional electromagnets to confine the fringe field.

The shim system is used to provide a means for magnetic field homogeneity. Homogeneity is expressed in units of either parts per million (ppm) or Hertz (Hz). Shimming can be accomplished actively or passively (like shielding). Passive shimming is accomplished with the use of metallic plates, strategically placed around the main magnet, known as shim plates. Active shimming is accomplished by shim coils. Shim coils are an additional set of electromagnetic coils, whereby current is added as needed.

Radiofrequency (RF) Subsystem

The RF subsystem consists of a transmitter and one or more receivers. The RF transmitter is used to produce RF energy required for excitation of the hydrogen protons. The RF transmitter coils use alternating current, and therefore produce an oscillating magnetic field known as the secondary magnetic field (B_1). The frequency of radiofrequency signals is expressed in units of megahertz (mHz). There is a specific frequency that is associated with each magnetic field strength, known as the **Larmor frequency**. In most MR imaging systems, there is a transmitter coil located within the imager itself. In other systems, the transmitter coil is positioned onto the patient during image acquisition. The RF receiver coil and its associated electronics are used to provide a means for detection of MR signals. As previously mentioned, some coils both transmit and receive while others may receive only. The determination of the type of coil configuration that is used is primarily a vendor preference.

In general, larger coils are uniform with regard to transmission, whereas smaller coils are more sensitive with regard to reception. Most MR systems have multiple types and shapes of RF coils designed for specific body parts. In general, one would select the RF coil that best fits the body part being imaged. Figure 42-3 shows various MR coils.

The main issue with MR coils is that we want the higher SNR provided by the smaller coils but often need the coverage provided by a larger coil. The current solution is referred to as *multi-channel* or *phased-array* coils. A typical coil array contains multiple small elements. Within the system electronics are multiple receivers (receiver channels).

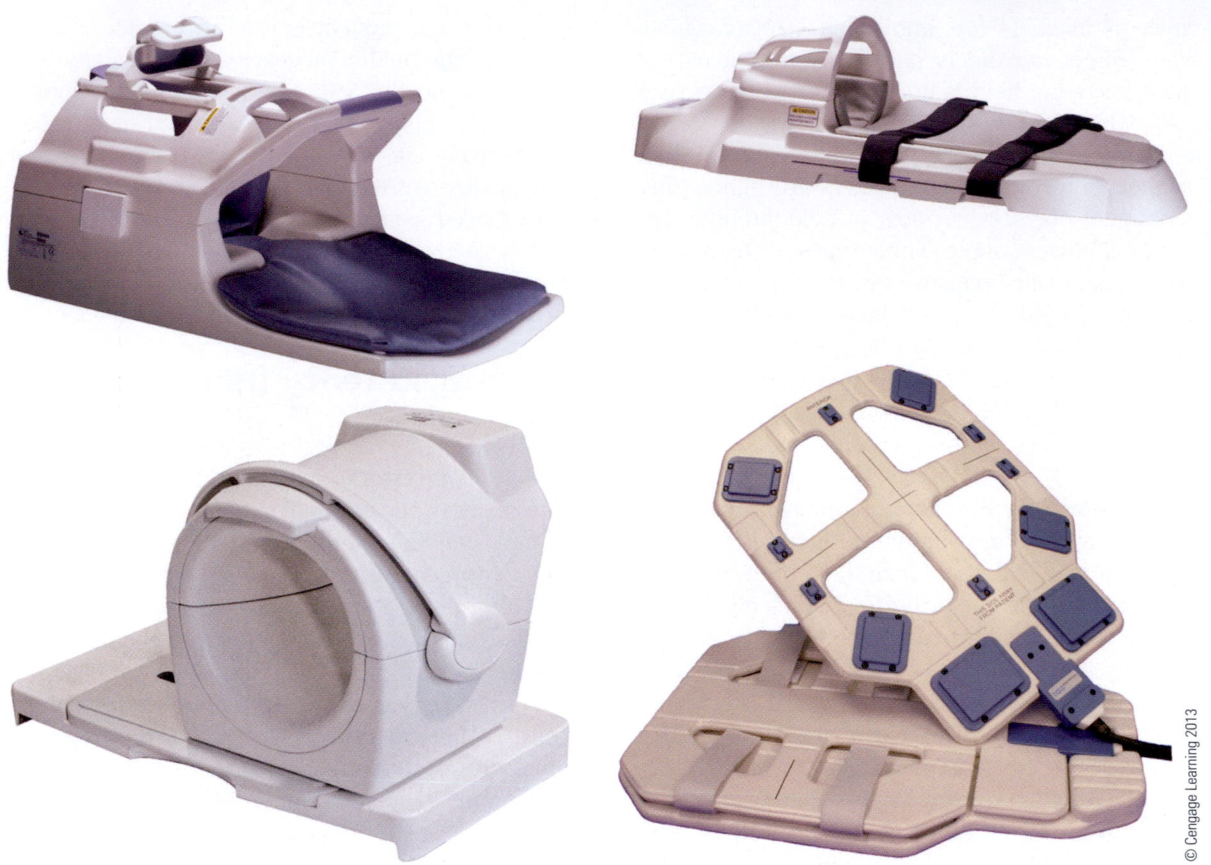

FIGURE 42-3. MR coils.

As an example, in an eight-channel MR system, there would be eight receiving channels. This would allow for up to eight coil elements to be utilized as separate and independent receiving coils. The overall coverage would be equal to the total area covered by the elements but the SNR would be related to the size of each individual element in the array. Multi-channel coils are instrumental in providing the high SNR required for high-spatial-resolution images or rapid data acquisition techniques. MR manufacturers continue to increase the number of receiver channels available for MR systems.

RF Shielding. Given that MRI utilizes radiofrequencies in TV and FM radio ranges, RF shielding is required to shield the sensitive receivers from detecting extraneous RF signals from the outside environment. This is done by lining the entire MR scan room with copper, effectively creating a Faraday cage (Figure 42-4).

Gradient Coils. Within the magnet enclosure (or bolted to the face of vertical field systems) are the gradient coils. The word *gradient* can be defined as expressing a slope or a rate of increase or decrease. The gradient magnetic field produced by the gradient coils is just that—a magnetic field that increases or decreases (slopes) over distance. The gradient fields are superimposed over the main magnetic field (B_0). The main purpose of the gradient magnetic fields is to provide or encode spatial information in the received MR signals. This is required for the production of images.

There are three sets of gradient coil windings within the coil itself (Figure 42-5). They produce a gradient magnetic field along the three orthogonal

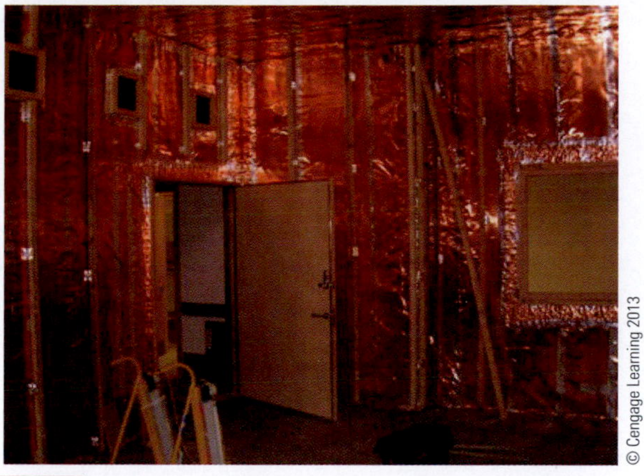

FIGURE 42-4. Copper RF Shielding Faraday Cage being built into an MRI room.

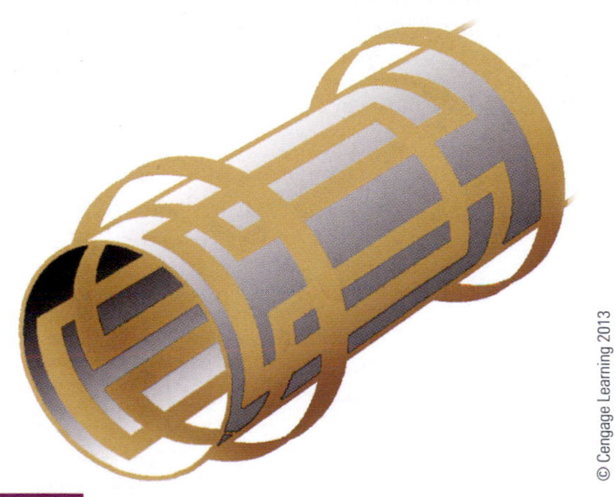

FIGURE 42-5. Gradient coil windings within the magnetic enclosure.

planes or directions of the body. They are annotated based on the direction in which their respective gradient field is produced. The coil that produces a gradient field along the head-foot direction of the patient/magnet is annotated as the z-gradient coil. The coil that produces a gradient field along the right-left direction of the patient/magnet is annotated as the x-gradient coil. The coil that produces a gradient field along the anterior-posterior direction of the patient/magnet is annotated as the y-gradient coil. Gradient coils are powered by gradient amplifiers, which are most likely located in an equipment room adjacent to or nearby the MR suite.

During the scan, the gradient coils are turned on and off rapidly by the scanning software and, as a result, vibrate within their housing/enclosure. This results in the sounds heard during the scan. In many systems, particularly higher-field systems, this noise is significant (i.e., greater than 99 dB) and hearing protection is required for the patient or anyone else in the scan room.

The gradient coils vary in intensity/strength not only over distance but also change over time. For this reason the field they produce may also be referred to as a *time-varying magnetic field.* As previously mentioned, the gradient coils are essential for encoding the MR signals required for the production of images.

MRI PHYSICS

Early in the evolution of the modality, the term *nuclear magnetic resonance*, or NMR, was widely used. In reality, it is still used in relation to chemical analysis. However, for medical imaging purposes, the term *magnetic resonance imaging*, or MRI, has been adopted. The term *nuclear* does not refer to radioactivity but rather to the nucleus of atoms.

Certain nuclei have properties that cause them to exhibit magnetic characteristics—that is, having an odd number of particles (protons and neutrons) in their nucleus. The sum of the nuclear particles is known as the atomic mass number, and these nuclei are considered to be magnetically active. The nuclear elements in these magnetically active nuclei are often referred to as *spins.* They exhibit a magnetic field known as a *magnetic moment.* In MRI, we utilize the magnetic properties of the hydrogen nucleus. Hydrogen has a single proton in its nucleus. Additionally, it is nearly 100 percent abundant in the human body, meaning that nearly all tissues and substances within the body contain hydrogen in their molecules. The hydrogen protons (or spins) behave as tiny bar magnets. A bar magnet has two poles and is referred to as a *dipole.*

Normally, the magnetic moments of the hydrogen protons are randomly aligned. However, when placed in a large externally applied magnetic field (B_0), their magnetic moments "align" either with (parallel) or against (anti-parallel) the direction of

B_0. In reality, they assume one of two energy levels or spin states. The low-energy state is represented by the parallel alignment and the high-energy state is represented by the anti-parallel alignment. After a few seconds, a slight majority of the spins will align their magnetic moments parallel with the externally applied magnetic field (B_0). As a slightly higher number of the spins are in the low-energy state (parallel alignment), the tissue will exhibit a bulk or net magnetization vector aligned parallel with the direction of B_0. This state is known as thermal equilibrium.

The alignment of the net magnetization is most often illustrated using a three-dimensional Cartesian coordinate system (Figure 42-6). The vertical axis of the graph is annotated with the letter z, and the horizontal (or transverse) axis is annotated with the letters x and y. When the patient is placed in the magnet of the scanner, the tissue magnetization will be aligned parallel with B_0, and will be illustrated as being along the z-axis of the three-dimensional Cartesian graph. Magnetization along this direction (z) is referred to as *longitudinal magnetization*. Longitudinal magnetization cannot be measured (or sampled). In order to measure an MR signal, the tissue's net magnetization must be "tipped" into the x-y or transverse plane. Only magnetization in the transverse plane can be measured or sampled.

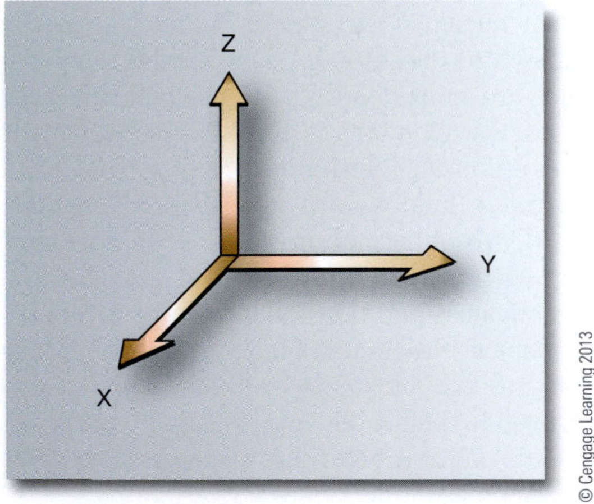

FIGURE 42-6. Alignment of net magnetization. The vertical axis of the graph is annotated with the letter "Z" while the horizontal (or transverse) axis is annotated with the letters "X and Y".

In order to do this, a secondary magnetic field is briefly applied. This is the RF or radiofrequency field. The way it is utilized in MRI is as a pulsed magnetic field (the B_1 field).

The hydrogen protons precess about the direction of B_0 in much the same fashion as a top wobbles as it spins (Figure 42-7). The rate at which the hydrogen protons precess is dependent upon the strength of B_0. This precessional or resonant frequency is known as the Larmor frequency, ω_0:

$$\omega_0 = \gamma B_0$$

where γ is the *gyromagnetic ratio* and B_0 is the strength of the applied magnetic field.

The symbol γ (gamma) is a constant known as the **gyromagnetic ratio**. For the hydrogen proton, its value is 42.6 MHz/tesla. As an example, if B_0 is 1.5 T, then the resonant or Larmor frequency is approximately 64 MHz (1.5 T × 42.6 MHz/T). In reality, at thermal equilibrium, the individual protons do not precess in phase (i.e., not at the same frequency). One reason is that the magnetic field is not uniform (homogeneous), particularly after the patient is placed in the magnetic field. Additionally, hydrogen protons in water molecules precess at a slightly

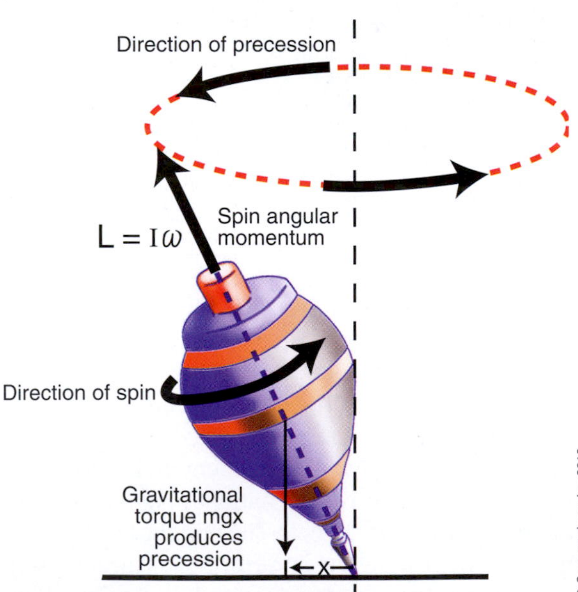

FIGURE 42-7. A spinning top illustrates how the hydrogen protons precess about the direction of B_0.

higher frequency than those in fat molecules. This difference in frequency based on the chemical environment is known as chemical shift. The difference in hertz between the frequency of hydrogen in water compared to fat depends on the field strength (B_0). Increasing B_0 increases chemical shift.

The B_1 or RF field used in MRI is much weaker than B_0. In order to tip the tissue's net magnetization from the longitudinal and into the transverse plane, the frequency of the RF pulse (B_1 field) must be centered about the Larmor or resonant frequency of the spins. If it were not "tuned" to the specific Larmor frequency, the net magnetization of the tissues would not be affected. When tuned to the Larmor (or resonant) frequency of the spins, there is a very efficient transfer of energy to the spins. The spins begin to precess in phase. At the same time, some of the spins in the low-energy state absorb energy from the RF field (B_1) and move from the low- to the high-energy state. As a result, the net magnetization rotates and tips outward toward the transverse plane. The greater the amount of RF power applied, the further the net vector tips away from its longitudinal alignment and into the transverse plane (Figure 42-8).

For our purposes, we will assume that an RF pulse of sufficient energy and duration is applied to tip the tissue net magnetization 90 degrees (fully into the transverse plane). The actual amplitude and duration of the RF pulse will vary with the specific sequence being performed. However, the duration of the RF pulse is generally only around 8 milliseconds (8 msec). Once the B_1 field is removed

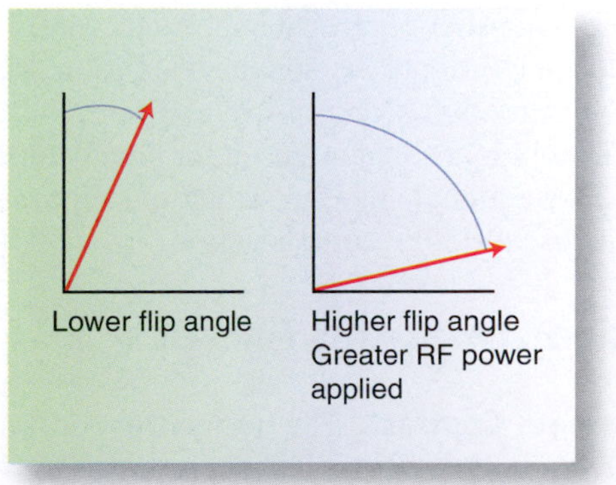

FIGURE 42-8. FLIP angle.

(stopped), the net magnetization is now precessing through the transverse plane. Our receiver coils are so designed that the net magnetization vector of the tissue is now precessing through a loop of conductive material (copper). Faraday's Law of Induction states that if a magnetic field moves through a loop of conductive material, it will induce a current in that conductor. In this way, the patient's magnetization induces the MR signal in the receiver coils. The receiver electronics (A/D converter) sample or measure the MR signal.

Upon removal of the B_1 field, however, the spins will begin to "relax" back to where we began, at thermal equilibrium. This relaxation process consists of two simultaneous yet independent processes: **T_2-** and **T_1-relaxation**. T_2-relaxation occurs due to an exchange of energy among the spins (hydrogen protons) and is referred to as spin-spin interaction. This exchange of energy results in the spins losing phase coherence. Additionally, field inhomogeneities and chemical shift further increase the loss of coherence among the spins. The result is an exponential decrease in detectable transverse magnetization and thus an exponential decrease in detectable MR signal. The rate of transverse magnetization decay varies with tissue type. Fat protons dephase much more quickly than water protons. Therefore, the signal from fat decays more quickly than that of water. The rate at which T_2-relaxation occurs for any given tissues is expressed by the T_2-relaxation time. Given that T_2-relaxation is exponential, the T_2-relaxation time for a given tissue is defined as when 63 percent of the transverse magnetization has decayed. T_2-relaxation times for all tissues are relatively quick and are expressed in milliseconds (msec). Although it is not necessary to remember T_2-relaxation times of tissues, as this is not used clinically, for purposes of understanding, the T_2-relaxation time of fat is approximately 50 msec at 1.5 T and water is approximately 200 msec at 1.5 T. The field strength is mentioned, as T_2-relaxation times are slightly affected by field strength.

If we were to look at the rate of decay based on T_2-relaxation alone, our signal decay would appear somewhat as shown in Figure 42-9. However, once the RF pulse ends, inhomogeneities in the magnet field and chemical shift (frequency differences between water and fat protons) immediately

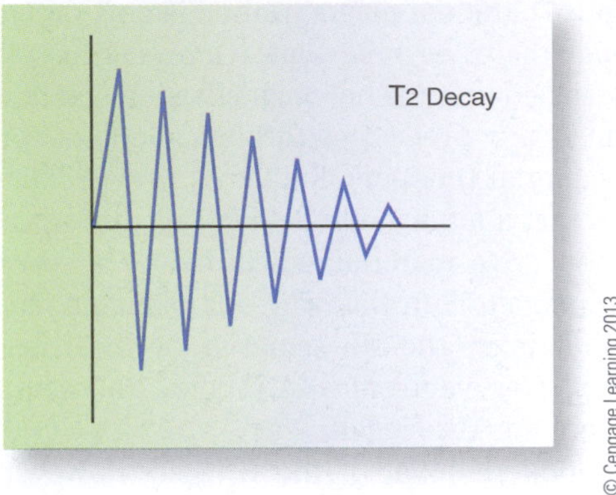

FIGURE 42-9. Rate of decay for T_2 relaxation alone.

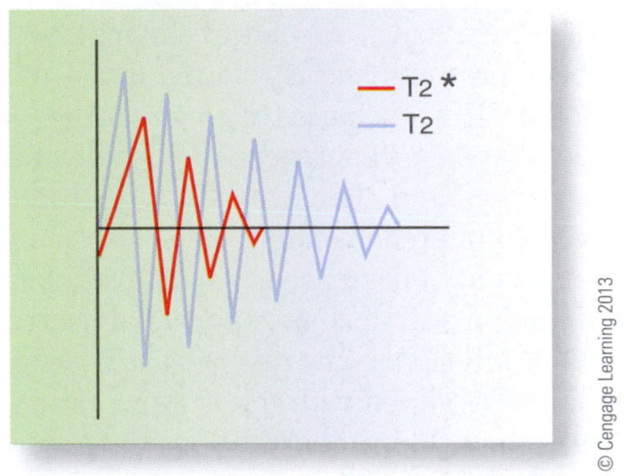

FIGURE 42-10. Rate of decay for T_2* relaxation.

begin to affect the spins, and this results in a more rapid decay of transverse magnetization. The rate of decay based on T_2-relaxation (i.e., spin-spin interaction) and these off-resonance effects (inhomogeneities and chemical shift) is known as T_2* (pronounced: "T_2-star"), as is illustrated in Figure 42-10. We can choose to correct for a majority of the off-resonant effects, or not, by way of selecting a certain type of imaging (or pulse) sequence. This will be discussed in more detail later.

At the same time (as T_2-relaxation is occurring), but independently, some of the spins in the high-energy state will lose their energy to their molecular lattice. This results in the tissue's net magnetization regrowing along the longitudinal or z axis and is known as T_1-recovery. This recovery of longitudinal magnetization is exponential and therefore the T_1-recovery time of a given tissue is defined as when 63 percent of longitudinal magnetization has recovered. As with T_2-relaxation times, T_1-relaxation times vary with tissue type. Fat protons have a short T_1-relaxation time of approximately 150 msec at 1.5 T. Water-based protons have a relatively long T_1-relaxation time of approximately 2,000 msec (2 seconds) at 1.5 T. T_1-relaxation times are very much affected by field strength (more so than T_2-relaxation times). As field strength increases, T_1-relaxation times of tissues lengthen. It is not, however, a linear relationship. For example, doubling B_0 does not double the T_1-relaxation time of a tissue. T_1-relaxation times are also dependent on temperature. Again, it is not important to memorize T_1- and T_2-relaxation times of tissues. It is only necessary to remember that fat protons have short T_1- and T_2-relaxation times while water protons have long T_1- and T_2-relaxation times.

Most pathology is associated with an increase in water content. Therefore, generally speaking, when tissue becomes diseased, the T_1- and T_2-relaxation times increase (assuming an increase in water content related to the pathology). The differences and changes to the T_1- and T_2-relaxation times of the tissues are major mechanisms by which we can visualize contrast between tissues on MR images.

MRI

MRI has a number of critical imaging factors. These include image contrast, spatial resolution, signal-to-noise ratio, and scan time. In addition, there are several techniques that are used for image improvement. These include motion reduction, suppression techniques, and flow compensation.

Critical Imaging Factors

MR Image Contrast. The properties of tissues within the body that can affect the contrast of an MR image are referred to as *intrinsic parameters*. They include: T_1-relaxation, T_2-relaxation, proton (or spin) density, flow, diffusion, perfusion, and magnetization transfer. The parameters selected by the operator at the MRI console to control the contrast of the MR image are referred to as *extrinsic parameters*. These include: time of repetition (TR), time to echo (TE), **time of inversion (TI)**, flip angle, b-value, and velocity encoding (VENC).

Also key to the contrast of an MR image is the pulse sequence selection. Pulse sequences are the acquisition techniques by which the protons are excited and the resultant signals are measured (sampled). As the name implies, they are specially programmed sequences of RF pulses and gradient field applications that excite the protons and spatially encode the MR signals. The operator will select the overall sequence type and set the timing parameters specific to that sequence. These selections will affect the contrast weighting, spatial resolution, and signal-to-noise of the resultant MR image. Generally speaking, the MR radiologists working with the MRI technologists will have predefined the particular sequences and general timing parameters required for the particular patient and/or MRI exam. However, it is not uncommon for the MRI technologist to make modifications to the sequence and its parameters to optimize the acquisition based on the patient's needs or condition.

There are two main types of pulse sequences utilized in MRI, spin echo (SE) and gradient recalled echo (GRE). GRE sequences are often utilized for very rapid acquisition techniques. Using GRE sequences, images can be acquired while a patient holds his or her breath. This is useful for examinations of the body (in particular the liver and kidneys) as well as cardiac studies (Figures 42-11 and 42-12). Flowing blood normally appears hyperintense (bright) relative to surrounding tissues when using GRE sequences. Therefore, GRE is often used for so-called MR angiograms (MRA) without the need for the injection of contrast media (Figure 42-13). Contrast media (in particular gadolinium-based MR contrast agents) is sometimes required for MRA studies. In these contrast-enhanced MRA studies, the images are generally acquired using GRE sequences due to their ability to acquire data rapidly during a breath-hold. Due to the way the MR signal is produced in a GRE sequence, there is high sensitivity to inhomogeneities in the local magnetic field within the tissues. In the brain and spinal cord, hemorrhagic lesions are well visualized using GRE sequences due to the iron-based components in blood (hemosiderin) and the disruption to the local magnetic fields caused by its presence (Figure 42-14).

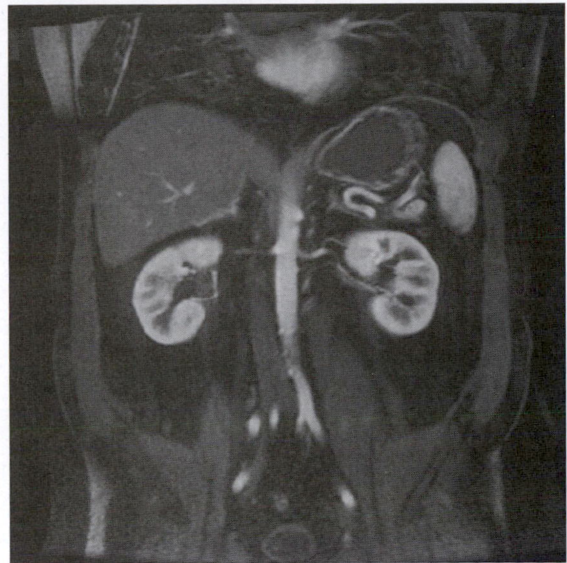

FIGURE 42-11. Abdominal GRE image following IV injection of Gd based contrast media.

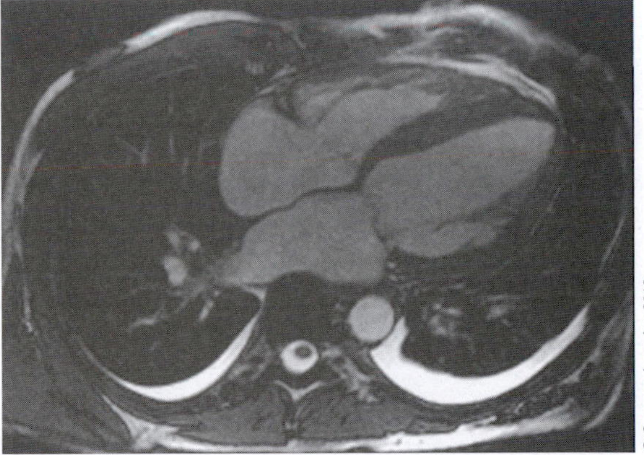

FIGURE 42-12. A balanced GRE cardiac image.

There are various types of GRE sequences. They will vary system to system depending on the vendor and model of the MRI system. Additionally,

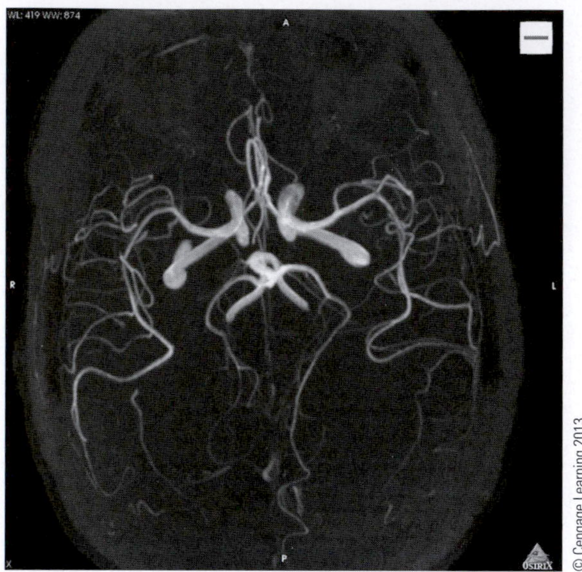

FIGURE 42-13. MRA of the Circle of Willis acquired using a GRE technique without the use of injected contrast media.

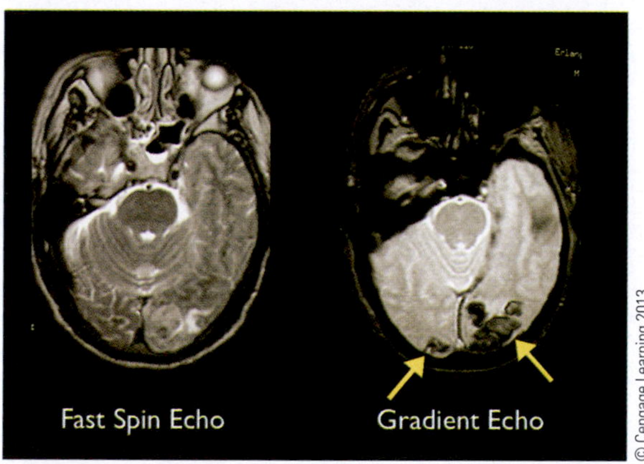

FIGURE 42-14. Hemorrhagic lesion well visualized through a GRE sequence.

although all GRE sequences are essentially the same, vendors use different acronyms or names for their particular sequences. This can be a source of confusion for the technologists and radiologists. However, regardless of the type of GRE sequence chosen, the main parameters that control the image contrast are TR, TE, and flip angle.

Regardless of the type of sequence used to acquire the MR data, the MR imaging process consists of several steps repeated over the course of the scan. After placing the patient in the external magnetic field to magnetize the tissue, the process begins as the protons are excited with an RF pulse; the resultant MR signal that is induced in the receiver coil is sampled. The tissue's magnetization is allowed to recover for some time period, at which point the process beginning with the excitation pulse is repeated. TR stands for *time of repetition*. It represents the time period between repetitions of the excitation pulse. TE stands for *time to echo*, and it represents the time period between excitation and sampling of the induced signal. The flip angle affects the magnitude (or power) of the RF excitation pulse. With a gradient echo sequence, both the TR and flip angle will affect the T_1-weighting of the image. The TE will determine the amount of T_2*-weighting in the image. T_2* (pronounced: "T_2-star") is the term used when a GRE sequence is utilized (this will be further explained in the next section dealing with spin echo sequences). Again, the particular type of GRE sequence selected as well as the particular parameters (TR, TE, flip angle) depend on the type of contrast weighting desired.

A spin echo (SE) pulse sequence utilizes two RF pulses prior to sampling the MR signal (the echo). A SE sequence begins with a 90° RF pulse and is followed by a 180° RF pulse (sometimes referred to as a refocusing pulse). In an SE sequence, the TE is the time between the 90° RF pulse and the center of the resultant echo. The 180° pulse will be applied halfway between the 90° pulse and the echo. The purpose of the 180° RF pulse is to correct for local inhomogenities and slight resonant frequency differences between water-based protons and fat-based protons (chemical shift). These "off-resonant" effects are responsible for the main contrast differences one sees between images acquired with GRE sequences, which does not utilize the refocusing pulse, as opposed to SE sequences, which do. When producing images using an SE sequence, the TR will affect the T_1-weighting of the resultant image and the TE will determine the T_2-weighting of the image. You will note that in the

GRE section, the term T_2* was used as opposed to T_2. This is because in a GRE the off-resonance effects are not corrected for, which results in a more rapid decay of the MR signal over time. T_2* is the result of T_2-decay plus the off-resonance effects (inhomogenities and chemical shift). For this reason, small hemorrhagic lesions are often not visualized as well with SE sequences as opposed to GRE sequences (Figure 42-14). However, larger areas of inhomogeneities such as those produced by metallic implants or devices are less problematic with SE sequences (Figure 42-15). In general, SE scan times are longer compared to GRE. There are, however, fast versions of SE sequences known as fast spin echo (FSE) or turbo spin echo (TSE). These versions of the SE sequence, introduced clinically in the early 1990s, resulted in dramatic reduction is scan times when using SE. In fact, FSE sequences have almost completely replaced conventional SE in clinical imaging today.

FSE sequences require the selection of an additional parameter, the echo train length (ETL). The ETL represents the number of differently encoded echoes sampled per TR period. Scan time decreases as the ETL increases. The TE selected with an FSE sequence is more correctly referred to as the effective TE (effTE). The effective TE will be encoded for the portion of the MR raw data that will have the greatest effect on the resultant image contrast. When acquiring FSE sequences with short effTE times, a short ETL is generally selected. Although it may vary with the system and its capabilities, for T_1-weighted FSE sequences, an ETL of 2–3 is generally selected. For PD-weighted sequences, the ETL may be as high as 8. For T_2-weighted images, a much higher ETL may be selected. While increasing the ETL results in shorter scan times, it is not without penalty. Increasing the ETL can, and often does, result in blurring in the image. This blurring is more obvious when a short effTE time is selected, which is why a shorter ETL is selected (as previously mentioned). Improvements to MR system hardware, in particular the gradient coil's electronics, have allowed for the use of higher ETLs with minimal FSE blurring.

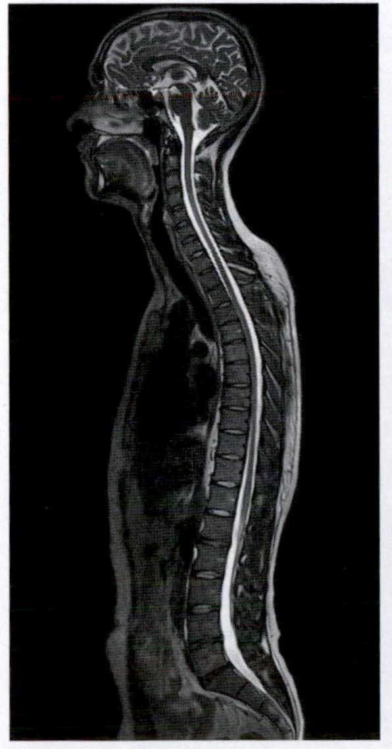

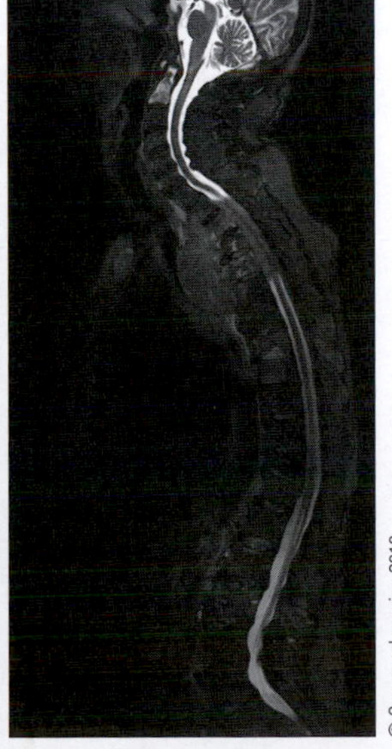

FIGURE 42-15. The SE sequence shown on the left displays less magnetic susceptibility artifact resulting from surgically placed wires as opposed to the Gd image on the right.

Spin-echo-based sequences that begin with a 180° "inversion" pulse are known as inversion recovery (IR). The purpose of using a sequence that begins with an inversion pulse is to null (or suppress) the signal from a particular tissue or substance. Because MRI images hydrogen existing primarily in fat and water, IR sequences are most often utilized to null the signal from fat or water. The time period between the 180° inversion pulse and the 90° excitation pulse in an IR sequence is most often referred to as TI (time of inversion). Selecting a TI time that is 69 percent of a tissue's T_1-relaxation time will result in the signal from that tissue being nulled.

The TI period is sometimes annotated by the Greek letter tau. Based on that, when using an IR sequence to null the signal from fat, the sequence is referred to as STIR (short tau inversion recovery). STIR sequences are most useful in imaging the musculoskeletal (MSK) system due to the high presence of fat, which may obscure water-based pathology.

In the brain, pathology is often best visualized using T_2-weighted sequences. However, the high signal from CSF in such images may obscure or limit the visualization of pathologic fluid. Using an IR sequence with an appropriately chosen TI, one can null the signal from CSF. This type of IR sequence is termed *FLAIR* (fluid attenuated inversion recovery). The acronym FLAIR is somewhat misleading in that CSF is what is null, as opposed to all fluid. Depending on the TR and TE selected, FLAIR sequences can be acquired with primarily T_2-weighting or T_1-weighting. In both instances, the signal from CSF is nulled (Figures 42-16, 42-17, 42-18).

Spatial Resolution. Spatial resolution can be defined as the ability to distinguish two structures as separate and distinct from each other. In any digital image, the smallest component is the pixel. The pixel size is determined by the selection of the field of view (FOV) and the acquisition matrix. Together this will determine the in-plane resolution. Based on the method currently used to reconstruct the MR image (Fourier transform), the acquisition matrix is often referred to by the two

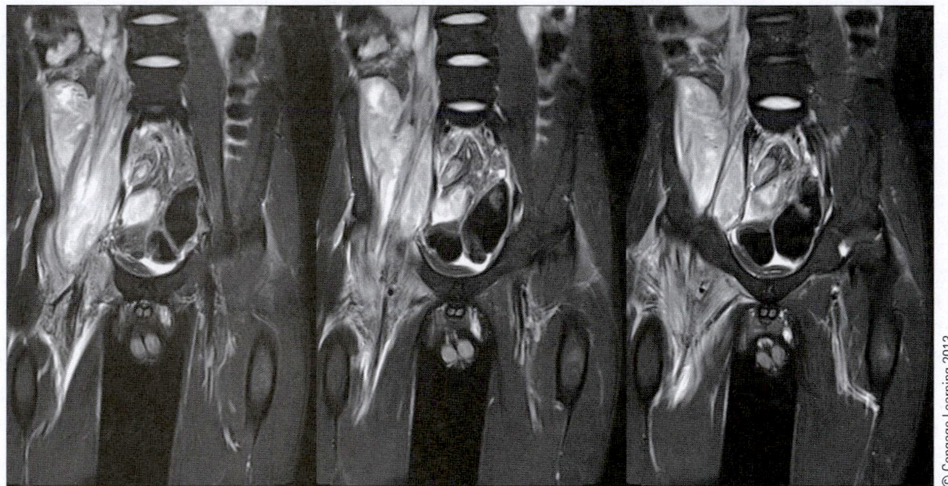

FIGURE 42-16. STIR image of a pelvic Infection from a 3-T MR unit.

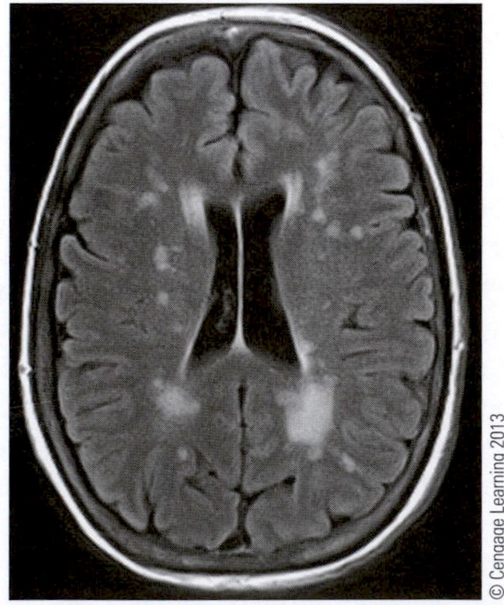

FIGURE 42-17. T2 FLAIR image.

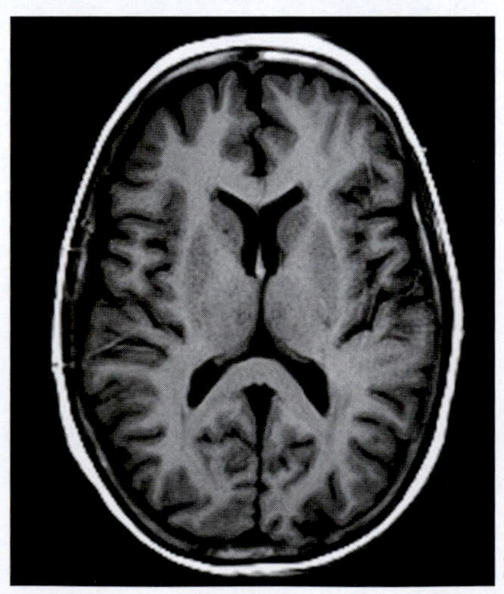

FIGURE 42-18. T1 FLAIR image.

directions of encoding: phase and frequency. When the number relating to the acquisition matrix is increased (for example, going from 256 × 256 to 512 × 512), the pixel size is reduced (assuming the FOV is unchanged). The smaller pixel size results in improved spatial resolution. The FOV affects the pixel size in two dimensions. Changes to the FOV dramatically affect the spatial resolution of an MR image.

MR images, however, represent "slices." The voxel is the three-dimensional element of the digital image, with the third dimension being represented by the slice thickness. As the slice thickness is reduced, the spatial resolution is increased. To summarize, the spatial resolution of an MR image is expressed either by the in-plane resolution (FOV and acquisition matrix) or voxel volume (FOV, acquisition matrix, and slice thickness).

In general, operator-selectable MRI parameters are closely interrelated. Reducing the acquired voxel volume reduces partial volume averaging, and therefore increases spatial resolution. However, given that the tissues in the voxel are the source of the MR signal, reducing the voxel volume so as to improve spatial resolution results in a reduction in MR signal (reduced signal-to-noise ratio). Additionally, due to the use of Fourier mathematics for image reconstruction, increasing the number of the phase matrix to improve spatial resolution will result in a direct increase in scan time.

Signal-to-Noise Ratio. MR signal-to-noise ratio (SNR) is as the name implies, a ratio of the signal in an acquired voxel to the noise in an acquired voxel. As previously mentioned, the size of the acquired voxel affects the signal. Doubling the voxel volume by doubling the slice thickness, as an example, will result in a two-fold increase in MR signal. This will, however, result in reduced spatial resolution. Given that the FOV affects the voxel volume in two dimensions, changes to the FOV dramatically impact the SNR. For example, a 20 percent reduction in the FOV will result in a 40 percent reduction in the SNR. The use of higher matrix values improves spatial resolution but also results in reduced SNR.

MR signal is directly proportional to the strength of the external field (B_0). Increasing B_0 increases the number of protons preferentially aligned parallel to the direction of the main magnetic field and therefore increases the magnitude (strength) of the tissue's net magnetization. Increased SNR is a major advantage of a higher-field-strength magnetic. Although it is a very complex issue as there are other factors influencing SNR, doubling the field strength (going from 1.5 T to 3.0 T as an example) while keeping all other factors constant results in a two-fold increase in available MR signal.

It should also be noted that improvements in receiving coil technology, in particular the increased number of elements and receiving channels available for multi-coil systems, greatly improves their efficiency. This increased coil efficiency directly improves overall SNR.

Noise contribution is complex, as there are several sources of noise. Noise can come from the environment. For this reason, it is imperative that the RF shielding of the scan room be optimally designed and maintained. Devices, such as those used for patient monitoring, must be specifically designed for safe and effective use in an MR environment. Lighting systems not designed for an MR environment can be significantly detrimental to SNR.

System electronics can also contribute to the overall noise level. Technology improvements such as the use of digital RF, fiber optics, and improved receiving coil technology have resulted in significant reductions in MR system noise.

With regard to the MR acquisition parameters, those that affect the time spent sampling or collecting MR signal affect noise. In general, the less time spent sampling or collecting MR signal, the higher the noise level. While MR signal is at the Larmor frequency, noise is random and occurs across all frequencies. As a result, MR noise is related to the square root of sampling time. There are several techniques and options that will not affect the voxel size but simply relate to the time spent sampling and collecting data. The exact techniques and options depend on the capabilities of the individual MR systems. However, the one that is common to all systems is the number of signal averages (NSA). As with some other user-selectable parameters and options, NSA may be referred to by other names depending on the system manufacturer.

The NSA is essentially the number of times the data required for a complete image is sampled and collected. It is somewhat analogous to the number of coats of paint applied when painting a wall. If one doubles the NSA, the data for the image will be sampled and collected twice, effectively doubling the scan time. Given that the NSA affects noise and not signal, increasing the NSA by a factor of two will increase the SNR by a factor of the square root of 2 (1.41). In order to double the SNR by increasing the NSA, one would have to increase the NSA by a factor of 4 (square root of 4 equals 2), which would also result in a four-fold increase in scan time.

A major limitation of a two-dimensional Fourier transform (2D-FT) technique is poor SNR when thin slices are desired for high spatial resolution. Additionally, gap between slices is necessary to minimize interference between the slices. This so-called "cross-talk" results in reduced signal and tissue contrast. These limitations can be overcome by acquiring the data using a three-dimensional Fourier transform (3D-FT), or volume acquisition technique. In a 3D-FT acquisition, slices are not selectively excited but rather reconstructed by "partitioning" the acquired volume by means of an additional phase encoding applied along the slice direction. The benefits of a 3D-FT acquisition are tremendous. In general, 3D-FT acquisitions provide for high SNR yet very thin slices are possible. If the acquired voxel is equal in all dimensions (isotropic voxel), slices may be retrospectively reformatted to produce high-quality images in any plane.

As MRI techniques continue to evolve toward more rapid data acquisition capabilities for physiologic imaging, it is important to understand the impact on MR SNR. In essence, all advanced MR techniques are "signal-to-noise starved" due to the rapid data collection techniques required. This highlights the importance of higher field strength and improved receiving coil technology to offset the SNR impact of rapid scanning techniques.

Scan Time. The time of an MRI acquisition (or scan) depends on the acquisition method utilized. In general, MR data may be acquired using a 2D-FT technique or a 3D-FT technique (Figure 42-19). For a 2D-FT acquisition, the scan time is calculated by the following formula: TR × Phase Encodings × NSA.

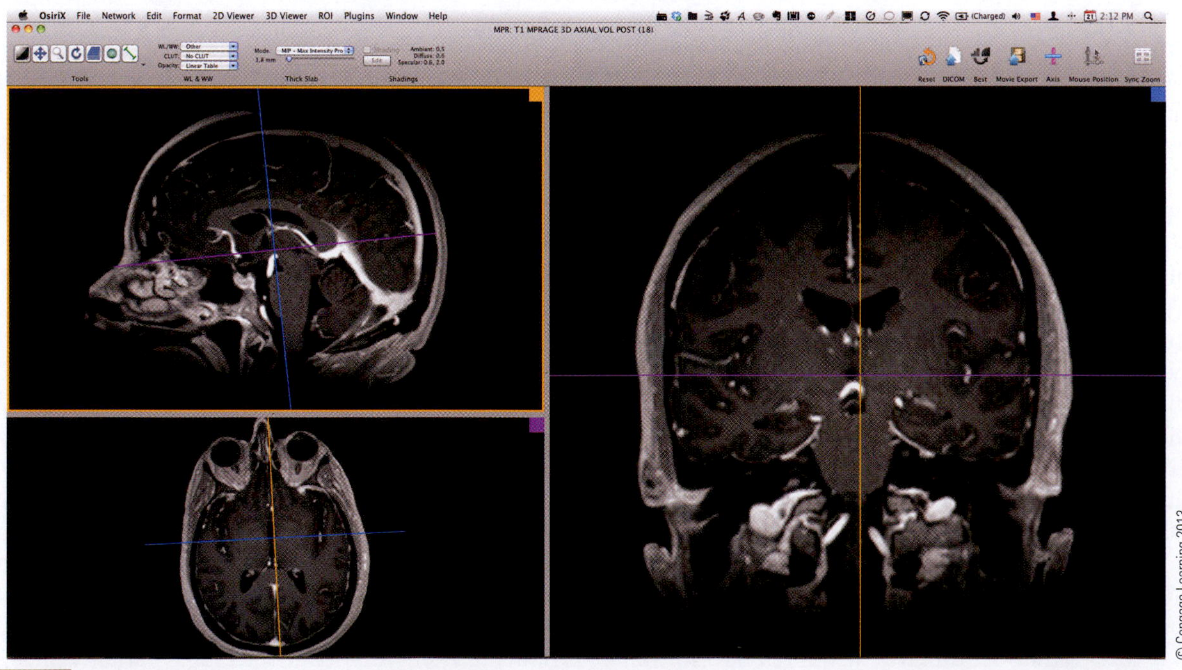

FIGURE 42-19. A 3D FT (Fourier transform) technique.

With this type of acquisition technique, changes to any of the parameters will result in changes to the overall image appearance and quality. Reducing the NSA in order to shorten scan times results in a reduction in the SNR. Reducing the number of phase encodings (phase matrix) will reduce the spatial resolution. The frequency matrix does not affect scan time. Therefore it is not uncommon to use a higher-frequency matrix compared to a phase matrix.

Reducing the TR will alter the image's contrast. Limitations with regard to the TR are more problematic when using spin-echo-based sequences (SE and FSE). Gradient echo sequences allow for selection of the flip angle in addition to the TR in order to control the contrast-weighting of an MR image. Using a reduced flip angle allows for the use of very short TR times, highlighting one of the advantages of GRE sequences. In addition to overall scan time, the TR determines the number of slices one can acquire within a given acquisition, or scan. The number of slices allowed will decrease as the TR is reduced.

As previously mentioned, fast spin echo (FSE) sequences acquire more data per TR than conventional SE techniques. The parameter that determines how many phase views are acquired in a given TR period is the echo train length (ETL). The scan time for a 2D-FT FSE acquisition is determined by the standard scan time formula (TR × Phase Encodings × NSA). For a 2D-FT FSE technique, that value is divided by the ETL. As an example, a conventional SE acquisition that takes 12 minutes to acquire would take only 1 minute using an FSE sequence with an ETL of 12. This illustrates why FSE rather than conventional SE is utilized, particularly with acquisitions requiring a long TR (T_2-weighted and PD-weighted).

In a 3D-FT acquisition, slices are not selectively excited but rather reconstructed by "partitioning" the acquired volume by means of an additional phase encodings applied along the slice direction. Therefore, with a 3D-FT acquisition, the number of slices will also affect scan time. For a 3D-FT acquisition, scan time is calculated as follows: TR × Phase Encodings × NSA × # of Slices. Fast scanning sequences, such as short TR GRE or FSE sequences with high ETL values, are utilized when acquiring data in a 3D sequence in order to obtain reasonable scan times.

There are various techniques often utilized to reduce acquisition time. However, it is important to remember that reducing the time of the acquisition more often than not results in a reduction in spatial resolution or SNR.

MR image quality is contrast, detail (spatial resolution), as a function of time. The time is the time spent sampling or collecting data. The greater the time spent sampling for a given voxel volume, the lower the noise (increase in SNR). The interrelationships of the various scanning parameters affecting image contrast, spatial resolution, and SNR are very complex. It should be fairly obvious that knowledge and skill is required of the MRI technologist to balance these parameters so that optimal image quality is obtained.

Image Improvement Techniques

Motion Reduction Techniques. Conventional MRI techniques acquire data in such a fashion that motion (whether voluntary or involuntary) becomes problematic. Motion can be divided into two major categories: periodic and aperiodic. Aperiodic refers to random motions such as peristalsis and is somewhat difficult to eliminate, particularly with conventional MR techniques. Periodic motion (such as respiratory and cardiac motion) is more easily compensated because it occurs at fairly regular intervals and can be monitored and detected (Figure 42-20).

To reduce or eliminate aperiodic motion, increasing the NSA can be an effective tool. However, the NSA directly affects scan time and longer scan times can result in general patient motion. Scanning very rapidly so that the images are acquired during a breath-hold is common. Additionally, imaging the patient in the prone position and/or using antispasmodic drugs such as glucagon can also be effective means of reducing such motion.

Respiratory and/or cardiac motion can be effectively managed by the use of triggering techniques. Cardiac triggering may be accomplished by the use of ECG monitoring or pulse oximetry. The system software times the scan sequence such that data is acquired either when there is minimal or no motion or data are acquired at the same point in time within the cardiac or respiratory cycles. The exact

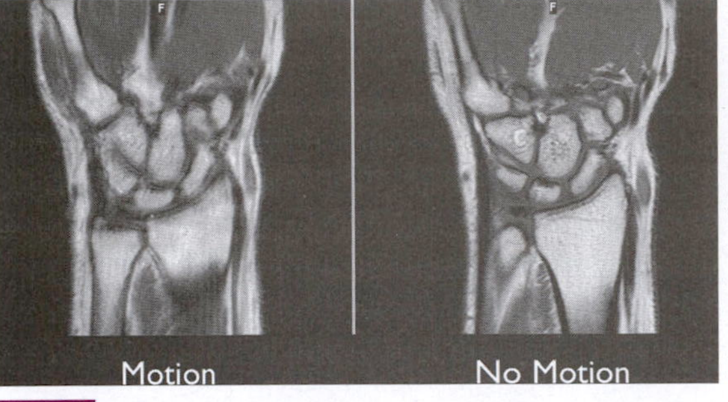

FIGURE 42-20. The effect of patient motion on MR image quality.

techniques utilized will depend on the system's capabilities as well as manufacturer preferences.

Suppression Techniques. In MRI, the term *saturation* refers to a condition in which longitudinal magnetization is not allowed to recover between excitations. The greater the saturation, the lower the detected signal from that tissue. There are two main types of saturation techniques commonly used in MRI: spectral and spatial (Figure 42-21).

Spectral saturation techniques are based on the fact that hydrogen protons in water and fat have different resonant frequencies (chemical shift). Using spectral saturation techniques, one can "tune" RF pulses to specific frequencies so that the magnetization, and therefore signal contribution, is reduced or eliminated from either fat-based or water-based hydrogen protons. These techniques are often referred to as fat saturation or water saturation. Frequency-based fat saturation techniques are often used after the injection of gadolinium-based contrast agents, particularly when fat-containing structures would mask gadolinium-enhanced water protons.

Spatial presaturation techniques apply an additional RF pulse in a particular location. This may be either outside or within the imaging slices or volume. When used outside the imaging slices or volume, it is most often used to reduce artifacts caused by blood flow, effectively eliminating the signal in vessels with flowing blood. Placing the saturation pulse within the imaging volume will reduce or eliminate the signal from moving tissues or structures in that area, effectively reducing motion artifacts.

Flow Compensation. In certain instances, high signal from flowing blood is desired. This is somewhat problematic given that the blood protons are moving. It is further complicated by the fact that blood protons are moving in the presence of gradient magnetic fields. In this situation, an imaging option known as gradient moment nulling or simply flow

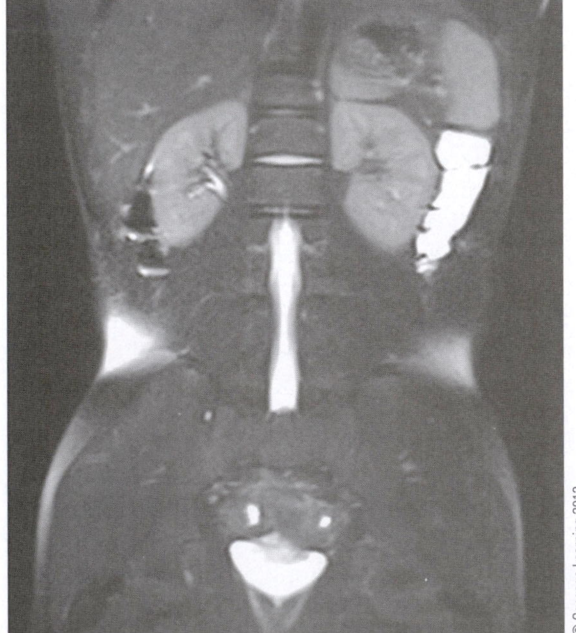

FIGURE 42-21A. Coronal abdomen with fat saturation.

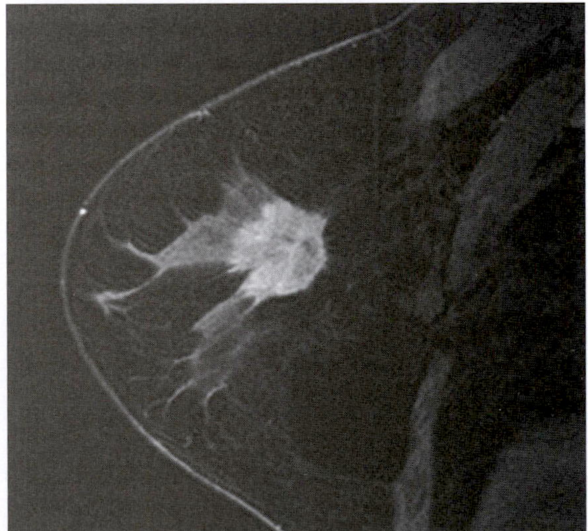

FIGURE 42-21B. Breast with fat saturation.

compensation may be utilized. This option compensates for signal loss from flowing protons and results in high signal from those protons (flowing blood). Flow compensation only compensates for constant velocities, and works best for slower flow and when short TE times are selected. Accelerated and/or turbulent flow is not compensated.

MR Contrast Agents

Various types of materials, such as air and fluid, can act as contrast agents in MR. There are also contrast agents that are iron-based. Most contrast agents currently used clinically in MRI are gadolinium-based agents. They will be the focus of this section.

Gadolinium-based contrast agents (GBCAs) work by altering the relaxation times (T_1, T_2, and T_2*) of tissues. The majority of these agents are extracellular fluid (EFC) agents. These agents, following their injection (IV), disperse to the extracellular fluid spaces. They do not remain in the blood system. A blood-pool agent, on the other hand, will exhibit a temporary binding to protein in the albumin and therefore remain in the blood stream for an extended period of time (several hours). Most GBCAs are excreted via the kidneys. Assuming normal renal function, the half-life for the renal excretion of an ECF agent is approximately 1.5 hours. Some of the ECF agents have dual excretion pathways being eliminated by the biliary system. These agents allow for the acquisition of images in the hepatobiliary phase. The time one would wait for the delayed hepatobiliary phase depends on the amount of biliary excretion and the patient's liver function (Figure 42-22).

Gadolinium is a heavy metal (lanthanide). It is not a trace element found normally in the body. As with any such metal, it is highly toxic to humans if injected in its pure form. Free gadolinium is not excreted by the kidneys. It will deposit in the liver and bone marrow. In order for the gadolinium to be eliminated by the kidneys (or liver as the case may be), the gadolinium ion (Gd^{3+}) is bound to a chemical known as a chelate. The word *chelate* comes from a Greek word that translates "claw." It should be rather obvious that it is desirable to have a gadolinium agent with a very strong bond between the gadolinium ion and its chelating agent. Current agents fall into two major categories of molecule structure,

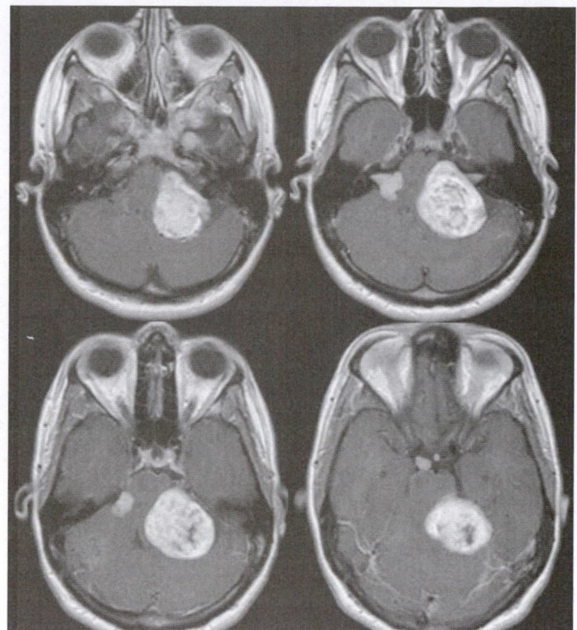

FIGURE 42-22. Bilateral neurofibromas post Gd injection.

macrocyclic or linear. Macrocyclic agents are a rigid ring-like design and are the most stable. Linear agents have fewer binding points and are generally less stable. However, if the liner design molecule is non-ionic, it has even lower stability. Nephrogenic systemic fibrosis (NSF) is a rare but debilitating disease first described in 1997. NSF is a fibrosing disease, primarily seen in the skin and subcutaneous tissues, most often in dependent extremities. It has also been found in other organs, such as the lungs, esophagus, heart, and skeletal muscles. In 2006 the first scientific papers were published linking NSF to patients in stage 4 and 5 renal disease who had received certain gadolinium-based contrast agents. It was also noted that in most cases, the patients had received high doses and repeat doses of the agents with lower-stability constants. As a result, the Food and Drug Administration (FDA) has required the manufactures of some of the agents to change their package insert information to reflect that they are contraindicated in patients in stage 4 or 5 renal disease. When renal disease is known or suspected, patients should have their renal function assessed prior to the administration of a gadolinium-based

MR contrast agent. Currently, the lab test most commonly used to assess a patient's renal function is eGFR (estimated glomerular filtration rate).

As with any contrast media, there is a small risk of an adverse event (AE), also known as an allergic-like reaction. GBMAs are no exception. Although not as frequent as AEs associated with iodinated contrast media, there is a slight risk. According to the published literature, the AE rate of all currently available GBCAs is similar for all types of "allergic-type" reactions; this ranges from 0.07 to 2.4 percent. For the most commonly observed AEs (hives, nausea with or without vomiting), the rate is between 0.04 and 0.07 percent. Severe and even fatal events are rare but do occur (0.001 to 0.01 percent). It has been shown, however, that some patients are at an increased risk for an adverse event. This would include patients who are asthmatic, who have a significant history of allergies, or who have had a previous AE following an injection of an iodinated contrast agent (as high as 3.7 percent). Additionally, it has been shown that patients who have experienced a previous AE following the injection of a GBCA are approximately eight times as likely to experience another AE that may be more severe than the first. One should therefore always closely monitor patients following the injection of a contrast agent and always be prepared to respond to and treat an adverse event. As with iodinated contrast media, GBCAs should not be injected without a physician immediately available to treat an adverse event.

As previously mentioned, GBCAs work by shortening the relaxation rates of water-based hydrogen protons. The relaxation rate of tissues is, in large part, based on the rate at which the molecules tumble. The larger the molecule, the slower the molecular tumbling rate; the smaller the molecule, the faster the molecular tumbling rate. Larger molecules, such as fat, have a relatively slow molecular tumbling rate and therefore exhibit rapid relaxation rates (T_1 and T_2). The much smaller water molecule has a very rapid molecular tumbling rate and therefore exhibits longer relaxation times. Gadolinium has seven unpaired electrons and, as such, is paramagnetic. Paramagnetic substances become magnetized when in a magnetic field. Given that the gadolinium ion is bound to the chelate, this results in a large, slow-tumbling magnet. When the gadolinium molecule gets within 3 angstroms of a water molecule, the molecular tumbling rate of the water molecule is reduced. This results in a shortening of the relaxation times of the water-based hydrogen protons. The measure of this effect is expressed by the relaxivity of the gadolinium agent. The higher the relaxivity, the greater the shortening of the T_1- and T_2-relaxation times. The effects on the T_1-relaxation rates are more dominant unless the gadolinium agent is in high concentration. In that case, the T_2-shortening effects begin to dominate.

When acquiring T_1-weighted images, any tissues/substances with short T_1-relaxation times will exhibit high signal. Therefore, water-based protons whose T_1-relaxation time has been shortened by the paramagnetic effects of the gadolinium-based MR contrast agent will appear as high signal on T_1-weighted images, compared to "unenhanced" or background tissue. The higher the relaxivity of the agent, the greater the contrast between the lesion and surrounding tissue. In the event the decision is made to reduce the dose, due to the patient's renal function, the use of an agent with higher relaxivity has been shown to mitigate the reduction in dose.

In general, the use of a GBCA improves the detection of disease by increasing sensitivity and improving the ability to fully identify the extent of disease. This is particularly important as treatment and surgical options for patients increase. Increased specificity is realized by way of evaluating the patterns of enhancement. As MR data acquisition speeds increase, contrast agents allow for the demonstration of pathophysiology by way of their perfusion and clearance. As more efficient and unique MR contrast agents are developed, the diagnostic power of MRI will undoubtedly increase.

MR SAFETY

Static Magnetic Field (B_0)

The "heart" of an MRI system is the magnet itself. The magnetic field generated is very powerful. Currently, the most commonly utilized field strength is 1.5 tesla. This equates to 15,000 Gauss. The earth's field strength is approximately 0.5 Gauss. Therefore, the magnetic field generated by a 1.5-T magnet is 30,000 times that of the earth's magnetic field. A 3.0-T magnet generates a field 60,000 times that of the earth's magnetic field. The magnetic field of the MRI system is always on. Any loose ferromagnetic objects can be drawn into the magnet with tremendous speed and force. As an example, a paper clip can have a terminal velocity of over 40 miles per hour in a 1.5-T field. Therefore, access to the MRI scan room should be tightly controlled and loose ferromagnetic objects should never be brought into an MRI scan room. In 2001, a 6-year-old child died as a result of the trauma of being struck in the head by a ferromagnetic oxygen tank that was brought into the scan room.

Additionally, the magnetic field of the imager may adversely affect or inhibit the operation of certain implants or devices in patients. Rigorous screening of all persons entering the scan room is always required.

Gradient Magnetic Fields

The gradient magnetic fields, used primarily to provide spatial encoding of the detected MR signals, are switched off and on very rapidly during the MRI process. The rapid switching of these gradient magnetic fields can induce current in loops of conductive materials (based on Faraday's Law of Induction). This can result in rapid and significant heating, which could result in a fire or a patient burn. As such, the formation of large loops with the wires associated with **surface coils** and/or leads used for cardiac triggering is always to be avoided. Some sequences, particularly the most rapid scanning techniques, may result in the patient experiencing peripheral nerve stimulation (PNS). This would present as a tingling sensation. Although not usually painful, it could be uncomfortable. As such, having patients not cross their hands in front of them or cross their ankles minimizes the likelihood of PNS.

Radiofrequency Field (B_1)

The pulsed RF fields used in MRI can result in heating in both conductive materials and patients. With regard to metals, even though the material may not be ferromagnetic, it may still be conductive. Exposure to RF at the proper frequency can induce significant heating in conductive materials. The increase in temperature can be very rapid, resulting in a significant burn in a matter of seconds.

Patients should be positioned so as not to touch the sides of the MR system's bore. The RF coil is just inside the covers. There should be space between the patient and the bore or insulating padding should be in place. Additionally, skin-to-skin contact should also be avoided. Severe burns have occurred when these precautions are not followed.

The amount of RF power absorbed by the body is given by the **specific absorption rate (SAR).** It is expressed in units of watts per kg of body weight. Current FDA guidelines limit SAR to 4 w/kg averaged over the whole body and 3.2 w/kg for the head. The body dissipates the RF energy by cooling. When the power input is greater than the output, heating occurs. Patient cooling is influenced by several factors, such as: ambient room temperature and humidity, air flow rate through the bore, perspiration, and blood flow. Patients taking certain medications such as beta-blockers or those with certain medical conditions such congestive heart failure are unable to efficiently dissipate heat, thus affecting their ability to tolerate a thermal challenge. Careful monitoring of SAR levels and the patient's comfort is therefore important.

Device Labeling

The ASTM Standard F2503 established labeling for objects and devices relative to MRI. The MR-Safe labeling means the object or device is completely safe in any MR environment and would pose no hazard whatsoever regardless of the field strength of the magnet. MR-Unsafe labeling means the object or device is unsafe in all MR environments and should never be allowed into the MR scan room under any circumstances. MR-Conditional labeling means the object or device can safely be used in, or will safely and effectively function in, an MR environment under certain well-defined conditions. These conditions may include limits on the static magnetic, maximum spatial field gradient,

SAR, and/or type of coil. Implanted devices that are electronic in nature will most likely have the most conditions.

MRI is a very powerful diagnostic tool. The many unique intrinsic contrast mechanisms of tissues along with various imaging techniques provide us with many ways to image and diagnose our patient's diseases. Although no ionizing radiation is used, there can be significant safety issues that must be considered.

SUMMARY

Magnetic resonance imaging (MRI) had its beginning as nuclear magnetic resonance (NMR), which was primarily used by chemists. Felix Bock and Edward Purcell (Harvard University) received the Nobel Prize for Physics for their work in developing the instruments to measure magnetic resonance, and Raymond Damadian and Paul Lauterbur were the first to produce two-dimensional images using back-projection. Beginning with the first commercial scanners installed during the 1980s, magnetic resonance imaging (as it is now known) has become a major method for imaging not only anatomic structures but physiologic functions of the human body.

MRI uses the magnetic properties of hydrogen (^1H) to produce images of the body. It requires the patient to be placed within a large externally applied magnetic field in order to magnetize the tissue. Radiofrequency (RF) coils produce a pulsed magnetic field (radio waves) to rotate the magnetic field of the tissues through a receiving coil (antenna), inducing an MR signal. Currently, the most widely used technique for MR image reconstruction is fast Fourier transform (FFT). The contrast of the resultant MR images is a function of the particular type of technique or sequence used to acquire the data and the type and timing of the RF pulses. Contrast agents based on materials with magnetic properties can be utilized to enhance visualization of structures and/or lesions. The main components of an MRI unit include: the main magnet, the radiofrequency subsystem, and the gradient coil subsystem.

Most pathology is associated with an increase in water content. Therefore, generally speaking, when tissue becomes diseased, the T_1- and T_2-relaxation times increase (assuming an increase in water content related to the pathology). The differences and changes to the T_1- and T_2-relaxation times of the tissues are major mechanisms by which we can visualize contrast between tissues on MR images.

MRI imaging has a number of critical imaging factors. These include image contrast, spatial resolution, signal-to-noise ratio, and scan time. In addition, there are several techniques that are used for image improvement. These include motion reduction, suppression techniques, and flow compensation. Various types of materials, such as air and fluid, can act as contrast agents in MR. There are also iron-based contrast agents. Most contrast agents currently used clinically in MRI are gadolinium-based agents.

The heart of an MRI system is the magnet itself. The magnetic field generated is very powerful. Currently, the most commonly utilized field strength is 1.5 tesla. This equates to 15,000 Gauss. The magnetic field generated by a 1.5-T magnet is 30,000 times that of the earth's magnetic field. A 3.0-T magnet generates a field 60,000 times that of the earth's magnetic field. The magnetic field of the MRI system is always on. Any loose ferromagnetic objects can be drawn into the magnet with tremendous speed and force. Therefore, access to the MRI scan room should be tightly controlled and loose ferromagnetic objects should never be brought into an MRI scan room. Additionally, the magnetic field of the imager may adversely affect or inhibit the operation of certain implants or devices in patients. Rigorous screening of all persons entering the scan room is always required. Although no ionizing radiation is used in MRI, there can be significant safety issues that must be considered. ■

REVIEW QUESTIONS

1. What is the source of the magnetic fields within the body that are used during MRI?
2. What is precession?
3. What is TI? TR? TE? T_1? T_2?
4. How do the gradient coils select an image section?
5. What is accomplished by an RF pulse during a pulse sequence?
6. What is the most common pulse sequence?
7. How can MR image noise be reduced by improving the S/N?
8. How is MR image contrast increased? decreased?
9. Describe appropriate safety measures for protection of all persons who approach the MRI unit magnetic field.

REFERENCES AND RECOMMENDED READING

Andrew, E. R. (1982). Nuclear magnetic resonance imaging. In P. N. T. Wells (Ed.), *Scientific basis of medical imaging.* Edinburgh: Churchill Livingstone.

Atkinson, D. J. (1990). Pulse sequence design. In R. R. Edelman & J. R. Hesselink (Eds.), *Clinical magnetic resonance imaging.* Philadelphia: W. B. Saunders.

Axel, L. (1988). Chemical shift imaging. In D. D. Stark & W. G. Bradley (Eds.), *Magnetic resonance imaging.* St. Louis, MO: Elsevier/C. V. Mosby.

Ayton, V. T., Smith, M. A., & Bingham, J. B. (1989). Practical consideration for patient investigation using a high field magnetic resonance system. *Radiography Today, 55*(620), 12.

Barrafate, D. (1985). MRI: A technologist's perspective. *The Canadian Journal of Medical Radiation Technology, 16*(3), 73.

Barrafate, D., & Henkelman, M. (1985). MRI and surgical clips. *The Canadian Journal of Medical Radiation Technology, 16*(3), 101.

Bloch, F. (1946). Nuclear induction. *Physics Review, 70,* 460–474.

Bloch, F. (1998). The principle of nuclear induction. In *Nobel Lectures in Physics: 1901–1995.* New York: World Scientific Publishers.

Bloch, F., Hansen, W. W., & Packard, M. E. (1946). Nuclear induction. *Physics Review, 69,* 127.

Bushberg, J. T., Seibert, J. A., Leidholdt, E. M., & Boone, J. M. (2002). *The essential physics of medical imaging* (2nd ed.). Philadelphia: Lippincott Williams & Wilkins.

Bushong, S. C. (1996). *Magnetic resonance imaging: Physical and biological principles* (2nd ed.). St. Louis, MO: Elsevier/C. V. Mosby.

Bushong, S. C. (2008). *Radiologic science for technologists: Physics, biology, and protection* (9th ed.). St. Louis, MO: Elsevier/C. V. Mosby.

Damadian, R. (1971). Tumor detection by nuclear magnetic resonance. *Science, 171,* 1151–1153.

Damadian, R. 1981. *NMR in medicine.* Berlin: Springer-Verlag.

Damadian, R., Goldsmith, M., & Minkoff, L. (1977). NMR in cancer XVI: FONAR image of the live human body. *Physiological Chemistry and Physics, 9,* 97–100.

Damadian, R., Zaner, K., Hor, D., DiMaio, T., Minkoff, L., & Goldsmith, M. (1973). Nuclear magnetic resonance as a new tool in cancer research: Human tumors by NMR. *Annals of the New York Academy of Science, 222,* 1048–1076.

Davis, P. (1981). Potential hazards in NMR imaging: Heating effects of changing magnetic fields and RF fields on small metallic implants. *American Journal of Roentgenology, 137,* 857–860.

Edelman, R. R., & Hesselink, J. R. (1990). *Clinical magnetic resonance imaging.* Philadelphia: W. B. Saunders.

Elster, A. D. (1986). *Magnetic resonance imaging: A reference guide and atlas.* Philadelphia: J. B. Lippincott.

Fitzsimmons, J. R., & Mick, R. C. (1985). Image quality and magnetic field strength in NMR imaging. *Applied Radiology, 14*(2), 52.

Fodor, J., & Mallot, J. (1984). MRI: A new imaging modality. *Radiologic Technology, 56*(1), 17.

Forster, E. (1985). *Equipment for diagnostic radiography.* Lancaster, UK: MTP Press.

Friedman, B. R., Jones, J. P., Chaves-Munoz, G., Salmon, A. P., & Merritt, C. R. B. (1989). *Principles of MRI.* New York: McGraw-Hill.

Grey, M. L., & Coffey, C. W. (1987). Methods for evaluating image quality in magnetic resonance imaging. *Radiologic Technology, 58*(4), 339.

Haacke, E. M., Brown, R. W., Thompson, M. R., & Brown, R. V. (Eds.). (1999). *Magnetic resonance imaging: Physical principles and sequence design* (2nd ed.). New York: Wiley-Liss.

Heiken, J. P., & Brown, J. J. (Eds.). (1991). *Manual of clinical magnetic resonance imaging* (2nd ed.). New York: Raven.

Hendee, W. R., & Ritenour, R. (1993). *Medical imaging physics* (3rd ed.). St. Louis, MO: C. V. Mosby.

Hinshaw, W. S., Bottomley, P. A., & Holland, G. N. (1977). Radiographic thin-section image of the human wrist by nuclear magnetic resonance. *Nature, 270*(22/29), 722–723.

Huettel, S., Song, A., & McCarthy, G. (2008). *Functional magnetic resonance imaging* (2nd ed.). Sunderland, MA: Sinauer Associates, Inc.

Kaut, C. (1992). *MRI workbook for technologists.* New York: Raven.

Lauterbur, P. C. (1973). Image formation by induced local interactions: Examples employing nuclear magnetic resonance. *Nature, 242*, 190–191.

Lipcamon, J. D., Chiu, L. C., Phillips, J. J., & Pottany, P. M. (1988). MRI of the upper abdomen using motion artifact suppression technique. *Radiologic Technology, 59*(5), 415.

Lufkin, R. B. (1990). *The MRI manual.* St. Louis, MO: Elsevier/C. V. Mosby.

Morgan, C. J., & Hendee, W. R. (1984). *Introduction to magnetic resonance imaging.* Denver: Multi-Media.

Nelson, T. R., Ritenour, E. R., Davis, K., & Pretorius, D. H. (1985a). MRI: The basic physical and clinical concepts Part 1. *Radiologic Technology, 56*(6), 410.

Nelson, T. R, Ritenour, E. R., Davis, K., & Pretorius, D. H. (1985b). MRI: The basic physical and clinical concepts Part 2. *Radiologic Technology, 57*(1), 26.

Nelson, T. R., Ritenour, E. R., Davis, K., Pretorius, D. H., & Hendrick, R. E. (1985). MRI: The basic physical and clinical concepts Part 3. *Radiologic Technology, 57*(2), 142.

Olendorf, W., & Olendorf, W., Jr. (1991). *MRI primer.* New York: Raven.

Philips Medical Systems. (1984). *Principles of MR imaging* (Publication 1984–11). The Netherlands: Author.

Purcell, E. (1998). Research in nuclear magnetism. *Nobel lectures in physics: 1901–1995.* New York: World Scientific Publishers.

Purcell, E. M., Torrey, H. C., & Pound, R. V. (1946). Resonance absorption by nuclear magnetic moments in a solid. *Physics Review, 69*, 37–83.

Rollo, F. D., & Patton, J. A. (1981). Nuclear magnetic resonance imaging. Radiographic films and screen-film systems. In C. M. Coulam, J. J. Erickson, F. D. Rollo, & A. E. James (Eds.), *The physical basis of medical imaging.* New York: Appleton-Century-Crofts.

Russel, R., Dallas-Hultema, C., & Cohen, M. D. (1986). MRI techniques in children. *Radiologic Technology, 57*(5), 428.

Schellock, F. G., & Kanal, E. (1994). *Magnetic resonance bioeffects, safety, and patient management.* New York: Raven.

Seeram, E. (1985). *X-ray imaging equipment: An introduction.* Springfield, IL: Charles C Thomas.

Sigal, R. (1988). *Magnetic resonance imaging: Basis for interpretation.* Berlin: Springer-Verlag.

Smith, H., & Ranallo, F. N. (1989). *A non-mathematical approach to basic MRI.* Madison, WI: Medical Physics.

Sobol, W. T. (1994). Artifacts in magnetic resonance imaging. *Applied Radiology, 23*(8), 11–16.

Stark, D. D., & Bradley, W. (Eds.). (1988). *Magnetic resonance imaging.* St. Louis, MO: C. V. Mosby.

Weishaupt, D., Koechli, V., & Marincek, B. (2006). *How does MRI work?: An introduction to the physics and function of magnetic resonance imaging* (2nd ed.). New York: Springer.

Westbrook, C. (2008). *Handbook of MRI technique* (3rd ed.). Oxford: Wiley-Blackwell.

Westbrook, C., Kaut, C., & Talbot, J. (2011). *MRI in practice* (4th ed.). Oxford: Wiley-Blackwell.

Wolbarst, A. B. (1993). *Physics of radiology.* Norwalk, CT: Appleton & Lange.

Wolfe, G., & Popp, C. (1984). *NMR: A primer for medical imaging.* Thorofare, NJ: Slack Book Division.

Woodward, P., & Freimarck, R. D. (1995). *MRI for technologists.* New York: McGraw-Hill.

Young, S. W. (1984). *Nuclear magnetic resonance imaging: Basic principles.* New York: Raven.

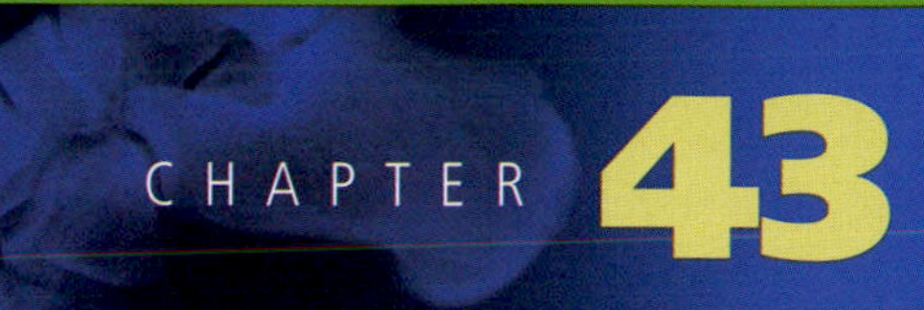

Nuclear Medicine and PET Scanning

Christina Truluck, PhD, CNMT, RT(N)

KEY TERMS

coregistration
dose calibrator
effective half-life (Te)
gamma camera
Geiger-Mueller counter
isotopes
PET
physical half-life (Tp)
radioactivity
radionuclide generator
radiopharmaceutical
scintillation detector
SPECT
technetium (Tc)

"He had me put my hand around a Geiger counter," recalled Oppenheimer, "and gave me a glass of water in which part of the salt had radioactive sodium in it. For the first half minute all was quiet, but about fifty seconds after I drank, there was a great clattering of the Geiger counter. This was supposed to show that in at least one complex physiochemical system, the salt had diffused from my mouth through my bloodstream to the tip of my fingers and that the time scale for this was fifty seconds."

An early experiment using radiotracers in a human subject. Performed at Berkeley in 1935 by Ernest O. Lawrence on his friend and colleague J. Robert Oppenheimer.

Cited in: George L. Voelz and Donald Petersen, 1995, "Tracer Studies at Los Alamos and the Birth of Nuclear Medicine." Los Alamos Science, 23, 257–279.

OBJECTIVES

Upon completion of this chapter, the student should be able to:

- Define the term radioactivity. Give examples of isotopes.
- Differentiate physical, biological, and effective half-lives.
- Explain the synthesis of radioisotopes in radionuclide generators.
- Explain why technetium-99m might be described as the "ideal radionuclide."
- Describe the creation of a nuclear medicine image from scintillation to image matrix.

OBJECTIVES (continued)

- Discuss the similarities and differences between SPECT and PET.
- Give examples of scintillation detectors and gas-filled detectors.
- Describe practical methods for reducing radiation exposure to staff and public in the nuclear medicine department.
- Explain the utility and role of nuclear medicine and compare to other diagnostic imaging modalities.

NUCLEAR PHYSICS

Nuclear Stability

Nuclear stability means that a nucleus has an optimal neutron-to-proton ratio. The stable ratio is 1:1 for lighter elements and greater than 1:1 for mid-weight elements. This ratio is frequently displayed as the nuclear line of stability.

Stable (nonradioactive) nuclei exist for all elements with atomic (Z) numbers up to 83 (bismuth), except for **technetium** (Z = 43) and promethium (Z = 61).

Isotopes, Isotones, Isobars, and Isomers

Isotopes are atoms of the same element. They have the same number of protons (Z), but different numbers of neutrons (N). Thus, their atomic masses (Z + N) are different. Iodine-123, iodine-125, and iodine-127 are examples of isotopes. Isotones are atoms of different elements. They have the same neutron number, but different numbers of protons. Silicon-31, phosphorus-32, and sulfur-33 are examples of isotones. Isobars are atoms of different elements that have the same atomic mass, such as potassium-45, calcium-45, and scandium-45.

Isomers are atoms of the same nuclide that are identical in atomic structure. One isomer has more energy compared to the other, and is said to be excited. The excited state is termed "metastable" (m), and can exist for a short (but measurable) duration before decaying by gamma emission or internal conversion to the lower-energy state, an isomeric transition. Technetium-99 and technetium-99m are examples of isomers.

RADIOACTIVE DECAY

Nuclear Instability

An unstable nuclide, termed a radionuclide, will try to become stable by undergoing radioactive decay. This involves emission of electromagnetic radiation or charged particles by alpha decay, beta decay, positron decay, electron capture, isomeric transition, gamma decay, and internal conversion.

Nuclear medicine imaging is the process by which some of these energetic particles and photons are detected.

Radioactivity Units

Radioactivity (or activity) is defined as the number of nuclear disintegrations per unit time. In Système International (SI) units, the unit of radioactivity is the becquerel (Bq). A becquerel is defined as the radioactivity of a sample that is decaying at a rate of 1 disintegration per second (dps):

$$1 \text{ Bq} = 1 \text{ dps}$$
$$1 \text{ KBq} = 10^3 \text{ dps}$$
$$1 \text{ MBq} = 10^6 \text{ dps}$$
$$1 \text{ GBq} = 10^9 \text{ dps}$$

In the United States, in clinical nuclear medicine, it is still common to use the older CGS (centimeter-gram-second) system of units, where the unit of radioactivity is the curie (Ci). A curie is defined as the radioactivity of a sample that is disintegrating at a rate of 3.7×10^{10} disintegrations per second:

$$1 \text{ Ci} = 3.7 \times 10^{10} \text{ dps}$$
$$1 \text{ mCi} = 3.7 \times 10^{7} \text{ dps}$$
$$1 \text{ µCi} = 3.7 \times 10^{4} \text{ dps}$$
$$1 \text{ nCi} = 3.7 \times 10 \text{ dps}$$
$$1 \text{ pCi} = 3.7 \times 10^{-2} \text{ dps}$$

It is useful to be able to convert between units of becquerels and units of curies. The following conversion is particularly valuable in the clinical nuclear medicine laboratory, given the usual magnitude of radiation dosages:

$$1 \text{ mCi} = 37 \text{ MBq}$$

Half-life (T½)

Radioactivity is a random phenomenon. It is not possible to predict exactly when a radioactive atom will decay, and atoms within a sample of a radionuclide will all decay at slightly different times. However, it is possible to predict the average behavior of a radionuclide sample containing billions of atoms.

Half-life (T½) is defined as the time it takes for half of the atoms to decay. The time taken for half of the remaining atoms to decay is also T½. After multiple subsequent half-lives, the radioactivity of the sample is close to zero. The progressive replacement of radioactive atoms by stable atoms produces an exponential decay curve. Each radionuclide has its own unique half-life.

Decay Equation

Mathematically, the average behavior of a sample of radioactive atoms can be described by the decay equation:

$$A_t = A_0 e^{-\lambda t}$$

where: A_0 is the initial number of radioactive atoms, A_t is the number of radioactive atoms remaining at time t, t is the elapsed time, and λ is the decay constant and is unique for each radionuclide.

Tables of decay factors ($e^{-\lambda t}$) have been compiled for many radionuclides, and may be used to simplify calculation of A_t.

Biologic Half-life (Tb)

The half-life of a radionuclide (T½) should more correctly be called the physical half-life (Tp). As previously stated, it is unique to each radionuclide, and cannot be altered by any physical, chemical, or biological means.

In nuclear medicine, we are concerned with the behavior of a radionuclide inside the human body, a living system, and must consider how the body handles the radionuclide. The term *biologic half-life* (Tb) refers to any material within the body, radioactive or not, and is defined as the time required for half of the material to be excreted from the body, or from an organ of the body.

Effective Half-life (Te)

The term **effective half-life (Te)** is a combination of **physical half-life (Tp)** and biologic half-life (Tb), and is defined as the time required for half of the initial radioactivity to disappear from an organ or body by a combination of excretion and physical decay. The effective half-life is always shorter than either the physical half-life or biologic half-life, and can be calculated as follows:

$$T_e = \frac{T_b \times T_p}{T_b + T_p} \quad or \quad \frac{1}{T_e} = \frac{1}{T_b} + \frac{1}{T_p}$$

RADIOCHEMISTRY AND RADIOPHARMACEUTICALS

History and Development

The earth has been radioactive ever since its formation into a solid mass, over 4½ billion years ago, but we have only known about radiation and radioactivity since 1895, when Wilhelm Roentgen discovered x-rays. Shortly after, in 1896, Antoine Becquerel was the first person to demonstrate the spontaneous emission of radiation from a substance without an external source. This was termed "radioactivity" by Marie Curie, in 1898.

Shortly after, Ernest Rutherford discovered that there were two types of natural radioactive emissions—alpha and beta—and Paul Villard described a third type: "rays non-deviable in character, but of very great penetrating power," gamma radiation.

One of the earliest radiotracer experiments appears to have been in 1911, by George de Hevesy, a Hungarian radiochemist, who suspected that his landlady was recycling leftover food. He supposedly added a radioisotope of lead to some meat pie on Sunday and proved that it showed up again in a meal on Wednesday.

In the early 1930s, following the discovery of artificial radioactivity by Irene and Frederic Joliot-Curie, Ernest Lawrence built the first cyclotron and began producing artificial radioisotopes of great value to biomedical science.

In 1941, Enrico Fermi built Chicago Pile 1, the world's first nuclear reactor, in an unused squash court under the old Stag Field at the University of Chicago. He achieved the first controlled nuclear chain reaction in 1942. Soon, reactor-produced radionuclides were plentiful and cheap.

A major development in nuclear medicine was the discovery of technetium in 1937 by Carlo Perrier and Emilio Segré. Technetium was the first element to be artificially produced, and was shown, in 1939, by Glenn Seaborg and Segré to have "an excited state. . .which reverts to the ground state by the emission of conversion electrons and gamma rays with a half-life of 6 hours." This isotope of technetium (Tc-99m) possesses the characteristics of an ideal radiopharmaceutical. Following invention of the **radionuclide generator** at Brookhaven National Laboratory in 1957, Tc-99m became conveniently and economically available on a daily basis, and nuclear medicine, as we know it today, was born.

Over the intervening years there has been a steady development in radiopharmaceuticals, allowing a very wide range of disease processes to be investigated. Gamma detection instrumentation has taken an evolutionary path of its own, culminating in the **SPECT** (single photon emission computed tomography), **PET** (positron emission tomography), and integrated PET/CT and SPECT/CT scanners that are commonly found in contemporary nuclear medicine laboratories.

Synthesis of Radionuclides

Currently, more than 2,700 radioisotopes have been artificially produced in reactors, cyclotrons, linear accelerators, and generators. Radionuclides used in nuclear medicine are mostly artificial, produced in cyclotrons, reactors, or generators (Table 43-1).

The radionuclide generator was developed for efficient and convenient production of short-lived radionuclides. A radionuclide generator makes use of the decay-growth relationship between a long-lived parent radionuclide and its short-lived daughter radionuclide. The parent radionuclide is loaded inside the generator and allowed to decay to the short-lived daughter, which is chemically separated from the parent and removed from the generator.

The Mo-99/Tc-99m generator for producing the technetium-99m daughter from a molybdenum-99 parent is invaluable in modern nuclear medicine. It is transportable, relatively inexpensive and easy to operate, and occupies a key position in many institutional nuclear medicine radiopharmacies (Figure 43-1).

The difference between the half-lives of the parent (66 hours for Mo-99) and the daughter (6 hours for Tc-99m) is such that the relative quantities of each inside the generator exist in transient equilibrium. Tc-99m activity builds up until it reaches approximately 90 percent of the Mo-99 activity in the generator, then Tc-99m appears to decay at the same rate as its parent. By fortuitous coincidence, maximum activity of Tc-99m occurs after four half-lives (approximately 24 hours), meaning that the maximum yield of Tc-99m can be removed from the generator at the start of every business day.

The process of removing Tc-99m from the Mo-99/Tc-99m generator is known as elution. The eluting solvent (eluant), sodium chloride solution, is drawn through the system using a vacuum, and the eluate (Tc-99m) is extracted in the form of sodium pertechnetate ($Na^{99m}TcO_4$) solution. Before use in patients, or for making Tc-99m–labeled radiopharmaceuticals, the eluate must undergo quality control testing.

Diagnostic Radiopharmaceuticals

A **radiopharmaceutical** is a radioactive prescription drug. It is internally administered, and may be intended for use in diagnosis and/or treatment of disease. The term includes nonradioactive

TABLE 43-1. The Half-Lives, Gamma Energies, Production Methods, and Usages of Radionuclides Nuclear Medicine

Radionuclide	Half-life	Gamma energy (KeV)	Production method	Usage
Carbon-11	20.4 min	511	Cyclotron	PET
Cesium-137	30 y	662	Reactor	Sealed sources
Cobalt-57	270 d	122	Cyclotron	Sealed sources and *in vitro* NM
Fluorine-18	110 min	511 (β^+)	Cyclotron	PET
Gallium-67	78 h	93, 185, 296	Cyclotron	Diagnostic NM
Gallium-68	68 min	511 (β^+)	Generator	Sealed sources
Indium-111	70 h	173, 247	Cyclotron	Diagnostic NM
Iodine-123	13 h	159	Cyclotron	Diagnostic NM
Iodine-125	59.4 d	35	Reactor	*In vitro* NM
Iodine-131	8.06 d	364 (β^-)	Reactor	Diagnostic NM and radionuclide therapy
Krypton-81m	13 s	190	Generator	Diagnostic NM
Molybdenum-99	66 h	740, 780	Reactor	Mo/Tc generators
Nitrogen-13	10 min	511 (β^+)	Cyclotron	PET
Oxygen-15	2 min	511 (β^+)	Cyclotron	PET
Phosphorus-32	14.3 d	none (β^-)	Reactor	Radionuclide therapy
Rubidium-82	76 s	511 (β^+)	Generator	PET
Samarium-153	46.3 h	none (β^-)	Reactor	Radionuclide therapy
Strontium-89	50.6 d	none (β^-)	Reactor	Radionuclide therapy
Technetium-99m	6 h	140	Generator	Diagnostic NM
Thallium-201	73 h	135, 167	Cyclotron	Diagnostic NM
Xenon-133	5.27 d	81	Reactor	Diagnostic NM
Yttrium-90	2.7 d	none (β^-)	Reactor	Radionuclide therapy

radiopharmaceutical reagent kits, as well as radionuclide generators. It does not include substances containing trace quantities of naturally occurring radionuclides or sealed sources used for radiotherapy.

Technetium. Technetium is the most commonly used radionuclide for nuclear medicine gamma imaging. With atomic number 43, it is a transition metal, possessing properties similar to those of manganese and rhenium. There are no stable isotopes of technetium. Sixteen radioisotopes exist, with mass numbers ranging from 92 to 107, but only one, technetium-99m (Tc-99m), is suitable for clinical use.

Advantages of Tc-99m include its half-life, decay mode, and gamma energy. At 6 hours, the half-life is sufficiently short to minimize radiation exposure to patients, and long enough to be a good match to natural clearance times in many metabolic processes. Tc-99m decays by isomeric transmission, with a gamma energy of 140 KeV, which is ideal for imaging. The gamma ray energy is high enough that there is minimal photoelectric absorption within the body, but low enough to be effectively shielded by lead.

Tc-99m can be manufactured quite cheaply and conveniently in a chemical generator by decay from molybdenum-99. The product, Tc-99m, is in the chemical form of sodium pertechnetate ($Na^{99m}TcO_4$). It can be manipulated chemically to

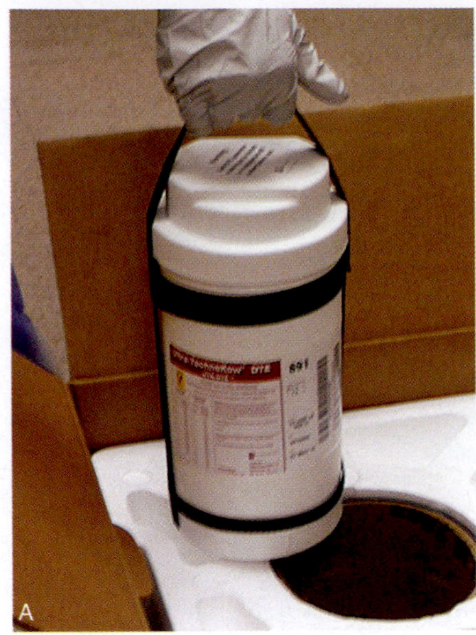

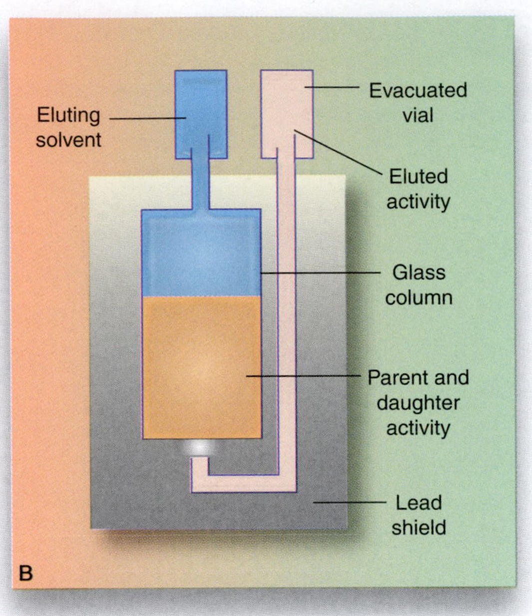

FIGURE 43-1. Radionuclide generator (A) and schematic (B). An evacuated vial is used to draw the eluting solvent through the column. The solvent selectively washes off the daughter isotope and carries it into the evacuated vial. The parent isotope remains on the column for further decay.

TABLE 43-2. Technetium-99m–Labeled Radiopharmaceuticals and Their Uses

Radiopharmaceutical	Chemical name	Major imaging application
Tc-99m MDP	Methylene diphosphonate	Skeletal system
Tc-99m MAA	Macroaggregated albumin	Regional lung perfusion
Tc-99m Sestamibi	Methoxyisobutylisonitrile	Myocardial perfusion
Tc-99m SC	Sulfur colloid	Reticuloendothelial system
Tc-99m IDA	Iminodiacetic acid	Hepatobiliary system
Tc-99m DTPA	Diethylene triamine pentaacetic acid	Renal system
Tc-99m MAG3	Mercaptoacetyl triglycine	Renal system
Tc-99m HMPAO	Hexamethylpropylene amine oxime	Regional cerebral perfusion
Tc-99m labeled RBCs	Labeled red blood cells	Cardiac blood pool
Tc-99m labeled WBCs	Labeled white blood cells	Inflammations and infections

form a wide variety of different radiopharmaceuticals and serve many applications (Table 43-2).

Due to their short-lived nature, and for ease of preparation, many technetium radiopharmaceuticals are manufactured in kit form. Kits contain the pharmaceutical ligand and any required reagents (reducing agents, stabilizers, buffers, etc.) as a lyophilized (freeze-dried) powder that is reconstituted by adding sodium pertechnetate. Some kits require simple processing steps, such as boiling or filtering. All radiopharmaceuticals must undergo quality control testing before use in patients.

Other Commonly Used Radionuclides. There are several other commonly used radionuclides in diagnostic nuclear medicine.

Iodine-123, iodine-125, iodine-131. Iodine is a reactive halogen, found naturally in many biological molecules. The radioiodination of molecules is a relatively simple process, and there are several radioisotopes of iodine from which to select. Iodine-123 is a pure gamma emitter, with a gamma energy of 159 KeV and a half-life of 13 hours. Although its physical characteristics are compatible with gamma imaging, use is limited because production requires particle bombardment in a cyclotron, which is expensive.

Iodine-125 is also a pure gamma emitter. However, its long half-life (59 days) and very low gamma energy (35 KeV) render it unsuitable for use in gamma imaging. It does have some non-imaging, or *in vitro*, applications.

Iodine-131 (I-131) has a half-life of 8 days and decays by a combination of beta and gamma emission. The gamma energy is 364 KeV, which is considered high energy and means that I-131 is difficult to collimate and images may be of suboptimal quality. The high-energy gamma coupled with beta particle emission limits the permissible activity dosage and compounds the problem of suboptimal image quality. Notwithstanding these disadvantages, I-131 has been used since the earliest days of nuclear medicine to label radiopharmaceuticals for diagnostic and therapeutic applications (Table 43-3).

Fluorine-18. Fluorine-18 (F-18) is one of the most commonly used isotopes in PET imaging. F-18 is a positron emitter and has a half-life of 110 minutes. It is manufactured in a cyclotron, which, owing to the short half-life of F-18, must be geographically close to the imaging center. The most common use for F-18 is synthesis of F-18 fluorodeoxyglucose (FDG), used to demonstrate glucose metabolism in the heart, brain, and oncologic processes.

TABLE 43-3. Non–Tc-99m Radiopharmaceuticals and Their Uses

Radiopharmaceutical	Chemical name	Imaging/therapeutic application
I-123 NaI	Sodium iodide	Thyroid imaging and uptake measurement
I-131 NaI	Sodium iodide	Thyroid uptake measurement, hyperthyroidism treatment, metastatic thyroid carcinoma survey, differentiated thyroid carcinoma treatment
I-125 HSA (RISA)	Human serum albumin (Radioiodinated serum albumin)	Measurement of blood and plasma volumes
I-123/131 MIBG	Metaiodobenzyl guanidine	Adrenal medullary imaging
I-125 Glofil	Iothalamate	Measurement of glomerular filtration rate
F-18 FDG	Fluorodeoxyglucose	Glucose metabolism of tumors, brain, myocardium, infections and inflammatory diseases
Tl-201	Thallous chloride	Myocardial perfusion and viability
Ga-67	Gallium citrate	Tumors (lymphoma, hepatoma), infectious processes (sarcoidosis, osteomyelitis)
In-111 WBCs	Indium oxine labeled white blood cells	Infectious/inflammatory processes (inflammatory bowel, vascular/orthopedic prostheses)
In-111 DTPA	Diethylene triamine pentaacetic acid	Communicating hydrocephalus, normal pressure hydrocephalus, CSF shunts, CSF leakage
In-111 ProstaScint	Capromab pendetide	Occult and metastatic prostate cancer
In-111 OncoScint	Satumomab pendetide	Metastatic colorectal and ovarian cancers
In-111 Zevalin	Ibritumomab	Uptake and distribution mapping in patients with B-cell lymphoma prior to treatment with Y-90 Zevalin

Thallium-201. Thallium-201 (Tl-201) is cyclotron-produced and decays by electron capture, emitting gamma rays with energies of 135 KeV and 167 KeV and mercury characteristic x-rays of 68–80 KeV. Its half-life is 73 hours. Tl-201 is used to synthesize Tl-201 thallous chloride. After intravenous injection, Tl-201 thallous chloride accumulates in viable myocardium in a manner analogous to that of potassium; thus it has been used since the 1970s to evaluate myocardial perfusion (Table 43-3).

Gallium-67. Gallium-67 (Ga-67) is cyclotron-produced and decays by electron capture, with a half-life of 78 hours and emitting gamma rays with energies of 93, 185, 296, and 388 KeV. Ga-67 is used to synthesize Ga-67 gallium citrate, which, after intravenous injection, attaches to iron-binding serum proteins for transportation around the body, and accumulates in certain tumors, infections, and inflammations (Table 43-3).

Indium-111. Indium-111 (In-111) is cyclotron-produced and decays by electron capture, with a half-life of 67 hours and emitting gamma rays with energies of 173 and 247 KeV and cadmium characteristic x-rays of 26 KeV. In-111 can be used to synthesize several clinically useful radiopharmaceuticals (Table 43-3).

Therapeutic Radiopharmaceuticals

Some radionuclides emit particulate radiation such as beta particles. This property can be used to directly destroy or ablate malignant disease processes. Some therapeutic radiopharmaceuticals and their applications are shown in Table 43-4.

Quality Control Testing of Radiopharmaceuticals

Quality control testing is carried out by commercial manufacturers of radiopharmaceuticals, and this is sufficient for those radiopharmaceuticals that have been purchased in a ready-to-use formulation. However, most institutional radiopharmacies ("hot labs") prepare radiopharmaceuticals for human use on an as-needed basis, at least occasionally. Therefore, nuclear medicine technologists must be competent at testing in-house preparations (Table 43-5).

Nuclear Pharmacy

Design of a Nuclear Pharmacy. Design of a nuclear pharmacy (radiopharmacy, "hot lab") should take into account protection of personnel and general

TABLE 43-4. Radiopharmaceuticals Used for Radionuclide Therapy

Radionuclide	Chemical form	Therapeutic applications
I-131	Sodium iodide	Treatment of hyperthyroidism (Graves' disease) and differentiated thyroid cancer
I-131	Tositumomab	Treatment of B-cell non-Hodgkin's lymphoma
P-32	Sodium phosphate	Treatment of polycythemia vera, palliation of painful bone metastases
P-32	Chromic phosphate	Palliation of joint pain (radiosynoviorthesis), intracavitary treatment of malignant peritoneal and pleural effusions
Sr-89	Strontium chloride	Palliation of painful bone metastases
Sm-153	Samarium EDTA	Palliation of painful bone metastases
Y-90	Ibritumomab tiuxetan	Treatment of B-cell non-Hodgkin's lymphoma
Y-90	Pentetreotide	Treatment of neuroendocrine tumors
Y-90	Coated microspheres	Treatment of hepatocellular carcinoma or liver metastases from primary colorectal cancer
Dy-165	Ferric hydroxide macroaggregate	Palliation of joint pain (radiosynoviorthesis)

TABLE 43-5. Radiopharmaceutical Quality Control Tests

Physical characteristics	Visual inspection for color and clarity of solution. Particle number and particle size of colloidal or aggregated preparations measured using hemocytometer. Checked by manufacturer and technologist.
pH and osmolality	Checked by manufacturer and maintained by technologist by adherence to guidelines for reconstitution of kits and dilution of doses.
Radionuclidic purity	Measurement of contamination of Tc-99m radiopharmaceutical with other radionuclides, which may alter biodistribution, dosimetry, and image quality. Checked by manufacturer and technologist by spectroscopy.
Radiochemical purity	Measurement of contamination of Tc-99m radiopharmaceutical with other radiochemical forms of Tc-99m, which may alter biodistribution, dosimetry, and image quality. Checked by manufacturer and technologist by instant thin-layer chromatography.
Chemical purity	Measurement of contamination of Tc-99m radiopharmaceutical with other (nonradioactive) chemicals, which may alter biodistribution, dosimetry, and image quality. Checked by manufacturer and technologist by colorimetry.
Sterility	Absence of viable bacteria or microorganisms. All radiopharmaceuticals for human use must be sterilized by autoclaving or by membrane filtration. Sterility checked by manufacturer and maintained by technologist by use of sterile techniques.
Apyrogenicity	Absence of fever-inducing proteins and polysaccharides (pyrogens) produced by metabolism of microorganisms. Checked by manufacturer by observing febrile response in test rabbits, or by use of limulus amoebocyte lysate test kit. Manufacturers and technologists endeavor to maintain apyrogenicity by maintaining sterility.
Toxicity	Toxic effects and safe dosage of radiopharmaceutical are established by manufacturer before FDA grants approval for manufacture and use.

public from radiation hazard, avoidance of contamination of work area and instrumentation, and disposal of radioactive waste (Figure 43-2).

Design features include:

- Situation out of main traffic area, with minimal access by public and patients.
- Designated areas for compounding/dispensing and radioactive waste storage/disposal.
- Use of materials that are easy to decontaminate after radioactive spills.
- Lead-lined storage areas and waste receptacles.
- Deep, stainless steel sink for dilution and cleanup.
- Exhaust fume-hood for storing and dispensing volatile radiopharmaceuticals.
- Eye-wash station and shower in case of major body contamination.

Nuclear Pharmacy Equipment. Nuclear pharmacy equipment includes the following items:

- **Dose calibrator** (Figure 43-3A-C) for measuring various types and quantities of radioactivity during radiopharmaceutical preparation and before dispensing.
- Radiation survey meters (Figure 43-3D and E) for daily exposure rate surveys and contamination detection.
- **Scintillation detector** with multichannel analyzer for detecting radionuclidic contaminants in radiopharmaceuticals.
- Well-type scintillation counter (Figure 43-3F) for counting samples and wipe test swabs.
- Lead bricks and barrier shields for protecting personnel from exposure.
- Lead-lined refrigerator for storing kits and radiopharmaceuticals.
- Water-bath for heating radiopharmaceuticals during preparation.

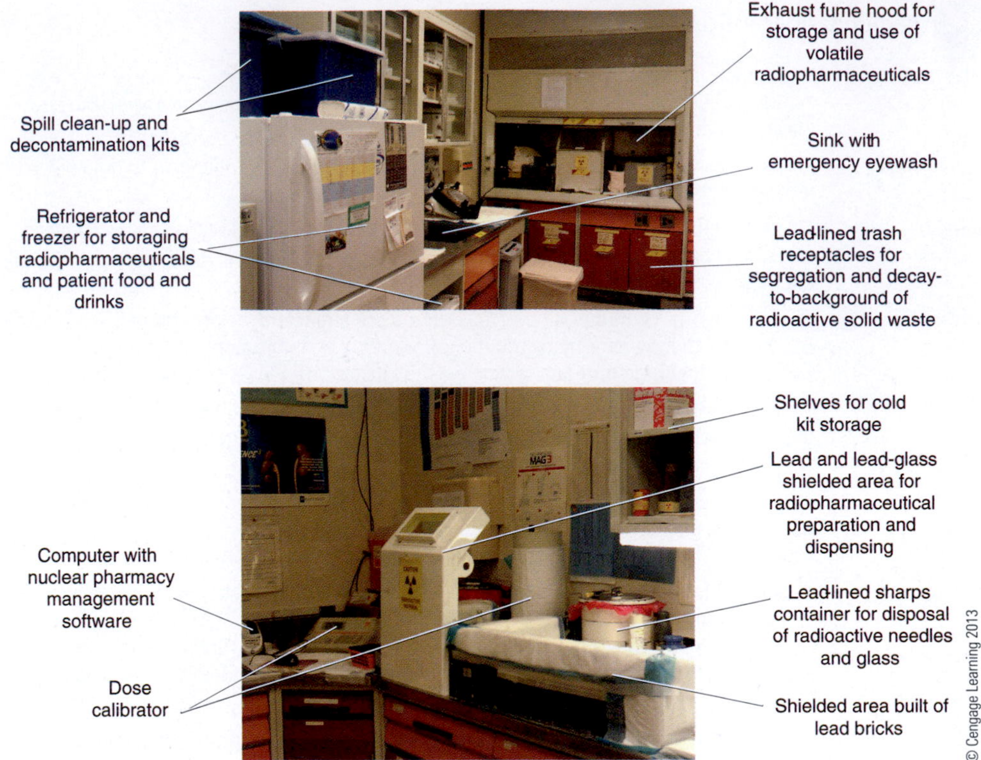

FIGURE 43-2. A radiopharmacy ("hot lab") should be laid out for optimal workflow and minimal personnel exposure. There must be shielded areas for compounding, storing, and dispensing radiopharmaceuticals, as well as for storage of radioactive waste while it decays to background.

- Lead vial and syringe shields (Figure 43-4C-E) for shielding radiopharmaceutical kits and doses during storage, transportation, handling, and administration.
- Basic laboratory equipment—glassware, pipettes, centrifuge, balance, calculator.
- Radiation warning labels and signage (Figure 43-5) for labeling radioactive items and areas.
- Equipment for quality control testing of radiopharmaceuticals.
- Personal protective equipment—lab coats, disposable gloves, safety glasses.
- Nuclear pharmacy management software package for radiopharmaceutical inventory and record keeping—shipments, radiopharmaceutical preparation, dispensing, waste disposal, survey and wipe test results, patient data, quality control test results.

Nuclear Pharmacy Operations. Each nuclear pharmacy has a variety of operations that must be performed. These operations are described next.

Instrument calibration. Calibration and operations checks of all instrumentation that will be used for detecting or measuring radioactivity must be performed daily—dose calibrators, survey meters, well counters, and rate meters.

Elution of Mo-99/Tc-99m generator. This is routinely performed early in the morning and usually provides enough Tc-99m for daily needs (Figure 43-6). Quality control testing must be performed on eluate before using it to prepare radiopharmaceuticals.

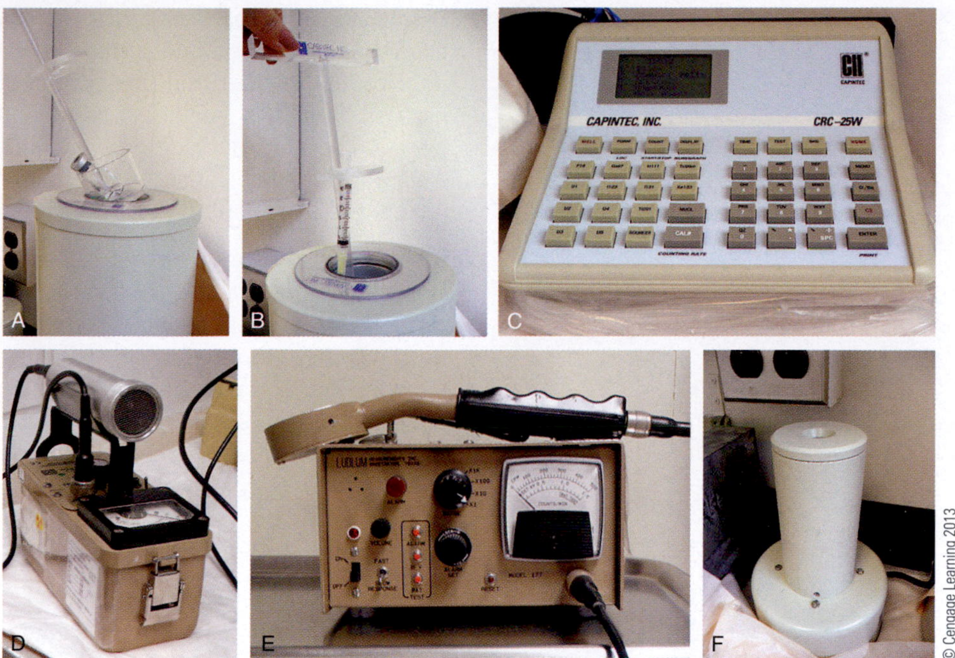

FIGURE 43-3. Nuclear pharmacy instrumentation. Dose calibrator used to measure (assay) the activity of radiopharmaceuticals in syringes and vials during compounding and before dispensing to patients (A, B, C). Geiger-Mueller counters with thin-end window (D) and pancake probe (E). Single-well well counter for measuring activity of samples contained in test-tubes (F).

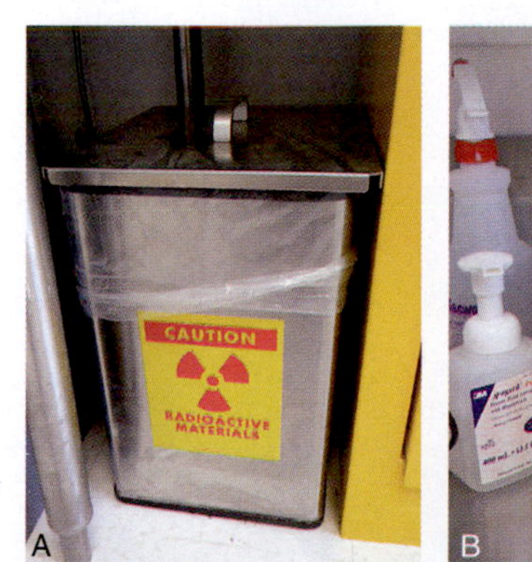

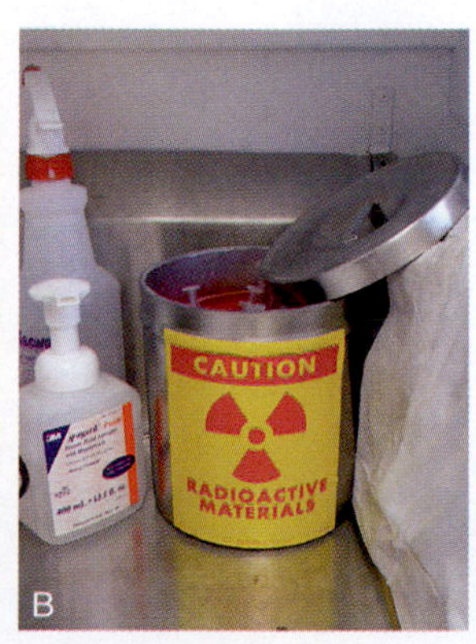

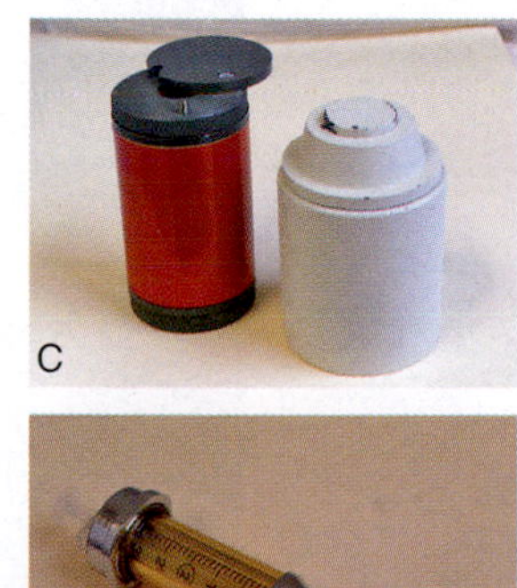

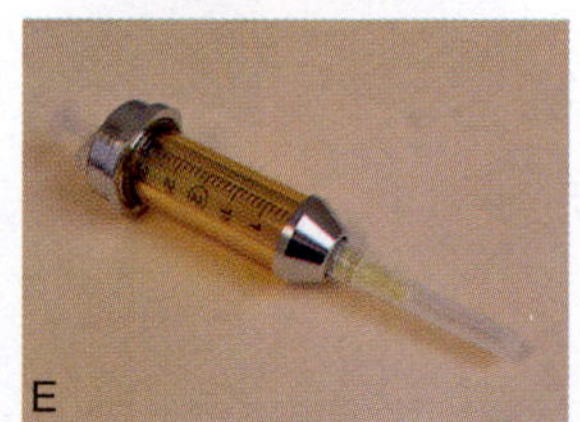

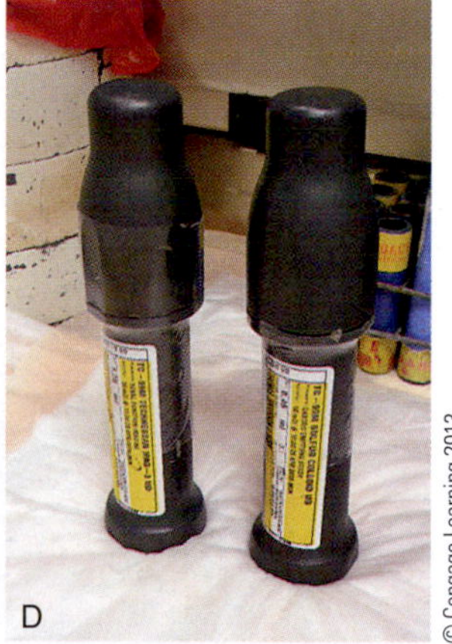

FIGURE 43-4. Nuclear pharmacy equipment. Lead and lead-lined storage containers and waste receptacles (A, B). Lead vial shields (C) and lead/lead-glass syringe shields (D, E).

Preparation of radiopharmaceuticals. Tc-99m-labeled radiopharmaceutical kits can be reconstituted as needed according to the patient schedule for the day. Kit manufacturers provide package inserts including instructions for preparing, quality control testing, and dispensing each radiopharmaceutical. The simplest preparations just require addition of the eluant and dilution with isotonic saline (Figure 43-7).

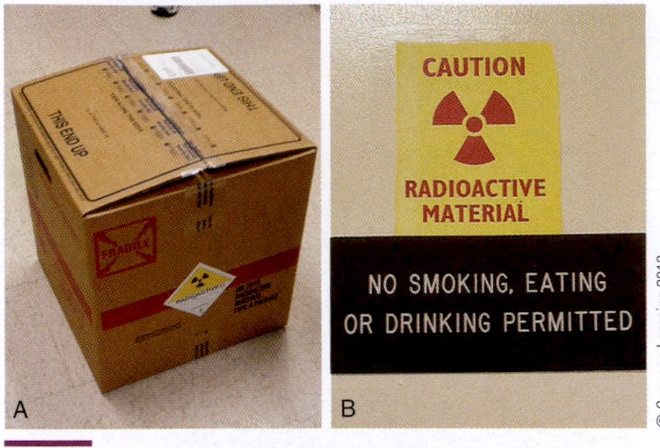

FIGURE 43-5. Radiation warning labels and signs.

Dispensing radiopharmaceuticals. Radiopharmaceuticals may be administered to patients only after receipt of a written prescription specifying a particular nuclear medicine study on a named patient. The indicated radiopharmaceutical is drawn from the kit vial (Figure 43-8), and the activity must be assayed carefully before administration.

Radioactive waste disposal. In the nuclear medicine clinic, most radioactive waste products have short half-lives and can be disposed of by decay-in-storage in appropriately labeled, leak-proof containers. When the radiation exposure rate from the waste is indistinguishable from the background radiation level, the waste container can be disposed of in the same way as nonradioactive waste.

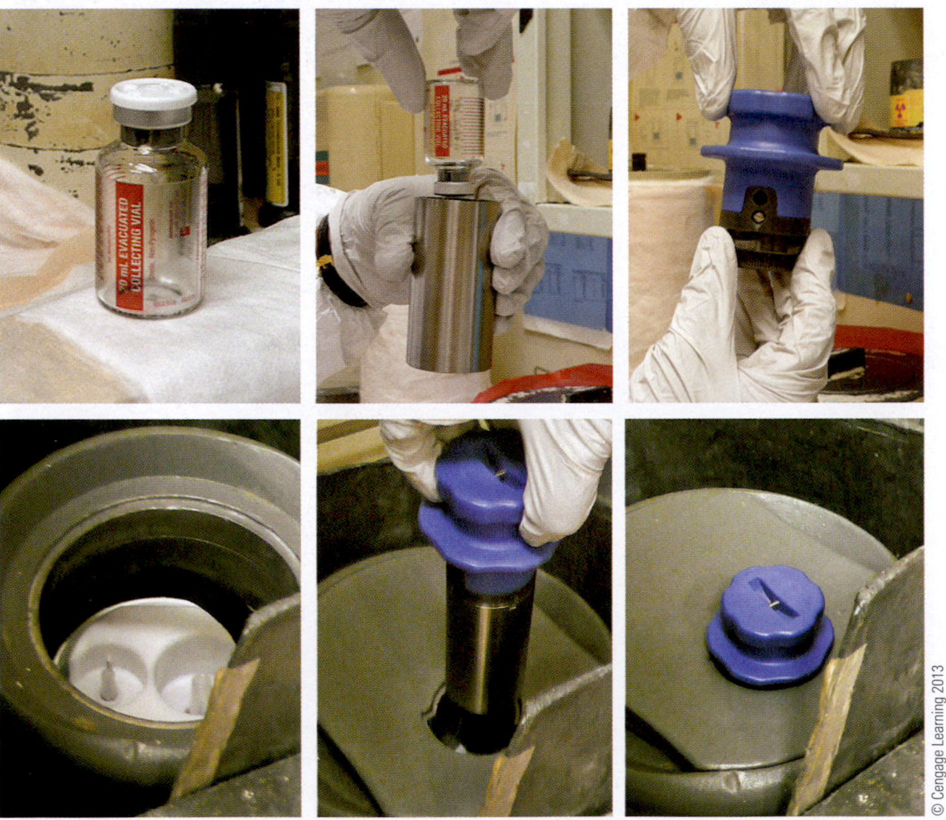

FIGURE 43-6. Eluting the radionuclide generator. The evacuated vial is placed inside a specially designed shield that fits onto the elution needle projecting from the top of the generator. After a few minutes the vial can be removed and will contain the generator eluate ready for quality control testing and patient use.

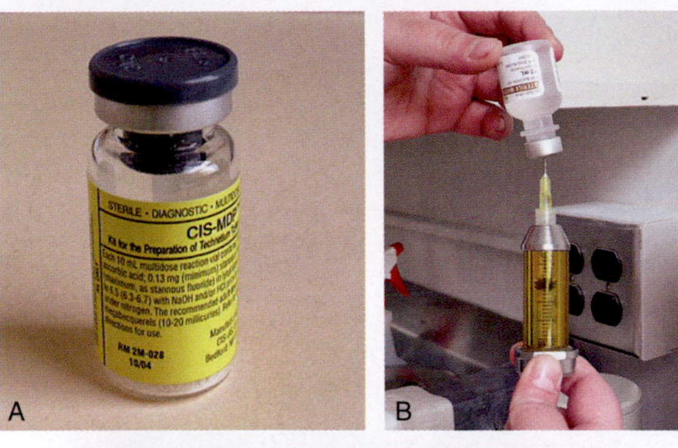

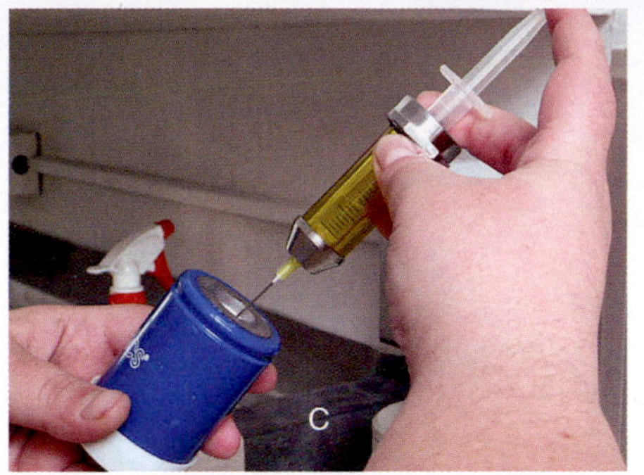

FIGURE 43-7. Preparing a radiopharmaceutical kit. (A) Cold kit vial. (B) Drawing up solvent. (C) Adding technetium-99m to the kit vial.

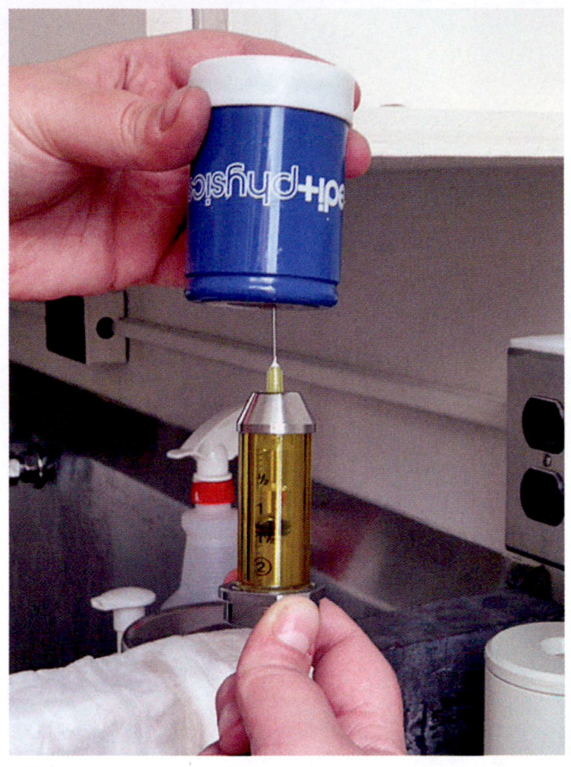

FIGURE 43-8. Drawing up a radiopharmaceutical dose.

IMAGING INSTRUMENTATION

Gamma Camera

Modern-day gamma imaging is performed using a **gamma camera**, also known as an Anger camera, named for the inventor, Hal Anger. Contemporary gamma cameras (Figure 43-9A) feature one, two, or three large field-of view scintillation detectors arranged in various configurations, and can be used for planar and SPECT (single photon emission computer tomography) acquisitions. Each camera is composed of a scintillation detector (crystal and photomultiplier tube assembly), a collimator, and a hardwired logic circuit for position-sensitive photon counting and energy analysis (Figure 43-9B).

Scintillation Detection. The term *scintillation detector* refers to the combination of a scintillation crystal and photomultiplier tubes that are capable of detecting scintillations (light flashes) and converting them into an electric signal, from which a digital image can be constructed.

Gamma photons from a patient containing a radiopharmaceutical exit the patient's body and strike the face of the scintillation crystal. Depending on the energies of the incident gamma photons, photoelectric effect and Compton scattering will take place in the crystal, resulting in production of visible light photons of 2 eV. The light photons pass through the crystal to the photocathodes of an array of photomultiplier (PM) tubes bonded to the back of the crystal.

Each 2-eV light photon is converted at the photocathode into a 2-eV electron, which is then drawn along a series of 10 dynodes before collection at the anode at the far end of the PM tube. At each dynode, the electron current is amplified. The electric current passing out of each PM tube

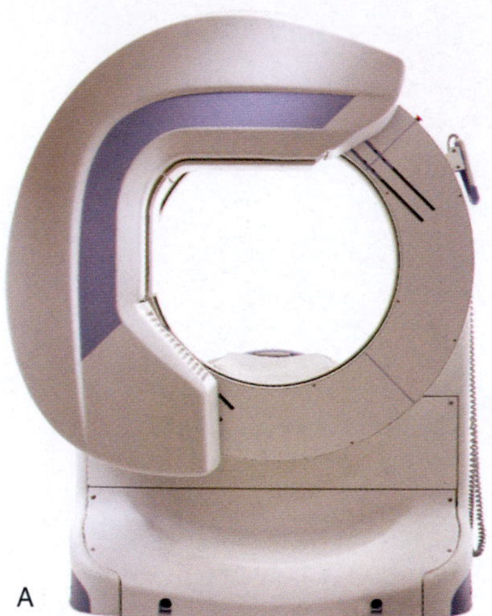

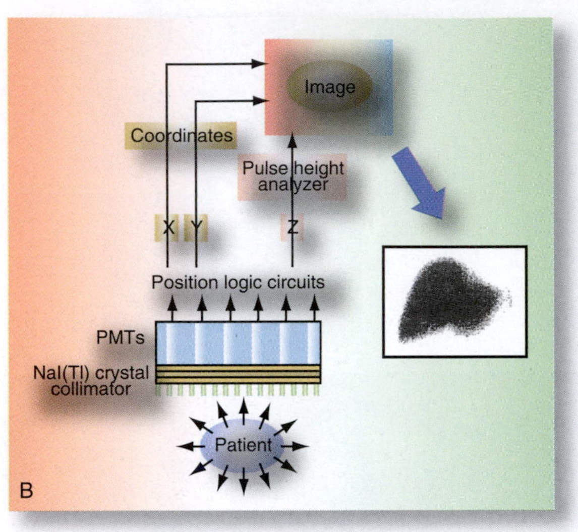

FIGURE 43-9. (A) A dual head gamma camera. (*Courtesy of GE Healthcare.*) (B) Schematic of gamma imaging. Gamma rays from the patient pass through the holes in the collimator and interact in the NaI(Tl) crystal. The scintillations are picked up at the photocathodes of the photomultiplier tubes and pass back to the anode, being multiplied at each dynode. The electric current leaving each PM tube passes through positioning logic circuitry for plotting of x, y coordinates, and a pulse height analyser for energy discrimination. The resulting image is a map of count distribution displayed in a matrix.

has been amplified by a factor of 510, and is in the magnitude of millivolts.

Scintillation Crystal. The scintillation crystal is a single crystal sheet, typically 10 mm thick and 30–50 cm across. For most nuclear medicine applications the crystal is thallium-activated sodium iodide, NaI(Tl).

Choice of scintillator material involves a trade-off between sensitivity for detection and decay time of the scintillation. NaI(Tl) is chosen for the efficiency with which it converts an ionization event into visible light, its long decay time, and high light output. Also, there is a linear relationship between the energies of the gamma photons striking the crystal and the amount of visible light produced, which allows for energy discrimination by the detector and results ultimately in a less noisy image.

Collimator. The most commonly used collimator is called a parallel-hole collimator. It is a lead plate, approximately 2–3 cm thick, that covers the entire surface of the crystal. The lead is pierced by thousands of parallel-oriented holes, each less than 1 mm in diameter. Each hole must be at least 10 times as long as it is wide.

The collimator is positioned between the radioactive source (patient) and the detector crystal, to reduce the number of gamma photons incident on the crystal. Collimator transmission is typically in the order of 0.1 percent of incident photons. The collimator defines a line of sight. The tubular holes through the parallel-hole collimator only allow through those photons travelling close to the axis of the hole, perpendicular to the crystal face. Photons traveling at oblique angles are absorbed by the lead septa forming the walls of the collimator holes.

Several different collimator designs are available for various special applications: converging, diverging, fan beam, slant hole, and pin hole.

Collimators can be categorized according to sensitivity or spatial resolution: high sensitivity, all-purpose, and high resolution. An appropriate collimator must be selected according to the energies of the gamma photons of the radionuclide in use. Low-energy collimators are suitable for use with 0- to 200-KeV gammas, medium-energy collimators for 200- to 400-KeV gammas, and high-energy collimators for 400- to 600-KeV gammas.

Output Analysis. In order to produce a meaningful image, the electronic signals from the PM tubes must be processed to determine the XY location of each scintillation in the crystal, which results in the location of each count in the corresponding pixel of the digital image matrix. This is performed by positioning circuitry, sometimes known as Anger logic (named for the inventor, Hal Anger).

Recall that the back surface of the NaI(Tl) crystal is connected to PM tubes—60 to 90 PM tubes in most modern cameras—closely packed and covering the entire surface of the crystal. Visible light from a scintillation within the crystal will be received at all PM tubes making up the array, but the PM tubes closest to where the light flash occurred will receive the most light. Each PM tube is connected to four amplifiers, X+, X−, Y+ and Y−, which sum the outputs from all PM tubes and scale it according to the tube's position. The X and Y positions of the scintillation can be estimated to within about 5 mm.

In addition to XY positioning, the PM tube outputs also undergo Z summing and pulse height analysis. The electrical currents from all the PM tubes in a detector are summed together into one Z pulse, which passes to the pulse height analyzer(PHA) for inspection. Z pulses that correspond to the preset gamma energy of interest are accepted by the PHA. Operation of the PHA is controlled by adjusting high voltage, gain of the amplifier, peak energy setting, and energy window width. A multichannel analyzer (MCA) permits selection of 2 or 3 gamma rays of different energies simultaneously.

Digital Image. For each Z pulse that is accepted by the pulse height analyzer, a count is added to the pixel of the image matrix corresponding to its XY location determined by the positioning circuitry.

The technologist can select the matrix configuration and number of pixels: 64 × 64, 128 × 128, and 256 × 256 are examples of square matrices, and the numbers refer to how many columns and rows of pixels there are in each matrix, the product of which is the pixel number. A 64 × 64 matrix contains 4,096 pixels. A 256 × 256 matrix contains 65,536 pixels. The greater the number of pixels, the smaller each pixel is and the better the resolution of the image.

For highly detailed static images a small pixel size should be used. For whole-body images the image matrix is typically 128 × 512. For rapid dynamic images or gated images, where a lot of counts are collected in a very short time, larger pixel size should be used (64 × 64).

Image Acquisition

A gamma camera can be used for planar imaging or for SPECT.

Planar Imaging. Planar static imaging (Figure 43-10A) involves counting gamma photons while keeping the camera in a fixed position and orientation relative to the patient. The image is a two-dimensional projection of all the activity throughout the entire thickness of that part of the patient's body in front of the camera. The camera is usually preset to acquire counts until a certain time has elapsed or a certain number of counts has been collected in the image matrix.

Whole-body images (Figure 43-10B) are planar images acquired by moving the gamma camera at a slow, steady speed (10–15 cm/min) along the length of the patient's body. Most commonly, whole-body imaging is performed using a dual-headed gamma camera, operating with one camera above and one camera below the imaging table, so that anterior and posterior views of the patient are acquired simultaneously.

Dynamic imaging (Figure 43-10C) refers to multiple, rapid, sequential images used to record changes in distribution of radiopharmaceutical in the body over a period of time. Each frame in the imaging sequence may last for less than 1 second or up to 30 seconds.

Gated images (Figure 43-10D) are a type of dynamic imaging used with rhythmically moving organs, generally the heart. The heart is imaged continuously for 500–600 beats, and the data is coordinated with the heart beat, recorded by an ECG machine. The heart beat (R-to-R interval) is divided into a number of equal time frames and each time a new R wave occurs, collection of new set of data frames begins. The R-to-R image sets from 500–600 heart beats are summed to create a composite image cycle. The images from each time frame of the R to R demonstrate different phases in contraction of the heart.

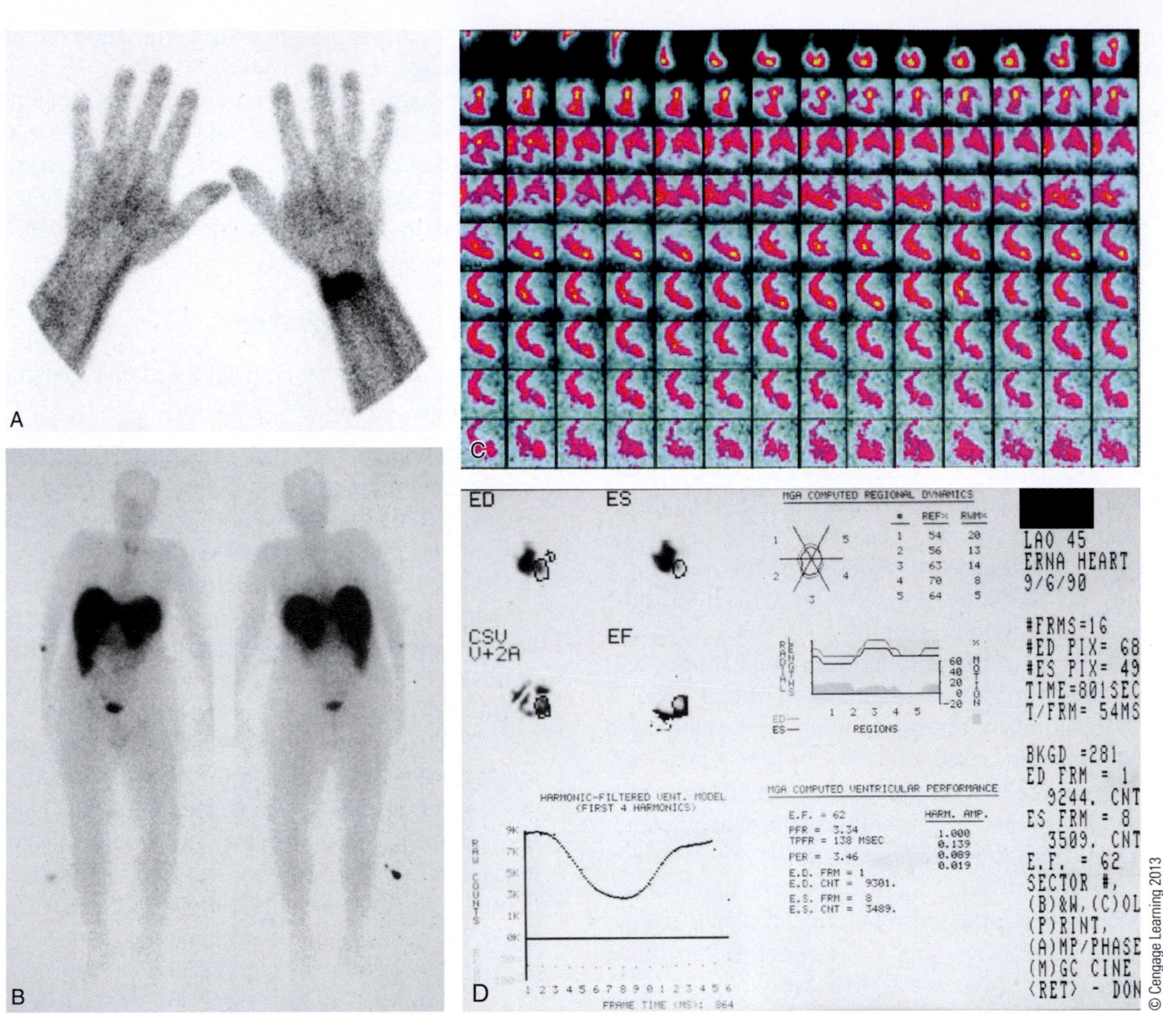

FIGURE 43-10. Image acquisition modes. (A) Planar static image. Palmar view of the wrists and hands showing left radial fracture. Radiopharmaceutical is Tc-99m methylene diphosphonate (MDP). (B) Planar whole-body scan. Anterior and posterior views of patient with metastatic pancreatic cancer. Radiopharmaceutical is In-111 pentetreotide. (C) Planar dynamic images. Cardiac first-pass study demonstrating chambers of the heart. Radiopharmaceutical is Tc-99m diethylene triamine pentaacetic acid (DTPA). (D) Planar gated imaging. Cardiac study showing ventricular function. When viewed in cine mode the study shows movement of the blood volume inside the left ventricle due to contraction of the myocardium. Radiopharmaceutical is Tc-99m–labeled autologous red blood cells.

Single Photon Emission Computed Tomography (SPECT). During SPECT, the gamma camera is rotated around the patient's body, taking a sequence of two-dimensional (2D) projections that are then processed mathematically to create a cross-sectional view of the organ of interest.

For 360° coverage of the patient, a single-headed camera must rotate 360°. Each head of a two-headed camera system will only need to rotate 180°, and each head of a three-headed system only 120°. Two-headed systems are most common, and are available with fixed (parallel configuration) or adjustable (perpendicular configuration) heads for additional versatility.

Operational parameters to consider when acquiring SPECT projections include the acquisition arc, number of projections, time per projection, type of angular motion, and orbit of rotation. These parameters are selected by the operator, and are specific to the body part being imaged, radiopharmaceutical and activity administered, features of the scanner, and body habitus of the patient.

Data Storage

Projection data storage is in the form of a sinogram, which is a stack of slices of projection views. When an acquisition is complete, and before dismissing the patient, the sinogram should be carefully inspected for signs of patient motion. Small amounts of motion can be improved using corrective algorithms, or repeat acquisition may be needed.

Data Reconstruction

There are two methods of reconstruction commonly used for transforming SPECT projection data into transaxial (transverse) slices.

Filtered Back-Projection. Due to the random nature of radioactivity, projection data is very noisy. Also the process of (unfiltered) back-projection introduces a star-shaped artifact into reconstructed data. Therefore, the projection data must be filtered before reconstruction. Filtering is a mathematical technique applied to improve the appearance of the images. During filtered back-projection, a high-pass (Ramp) filter is used to reduce noise and the star artifact.

After filtering, back-projection is performed by projecting each 2D projection back in the direction from which it came and into the pixels of a blank matrix.

Iterative Reconstruction. The computer starts out with an estimate of the data to produce a set of transaxial slices. These slices are used to create a second set of projection views, which are compared to the original ones acquired from the patient.

The computer estimate is tweaked and modified, and recompared to the original patient projections. This process is repeated multiple times, until the difference between the estimated views and original views is below a predetermined threshold.

The two most common mathematical techniques for iterative reconstruction are maximum likelihood expectation maximization (MLEM) and ordered subsets expectation maximization (OSEM).

Pre- and Post-reconstruction Filtering. Use of filters pre- and post-reconstruction depends on the characteristics of the data and the preference of the user. Low-pass filters, such as Butterworth, Hann, and Hamming filters, remove noise, creating smoother, but less-detailed images. High-pass filters, such as Ramp filters, can be used to remove blur, creating noisier, “grainy” images.

Attenuation Correction. Gamma photons originating deep within the body are more likely to be scattered or absorbed before reaching the camera than gamma photons originating near the surface of the body. Attenuated parts of the body will show reduced counts in images, which may be mistaken for pathology.

Attenuation correction can be performed by two methods:

- Calculated attenuation correction

A correction factor is applied, which takes into account tissue thickness and tissue attenuation coefficients. This technique is inaccurate for body parts such as the chest, which contains a variety of tissue types of different densities.

- Transmission attenuation correction

For each SPECT acquisition, a matrix of correction factors is created using a transmission image of the patient acquired using an external gamma source or a computed tomography (CT) scan.

Image Processing and Display. Following construction of the transaxial (transverse) images, image processing can be performed and additional images generated. Commonly, 2D tomograms are displayed in sagittal, coronal, and oblique views (Figure 43-11A–D).Cardiac images are in horizontal long axis, vertical long axis, and short axis views (Figure 43-11E–H). The 3D volume image can be manipulated to enhance certain features, for example, surface rendering or volume rendering.

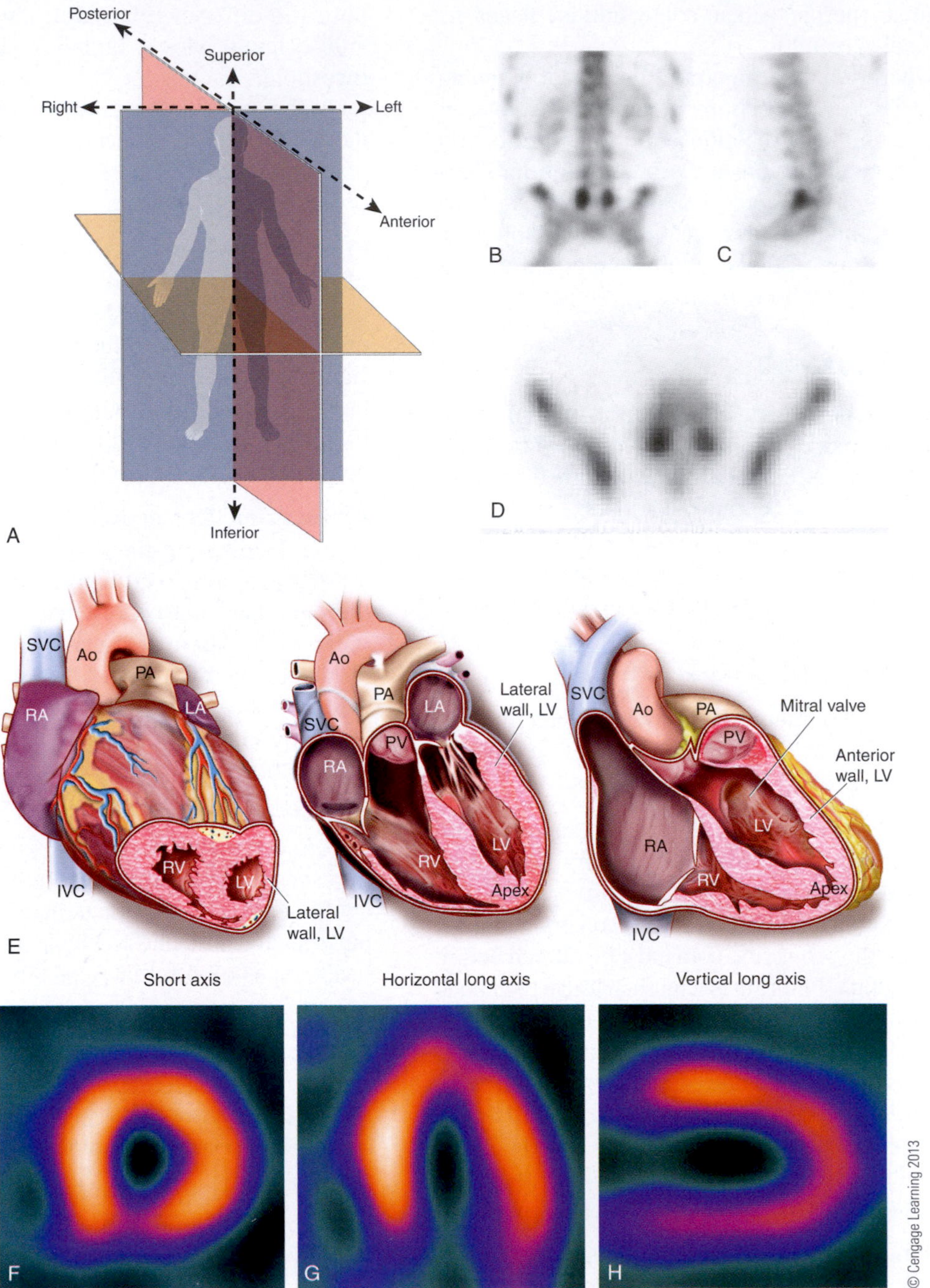

FIGURE 43-11. SPECT image display planes (A): coronal (B), sagittal (C), and transverse (D) slices through the spine on a bone scan using Tc-99m methylene diphosphonate (MDP). (*http://www.vhlab.umn.edu/atlas/anatutorial/anatutorial1.shtml*) SPECT planes used for the heart. SPECT myocardial perfusion slices (E): short axis (F), horizontal long axis (G), and vertical long axis (H). Radiopharmaceutical is Tc-99m sestamibi. (*http://www.med.yale.edu/intmed/cardio/imaging/techniques/spect_anatomy/index.html*)

POSITRON EMISSION TOMOGRAPHY (PET)

Positron emission tomography (PET) is a modification of gamma imaging that detects annihilation photons. The positron emitted from the nucleus of a proton-rich radionuclide atom travels a short distance from the point of emission before encountering an orbital electron and being annihilated. Annihilation results in the simultaneous creation of two gamma photons, each of 511 KeV, traveling in opposite directions.

The PET scanner (Figure 43-12) employs the technique of coincidence detection. With the patient encircled by a ring of detectors, a true event is defined as two interactions occurring simultaneously in two detectors on opposite sides of the ring. The line joining these two detectors represents a line of response (LOR) through the patient, somewhere along which the annihilation took place. Many pairs of events are detected at all angles around the patient, so that the site of annihilation can be determined.

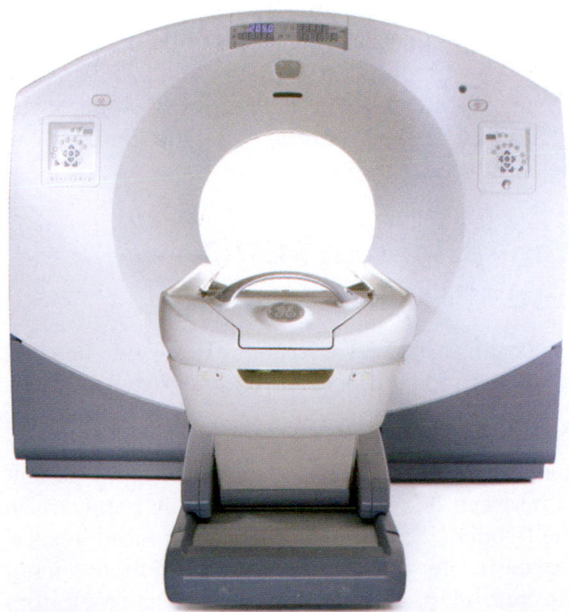

FIGURE 43-12. PET scanner. *(Courtesy of GE Healthcare.)*

PET Scanner

The most common PET scanner design features a tubular array of detectors inside which the patient is positioned for scanning. Individual crystal scintillation detectors, 3–4 mm in cross-section, are grouped into blocks, each backed by four photomultiplier (PM) tubes. The blocks are arranged into rings and the rings are stacked into a cylinder.

The NaI(Tl) crystal used in gamma cameras is generally considered too low density for adequately stopping 511-KeV gamma photons, so denser materials such as lutetium orthosilicate (LSO), gadolinium orthosilicate (GSO), and bismuth germinate oxide (BGO) are used. The role of the PM tubes in the PET scanner is the same as that of those in a gamma camera.

In planar or SPECT gamma imaging the line of sight for the projection images is established using collimators. In PET the line of sight is established by coincidence detection, and collimators are unnecessary. However, ring-shaped septa of lead or tungsten are sometimes positioned between the rings of detector blocks to decrease gamma ray scatter and improve resolution.

PET images are stored as sinograms, reconstructed using iterative reconstruction, and displayed as sagittal, coronal, and transaxial (transverse) slices. Attenuation correction is usually performed by means of transmission images.

Advantages of PET over SPECT

High Sensitivity. Because a PET scanner does not require a collimator, it is 100 times more sensitive than a SPECT scanner, and has a higher count rate for similar quantities of radioactivity.

High Resolution. Recall that true coincidence events are defined as simultaneous interactions in two detector crystals joined by a line of response. Sometimes two random or single gamma photons may strike crystals simultaneously and be misinterpreted as coincidence events. Scatter and random events are undesirable because they cause a reduction in image contrast. Modern PET scanners may make use of time of flight (TOF) technology to enhance detection of only true coincidence events, although this often results in reduced spatial resolution.

PET Radiopharmaceuticals. Positron-emitting isotopes can be synthesized for a large number of low-atomic-number elements, and can be incorporated into many biologically useful compounds and used for demonstrating very specific physiologic properties of organs and tissues. For example, glucose metabolism can be imaged with F-18 fluorodeoxyglucose.

HYBRID SPECT/CT AND PET/CT IMAGING

PET and SPECT imaging have the advantage over CT and MRI of very high sensitivity, with the ability to detect picomolar amounts of radiopharmaceutical. However, spatial resolution of PET and SPECT is low and interpretation of PET and SPECT images can be difficult because they contain few anatomical landmarks.

Coregistration or fusion of PET or SPECT with CT or MRI acquired in separate imaging sessions has been used as a method of providing anatomical context to functional/metabolic images. Until the late 1990s, software fusion was used, with a limited amount of success. Unless patient positioning was identical on the two scans, the images would not match up exactly when fused, and the anatomical location of functional abnormalities was incorrectly determined.

In the late 1990s, David Townsend developed a hybrid PET/CT scanner in which the patient stayed on the same imaging table and underwent PET and CT in the same session, within minutes of each other. This resulted in considerably more successful image fusion and improved patient outcomes, particularly in the field of oncology.

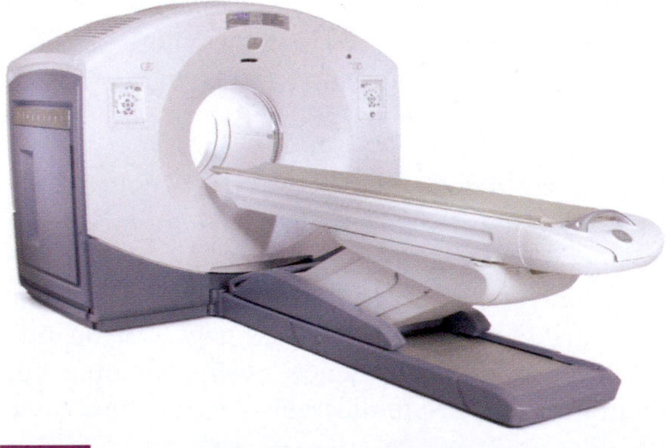

FIGURE 43-13. Hybrid scanner, A PET/CT unit. *(Courtesy of GE Healthcare.)*

Hybrid PET/CT and SPECT/CT Scanners

Most hybrid scanners (Figure 43-13) make use of a third-generation CT scanner in which the x-ray tube rotates around the gantry diametrically opposed to an arc-shaped, rotating detector array. Spiral or helical CT imaging is performed by moving the patient table through the gantry while the x-ray tube and detectors rotate. Use of slip-ring technology means that rotation is not limited.

After a scout or topogram CT image to set the scan area, a non-contrast CT scan is performed. This is followed by a PET or SPECT image of the same body part. The CT image is used to generate a matrix of attenuation coefficients, which is then used for attenuation correction of the PET/SPECT data. The attenuation-corrected PET/SPECT and CT images are fused. Following acquisition of the PET or SPECT, an optional CT with contrast can be performed.

Limitations in PET/CT and SPECT/CT Imaging

Limitations in PET/CT and SPECT/CT imaging include motion artifacts and contrast agent artifacts.

Motion Artifacts. Performance of the CT scan and the PET or SPECT without moving the patient in between has led to a considerable reduction in the frequency of motion artifacts on fused images. However, certain internal organ motion cannot be controlled. The biggest problem is respiratory motion. Conventionally, chest CT is acquired with the patient in breath-hold, whereas PET or SPECT requires the patient to breathe normally. Fusion of these images can result in serious misalignment of the lungs, diaphragm, and liver. To overcome this problem, some imaging departments instruct patients to breathe normally for both the CT and the PET/SPECT. Other institutions may employ respiratory gating techniques.

Contrast Agent Artifacts. Use of contrast agents (intravenous and oral) can increase the diagnostic value of the CT and also improve anatomic localization of PET or SPECT abnormalities. However, because contrast agents are dense by nature, they can alter the attenuation coefficients in contrast-containing areas of anatomy, and result in uptake artifacts on attenuation-corrected PET or SPECT images. Therefore CT with contrast, if required, should not be acquired until after non-contrast images for attenuation correction.

Quality Control Testing

It is extremely important to follow a quality control (QC) testing routine in order to detect changes in imaging system performance that may adversely affect the interpretation of clinical studies. Table 43-6 explains the basic quality control requirements for planar, SPECT, and PET imaging systems. Images of common QC tests are shown in Figure 43-14.

TABLE 43-6. Quality Control Testing of Imaging Instrumentation

PLANAR	**Photopeak**	Daily check to center range of acceptable photon energies
	Uniformity	Uniform source should produce uniform image. Check daily using sheet source for extrinsic uniformity (collimator on); point source for intrinsic (collimator off). (Figure 43-14)
	Spatial resolution	Check weekly using bar phantom and uniformity source. Visually assess images for resolution degradation. (Figure 43-14)
	Spatial linearity	Check weekly using bar phantom and uniformity source. Visually assess images to make sure lead bars appear as straight, unbroken lines. (Figure 43-14)
SPECT	**Uniformity**	A small non-uniformity in the flood field on planar imaging can become a serious bull's-eye artifact on reconstructed SPECT images, so it is very important to acquire good quality, high count flood uniformity correction data.
	Center of rotation	SPECT performance depends on a match between the electronic center of the path of orbital rotation and the mechanical center, and assumes that the camera heads will rotate in a perfect circle (or ellipse) and that the heads will remain precisely aligned opposite each other. Deviation from the above is seen as a displacement of the center of rotation (COR) and degrades image quality.
	Lucite phantoms	SPECT phantom is lucite cylinder containing different sized lucite rods, cylinders and cones. Filled with water containing small amount of radioactivity; for example, Jaszczak phantom. Used to perform acceptance testing and routine evaluation of system performance.
PET	**Blank scan**	Daily quality control procedure. Performed using transmission source without patient in the scanner. Data displayed as sinograms. Visually inspect to locate defective detectors.
	PM tube gain	Output from each PM tube checked daily or weekly to assure uniform response across all, and no fluctuations due to temperature and humidity.
	Normalization	Performed quarterly to adjust PM tube gain.
	Absolute calibration	Performed quarterly so that a certain number of counts within a pixel can be converted to average activity concentration for that pixel. Necessary calibration for using quantitative measurement of radiopharmaceutical uptake, e.g., standard uptake value (SUV).

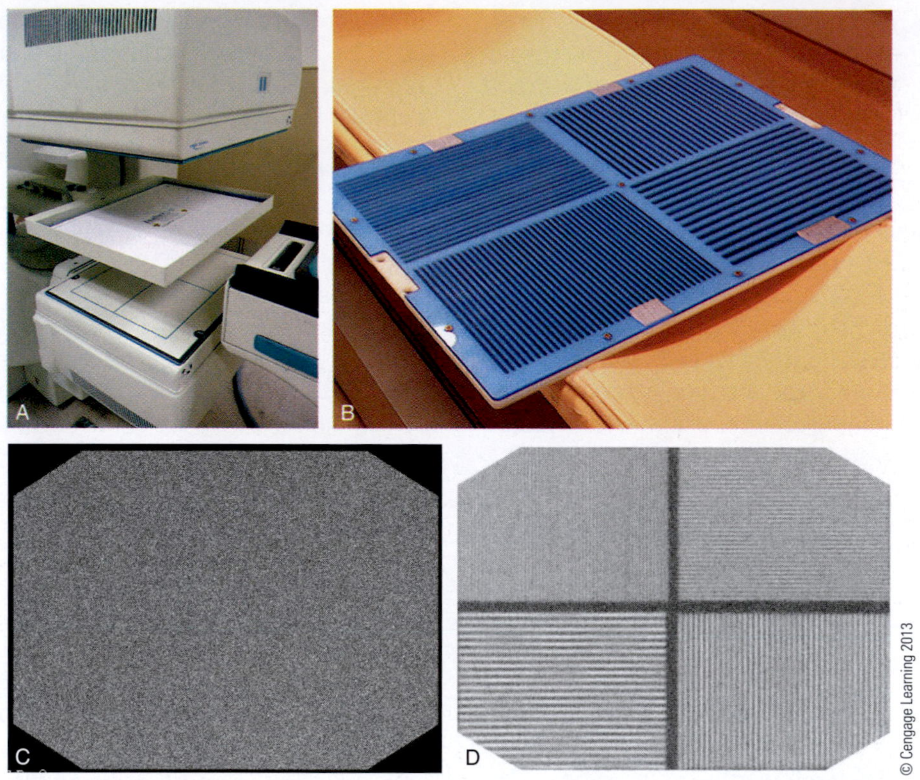

FIGURE 43-14. Gamma camera quality control testing. Flood source in place for acquisition of extrinsic uniformity test (A). Bar phantom for spatial resolution and linearity tests (B). Uniformity flood image (C). Bar phantom image (D).

NONIMAGING INSTRUMENTATION

Several other important pieces of instrumentation are found in the nuclear medicine department and are not used for imaging. Some are based on the same scintillation detector technology as gamma cameras. Others are gas-filled detectors, specifically ionization chambers.

Geiger Counter

A **Geiger-Mueller counter**, commonly called a Geiger counter or GM meter, is a portable ionization chamber (see Figure 43-3D). It consists of a gas-filled cylinder attached to a readout meter and a battery pack. A wire protrudes into the center of the cylinder. Electrical current from the battery establishes a potential difference, such that the wire becomes a positively charged anode and the wall of the chamber becomes a negatively charged cathode. The end of the cylinder is closed with a mica window and mesh screen.

Photons pass through the window into the chamber and ionize the argon gas inside. Positively charged ions are collected at the cathode and negatively charged ions are collected at the anode. The meter readout is proportional to the number of photons entering the chamber. In the nuclear medicine clinic, Geiger counters are used to monitor areas for radiation and detect contamination of items and people. The meter must be calibrated regularly to ensure proper function.

Dose Calibrator

The dose calibrator is a tabletop ionization chamber. The shape of the cylindrical chamber has been modified into that of a deep, open well. A dipper is used to lift vials and syringes in and out of the well (see Figure 43–3A–C).

The dose calibrator is used to measure the activity of radiopharmaceuticals before administration to patients. For ease of use, the chamber is connected to a digital readout meter with an array of buttons precalibrated to the energies of all the commonly used radionuclides. The dose calibrator must be calibrated at installation, and undergo regular quality control testing for accuracy, constancy, linearity of response, and effect of sample geometry.

Uptake Probe

The uptake probe is a scintillation detector (Figure 43-15). It consists of a scintillation crystal and cylindrical (flat field) collimator. Behind the NaI(Tl) crystal is one photomultiplier tube, the output from which passes to a preamplifier, amplifier, and pulse height analyzer to a digital readout. The probe is mounted on a stand with an adjustable arm for versatility of positioning. The most common use for the uptake probe is measurement of radioactive iodine uptake in the thyroid gland. The probe must be calibrated regularly to ensure proper functioning.

Well Counter

The well counter is a scintillation detector in which the NaI(Tl) crystal has been drilled out to contain a cylindrical well into which a vial or test tube can fit (see Figure 43-3F). The well counter is connected to a digital readout. Some well counters are designed to handle multiple samples. In the nuclear medicine laboratory a well counter is commonly used for looking for radioactive contamination on swabs used for wipe testing. It can also be used to measure the radioactivity of body fluid samples. The well counter must be calibrated regularly to ensure proper function.

RADIATION PROTECTION

Radiobiologic Effect

In terms of radiobiologic damage, different types of ionizing radiation are more or less damaging depending on whether they are outside the body or taken internally.

Alpha and beta radiation possess charge and mass. They cause ionizations in tissue and are non-penetrating. We make use of these properties for radiation therapy using internalized radionuclides. However, alpha and beta sources external to the

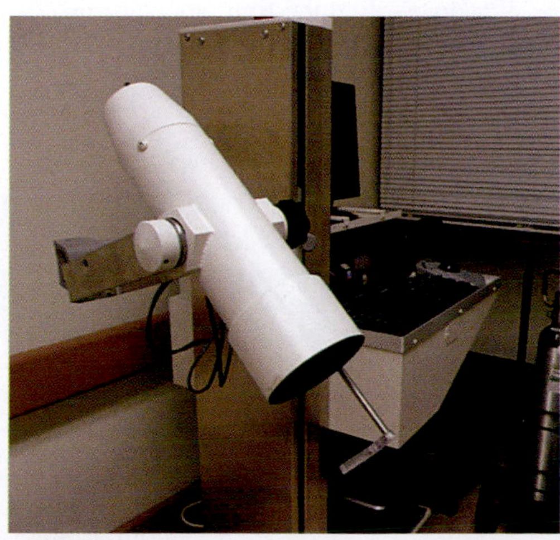

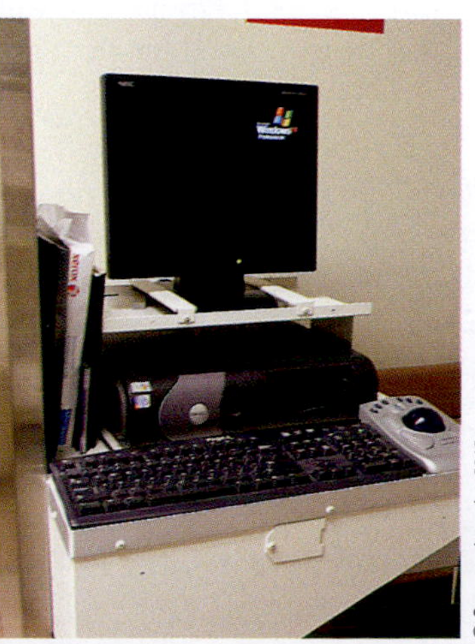

FIGURE 43-15. Uptake probe.

body are relatively safe (depending on their energy) because they are unable to penetrate the body's layer of dead skin cells. Gamma and x-rays have no electrical charge or mass. Therefore they are penetrating, although they cause fewer ionizations in tissue and are less damaging.

Regulation of Radioactive Materials

To minimize radiation hazards, international and national organizations have been established to set guidelines for safe handling of radioactive materials. The International Commission on Radiological Protection (ICRP) provides recommendations and guidance on all aspects of protection against ionizing radiation. The National Council on Radiological Protection and Measurements (NCRP) disseminates information, guidance, and recommendations on radiation protection and measurements that represent the consensus of leading scientific thinking.

The U.S. Nuclear Regulatory Commission (NRC) protects the health and safety of the public and the environment by licensing and regulating the civilian uses of source material (uranium and thorium), special nuclear material (enriched uranium and plutonium), and reactor by-product material (Table 43-7).

Under certain conditions, the NRC enters into agreements with state governors that authorize individual states to regulate their own use of specific radioactive materials used in medicine and industry. Generally, the agreement states regulate the sources of radiation that the NRC does not: all naturally occurring radioactive materials (radium and radon), radiation-producing machines (x-ray machines and particle accelerators), and radionuclides produced by particle accelerators.

Radiation Protection Principles

The ALARA (as low as reasonably achievable) concept was instituted by the NRC to reduce radiation exposure to individuals to a minimum. Techniques, equipment, and procedures should all be evaluated critically. ALARA action levels indicate high occupational exposures that merit investigation and/or corrective action. Variables associated with radiation dose exposure in a nuclear medicine facility include time, distance, shielding, and contamination control.

Time. The total radiation exposure to an individual is directly proportional to the time of exposure to the radiation source. Keep exposure ALARA by spending no more time than necessary near radiation sources. In the nuclear medicine clinic, the injected patient is the greatest source of exposure to personnel. Consider ways to reduce exposure by becoming fast and efficient at radiopharmacy procedures such as eluting the generator and preparing doses. Reduce time spent in proximity to injected patients by careful selection of a study protocol and

TABLE 43-7. Highlights of NRC Regulations Pertaining to Operation of a Nuclear Medicine Facility; Title 10 of the Code of Federal Regulations, Part 20 Addresses Radiation Protection Requirements; Part 35 Addresses Medical Uses of Byproduct Material

10CFR20 Radiation protection requirements	10CFR35 Medical uses of byproduct material
Dose limits for radiation workers and general public	Licensing requirements
Exposure limits for individual workers	Training of personnel (radiation safety officer, medical physicist, nuclear pharmacist, authorized user)
Monitoring and labeling radioactive materials	Survey instruments (possession, use, calibration)
Posting signs in and around radiation areas	Use of unsealed byproduct material
Reporting theft or loss of radioactive material	Use of sealed sources
Penalties for not complying with NRC regulations	Record-keeping

by explaining the procedure to the patient before he or she is injected.

Distance. The intensity of a radiation source, and thus radiation exposure, varies inversely as the square of the distance from the source to the point of exposure (i.e., the inverse square law). Keep exposure ALARA by staying as far away as possible from the radiation source. Consider where a radiopharmaceutical injection will be performed, where patients will wait during uptake, and try to monitor patients from a distance.

Shielding. Penetrating ionizing radiation such as gamma photons requires shielding with high-atomic-number materials such as lead, which will absorb the radiation by photoelectric effect. In order to keep exposure ALARA, gamma-emitting radionuclides should always be stored in lead containers and injected using syringe shields. Radioactive waste should be stored until it decays to background in lead-lined waste bins. Pure beta-emitting radionuclides should be stored in containers of low-atomic-number materials, such as plastic or aluminum, otherwise they will produce highly penetrating bremsstrahlung radiation.

Contamination Control. It is difficult to optimize the effects of time, distance, and shielding and maintain an ALARA environment if there are unidentified areas of radioactive contamination. Therefore, a nuclear medicine facility should follow NRC guidelines for routine measurement of ambient radiation levels and spot checking (wipe testing) for removal contamination. Personnel should survey themselves regularly for contamination of their hands, feet, and clothing. If items and/or personnel are found to be contaminated, the recommended procedures for restricting spread of contamination and decontamination should be followed, under the guidance of the institutional radiation safety officer.

NRC-Mandated Radiation Safety Procedures

There are several mandated NRC safety procedures required in nuclear medicine, as described next.

Measurement of Ambient and Area Exposure Rates. Using a GM meter, perform daily surveys of all areas where radiopharmaceuticals are prepared or administered, and weekly surveys of all areas where radiopharmaceuticals or radioactive waste are stored (Figure 43-16A).

Wipe Testing. Wipe 100-cm^2 areas with absorbent swabs and count swabs in well counter. Perform weekly testing of all areas where radiopharmaceuticals are prepared, administered, or stored (Figure 43-16C-D).

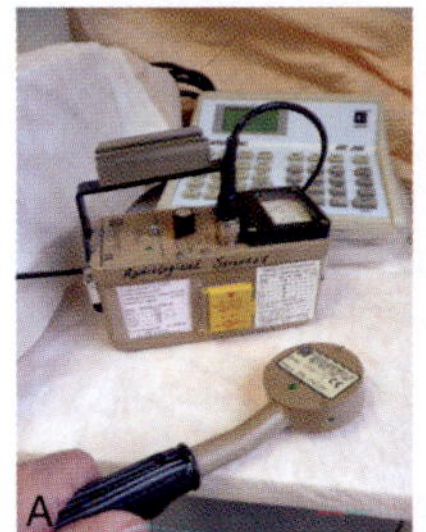

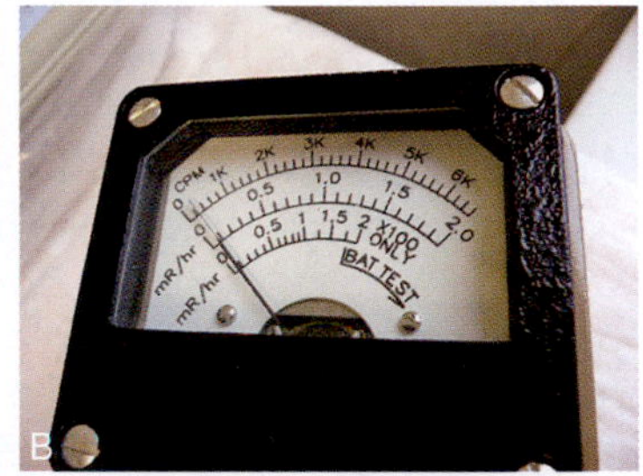

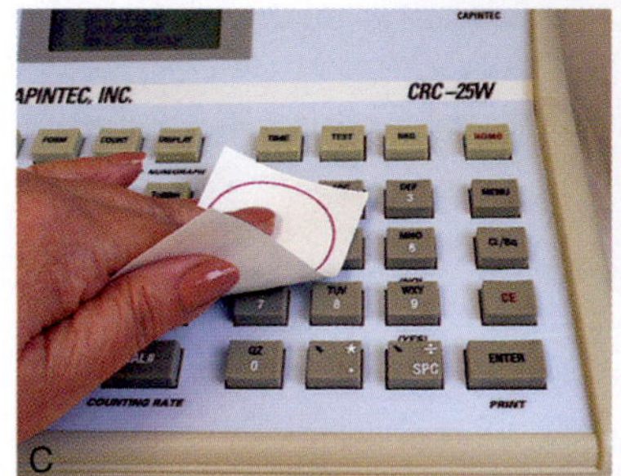

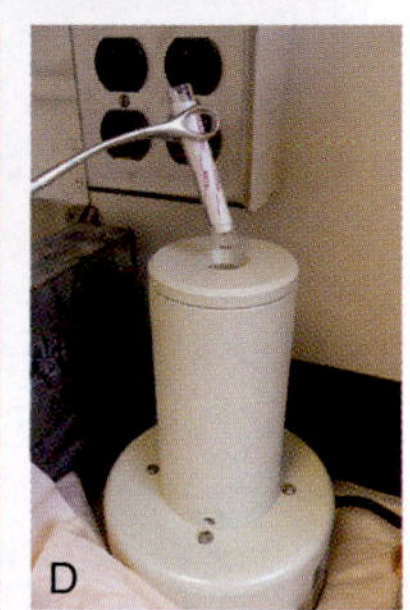

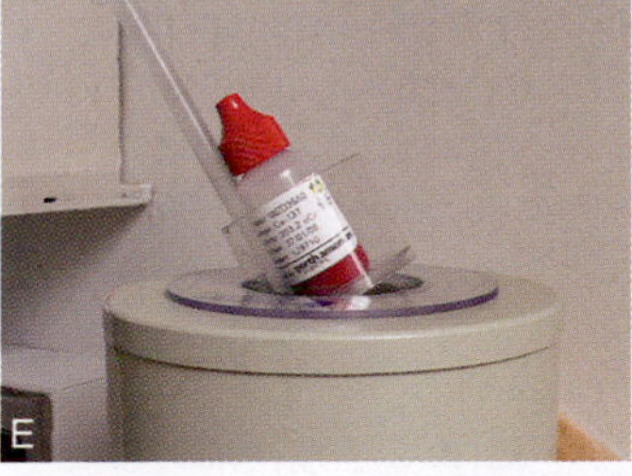

FIGURE 43-16. Contamination surveys. Daily check with GM meter of all areas where radiopharmaceuticals are prepared or administered (A). Daily constancy check of GM meter (B). Wipe test for removable contamination (C). Measurement of used swab in well counter (D). Calibration of dose calibrator with long-lived sources of radioactivity (E).

Dose Calibrator Calibration. Using certified sealed sources of long-lived radionuclides, perform a yearly accuracy test and a daily constancy test (Figure 43-16E). Using Tc-99m, perform a quarterly test for linearity of response. All tests must be performed, including a test for the effect of sample geometry, when a dose calibrator is installed or after it is sent out for service or repair.

Survey Meter Calibration. The survey meter used must be capable of detecting exposure rates from 1 μSv/hr (0.1 mrem/hr) to 1 mSv/hr (100 mrem/hr). Using certified sealed sources of long-lived radionuclides, the meter should be calibrated annually. A daily calibration check should be performed, using the long-lived sealed source on the meter.

Signs, Symbols, and Labels. Radiation warning signs and labels with magenta/black symbols and writing on a yellow background should be used to warn people of possible danger of radiation exposure. Signs indicating the potential exposure level must be posted on doors, and labels must be used on all containers of radioactive material. Specific U.S. Department of Transportation (D.O.T) labels are used when transporting radioactive materials (see Figure 43-5).

Receipt of Radioactive Packages. Received packages of radiopharmaceuticals must be unpacked and attended to as soon as possible after delivery. Each package must be visually inspected for damage and leakage. The external exposure rate of packages should be measured using a GM meter and the package surface and contents should be wipe tested for detection of removable contamination. The contents of the package must be logged into the inventory and stored behind lead in a secure area.

Record Keeping. Records must be maintained for receipt, storage, use, and disposal of all radioactive materials, and for activities performed in the nuclear medicine department, including elutions, kit preparation, dose administration, instrumentation calibration and quality control, inventory checks, sealed sources, ambient surveys, wipe tests, written directives, therapeutic administrations, accidents, and medical events. The NRC is specific on the exact contents of each type of record and the length of time that each must be kept.

CLINICAL APPLICATIONS

The clinical nuclear medicine repertoire includes diagnostic studies for just about every major body organ and system. Additionally, nuclear medicine includes radionuclide therapy applications and some nonimaging (*in vitro*) diagnostic tests. Procedural details are beyond the scope of this book chapter, but a short explanation of the most common techniques is appropriate.

Skeletal Imaging

Uptake of Tc-99m MDP (methylene diphosphonate) reflects bone metabolism and blood flow, and allows functional analysis of bone turnover (Figure 43-17A). A bone scan can detect lesions such as bone metastasis and neoplasia, metabolic bone diseases (e.g. Paget's disease), bone infections and inflammations (e.g., arthritis, osteomyelitis), and bone fractures.

Lung Imaging

In nuclear medicine the term *V/Q scan* is used to refer to a diagnostic study including a lung ventilation scan (V) and a lung perfusion scan (Q). During a lung ventilation scan, a radioactive gas or aerosol is inhaled, demonstrating regional pulmonary ventilation. During the lung perfusion scan, Tc-99m MAA (macroaggregated albumin) is trapped in the pulmonary alveolar microcirculation, demonstrating regional pulmonary blood flow. A V/Q scan is used most often to diagnose and evaluate pulmonary emboli (Figure 43-17B).

Thyroid Studies

Radioactive iodine uptake measurement refers to the use of I-123 or I-131 sodium iodide, administered as a capsule, to evaluate thyroid function

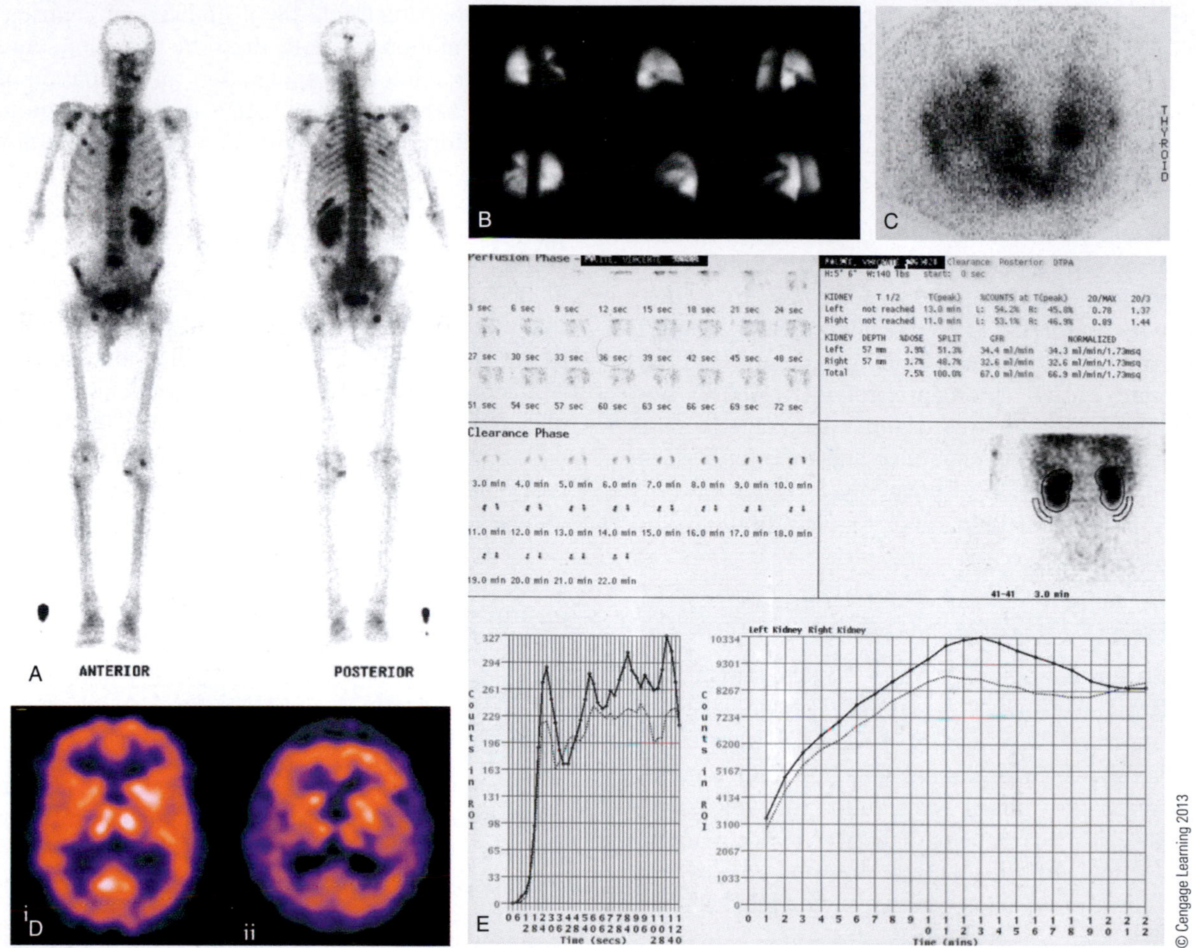

FIGURE 43-17. Clinical applications: (A) Tc-99m MDP (methylene diphosphonate) whole-body scan showing widespread focal areas of increased uptake indicative of skeletal metastases. (B) Lung perfusion scan using Tc-99m MAA (macroaggregated albumin). Large wedge-shaped defects in both lungs are highly suspicious for pulmonary embolism. (C) Pinhole image of thryoid gland using Tc-99m pertechnetate shows toxic multinodular goiter. (D) Regional cerebral perfusion scans using Tc-99m HMPAO (hexamethylpropylene amine oxime). Normal perfusion (left). Typical appearance of Alzheimer's disease—atrophied cerebral cortex, decreased uptake in bilateral temporal and parietal lobes (right). (E) Renography using Tc-99m DTPA (diethylene triamine pentaacetic acid) showing decreased perfusion, uptake and excretion of both kidneys.

in terms of iodide trapping and organification. A thyroid scan (Figure 43-17C) can be performed using I-123 sodium iodide or Tc-99m pertechnetate to evaluate morphology and function of the thyroid gland. Together, the uptake and scan are commonly used to evaluate thyrotoxicosis and plan dosimetry for thyroid ablation.

Brain Imaging

After intravenous injection, Tc-99m HMPAO (hexamethyl propylene amine oxime) and Tc-99m ECD (ethyl cysteinate dimer) are retained predominately in the gray matter of the brain, reflecting regional cerebral blood flow (Figure 43-17D). Both can be used to enhance detection of brain dementias (e.g., Alzheimer's disease), localize seizure foci, and evaluate cerebral ischemia, trauma, and brain death.

Kidney Imaging

Dynamic renal scintigraphy (renography) is used to demonstrate renal perfusion, tracer uptake, and excretion. The term *renogram* refers to a time-activity graph that is used to quantify and compare left and right kidney function (Figure 43-17E). Tc-99m MAG3 (mercaptoacetyl triglycine) and Tc-99m DTPA (diethyl triamine pentaacetic acid) are used for renal clearance and function assessment. Tc-99m DMSA (dimercapto succinic acid) is used to show renal parenchymal morphology and function.

Hepatobiliary Studies

After intravenous injection, Tc-99m HIDA (hydroxyiminodiacetic acid) and Tc-99m DISIDA (diisopropyl iminodiacetic acid) are taken up by hepatocytes, incorporated into bile, and secreted through the biliary tree into the duodenum (Figure 43-18A). A hepatobiliary scan is commonly performed to differentiate between acute and chronic cholecystitis, and to evaluate bile leaks.

Gastrointestinal Studies

To evaluate functions such as transit time in various parts of the gastrointestinal tract, Tc-99m radiopharmaceuticals can be added to foods or drinks for patient consumption. A common example is the gastric emptying study, where Tc-99m SC (sulfur colloid) is mixed into scrambled eggs, and its passage is tracked from the patient's stomach into the small intestine (Figure 43-18B).

MUGA Scan

A MUGA (multiple gated acquisition) makes use of Tc-99m–labeled autologous red blood cells to image the blood pool inside the heart. Image acquisition is synchronized to the heart beat (i.e., gated), and shows dynamic blood volume count rate changes, enabling left and right ventricular blood volume quantitation (Figure 43-18C). Analysis of ventricular wall motion, systolic-diastolic function, and ejection fraction have application for evaluation of coronary artery disease (CAD), risk stratification, and monitoring of cardiotoxicity in chemotherapy patients.

Myocardial Perfusion Scan

Tc-99m sestamibi, Tc-99m tetrofosmin, and Tl-201 thallous chloride accumulation in the myocardium depends on blood flow and cellular metabolism. Uptake reflects regional perfusion and, in the case of Tl-201, myocardial viability. In the evaluation of a patient with suspected or known CAD, a stress test is performed. Myocardial perfusion images of the heart under conditions of maximum stress are compared with images of the myocardium at rest. Areas of myocardial ischemia and infarct can be identified and localized (Figure 43-18D).

Infection and Inflammation Imaging

Autologous white blood cells labeled with Tc-99m HMPAO or In-111 oxine can be used to localize and evaluate sites of infection and inflammation (Figure 43-18E). Typical indications include abdominal (e.g., colitis, Crohn's disease), pulmonary (e.g., sarcoidosis, pneumonia), musculoskeletal (e.g., osteomyelitis, joint prostheses), abscesses, fevers of unknown origin, and opportunistic infections.

Tumor Imaging

Many radiopharmaceuticals are available for diagnosing and evaluating tumors (Figure 43-19). The list includes:

- I-131 sodium iodide for papillary/follicular thyroid carcinoma
- Tc-99m sestamibi for parathyroid adenoma
- I-123 or I-131 MIBG (methyliodobenzyl guanidine) for adrenergic tumors
- Ga-67 gallium citrate for lymphoma, hepatoma, bronchogenic carcinoma, and osteosarcoma
- F-18 FDG for PET of multiple cancer types

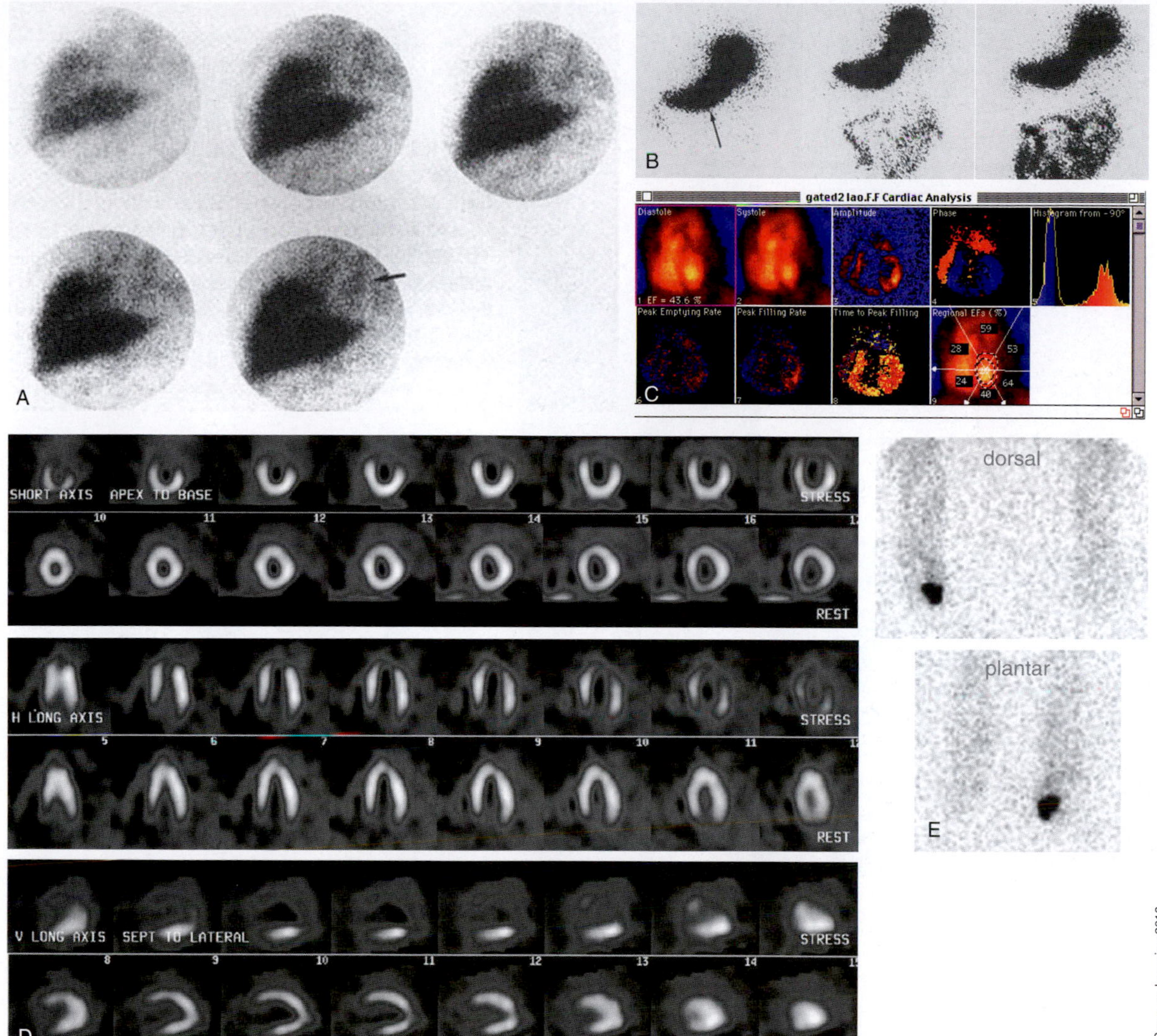

FIGURE 43-18. Clinical applications: (A) Hepatobiliary scan using Tc-99m DISIDA (diisopropyl iminodiacetic acid), showing complete obstruction of the common bile duct. (B) Normal gastric emptying study. Patient was dosed with Tc-99m SC (sulfur colloid) in a scrambled egg and toast sandwich. Images were taken at 0, 15, and 30 minutes after ingestion of the dose, and show passage of the stomach contents into the small intestine. (C) Normal MUGA scan. Tc-99m–labeled red blood cell gated images show left ventricle at end diastole and end systole (top), pixel-by-pixel analysis of left ventricular contraction phase and amplitude (middle), global left ventricular ejection fraction of 61 percent, and regional left ventricular ejection fraction and wall motion (bottom). (D) Myocardial perfusion scan using Tc-99m sestamibi—short axis (top), horizontal long axis (middle), vertical long axis (bottom). Images demonstrate ischemia of the anteroapical wall of the left ventricle. (E) Infection imaging with In-111-oxine–labeled white blood cells, shows osteomyelitis of the great toe of the right foot.

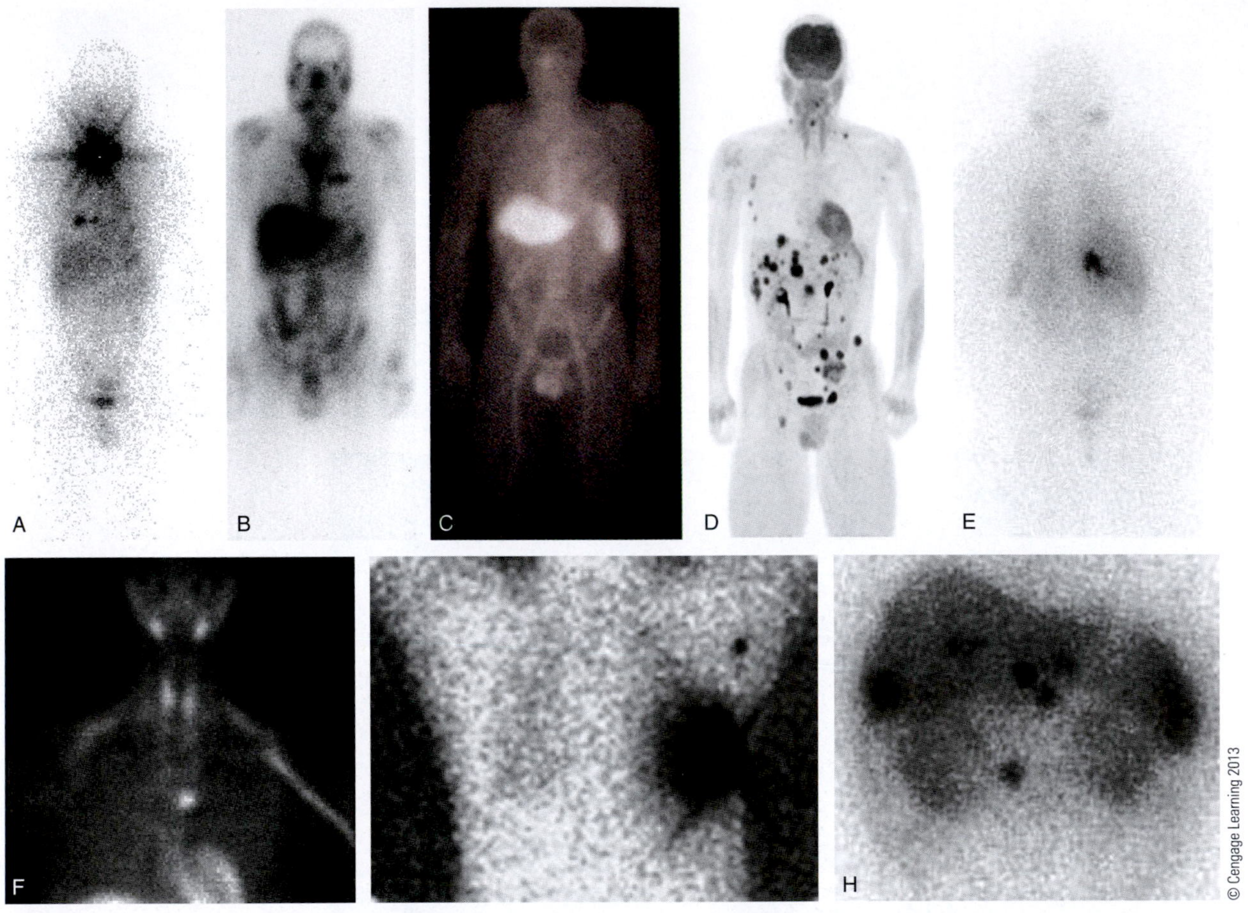

FIGURE 43-19. Tumor imaging: (A) I-131 sodium iodide scan showing metastatic thyroid carcinoma. (B) Ga-67 gallium citrate scan showing lymphoma. (C) In-111 satumomab pendetide (OncoScint®)—a radiolabeled antibody against colorectal cancer. (D) F-18 FDG (fluorodeoxyglucose) PET scan showing metastatic melanoma. (E) I-131 MIBG (metaiodobenzyl guanidine) scan showing pheochromocytoma. (F) Tc-99m sestamibi scan showing parathyroid adenoma. (G) Tc-99m SC (sulfur colloid) scan showing sentinel lymph node in patient with breast cancer. (H) In-111 pentetreotide scan showing gastrinoma.

SUMMARY

Nuclear medicine involves the administration of a radiopharmaceutical—a carrier substance labeled with a radioisotope. The radiopharmaceutical is dispersed throughout the body, and concentrates preferentially in a designated target organ or particular disease process by participation in local metabolic processes.

The most common clinically used radioisotope is technetium-99m (Tc-99m), which possesses many qualities that make it ideal for imaging nuclear

SUMMARY (continued)

medicine applications. Other frequently used radioisotopes include iodine-123 and iodine-131, indium-111, thallium-201, and gallium-67. For positron emission tomography (PET), fluorine-18 is most often used.

The possession, usage, and disposal of radioactive materials is carefully controlled by the U.S. Nuclear Regulatory Commission (NRC) and/or agreement states. Every procedure performed in nuclear medicine must follow recommended protocols and be documented, to ensure maximal protection of the patient, the general public, and the staff.

The radioisotope used emits gamma rays that pass out of the body and can be collected by a gamma camera, which incorporates a scintillation detector, photomultiplier tubes, amplifiers, and positioning and energy discrimination circuitry. The resulting image is a map of the distribution of the radioisotope throughout the patient's body. Images may be limited to a particular body part, may show the whole body, or may be tomographic (SPECT). PET systems include modifications for detection of annihilation photons. Additional radiation counting and measuring equipment in the nuclear medicine department, such as dose calibrators and survey meters, employs scintillation or gas-filled detection technology. All equipment needs to undergo regular quality control testing.

In contrast with computed tomography and magnetic resonance imaging, nuclear scintigraphy has relatively poor spatial resolution and low signal-to-noise ratio. The amount of radioisotope injected, and hence the gamma photon flux, is limited by the radiation dose conferred on the patient. This results in a considerable amount of noise in the images, which is confounded by the absorption and scatter that the gamma rays are subjected to as they pass out of the patient and into the detector.

Nuclear medicine does not attempt to compete with high-spatial-resolution imaging (CT and MRI). Rather, its utility is its ability to image metabolic processes with very high sensitivity. Nuclear medicine images are almost entirely functional in nature. Some radioisotopes, emitters of particulate (alpha or beta) radiation, have a role in radionuclide therapy. ■

REVIEW QUESTIONS

1. In the molybdenum-99/technetium-99m generator system, which is the parent radioisotope and which is the daughter?
2. What is the usual method in a nuclear pharmacy for disposing of radioactive waste materials?
3. What is meant by the term *pulse height analysis*?
4. What is the purpose of wipe testing?
5. What type of phantom is used for testing the spatial resolution of a gamma camera?
6. What is the role of a high-pass filter in SPECT image analysis?
7. What are the two uses for the computed tomography (CT) scan acquired by a hybrid SPECT/CT or PET/CT scanner?
8. Name:
   (a) A Tc-99m radiopharmaceutical that can be used for cardiac imaging.
   (b) A PET radiopharmaceutical used for tumor imaging.
   (c) A radiopharmaceutical used for thyroid cancer therapy.

REFERENCES AND RECOMMENDED READING

Aquilina, M. A. (2008). The expanding role of nuclear medicine in therapeutic strategies. *Malta Medical Journal*, *20*, 8–12.

Bolus, N. E. (2008). Review of common occupational hazards and safety concerns for nuclear medicine technologists. *Journal of Nuclear Medicine Technology*, *36*, 11–17.

Bybel, B., Brunken, R. C., DiFilippo, F. P., Neumann, D. R., Wu, G., & Cerqueira, M. D. (2008). SPECT/CT imaging: Clinical utility of an emerging technology. *Radio-Graphics*, 28, 1097–1113.

Hicks, R. J., Lau, E. W. F., & Binns, D. S. (2007). Hybrid imaging is the future of molecular imaging. *Biomedical Imaging and Intervention Journal*, *3*, e49.

Lin, E. C., & Alavi, A. (2009). *PET and PET/CT: A clinical guide* (2nd ed.). New York: Thieme Medical Publishers.

Ponto, J. A. (1998). Radiopharmaceuticals. *RadioGraphics*, *18*, 1395–1404.

Powsner, R. A., & Powsner, E. R. (2006). *Essentials of nuclear medicine physics* (2nd ed.). Malden, MA: Blackwell Publishing.

Prekeges, J. (2011). *Nuclear medicine instrumentation*. Sudbury, MA: Jones & Bartlet Publishers.

Prvulovich, E. M., & Bomanji, J. B. (1998). Fortnightly review: The role of nuclear medicine in clinical investigation. *British Journal of Medicine*, *316*, 1140–1146.

Saha, G. B. (2004). *Fundamentals of nuclear pharmacy* (5th ed.). New York: Springer.

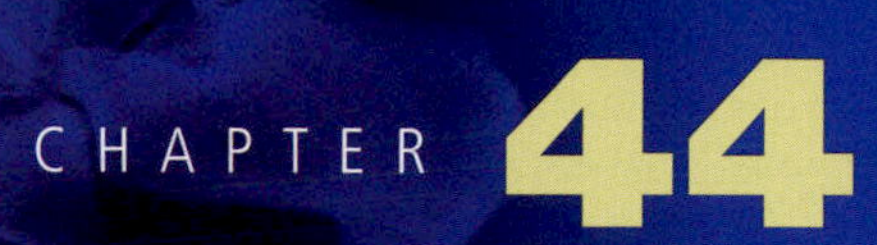

Radiation Therapy

Julie Hollenbeck, BS, RT(T)

KEY TERMS

clinical target volume (CTV)
cone beam CT (CBCT)
contouring
gross tumor volume (GTV)
image guided radiation therapy (IGRT)
isocenter
linear accelerator
planning target volume (PTV)
portal radiograph
proton therapy
stereotactic irradiation

> Once you choose hope, anything's possible.
>
> *Christopher Reeve*

OBJECTIVES

Upon completion of this chapter, the student should be able to:

- Explain the historical development of the use of radiation for therapeutic purposes.
- Describe the difference between portal imaging and image guided radiation therapy.
- Define the major components of a linear accelerator.
- Distinguish between image fusion and hybrid imaging.
- Describe various specialized units and treatment methods.

HISTORICAL OVERVIEW

The use of x-rays for therapeutic purposes started only a few months after Roentgen's great discovery. The first therapeutic treatments were used mainly for non-malignant conditions such as ringworm of the scalp, which was quite common in Victorian cities, or certain skin conditions. Some superficial lesions were also treated but it wasn't until after Coolidge tubes were invented that deep-seated tumors could be reached. Coolidge tubes allowed the delivery of higher-kilovoltage x-rays that could penetrate tissues. In the United States a medical student in Chicago, Emil H. Grubbe, was one of the first documented individuals to treat cancer with therapeutic x-rays. Grubbe treated a woman's left breast in 1896; though it was not successful, he was the first to shield healthy parts of the patient's body. He did this remembering the dermatitis he experienced on his hands from working with x-rays. It wasn't until 1956 at Stanford University that Dr. Henry Kaplan and his staff of physicists created the first linear accelerator. The machine stood 6 feet high, weighed 2 tons, and was harnessed from the ceiling. The first patient treated was a 2-year-old boy who was diagnosed with retinoblastoma. The boy had already lost sight in one eye due to the disease, so the first goal for radiation therapy treatment was to preserve the boy's sight and destroy the growing tumor. Day after day for 6 weeks they positioned a lead block that had a pinhole drilled through it. The block was so heavy they borrowed an automobile jack from a local garage to position the block so that the rest of the delicate eye was shielded except for the tumor. Treatment was successful. The boy's sight was saved and he went on to live a long full life.

The invention of computers and new technology has helped researchers create sophisticated machines used to treat cancer. Clinical trials have helped researchers create a language and a history for every type of malignancy. Working with others and being part of new therapies has allowed great increases in cancer survival rates and lower morbidity. In 1962 radiation therapy became a separate specialization with its own professional society and registration and accreditation agencies. The goals of radiation therapy are to protect healthy tissue as much as possible, preserve function of the structure or structures surrounding the tumor, eradicate the tumor, and minimize side effects. These goals take a network of trained, educated medical professionals who all have the patients' best interest in mind. Figure 44-1 illustrates the processes involved in treating a patient in a radiation therapy department.

CONSULTATION

Most patients are in the radiation oncology department for a malignancy and are typically referred to the radiation oncologist by surgeons, neurologists, urologists, primary care physicians, or medical oncologists. The first step for a patient in the radiation oncology department is to meet with the physician for consultation. Before the consultation, the physician has reviewed the patient's medical chart, his or her history and physical, all diagnostic examinations, pathology reports, and other procedure reports and consultations. From this information a decision will be made to determine if the patient is a candidate for radiation therapy. This is followed by the creation of a radiation treatment plan that is specific for each individual patient. To create this plan, the oncology team uses all of the patient's medical information, research from clinical trials, and the team members' expertise. The foundation of this radiation treatment plan is called the prescription. The prescription is precise, detailed, serves as the physician's orders for treatment, and must include the physician's signature. It must include:

- Anatomic site to be treated
- Total radiation dose
- Individual treatment dose (fractionation)
- Time over which the total dose is delivered (protraction)
- The treatment technique being used
- Number of treatment fields
- Treatment field angles

Other components that may be included are the beam energy, treatment field sizes, and beam modifiers. Dose is written in gray (Gy), which is

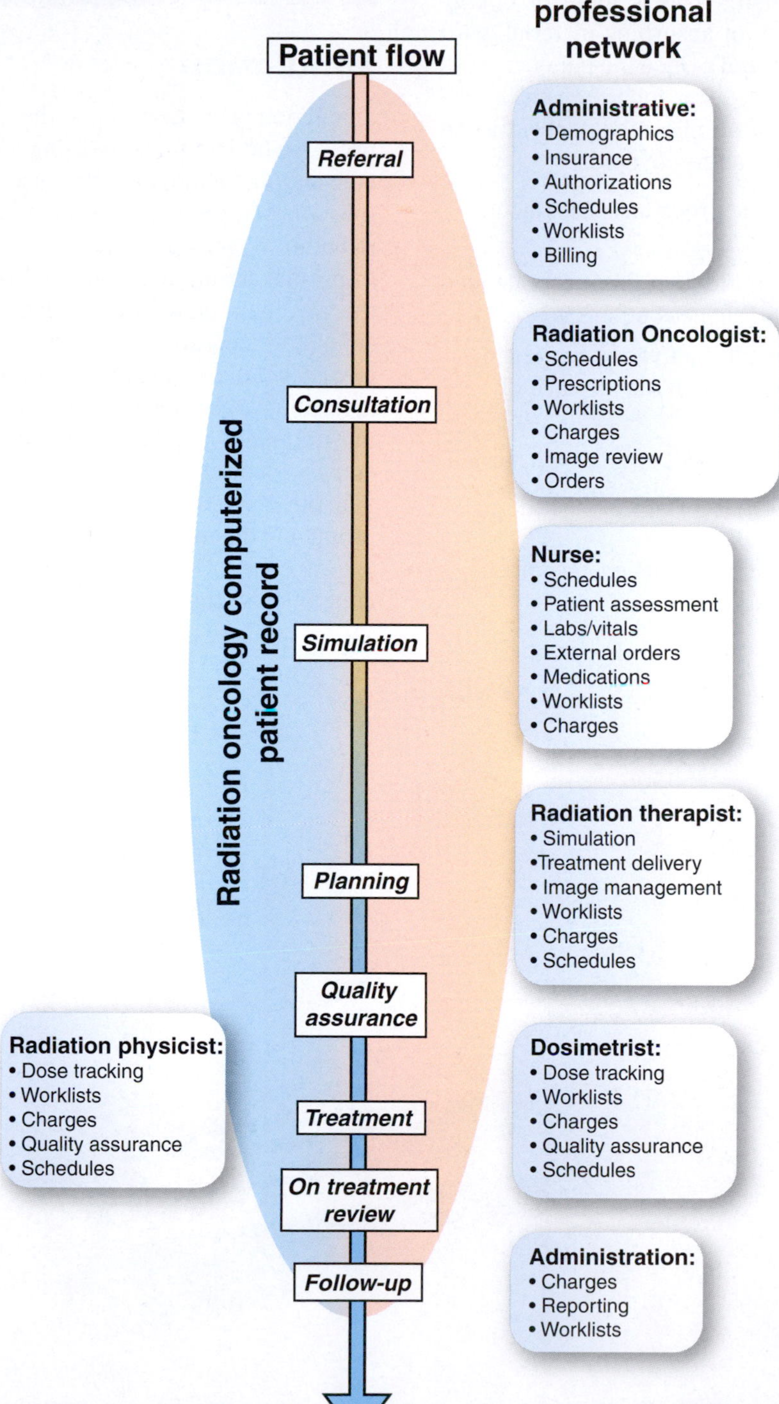

FIGURE 44-1. The processes involved in treating a radiation therapy patient.

the SI equivalent of the rad (radiation absorbed dose). The gray is defined as 1 joule of energy absorbed per kilogram of absorbing material, with 1 Gy = 100 (cGy = 100 rad). Once the patient agrees on radiation therapy, consent for treatment is discussed and signed. For an informed consent to be valid, it must have four areas covered:

- It must describe the procedure, treatment, and disease.
- It must state the outlook of the recommended treatment and the chances of success.
- It must also have alternatives to treatment and the likely outcome in the absence of treatment.
- It must state known risk factors, such as side effects that could be possible with this form of treatment

Once the patient signs the consent, he or she is scheduled for a simulation.

TREATMENT PLANNING

Simulation

Simulation is the first step in the treatment planning process and can be done using a CT simulator or a conventional simulator. Because the main purpose for radiation therapy treatment is to give a dose of radiation to malignant tissue and reduce the dose to normal tissue, accuracy and reproducibility are the two main goals for simulation. A conventional simulator (Figure 44-2) is a replica of the treatment machine or linear accelerator with the same mechanical, geometrical, and optical operations as the treatment machine. The difference between a conventional simulator and a linear accelerator is that the conventional simulator is only capable of producing diagnostic-level ionizing radiation.

A conventional simulator has all of the same components that make up a linear accelerator,

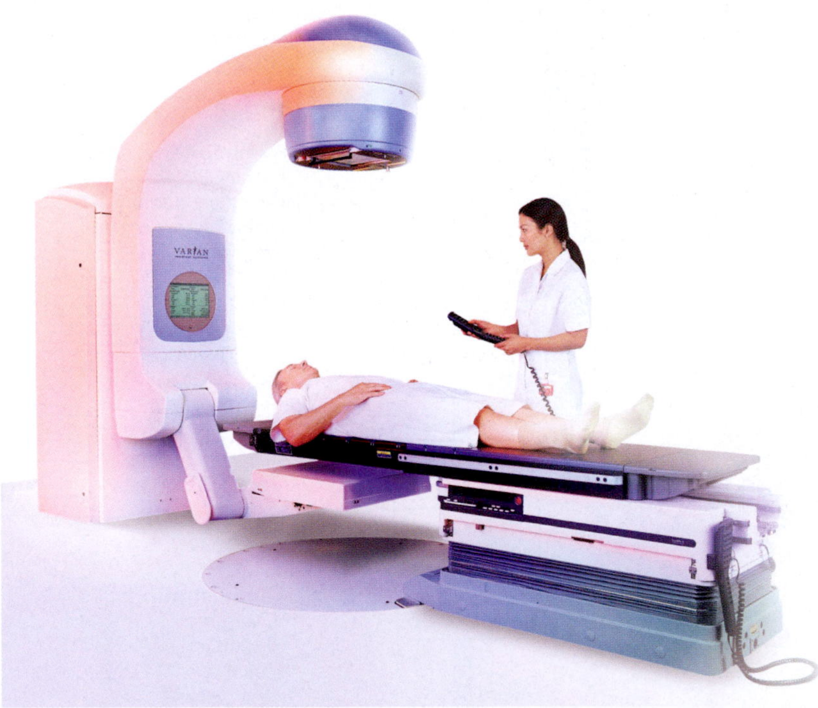

FIGURE 44-2. A conventional radiation therapy simulator. This unit is designed to replicate a linear accelerator treatment machine. This unit produces radiation in the kilovoltage range, not in the megavoltage treatment range. *(Image courtesy of Varian Medical Systems, Inc. All rights reserved.)*

which will be discussed later, plus two other features to help with the simulation process: field defining wires (Figure 44-3) and an image intensifier system (Figure 44-4). Field defining wires are located in the gantry head, and define the treatment field borders that are established by the radiation oncologist. There are four thin wires, two for the x axis, and two for the y axis. They can move dependently or independently of each other. The image intensifier system is located on the opposite side of the arm that is connected to the gantry head. The image intensifier unit can house a cassette for hard-copy films as well as be used for fluoroscopic purposes. The intensifier has its own independent movement for optimal image quality. It can move on a vertical, longitudinal, and lateral axis.

A CT scanner is used for CT simulation, and whether the department uses a conventional simulator or a CT scanner, the same set of information needs to be obtained. To achieve reproducibility the patient needs to be immobilized; this allows for the therapists on the treatment machine to set the patient up using the same immobilization device (Figure 44-5) every day to help confirm accuracy and consistency. This is critical because patients receive multiple radiation treatments. For palliative intent, 10 to 20 treatments are usually given, and for curative intent, 30 to 40 treatments are typical. Immobilization devices depend on the area of the body that is being treated as well as the patient. The second goal of simulation is accuracy. The tumor needs to be localized. To create an accurate treatment plan, the area of the tumor needs to be identified, including the volume, extent, and lymphatics or regional involvement. For conventional simulation this is done with fluoroscopy; for CT, a CT scan is preformed. After the area is localized the simulation therapist creates a coordinate system on the patient's external surface for reproducibility and accuracy during treatment.

Marking the coordinates on the patient is necessary for both CT and conventional simulation but they are performed at different times in each scenario. The coordinate system is a series of marks that are placed on the patient that are references to the radiation therapist to set the patient

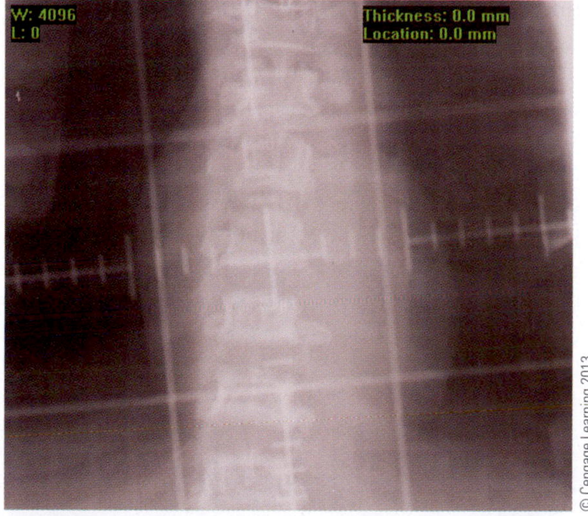

FIGURE 44-3. Defining wire used for patient setup.

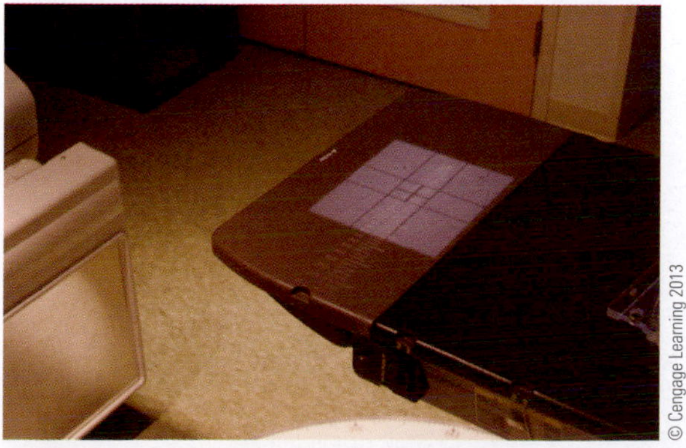

FIGURE 44-4. Receptor unit for a simulator.

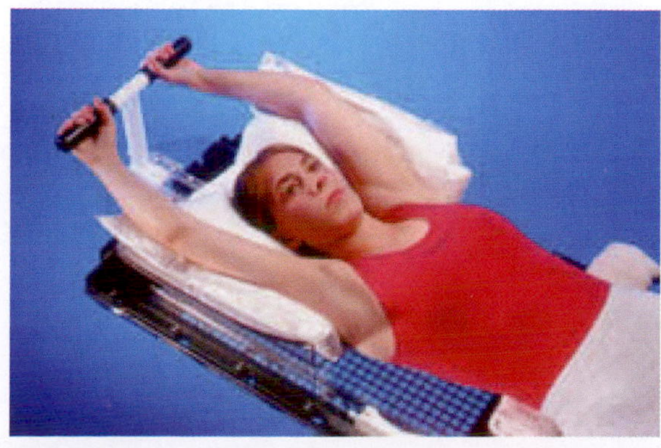

FIGURE 44-5. A radiation therapy immobilization device. *(Photo courtesy of CIVCO.)*

up accurately on the treatment machine. They are created from a laser system that is installed in every simulation and treatment room. Lasers are placed on either side of the machine to line the body longitudinally (superior, inferior) and vertically (anterior, posterior). A laser is also placed on the ceiling, which helps line the body longitudinally again and laterally (right, left). All lasers meet at one center, which is called the **isocenter**. The isocenter is the point where all three rotational axes intersect from the simulator and for the treatment machine. Great care is given each day to make sure that the laser coordinate system intersects at the isocenter. These reference points for conventional simulation are usually made after an immobilization device is created and the tumor is localized under fluoroscopy. Marks are either permanent or non-permanent at this point. For CT, simulation marks are made prior to a CT scan and small metal BBs are placed on the marks for treatment planning purposes. Once these preliminary marks are made the physician needs to establish where the isocenter will be inside the volume being treated. This process can be done during simulation or during the treatment planning process. Once the patient has been marked, immobilized, and images have been created for tumor localization, the simulation therapist records parameters associated with the patient's set-up, photographs are taken to ensure proper set-up, charges are made, and documentation of the procedure is completed. The patient is then given a return appointment time to start the first day of treatment and is asked not to remove the temporary marks. The CT scan is then transferred to a treatment planning computer system and for conventional simulation. Radiographs and a physical contour of the patient's body are given to the medical dosimetrists. Whether images are obtained using a conventional simulator or a CT scanner, they are used to create the patient's unique treatment plan and are referenced throughout the treatment process.

Image Fusion

The development of positron emission tomography (PET) in the 1990s has provided oncologists the information to metabolically trace malignancies and more accurately manage their treatment. Single photon emission computed tomography (SPECT) and PET use specific radiotracers to create functional images that display physiologic images. This new insight has allowed radiation oncologists to more accurately define the tumor volume, lymph node involvement, and detect metastases at an early stage. The disadvantage to functional images is that they lack the structural framework of the patient. The patients' anatomy is best represented in magnetic resonance imaging (MRI) and computed tomography (CT).

Image fusion (Figure 44-6) is the process of integrating structural images, MRI or CT, with functional images, PET or SPECT. The images are essentially fused together to create another series of images and display characteristics of each. This has been very beneficial in radiation oncology. These images are fused together through a process called registration. There are many methods that can be used to register these fused images; one of the most advanced forms is through hybrid imaging. Hybrid imaging uses a multimodality unit such as PET/CT or PET/MR. The scans are performed during the same visit, with the patient staying on the table. The advantage to hybrid imaging is the

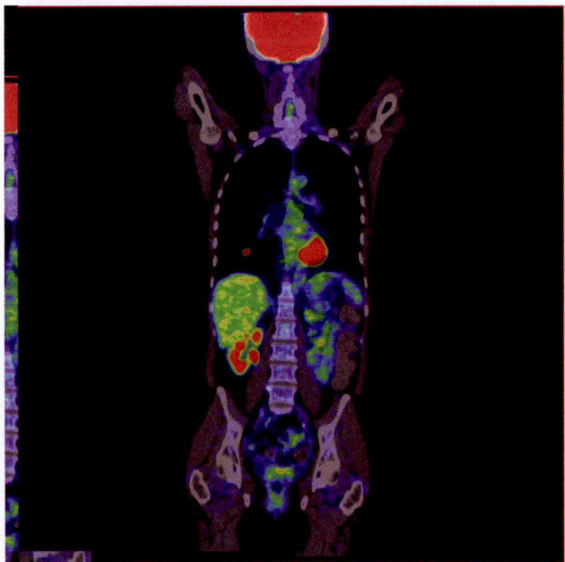

FIGURE 44-6. A PET scan fusion image. *(Image by permission of GE Healthcare.)*

accuracy of the registration process. With minimal patient movement along with the creation of the data sets during the same visit, the margin for error is diminished with hybrid imaging. Staging of disease, surgical and radiation therapy planning, and assessment of tumor response are some of the benefits of image fusion.

Treatment Planning Systems

Treatment planning is the primary responsibility of the medical dosimetrist. Under the physician's direction, the dosimetrist identifies an isocenter, the volume of tissue to be treated, radiation beam arrangements, and creates an acceptable isodose distribution. These four tasks are accomplished by reviewing the physician's prescription, viewing other diagnostic imaging studies, and using the simulation data. There are a number of treatment planning (TP) systems commercially available, as well as oncology centers that have created their own unique systems. All TP systems have different features but ultimately achieve the same goal, to create a treatment plan that is designed for a particular patient.

Once the dosimetrist reviews all materials and finds the coordinate metal BB points, an isocenter needs to be placed and a treatment volume needs to be defined. The process of **contouring** is used to achieve these first two goals. Contouring (Figure 44-7) is a tracing of the shape of the tumor volume as well as structures near the tumor volume that the radiation dose will affect. Depending on the treatment planning system and the type and extent of disease, this task can take from a few seconds to a few hours.

To establish the volume of tissue (Figure 44-8) that will be irradiated, a contour of the **gross tumor volume (GTV), clinical target volume (CTV),** and **planning target volume (PTV)** must be created. Also, any structure that is in the path of radiation either before entering the GTV, CTV, or PTV or after needs to be contoured to calculate how much radiation dose the patient will be receiving. The gross tumor volume, or GTV, is defined as the palpable or visible growth of the malignant tumor. It is considered the primary location of the tumor, and any lymphatic or other metastatic spread. If the patient's tumor has been removed or eradicated prior to radiation therapy, no GTV is defined. The clinical target volume, or CTV, always includes the GTV and a volume of tissue that contains microscopic subclinical disease. If the tumor was removed prior, the CTV would include the tumor bed and tissue surrounding the tumor bed. The planning target volume, or PTV, includes the GTV and CTV and includes lymph nodes adjacent to the primary tumor that have evidence of disease. The CTV also is used for patient movement and set-up errors.

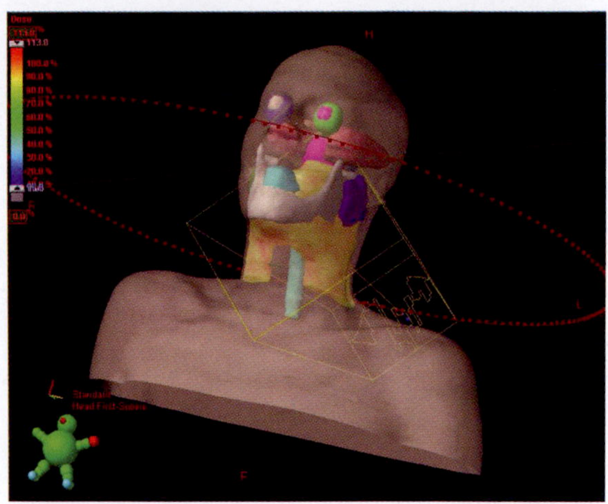

FIGURE 44-7. A contouring image that is used to determine the ixocenter and treatment volume prior to beginning treatment. *(Image courtesy of Varian Medical Systems, Inc. All rights reserved.)*

The isocenter is a point that the radiation oncologist chooses that receives 100 percent of the radiation dose that is prescribed. It is a fixed point that corresponds with all rotational axes associated with the treatment machine. The radiation oncologist places this point usually inside the GTV or PTV. For example, with a left lung tumor that needs to be treated, the physician will set the isocenter inside the area to be treated and the dosimetrist places a margin or contour around the area. Depending on the area, these margins can be very small or large. If a lung tumor is located in the center of the left lung and the tumor is 1 cm in diameter, that would be the GTV. The radiation oncologist might want to add another 1 cm around the GTV for subclinical disease. This is the CTV. As the chest rises and

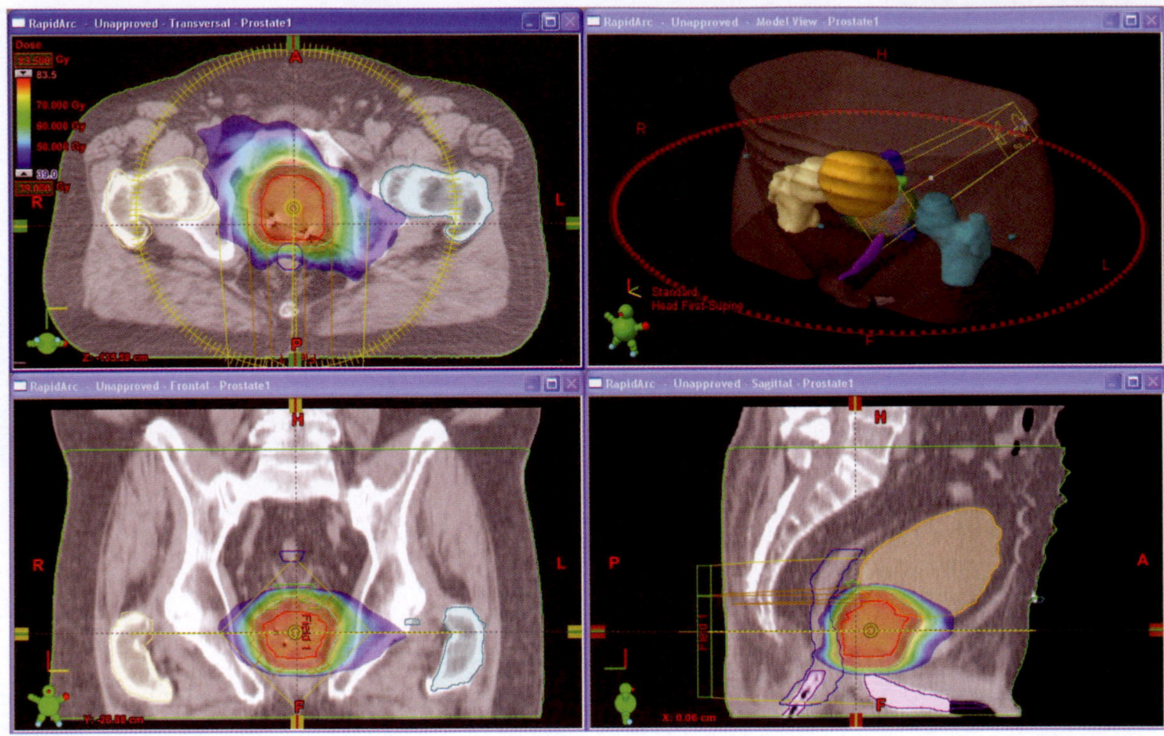

FIGURE 44-8. Treatment planning system images for a prostate cancer patient showing gross tumor volume, clinical target volume, and planning target volume. A three-dimensional image is also produced. These images allow the treatment planning system to calculate radiation doses to various critical anatomical structures. *(Image courtesy of Varian Medical Systems, Inc. All rights reserved.)*

falls with every breath, the radiation beam needs to be large enough that the tumor is treated regardless of whether the patient is exhaling or inhaling. That could be another 1.5- to 2 cm margin, and this would be the PTV. Consequently, the total field size to treat a 1 cm tumor could be 3.5 to 4 cm in diameter. The dose that the lung absorbs before the beam reaches the PTV must also be considered, as must the dose to healthy lung tissue, the heart, spinal cord, and great vessels. These structures are called critical structures and they also need to be contoured by the dosimetrist so the computer knows to calculate what dose they will get as well. The challenge is that the dosimetrist must make sure the PTV receives the prescribed dose and that the structures surrounding the PTV receive as little dose as possible. To assist with this goal, the dosimetrist manipulates the radiation beam. By using multiple beam angles, less dose is received by surrounding structures, with the PTV still receiving 100 percent of the prescribed dose.

Beam angles are formed by manipulating the gantry, angle, and couch angles. The traditionally flat, symmetrical beam can also be adjusted by having beam modification devices inserted into its pathway; this creates a three-dimensional angle of dose distribution inside the body. This aids in achieving an even dose distribution in irregular body compositions or in avoiding surrounding structures. Since the 1990s, treatment planning systems have been further developed to provide accuracy in radiation therapy treatment. Most treatment planning systems are capable of three-dimensional treatment planning (see Figure 44-8). This allows dosimetrists and physicians to view the treatment plan in the coronal, sagittal, and transverse planes, allowing for more precise treatment plans. Once an isocenter is chosen, the target volume is defined, and then the beam is arranged so that the computer can calculate the dose to all pertinent volumes and structures.

Using machine data, an isodose distribution can be defined based on the prescribed dose, the treatment volume, and patient composition. This graphic representation (Figure 44-9) of the radiation beam gives the dosimetrist the ability to visually see what percentage of the prescribed dose is being received to a particular volume. It can then be determined if the PTV is receiving enough dose and how much dose surrounding structures are receiving as well. If the isodose distribution needs to be adjusted, the treatment beams can be changed to implement the most favorable treatment plan. Once approved by the radiation oncologist, the treatment plan is uploaded to the treatment machine and important information is passed on to the physicist and the therapists. The physicist checks the plan, reviews all of its parameters, and makes sure the plan is also accurate at the treatment machine. The physicist then can perform quality assurance tests on the treatment machine to make sure the dose distribution is accurate. The radiation therapist reviews the treatment plan and also makes sure the set-up of the treatment is accurate. The therapist looks at the field location and size, marked coordinate points, and the planned coordinate shifts to line up to isocenter, beam angles, and depth measurements.

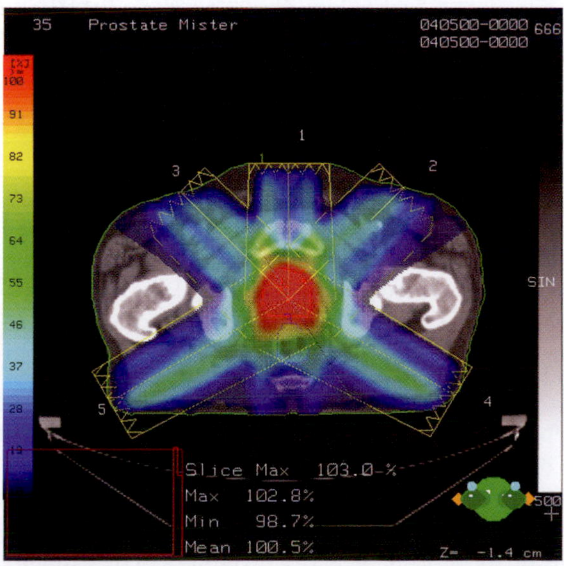

FIGURE 44-9. An isodose disbribution image of a five field prostate cancer treatment plan. *(Image courtesy of Varian Medical Systems, Inc. All rights reserved.)*

TREATMENT

Once the simulation visit has been completed and a treatment plan produced, radiation treatment can be administered. Radiation therapists work on the treatment machine to perform this. Like the simulation room, the treatment room is equipped with a laser system that is aligned with the treatment machine's isocenter. Before treatment begins, the therapists review the patient's prescription, simulation notes, and the treatment plan, which includes digital reconstructed radiographs (DRRs) or hard-copy simulation films. DRRs (Figure 44-10) bear a resemblance to radiographs and are acquired from the simulation CT scan. They include the anatomy of the patient, treatment field, and other pertinent information. The therapists also review the patient's history and physical and identification information. During the first visit, the therapist explains the process to the patient and gives the patient time to

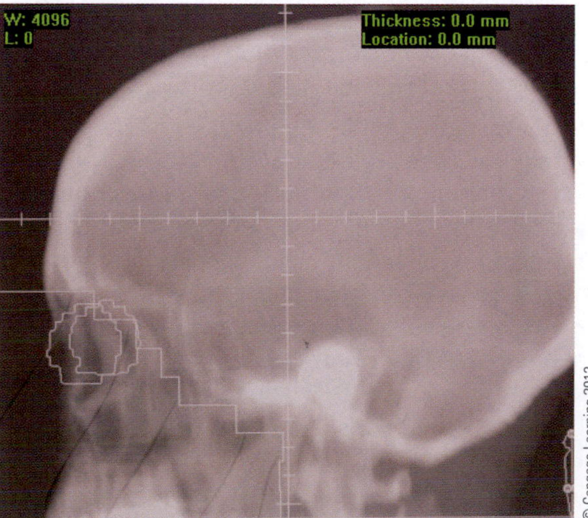

FIGURE 44-10. A digital reconstructed radiograph (DRR) from a simulation CT scan.

ask any questions. The treatment couch is set up to include any immobilization devices that were constructed for the patient as well as other devices used during simulation. The patient is placed on the table and the external marks that were made during simulation are lined up to the laser coordinate system. Once the patient is lined up, the therapist references the treatment plan to move the patient to the planned treatment isocenter. Once the patient is set up, the therapists ask the patient not to readjust and to breathe normally throughout the process. During the first treatment, x-rays are taken to verify patient placement. This can be accomplished through portal imaging or by **image guided radiation therapy (IGRT).** These images are taken outside the room at the control console and are compared to the DRRs or simulation films associated with the treatment plan. The therapist and/or oncologist then analyzes the new image and makes appropriate adjustments to the couch and/or patient to make sure treatment is centered on the treatment isocenter. Once the patient is set up accurately, the therapists make adjustments to the marks on the patient and record appropriate steps that need to be taken to align perfectly to the treatment isocenter. The therapist may also take set-up photos of the patient and the treatment fields to help with proper set-up. At this point, radiation treatment can be administered. The treatment plan is downloaded into the treatment machine and all machine parameters are adjusted for treatment of the field.

X-rays in the therapeutic range are measured in megavoltage (MV). Interactions in this energy range are from coherent scattering, photoelectric effect, Compton scattering, pair production, and photodisintegration. As the x-ray beam travels through the treatment machine it is polyenergetic, and lower energies not in therapeutic range need to be filtered out before reaching the patient. To achieve this, filters are placed within the gantry head to attenuate lower energies out of the x-ray beam, thus hardening the beam to MV range. The beam is also shaped to the treatment field and exits the gantry head into the patient, directed at the isocenter where interactions with tissue and radiation occur. A typical treatment field is measured in monitor units (MUs) and usually takes seconds to treat. Once the treatment is administered the next field can be treated. The parameters are changed and checked and radiation is administered again. Patients can be treated using one treatment field or multiple fields depending on the treatment plan. Once treatment is completed, the therapist enters the treatment room, lowers the treatment couch, and assists the patient off the table.

Image Acquisition

The image acquisition process in radiation oncology is the same as the diagnostic process in terms of creating the beam and creating the image. The form in which the image is displayed is unique to each radiation oncology department depending on the age and features of the department's particular equipment. Some departments use conventional film/screen imaging, whereas many use digital imaging. In the simulation process, a conventional simulator will use film/screen imaging that can produce either hard-copy film or display images on a monitor (soft copy). For CT simulation, images are viewed on a monitor. Megavoltage (MV) imaging, kilovoltage (KV) imaging, and **cone beam computed tomography (CBCT)** imaging are processes that are used on the radiation therapy treatment machine. Depending on the age and type of machine, one or all of the processes are available, and each is described next.

To ensure accuracy of treatment, being able to image treatment fields throughout the patient's treatment regimen is critical. Imaging gives the radiation therapist and oncologist the ability to compare the planned treatment field with the anatomy of the patient. Changes can then be made either during treatment set-up or to the treatment plan, thus ensuring that the treatment is accurate. Imaging is the most common technique available to measure and document this accuracy.

Portal Imaging. The American Association of Physicists in Medicine defines a **portal radiograph**[1] as "a radiograph produced by exposing the image receptor to the radiation beam which emanates from the portal of a therapy unit." Traditionally, MV imaging (Figure 44-11) is used to visualize the target. Images produced with MV beams suffer from low subject contrast, and they can be difficult to read for making accurate adjustments.

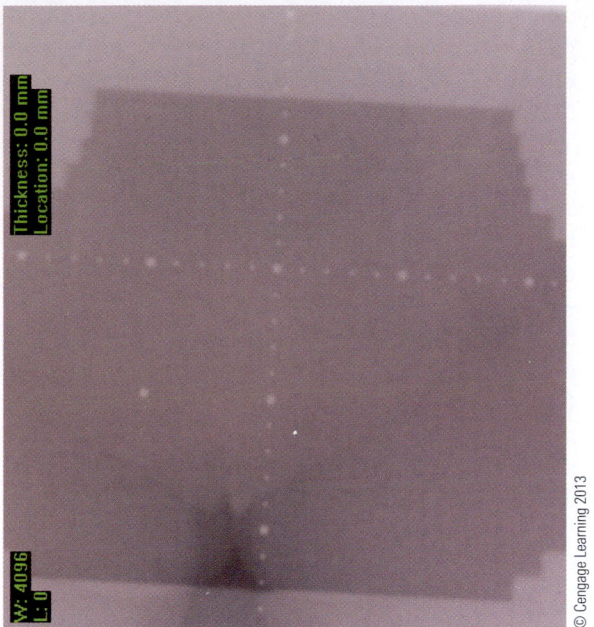

FIGURE 44-11. A portal image produced with a megavoltage energy beam.

Megavoltage images are subject to Compton scattering as well as some increase in pair production. This decreases the quality of the image, making it difficult to read. Many other factors contribute to the poor quality of images in MV portal imaging, including the performance of the image receptor and scatter. MV portal images can be captured with either a radiographic film and then processed conventionally or with an electronic portal imaging device (EPID). Norman Baily introduced electronic portal imaging devices in the 1980s. The EPID (Figure 44-12) is attached to the gantry of a treatment machine so it can capture an image at any gantry angle. It retracts into the gantry to accommodate patient access. EPIDs are commonly used in the clinical setting and have many advantages over hard-copy film. The images obtained by EPIDs are immediately available and can be used interactively to adjust patient or field position during treatment. The images are digital, which aids in image processing, contrast enhancement, and image matching. Moreover, digital archiving saves space and allows for rapid recall of images over a network.

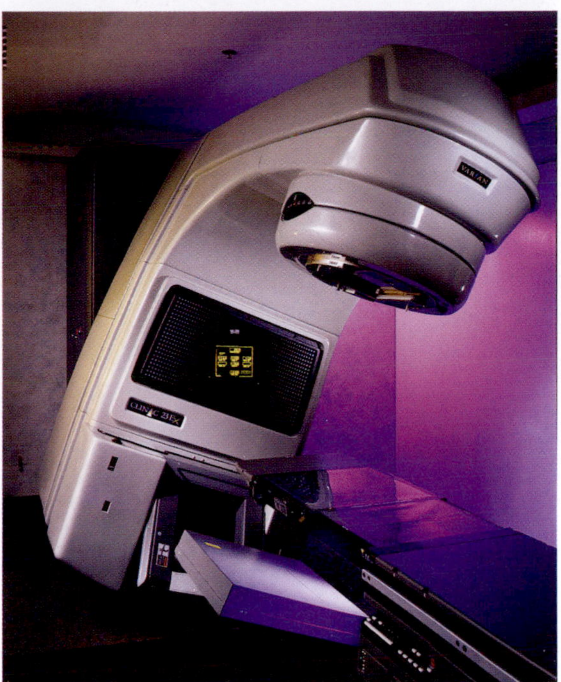

FIGURE 44-12. An electronic portal image device (EPID) attached to the gantry of a linear accelerator treatment unit. *(Image courtesy of Varian Medical Systems, Inc. All rights reserved.)*

Image Guided Radiation Therapy. With advancements in treatment techniques, such as intensity modulated radiation therapy (IMRT), stereotactic radiosurgery (SRS), and stereotactic therapy (SRT), the need for quality images with good soft tissue contrast and quick image processing has developed at a rapid pace. Image guided radiation therapy (IGRT) allows for quick corrections of patient positioning errors and patient movement before a radiation treatment is administered or during treatment. Tumors are not stationary, unchanging targets; they move between and during treatments. IGRT uses daily imaging techniques such as KV-imaging and cone beam CT (CBCT) to create three-dimensional images that pinpoint the exact size, location, and coordinates of the treatment isocenter. In the past, oncologists have had to compensate for tumor movements by making the radiation beam larger, exposing a significant volume of healthy tissue to radiation. With IGRT (Figure 44-13), two robotically controlled "arms" capture CT, fluoroscopic, and x-ray images on a daily basis, pinpointing the position of the tumor just prior to or during treatment. This increased precision allows for higher doses of radiation, ultimately leading to higher cure rates. Registration of the images happens at the control console, where they are fused with the DRRs from the patient's treatment plan (Figure 44-14). The therapist can then adjust the image that was acquired before daily treatment to match the image taken at time of simulation. Within minutes the images can be analyzed in multiple planes to precisely pinpoint the treatment isocenter. The couch then moves to the appropriate position for that treatment and the patient is treated. This accuracy has allowed for treatment plans to conform closer to the target volume and sparing surrounding healthy tissues. With a patient who has prostate cancer, the prostate is roughly the size of a walnut and is located posterior to the bladder and anterior to the rectum. The prostate is located between two organs that change shape depending on how full or empty they are. This changes the location of the prostate considerably. The goal of radiation therapy is to give 100 percent of the dose to the diseased prostate while giving as little dose as possible to the bladder and rectum. This could cause the prostate to be completely missed during treatment. With IGRT the patient can be imaged each day before treatment. The images are registered and fused with the DRRs from simulation and the prostate can be adjusted to be aligned to its treatment-planned location. Once the radiation therapist analyzes the images, the couch will adjust to match the planned treatment isocenter. This can be preformed quickly before each radiation treatment and makes treatment of the prostate more accurate with smaller treatment fields and less dose to the bladder and rectum, resulting in fewer side effects.

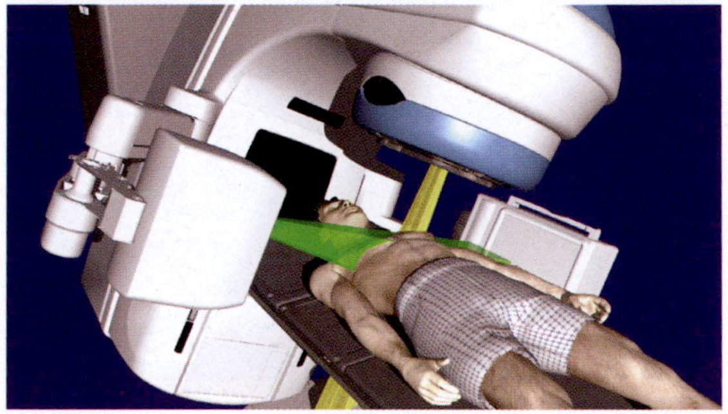

FIGURE 44-13. Image guided radiation therapy (IGRT) allows corrections of patient positioning prior to treatment. The treatment beam is shown in yellow and the IGRT beam is shown in green. *(Image courtesy of Varian Medical Systems, Inc. All rights reserved.)*

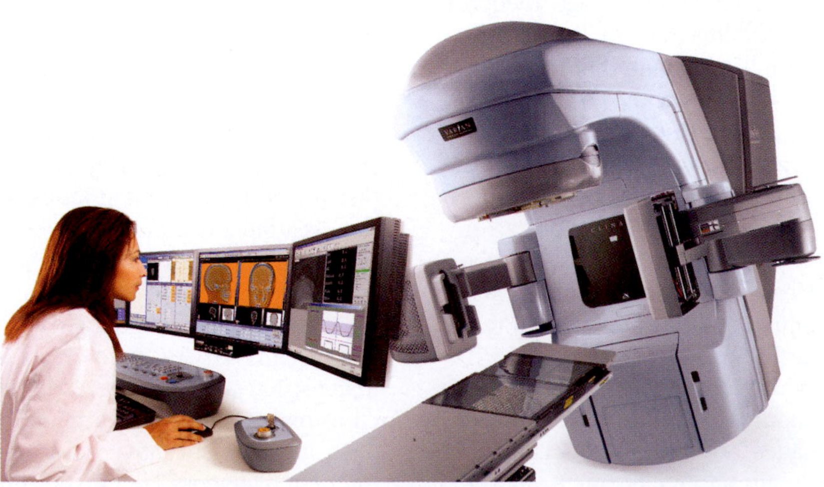

FIGURE 44-14. A linear accelerator unit and patient couch shown with the operator's console where images are fused with the patient treatment plan prior to initiating treatment. *(Image courtesy of Varian Medical Systems, Inc. All rights reserved.)*

There are many IGRT techniques that are being used and are currently under research. One technique of IGRT is optical tracking, where fiducial markers are placed internally or externally on the patient. A fiducial is an object that appears in the image being produced and can be used as a point of reference. These fiducials must be present during the patient's simulation. When the treatment plan is being created the dosimetrist plans the coordinate system using the fiducials in regard to the treatment isocenter. The fiducials are calibrated to a tracking device located in the treatment room. If movement occurs during treatment, the radiation therapist can pause the treatment, adjust the patient into the treatment range, and then continue treatment.

Respiratory gating is another form of IGRT that can be used for lung, breast, and upper abdominal sites. It tracks target volume movement due to respiration throughout radiation treatment. If the target moves out of the treatment field, the machine will pause treatment until the target is moved back into the radiation field. These techniques and many more are being developed and researched with the hope of increasing radiation dose to the diseased area and lessening dose to healthy tissue.

Linear Accelerator

The **linear accelerator** (Figure 44-15) is made up of the drive stand, gantry, treatment couch, control console, and modulator cabinet.

Drive Stand. The drive stand is a large cabinet that is secured to the floor in the treatment room. The gantry, which is a feature that rotates 360 degrees around the treatment couch, is connected to the drive stand and its rotational components are housed within the stand. The drive stand includes a cooling system, circulator, waveguide, and klystron (Figure 44-16). The klystron generates the

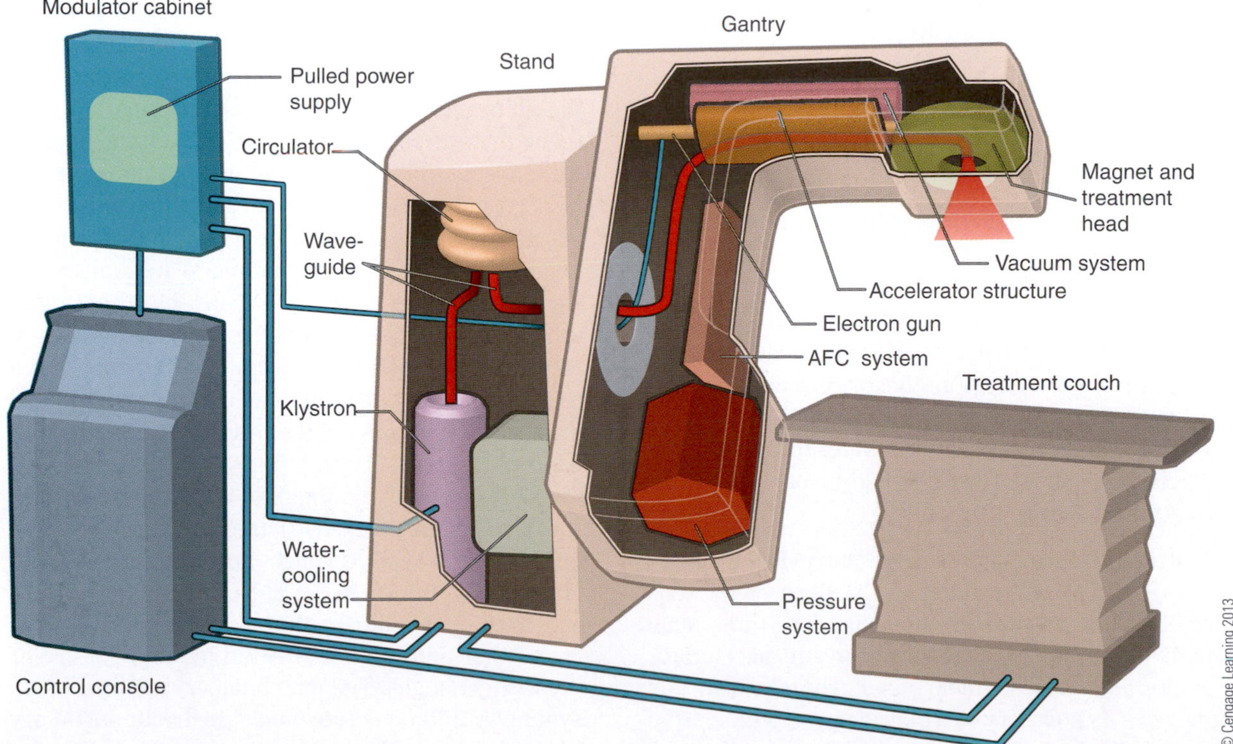

FIGURE 44-15. A linear accelerator with drive stand, gantry, treatment couch, and control console.

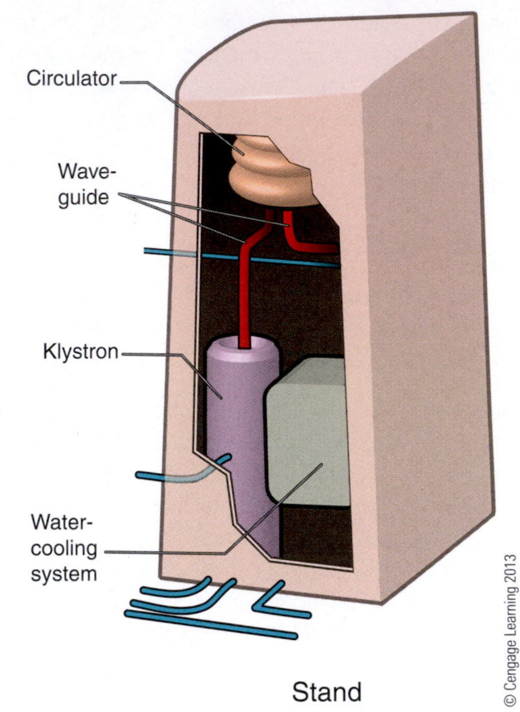

FIGURE 44-16. A linear accelerator drive stand.

microwave power that is used to excite or accelerate the electrons. This energy is then transferred to a waveguide, which runs into a circulator that acts as a holding area for the microwave energy. This does not allow it to be pushed back into the klystron. The other side of the circulator is also connected to a waveguide, which is a hollow tube that is used to transport the radiofrequency (RF) energy. Also located in the drive stand is a cooling system that circulates chilled water throughout the machine, particularly to the klystron, circulator, target, and accelerator guide.

Gantry. The primary job of the gantry (Figure 44-17) is to direct energy, either in the form of photons or electrons, toward the isocenter. The three main parts of the gantry are the electron gun, accelerator guide, and the treatment head. The electron gun receives its power from a pulsed power supply from the modulator cabinet. The electron gun produces electrons and directs them into the accelerator guide. Electron production by the electron gun is similar to a diagnostic x-ray tube. The cathode is made of a high atomic number material, usually tungsten, and is circular in shape. The anode is separated from the cathode and the electrons pass through it into the accelerator guide.

The accelerator guide has electrons passing through it from the electron gun at approximately 50 keV. Microwave energy produced by the klystron is directed by the waveguide. The electrons interact with the electromagnetic field from the microwaves and gain energy as they travel through the accelerator guide. The accelerator guide structure looks like a tube. If the accelerator guide is cut in half it would show an S shape that is designed to speed up and concentrate the electrons. Once the electrons travel through the accelerator guide, they enter the treatment or gantry head.

The gantry head is where the photon or electron beam is shaped and monitored. For photon energy the electron pathway travels to a bending magnet, then an x-ray target, a primary collimator, a beam flattening filter, the ion chamber, and finally the secondary collimators. It is also possible to add beam modification devices outside the gantry head. The bending magnet's purpose is to take the electrons from the accelerator guide and aim them toward the patient. If the bending magnet were absent, the electrons would continue to travel in a straight line. The bending magnet creates a 90- to 270-degree angle in the traveling electrons, which steers them in a downward motion to the x-ray target. Once the electrons hit the target, x-rays are produced. Once the x-rays are emitted, they pass through primary collimators that serve to form the x-ray beam into an intended shape. The primary collimators are the first step in shaping the beam to the patient's treatment plan.

After primary collimation the x-ray beam then travels through the beam-flattening filter. The x-ray beam then travels through an ion chamber that checks it symmetry in the X, Y, and Z planes. There are two ion chambers that work independent of each other and are not affected by temperature or pressure changes. The ion chambers monitor beam symmetry and dose rate. Once the beam dosimetry has been cleared by the ion chambers, it is deemed stable. The beam then travels to secondary collimators that have asymmetric jaws that shape it to the

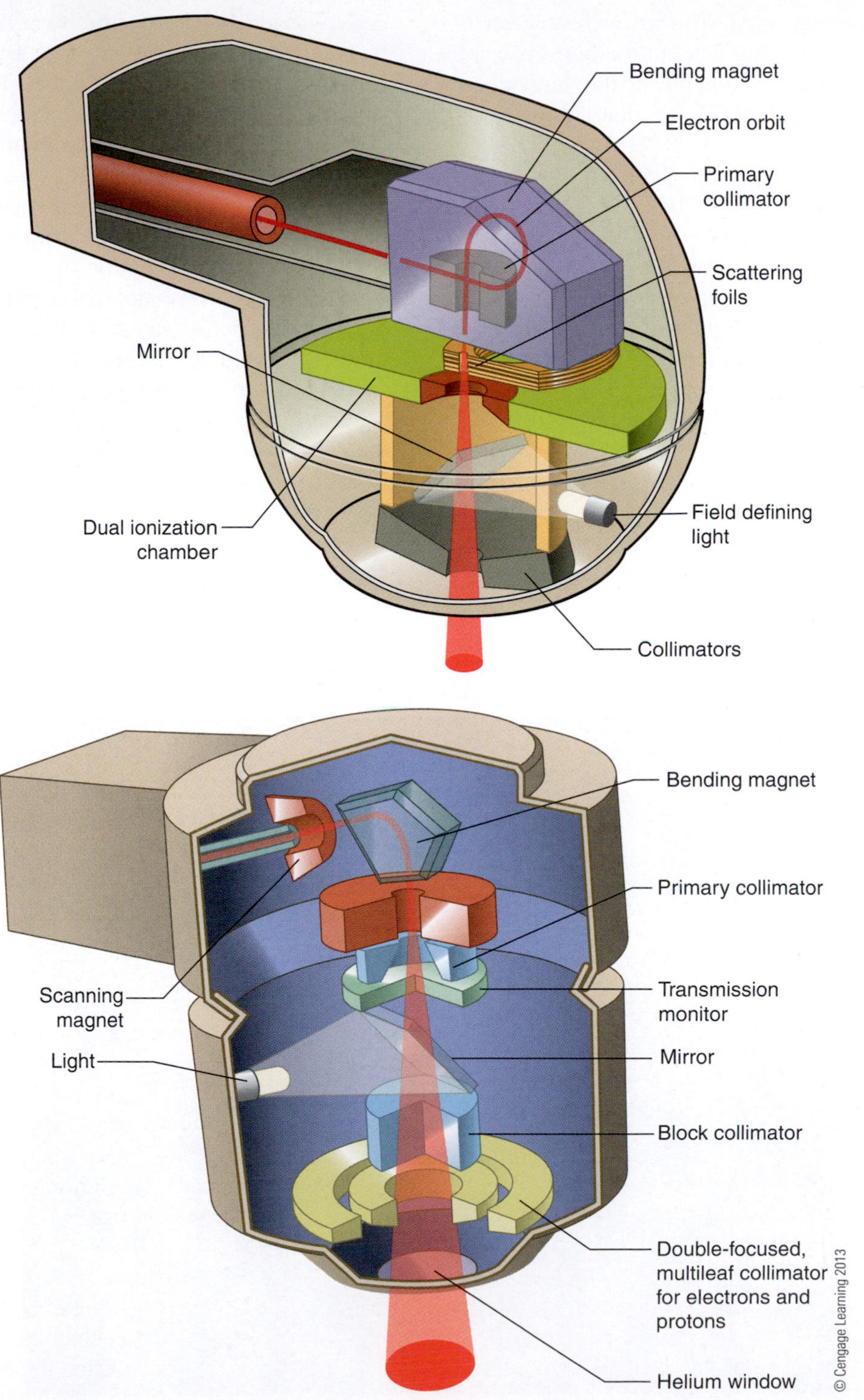

FIGURE 44-17. A linear accelerator gantry.

patient's treatment plan. The x-ray beam can be further shaped by either custom made Cerrobend® blocks inserted on the outside of the gantry head or multi-leaf collimators (MLCs) that are located in the gantry head.

For electron energy, the electrons from the accelerator guide move through the bending magnet first. The target is moved out of the path and an electron scattering foil is moved into the pathway. The scattering foil is responsible for creating a homogenous dose and causing the beam to widen. Electrons then travel through the primary collimator, ion chambers, and secondary collimators. An outside attachment is placed onto the gantry head that allows a final level of collimation known as tertiary collimation. Electron beams need to be more controlled and require a fixed direction close to the patient. These outside attachments are called electron cones and are available in many sizes. At the bottom of the electron cone, close to the patient's skin, a custom Cerrobend® insert is made that shapes the beam to the patient's treatment volume.

Also located inside the gantry head is a light that is projected using mirrors that display the radiation treatment field shape. This field light (Figure 44-18) displays on the patient's skin and is used by the radiation therapist to accurately set up treatments. Another light called the optical distance indicator (ODI) (Figure 44-19) projects a scale that indicates treatment distance from the target to the central axis of the radiation beam. An intersecting line called the crosshairs or central axis is located on a reticle in the gantry head. As the field light projects through the reticle, it casts the central axis shadow on the patient's skin, indicating the central portion of the beam. Typically, the central axis or crosshairs are set up to a mark on the patient's skin in the directed path leading to the treatment isocenter.

Treatment Couch. The treatment couch is also referred to as a patient support assembly. This is where the patient is positioned and receives treatment (see Figure 44-19). Couches move on

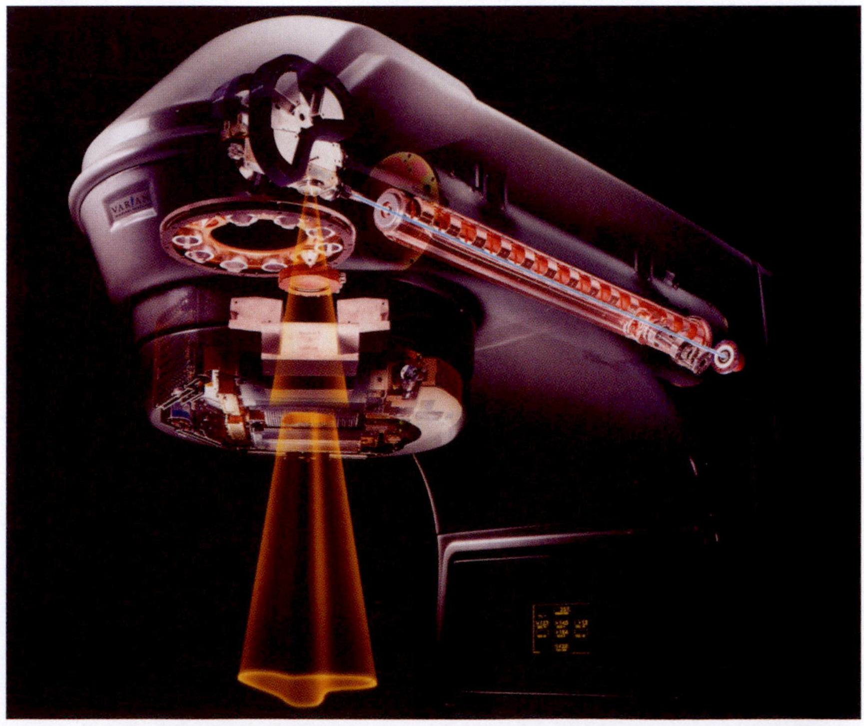

FIGURE 44-18. A custom shaped field light from a linear accelerator. *(Image courtesy of Varian Medical Systems, Inc. All rights reserved.)*

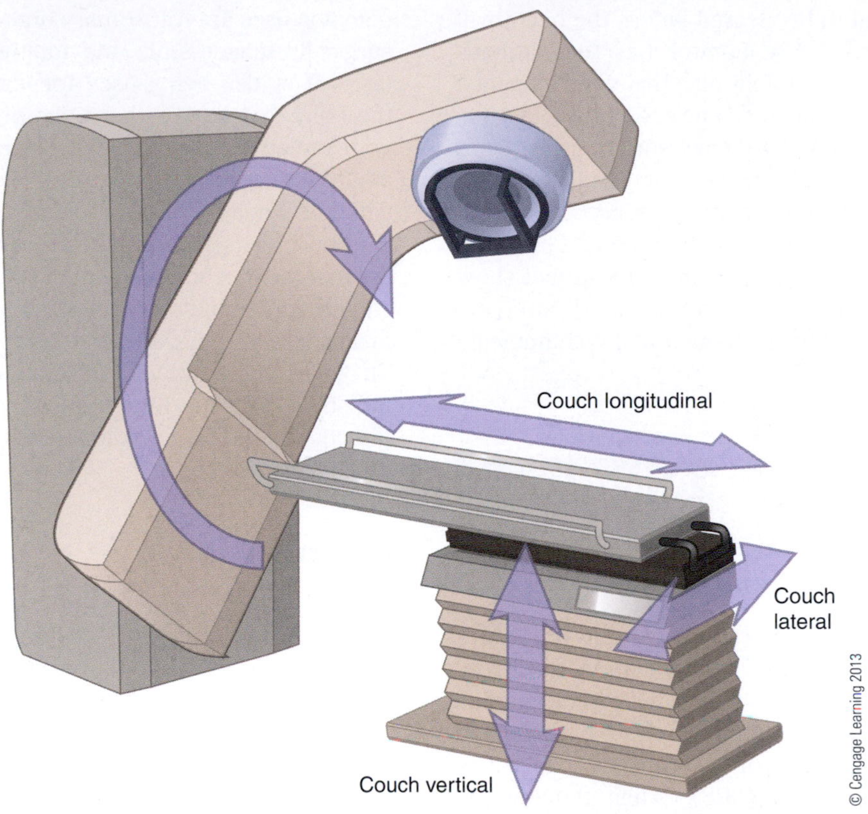

FIGURE 44-19. The field light and optical distance indicator (ODI) used to provide patient setup accuracy.

multiple planes to line the patient up to the marks placed at the time of simulation. Couches move vertically (up/down), longitudinally (in/out), and laterally (left/right) around the isocenter. To allow the radiation treatment beam to enter the patient without attenuating material in its path, a clear Mylar-covered section resembling a grid is part of the treatment tabletop. Couches can typically handle 450 lbs (200 kg) and are about 45 to 50 cm in width. Couches also have appendicles for attachment of immobilization devices. Also located on the couch are controls used by the radiation therapist to manipulate the table parameters to assist in setting the patient to the isocenter. Depending on the manufacturer, a pendant is attached to the treatment machine that allows the therapists to move certain parameters of the machine. The pendent also allows for room lights to be dimmed, and turns on or off the field light and ODI. If the treatment machine has an imaging device attached to it, the pendent will control that as well.

Modulator Cabinet. The modulator cabinet is usually located in the treatment room and contains the primary power distribution system, auxiliary power distribution system, and fan control. Primary power gives power to the treatment machine. The auxiliary power distribution system gives power to the emergency off switches that shut the treatment machine down immediately. The fan turns on and off when the power systems need to be cooled.

Control Console. The control console is located outside of the treatment room. It is where radiation therapists monitor and control the treatment machine as well as monitor the patient. The machine parameters are located on a monitor and all interlocks need to be cleared before the beam will be activated. Another monitor has the patient's information and treatment plan that can be opened and loaded into the machine's software. All parameters are checked to make sure the machine's parameters match the patient's treatment plan. A paper chart or another monitor is used to record and verify the accuracy of treatment. There are also cameras within the treatment room that show the patient from different angles and an intercom system so the therapist can hear and communicate with the patient at all times.

SPECIALIZED TREATMENTS AND UNITS

Stereotactic Irradiation

Stereotactic irradiation is a noninvasive procedure that delivers a high dose of radiation to a very conformed stereotactically defined target volume. When the total dose of radiation is delivered in one treatment session or fraction it is called stereotactic radiosurgery (SRS). When the dose is broken into multiple treatment fractions it is called stereotactic radiotherapy (SRT). Stereotactic irradiation can be performed using a variety of linear-accelerator-based systems or radioisotope units. Its common uses are for primary brain lesions that are surgically inaccessible and multiple brain metastases. It is also being used for lesions throughout the body that have either been previously treated with radiation, are surgically inaccessible, or are adjacent to a critical structure that would decrease a patient's quality of life if damaged. In addition to cancer, it has also been shown to be beneficial for the treatment of some non-malignant conditions, including functional disorders such as arteriovenous malformations (AVMs) and trigeminal neuralgia. The goals of stereotactic irradiation are rapid dose fall-off outside the target volume, conformality of the dose to the target volume, and flawless repositioning accuracy.

Proton Therapy

Proton therapy (Figure 44-20) for the treatment of deep-seated targets is undergoing tremendous worldwide growth. In the early 1990s, when the Loma Linda University Medical Center in California opened as the first high-volume hospital-based proton-therapy facility, fewer than 1,000 patients per year were treated with high-energy protons. At that time, such proton beams were only otherwise available at laboratory-based nuclear physics facilities. Protons are positively charged particles that reside in the nucleus of all atoms. The advantage of proton

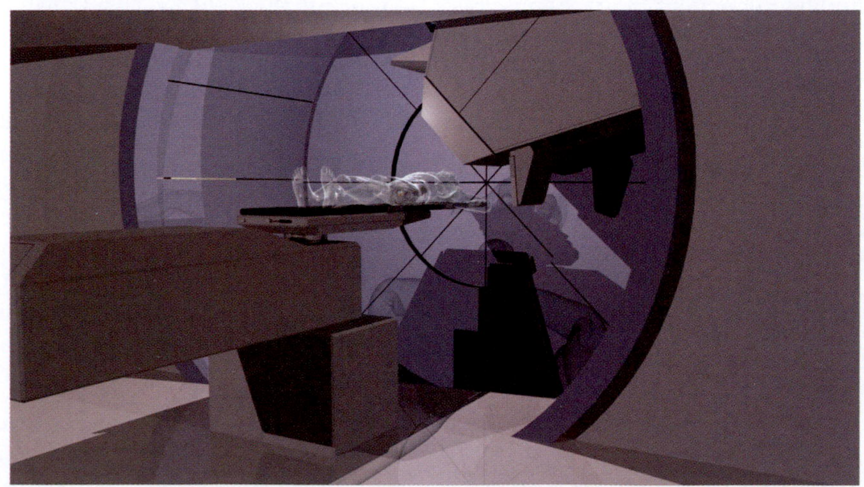

FIGURE 44-20. A proton therapy unit. *(Image courtesy of Varian Medical Systems, Inc. All rights reserved.)*

therapy is its ability to conform the deposited energy, or dose, to the intended target. Basically, protons are clinically useful because they are easy to control, and there is minimal scattering involved. Another clinical advantage of protons is the process by which they deposit energy in relation to depth. This is referred to as the Bragg peak (Figure 44-21). Most of the energy that is deposited by protons is done at the end of their range, where the dose deposited is almost 100 percent and then drops off rapidly to zero. This scenario is in sharp contrast to the dose deposited by an X-ray beam, which is attenuated exponentially as it passes through matter. The process of producing therapeutic protons starts with protons being stripped from atoms and accelerated with a cyclotron or a synchrocyclotron. The protons are then directed through a pipe to the treatment machine. Proton therapy is used to treat both benign and malignant lesions, such as prostate cancer, pituitary adenomas, pediatric tumors, and tumors of the head and neck.

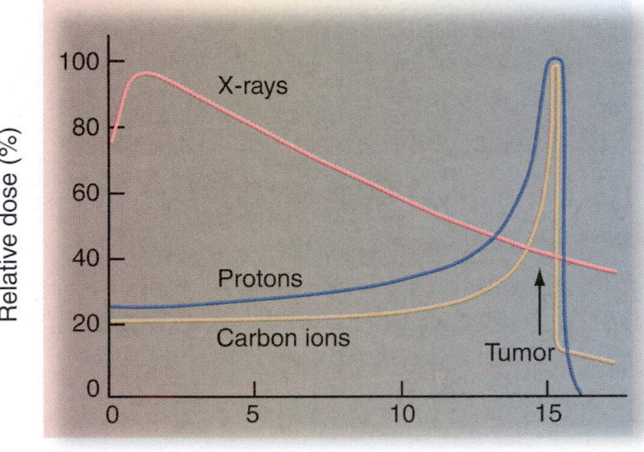

FIGURE 44-21. A treatment plan for proton therapy for a prostate cancer patient. Note the red areas where the proton Bragg peak process deposits nearly all the energy in a small tissue volume.

TomoTherapy®

TomoTherapy® is a helical treatment unit that combines the capabilities of a CT scanner with a linear accelerator. The unit looks very similar to a CT scanner. There is a gantry in which the waveguide component of a linear accelerator and the MV detector subsystem of a CT scanner are located. The gantry continuously rotates and the treatment couch moves throughout the treatment, allowing for helical treatment arcs. TomoTherapy® uses IMRT, SRS, or SRT to conform the dose to a very precise area, thus allowing for minimal side effects and smaller treatment fields. In TomoTherapy® the patient is set up to established marks and an MV CT scan is performed. The CT images are registered and fused with the CT-simulated images used to create the patient's treatment plan. The patient's anatomy is adjusted to match the CT simulation images. Once they are matched, the couch moves to align with the exact planned isocenter and then treatment can begin. TomoTherapy® can be used on all malignancies.

SUMMARY

The use of x-rays for therapeutic purposes began shortly after Roentgen's discovery. The first documented treatment of cancer was in 1896 on a woman's left breast. In 1962 radiation therapy began as a separate specialization. The goals of radiation therapy are to protect healthy tissue as much as possible, preserve function of the structure or structures surrounding the tumor, eradicate the tumor, and minimize side effects.

The first step for a patient in a radiation oncology department is to meet for a consultation. If the patient is a candidate for radiation therapy, a treatment plan is determined. The foundation of this treatment plan is called the prescription.

SUMMARY (continued)

The first step in treatment planning is simulation. This can be done using a CT simulation or a conventional simulator. The main goals for simulation are to give a dose of radiation to malignant tissues and reduce the dose to normal tissue. Treatment planning is the primary responsibility of the dosimetrist. The dosimetrist identifies an isocenter, the volume of tissue to be treated, radiation beam arrangements, and the creation of an acceptable isodose distribution. To establish the volume of tissue that will be irradiated, a contour of the gross tumor volume (GTV), clinical target volume (CTV), and planning target volume (PTV) must be created. Once the simulation visit has been completed and a treatment plan produced, radiation treatment can be administered. To ensure accuracy of treatment, the ongoing imaging of treatment fields is critical. This is accomplished through either portal imaging or image guided radiation therapy (IGRT).

The most common radiation therapy unit is the linear accelerator. It consists of drive stand, gantry, treatment couch, control console, and modulator cabinet. Other specialized treatment units include stereotactic irradiation, proton therapy, and TomoTherapy®. ■

REVIEW QUESTIONS

1. What needs to be included in a radiation therapy treatment prescription?
2. What are the two goals of simulation?
3. Differentiate between the treatment and machine isocenter.
4. What are some benefits of image fusion?
5. Explain the difference between GTV, CTV, and PTV.
6. Why are MV portal images so difficult to read?
7. Why is IGRT beneficial?
8. Describe the path an electron takes in a linear accelerator to become a photon.
9. What are the goals of stereotactic irradiation?
10. Describe three clinical advantages of proton therapy.

REFERENCES AND RECOMMENDED READING

Amies, C., Bani-Hashemi, A., Celi, J., Grousset, G.., Ghelmansarai, F., Hristov, D., Lane, D., Mitschke, M., Singh, A., Shukla, H., Stein, J., & Wofford, M. (2006). A multi-platform approach to image guided radiation therapy (IGRT). *Medical Dosimetry, 31*(1), 12–19. doi:10.1016/j.meddos.2005.12.013

Baker, M. (2007, April 18). Medical linear accelerator celebrates 50 years of treating cancer. *Stanford Report.* Retrieved from http://news-service.stanford.edu/news/2007/april18/med-accelerator-041807.html.

Bar-Shalom, R., Yefremov, N., Guralnik, L., Gaitini, D., Frenkel, A., Kuten, A., Altman, H., Keidar, Z., & Israel, O. (2003). Clinical performance of pet/ct in evaluation of cancer: Additional value for diagnostic imaging and patient management. *The Journal of Nuclear Medicine, 44*(8), 1200–1209.

Beavis, A. W. (2004). Is tomotherapy the future of IMRT? *British Journal of Radiology, 77*, 285–295. doi: 10.1259/bjr/22666727

Bentel, G. C. (1996) *Radiation therapy planning* (2nd ed.). Columbus, OH: McGraw-Hill.

Frame, P. (2011). Tales from the atomic age: The legend of Emil H. Grubbe. Retrieved from http://www.orau.org/ptp/articlesstories/grubbe.htm.

Kaplan, H. S., & Bagshaw, M.A. (1963). Radiation therapy program at Stanford University. *CA: A Cancer Journal for Clinicians, 13*, 242–243. doi: 10.3322/canjclin.13.6.242

Leibel, S., & Phillips, T. (2000) *Textbook of radiation oncology* (2nd ed.). Philadelphia: Saunders.

McDonough, J. (2008, May 20). Proton-therapy technology: Developing at pace. *Medical Physics Web.*

Retrieved from http://medicalphysicsweb.org/cws/article/opinion/34237.

Nobel lectures, physics 1901–1921. (1967a). Amsterdam: Elsevier. Retrieved from http://nobelprize.org/nobel_prizes/physics/articles/curie/index.html.

Nobel lectures, physics 1901–1921. (1967b). Amsterdam: Elsevier. Retrieved from http://nobelprize.org/cgibin/print?from=%2Fnobel_prizes%2Fphysics%2Flaureates%2F1901%2Frontgen-bio.html.

Oelfke, U., Tucking, T., Nill, S., Seeber, A., Hesse, B., Huber, P., & Thilmann, C. (2006). Linac-integrated kV-cone beam ct: Technical features and first applications. *Medical Dosimetry*, *31*(1), 62–70. doi:10.1016/j.meddos.2005.12.008

Perez, C. A., Halperin, E. C., Brady, L. W., & Schmidt-Ulirich, R. K. (2004). *Principles and practice of radiation oncology* (4th ed.). Philadelphia: Saunders.

Rubin, P. (2001). *Clinical oncology: A multidisciplinary approach for physicians and students* (8th ed.). Philadelphia: Saunders.

Schillaci, O., & Simonetti, G. (2004). Fusion imaging in nuclear medicine-applications of dual-modality systems in oncology. *Cancer Biotherapy & Radiopharmaceuticals*, *19*(1), 1–10.

Washington, C. M., & Leaver, D. (2004). *Principles and practice of radiation therapy* (2nd ed.). St. Louis: Mosby.

Wishart, A. (2007). *One and three: A son's journey into the history and science of cancer*. New York: Grove.

Xing, L., Thorndyke, B., Schreibmann, E., Yang, Y., Li, T., Kim, G.., Luxton, G.., & Koong, A. (2006). Overview of image-guided radiation therapy. *Medical Dosimetry*, *31*(2), 91–112. doi:10.1016/jmeddos.2005.12.004

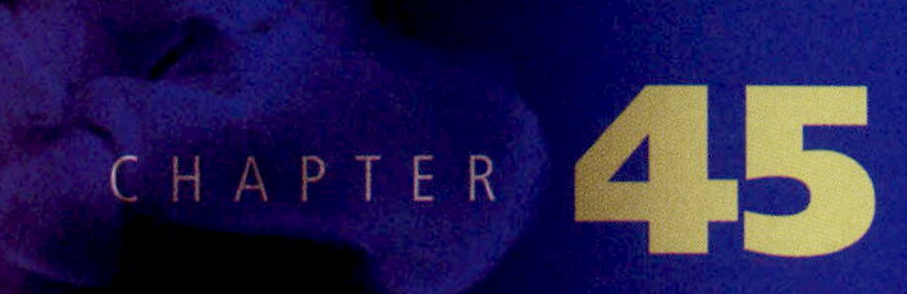

Diagnostic Medical Sonography

Sharon Lakia, MS, RT(R), RDMS, RVT

KEY TERMS

acoustic impedance
compression
continuous wave
Doppler
frequency
harmonics
Huygen's Principle
period
piezoelectric effect
propagation speed
pulse duration
pulse repetition frequency
pulse repetition period
pulse wave
rarefaction
transducer
wavelength

The shadow of a sound,—a voice without a mouth, and words without a tongue.

—Paul Chatfield (a/k/a Horace Smith), http://www.giga-usa.com/quotes/topics/echo_t001.htm (retrieved March 27, 2010)

OBJECTIVES

Upon completion of this chapter, the student should be able to:

- Explain ultrasonographic orientations as seen on the monitor.
- Determine the variables that affect the sound wave.
- Explain the difference between continuous wave and pulse wave.
- Identify the pulse wave parameters.
- Explain attenuation and acoustic impedance.
- List the components found in the transducer housing.
- Explain the sound wave field.
- Define Doppler.
- Explain the different types of transducers.
- Explain basic instrumentation of a diagnostic ultrasound machine.
- Explain basic harmonics.

INTRODUCTION

Diagnostic medical sonography incorporates sound waves to generate images capable of diagnosing pathology found within the human body. In order to perform proper imaging, an understanding of sound waves and how they interact with the human body is an integral part of the modality. In addition, a sonographer must have knowledge of the ultrasound machine, instrumentation, and how to produce quality images that show correct anatomical representation of the area being imaged. Physicians rely heavily on the expertise of the sonographer in obtaining images necessary for proper diagnosis.

The field of diagnostic medical sonography (DMS) has its own registry and governing agencies. The American Institute of Ultrasound in Medicine (AIUM) determines the parameters used for diagnostic ultrasound machines and makes recommendations as to the prudent use of these machines. The American Registry of Diagnostic Medical Sonography (ARDMS) implements the national credentialing examinations that sonographers may take. The ARDMS is internationally recognized as the gold standard in DMS credentialing. In addition, the American Registry of Radiologic Technologists (ARRT) offers sonography credentialing. The ARDMS offers three credentials, Registered Diagnostic Medical Sonographer (RDMS), Registered Vascular Technologist (RVT), and Registered Diagnostic Cardiac Sonographer (RDCS).

Historical Overview

The ability to use sound waves in locating objects under water was realized during World War I, but it was not discovered in time for use by the military during that war. Sonar was first used by the military during World War II in the location of submarines. With the ending of the war, medical science began discovering new ways to utilize ultrasound in the diagnosing of pathology. By the 1950s research was ongoing; however, the United States chose to drop out of the research while the European nations continued forward. In the 1960s, ultrasound applications were increasing at such a pace that the United States returned to the research of ultrasound and has been instrumental in helping to make it one of the fastest growing modalities found in the diagnostic department. Today, ultrasound is used in imaging most aspects of the body, such as abdominal structures, pelvic structures, obstetrics, and the vascular system.

Orientation

Unlike other diagnostic modalities, sonograms or real-time monitors are viewed differently. Most other images assume the anatomical position and are viewed accordingly. Sonography does not. In order to view ultrasound images correctly, a clear understanding of the orientation is required.

Ultrasound utilizes two planes, longitudinal and transverse, when scanning a patient. As with other modalities, the two fields or views are required in order to determine location and size of an area of interest. In most instances, placing the sound beam perpendicular to the field of interest is required as well. The sound beam is emitted by the **transducer**, which is held in position against the patient's body by the sonographer. Using two opposite planes allows the sonographer to determine if what is being imaged is real or not. Artifacts are an inherent aspect of scanning, and it requires a skilled sonographer to determine if what is being seen is real or an artifact that will dissipate by using a different imaging plane or by more efficient use of the instrumentation of the machine.

When a sonographer scans in the longitudinal/transverse plane, he or she may or may not be scanning longitudinal or transverse to the body. Organs are rarely positioned perfectly longitudinal or transverse within the body cavities; they often are at angles to each other in various planes. To compensate for that, the transducer must be placed according to the lay of the body part and not the patient's actual body. What may appear to be an oblique plane may actually show the organ in the proper longitudinal or transverse view. If an organ is not imaged properly, it may be foreshortened, leading to an inaccurate diagnosis.

Each transducer has built into it markings that designate orientation. The scan head should be placed such that the mark on the transducer is pointing toward the head of the patient when in the longitudinal view. When turning to the transverse plane, the mark is pointed toward the patient's right side. Correct orientation is shown in Figures 45-1 and 45-2. Should a sonographer inadvertently point the marked edge of the transducer toward the feet of the patient or turn it toward the patient's left side, the image on the screen and subsequent hard copies will be anatomically incorrect, as the organs will appear to be flipped (i.e., the liver will be seen on the left side of the body and the spleen will be seen on the right, or the superior dome of the liver will be seen on the inferior edge). Incorrect orientation is shown in Figures 45-3 and 45-4.

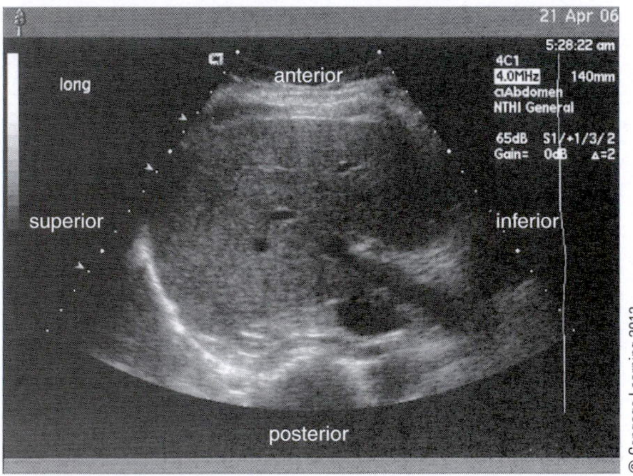

FIGURE 45-1. Correct orientation of the transducer for a longitudinal image.

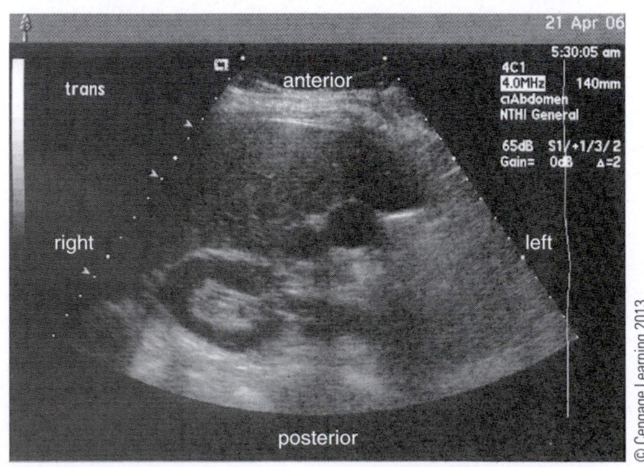

FIGURE 45-2. Correct orientation of the transducer for a transverse image.

SOUND WAVES

Sound waves operate in a cyclical fashion. They move forward and then back again rhythmically as they travel. A simple sine wave can be used to describe this movement. The forward movement is termed **compression** or condensation. It is the positive portion of the wave. The backward movement is termed **rarefaction** or rarefacts. This is the negative portion of the wave. Figure 45-5 shows

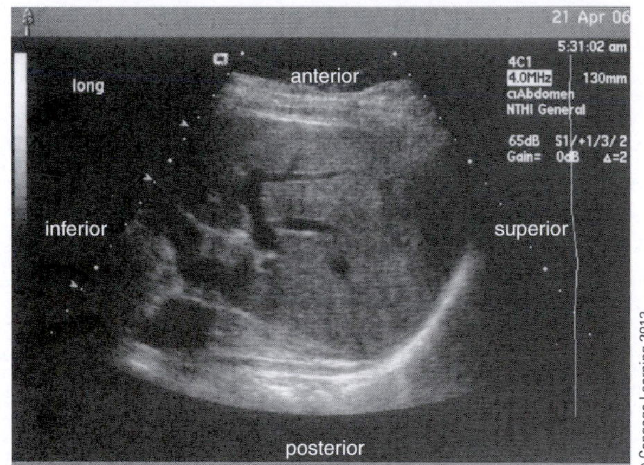

FIGURE 45-3. Incorrect positioning of the transducer in a longitudinal image. The orientation for superior/inferior is now flipped.

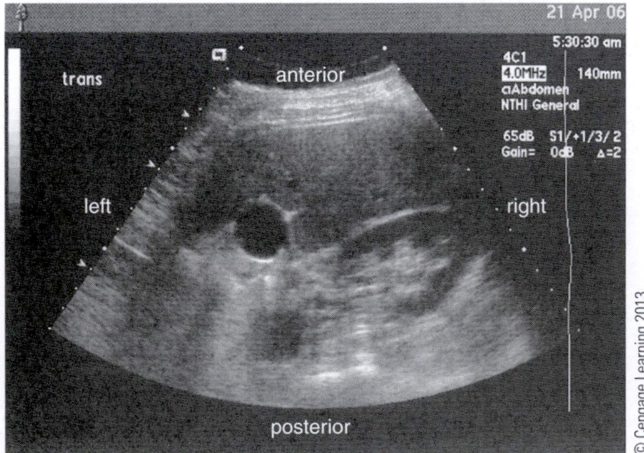

FIGURE 45-4. Incorrect positioning of the transducer in a transverse image. The orientation for right/left is now flipped.

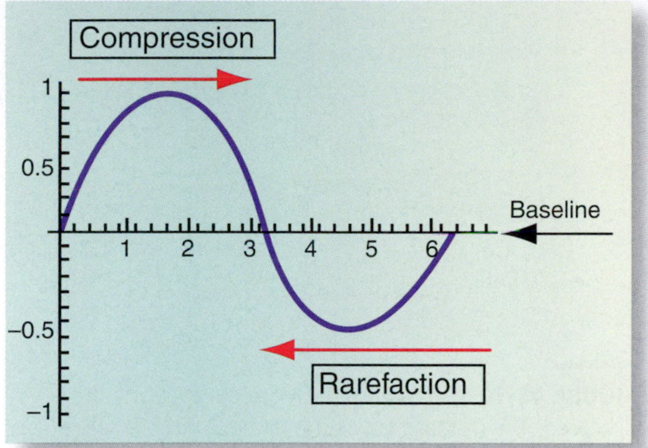

FIGURE 45-5. Above the baseline is showing the positive or compression portion of the sine wave. Below the baseline shows the negative or rarefaction portion of the sine wave.

the compression/rarefaction movement of the sound wave.

A sound wave requires particles to interact with in order to travel. If particles are not present, such as in a vacuum, there will be no sound. The particles found in a medium are what allow for the forward and backward movement of the wave. With each compression (forward movement) the particles are pushed forward, and with each rarefaction (backward movement) the particles return to their position. These particles will move forward/backward, parallel to the wave. This is termed a longitudinal wave and can be seen in Figures 45-6 and 45-7.

The Law of Conservation of Energy states that energy can neither be created nor destroyed, only converted to another form of energy. As the wave passes through a medium and interacts with the particles, it transfers some of its energy to the medium. This movement causes a by-product in the form of heat, which is then transferred into the medium. The transference of energy through movement is known as mechanical energy. Therefore, the sound wave is a mechanical wave as it transfers energy from one point to another.

Sound is a longitudinal, mechanical wave that compresses and rarefacts as it moves through a medium. It travels in a straight line and requires particles within a medium to travel. The main by-product of this movement is heat.

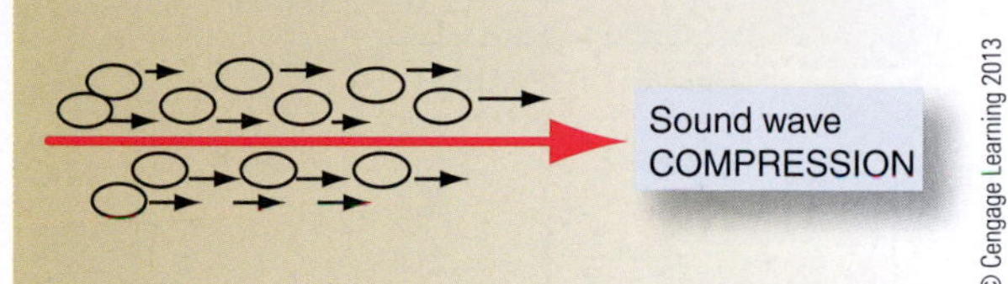

FIGURE 45-6. As the wave moves through the medium, it displaces particles. These particles will move in the direction of the wave. During compression there is forward movement of the particles.

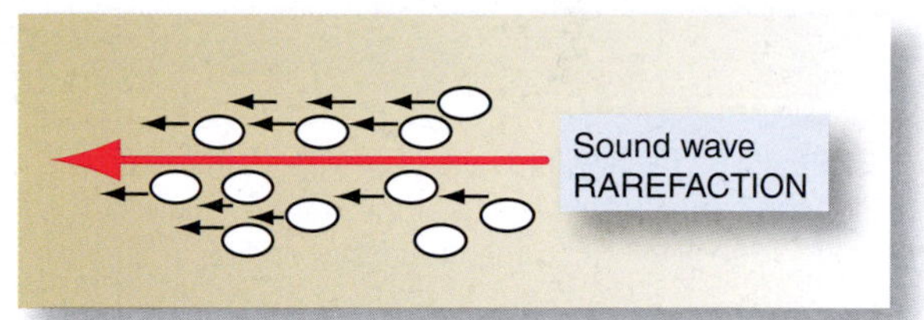

FIGURE 45-7. As the wave rarefacts of moves backwards, the particles return to their original positions.

Variables of Sound Waves

A number of variables affect the particles in the medium as a sound wave passes through it. These variables include pressure, tissue density, particle vibrations, and temperature.

Pressure. Pressure refers to the concentration of force over a given area. During compression, the wave puts pressure on the particles it is interacting with. This forces the particles against each other, thereby increasing the pressure between them. During the rarefaction portion, this pressure is lessened as the particles resume their normal spaces. The sine wave can be a tool to indicate the amount of pressure during the wave, showing both an increase (positive) and decrease (negative) in amounts of pressure. Figure 45-8 shows the positive and negative pressure as the wave travels through the medium.

Tissue Density. Density is the concentration of mass over volume. As the wave passes through the medium, such as tissue, it forces the particles together, causing a higher concentration of particles

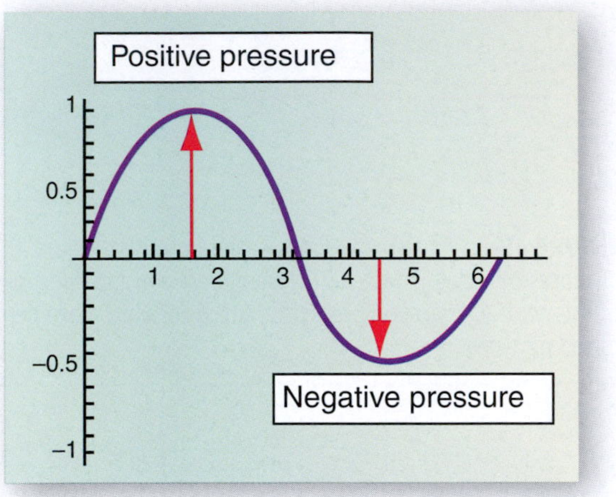

FIGURE 45-8. Positive pressure is applied to the medium during the compression portion of the wave. Negative pressure is applied during the rarefaction portion of the wave.

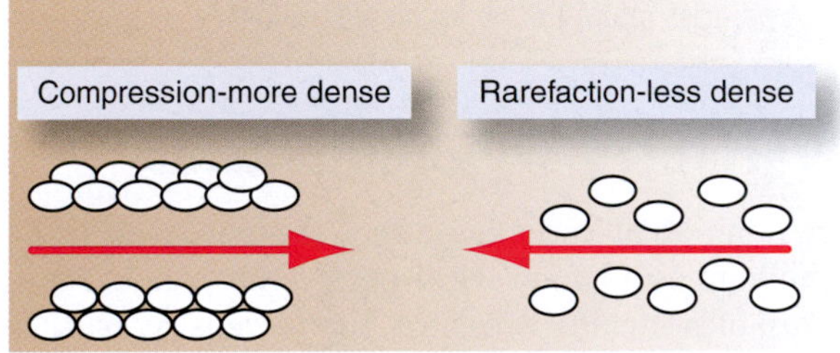

FIGURE 45-9. As the wave moves through a medium, particles are pushed together, thereby increasing the density in that area. As the wave rarefacts, the particles return to their original position, which returns the tissue to its original density.

within that space. As the wave rarefacts, the particles revert back to the density originally held. The sine wave can be used to describe this effect as well, with increased pressure seen as the positive portion of the wave and decreased pressure seen as the negative part of the wave. Figure 45-9 shows how the particles are pushed together during compression and the return to normal position during rarefaction.

Particle Vibration. As the oncoming sound wave hits the surrounding particles, they vibrate, causing

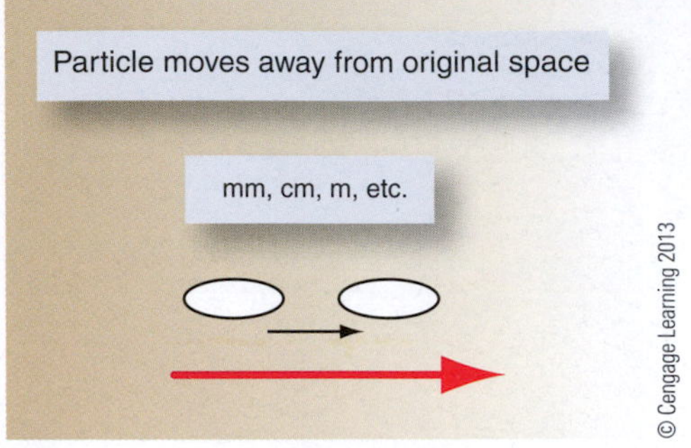

FIGURE 45-10. During compression, particles will be displaced. The distance traveled is termed *particle vibration*.

them to become displaced from their original spot. Figure 45-10 shows the displacement of the particles as the wave travels through.

Temperature. Temperature refers to the concentration of heat energy. Although temperature will affect a sound wave, it is not a dominant variable when analyzing a sound wave.

Parameters of Sound Waves

Parameters of the sound waves refer to the different facets of the wave. They are terms that reflect the composition of the wave and how each part will be affected by the medium in which it is traveling through. A clear understanding of these parameters helps the sonographer produce an optimal image.

Frequency. **Frequency** refers to the number of cycles occurring within a given point in time. The unit for frequency is the hertz (Hz), and 1 Hz refers to 1 cycle per second. Frequency is found in three ranges: 20–20,000 Hz (audible range), <20 Hz (infrasound), and >20,000 Hz (ultrasound). Both infrasound and ultrasound are beyond the human ear's capability for hearing. Diagnostic ultrasound uses frequencies in the megahertz (MHz) range; therefore each transducer is emitting at least 1 million cycles per second. For example, if a 3-MHz transducer is being used, the transducer is emitting a frequency of 3 million cycles per second. Figure 45-11 shows a 1-Hertz frequency and Figure 45-12 shows a 2-Hertz frequency.

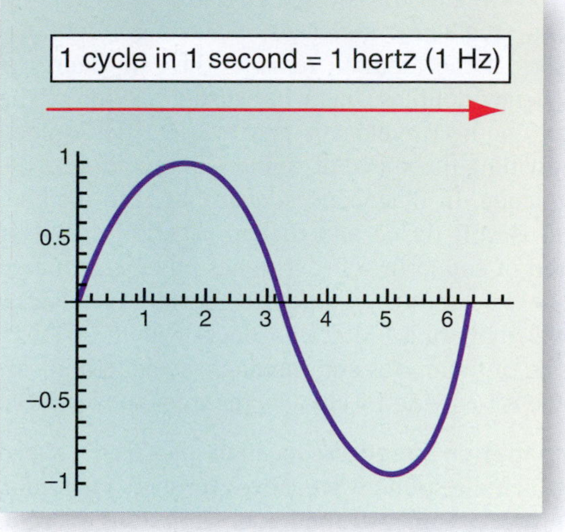

FIGURE 45-11. This diagram shows one sine wave during a 1-second time frame. This represents a 1-Hz frequency.

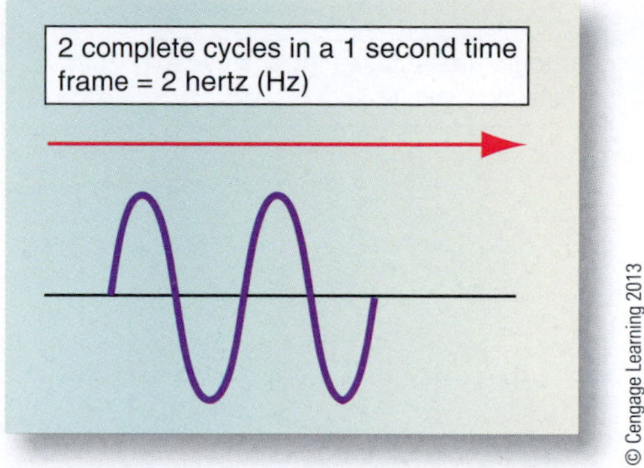

FIGURE 45-12. This diagram shows two complete since waves during a 1-second time frame. This represents a 2-Hz frequency.

The sonographer is not in control of frequency; it is an inherent feature within the transducer and is determined by the transducer's characteristics only. Frequency will determine axial resolution and penetration of the sound beam. By increasing the frequency used, the sonographer will increase the axial resolution of the image, thereby improving the quality of the image. Improved axial resolution is made at the expense of penetration, as a higher-frequency transducer cannot penetrate tissue as well as a lower-frequency transducer. The part being imaged will determine which transducer is to be used. For superficial structures, a high-frequency transducer is utilized in order to have the best possible axial resolution. For structures deep within the body, a lower frequency is best as the sound wave is better able to penetrate deeper; however, axial resolution will be lost (Figure 45-13).

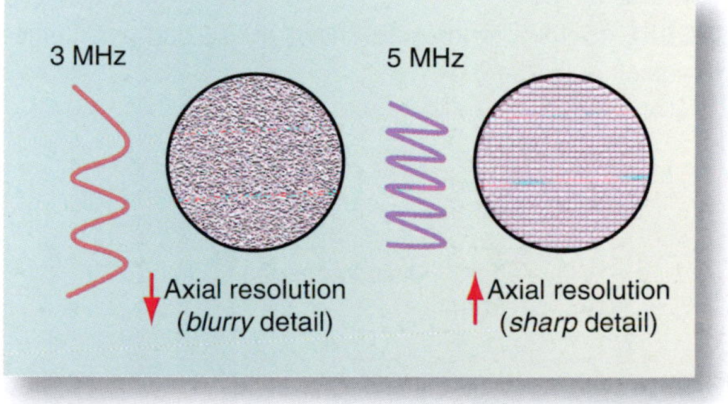

FIGURE 45-13. Axial resolution is the ability to resolve two adjacent spaces. The first image shows adjacent areas as being blurred. The second image shows distinct areas within the image. Higher-frequency transducers give better axial resolution.

Period. Period is the amount of time it takes to complete one cycle. The unit is any variation of time: seconds, microseconds, and so forth. Microseconds (μs) are typically used in diagnostic sonography (Figure 45-14). Period cannot be changed by the sonographer. As with frequency, the sonographer is not in control of period; it is inherent in the transducer. In order to change the period, frequency would have to change, and in order to change frequency, a new transducer would have to be used. Period is inversely related to frequency and is the reciprocal of frequency. If frequency is increased, then period will decrease. To determine period, divide the number one by the frequency.

Wavelength. Wavelength is the distance over which one cycle occurs. The units are variations of length: mm, cm, m, and so forth. In diagnostic sonography, mm are used (Figure 45-15). Wavelength cannot be changed by the sonographer. It is determined by the transducer and the medium in which it is traveling.

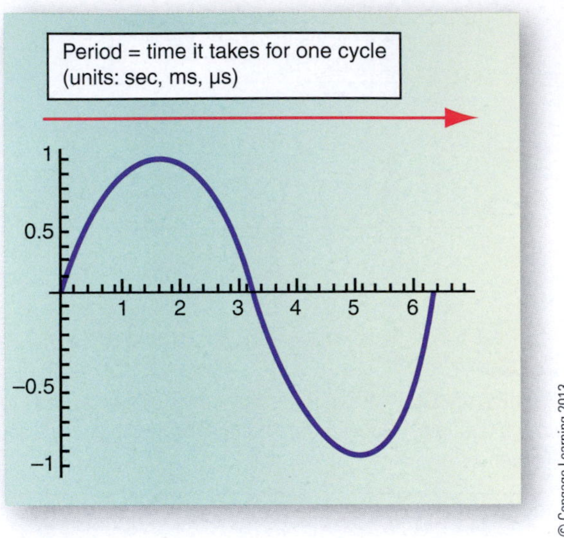

FIGURE 45-14. This diagram shows a 1-second time frame to complete one sine wave.

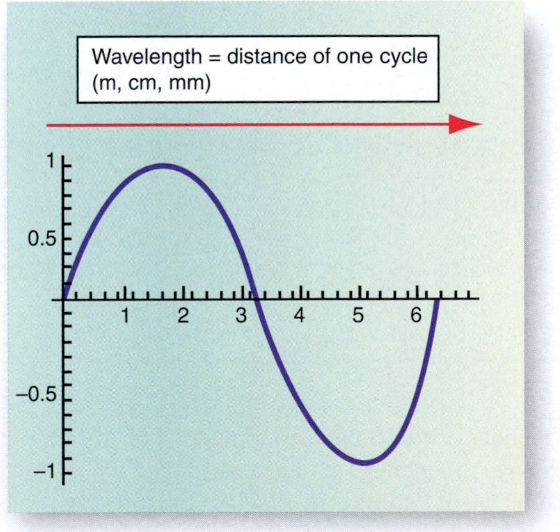

FIGURE 45-15. This diagram shows the distance for one complete sine wave.

As long as the transducer and the medium remain the same, wavelength will not change. If the sound wave interacts with a different medium, frequency remains the same but wavelength changes.

Wavelength is inversely related to frequency, so as frequency increases, wavelength will decrease. If the medium remains the same and the frequency doubles, this will cause a halving of the wavelength. Wavelength can also be determined by dividing the speed of sound in a medium by the frequency. In diagnostic sonography, the medium used is soft tissue and the propagation speed or speed of sound in soft tissue has been determined to be 1.54 mm/µs. Therefore, in soft tissue, the wavelength for a 1-MHz transducer will be 1.54 mm. A rule of thumb for determining wavelength in soft tissue is to divide 1.54 mm by the frequency in MHz.

Propagation Speed. **Propagation speed** is the speed at which the sound wave moves through a medium. The unit is mm/s or mm/µs or variations thereof. The medium determines the propagation speed and the sonographer cannot change it. The propagation speed in a medium will remain the same so long as the medium does not change. Propagation speed can be determined by multiplying frequency times the wavelength. Two factors affect propagation speed: the stiffness and density of the medium.

Stiffness. Stiffness refers to the hardness of the medium. Stiffness is inversely related to the compressibility and elasticity of the tissue. As the stiffness of a medium increases, the compressibility and elasticity will decrease. Stiffness and speed have a direct relationship. The harder or stiffer a material is, the higher the speed will be through the medium.

Density. Density refers to the concentration of matter. If you increase mass or the concentration of matter, you increase density. Speed and density are indirectly related. As the density of a medium increases, speed will decrease.

Propagation speed can be determined by multiplying frequency by the wavelength. By calculating the propagation speeds of various tissues, physicists have established that the average propagation speed for soft tissue is 1,540 meters/second (1,540 m/s or 1.54 km·s or 1.54 mm/µs). Diagnostic ultrasound machines are calibrated to this rate. Average propagation speeds for different types of tissue found in the body are listed in Table 45-1.

Amplitude. Amplitude refers to the strength of the wave. The unit to describe amplitude will vary

TABLE 45-1.

Type of Tissue	Average Propagation Speed
Air	330 m/s
Brain	1,520 m/s
Kidney	1,560 m/s
Liver	1,570 m/s
Muscle	1,630 m/s
Bone	3,500 m/s

depending on which variable it is referring to, such as pressure, density, particle motion, or temperature. Amplitude is determined by the machine, but can be changed by the sonographer. Initially, the voltage applied to the transducer will determine the amplitude, or strength, of the wave. Once the voltage has been applied, the sonographer can change the amplitude by changing power, dB, output, or transmit control knobs. These control knobs are found on the keyboard of the machine. By increasing one of these controls, the sonographer increases the amplitude (strength) of the sound wave or decreases the amplitude (strength) of the sound wave before it enters the body.

Amplitude, or the strength of the wave, will decrease as it travels through the medium. Amplitude is measured from the baseline to the peak, either in the positive or negative portion of the sine wave. You can also measure peak-to-peak amplitude, whereby you measure the distance from the positive peak to the negative peak. Figure 45-16 shows how amplitude is measured.

Power. Power is the rate at which work is performed or the rate that energy is transferred. The unit is the watt (W). Power is determined by the machine but can be changed by the sonographer. The sonographer can change power by using the output control on the machine's keyboard. Power is about equal to amplitude squared. If amplitude is doubled, then power will increase by four times. If amplitude is halved, then power is reduced to a quarter. Power also decreases as it travels through a medium.

Intensity. Intensity is the concentration of energy within the sound wave over a specified area. The unit for intensity is watts/cm^2. Intensity is

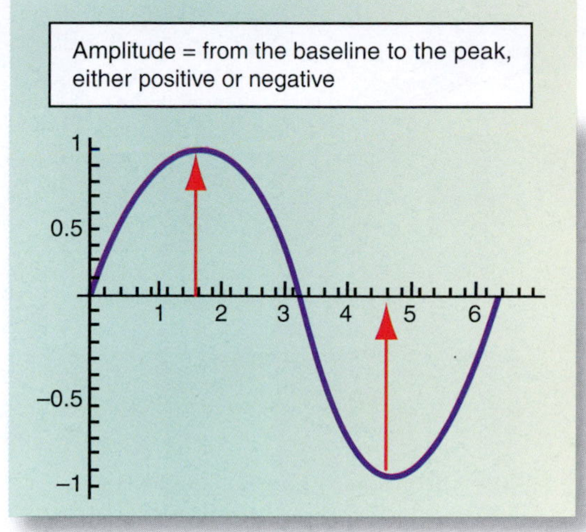

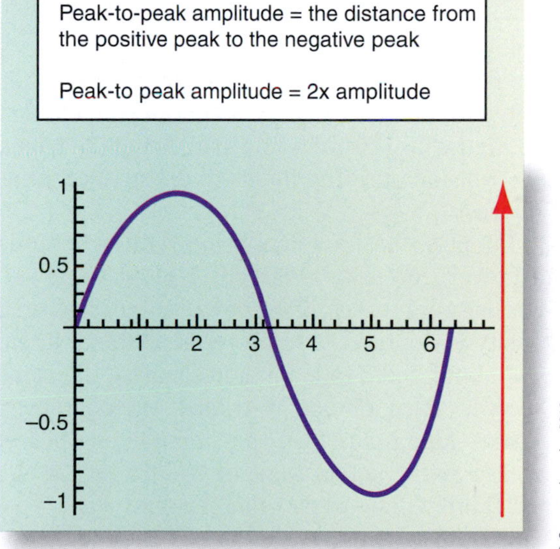

FIGURE 45-16. Amplitude is measured from the baseline to the peak, either in the positive or negative direction. It can also be measured from the positive peak to the negative peak.

determined by the machine and the transducer diameter. The sonographer can change the intensity by adding or decreasing focal zones. Focal zones are used to increase the intensity of the beam to a specific area. Intensity is greatest where the area

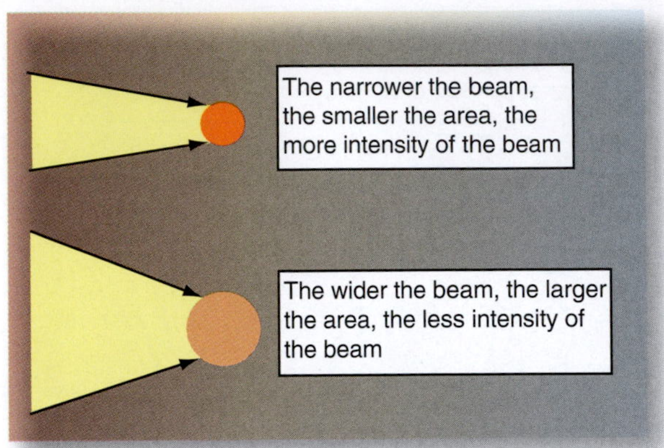

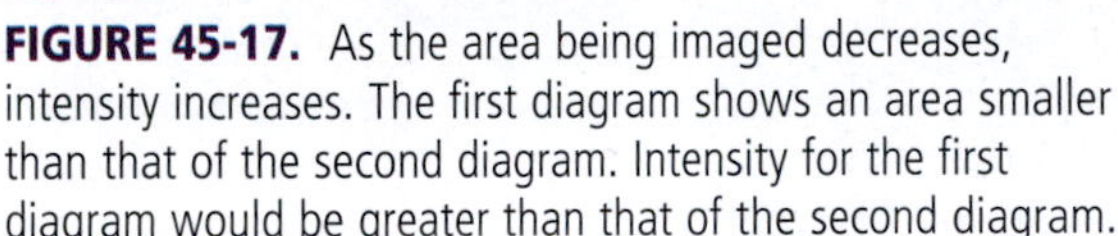

FIGURE 45-17. As the area being imaged decreases, intensity increases. The first diagram shows an area smaller than that of the second diagram. Intensity for the first diagram would be greater than that of the second diagram.

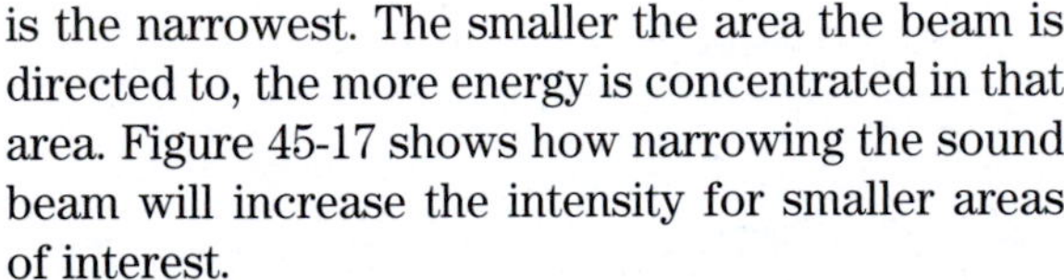

is the narrowest. The smaller the area the beam is directed to, the more energy is concentrated in that area. Figure 45-17 shows how narrowing the sound beam will increase the intensity for smaller areas of interest.

Intensity has a relationship with amplitude and power. Intensity is directly related to power. If intensity increases, then power increases, or if intensity is doubled, then power is doubled. Intensity is about equal to amplitude squared, the same as power. If amplitude is tripled, then intensity increases nine times. Just as amplitude and power decrease as the sound wave travels through a medium, there will be a loss of intensity as well.

Types of Sound Waves

Modern ultrasound machines utilize two different avenues of sending out sound waves. They are continuous waves or pulsed waves. Continuous-wave ultrasound emits more power than pulsed-wave ultrasound and does not create an image. It therefore has very specific usage during diagnostic exams.

Continuous Wave. **Continuous wave** means the sound wave never stops being emitted by the transducer (Figure 45-18). This process requires two crystals/transducers. One crystal is required to produce the sound wave and the other crystal is used to pick up the returning echo. Amplitude and frequency for a continuous wave will always be the same; there is no variation as it is always on. Continuous-wave ultrasound is used in therapeutic (physical therapy) ultrasound. A by product of ultrasound is heat. Continuous wave has the ability to produce heat in tissue, thereby increasing the blood supply to the area, which in turns helps with healing.

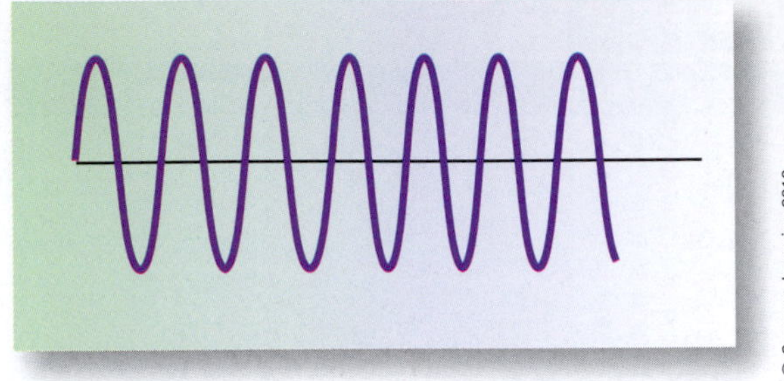

FIGURE 45-18. Continuous-wave ultrasound never stops. It is an endless cycle.

Pulsed Wave. Diagnostic ultrasound machines today utilize **pulsed wave**. Pulsed-wave ultrasound sends out short bursts of sound waves and then stops and waits for the returning echoes (Figure 45-19). It has a beginning and an end. Pulsed wave requires only one crystal (transducer) to operate. The crystal sends out the pulse, stops sending, and then

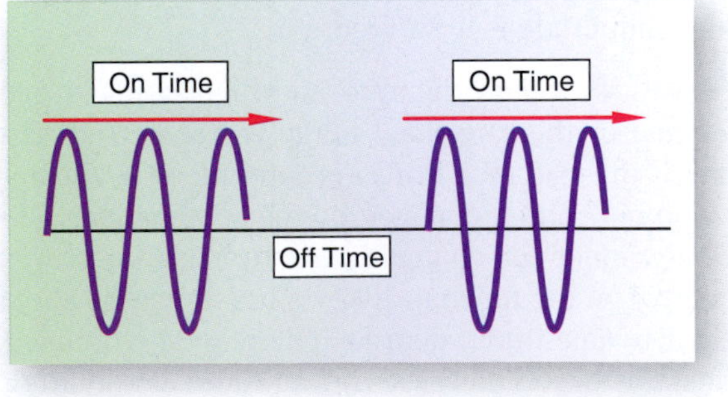

FIGURE 45-19. Pulsed-wave ultrasound has a beginning and an end. One pulse is transmitted, then the pulse is turned off and the transducer listens for the returning echo. Upon its arrival, another pulse is transmitted.

retrieves the returning echo as well. The following are the parameters for pulsed-wave ultrasound.

Pulse repetition frequency (PRF). The **pulsed repetition frequency (PRF)** is the rate at which a pulse is repeated in a given amount of time. The unit used is kHz. In diagnostic ultrasound an average pulse is comprised of two to four cycles (Figure 45-20). PRF is determined by the machine but can be changed by the sonographer. PRF includes the on time and the off time; it is the number of pulses in a given amount of time. This off time could also be referred to as listening time, as the machine is waiting for or listening for the returning echo. Off time is something the sonographer can change by altering depth. If depth is increased, the waiting/listening time is increased, thereby decreasing PRF. If depth is decreased, the waiting/listening time is shortened and PRF will increase. Although PRF can be changed, frequency does not change (Figure 45-21 and 45-22).

Pulse repetition period (PRP). The **pulse repetition period (PRP)** is the time it takes from the beginning of one pulse to the beginning of the next pulse (Figure 45-23). The unit is any increment of time. In ultrasound the microsecond is normally used (μs). Just as period is a reciprocal of frequency, PRP is the reciprocal of PRF. They are inversely related, so if the PRF increases then the PRP will decrease, and the PRP can be found by dividing 1 by the PRF.

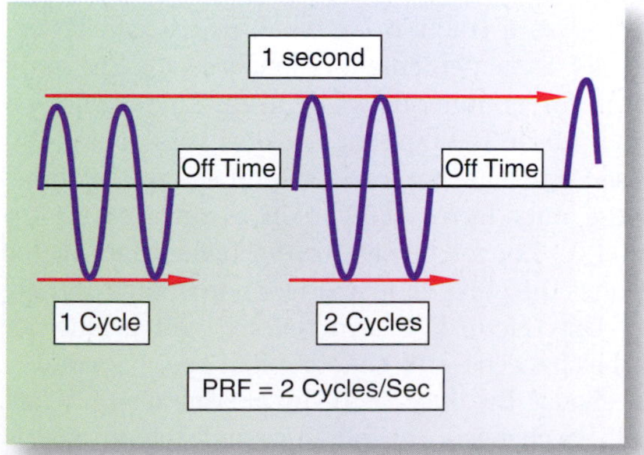

FIGURE 45-20. There are two cycles in a given point in time.

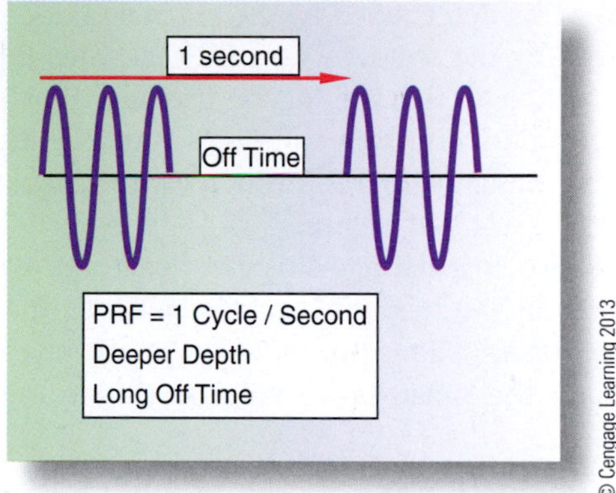

FIGURE 45-21. As image depth increases, it takes longer for the returning echo to arrive. This will increase the off time and decrease PRF.

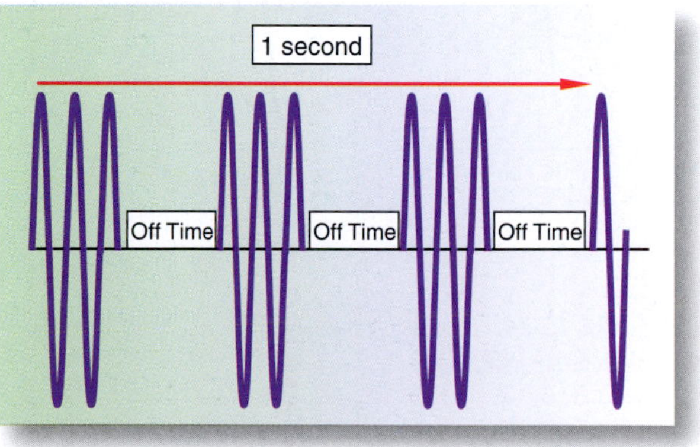

FIGURE 45-22. As image depth decreases, the off time is shortened and the echoes return more quickly. This will increase PRF.

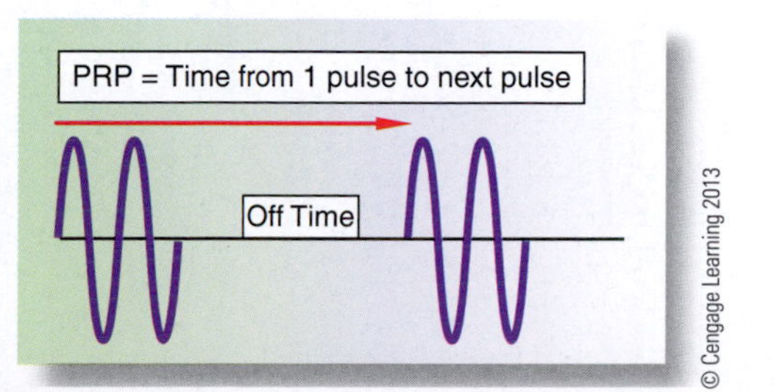

FIGURE 45-23. PRP is determined from the start of the pulse to the beginning of the next pulse. It includes the off time. Increasing or decreasing depth will help to determine PRP.

PRP is determined by the machine but can be changed by the sonographer. PRP includes the off time, which is the waiting or listening time. The sonographer controls this by altering depth, thereby changing the PRF, which then changes PRP (Figures 45-24 and Figure 45-25).

Pulse duration. **Pulse duration** is the time it takes from the beginning of the pulse to the end of the pulse. It does not include the off time, only the time the pulse is actually on (Figure 45-26).

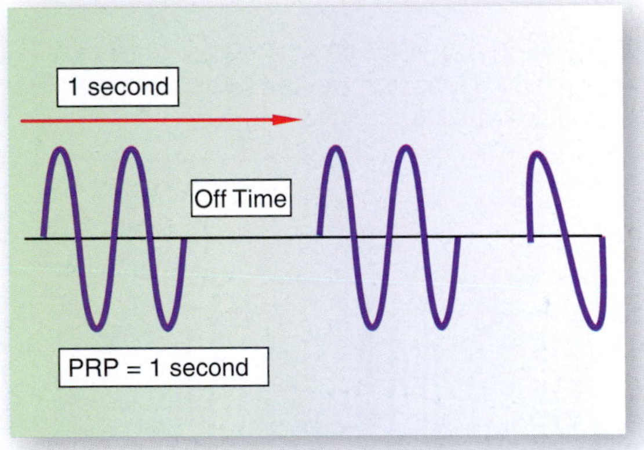

FIGURE 45-24. Increasing depth will increase off time and increase PRP.

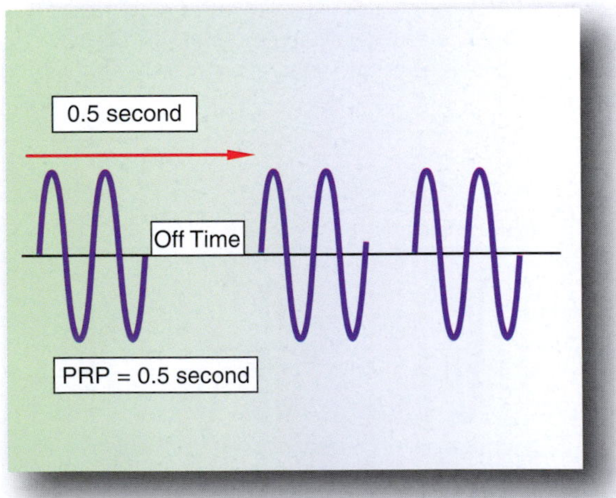

FIGURE 45-25. Decreasing depth will shorten off time and increase PRP.

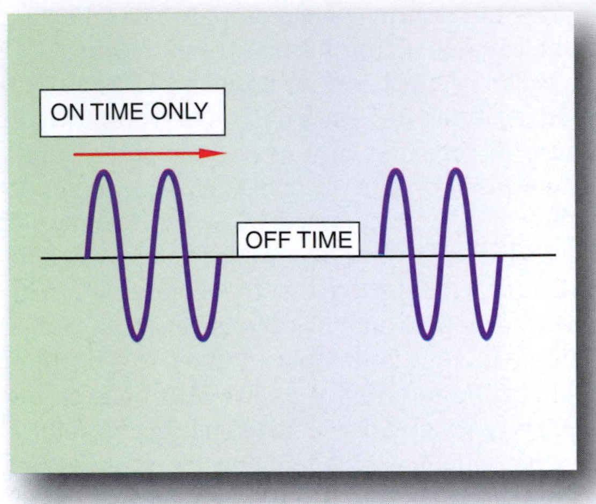

FIGURE 45-26. Pulse duration is the on time only. It does not include off time.

Pulse duration can be determined by multiplying the period by the number of cycles in the pulse. As the period decreases or the number of cycles in a pulse decreases, pulse duration will decrease. Shorter pulses produce better images. To obtain a shorter pulse, use a higher-frequency transducer. Pulse duration is determined by the machine and cannot be changed by the sonograhper. Off time is not included in pulse duration; the sonographer cannot change it by altering depth.

Duty factor. The duty factor is the fraction of time the pulse is on or the percentage of time the pulse is on. It is a unitless number. It can be expressed as a fraction (½ or .25) or it can be expressed as a percentage (25 percent). The duty factor for continuous-wave ultrasound would be either 1.0 or 100 percent because it is always on. Pulsed wave is not on 100 percent of the time, so the duty factor will be in a range of 0.1 up to <1.0. Longer pulses have a higher-duty factor because the pulse is on a longer percentage of time.

Duty factor is determined by the machine but can be changed by the sonographer. The sonographer can change the duty factor by altering depth. When depth is changed, the off time or listening time is changed, thereby changing the on time and ultimately changing the duty factor. Duty factor is inversely related to the PRP and directly related to pulse duration. Increased pulse duration will increase the duty

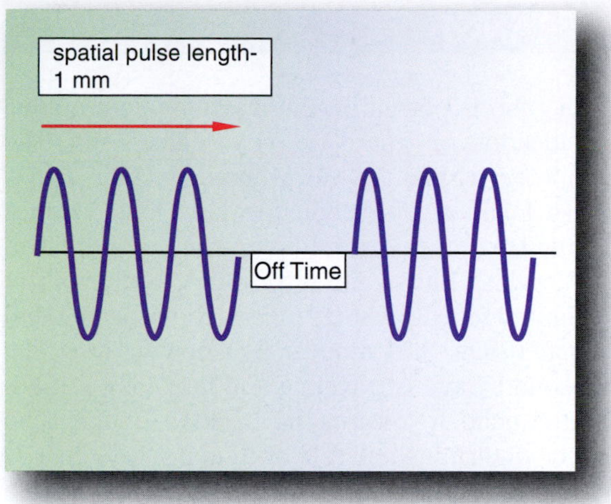

FIGURE 45-27. SPL shows the distance one pulse travels from the beginning of the pulse to the end of the pulse.

factor, which would require a new transducer as the sonographer cannot change duty factor.

Spatial pulse length (SPL). This is the distance from the beginning of the pulse to the end of the pulse. It does not include the off time. The unit would be any increment of length (Figure 45-27). Spatial pulse length is determined by the machine and the medium and cannot be changed by the sonographer. SPL does not include the off time; therefore changing depth will not change it. The spatial pulse length can be determined by multiplying wavelength times the number of cycles in the pulse. It is inversely related to frequency, so if frequency is increased, the SPL will decrease. The shorter the SPL, the better will be the axial resolution. SPL is the main determining factor for axial resolution.

ATTENUATION

Power, intensity, and amplitude all decrease as the sound wave travels through a medium. This reduction is termed *attenuation*. The unit for attenuation is the decibel (dB). Attenuation means a loss of information in the image. Either the returning echoes are so weak they provide very little data or there are no echoes produced at all. Two factors of attenuation are absorption and scatter. Absorption occurs when the sound wave is converted to heat and the energy is then absorbed into the surrounding tissue. Bone absorbs sound. Posterior to bone is an area of black, meaning no information. Scatter attenuates sound by causing the wave to be reflected in many different directions. Air scatters the sound wave. Posterior to a pocket of air are multiple shades of gray, masking what lies beneath. Higher frequencies and longer path lengths cause more attenuation. Increasing frequency or increasing path length will increase attenuation.

Decibels (dB)

The unit for attenuation is the decibel (dB), and a decibel is 1/10 of a Bel. It is a ratio or the relationship between two sound values. Decibels describe the difference between the beginning and end intensity, or how much was lost. The sonographer can change the intensity/power/amplitude of a wave by altering the dBs.

The output or power buttons on the control panel allow the sonographer to alter the amount of power being transmitted into the body. Using the gain or time gain compensation (TGC) buttons will alter the returning echoes. By working with the sound wave, the sonographer can cause a darkening or lightening of the image, depending upon the desired effect.

Attenuation Coefficient

The attenuation coefficient describes how much of the sound wave is lost per centimeter traveled. In soft tissue, attenuation of the beam occurs at a rate of ½ dB per centimeter per MHz used. If frequency is increased, the attenuation coefficient increases. A general rule of thumb for soft tissue is to divide the MHz used by 2 to obtain the attenuation coefficient.

Acoustic Impedance (AI)

Acoustic impedance determines the resistance a material has to the oncoming sound wave. It is related to the acoustic pressure and the speed of the particle vibrations in the sound wave. It is a characteristic of the medium only. The unit is the Rayls (Z) and can be determined by multiplying the speed of sound by the density of the medium. If the propagation speed or density of the medium increases, the acoustic impedance will increase.

As the sound wave travels through a medium, it interacts with a variety of boundaries or interfaces. Each new interface may have a different acoustic impedance depending on the properties of that tissue. If the acoustic impedances of two adjacent tissues are equal and the sound wave hits at a perpendicular angle, the wave will be transmitted, resulting in no reflection (echo). The transmitted intensity will equal the incident (original) intensity. If there is a difference of acoustic impedances and the wave hits the boundary at a perpendicular angle, then reflection may occur. The difference between the acoustic impedance found in the adjacent interfaces will determine the strength of the returning echo. The greater the difference, the higher will be the amplitude of the returning echoes. The higher the amplitude of the returning echo, the brighter the image will be.

Acoustic impedance for soft tissue is about 1.53 Z and the machine is calibrated for soft tissue. Bone is much higher at 7.8 Z and air is 0.0004 Z. When a sound wave interacts with either of these tissues, the resulting image will show bright white due to the great differences of AI compared to soft tissue. There are more subtle differences when imaging soft tissues found within the body. Though they are not huge differences as seen with air and bone, they are still differences. This gives the various shades of gray seen on the image.

In order to have reflection, a difference of acoustic impedance is required, as well as a perpendicular sound wave. Should the sound beam hit an interface at an oblique angle, reflection may or may not occur. In order to produce the best possible image, there must be a difference of acoustic impedances and a perpendicular angle used (Figure 45-28).

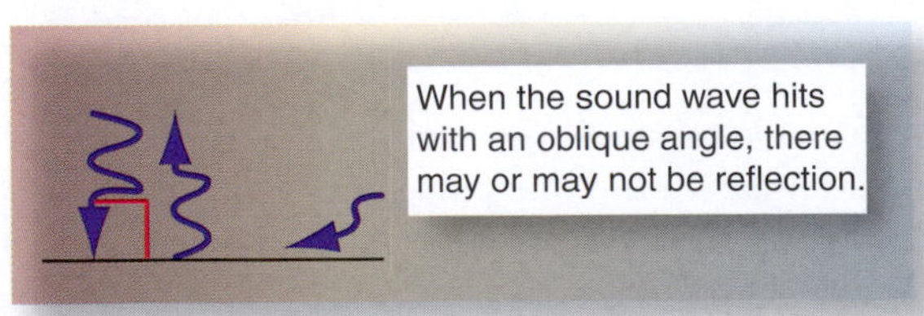

FIGURE 45-28. When an incident wave hits an interface at a perpendicular angle and there is a difference in acoustic impedance, there will be reflection known as an echo.

RANGE

Each echo is placed on the image by determining the location of where the echo came from. The computer within the ultrasound machine determines location by calculating how long it takes for the echo to return to the crystal that produced the original pulse. All ultrasound machines are calibrated for the average propagation speed found in soft tissue, 1.54 mm/µs. By knowing how fast the sound wave is traveling and how long it takes for the echo to return, the location of the echo can be determined. A rule of thumb for diagnostic ultrasound equipment is that it will take 13 µs for a pulse to travel 1 cm deep into the tissue and travel back 1 cm to return to the crystal; total centimeters traveled is 2. If the pulse were to travel 2 cm deep and return to the crystal, it would take 26 µs, and so on.

FIELD

Huygen's Principle explains a sound wave as having the shape of an hourglass. The wave narrows as it moves forward and then widens back out. At the origin, the beam width is equal to the diameter of the transducer. At its narrowest point, the beam width is ½ the original value when an unfocused transducer is being used. From that point it continues to widen as it travels forward and eventually becomes the original width and then travels and widens beyond that.

The area from the origin, or transducer, to the narrowest point is termed the near field. The narrowest area is termed the transition or focal zone. From the transition zone to the point where the beam is once again the original width is termed the far field. The area beyond the far field is of no value in forming an image as the beam becomes too weak. In diagnostic ultrasound, the beam is useful to about 2 near field lengths (NFLs), which is the equivalent of the near field, transition, and far field. The NFL determines how far the beam can be focused. Focal depth is measured from the transducer to the focal zone (Figure 45-29).

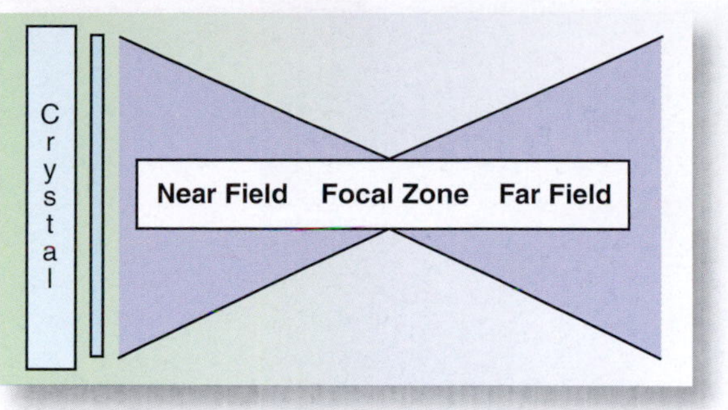

FIGURE 45-29. Huygen's Principle—sound travels in the shape of an hourglass.

DOPPLER

Doppler is used to detect and/or evaluate blood flow. It can be used with continuous wave (CW), pulsed wave (PW), or color flow imaging. In order to implement Doppler, there must be a moving object. When imaging a blood vessel, the moving object being evaluated is the red blood cell (RBC). The incident (original) frequency is transmitted into the body and interacts with an RBC. The reflected wave returns to the transducer at a different frequency. The difference between the incident frequency and the reflected frequency is the Doppler shift. The Doppler shift is the amount of change in the frequencies. It can also be said that the greater the difference in frequencies, the greater the Doppler shift, and the greater the velocity of the RBCs, the greater the Doppler shift.

The Doppler shift is within the 20- to 20,000-Hz range; therefore, it is within the audible range of sound. This allows the sonographer to hear the shift to help differentiate between blood vessels, as each have a unique sound to them. This can be very helpful when performing a carotid Doppler exam and the internal and external carotid arteries need to be identified.

The direction of the moving RBCs will determine if the Doppler shift is positive or negative. If the RBC is coming toward the transducer, the reflected wave will have a higher frequency than the incident (original) frequency and a positive shift will occur. Should the RBC be traveling away from the transducer, the opposite effect will happen and the reflected frequency will be lower than the incident (original) frequency, causing a negative Doppler shift.

A variety of colors may be used to designate a positive or negative Doppler shift. On the display image is a box designating which color is representing flow toward the transducer and flow away from the transducer. The color in the top of the box represents forward or positive flow and the color in the bottom of the box designates flow away from the transducer. This box can be inverted to properly identify vessels. Red traditionally indicates an artery and blue is used for veins, so the color box is set up to reflect this. Figure 45-30 shows an image of the common carotid artery and the internal jugular vein.

Doppler measures velocity as opposed to speed. Velocity is magnitude and direction, whereas speed is magnitude only. Doppler is able to determine the speed at which blood is flowing, as well as the direction it is flowing. This is extremely helpful when diagnosing a stenosis or occlusion within a vessel.

HARMONICS

The sound wave can be manipulated from the traditional sinusoidal wave into a bent shape. These waves are referred to as **harmonics** or sawtooth waves (Figure 45-31). These harmonic waves become stronger as the sine wave becomes less sinusoidal, or more bent. Using these harmonic waves gives a better image quality by doubling the frequency of the transducer without losing penetration. In Figure 45-32 a gallbladder is being imaged using a lower-MHz transducer in order to penetrate to the part. The gallbladder has echoes within it that could be mistaken for pathology. Harmonics is then applied, the resolution or image quality is increased, and the gallbladder is free of the echoes, thereby giving a more accurate viewing of the gallbladder.

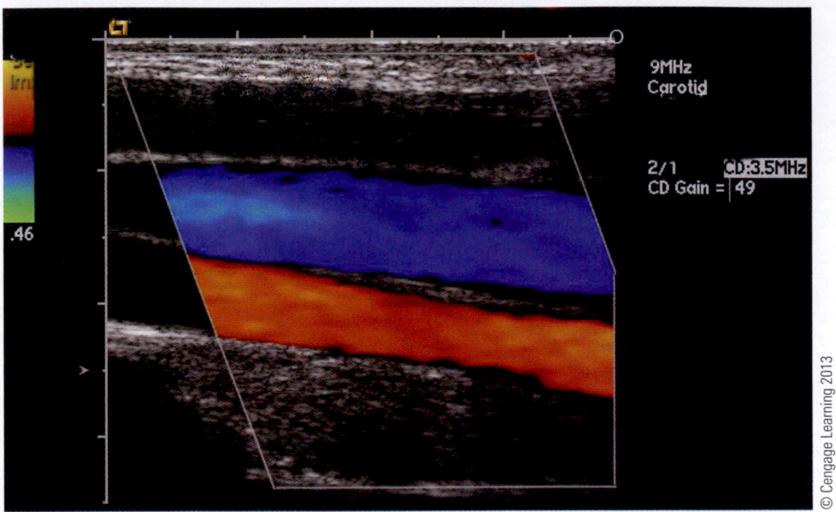

FIGURE 45-30. The red vessel is showing a positive Doppler shift and is flowing toward the transducer. The blue vessel is showing a negative Doppler shift and is flowing away from the transducer.

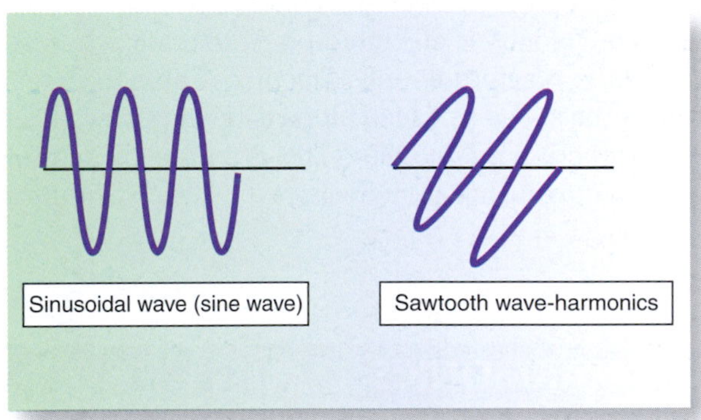

FIGURE 45-31. A typical sinusoidal wave and a sawtooth (bent) wave found when using harmonics.

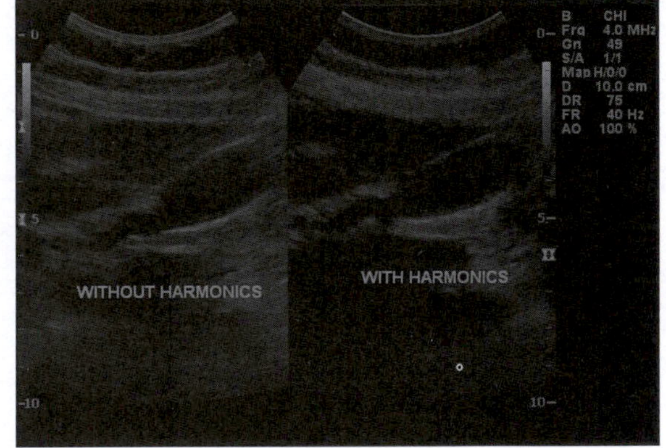

FIGURE 45-32. An image of the gallbladder with and without harmonics. Note how the image of the gallbladder is much blacker and "cleaner" when using harmonics.

TRANSDUCER AND COMPONENTS

Transducer Housing Components

The transducer housing is the actual piece of equipment the sonographer holds in his or her hand to obtain the image. It is what most think of as the transducer or the probe and is what is visibly seen during the course of the exam. Within this housing lie the real transducers and other essential parts (Figure 45-33).

Transducer. A transducer is any device that converts one form of energy into another form of energy. It is also known as the crystal or element. Within the plastic transducer housing are crystals

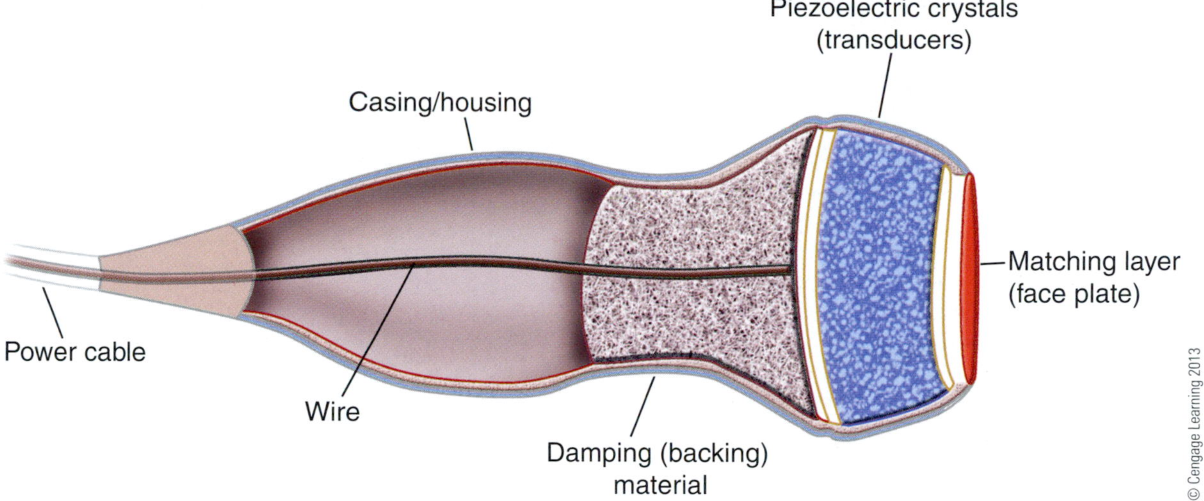

FIGURE 45-33. The components found in the transducer housing.

or ceramics. These crystals are the true transducers used in ultrasound, as they will convert one form on energy into another form.

The crystals or transducers used in ultrasound convert electrical energy into mechanical energy and mechanical energy into electrical energy. This is termed the piezoelectric and reverse **piezoelectric effect**. An electrical voltage is applied to the crystal, which causes the crystal to convert the energy to mechanical energy. The sound wave enters the body, hits an interface, is reflected back to the transducer as an echo (mechanical energy still), and hits the crystal. The crystal then converts the mechanical energy back into electrical energy, which is sent to the machine's computer for the production of the image.

Most crystals used today are man-made and use lead, zirconate and titanate, or PZT. Achieving the piezoelectric and reverse piezoelectric effect requires the crystals to be heated to a very high temperature and then exposed to a magnetic field. Reheating the crystal to the high temperature, once polarization has occurred, will cause the crystal to depolarize and lose the piezoelectric effect. Transducers/crystals cannot be sterilized in an autoclave, as the temperatures are too high and will cause depolarization and render the transducer useless. Cleansing of the probes requires an application of chemical disinfectants.

The crystals are usually spherical in shape and have two flat parallel surfaces. The surfaces are coated with a thin electrode, which serves as the electrical link to and from the crystal.

Damping Material. The damping material is also known as the backing material. It is placed directly behind the crystal. When a pulse is sent out, not all waves travel forward. Some are reflected back to the transducer's surface. The damping material absorbs these unwanted waves and limits the number of pulses in the wave. It will also reduce the amplitude of the wave, which is a disadvantage. Damping material reduces the spatial pulse length, which in turn increases resolution, which is a major benefit. A damped transducer improves axial resolution.

Matching Layer. The matching layer is the face plate. It comes in direct contact with the patient. Behind it, within the housing, are the crystals. The matching layer helps to protect the crystals and acts as an interface between the patient and the crystals. In order to maximize transmission of the sound wave, the matching layer must have a propagation speed close to 1,540 m/s in order for transmission to occur.

Coupling Medium. Between the matching layer and the patient's skin is air. A coupling agent is required between the matching layer and the tissue in order for transmission to occur. In most cases, gel is applied, although water is effective as well. This eliminates the matching plate/air or air/tissue interface. It ensures the transmission of the beam.

Casing/Housing. The casing/housing is the plastic case in which the internal parts are housed. It protects the internal parts of the transducer. It also insulates the patient from electrical shock. If a casing is cracked the transducer should not be used. The manufacturer determines the shape of the transducer, taking into account what it will be used for.

Wire. An electrical charge must be utilized in order to activate the crystals. The wire conveys the electrical charge to the crystal. It also receives the electrical charge of the converted mechanical echo. It then conveys this charge back to the machine to form the image.

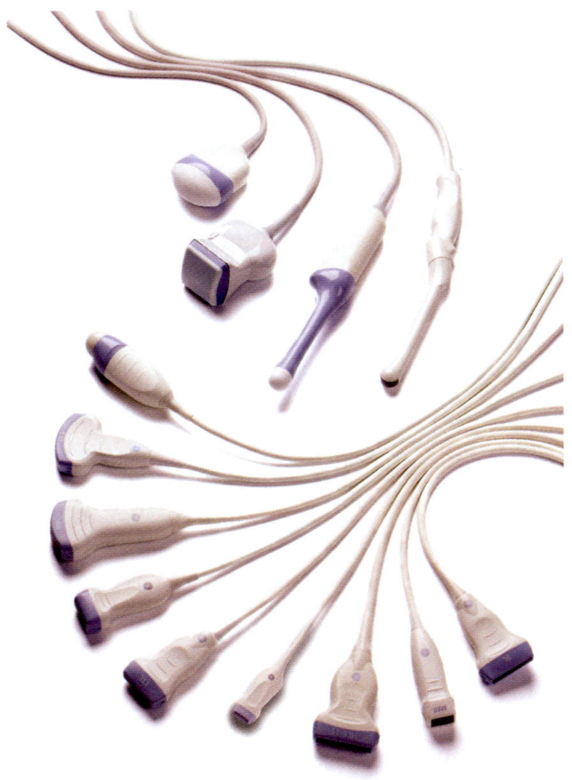

FIGURE 45-34. A variety of transducer probes commonly used in ultrasound imaging. *(Courtesy of GE Healthcare.)*

Types of Transducers

There are a variety of transducers. Each is unique and has a specific diagnostic value. Some are shaped for the organ systems they examine and each has a range of frequencies for the best possible image. The exam type and patient habitus will determine which transducer is used for an exam (Figure 45-34).

Mechanical Transducer. Mechanical transducers can be curved or linear in shape. They have a single circular disc-shaped active element. Curvature of the crystal or adding a lens is what focuses the beam at a specific depth. In order to change a focus, the sonographer must change the scanhead. These scanners give a fan or sector-shaped image, and a defective crystal will destroy the entire image.

Arrays. An array contains a collection of elements (crystals) in a single transducer. Each element is connected to its own electronic circuitry called channels. Scanning of the beam is done electronically. As the scanner sweeps across the part, frames of images are acquired. Types of arrays include linear arrays, phased arrays, convexed arrays, annular phased arrays, and vector arrays. Most transducers in use today are arrays.

Linear array. The elements in a linear array are in a line and are fired sequentially. There is no steering involved. The elements are lined up in a straight line that gives a rectangular-shaped image. The width of the image is approximately equal to the length of the array. It has fixed focusing.

Phased array. Phased array transducers can be focused and steered. The crystals are fired almost simultaneously. They can be fired in different patterns that focus and steer the beam. Electronic curvature focuses the beam. Electronic slope steers the beam. They produce a fan-shaped or sector-shaped image.

Convexed array. The crystals in this array are arranged in a curve. They can be a sequential or phased array. The transducer is usually large with a large footprint. Convexed arrays produce a sector-type image.

Annular phased array. Annular phased arrays contain concentric rings cut from the same circular slab of piezoelectric material. The elements are arranged in an arc. Small-diameter rings have a shorter focus but will diverge quickly. Large rings have a deep focal length. They have electronic focusing in all planes at all depths. They are mechanically steered. An annular phased array produces a fan-or sector-shaped image.

Vector arrays. Vector arrays have groups of elements that are fired together to steer the pulses in various directions. The image format can change from rectangular to sector. The footprint is smaller than the convex and the top of the display is flat. They can be used for linear where the elements are fired in different directions and not straight down. The rectangular display can be changed to a parallelogram or a trapezoidal shape.

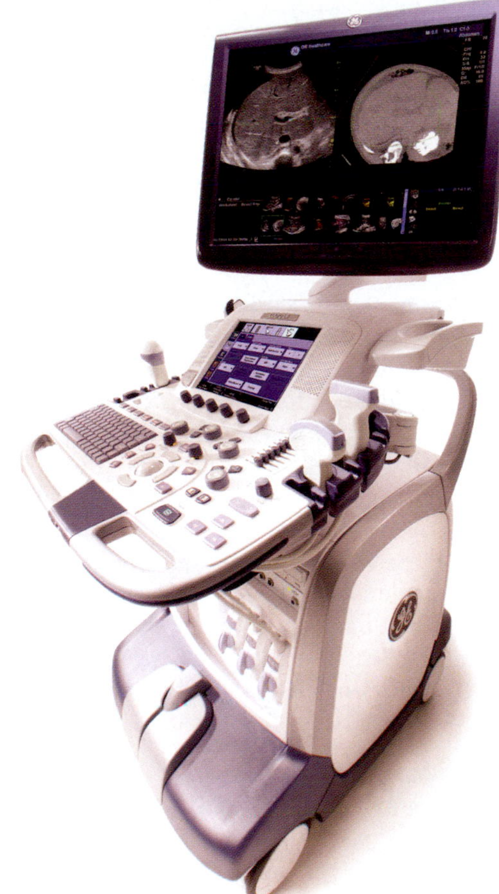

FIGURE 45-35. A typical ultrasound unit. *(Courtesy of GE Healthcare.)*

INSTRUMENTATION

In order for the sonographer to properly image the human body, knowledge of the machine is imperative. By knowing the internal and external components of the ultrasound machine, diagnostic-quality imaging can be performed. Figure 45-35 shows a typical ultrasound machine used in today's sonography department.

Pulser

The pulser produces the electrical signal that excites the crystal into producing the sound wave. It will determine the PRF, PRP, and the pulse amplitude. It also determines the firing sequence for a phased array. The frequency of the voltage applied to the crystal will determine the resonant frequency of the transducer. Each time voltage is applied to the crystal, it produces a pulse. The greater the voltage amplitude, the greater will be the intensity and power in the beam. The sonographer can control the pulser by changing depth and increasing/decreasing power. Components found in the pulser include a clock generator, a high-voltage pulse generator, and the transducer. The clock generator controls the number of voltage pulses, which activates the crystals. It starts the pulse cycle. It sends the timing signals to the pulse generator, TGC (time gain compensation) circuitry, and memory. The high-voltage pulse generator delivers short, high-amplitude signals to the transducer, which receives the voltage generated by the pulser.

Receiver

The returning echoes are converted back into an electrical form by the transducer and the signal then goes to the receiver. The receiver turns these signals into a form to be used in a display unit. Components of the receiver include amplification, compensation, compression, demodulation, and rejection.

Amplification. Amplification is also known as overall gain. This part of the receiver will amplify the weaker voltage signals. The sonographer can change the amplification by increasing/decreasing the overall gain knob. Each signal is treated equally; therefore the entire image is affected. If amplification is increased too much, there will be a loss of axial and lateral resolution. If amplification is decreased too much, there will be a loss of the lower-amplitude echoes, which would mean a loss of information. Overall gain will not produce a uniform image, as it treats all echoes equally. The image will either be bright or the image will be dark; there will be no uniformity to it.

Compensation. Compensation is also known as time gain compensation (TGC). This part of the receiver makes all returning echoes appear the same, regardless of the depth from which they've returned. The sonographer can change compensation by using the TGC pods on the control panel. When a higher-frequency transducer is used, more attenuation occurs; therefore, more compensation is required. The sonographer is able to compensate for the attenuation by applying more amplitude to the weaker signals. Compensation creates a more uniform image.

Compression. Compression reduces the overall total range of the signal from smallest to largest. It reduces the dynamic range of the unit. It keeps the range within the operating range of the machine. The sonographer cannot change it.

Demodulation. Once the receiver obtains the echoes in electrical form, it must change the signal to one suitable for display on a cathode ray tube (CRT). The CRT is a TV monitor. Demodulation is inherent in the machine and cannot be changed by the sonographer. There are two steps in this process, rectification and smoothing. Rectification eliminates the negative signals and turns them into positive signals. Smoothing will even out all the rough edges.

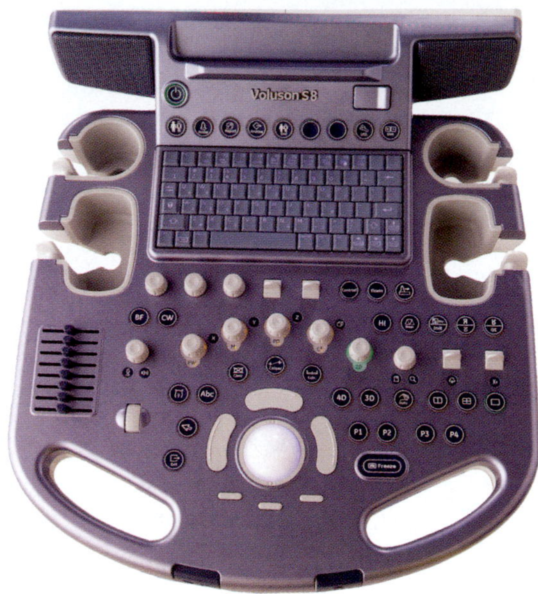

FIGURE 45-36. An instrument panel for an ultrasound unit. *(Courtesy of GE Healthcare.)*

Rejection. Rejection involves eliminating the very-low-level echoes associated with noise. The sonographer can change this by increasing the low-level signals or reducing them. Rejection only affects the low levels. Figure 45-36 shows a typical instrument panel with the control knobs used by the sonographers.

Scan Converter

The scan converter is a device that electronically stores the image. It is a memory component. It accepts data in one format and converts it to another format. It accepts data in the form of electrons (electricity) and then converts the electrons to light. The light is then projected onto the CRT screen. Data is placed on the screen by using a line raster system. Scan converters can also transmit the image via a cable to a remote monitor. This allows viewing of the images at external work stations without having to be physically present in the room. There are two types of scan converter, digital and analog.

Digital Scan Converter. A digital scan converter converts a digital signal into analog. It has a limited range of values and uses solid-state computer components. Shades of gray found in an image are converted to numbers and the numbers are stored in the memory. The numbers can be manipulated and then displayed. Once data is acquired, it can be manipulated in two ways, through preprocessing and/or post-processing. After the data is acquired but before it goes into the scan converter it can undergo preprocessing. This process reduces the area being imaged prior to the storage of the image. After the data is acquired and has been stored in the scan converter but before it is displayed, it can undergo post-processing. An example of post-processing would be magnifying a specific area. Processing of a frozen image is always post-processing.

Analog Scan Converter. The analog scan converter converts an analog signal into digital. It has a wide range of values. It is what originally made grayscale images possible. The picture is divided into a matrix with electrical storage elements found within. Electrons from a CRT strike the dielectric matrix and the charge is stored. These stored charges are then read out for display.

Display

The display component is a device that presents the processed data in a form that is readable. A TV monitor or CRT is normally what is used. It turns electrons into light. Different levels of brightness or shades of gray are possible. There are control knobs to determine the brightness of the display and the contrast. Contrast is the range of weakest to strongest signals. Types of display modes include A-mode, B-mode, M-mode, B-scan, and Real time.

A-mode (Amplitude Mode). A line or dot moves across the screen at a constant rate. The upward deflection off of the baseline is related to the amplitude of the echo. The horizontal path reflects the depth. This mode is not in common use today.

B-mode (Brightness Mode). The returning echoes are seen as dots on a line. Amplitude is determined by the brightness of the dot. Location of the dot determines the depth and which crystal the pulse came from. This mode is used with real-time scanning. It is the process by which images are displayed on current machines.

M-mode (Motion Mode). Motion is displayed as a wavy or moving baseline as motion occurs. M-mode is used when assessing fetal heart tones.

B-scan. This displays echoes along a straight line and is not in use today. The sonographer moved the transducer along a pathway and the echoes were then acquired as static images. B-scan has the advantage of a large field of view (FOV) with good resolution. However, it was time consuming and patient and structural movement were problem.

Real Time. Real time came about to make up for the disadvantages of B-scanning. Real-time scanning uses B-mode and allows the sonographer to view structures in real or current time. This is the current display mode used in ultrasound today. It can image moving structures and is capable of Doppler. Anatomic structures display on the monitor as two-dimensional images. When a sonographer wishes to acquire an image, the image frame on the monitor can be frozen and stored. Through software, the two-dimensional acquired images can be rendered into three-dimensional images, although this is time consuming. Some state-of-the art equipment is capable of taking three-dimensional imaging in real time. This is known as 4-D imaging, with time as the fourth dimension.

Storage Media

Once an image has been acquired, the sonographer has the capability to store the image as a hard copy on such media as paper, film, videotape, magnetic discs, or CDs. Today, most images are stored through a picture archiving and communications system (PACS) so they can easily be sent to the physician for interpretation.

SUMMARY

Diagnostic medical sonography is a vital component in the diagnostic field. By utilizing sound waves, physicians are able to diagnose pathologies and abnormalities quickly and efficiently. Ultrasound utilizes two planes, longitudinal and transverse, when scanning a patient. As with other modalities, the two fields are required in order to determine location and size of an area of interest. Sound waves move forward and then back again rhythmically as they travel. A simple sine wave can be used to describe this movement. The forward movement is termed compression and the backward movement is termed rarefaction. Variables of sound include pressure, tissue density, particle vibration, and temperature. Parameters of sound waves include frequency, period, wavelength, propagation speed, amplitude, power, and intensity. Power, intensity, and amplitude all decrease as the sound wave travels through a medium. This reduction is termed attenuation. The unit is the decibel (dB).

Transducers are devices that convert one form of energy to another. The ultrasound transducer receives the sound wave and converts it to electrical energy. There are two types of transducers, mechanical and array. The instrumentation in a diagnostic ultrasound machine includes a pulser, a receiver, a scan converter, and image display and storage. ■

REVIEW QUESTIONS

1. A 5-MHz sound wave is transmitted into the body. As it travels, it passes through fat, liver, and muscle. What will the frequency be for the returning echo?
2. A sound wave is transmitted into the body and interacts in liver tissue and then in muscle tissue. It hits these boundaries with a perpendicular incidence. Will there be reflection?
3. How many decibels would it take to reduce 100 percent intensity by 87.5 percent?
4. What would happen if an ultrasound transducer were sterilized in an autoclave?
5. Does Doppler shift measure speed?
6. Are the crystals in phased array transducers fired simultaneously?
7. In order to reduce exposure to a patient, what should the sonographer do with the overall gain and power?
8. What device stores the image for display?
9. What mode of ultrasound is used in real-time imaging?
10. During the course of an exam, the sonographer turns harmonics on to image the gall bladder. A 4-MHz transducer is being used. What will the frequency be for the harmonic image being produced?

REFERENCES AND RECOMMENDED READINGS

Edelman, S. K. (2007). *Understanding ultrasound physics* (3rd ed.). Woodlands, TX: ESP, Inc.

Hedrick, W. R., Hykes, D. L., Starchman, D. E. (2005). *Ultrasound physics and instrumentation* (4th ed.). St. Louis, MO: Elsevier Mosby.

Kremkau, F. W. (2006). *Diagnostic ultrasound principles and instruments* (7th ed.). St. Louis, MO: Saunders Elsevier.

Miele, F. R. (2006). *Ultrasound physics and instrumentation* (4th ed.). Forney, TX: Pegasus Lectures.

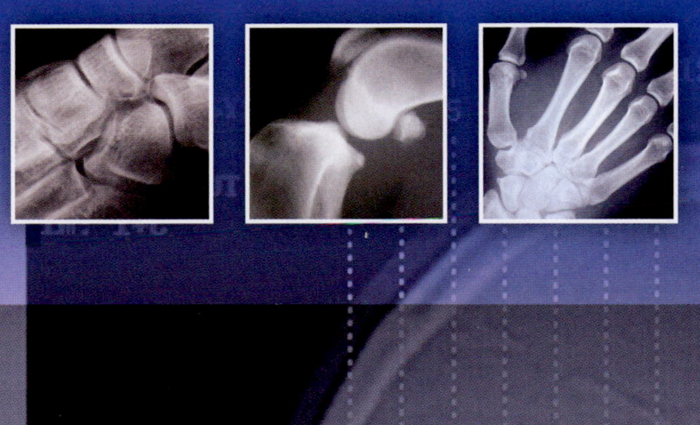

Appendix A On a New Kind of Rays* by W. C. Röntgen

(1) A discharge from a large induction coil is passed through a Hittorf's vacuum tube, or through a well-exhausted Crookes' or Lenard's tube. The tube is surrounded by a fairly close-fitting shield of black paper; it is then possible to see, in a completely darkened room, that paper covered on one side with barium platinocyanide lights up with brilliant fluorescence when brought into the neighbourhood of the tube, whether the painted side or the other be turned towards the tube. The fluorescence is still visible at two metres distance. It is easy to show that the origin of the fluorescence lies within the vacuum tube.

(2) It is seen, therefore, that some agent is capable of penetrating black cardboard which is quite opaque to ultra-violet light, sunlight, or arc-light. It is therefore of interest to investigate how far other bodies can be penetrated by the same agent. It is readily shown that all bodies possess this same transparency, but in very varying degrees. For example, paper is very transparent; the fluorescent screen will light up when placed behind a book of a thousand pages; printer's ink offers no marked resistance. Similarly the fluorescence shows behind two packs of cards; a single card does not visibly diminish the brilliancy of the light. So, again, a single thickness of tinfoil hardly casts a shadow on the screen; several have to be superposed to produce a marked effect. Thick blocks of wood are still transparent. Boards of pine two or three centimetres thick absorb only very little. A piece of sheet aluminium, 15 mm. thick, still allowed the x-rays (as I will call the rays, for the sake of brevity) to pass, but greatly reduced the fluorescence. Glass plates of similar thickness behave similarly; lead glass is, however, much more opaque than glass free from lead. Ebonite several centimetres thick is transparent. If the hand be held before the fluorescent screen, the shadow shows the bones darkly, with only faint outlines of the surrounding tissues.

Water and several other fluids are very transparent. Hydrogen is not markedly more permeable than air. Plates of copper, silver, lead, gold, and platinum also allow the rays to pass, but only when the metal is thin. Platinum .2 mm. thick allows some rays to pass; silver and copper are more transparent. Lead 1.5 mm. thick is practically opaque. If a square rod of wood 20 mm. in the side be painted on one face with white lead, it casts little shadow when it is so turned that the painted face is parallel to the x-rays, but a strong shadow if the rays have to pass through the painted side. The salts of the metals, either solid or in solution, behave generally as the metals themselves.

(3) The preceding experiments lead to the conclusion that the density of the bodies is the property whose variation mainly affects their permeability. At least no other property seems so marked in

*This article was reprinted from Nature, No. 1369, Vol. 53, January 23, 1896. By W. C. Röntgen. Translated by Arthur Stanton from the *Sitsungsberichte der Würsburger Physikmedic. Gesellschaft*, 1895.

this connection. But that the density alone does not determine the transparency is shown by an experiment wherein plates of similar thickness of Iceland spar, glass, aluminium, and quartz were employed as screens. Then the Iceland spar showed itself much less transparent than the other bodies, though of approximately the same density. I have not remarked any strong fluorescence of Iceland spar compared with glass (see below, No. 4).

(4) Increasing thickness increases the hindrance offered to the rays by all bodies. A picture has been impressed on a photographic plate of a number of superposed layers of tinfoil, like steps, presenting thus a regularly increasing thickness. This is to be submitted to photometric processes when a suitable instrument is available.

(5) Pieces of platinum, lead, zinc, and aluminium foil were so arranged as to produce the same weakening of the effect. The annexed table shows the relative thickness and density of the equivalent sheets of metal.

	Thickness	Relative Thickness	Density
platinum	.08 mm	1	21.5
lead	.050 "	3	11.3
zinc	.100 "	6	7.1
aluminum	3.500 "	200	2.6

From these values it is clear that in no case can we obtain the transparency of a body from the product of its density and thickness. The transparency increases much more rapidly than the product decreases.

(6) The fluorescence of barium platinocyanide is not the only noticeable action of the x-rays. It is to be observed that other bodies exhibit fluorescence, e.g. calcium sulphide, uranium glass, Iceland spar, rock-salt, etc.

Of special interest in this connection is the fact that photographic dry plates are sensitive to the x-rays. It is thus possible to exhibit the phenomena so as to exclude the danger of error. I have thus confirmed many observations originally made by eye observation with the fluorescent screen. Here the power of the x-rays to pass through wood or cardboard becomes useful. The photographic plate can be exposed to the action without removal of the shutter of the dark slide or other protecting case, so that the experiment need not be conducted in darkness. Manifestly, unexposed plates must not be left in their box near the vacuum tube.

It seems now questionable whether the impression on the plate is a direct effect of the x-rays, or a secondary result induced by the fluorescence of the material of the plate. Films can receive the impression as well as ordinary dry plates.

I have not been able to show experimentally that the x-rays give rise to any calorific effects. These, however, may be assumed, for the phenomena of fluorescence show that the x-rays are capable of transformation. It is also certain that all the x-rays falling on a body do not leave it as such.

The retina of the eye is quite insensitive to these rays: the eye placed close to the apparatus sees nothing. It is clear from the experiments that this is not due to want of permeability on the part of the structures of the eye.

(7) After my experiments on the transparency of increasing thicknesses of different media, I proceeded to investigate whether the x-rays could be deflected by a prism. Investigations with water and carbon bisulphide on mica prisms of 30° showed no deviation either on the photographic or the fluorescent plate. For comparison, light rays were allowed to fall on the prism as the apparatus was set up for the experiment. They were deviated 10 mm. and 20 mm. respectively in the case of the two prisms.

With prisms of ebonite and aluminium, I have obtained images on the photographic plate, which point to a possible deviation. It is, however, uncertain, and at most would point to a refractive index 1.05. No deviation can be observed by means of the fluorescent screen. Investigations with the heavier metals have not as yet led to any result, because of their small transparency and the consequent enfeebling of the transmitted rays.

On account of the importance of the question it is desirable to try in other ways whether the x-rays are susceptible of refraction. Finely powdered bodies allow in thick layers but little of the incident light to pass through, in consequence of refraction and reflection. In the case of the x-rays, however, such layers of powder are for equal masses of substance equally transparent with the coherent solid itself. Hence we cannot conclude any regular reflection or refraction of the x-rays. The research was conducted by the aid of finely-powdered rock-salt, fine electrolytic silver powder, and zinc dust already many times employed in chemical work. In all these cases the result, whether by the fluorescent screen or the photographic method, indicated no difference in transparency between the powder and the coherent solid.

It is, hence, obvious that lenses cannot be looked upon as capable of concentrating the x-rays; in effect, both an ebonite and a glass lens of large size prove to be without action. The shadow photograph of a round rod is darker in the middle than at the edge; the image of a cylinder filled with a body more transparent than its walls exhibits the middle brighter than the edge.

(8) The preceding experiments, and others which I pass over, point to the rays being incapable of regular reflection. It is, however, well to detail an observation which at first sight seemed to lead to an opposite conclusion.

I exposed a plate, protected by a black paper sheath, to the x-rays, so that the glass side lay next to the vacuum tube. The sensitive film was partly covered with star-shaped pieces of platinum, lead, zinc, and aluminium. On the developed negative the star-shaped impression showed dark under platinum, lead, and more markedly, under zinc; the aluminium gave no image. It seems, therefore, that these three metals can reflect the x-rays; as, however, another explanation is possible, I repeated the experiment with this only difference, that a film of thin aluminium foil was interposed between the sensitive film and the metal stars. Such an aluminium plate is opaque to ultra-violet rays, but transparent to x-rays. In the result the images appeared as before, this pointing still to the existence of reflection at metal surfaces.

If one considers this observation in connection with others, namely, on the transparency of powders, and on the state of the surface not being effective in altering the passage of the x-rays through a body, it leads to the probable conclusion that regular reflection does not exist, but that bodies behave to the x-rays as turbid media to light.

Since I have obtained no evidence of refraction at the surface of different media, it seems probable that the x-rays move with the same velocity in all bodies, and in a medium which penetrates everything, and in which the molecules of bodies are embedded. The molecules obstruct the x-rays, the more effectively as the density of the body concerned is greater.

(9) It seemed possible that the geometrical arrangement of the molecules might affect the action of a body upon the x-rays, so that, for example, Iceland spar might exhibit different phenomena according to the relation of the surface of the plate to the axis of the crystal. Experiments with quartz and Iceland spar on this point lead to a negative result.

(10) It is known that Lenard, in his investigations on kathode rays, has shown that they belong to the ether, and can pass through all bodies. Concerning the x-rays the same may be said.

In his latest work, Lenard has investigated the absorption coefficients of various bodies for the kathode rays, including air at atmospheric pressure, which gives 4.10, 3.40, 3.10 for 1 cm., according to the degree of exhaustion of the gas in discharge tube. To judge from the nature of the discharge, I have worked at about the same pressure, but occasionally at greater or smaller pressures. I find, using a Weber's photometer, that the intensity of the fluorescent light varies nearly as the inverse square of the distance between screen and discharge tube. This result is obtained from three very consistent sets of observations at distances of 100 and 200 mm. Hence air absorbs the x-rays much less than the kathode rays. This result is in complete agreement with the previously described result, that the fluorescence of the screen can be still observed at 2 metres from the vacuum tube. In general, other bodies behave like air; they are more transparent for the x-rays than for the kathode rays.

(11) A further distinction, and a noteworthy one, results from the action of a magnet. I have not succeeded in observing any deviation of the x-rays even in very strong magnetic fields.

The deviation of kathode rays by the magnet is one of their peculiar characteristics; it has been observed by Hertz and Lenard, that several kinds of kathode rays exist, which differ by their power of exciting phosphorescence, their susceptibility of absorption, and their deviation by the magnet; but a notable deviation has been observed in all cases which have yet been investigated, and I think that such deviation affords a characteristic not to be set aside lightly.

(12) As the result of many researches, it appears that the place of most brilliant phosphorescence of the walls of the discharge-tube is the chief seat whence the x-rays originate and spread in all directions; that is, the x-rays proceed from the front where the kathode rays strike the glass. If one deviates the kathode rays within the tube by means of a magnet, it is seen that the x-rays proceed from a new point, *i.e.* again from the end of the kathode rays.

Also for this reason the x-rays, which are not deflected by a magnet, cannot be regarded as kathode rays which have passed through the glass, for that passage cannot, according to Lenard, be the cause of the different deflection of the rays. Hence I conclude that the x-rays are not identical with the kathode rays, but are produced from the kathode rays at the glass surface of the tube.

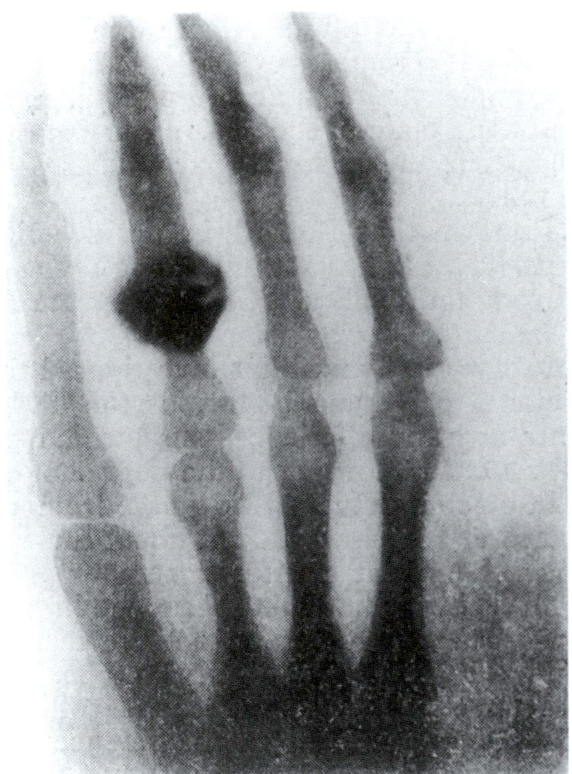

FIGURE A-1. Photograph of the bones in the fingers of a living human hand. The third finger has a ring upon it. *(Courtesy of the American College of Radiology.)*

(13) The rays are generated not only in glass. I have obtained them in an apparatus closed by an aluminium plate 2 mm. thick. I purpose later to investigate the behaviour of other substances.

(14) The justification of the term "rays," applied to the phenomena, lies partly in the regular shadow pictures produced by the interposition of a more or less permeable body between the source and a photographic plate or fluorescent screen.

I have observed and photographed many such shadow pictures. Thus, I have an outline of part of a door covered with lead paint; the image was produced by placing the discharge-tube on one side of the door, and the sensitive plate on the other. I have also a shadow of the bones of the hand (Figure A-1), of a wire wound upon a bobbin, of a set of weights in a box, of a compass card and needle completely enclosed in a metal case (Figure A-2), of a piece of metal where the x-rays show the want of homogeneity, and of other things.

For the rectilinear propagation of the rays, I have a pin-hole photograph of the discharge apparatus covered with black paper. It is faint but unmistakable.

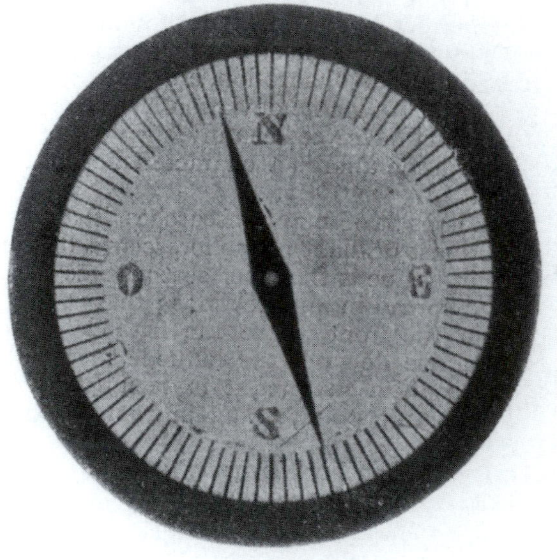

FIGURE A-2. Photograph of a compass card and needle completely enclosed in a metal case.

(15) I have sought for interference effects of the x-rays, but possibly, in consequence of their small intensity, without result.

(16) Researches to investigate whether electrostatic forces act on the x-rays are begun but not yet concluded.

(17) If one asks, what then are these x-rays; since they are not kathode rays, one might suppose, from their power of exciting fluorescence and chemical action, them to be due to ultra-violet light. In opposition to this view a weighty set of considerations presents itself. If x-rays be indeed ultra-violet light, then that light must possess the following properties.

(a) It is not refracted in passing from air into water, carbon bisulphide, aluminium, rock-salt, glass or zinc.

(b) It is incapable of regular reflection at the surfaces of the above bodies.

(c) It cannot be polarised by any ordinary polarising media.

(d) The absorption by various bodies must depend chiefly on their density.

That is to say, these ultra-violet rays must behave quite differently from the visible, infrared, and hitherto known ultra-violet rays.

These things appear so unlikely that I have sought for another hypothesis.

A kind of relationship between the new rays and light rays appears to exist; at least the formation of shadows, fluorescence, and the production of chemical action point in this direction. Now it has been known for a long time, that besides the transverse vibrations which account for the phenomena of light, it is possible that longitudinal vibrations should exist in the ether, and, according to the view of some physicists, must exist. It is granted that their existence has not yet been made clear, and their properties are not experimentally demonstrated. Should not the new rays be ascribed to longitudinal waves in the ether?

I must confess that I have in the course of this research made myself more and more familiar with this thought, and venture to put the opinion forward, while I am quite conscious that the hypothesis advanced still requires a more solid foundation.

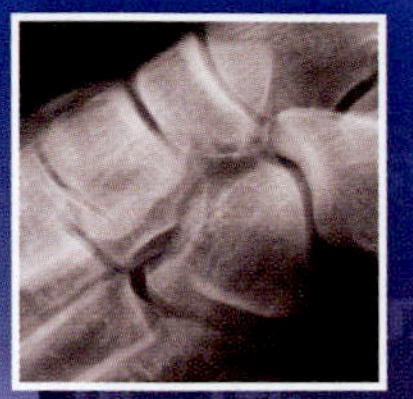
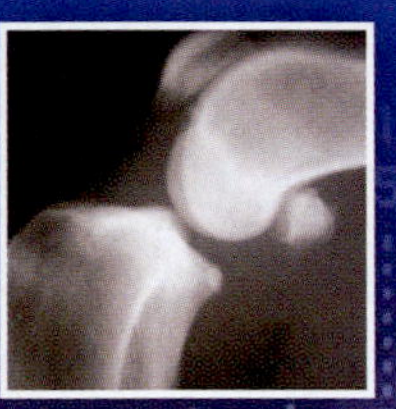
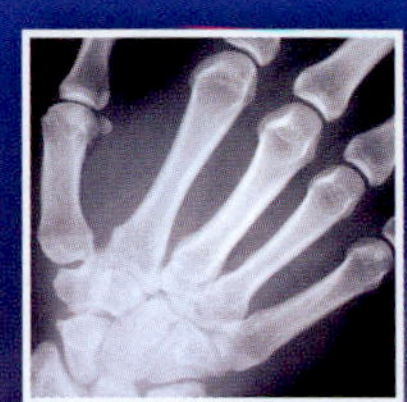

Appendix B *Answers to Case Studies*

THE CASE OF THE MYSTERIOUS MAMMALS

Chapter 1, p. 19
Bats

THE CASE OF THE UNIDENTIFIED FLYING OBJECT IN THE SKULL

Chapter 5, p. 107
This patient was shot in the left temporal region by an arrow. The shaft was broken off prior to the time the radiograph was taken.

THE CASE OF LUMPY

Chapter 11, p. 190
Theodore Bear

THE CASE OF THE MISSING LOWER PELVIS

Chapter 14, p. 232
This patient is quite obese and the large volume of soft tissue that has fallen down over the pelvis is demonstrated with an appropriate density. However, these technical factors produce much too much density for the pelvis. A second radiograph to demonstrate the pelvis, shown here, fails to demonstrate the abdomen. A case of "You can't have your cake and eat it too."

THE CASE OF THE INJURED ANIMAL

Chapter 16, p. 245
This is a rodent, a muskrat. The cause of death was a severed thoracic vertebral column, the result of being caught in a trap in the Ohio woods.

THE CASE OF THE WHITE SNAKES

Chapter 18, p. 272
The radiographer failed to observe that the high-voltage cables were within the primary beam field. Observe the sheath of grounding net inside the upper cable.

THE CASE OF THE COLON IN THE SPIDER'S WEB

Chapter 20, p. 293
This patient was unable to hold the barium within the colon and the sheet has become barium soaked. The wrinkled sheet is dense enough to make a distinct image under the patient.

THE CASE OF THE ANIMAL WITH THE LARGE CALCIFIED TUMOR-LIKE MASS

Chapter 27, p. 423
A chicken's egg about to be laid

THE CASE OF THE LINE IN THE STOMACH

Chapter 29, p. 457
The stomach is half filled with liquid barium. The line is an air-fluid level between the air and barium.

THE CASE OF THE DEEP SEA RODEO

Chapter 31, p. 484
A seahorse

THE CASE OF THE DRIPPING FILM

Chapter 34, p. 520
The horizontal lines are pi lines, so called because they are spaced apart by pi times the diameter of the first film processing roller. They are caused when developer precipitates onto the top rollers at the level of the chemistry when left in the tank overnight. When the first film is processed, the precipitate is deposited on the film emulsion each time the roller turns. The drip marks are most likely from developer solution that was splattered onto the film while it was being held vertically before processing.

THE CASE OF THE LAST DINNER

Chapter 36, p. 547
There are no skeletal remains of the snake's last dinner on this image, but it's good practice to always examine your radiographs with careful attention to detail; the last dinner could have been demonstrated if it had been eaten more recently.

THE CASE OF THE GHOSTLY PLANTS

Chapter 37, p. 560
A peony

THE CASE OF THE MYSTERIOUS MAMMAL

Chapter 39, p. 603
Loggerhead turtle *(Caretta, caretta)*

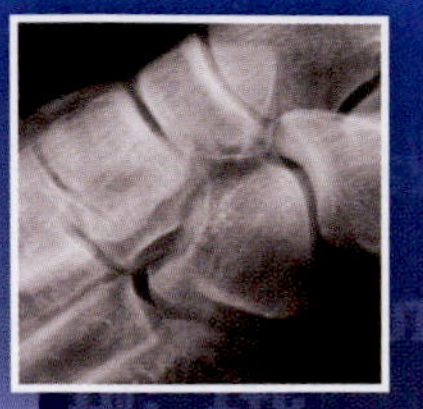
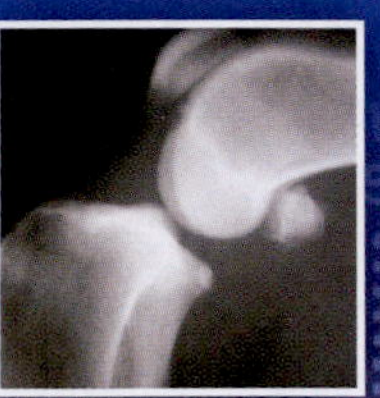
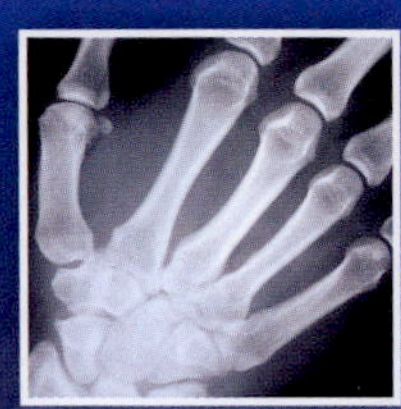

Appendix C *Epigraph Sources and Credits*

Chapter 1 attributed to Albert Einstein

Chapters 2, 3, 7, 8, 9, and 34 from Otto Glasser, *Dr. W. C. Röntgen*, 2nd edition, 1972. Courtesy of Charles C Thomas, Publisher, Springfield, Illinois.

Chapters 4 and 29 from *The Magic Mountain (Der Zauberberg)* by Thomas Mann, originally published by S. Fischer Verlag, Berlin, 1924; translated from the German by H. T. Lowe-Porter, New York: Alfred A. Knopf, 1965.

Chapter 5 by permission from "One More Time," copyright, Patricia Goedicke.

Chapters 6, 13, and 27 from W. D. Coolidge, "Experiences with the Roentgen-Ray Tube," *American Journal of Roentgenology, 54*, 6, 1945.

Chapter 10 by permission, copyright Celia Gilbert, "X-Ray" from *Queen of Darkness*, Viking Press, New York, NY, 1977.

Chapters 11, 26, and 30 from E. C. Jerman, "An Analysis of the End-Result: The Radiograph," *Radiology, 6*, 59–62, 1926.

Chapter 12 from A. H. Compton in the preface to the first edition of *X-Rays and Electrons*, reprinted in *X-Rays in Theory and Experiment*, by A. H. Compton and H. K. Allison, 2nd edition, New York: Van Nostrand and Company, 1935.

Chapter 14 by Lawrence K. Russell, *Life*, March 12, 1896.

Chapter 15 lyrics from the song "X-Ray Vision" from the Capitol-EMI album *Mystery Ticket*, by Moon Martin, Pete Sinfield, and Terry Taylor, copyright 1982, Paper Music, Ltd.

Chapter 16 from William Carlos Williams, *The Autobiography of William Carlos Williams*, copyright 1951, William Carlos Williams. Reprinted by permission of New Directions Publishing Corporation.

Chapter 17 lyrics from the song "I'm Looking through You" from the Capitol-EMI Records, Inc. album, *Rubber Soul*, by John Lennon and Paul McCartney, Northern Songs, Ltd., copyright 1965, EMI Records, Inc.

Chapter 18 from Hollis E. Potter, "The Bucky Diaphragm Principle Applied to Roentgenography," *The American Journal of Roentgenology, 7*, 292–295, 1920.

Chapter 19 quoted from the Jerman Memorial Lecture given by Arthur W. Fuchs during the 1950 Annual Meeting of the American Society of X-Ray Technicians in Cincinnati, Ohio.

Chapter 20 reprinted by permission of Margaret Atwood, from *Selected Poems I*, published by Houghton Mifflin, U.S.A and *Selected Poems 1966–1984*, published by McClelland and Stewart, Canada, copyright 1968.

Chapter 21 reprinted by permission of the estate of Howard Moss from "In The X-Ray Room" from *New Selected Poems*, Antheneum Press, copyright MacMillan Publishing Company, 1985.

Chapter 22 as quoted from *Pall Mall Gazette*, March, 1986 by Arthur W. Fuchs in "Radiography of 1896," Image 9: 4–17, 1960.

Chapter 23 from William Shakespeare, Sonnet XXIV.

Chapter 24 attributed to Oscar Wilde.

Chapter 25 from Gerhart S. Schwarz, *Unit-Step Radiography*, 1961. Courtesy of Charles C Thomas, Publisher, Springfield, Illinois.

Chapter 28 quoted from Merrill C. Sosman.

Chapter 31 William B. Hendee and Raymond P. Rossi in *Quality Assurance for Radiographic X-Ray Units and Associated Equipment*, Rockville, MD: U.S. Department of Health, Education, and

Welfare, Public Health Service, Food and Drug Administration, Bureau of Radiological Health, HEW Publication FDA 79–8094, 1979.

Chapter 32 from Arthur W. Fuchs in the Preface to *Principles of Radiographic Exposure and Processing*, 1st edition, 1949. Charles C Thomas, Publisher, Springfield, Illinois.

Chapter 33 from the text of the chapter.

Chapter 35 from William Shakespeare, *Hamlet*, III, iv, 18.

Chapter 36 Arthur W. Fuchs, "Edison and Roentgenology," *The American Journal of Roentgenology and Radium Therapy*, *57*, (2), 145–156, 1947.

Chapter 37 from French patent 536464, June 3, 1921 by Andre-Edmund-Marie-Bocage, entitled "Method of, and Apparatus for, Radiography on a Moving Plate," as quoted by J. T. Littleton in *Tomography: Physical Principles and Clinical Applications*. Section 17: Golden's Diagnostic Radiology Series. Baltimore, MD: Williams & Wilkins, 1976.

Chapter 38 attributed to Hippocrates.

Chapter 39 attributed to Francois Rabelais

Chapter 40 from Margaret Hoing (The First Lady of Radiologic Technology) in *A History of the American Society of X-Ray Technicians*, Chicago: American Society of Radiologic Technologists, 1952.

Chapter 41 quoted from Allan Cormack, upon being informed that he and Godfrey Hounsfield were to share the 1979 Nobel Prize for Medicine for the invention of computed tomography.

Chapter 42 from Edward M. Purcell, "Research in Nuclear Magnetism," *Nobel Lectures: Physics 1901–1995*, New York: World Scientific Publishing, 1998.

Chapter 43 by permission from Voetz G and Petersen D. (1995) Tracer Studies at Los Alamos and the Birth of Nuclear Medicine. Los Alamos Science. 23: 257–279.

Chapter 44 attributed to Christopher Reeve.

Chapter 45 from Paul Chatfield (aka Horace Smith) as given at www.giga-usa.com/quotes/topics/echo_t001.htm (retrieved March 27, 2010)

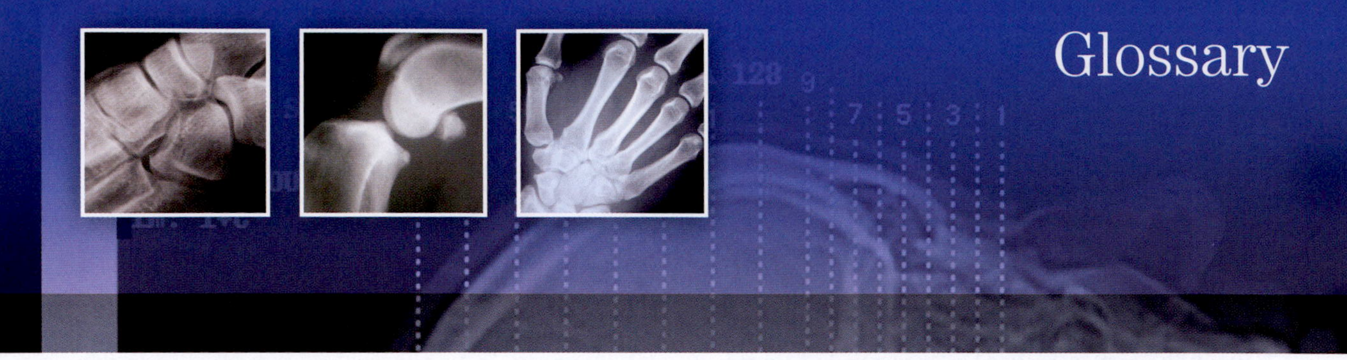

Glossary

A

abscess An encapsulated infection.

absolute value The meaning of a number equal to the distance of that number from zero on the number line.

acceptance limits The range of images determined to be of good quality by a given individual or department.

acoustic impedance Determines the resistance a material has to the oncoming sound wave.

acromegaly An overgrowth of the hands, feet, face, and jaw resulting from hypersecretion of growth hormones.

activator A chemical used in film developing in the fixer solution to maintain an acidic pH to enhance the functioning of the clearing agent.

active osteomyelitis Initial loss in bone tissue resulting from a bone infection.

activity Describes the quantity of radioactive material; expressed as the number of radioactive atoms that undergo decay per unit time.

actual focal spot The physical area of the focal track that is impacted.

added filtration Any filtration that occurs outside the tube and housing before the image receptor.

additive condition A disease that causes body tissues to thicken, increase in atomic number, or increase in density, requiring an increase in technical factors to achieve proper image receptor exposure.

adhesive A thin coating applied to the base material before it is coated with the emulsion to prevent bubbles or other distortion during processing or handling.

admittance The measure of resistance in an AC current when the expression 1/R is used.

aerophagia A psychological disorder resulting in abnormal swallowing of air.

afterglow Delayed phosphorescent emission; also called screen lag.

air-core transformer Arrangement of two coils of wire in proximity to facilitate induction.

air kerma The kinetic energy released per unit of mass air.

ALARA As low as reasonably achievable.

algebraic expression A mathematical sentence or term consisting of letters and/or numbers that are multiplied, divided, added, subtracted, or raised to a power.

aliasing Occurs when spatial frequency exceeds the Nyquist frequency and the incoming data are sampled less than twice per cycle.

alpha particle Contains two protons and two neutrons, is equivalent to a helium nucleus, and is emitted from the nuclei of heavy elements as they undergo radioactive decay. It has a great mass and a positive charge.

alternating current (AC) Electrons move first in one direction and then reverse and move in the opposite direction.

ammeter A device used to measure current connected in a series; measured in amperes.

amp (A) The unit of current; also known as the ampere.

ampere (A) The unit of current; also known as the amp.

amplitude The intensity of the wave defined by its maximal height.

anatomically programmed radiography A computerized exposure control system; technique charts using existing exposure systems that are stored in the data memory banks.

annihilation reaction Matter being converted back into energy as a result of a positron combining with a negative electron, which creates two photons moving in opposite directions.

anode The positive side of the x-ray tube; serves as a target surface for high-voltage electrons from the filament, conducts the high voltage from the cathode back into the x-ray generator circuitry, and serves as the primary thermal conductor.

anode assembly Consists of the anode, stator, and rotor.

anode cooling chart Permits the calculation of the time necessary for the anode to cool enough for additional exposures to be taken.

anode heel effect Due to the geometry of the angled anode target, the radiation intensity is greater on the cathode side.

anorexia nervosa A psychological eating disorder resulting in extreme weight loss.

antihalation coating A substance applied to the back of a single-emulsion film designed to absorb light coming from the emulsion and preventing backscatter.

aortic aneurysm A large dilation of the aorta.

approximate entrance skin dose An estimate of the quantity of radiation that will be measured at initial entrance to the body.

approximate entrance skin exposure An estimation of the dose of radiation related to a specific type of radiologic exam or procedure.

armature A coil of wire that acts as a conductor.

artificial permanent magnet Manufactured from steel alloy called alnico, composed of aluminum, nickel, and cobalt.

ascites Fluid accumulation within the peritoneal cavity.

aseptic necrosis Death of tissue.

atelectasis Collapse of the lung.

atom The smallest particle of an element that still possesses the chemical properties of that element.

atomic mass number (A) The mass of an atom; used when precision is not necessary; is equal to the number of protons and neutrons in the nucleus of an atom.

atomic mass unit (amu) The mass of the particles of an atom.

atomic number The number of nuclear protons in an atom unique to each element; also known as the Z number.

atomic reactor A device that converts nuclear energy to electrical energy.

atrophy A wasting away of body tissue with diminished cell proliferation.

attenuation The reduction in the number of x-ray photons in the beam, and subsequent loss of energy, as the beam passes through matter.

automatic exposure control A device programmed to terminate the radiographic exposure time; also called automatic exposure device.

automatic exposure device A device programmed to terminate the radiographic exposure time; also called automatic exposure control.

autotransformer A transformer that automatically sets by adjustments.

average gradient The average slope of the D log E curve at the straight-line portion of the curve.

B

backscatter radiation Photons that deflect back toward the source, traveling in the opposite direction of the incident photon.

backup time Establishes the maximum exposure time for the system in order to prevent overexposure.

base The base material that the film is made from; it is usually polyester, tough, stable, rigid, and uniformly lucent; it usually contains a blue tint.

base plus fog The density at no exposure; the density that is inherent in the film.

battery A device that converts chemical energy into electrical energy.

becquerel The SI unit for activity.

beta particle Identical to an electron, except it is emitted from the nuclei of radioactive materials; it is very light and negatively charged.

bias focusing Engagement of a small focal spot while a negative voltage that is applied to the focusing cup acts to reduce the size of the electron stream, creating a smaller focal spot.

biomedical informatics (BMI) Platforms that are used for medical purposes, such as patient care, and for biological applications and activities related to health care, including both preclinical research (studying disease or treatments in cells and animals) and clinical research (e.g., testing new drugs on patients or analyzing health-care statistics).

bit Binary digits.

blur The streaking or smearing that results in the loss of nearly all recorded detail of objects outside the focal plane.

bone densitometry A noninvasive procedure for the measurement of bone mineral density (BMD) that plays an important role in the early diagnosis of osteoporosis, monitoring therapy, and predicting fracture risk.

bone mineral density (BMD) Measurement of bone mass that plays an important role in the early diagnosis of osteoporosis.

bowel obstruction Abnormal accumulation of air and fluid resulting from a blockage in the bowel.

bremsstrahlung interaction An incident electron interacts with the force field of the nucleus, causing the incident electron to slow down, thus diverting the electron's course. The electron loses energy and changes direction. The energy lost is a bremsstrahlung photon, and the photon energy is half the difference between the entering and exiting kinetic energy of the electron.

brightness The concept of density as it is displayed on a soft-copy monitor for digital images.

bronchiectasis Chronic dilation of the bronchi.

brush A device, attached to slip rings, that allows the circuit to remain stationary while the armature rotates without breaking the electrical contact between them.

byte An 8-bit word.

C

calcified stones Calcium deposits in the form of stones that can be found in the gallbladder and kidneys.

calibrate To adjust a tool of measurement to zero.

caliper A device used to measure part thickness.

capacitor A device capable of accumulating and storing an electrical charge.

carcinoma Malignancy.

cardiomegaly Enlargement of the heart.

c-arm tube suspension system A type of radiography equipment that utilizes a c-shaped arm device to support the tube and the image receptor that allows the tube and image receptor to be rotated to new positions.

carriage The arm that supports the fluoroscopic equipment suspended over the table.

cathode The negative side of the x-ray tube; produces a thermionic cloud, conducts the high voltage to the gap between the cathode and anode, and focuses the electron stream as it heads for the anode.

cathode assembly Consists of the filament, focusing cup, and associated wiring.

caudad Longitudinal angulation in which the tube is angled toward the patient's feet.

cephalad Longitudinal angulation in which the tube is angled toward the patient's head.

characteristic cascade The reaction of electrons dropping into the holes created during a characteristic interaction until there is only a hole in the outer shell.

characteristic curve A radiographic relationship between the amount of exposure and the resultant density on the film; also known as D log E curve, sensitometric curve, and Hurter and Driffield curve.

characteristic interaction The incident electron interacts with an inner-shell electron, knocking out the inner-shell electron and continuing in a slightly different direction, which creates a hole in the inner shell, making the shell unstable.

characteristic peak Occurs when K-shell emissions reach their effective energy range of 69 keV.

characteristic photon An x-ray photon created by the electron transfer from one shell to another.

chemical energy The form of energy released during a chemical reaction.

chemical fog The effect on a film when unexposed silver halides are reduced.

chronic osteomyelitis New bone growth at the site of a chronic bone infection.

circuit breaker A device constructed to interrupt a circuit before a dangerous temperature is reached.

circulation system A part of the automatic processing system designed to stabilize temperatures, agitate solutions, mix the chemistry, and filter the solutions.

cirrhosis Fibrotic changes in the liver causing the liver to enlarge and ascites to develop.

clearing agent The primary agent of the fixer.

clearing time Twice the time necessary for the milky appearance of the film to disappear.

clinical target volume (CTV) Includes the GTV and a volume of tissue that contains microscopic subclinical disease.

closed-core transformer Arrangement of two coils of wire each filled with an iron core in proximity to facilitate induction that converges the inside and outside lines of force through the core.

coating The phase of the film production process in which the adhesive layer is applied to the base, then the emulsion, and, finally, the supercoat.

coercivity The energy that causes reorientation of the magnetic dipoles.

coherent scatter An interaction between x-rays and matter characterized by interaction between a very-low-energy x-ray photon and matter causing the electron to vibrate at the same frequency as the incident photon, which then produces a secondary photon with the same energy and wavelength as the incident photon but that travels in a different direction; also called classical scatter or unmodified scatter.

collimator A set of lead shutters at right angles to one another that move in opposing pairs.

collimator pitch The pitch of a single detector within an MDCT array of image receptors.

commutator ring A single ring that is divided in half, with each half connected to one end of the armature wire.

compensating filter Used to even out unequal densities.

compound A complex substance; two or more elements that are chemically united in a definite proportion.

compound filter The use of two or more materials to complement one another in their absorbing abilities; also known as K-edge filters.

compression The positive portion of the sound wave.

compression band A piece of equipment used to restrain a patient or compress abdominal tissue.

Compton effect An interaction between x-rays and matter characterized by an incident x-ray photon interacting with a loosely bound outer-shell electron, resulting in removal of the electron from the shell, which then proceeds in a different direction as a scattered photon; also known as Compton scattering.

Compton (or recoil) electron The dislodged electron resulting from Compton scattering; also called a recoil electron.

Compton scattered photon The photon that exits the atom in a different direction as a result of Compton scattering.

Compton scattering An interaction between x-rays and matter characterized by an incident x-ray photon interacting with a loosely bound outer-shell electron, resulting in removal of the electron from the shell, which then proceeds in a different direction as a scattered photon; also known as Compton effect.

computed radiography (CR) A type of indirect digital radiography; the radiographer must usually move the detector, that is most often housed in a cassette, between image acquisition and display.

computed tomography unit Specialized radiography equipment that allows the taking of sectional images.

concentration Law of electrostatics that states the greatest intensity of charge will be on the surface where the curvature is the sharpest.

conductance The measure of resistance in a DC current when the expression 1/R is used.

conduction band An area within the force field of an atom beyond the valence band.

conductor A material that allows electrons to flow freely.

cone beam CT (CBCT) Process used in IGRT to create three-dimensional images that pinpoint the exact size, location, and coordinates of the treatment isocenter.

cone cells Cells in the retina of the eye that are responsible for color vision.

congestive heart failure Increased venous congestion in the heart resulting from diminished cardiac output.

contact Electrification by contact occurs when two objects touch, permitting electrons to move from one to the other.

continuous wave The sound wave never stops being emitted by the transducer

contouring A tracing of the shape of the tumor volume as well as nearby structures that the radiation dose will affect.

contrast One of the properties that comprise visibility of detail; the difference between adjacent densities.

contrast medium injection device Type of instrument that is used to inject contrast media into vessels for radiographic studies.

contrast perception The ability to visually distinguish differences in density or contrast.

conversion efficiency The ability of the phosphor to emit as much light per x-ray photon interaction as possible, which is related to the screen speed.

convolution The process of modifying pixel values by a mathematical formula; also referred to as mask.

coregistration Fusion of PET or SPECT with CT or MRI acquired in separate imaging sessions; used as a method of providing anatomical context to functional/metabolic images.

coulomb per kilogram A radiographically derived unit of the SI system, abbreviated as C/kg, formerly known as the roentgen.

criss-cross grid Two linear grids placed on top of one another so that the lead strips form a criss-cross pattern.

cross-hatched grid Two linear grids placed on top of one another so that the lead strips form a criss-cross pattern.

crossover effect Blurring of the image caused by light from one screen crossing into the light from another screen.

cryogen Cooling agent.

crystal production The part of the film manufacturing process that must be done in total darkness. Silver nitrate and potassium bromide are combined in the presence of gelatin; the silver bromide precipitates out and the potassium nitrate can be washed away as a waste product.

curie (Ci) The unit of activity.

current The quantity or the number of electrons flowing.

D

D log E curve A radiographic relationship between the amount of exposure and the resultant density on the film; also known as characteristic curve, sensitometric curve, and Hurter and Driffield curve.

D_{max} The maximum density the film is capable of recording.

deconvolution The process of returning the pixel values to their original level by a reverse process.

definition One of the geometric properties of image quality; the degree of geometric sharpness or accuracy of structural lines actually recorded in the image; also referred to as detail, recorded detail, sharpness, and spatial resolution.

degenerative arthritis Inflammation of the joints resulting in destruction of adjoining joint tissue.

densitometer An instrument that provides a readout of the amount of blackening (density) on a film.

density One of the photographic properties that comprise visibility of detail; the degree of overall blackening of the film.

destructive condition A disease that causes body tissues to thin, decrease in atomic number, or decrease in density, requiring a decrease in technical factors to achieve proper image receptor exposure.

detail One of the geometric properties of image quality; the degree of geometric sharpness or accuracy of structural lines actually recorded in the image; also referred to as recorded detail, definition, sharpness, and spatial resolution.

detective quantum efficiency (DQE) Measure of the sensitivity and accuracy by which the image receptor converts the incoming data to the output viewing device.

deterministic effect Results of radiation exposure for which a threshold dose of radiation is assumed (e.g., cataracts, sterility).

developing The step in film processing; silver is deposited at the latent image sites and an image becomes visible.

deviation index (DI) An indicator as to whether the detector response of a specified image K_{IND} agrees with K_{TGT}.

diagnostic Methods used to determine the source or cause of a disease, disorder, or traumatic injury.

diamagnetic Materials weakly repelled by all magnetic fields (e.g., beryllium, bismuth, lead).

dielectric The insulation between two plates in a capacitor.

differential attenuation The result of differences in transmission of the beam as it passes through the patient resulting in signal differences to the digital detector.

digital angiography Produces one image similar to the last fluoroscopy hold vascular image; also called spot imaging.

digital cineradiography Takes numerous exposures (frames) in a second of time.

digital imaging and communication in medicine (DICOM) An acronym for the Digital Imaging and Communications in Medicine standard; originated in the 1980s as a collaborative effort between the American College of Radiology (ACR) and the National Electrical Manufacturers' Association (NEMA) to establish a universal, standardized public format and protocol for communicating biomedical imaging files; it is periodically upgraded.

digital mammography unit A dedicated breast imaging machine that utilizes a CR/DR image receptor system.

digital radiography (DR) Imaging systems that replace traditional film with a reusable detector.

digital subtraction angiography Eliminates bone and soft tissue structures from an image so that only the contrast-filled vessels remain.

digital tomosynthesis Digital radiographic tomography.

diode A rectifying semiconductor made by sandwiching p-type crystal with an n-type to form a p-n junction.

direct conversion Direct conversion of incoming x-ray photons to an electronic signal without scintillation.

direct current (DC) All electrons travel in the same direction.

direct square law A direct relationship is necessary to compensate for the changes in intensity and film density.

direct variation One quantity is a multiple of a second quantity.

distortion One of the geometric properties affecting radiographic image quality; a misrepresentation of the size and shape of the structures being examined.

distribution Law of electrostatics that states charges reside on the surfaces of conductors but are evenly distributed throughout nonconductors.

Doppler Used to detect and/or evaluate blood flow; can be used with continuous wave (CW), pulsed wave (PW), or color flow imaging.

dose calibrator Used for measuring various types and quantities of radioactivity during radiopharmaceutical preparation and before dispensing.

dose limit Radiation exposure limits that are pertinent to the protection of radiation workers.

dosimeter A mechanism that can measure amounts of radiation.

dryer system The final stage of film processing that removes the excess water, cools and dries the film, and seals the film for viewing and storage.

drying The process of film developing in which hot air is forced over both sides of the film as it exits the processor.

dual focus A two-filament arrangement within the x-ray tube.

dual photon absorptiometry (DPA) The first dual energy bone densitometer that made possible the measurement of the hip and spine; used a radioactive source (Gd 153) that naturally emitted photons of two different energies (40 and 100 KEV).

dual x-ray absorptiometry (DXA) The gold standard of noninvasive bone mineral density (BMD) determination. DXA units use two x-ray beams of different energy levels. After soft tissue absorption is subtracted out, the BMD can be calculated.

duplication film A type of film designed to provide an exact image of the original film.

duplitized Describes a film that is coated with emulsion on both sides.

dynamic range The concept of contrast as it is displayed on a soft-copy monitor for digital images; range of density/brightness of the display monitor light emission.

dynamometer Used to measure alternating current when electromagnets are used.

E

eddy current loss Result of currents opposing the cause that produced them.

edema Swelling.

edge enhancement Increase in contrast due to high-pass filtering; also known as sharpening.

edge spread function (ESF) Expression of the boundaries of an image.

effective dose The sum of the weighted equivalent doses for all irradiated tissues and organs; used to measure the radiation and organ-system-specific damage in humans.

effective focal spot The area of the focal spot that is projected out of the tube toward the object being radiographed.

effective half-life (Te) The time required for half of the initial radioactivity to disappear from an organ or body by a combination of excretion and physical decay.

effective target angle In mammography, measured from the vertical central ray point.

electric current Electrons that are moving in predominantly the same direction.

electric field A force field; the result of the composite forces of the charges residing within an object.

electric timers Capable of accurate exposures as short as 0.001 second with only a 1-msec delay.

electrical circuit A pathway that permits electrons to move in a complete circle from their source, through resisting electrical devices and back to the source.

electrical energy The result of movement of electrons; also known as electricity.

electricity The result of movement of electrons; also known as electrical energy.

electrification Describes the process of electron charges being added to or subtracted from an object.

electromagnet Temporary magnet produced by moving electric current.

electromagnetic energy A form of energy resulting from electric and magnetic disturbances in space.

electromagnetic radiation (EM) A form of energy that is the result of electric and magnetic disturbances in space.

electromagnetic relay A device used to protect the radiographer from electric shock by isolating control buttons on the x-ray console from the actual circuit in which high voltage is flowing; similar to a circuit breaker.

electromagnetic spectrum Describes the different forms of electromagnetic radiation.

electromotive force (emf) The force or strength of electron flow; also known as potential difference.

electron (e^-) Negatively charged subatomic particle of an atom.

electron binding energy (E_b) The amount of energy needed to remove the electron from the atom.

electron volt (eV) Measurement of the binding energy of an electron; the energy one electron will have when it is accelerated by an electrical potential of 1 volt.

electronic health-care (or health) record (EHR) An electronic version of an individual patient's collection of medical documents.

electronic medical record (EMR) All patient medical documentation stored in electronic format.

electrostatics The study of the distribution of fixed charges, or electrons, that are at rest.

element A simple substance; it cannot be broken down into any simpler substances by ordinary means.

elongation Projection of an object, making it appear longer than it really is.

emaciation A generalized wasting of body tissue.

emphysema The overdistention of lung tissues by air.

empyema Pus in the thoracic cavity.

emulsion with crystals A gelatin in which photosensitive silver halide crystals are suspended. It is an extremely thin coating that acts as a neutral lucent suspension medium for the silver halide crystals to separate and allow chemicals to interact with them.

energy-switching system A system that switches the kVp between 100 and 140, resulting in a primary beam with two different energy peaks (near 40 and 80 keV).

entrance roller Specially designed crossover network to begin the film traveling from the feed tray down into the developer section.

entrance skin exposure The area where the maximum exposure received by the patient lies.

envelope The entire cathode and anode assembly is housed within this glass or metal structure.

equation A statement that contains an equal sign.

equivalent equation Equations that have the same solutions.

excitation Process in which electrons in an atom are moved to a higher-energy state without actually being removed from the atom.

exposure Subjecting something to bombardment by x-ray photons or another type of irradiation. The term is also used to represent a measurement of the value of such bombardment.

exposure amplitude The total distance the tube travels during the tomographic exposure.

exposure maintenance formula A direct square law; mAs must increase when distance increases, and vice versa, in order to maintain image receptor exposure.

exposure switch A remote control device that permits current to flow through the circuit.

external beam evaluation The measurement of the quantity and quality of the external radiation beam.

extrafocal radiation Photons that were not produced at the focal spot; also called off-focus radiation.

F

farad (f) The unit of capacitance.

ferromagnetic Materials that are highly permeable and susceptible to induction (e.g., iron, cobalt, nickel).

fibrosarcoma Malignant tumor of the metaphysis of bone resulting in reduction of bone composition.

field survey instrument Portable device used to measure radiation in a given location.

15 percent rule An increase in kVp by 15 percent that causes a doubling in exposure, and vice versa.

filament A small coil of thin thoriated tungsten wire.

filament circuit Supplies the filament of the x-ray tube with properly modified power.

film badge dosimeter Two pieces of film having different sensitivities to x-rays contained within a light, tight envelope; the film emulsion darkens in response to the radiation exposure received.

film processing system The equipment used to process radiographic film for viewing of the radiographic image

filter Any material designed to effectively absorb photons from the x-ray beam.

fixed A piece of equipment that remains in one place and is not movable.

fixing The process of removing undeveloped silver halides to make the image permanent for viewing.

flat panel detector Descriptive term used for the plates used in both direct and indirect DR digital systems.

Fleming's hand rules A series of easily remembered aids to help with the relationship between electricity and magnetism.

floor suspension system A type of radiography unit that uses a tube support column mounted on the floor.

floor-to-ceiling suspension system A type of radiography unit that uses a pair of rails for longitudinal positioning.

fluorescence The ability of a material to emit light instantaneously in responses to excitation within 1 nanosecond.

fluoroscopic screen A specialized x-ray tube with an image receptor which can be viewed during an x-ray exposure.

Fluoroscopy A dynamic radiographic examination; involves active diagnosis during an examination.

flux density Determined by field strength and the arc in which the lines of flux are located.

flux gain A measurement of the increase in light photons due to the conversion efficiency of the output screen.

focal plane The section; also section level, layer height, object plane, and depth of focus.

focal point The portion of the anode where the high-voltage electron stream will impact.

focal spot The portion of the anode where the high-voltage electron stream will impact.

focal track The portion of the anode where the high-voltage electron stream will impact. When discussing a rotating anode, this describes the circular path that will be impacted by the electron beam.

focus The portion of the anode where the high-voltage electron stream will impact.

focused grid A grid created with the central grid strips parallel with the strips and becoming more inclined as they move away from the central axis; the lines would intersect along a point in space called the line of convergence.

focusing cup A shallow depression in the cathode assembly designed to house the filament.

footboard A piece of equipment used with a tilting table that allows the patient to stand when the table is upright.

foreshortening Projection of an object, making it appear shorter than it really is.

fractional focal spot A very small focal spot; usually a fraction of a millimeter in size.

frequency The number of waves that passes a particular point in a given time frame.

friction Electrification that occurs when one object is rubbed against another and, due to differences in the number of electrons available on each, electrons travel from one to the other.

fulcrum The pivot point around which the motions of the tube and the image receptor are centered.

full-wave rectification The conversion of the opposing half of the incoming electron flow to always move in the same direction, instead of discarding half the cycle.

fuse A device constructed to interrupt a circuit before a dangerous temperature is reached.

G

galvanometer Used to measure direct current when permanent magnets are used.

gamma A measure of the slope of the straight-line portion of the D log E curve at the speed point.

gamma camera Feature one, two, or three large field-of-view scintillation detectors arranged in various configurations, and can be used for planar and SPECT (single photon emission computed tomography) acquisitions; also known as an Anger camera, named for the inventor, Hal Anger.

gantry The movable frame of the CT unit.

gasses A light mixture that has neither shape nor volume.

gauss (G) The unit used for measuring magnetic flux density.

Geiger-Mueller counter A portable ionization chamber; commonly called a Geiger counter or GM meter.

generator A device that converts mechanical energy to electrical energy using moving lines of flux in relationship to a conductor to induce current; also known as a dynamo.

genetic Describes the effects of radiation that appear in the descendants of the individual being irradiated.

gout A metabolic disease that can cause a reduction in bone composition.

gradient point The slope of any portion of the D log E curve.

gray (Gy) Unit of absorbed energy or dose; 1 joule of energy absorbed in each kilogram of absorbing material.

grayscale [27] The number of shades of gray in a radiographic image

grayscale bit depth The number of shades of gray; ranges from 8 bits to 32 bits. A grayscale bit depth of 8–32 equals a range of 1–4 bytes of storage that would be required per pixel in the image matrix. A grayscale bit depth of 12 produces 2^{12} gray levels. This represents 4,096 different shades of gray.

grid A device used to improve contrast of the radiographic image.

grid-biased A type of tube that quickly regulates the flow of electrons, producing x-ray photons.

grid-controlled A type of tube that quickly regulates the flow of electrons, producing x-ray photons.

grid cut-off The result of the primary beam being angled into the lead strips.

grid frequency The number of grid lines per inch or centimeter.

grid-pulsed A type of tube that quickly regulates the flow of electrons producing x-ray photons.

grid ratio The ratio of the height of the lead strips to the distance between the strips.

gross tumor volume (GTV) The palpable or visible growth of the malignant tumor. It is considered the primary location of the tumor, and any lymphatic or other metastatic spread.

gyromagnetic ratio The ratio of the magnetic moment to the moment of inertia.

H

halation An effect on a radiographic image caused when light that is reflected from the air interfaces on the back of the base material.

half-value layer (HVL) The amount of absorbing material that will reduce the intensity of the primary beam to one-half its original value.

half-wave rectification Suppressed rectification resulting from only half of the incoming alternating current being converted to pulsating direct current; called self-rectification.

handgrip A piece of equipment that allows the patient to grip when the table is being tilted for added support and reassurance.

hard copy Images that are visualized on film.

hardener A chemical used in film processing that controls the swelling of the gelatin to prevent scratches and abrasions to the emulsion during processing; in a fixer solution, must function in an acidic environment.

harmonics Manipulation of a sound wave from the traditional sinusoidal wave into a bent shape; also called sawtooth waves.

head unit Specialized radiography equipment used to conduct cranial studies.

heat The result of the motion of atoms and molecules; also known as thermal energy.

hemothorax The filling of the pleural cavity with blood.

high-pass filtering Amplifies or deletes all but the high frequencies.

histogram Generated by dividing a scanned area into pixels and determining the signal intensity for each pixel; can be calculated for specific anatomy and procedures.

hospital information system (HIS) The electronic database used in the hospital to store, generate, and retrieve information on patients.

housing cooling chart Permits the calculation of the time necessary for the housing to cool enough for additional exposures to be made.

Hurter and Driffield (H&D) curve A radiographic relationship between the amount of exposure and the resultant density on the film; also known as characteristic curve, sensitometric curve, and D log E curve.

Huygen's Principle Explains a sound wave as having the shape of an hourglass.

hydrocephalus Dilatation of fluid-filled cerebral ventricles resulting in enlargement of the head.

hydrothorax The filling of the pleural cavity with serous fluid.

hyperparathyroidism Oversecretion of the parathyroid hormone, causing calcium to leave bone and enter the bloodstream.

hysteresis loss Results from energy expended as the continually changing AC current magnetizes, demagnetizes, and remagnetizes the core material; also called lagging loss.

I

I^2R loss Results from the inherent resistance to current flow that is found in all conductors; power lost from resistance is proportional to the square of current; sometimes called copper loss.

identity An equation in which all numeric values substituted for the unknown will give a true statement.

image guided radiation therapy (IGRT) Acronym for image guided radiation therapy.

image intensification tube Video camera and monitor used to view fluoroscopic images.

image receptor contrast The total amount of contrast acquired from the image receptor.

imaging noise Background information that the imaging receptor receives.

incident electron The electrons from the thermionic cloud that arrive at the anode target.

incoming-line current The alternating current that is supplied to buildings; usually supplied in three-phase power cycle; also called the mains.

indirect conversion A two-part process involving a scintillator (which converts incoming x-ray photons to light) and a photodetector (which converts light into an electronic signal).

induction The process of electrical fields acting on one another without contact.

inductive reactance The ability of an alternating current to switch directions, causing the opposing potential difference to induce against the incoming supply of electrons; measured in ohms of resistance.

informatics A body of ideas, devices, and processes related to handling multiple types of information.

inherent filtration Results from the composition of the tube and housing.

insulator A material that inhibits electron flow.

integral dose The total amount of energy imparted to matter; the product of dose and the mass over which the energy is imparted.

intensification factor The most accurate factor that measures the speed or sensitivity of an intensifying screen; a measurement of the amplification of the image that occurs due to the screen's ability to convert x-ray photons to light.

intensifying screen Device used to amplify the incoming x-ray beam and reduce patient radiation dose.

inverse square law Law of electrostatics that states the force between two charges is directly proportional to the product of their magnitudes and inversely proportional to the square of the distance between them.

inverse variation When two quantities are multiplied, their product is a constant.

ion An atom that has gained or lost an electron.

ionic solution Charged particles dissolved within a solution.

ionization The process of adding or removing an electron from an atom.

ionization chamber An automatic exposure control device used to terminate the exposure after a desired exposure has been reached.

IR exposure One of the two photographic properties that comprise visibility of detail. In digital imaging it is the critical quality factor to assess and comparable to density in the film/screen environment.

isocenter The point where all three rotational axes intersect from the simulator and the treatment machine.

isotope Atoms that have the same number of protons in the nucleus but differ in the number of neutrons.

K

K-edge filter The use of two or more materials to complement one another in their absorbing abilities; also known as compound filters.

kerma Kinetic energy released in matter; the energy imparted directly to electrons per unit mass.

kilogram The standard unit of mass, abbreviated as kg.

kinetic energy The energy of motion.

K-shell The orbital shell closest to the nucleus.

K-shell absorption edge When the incident x-ray photons match the K-shell binding energy of the phosphor, there is an increase in characteristic production within the screen.

L

lambda The Greek letter that represents the measurement of a wavelength.

Larmor frequency In a static homogenous magnetic field, all protons in a nucleus of a given type of element will rotate with exactly the same frequency.

latitude The range of exposures that will produce densities within the diagnostic range.

laws of electrostatics Rules relating how objects are electrified.

leakage radiation Any photons that escape from the housing except at the port.

like terms Terms (numbers) with identical literal factors (usually noted by a letter).

line spread function (LSF) Measurement of recorded detail, sharpness, and resolution; the ability of a film/screen system to accurately measure the boundaries of an image.

linear accelerator Made up of the drive stand, gantry, treatment couch, control console, and modulator cabinet.

linear grid A grid with lead strips running in only one direction.

line-focus principle Used to reduce the effective area of the focal spot.

lines of flux The force fields that are created when magnetic dipoles orient to create a magnet; also called lines of force and magnetic field.

lines of force The force fields that are created when magnetic dipoles orient to create a magnet; also called lines of flux and magnetic field.

line pairs per millimeter (lp/mm) Measurement of recorded detail, sharpness, and resolution; the minimum size and space between objects that can be visualized on the final image.

look-up table (LUT) Data that are stored to substitute new values for each pixel during processing.

low-pass filtering Amplifies or deletes all but the low frequencies.

luminescence The ability of a material to emit light in response to excitation.

M

M theory Electrons and quarks may not be particles, but instead may be extremely small loops of rapidly vibrating string-like matter.

Mach effect Each time the eye sees a change in density, there is a change in the intensity of the impulses sent to the brain.

magnet An object that exhibits a uniformly strong magnetic field.

magnetic dipole Groups of atoms with their net magnetic field moving in the same direction; also know as magnetic domains.

magnetic domain Groups of atoms with their net magnetic field moving in the same direction; also know as magnetic dipoles.

magnetic field The force fields that are created when magnetic dipoles orient to create a magnet; also called lines of flux and lines of force.

main circuit Supplies the x-ray tube with properly modified power.

main switch The switch that generates the power to the x-ray tube.

mains The alternating current that is supplied to buildings; usually supplied in three-phase power cycle; also called the incoming-line current.

mammography unit Specialized radiography equipment for studies and imaging of the breast tissues.

mask The process of modifying pixel values by a mathematical formula; also referred to as convolution.

mass The quantity of matter contained in an object.

matrix A square series of boxes that gives form to the image.

mechanical energy The result of the action of machines or physical movement; can be potential or kinetic.

metallic conductor The most common pathway for the movement of electrical current (e.g., copper).

meter The standard unit of length, abbreviated as m.

milliamperage (mA) A measurement of x-ray tube current—the number of electrons crossing the tube from cathode to anode per second.

milliamperage-second (mAs) The product of tube current and exposure time.

milliampere-second timer A device used in falling-load generators and some capacitor units to monitor the product of mA and time on the secondary side of the high-voltage step-up transformer.

minification gain Resulting from the same number of electrons that were produced at the large input screen being compressed into the area of the small output screen.

minimum reaction (or response) time The length of time necessary for the AEC to respond to the radiation and for the generator to terminate the exposure.

minimum response time The length of time necessary for the AEC to respond to the ionization and send a signal to terminate the exposure.

mixing The period of film production in which the shredded emulsion is melted at a precise temperature to properly sensitize the crystals.

mixture The combination of two or more substances.

mobile system A type of radiography equipment that can be brought to the patient anywhere the patient may be.

modulation transfer function (MTF) Measurement of recorded detail, sharpness, and resolution; measures the resolving ability of a film/screen combination.

molecule Two or more atoms chemically united; the smallest particle of a compound that still possesses the characteristics of the compound.

molybdenum In mammography, the anode is made of this element.

motor A device that is supplied with electrical current to produce mechanical motion.

movement Second law of electrostatics that states only negative charges move along solid conductors.

multiple myeloma A malignant tumor arising from plasma cells of bone marrow, causing a reduction in bone composition.

multiphase power Combination of several waveforms of current slightly out of step with one another.

mutual induction The result of two coils being placed in close proximity with a varying current supplied to the first coil, which then induces a similar flow in the second coil.

N

natural magnet Created when iron oxide remains in the earth's magnetic field for ages, slowly orienting the magnetic dipoles in the same direction (e.g., lodestones).

negative charge Charge of the electron, which is located outside the nucleus, bound by relatively weak forces.

negatron A negatively charged electron resulting from pair production.

neutron (n^0) Subatomic particle of an atom containing no charge.

nonmagnetic Materials not affected by magnetic fields and that cannot be magnetized (e.g., wood, glass, rubber, plastic).

nu Greek letter used to denote the number of cycles per second.

nuclear energy The energy stored in the bond of the nucleus of an atom.

nucleon The protons and neutrons that make up the nucleus.

nucleus The small dense center of an atom; consists of protons and neutrons.

Nyquist criterion The sampling of the spatial resolution frequency signal twice from each cycle in digital systems.

O

occasionally exposed worker Workers whose duties may occasionally bring them into areas where radiation exposure may occur.

occupationally exposed worker Workers who have a significant potential for exposure to radiation in the course of their employment.

octet rule The number of electrons in the outermost shell never exceeds eight electrons.

off-focus radiation Photons that were not produced at the focal spot; also called extrafocal radiation.

ohm (Ω) The unit of resistance.

opacity The ability of a film to stop light.

open equation An equation that contains at least one unknown (variable).

open-core transformer Arrangement of two coils of wire each filled with an iron core in proximity to facilitate induction.

optical density numbers The numbers displayed by a densitometer.

optically stimulated luminescence (OSL) dosimeter Measures radiation that passes through a thin strip of aluminum oxide. A laser light simulates the aluminum oxide, which becomes luminescent in proportion to the amount of radiation exposure.

optimal kVp The maximum kVp level that will produce images with appropriate contrast that are consistently within acceptance limits.

orbital magnetic moment The motion of a charged particle creates a magnetic force field perpendicular to the motion.

orthochromatic A film that is not sensitive to the red spectrum.

osteitis deformans New bone growth resulting from an increase in bone cell activity.

osteoblastic metastases New bone growth resulting from the spread of cancer in bone.

osteochondroma A tumor in the bone and cartilage.

osteolytic metastases Destruction of bone due to malignancies that have spread to the bone.

osteomalacia A defect in bone mineralization, causing decreased composition.

osteoporosis A defect in bone production due to failure of osteoblasts to lay down bone matrix.

overhead suspension system A type of radiography unit that allows control of longitudinal and transverse positioning as well as vertical distance.

P

Paget's disease New bone growth resulting from an increase in bone cell activity.

pair production An interaction between x-rays and matter characterized by the conversion of the energy of an x-ray photon into matter in the form of two electrons.

panchromatic A film that is sensitive to all colors.

panoramic dental and facial unit Specialized radiography equipment for combined tomography of facial and dental structures.

pantomography A type of tomography that permits a slit scan of curved surfaces such as the face and head.

parallel circuit An electric circuit designed to send electrons through various resistance devices by giving each component its own branch.

parallel grid A grid created with the lead and interspace strips running parallel to one another; the lines will never intersect.

paramagnetic Materials that have a low permeability and weak attraction to magnetic fields (e.g., aluminum).

particulate radiation High-energy electrons, neutrons, and protons that produce ionization in matter by direct atomic collisions.

pathology The medical science concerned with all aspects of disease, including the structural and functional changes caused by a disease process.

patient equivalent phantom A dummy or surrogate device that can be imaged that will mimic the thickness of an actual patient; used to control quality and acceptance levels of radiographic images.

penetrability The ability of the x-ray to pass through structures and tissues.

penetrometer A series of increasingly thick, uniform absorbers.

penumbra A geometric unsharpness around the periphery of the image.

period The time required to complete one cycle of the wave.

peripheral quantitative computed tomography (pQCT) A smaller, dedicated CT unit for extremities only.

permeability The ease with which a material can be magnetized.

personnel monitoring device Instrument worn by health-care workers who work regularly in radiation-exposed environments.

PET Acronym for positron emission tomography.

phosphor layer A layer of material used in an intensifying screen that is capable of absorbing the energy of an incident x-ray photon and then emitting light photons.

phosphorescence The ability of a material to delay emission of light in response to excitation.

photodisintegration An interaction between x-rays and matter characterized by the interaction between a high-energy photon and the nucleus. The high-energy photon strikes the nucleus; the nucleus absorbs all the photon's energy and then emits a nuclear fragment.

photoelectric absorption An interaction between x-rays and matter characterized by an incident electron with slightly greater energy than the binding energy of the electrons in the inner shells, ejecting an electron from the inner shell while being absorbed in the reaction, resulting in an ionized atom.

photoelectron An ionized atom with a missing inner-shell electron resulting from ejection of the electron due to photoelectric absorption.

photon A small bundle of energy. The specific amount of energy depends on frequency; also known as a quantum.

photostimulable storage phosphor imaging plate Typically inside a cassette; used in computed radiography.

phototimer Often used to describe all automatic exposure controls; this type of AED is rarely used in modern radiography.

physical half-life (Tp) The half-life of a radionuclide (T½)

picture archiving and communication system (PACS) A computer system that can manage images in an electronic form.

piezoelectric effect The use of crystals or transducers used in ultrasound to convert electrical energy into mechanical energy and mechanical energy into electrical energy.

pitch The extension or contraction of the helix; the ratio of the distance the table moves during one 360-degree tube rotation to the total beam collimation.

pixel Picture elements; individual matrix boxes.

pixel pitch The physical distance between pixels; generally measured from center to center.

planning target volume (PTV) Includes the GTV and CTV and includes lymph nodes adjacent to the primary tumor that have evidence of disease.

pleural effusions The filling of the pleural cavity with blood or serous fluid.

pneumoconiosis The inhalation of dust particles, causing fibrotic scarring of the lungs.

pneumonectomy The removal of a lung.

pneumonia Inflammation of lung tissues, causing fluid to fill the alveolar spaces.

pneumonitis Inflammation of lung tissues, causing fluid to fill the alveolar spaces.

pneumothorax Free air in the pleural cavity that displaces lung tissue.

pocket dosimeter A personal-use ionization chamber. When exposed to radiation, ionization occurs in the chamber, which neutralizes a positively charged electrode that will appear as movement of an exposure scale.

point spread function (PSF) Expression of the boundaries of an image; determined by a mathematical measurement of an image produced at a single point.

portal radiograph A radiograph produced by exposing the image receptor to the radiation beam that emanates from the portal of a therapy unit.

positive beam limitation device (PBL) An automatic collimator that adjusts to the size and placement of the cassette.

positive charge Charge of the proton, which is locked within the nucleus by very strong forces.

positron A positively charged electron resulting from pair production.

potential difference The force or strength of electron flow; also known as electromotive force (emf).

potential energy The energy an object has because of its position.

potentiometer A variable resistor that permits a variable contact to slide along a series circuit of resistance coils.

power loss formula Calculation that can provide an understanding of the changes in resistance to heat output.

precession Rotation of the axis of rotation within a nucleus when it encounters a magnetic field; causes a loss in momentum.

preservative A chemical used in film processing to help decrease the oxidation of the reducing agents when they are combined with air; also used in fixer solution to aid in removal of silver from the emulsion.

primary barrier A shielding structure that can be struck by the primary x-ray beam exiting the x-ray tube.

primary coil The coil first supplied with the current.

prime factor Factors related to x-ray emission that are under the direct control of the radiographer; milliamperage, kilovoltage, and distance.

propagation speed The speed at which the sound wave moves through a medium.

Proportionally Corresponding to something else in a constant ratio to another quantity.

protective coat A layer of material used in an intensifying screen applied to the top of the phosphor layer to protect it from abrasions and stains; usually thick plastic.

protective device Items worn by the radiation worker to reduce exposure to radiation.

protective housing The entire cathode and anode assembly is housed within this metal structure.

proton (p^+) Positively charged subatomic particle of an atom.

proton therapy A method of radiation therapy treatment the uses a beam formed by the positive subatomic particles stripped from the nucleus and then accelerated through a cyclotron. The beam has remarkable qualities of the deposition of energy that dramatically decreases patient side effects.

pulmonary edema The filling of the interstitial lung tissues and alveoli with fluid.

pulse duration The time it takes from the beginning of the pulse to the end of the pulse.

pulse repetition frequency (PRF) The rate at which a pulse is repeated in a given amount of time.

pulse repetition period (PRP) The time it takes from the beginning of one pulse to the beginning of the next pulse.

pulsed wave Utilized in ultrasound; sends out short bursts of sound waves and then stops and waits for the returning echoes.

pyramid problem Acceptable images depend on many factors. If any of those factors are off, it can cause a problem in various other factors, thus a pyramid effect of problems is the result.

Q

quality assurance All activities that provide adequate confidence that a radiology service will render consistently high-quality images and services.

quality control The aspect of quality assurance that monitors technical equipment to maintain superior standards.

quality factor Radiation weighting factor, specific to specific types of radiation; accounts for the biological effectiveness of the specific radiation.

quantitative computed tomography (QCT) Special software applied to an existing CT scan to determine a true three-dimensional or volumetric (unit of measure g/cm^3) measurement of bone density as opposed to the two-dimensional or areal (unit of measure g/cm^2) provided by DXA.

quantitative ultrasound (QUS) A technique used in more recent years for determining the interrogation of bone.

quantum A small bundle of energy. The specific amount of energy depends on frequency; also known as a photon.

quantum mottle A lack of sufficient incoming data to process an image; also known as quantum noise.

quantum noise A lack of sufficient incoming data to process an image; also known as quantum mottle.

quark Subnuclear structure that makes up protons and neutrons.

R

rad Term used to describe the measurement related to the absorbed dose of radiation; unit of absorbed energy or dose applicable to any material; 100 ergs of energy absorbed in 1 gram of absorbing material.

radiation Energy emitted and transferred through matter.

radiation fog The result of scattered photons striking the radiographic film and placing a density on the film that is unrelated to the patient's anatomy.

radiation worker An individual who, through occupational risk, has a certain likelihood of exposure to ionizing radiation in the course of his or her normal duties.

radioactivity The number of nuclear disintegrations per unit time.

radiofrequency Coils that produce a pulsed magnetic field (radio waves) to rotate the magnetic field of the tissues through a receiving coil (antenna), inducing an MR signal.

radiographic tube rating chart A guide regarding the most common technical factor combinations that can be used without overloading the tube.

radiology information system (RIS) A database of images and patient records specific to the imaging department.

radionuclide generator A self-contained system housing a radionuclide parent/daughter equilibrium. It is designed to produce the daughter for a separate purpose (i.e., injection into a patient for a nuclear medicine study) while leaving the parent intact for additional daughter production.

radiopharmaceutical A radioactive prescription drug.

rarefaction The backward movement of a sound wave.

reciprocity law The density on an x-ray film should remain unchanged as long as the intensity and duration of the x-ray exposure remains unchanged.

reciprocity law failure Failure to maintain consistent exposures when extremely short or long exposure times are used.

recorded detail One of the geometric properties of image quality; the degree of geometric sharpness or accuracy of structural lines actually recorded in the image; also referred to as detail, definition, sharpness, spatial resolution.

rectification The process by which alternating current is changed to pulsating direct current.

reducing agent A chemical used in film developing that provides electrons to the silver ions attached to the sensitivity specks of the silver halide crystals.

reference axis The angled central ray as used in mammography.

reference axis target angle In mammography, measured from the center of the x-ray beam as in conventional radiography.

reflective layer A layer of material used in an intensifying screen to reflect light toward the film.

relative speed The most useful rating of intensifying screens; expressed with par-screens and film being arbitrarily assigned a relative speed number of 100 as a control point.

rem Term used to describe the measurement of the biologically equivalent dose.

remodeling cycle Maintenance of the balance between bone growth and breakdown.

replenishment system Replaces chemicals that are depleted through the chemical reactions of processing, oxidation, and evaporation.

repulsion-attraction Law of electrostatics that states like charges repel and unlike charges attract.

rescaling Correction of an exposure that is outside the range from underexposure or overexposure by shifting the histogram to the correct area.

resistance The amount of opposition to the current in the circuit.

resolution The ability to accurately image an object; measured by the ability to see pairs of lines.

resolving power The ability to accurately image an object; measured by the ability to see pairs of lines.

restrainer A chemical used in film processing added to the developer to restrict the reducing action to those crystals with sensitivity speck gates.

retentivity The ability of a material to stay magnetized.

reversal The process of reducing the intensity of the latent image, producing less density.

rheostat A device constructed to interrupt a circuit before a dangerous temperature is reached.

rhodium In mammography, newer anodes are made from this substance.

ripening The period of film production during which silver halides are allowed to grow.

rod cell Cells in the retina of the eye that are sensitive to dim light.

roentgen (R) Term used to describe the measurement related to exposure; the unit of exposure in air; the quantity of x-rays or gamma rays required to produce a given amount of ionization in a unit mass of air.

rotating anode An anode assembly that turns during exposure.

rotor A hollow copper cylinder or cuff that is attached to the anode disk by a molybdenum shaft.

S

saturation current As kVp increases, a greater percentage of the thermionically emitted electrons are driven toward the anode.

scale of contrast The number of useful visible densities or shades of gray.

scattering The interaction of x-ray photons and matter that causes a change in direction of the photons.

scintillation detector Uses a multichannel analyzer to detect radionuclidic contaminants in radiopharmaceuticals.

sclerosis An increase in bone hardening resulting from a chronic inflammation of the bone.

screen lag Delayed phosphorescent emission; also called afterglow.

second The standard unit of time, abbreviated as s.

secondary barrier A shielding structure that can be struck by scattered and leakage radiation.

secondary coil The coil in which a current is inducted by the primary coil.

secondary radiation A characteristic photon created by the electron transfer from one shell to another but occurring outside the x-ray target.

section interval The distance between the fulcrum levels.

section thickness The width of the focal plane, which is controlled by the exposure angle.

self-induction The ability of an alternating current to switch directions, causing an opposing potential difference to induce against the incoming supply of electrons; allows direct current to flow while at the same time hindering alternating current.

self-rectification Suppressed rectification resulting from only half of the incoming alternating current being converted to pulsating direct current; called half-wave rectification.

semiconductor A material that allows electrons to flow freely under certain conditions (conductor) or that inhibits electron flow under certain conditions (insulator).

sensitivity speck An impurity added to silver halide crystals (usually gold-silver sulfide) to act as an electrode that attracts free silver ions during latent image formation.

sensitometer An instrument designed to expose a reproducible, uniform, optical step wedge onto a film.

sensitometric curve A radiographic relationship between the amount of exposure and the resultant density on the film; also known as characteristic curve, D log E curve, and Hurter and Driffield curve.

sensitometry The measurement of the characteristic responses of film to exposure and processing.

series circuit An electric circuit designed to send electrons through various resistance devices by linking them one after the other.

sharpness One of the geometric properties of image quality; the degree of geometric sharpness or accuracy of structural lines actually recorded in the image; also referred to as detail, definition, recorded detail, and spatial resolution.

shell The energy level occupied by an electron determined by the distance from the nucleus.

shell-type transformer Arrangement of two coils of wire each filled with an iron core in proximity to facilitate induction.

shoulder supports A piece of equipment that keeps the patient from sliding off the table when the table is tilted head down.

sievert (Sv) The product of the absorbed dose in gray and the radiation weighting factor.

signal-to-noise ratio The quantity of incoming information compared to the level of random background information.

silicon-controlled rectifier (SCR) A complex semiconductor useful for high-speed switching of the primary high-voltage x-ray circuit; also known as a thyristor.

silver bromide Type of silver halide crystal used to create x-ray films.

silver chloride Type of silver halide crystal used to create x-ray films.

silver iodide Type of silver halide crystal used to create x-ray films.

silver iodobromide Type of silver halide crystal used to create x-ray films.

simulator unit Specialized radiography equipment that allows verification of radiation therapy prior to actual treatment.

sine wave The type of curve produced by an AC generator.

single-phase power Power supply that allows the potential difference to drop to zero with every change in the direction of current flow.

single-photon absorptiometry (SPA) The first bone densitometer to be used clinically; offered a single energy measurement and utilized a sealed radionuclide source (I^{125}).

single x-ray absorptiometry (SXA) A modification of the SPA forearm scanner, but instead of a radioactive source it used x-rays.

slip ring A device with attached brushes that allows the circuit to remain stationary while the armature rotates without breaking the electrical contact between them.

soft copy Images visualized on monitors, either flat panel technology or older cathode ray tubes.

solar converter A device that converts solar photons to electrical energy.

solarization The process of reducing the intensity of the latent image, producing less density.

solenoid A coil consisting of a series of loops, which serve to increase the flux density.

solvent Chemicals used in developing film suspended in water.

somatic Describes the effects of radiation that appear in the individual who was irradiated.

space charge cloud The ejection of electrons from the surface of the wire due to increased heat, causing an electron cloud; also called thermionic emission.

space charge effect As more and more electrons build up in the area of the filament, their negative charges begin to oppose the emission of additional electrons.

spatial resolution One of the geometric properties of image quality; the degree of geometric sharpness or accuracy of structural lines actually recorded in the image; also referred to as detail, definition, sharpness, and recoded detail. In digital images, it can be expressed in terms of three dimensions of the image.

specific absorption rate (SAR) The absorption of RF radiation.

SPECT Acronym for single photon emission computed tomography.

spectral emission An indication of the precise wavelength of light emitted by the phosphor.

speed exposure point The log exposure that will produce the speed point for a given film.

speed point The point on the D log E curve where a density of OD 1.0 + b + f is achieved.

spin magnetic moment The magnetic effect created by electrons spinning on their axes.

static discharge The result of electrons jumping the gap between two objects, one negatively charged and one positively charged, resulting in the equalization of the charges of the two objects.

stationary anode An anode assembly that is immobile.

stator Induction-motor electromagnets that turn the anode.

step wedge A type of penetrometer that is wedge shaped and has different levels or steps.

step-down transformer A device used to decrease the voltage from the primary to the secondary coil.

step-up transformer A device used to increase the voltage from the primary to the secondary coil.

stereotactic irradiation A noninvasive procedure that delivers a high dose of radiation to a very conformed stereotactically defined target volume.

stochastic effects Results of radiation exposure for which no threshold dose of radiation exists (e.g., cancer, genetic effects).

straight-line portion The useful range of densities on the D log E curve.

string theory The idea that matter behaves differently depending on the vibration of the string-like matter.

structural protective barriers Fixed x-ray facilities that are constructed of materials having effective x-ray attenuating properties and are of thickness sufficient to reduce exposures to desired levels.

subject contrast The degree of differential absorption resulting from the differing absorption characteristics of the tissues in the body.

subject density The impact the subject (patient) has on the resulting radiographic density.

subject detail The impact that the position of the structures of interest within the body has on the recorded detail.

subject distortion The impact that the position of the structures of interest within the body has on distortion.

substance A material that has a definite and constant composition.

superadditivity When two reducing agents are combined, forming a PQ developer, their reducing ability is the sum of their independent abilities.

supercoat A layer of hard, protective gelatin designed to prevent the soft emulsion underneath from being physically or chemically abused due to handling.

superconductor A material that allows electrons to flow freely.

surface coil An RF coil shaped to conform to the body part being imaged.

Système International d'Unités (SI units) An international system of units based on the metric system.

T

T_1 The time required for precessing spins to align with the constant external magnetic field to 63 percent of the maximum possible strength.

T_2 The time required after precessing spins have aligned at an angle to the external magnetic field due to an RF pulse for them to lose 63 percent of their coherence due to interactions between the spins.

target The portion of the anode where the high-voltage electron stream will impact.

target interaction The actions that take place when the electrons strike their target or focal spot.

targeting A magnification technique that permits an area of interest to be selected for reformatting.

technetium (Tc) An ideal radiopharmaceutical.

temperature A measure of thermal energy.

temperature control system The part of the automatic processing unit that maintains all three solutions at compatible temperatures.

10-day rule The practice of waiting 10 days after a woman's menstrual flow to conduct a radiographic examination or study.

tesla (T) The unit used for measuring magnetic flux density.

therapeutic Methods used to treat and rehabilitate a disease, disorder, or traumatic injury.

thermal energy The result of the motion of atoms and molecules; also known as heat.

thermionic emission The ejection of electrons from the surface of the wire due to increased heat, causing an electron cloud; also called the space charge cloud.

thermoluminescent dosimeter (TLD) Small chips of thermoluminescent material, usually lithium fluoride. When exposed to radiation, the chips enter a metastable state; when exposed to heat they give off visible light.

Thoreaus filter A type of compound filter consisting of tin, copper, and aluminum, in that order, typically used in radiation therapy.

three-phase six-pulse A full-wave rectification produces a voltage ripple that produces six usable pulses per cycle.

threshold detection A visual phenomenon involving the perception of extremely small or faint details.

thyristor A complex semiconductor useful for high-speed switching of the primary high-voltage x-ray circuit; also known as a silicon-controlled rectifier (SCR).

tilting A piece of equipment that is movable and can be angled according to need.

time of inversion The time period between the 180° inversion pulse and the 90° excitation pulse in an IR sequence.

timer Device used to end the exposure at an accurately measured preset time.

tomographic amplitude The total distance the tube travels; tomographic arc or tomographic angle.

tomography A radiographic technique that employs motion to show anatomical structures lying in a plane of tissue while blurring or eliminating the detail in images of structures above and below the plane of interest.

tomography unit Specialized radiography equipment that allows movement in an arc during exposure.

total brightness gain A measurement of the increase in image intensity achieved by an image intensification tube.

total filtration The sum of inherent and added filtration.

total repeat rate A figure that is calculated as a percentage of the total number of images produced during the period of the study.

transducer the device that emits and receives the a sound wave for use in ultrasound.

transformer A device in which two coils are placed near one another without electrical connection. The number of turns in the coils differs, causing a change in current in the secondary coil; this serves to either increase or decrease the voltage.

transformer law When the voltage is increased from primary to secondary it is called a step-up transformer. When the voltage is decreased from primary to secondary it is called a step-down transformer; expressed as

$$\frac{V_s}{V_p} = \frac{N_s}{N_p}.$$

transport system Part of the automatic processing system designed to move a film through the developer, fixer, wash, and dryer sections of the processor.

trough filter A type of compensating filter used to even out densities such as in the mediastinum.

T-score Marks how far a patient's BMD is deviated from the mean of a sex-matched young adult population (ages 20–35) of individuals who have reached their peak bone mass.

tube rating chart Provides a guide regarding the most common technical factor combinations that can be used without overloading the tube.

tuberculosis Infection by mycobacteria, causing inflammation of the lungs.

tumor An abnormal new growth in tissue.

U

unsharpness Lack of sharp definition of fine detail.

urologic unit Specialized radiography equipment that allows study of the urological and genital structures.

V

vacuum A space from which air has been removed.

valence The chemical combining characteristic of an element; determined by the number of electrons in the outermost shell.

valence energy band The outermost (sometimes the next-to-outermost) orbital shell.

visual acuity The ability of the eye to resolve detail.

volt (V) The unit of potential difference.

voltage (V) The unit of potential difference.

voltage ripple The net voltage produced during full-wave rectification.

voltmeter A device used to measure current connected in parallel; measures potential difference in volts.

W

washing The process of using water to remove as much of the fixer and developer solutions as possible.

wavelength The distance between two successive points on a wave.

Weber (Wb) SI unit used to measure magnetic flux.

wedge filter A type of compensating filter used to even out densities such as in the foot or lower extremities.

weight The force that an object exerts under the influence of gravity.

window A structure where the primary x-ray beams exits the envelope, which allows less absorption or scatter of photons.

window level The digital processing that produces changes in density/brightness.

window width The digital processing that produces changes in the range of density/brightness, which can be used to control contrast.

windowing A point processing operation that changes the contrast and brightness of the image on the monitor.

wiring The parts within the cathode assembly that connect the elements of the assembly together.

X

x-ray quality A measurement of the penetrating ability of the x-ray beam.

x-ray quantity A measure of the number of x-ray photons in the useful beam.

Z

Z number The number of nuclear protons in an atom, unique to each element; also known as the atomic number.

Z-score Marks how far a patient's BMD is deviated from the mean; conceptually similar to a T-score, except the reference population is matched by the patient's age.

zero potential A neutral reference point for discussing charges. The earth is defined as zero; also known as ground potential.

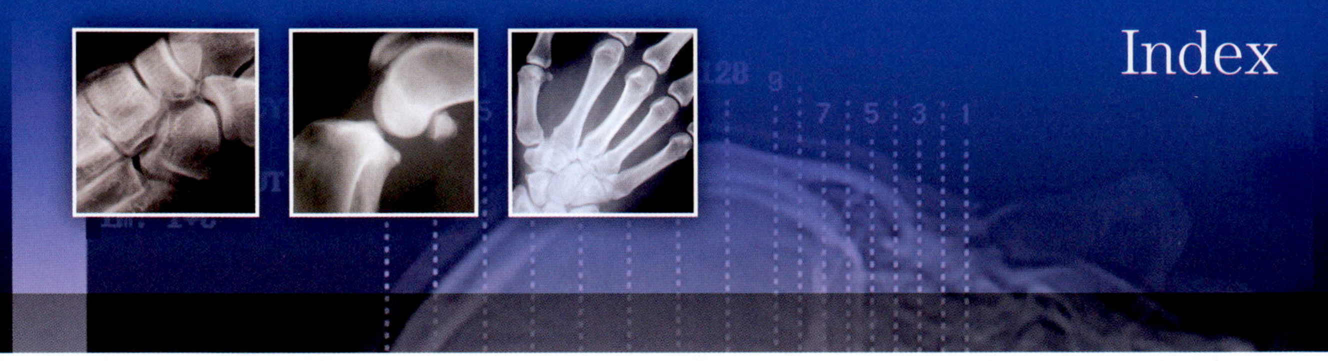

Index

A

A, 17
a, 17
ABC, 540
Abdominal radiography
  additive conditions, 252
  destructive conditions, 253–254
  human body as attenuator, 241–243
ABS, 540
Abscess, 250
Absolute value, 8
Absorbed dose, 1403
AC, 46
Acceptance limits, 381–384
Accreditation, 468
Acetic acid, 288
AC generator, 71
Acromegaly, 252
Activator
  developing, 287
  fixing, 288
Active osteomyelitis, 254
Activity, 146
Actual focal spot, 115
ADC, 540
Added filtration, 171
Addition and subtraction principle, 14
Addition sign (+), 9
Additive conditions, 247, 250–252
Adhesive, 276
Admittance, 49
Adult part thickness, 490
Advisory groups, 156
AEC systems, 490
  mammography, 570–571
  mobile radiography, 527
  performance monitoring, 475–476
Aerophagia, 253
Afterglow, 311
AGC, 540
Agfa relative speed film/screen combination chart, 317
Air, 242
Air core transformer, 79
Air-gap technique, 269–270
Air kerma, 143
ALARA, 158–159
Algebra, 8–16
Algebraic expressions, 10–12, 13
Aliasing, 429
Alignment, 449–453
Alpha particles, 141
Alternating current (AC), 47
Alternating-current induction motors, 75
Alternating-current motors, 76
Ammeter, 78
Ampère, André, 47
Ampere (A), 17, 47
Ampere (amp), 47
Amplitude, 34
amu, 26–27
Analyzing the image. *See also* individual subject headings
  art of image critique, 458–466
  contrast, 403–423
  density, 380–402
  distortion, 442–457

imaging process, 375–385
quality management, 467–484
recorded detail, 424–441
Anatomically programmed radiography (APR), 490
Anatomical part size (thickness). *See* Part size (thickness)
Angiographic tables, 611–612
Angstrom, 34
Angulation, 453
Annihilation reaction, 199
Anode, 45, 84, 113–118
Anode assembly, 113–120
Anode cooling charts, 125
Anode heel effect, 117–118, 394, 417
Anode warm-up procedure, 115
Anorexia nervosa, 253
Antihalation coating, 275
Antique full-body radiograph, 242
Aortic aneurysm, 252
Approximate values, 5
APR, 490
Archaeological radiography, 228–229
Archiving, 288
Arithmetic, 3–8
Armature, 71
Artifacts, 316
CT scan, 639, 641
Artificial permanent magnets, 62
Artistic radiography, 227
Art restoration, 228
Ascites, 252
Aseptic necrosis, 254
Asymmetrical screens, 314
Atelectasis, 251
Atom, 22
Atomic clock, 17
Atomic mass, 27–28
Atomic mass number, 27
Atomic mass unit (amu), 27
Atomic number, 25
Atomic particles, 25–27
Atomic theory, 24–32
Atrophy, 253
Attenuation, 241, 247. *See also* Pathological conditions
Attenuation unsharpness, 435
atto-, 17
Atwood, Margaret, 283
Automatic brightness control (ABC), 540
Automatic brightness stabilization (ABS), 540
Automatic collimation, 236–237
Automatic dose control (ADC), 540
Automatic exposure control. *See* AEC systems
anatomically programmed radiography, 511
collimation, 510
configurations, 507
creative positioning, 511
density control, 509
ionization chambers, 507–508
positioning skills, 509–512
subject density, 509–510
timing, 510
Automatic exposure controls, 104–107
Automatic exposure control timers, 98
Automatic film handling systems, 280–281
Automatic film processing, 288–290
circulation system, 290
dryer system, 289
replenishment system, 289–290
temperature control system, 290
transport system, 288–289
Automatic gain control (AGC), 540
Automatic radiographic processing chemicals, 285
Automatic radiographic processor systems, 289
Autotransformer, 80
Average gradient, 303

B

Back-projection, 635–636
Backscatter radiation, 197–198
Backup time, 105
Barium, 30
Barium-filled colon, 291
Base, 6, 275–276
Base plus fog, 298
Battery-operated mobile generator, 102–103
Beam hardening artifacts, 641
Beam restriction, 233–239, 396, 418
ancillary devices, 238
collimator, 236–237

Beam restriction (*continued*)
 cones and cylinders, 237–238
 controlling scatter, 234–236
 irradiated material, 235–236
 kilovoltage (kVp), 234–235
Becquerel (Bq), 17, 145
Beryllium, 578
Beta particles, 141
Bias focusing, 571–572
Bilateral pneumonia, 248
Binding energy, 27, 28, 30
Biological research, 227
Bit system, 488
Blooming, 368
Blur, 551
Blur edges, 551
Blur margins, 551
Bocage, André Edmund, 548, 549
Body section radiography, 549
Bohr, Niels, 24
Bone, 243
Bone densitometry, 589–603
 bone science, 591–592
 diagnostic criteria, 595
 DXA principles, 596, 597
 femur, 596–597
 forearm, 600–601
 historical overview, 589–590
 k-edge filtered, 596
 osteoporosis, 592–594
 quality control, 601
 radiation safety, 601
 scan analysis, 596
 spine, 598–600
Boundary effect, 224
Boveri, Theodor, 29
Bowel obstruction, 254
Bow tie filter, 644
Bq, 17, 145
Breast (anatomy), 569
Breast images. *See* Mammography
Bremsstrahlung interactions, 130–131
Bremsstrahlung photons, 131
Brightness, 387
Brightness control, 540
Brightness gain, 538
British (foot-pound-second) system, 16
Bronchiectasis, 251
Bucky, 263
Bucky, Gustav, 92, 259
"Bucky Diaphragm Principle Applied to Roentgenography, The" (Potter), 257
Bucky tray, 92
Bucky unit, 93

C

C, 17
c, 17
Calcified stones, 252
Caliper, 490
Candela (cd), 17
Capacitor, 81
Capacitor discharge mobile generator, 99
Carbon, 30
Carcinoma, 254
Cardiac Cine CT, 621
Cardiomegaly, 251
Carlton, Richard, 506
C-arm tube suspension system, 93
Carriage, 534–535
Carroll, Quinn, 488
Case studies
 barium-filled colon, 293
 calcified tumor-like mass (abdomen), 423
 dead animal, 245
 ghostly plant, 558
 horizontal lines/dripping marks, 520
 unidentified flying object in skull, 107
 white snakes, 272
Cassette cleaning, 476
Cassettes and holders, 315
Cassette spot imaging, 543
Cathode, 45, 84, 109
Cathode assembly, 109–113
Cathode focusing cup, 112–113
Cathode ray tube (CRT) imaging, 280
CAT scan. *See* Computed tomography (CT)
Caudad, 452

CCD, 541
cd, 17
CDRH, 468
Ceiling suspension, 92
Center for Devices and Radiological Health (CDRH), 468
centi-, 17
Centimeter (cm), 18
Central ray, 449–450
Cephalad, 452
CGS system, 16–18
Characteristic cascade, 196
Characteristic curve, 298
Characteristic interactions, 132–133
Characteristic peak, 134
Characteristic photons, 132, 194
Characteristic x-rays, 578
Charge-coupled device (CCD), 541
Chatfield, Paul, 724
Chemical energy, 32
Chemical fog, 284
Chemical precipitation silver recovery unit, 291
Chest radiography
  additive conditions, 251
  destructive conditions, 253
  distortion, 526
Chronic osteomyelitis, 252, 255
Ci, 17, 145
Cine CT, 622
Cine film systems, 542
Circuit breaker, 56
Circular tomographic motions, 555
Circulation system, 290
Cirrhosis, 252
Clearing agent, 288
Clearing time, 288
ClearPb, 174, 175
Closed-core transformer, 78
cm, 18
Coating, 278
Coercivity, 78
Coherent scattering, 196
Cold water processors, 290
Collimation, 163, 236–237
Collimator pitch, 622
Commutator, 71
Commutator ring, 71
Compensation filtration, 173–174
Compound filtration, 172–173
Compression band, 92
Compton, Arthur H., 191, 197–198
Compton effect, 196
Compton electron, 197–198
Compton interaction, 258
Compton scattered photon, 197–198
Compton scattering, 197–198, 199
Computation with values (numbers), 5
Computed radiography (CR), 324. *See* Digital radiography
Computed tomography (CT), 617–647
  algorithms, 641
  artifacts, 639, 641
  back-projection, 635–636
  computer, 631–632
  contrast, 638
  convolution, 636–638
  CTDI, 644
  CT number, 633
  deconvolution, 636–637
  density, 638
  detectors, 627–630
  3-D imaging, 633
  display console, 632–633
  exposure factors, 640–641
  Fourier transform, 635–636
  gantry, 626–627
  helical scanner, 622–625
  historical overview, 619–626
  Hounsfield unit (HU), 633
  image quality, 638–639
  image reconstruction, 636–638
  magnification, 639
  motion, 641
  MSAD, 644
  MSCT/MDCT units, 625–626
  noise, 639
  radiation protection, 643–644
  reformatting, 638
  resolution, 639
  scan field size, 641

Computed tomography (CT) (*continued*)
 scanner generations, 619–626
 scanogram/sinogram, 632
 section interval/thickness, 641
 table, 627
 x-ray tube s, 627
Computed tomography dose index (CTDI), 643
Conductance, 49
Conduction band, 49
Conductor, 46, 47
Cone, 237–238
Cone cell, 222
Cone field size, 237
Congestive heart failure, 251
Conklin, William, 227
Contact surgical radiography, 280
Contamination, 288
Continuing education, 470
Contrast, 301–305, 403–423
 anatomical part size, 418
 anode heel effect, 418
 beam restriction, 418
 defined, 404
 distance, 418
 evaluating, 411–416
 factors to consider, 416–419, 418
 filtration, 418
 focal spot size, 418
 grids, 418
 image receptor, 418
 image receptor contrast, 407–409
 irradiated material, 411
 kilovoltage (kVp), 409–411, 412–416, 416–419
 manipulating, 406–407
 mAs, 418
 processing, 418
 subject, 409–411
 terminology, 404–407
Contrast improvement factor (K), 265
Contrast index, 304
Contrast mask, 412
Contrast medium injection devices, 613–615
Contrast perception, 222, 225
Conversions. *See* Exposure conversion problems; Mathematical conversions
Convolution, 636–637
Coolidge, William D., 111, 204, 403
Coolidge tube, 111
Cooling curves, 125–126
Copper loss, 77
Cormack, Allan, 617
Corrective action adjustments, 462
Coulehan, Jack, 230
Coulomb (C), 17
Covalent bond, 28, 33
cps, 17, 71
Creating the image, 219–370. *See also* individual subject headings
 beam restriction, 233–239
 digital image management, 362–372
 film processing, 283–293
 film/screen combinations, 316–319
 film sensitometry, 294–307
 grid, 257–272
 human body as attenuator, 241–253
 intensifying screens, 308–322
 pathology problem, 246–256 (*See also* Pathological conditions)
 patient and image quality, 243–244
 patient as beam emitter, 240–245
 radiographic film, 273–282
 vision and perception, 220–232
Criss-cross grid, 262
Critiquing an image. *See* Image critique
Crossover effect, 275
Crossover network, 289
CR system. *See* Digital radiography
CRT monitor, 367–369, 541
Crystal production, 276–277
CT bow tie filter, 644
CT computer, 631–632
CT detectors, 627–630
CTDI, 643
CT imaging detail, 639
CT magnification, 639
CT number, 633
CT pitch formulas, 622–625
CT scan. *See* Computed tomography (CT)
CT solid-state detectors, 630–631
CT table, 627
Cupping artifacts, 641
Curie (Ci), 17, 145

Current, 47–48
Curvilinear tomography, 555
Cycles per second (cps), 17, 71
Cylinder, 237

D

d, 17
da, 17
Daguerre, Louis, 274
Dalton, John, 24
Darkroom, 290–291
Darkroom plan, 291
Darkroom safelights, 290–291
Daylight vision, 222
DC, 47
DC generator, 73
Dead animal, 245
deci-, 17
Decimal number place values, 4
Decimals, 4–5
Deconvolution, 636–637
Decreased attenuation, 250–252. *See also* Pathological conditions
Decreased contrast, 407
Definition. *See* Recorded detail
Degenerative arthritis, 254
Degree, 453
deka-, 17
Densitometer, 297
Density, 241, 380–402
  anatomical part size, 396–398
  anode heel effect, 394
  beam restriction, 396
  defined, 387
  distance, 394–396
  film processing, 399
  filtration, 396
  focal spot size, 394
  grids, 398
  image receptor, 398–399, 399
  kilovoltage (kVp), 391–393
  mAs, 388–391
Depletion, 288
Der Zauberberg (Mann), 59, 442
Destructive conditions, 247, 253–255
Detail. *See* Recorded detail
Detail extremity radiography, 280
Deterministic effects, 156
Developer contamination, 286–287
Developer hardener, 287–288
Developing the film, 284–287
Diagnosing/treating the image, 380–381
Diagnostic medical sonography
  acoustic impendance, 735–736
  attenuation, 735–736
  attenuation coefficient, 735
  decibels, 735
  display, 743
  Doppler, 737
  field, 736
  harmonics, 737
  historical overview, 725
  instrumentation, 741–743
  orientation, 725
  pulser, 741
  range, 736
  receiver, 742
  scan converter, 742–743
  sound waves
    parameters, 728–732
    types, 732–735
    variables, 727–728
  storage media, 743
  transducer, 738–741
Diagnostic x-ray console controls, 99
Diamagnetic materials, 65
Dielectric, 81
Digital angiography, 632
Digital cineradiography, 609
Digital fluoroscopy, 542, 543
Digital image histogram, 389
Digital image management, 362–372
  dry processor, 367
  hard-copy display, 366–367
  image acquisition, 363
  image display, 366–369
  image distribution, 365–366
  laser printer, 366
  monitor, 367–369
  PACS, 363

Digital image management (*continued*)
soft-copy display, 367–369
storage, 367–369
Digital image receptor systems, 213, 437
Digital imaging recorded detail. *See* Recorded detail
Digital mammography, 622–623
Digital radiography
artifacts, 356–358
computer radiography, 339–352
data manipulation, 345–352
data reading, 341–345
defective quamtum efficiency, 333
digital image characteristics, 325–326
digital image formation, 324–327
direct detectors, 353
exposure factor selection, 335–339
exposure index, 333–335
exposure indicators, 333–339
flat panel radigraphy, 353–355
grid use, 352
high-pass filtering, 330
historical overview, 324
image acquisition, 340
image processing operations, 327–332, 355
image quality, 332–333
indirect detectors, 353–355
latent image production, 340–341
local processing, 330–332
noise, 333
photostimulable imaging plates, 339–340
point processing, 327–330
resolution, 332–333
spatial domains, 327
Digital sampling, 427
Digital storage of images, 369–370
Digital subtraction angiography (DSA), 609, 632
Digital tomosynthesis, 555, 556
Dimensional analysis, 7–8
Diode, 82
Direct current (DC), 47
Direct-current motors, 75
Direct exposure film, 280
Direction, 452
Directly proportional, 16
Direct square law, 186
Direct variation, 16
Distance, 179–182
contrast, 418
density, 394–396
mobile radiography, 528–529
patient dose, 211
recorded detail, 432–433
size distortion, 446–447
Distortion, 244, 442–457
alignment, 449–453
anatomical part size, 450–452
angulation, 453
central ray, 449–450
defined, 443
degree, 453
direction, 452
distance, 446–447
image receptor, 452
OID, 445–446
shape, 449–453, 455
SID, 444
size, 443–448, 453
Distributive law, 10
D log E curve, 299, 407–408
Dmax, 299
Dose equivalent, 145, 157
Dose limits, 157
Dosimeter, 148–150
Dosimetry reporting, 152
Double-coated film, 276
Double wedge, 173
Drive system, 289
Dryer system, 289
Drying the film, 287
Dry processor, 367
DSA, 609, 632
Dual-field intensifiers, 538
Dual-filament wiring, 111
Dual focus, 110
Duplicating film, 280
Duplication process, 280
Duplitized, 276
Dwell time, 291
Dynamic range, 477
Dynamometer, 76

E

Eagan, Robert, 562
Eastman, Terry, 488
Eb, 27
EBT, 622
Eddy current loss, 78
Edema, 250
Edge enhancement, 224
Edge spread function (ESF), 425
Edison, Thomas A., 309, 534
"Edison and Roentgenology" (Fuchs), 533–547
Effective focal spot, 115
Einstein, Albert, 2, 22
Electrical circuit, 46
Electrical energy, 33
Electric current, 45
Electric fields, 44
Electricity, 33, 39–58
  current, 47–48
  electrical circuit, 45
  electrification, 41–44
  electrodynamics, 45–53
  electrostatics, 40–45
  Ohm's law, 51–53
  parallel circuits, 53–56
  potential difference, 48
  resistance, 48–50
  series circuits, 53–56
Electrification, 41–44
Electrification by contact, 43
Electrification by friction, 43
Electrification by induction, 44
Electrodynamics, 45–53
Electrolysis, 45
Electrolytic silver recovery unit, 291
Electromagnet, 62, 68
Electromagnetic energy, 33
Electromagnetic induction, 68–70
Electromagnetic radiation (EM), 33, 141
Electromagnetic relays, 68
Electromagnetic spectrum, 33, 34
Electromagnetism, 59–89
  autotransformer, 80–81
  capacitor, 81
  electromagnetic induction, 68–70
  Faraday's law, 68
  Fleming's hand rules, 66
  generator, 70–74
  Lenz's law, 69
  magnet, 62
  magnetic classification of materialism, 64
  magnetic induction, 63
  magnetism, 60–64
  motor, 74–76
  Oersted's experiment, 65
  rectification, 81–84
  solenoid, 68
  transformer, 76–80
Electromotive force (emf), 48
Electron, 25–27
Electron beam tomography (EBT), 622
Electron binding energy (Eb), 27
Electron volt (eV), 28
Electroscope, 43
Electrostatics, 40–45
Elliptical tomographic motions, 555
Elon, 285
Elongation, 448, 451
Emaciation, 253
Emission spectrum, 133–136, 316
Emphysema, 253
Empyema, 251
EM radiation, 33, 141
Emulsion, 276
Energy
  chemical, 32
  defined, 22
  electrical, 33 (*See also* Electricity)
  electromagnetic, 33
  heat, 32
  kinetic, 32
  mechanical, 32
  nuclear, 33
  potential, 32
  thermal, 32–33
Entrance rollers, 289
Entrance skin exposure (ESE), 208
Envelope, 120–121
Equation, 14–16
Equipment malfunctions, 463. *See* Troubleshooting
Equipment motion, 437

Equipment performance evaluation. *See* Monitoring equipment performance
Equivalence principles, 14
Equivalent dose, 146
Equivalent equations, 14
erg, 17
ESE, 208
ESF, 425
esu, 17
eV, 28
Evaluating algebraic expressions, 13
Exact values, 5
Excitation, 33
"Experiences with the Roentgen-ray tube" (Coolidge), 108
Exponent, 6
Exposure, 143
Exposure amplitude, 551
Exposure conversion problems, 515
Exposure maintenance formula, 395, 515
Exposure maintenance rules, 515
Exposure switch, 97–98
Exposure systems, 485–521
  anatomically programmed radiography, 490
  anatomical part thickness, 490
  automatic exposure control (AEC), 490
  complex exposure problems, 517–519
  conversion problems, 515
  fixed kVp systems, 492–496
  technique chart, 491
  variable kVp systems, 496–502 (*See also* Variable kilovoltage systems)
Exposure time reduction, 437–438, 438
Extended film processing, 620–621
External beam evaluation, 471
Extrafocal radiation, 122
Eye (anatomy), 222
Eye movement, 225

F

f, 17
Falling load generators, 103–104
Farad, 81
Faraday, Michael, 68
Faraday's law, 68, 655
Fast spin echo (FSE), 685–686
Fat, 242
Father of Radiologic Technology, The (Jerman), 386, 458
FDA, 156
femto-, 17
Fermi, Enrico, 674
Ferromagnetic materials, 63
Fibrosarcoma, 254
Field survey instruments, 147
15 percent rule, 183, 390, 515
Fifth generation CT units, 622
Figure eight, 555
Filament, 110–111
Filament circuit, 83, 98
Film. *See* Radiographic film
Film badge dosimeter, 149
Film base, 275–276
Film characteristics, 299–306
Film contrast, 301–305, 406. *See also* Contrast
Film density, 180–182. *See* Density
Film graininess, 299
Film identification, 281
Film laser camera, 366–369
Film processing, 283–293, 399
  activator, 287
  archiving, 287
  automatic processing, 288–290 (*See also* Automatic film processing)
  chemicals, 286
  clearing agent, 287
  contamination, 287
  darkroom, 290–291
  depletion, 287
  developing, 284–287
  drying, 287
  fixing, 287–288
  hardener, 287–288
  overview, 286
  preservative, 287
  reducing agents, 284–286
  restrainer, 287
  silver recovery systems, 291
  solvent, 287
  washing, 287

Film resolution, 299
Film/screen combinations, 316–319, 435–437
  contrast, 319
  emission spectra, 316
  latitude, 319
  resolution, 318–319
  speed, 316
Film/screen contact tests, 476
Film/screen image receptor systems, 212
Film sensitometry, 294–307
  densitometer, 297
  D log E curve, 299
  film characteristics, 299–306
  penetrometer, 295
  sensitometer, 295–297
Film speed, 299–301
Film storage and handling, 280
Filter, 171
Filtration, 162, 171–177, 212, 396, 418
  added, 171
  compensation, 174
  compound, 172–173
  defined, 171
  effect of, 175
  HVL, 171
  inherent, 172
  measurement, 171–172
  total, 175
Fine-detail intensifying screen, 312
First-generation CT scanners, 619–621
First law of electromagnetics, 69
Fixed kilovoltage systems, 488, 492–496
  advantages/disadvantages, 492–493
  optimal kilovoltage peak, 493
  technique chart, 496
Fixed kVp technique chart, 496
Fixed tables, 92
Fixer hardeners, 287
Fixing, 287–288
Fix-queue, 477
Flat contact shields, 163
Flat panel LCD monitor, 369–370
Fleming, John, 65
Fleming's hand rules, 66
Fleming's left-hand motor rule, 75
Fleming's right-hand generator rule, 70, 71
Fleming's right-hand thumb rule, 66
Flood replenishment, 289
Floor suspension system, 93
Floor-to-ceiling suspension system, 93
Fluorescence, 311
Fluoro carriage, 534–535
Fluoroscopic generators, 540
Fluoroscopic mA range, 535–536
Fluoroscopic R/min charts, 207
Fluoroscopic spot filming, 280
Fluoroscopic x-ray tubes, 535–536
Fluoroscopy (fluoro), 533–547
  anode/output screen, 538
  brightness control, 540
  CCD, 541
  cine film systems, 542
  contrast, 540
  digital fluoroscopy, 542, 543
  distortion, 541
  electrostatic lenses, 537–538
  generators, 540
  historical overview, 534
  image control, 540–541
  image intensification tubes, 536–540
  input screen, 536–537
  isodose curve, 544
  magnification tubes, 537–538
  mA range, 535–536
  mobile units, 543, 579
  performance monitoring, 473–474
  quantum mottle, 541
  radiation protection, 543–544
  recording the image, 542–543
  resolution, 540
  static spot imaging systems, 542–543
  total brightness gain, 538–539
  types of equipment, 534–535
  uses, 534
  video camera tube, 541–542
  video monitor, 542
  video recording, 542
  viewing systems, 541–542
  x-ray tubes, 535–536
Flux density, 62
Flux gain, 539
Focal plane, 552

Focal spot, 115
Focal spot size, 117–118, 394, 418, 433–435
Focal track, 1125
Focused grid, 262
Focusing cup, 112–113
FOCUS-PDCA method, 468
Fog, 410
FONAR, 649
Food and Drug Administration (FDA), 156
Forensic radiography, 228
Foreshortening, 448, 451
Forgiving film, 304
Formulae, 13
4-5 cm rule, 515
Fourier algorithm, 635–636
Fourier transform, 635–636
Fourth-generation CT units, 621–622
Fractional focal spot, 117–118
Fractions, 3
Frequency, 35
Fuchs, Arthur W., 273, 487, 488, 490
Fulcrum, 552
Full-wave rectification, 86–87
Fundamentals of Radiology (Squire), 226, 459
Fundamental units, 17
Fuse, 56

G

G, 17, 62
Gadolinium, 312
Gadolinium oxysulfide, 619
Galvanometer, 78
Gamma, 302
Gamma rays, 33, 141
Gauss, Johann, 62
Gauss (G), 17, 62
GCF, 264–265
Gd-DTPA, 696
Geiger-Mueller survey instruments, 147, 692–693
Gelatin, 276
Generator, 70–74, 99–104
Genetically significant dose (GSD), 142
Genetic effects, 142
Geometric problems, 461
giga-, 17
Gilbert, William, 64
Glare, 368
Glass envelope, 120
Glasser, Otto, 140, 155
Glutaraldehyde, 287, 290
Gonadal shielding, 163, 212
Good contrast, 404
Gout, 254
Gray (Gy), 17, 143
Gray scale bit depth, 365–366, 404
Grenz ray radiography, 228
Grid. *See also* Radiographic grid
  contrast, 418
  density, 398
  mammography, 617
  mobile radiography, 529–530
  patient dose, 213–214
Grid-biased tubes, 113
Grid cassette, 263
Grid conversion factor (GCF), 264–265
Grid cut-off, 262
Grid errors, 265–269
Grid frequency, 261–262
Grid ratio, 260–261
Grid ratio conversion, 516
Grid ratio conversion formula, 515
Grids, 162, 213–214
Grossman principle, 552
Grubbe, Emil H., 704
GSD, 142
Gurney-Mott theory, 278–279
Gy, 17, 143
Gyromagnetic (magnetogyric) ratio, 654

H

h, 17
Halation, 275
Halation effect, 275
Half-value layer (HVL), 171
Half-wave rectification, 84–85
Hamadryas baboon mummy, 229
Hamlet (Shakespeare), 523

Hand generator effect rules, 66
Hand motor principle rules, 66
Hand thumb rules, 66
Hard-copy display, 366–367
Hardener
developing, 287–288
fixing, 287
Hardening the beam, 171
Heat, 33, 51
Heat exchanger, 290
Heat production, 130
Heat unit (HU), 125
Heat unit rectification constants, 1215
hecto-, 17
Helical scanner, 622
Hemothorax, 251
Hendee, William R., 467
Hertz (Hz), 17, 35, 71
High contrast, 404, 407
High-frequency generators, 101–102
High-frequency grids, 263
High-speed intensifying screen, 312
Hippocrates, 561
HIS, 363
Histogram, 390
History of the American Society of X-Ray Technicians (Hoing), 627
Hittorf-Crookes tube, 36
Hospital information system (HIS), 363
Hounsfield, Godfrey N., 619, 633
Hounsfield unit (HU), 633
Housing cooling charts, 125–126, 126
HU, 125, 633
Human eye, 222
Human visual ability, 223
Hurter and Driffield (H&D) curves, 298
Hydrocephalus, 252
Hydrogen, 30, 31
Hydroquinone, 286–287, 290, 302
Hydrothorax, 251
Hyperparathyroidism, 255
Hypocycloidal motion, 555
Hypothesis activation, 381
Hypothesis evaluation, 381
Hysteresis loss, 77
Hz, 17, 35, 71

I

ICRP, 156
Identity, 14
Illuminator (view box), 476
Image acquisition, 376–370
Image analysis, 378–380. *See also* Analyzing the image
Image archiving, 377
Image contrast, 404. *See also* Contrast
Image control, 540–541
Image creation. *See* Creating the image
Image critique, 458–466
cause of problem, 459–460
classification of image, 459
corrective action adjustments, 463
form, 462
Image critique form, 462
Image density/brightness, 387. *See also* Density
Image display, 366–369, 377–378
Image intensification tubes, 536–540
Image perception, 221–226
Image processing, 377
Image receptor, 163–164
contrast, 418
density, 398–399, 399
digital system, 213
distortion, 452
mobile radiography, 530
recorded detail, 435–437
Image receptor contrast, 407–409
Image storage, 370
Imaging noise, 427
Imaging process, 375–385
acceptance limits, 381–384
diagnosing/treating the image, 380–381
image acquisition, 376–370
image analysis, 378–380
image archiving, 377
image display, 377–378
image processing, 377
pyramid problem, 380
"I'm Looking Through You" (Lennon/McCartney), 246
Immersion time, 301
Immobilization, 209, 438

Incident electrons, 130
Incoming line current, 94–95
Increased attenuation, 250–252. *See also* Pathological conditions
Increased contrast, 407
Induction, 44
Induction motors, 76
Inductive reactance, 69
Inefficiency of medical imaging, 223
Inherent filtration, 172
Initial phantom images, 491, 493, 500
Insulator, 46, 47
Integer, 6
Integral dose, 143
"Intemperance" (Bosch), 228
Intensification factor, 313
Intensifying screen, 213, 308–322
  artifacts, 316
  asymmetrical screens, 314
  atomic number, 311
  base, 309
  care, 316
  cassettes and holders, 315
  cleaning, 316
  contrast, 314
  conversion efficiency, 310
  K-shell absorption edge, 314
  latitude, 314
  loading and storage, 316
  luminescence, 311
  phosphor layer, 310
  phosphors, 311–312
  protective coat, 310
  quantum mottle, 312–313, 313
  rare earths, 311–312
  reflective layer, 310
  resolution, 312–313
  spectral emission, 311
  speed, 313–314
Intensifying screen film, 280
"In the X-Ray Room" (Moss), 294
Inverse Fourier transformation, 635
Inversely proportional, 16
Inverse square law, 41–42, 63, 185, 395
Inverse variation, 16
Involuntary motion, 438
Iodine, 30
Ion, 27
Ionic bond, 31
Ionic solutions, 45
Ionic stage, 278
Ionization, 27
Ionization chamber instruments, 147
Ionization chambers, 104
Ionization dosimeters, 148–150
Ionizing radiation, 141–142
I^2R loss, 77
Irradiated material, 411
Iso-exposure curves, 161
Isotope, 25

J

J, 17
JCAHO, 468
Jerman, Ed C., 178, 488
Johnson, Bradley C., 627
Joint Commission on the Accreditation of Healthcare Organizations (JCAHO), 468
Jones, Robin, 627
Joule (J), 17

K

K, 17
k, 17
Kaplan, Henry, 704
K-edge filters, 173
Kelvin (K), 17
Kerma, 143
keV, 28
K factor, 265
kg, 17
Kieffer, Jean, 549
kilo-, 17
Kilo-electron volt (keV), 28
Kilogram (kg), 17
Kilovoltage peak (kVp)
  beam restriction, 234–235
  contrast, 409–411, 412–416, 417

defined, 134
density, 391–393
15 percent rule, 390
fixed kVp system, 492–496
mammography, 569
patient dose, 209–211
variable kVp system, 496–502 (*See also* Variable kilovoltage systems)
Kilovolt (kV), 18
Kinetic energy, 32
K-shell, 27–28
K-shell absorption edge, 314
kV, 18
kVp. *See* Kilovoltage peak (kVp)

L

"Lady and the Chalice, The" (Rubin), 221
Lagging loss, 77
Lambda, 34
Laminography, 549
Lanthanum oxybromide, 312
Larmor, Joseph, 649
Laser films, 280
Laser printer, 366
Laser printer calibration film, 366
Latent image formation, 278–279
Latitude, 304
Lauterbur, Paul, 649
Law of concentration of charge, 42
Law of conservation, 22
Law of distribution of charge, 42
Lawrence, Ernest O., 671
Laws of electrostatics, 41–42
Laws of exponents, 12–13
LCD monitor, 367–369
Lead, 30
Leakage radiation, 121–122
Leborgne, Raul, 562
Lenard tube, 36
Length, 17
Lenz, Heinrich, 69
Lenz's law, 69
LiF, 149
Life (Russell), 220
Lightning, 44
Like terms, 11
Linear grid, 262
Linear tomography, 555
Line-focus principle, 115–117
Line pairs per millimeter (lp/mm), 317, 425
Lines of force, 62
Line spread function (LSF), 317, 425
Literal factor, 11
Lithium fluoride (LiF), 149
Lo Dose I, 564
Lo Dose II, 564
Long bone leg length study, 450
Longitudinal angulations, 452
Longitudinal magnetization, 654
Long scale contrast, 407
Low contrast, 404, 407
lp/mm, 317, 425
LSF, 317, 425
L-shell, 27–28
Luminescence, 311
Luxel OSL dosimeter, 148

M

M, 17
m, 17
mA, 18
mA changes, 135
Mach effect, 224–225
Magnet, 61, 62
Magnetic classification of materialism, 64
Magnetic dipoles, 61
Magnetic domains, 61
Magnetic induction, 63
Magnetic poles, 63
Magnetic resonance imaging (MRI), 648–670
contrast agents, 665–666
critical imaging factors, 656–663
device labeling, 667–668
flow compensation, 664–665
gradient coils, 652–653
gradient magnetic fields, 667
historical background, 649
image contrast, 656–660

Magnetic resonance imaging (MRI) (*continued*)
  image improvement techniques, 663–665
  magnet, 649–651
  motion reduction technique, 663–664
  permanent magnets, 650
  physics, 653–656
  radiofrequency field, 667
  radio frequency subsystem, 651–653
  resistive magnets, 650
  safety and biological hazards, 666–668
  scan time, 662–663
  shhielding, 652
  signal-to-noise ratio, 661–662
  spacial resolution, 660–661
  static magnetic field, 666–667
  superconducting magnets, 651
  suppression technique, 664
  T1, 655–656
  T2, 655–656
  T*, 655–656
Magnetism, 60–64
Magnification, 443–448, 454
Magnification factor, 448
Magnification tubes, 537–538
Mammography, 280, 561–588
  AEC system, 570–571
  anode configuration, 574–575
  anode material, 575–578
  breast (anatomy), 569
  cassettes, 619
  cathode, 571–572
  characteristic x-rays, 578
  compression device, 617–618
  conventional radiography, contrasted, 568
  digital, 622–623
  exposure time, 569–670
  extended film processing, 620–621
  film, 620–621
  filtration, 578
  generator characteristics, 567–571
  grids, 617
  heel effect, 571–572
  historical overview, 562–567
  kVp, 569
  legislation, 563
  magnification, 615–617
  noise, 616
  overview (table), 569
  quality control, 624
  resolution, 622
  screen, 619–620
  screen/film combination, 621–622
  x-ray tube, 571–572
Mammography film, 620–621
Mammography grids, 617
Mammography Quality Standards Act (MQSA), 566
Mammography screens, 619–620
Mammography x-ray tube, 571
Mammography x-ray tube configurations, 575
Man-made sources of radiation, 142
mAs, 178–190, 211, 388–391, 418
mAs formula, 515
Mass, 17
Mathematical conversions
  decimal to percent, 5
  fraction to decimal numbers, 5
  ordinary to scientific notation, 7
  percent to decimal, 5
  scientific to ordinary notation, 7
  units of measurement, 16–18
Mathematics, 2–18
  algebra, 8–16
  algebraic expressions, 10–12, 13
  arithmetic, 3–8
  computation with values (numbers), 5
  conversions (*See* Mathematical conversions)
  decimals, 4–5
  dimensional analysis, 7–8
  equation, 14–16
  evaluating algebraic expressions, 13
  fractions, 3
  fundamental units, 17
  laws of exponents, 12–13
  order of operation, 9–10
  powers of 10, 7
  scientific notation, 7
  signed numbers, 8–9
  SI units, 16–17
  units of measurement, 16–18
  variation, 16
Matter, 21–24
MDA scanners, 624

MDCT, 624
Mechanical energy, 32
Mechanical problems. *See* Troubleshooting
mega-, 17
Mendeleev, Dmitri, 24
Metal envelope, 120
Metallic conductors, 45
Metallic replacement silver recovery unit, 291
Metal (star) artifact, 641
Meter (m), 17
Metric system, 14–16
mGy, 18
micro-, 17
Middle gradient, 303
Miliary TB, 251
milli-, 17
Milliamperage (mA), 48
Milliamperage-second (mAs), 179–182, 211
Milliampere (mA), 18
Milliampere-seconds (mAs), 179–182, 211, 388–391, 418
Milliampere-second timers, 98
Milligray (mGy), 18
Minification gain, 538
Minimizing patient dose, 204–218
Minimum reaction time, 105
Min-R, 564
Mixing, 277–278
Mobil-AID, 527
Mobile radiography, 523–532
  AEC, 527
  distance, 528–529
  generators, 528
  grids, 529–530
  image receptor systems, 533
  kilovoltage, 528
  mAs, 528–529
  power drive, 528
  power supplies, 528
  radiation protection rules, 527
  special patient considerations, 527
  special technical factors, 528
Modulation transfer function (MTF), 319, 425, 427
Moire effect, 269
Moiré pattern, 429
Molecule, 22
Mole (mol), 17
Molybdenum, 30
Monitor, 367–369
Monitoring equipment performance, 470–476
  automatic exposure control (AEC units), 475–476
  cassette cleaning, 476
  diagnostic radiographic system, 472
  external beam evaluation, 471
  film/screen contact tests, 476
  fluoroscopic systems, 473–474
  monitors, 477
  objectives, 470
  PACS, 477
  processor monitoring, 471
  repeat image studies, 478–479
  tomographic systems, 474–476
  troubleshooting, 479–480 (*See also* Troubleshooting)
  view boxes, 476
Monitors, 477
Motion, 437–438
Motion unsharpness, 429
Motor, 74–76
Motor principle, 73, 75
MRI. *See also* Magnetic resonance imaging (MRI)
mR/mAs charts, 206–207
MSAD, 643
MSCT/MDCT units, 625–626
M-shell, 27–28
MTF, 319, 425, 427
M theory, 24
μ, 17
Multidetector computed tomography (MDCT), 624
Multifield intensifiers, 538
Multiple array solid-state detector, 630–631
Multiple detector array scanners (MDA), 624–625
Multiple myeloma, 255
Multiple scan average dose (MSAD), 643
Multiplication and division principle, 14
Multisection computed tomography (MSCT), 625–626
Muscle, 243
Mutual induction, 69

N

N, 17
n, 17
nano-, 17
Nanosecond (ns), 18
Narrow-angle tomography, 557
Narrowing the search, 380
NAS-BEIR, 156
Natural magnets, 63
Natural sources of radiation, 142
NCRP, 156
NCRP Report No. 116, 157
NDT, 227
Negative integer exponents, 7
Negative numbers, 8
Negatron, 199
Neutron, 25, 27
Newton (N), 17
NEXT study, 563
Nièpce, Joseph, 274
Night vision, 223
NIT, 477
NMR. *See* Magnetic resonance imaging (MRI)
Noise, 429
Nondestructive testing (NDT), 227
Nonmagnetic materials, 65
Nonscreen film, 280
Nonstochastic effects, 156
NRC regulation IOCFR20, 158
NRC regulations, 156
ns, 18
N-shell, 27–28
N-type materials, 81
Nuclear energy, 33
Nuclear magnetic resonance (NMR). *See* Magnetic resonance imaging (MRI)
Nuclear medicine
  biologic half-life, 673
  clinical applications, 696–700
  data reconstruction, 687–688
  data storage, 687
  decay equation, 673
  diagnostic radiopharmaceuticals, 674–678
  dose calibator, 693
  effective half-life, 673
  gamma camera, 683–685
  half-life, 673
  hybrid imaging, 690–691
  image acqusition, 685–687
  isobars, 672
  isomers, 672
  isotones, 672
  isotopes, 672
  nonimaging instrumentation, 692–693
  nuclear instability, 672
  nuclear pharmacy, 678–682
  nuclear physics, 672
  nuclear stability, 672
  position emission tomography, 689–690
  quality control, 678
  radiation protection, 693–696
  radioactive decay, 672–673
  radioactivity units, 672
  radiochemistry-682, 673
  radionuclides, 674
  therapeutic radiopharmaceuticals, 678
Nuclear Regulatory Commission (NRC), 158
Nucleon, 24
Nucleus, 24
Number line, 8
nu (n), 35
Nyquist criterion, 429

O

Object-to-image receptor distance (OID). *See also* Distance
  contrast, 418
  density, 396
  recorded detail, 432
  resolution, 433
  size distortion, 446–447
Occasionally exposed workers, 157
Occupationally exposed workers, 157
Octet rule, 27–28
OD number, 296, 298
Oersted, Hans, 65
Oersted's experiment, 64
Off-center grid error, 267
Off-focus grid error, 267

Off-focus radiation, 122
Off-level grid error, 265–266
Ohm, Georg, 48, 51
Ohm's law, 51–53
Ohm's law triangle, 51
Ohm (W), 49
OID. *See also* Object-to-image receptor distance (OID)
"Old Man with Stars Inside Him, The" (Coulehan), 230
"On a New Kind of Rays" (Röntgen), 36
Opacity, 296, 298
Open-core transformer, 79
Open equation, 14
Oppenheimer, J. Robert, 671
Optical density/brightness, 478
Optical density numbers, 296, 298
Optical step wedges, 225, 295
Optimal kilovoltage peak, 493
Optimal phantom image, 491, 493, 500
Orbital electrons, 27–28
Orbital magnetic moment, 61
Order of operation, 9–10
Orthochromatic films, 278
Orthopantomography, 557
Oscillating grid, 263
O-shell, 27–28, 28
OSL dosimeter, 148
Osteitis deformans, 252
Osteoblastic metastases, 252
Osteochondroma, 252
Osteolytic metastases, 255
Osteomalacia, 255
Osteoporosis, 255, 592–594
Overhead suspension system, 93
Oxidation, 287
Oxygen, 30, 31

P

p, 17
PA chest radiograph, 227
Packing density, 436
PACS, 363, 478
Paget's disease, 252
Pair production, 199
Panchromatic films, 278
Panoramic tomography, 557–558
Pantomography, 557
Parallel circuits, 53–56
Parallel grids, 262
Parallel-plate ionization chamber AEC, 105
Paramagnetic materials, 65
Parentheses, 11
Partial volume effect, 642, 643
Particle theory, 35
Particulate radiation, 141
Part size (thickness)
  contrast, 418
  density, 396–398
  distortion, 450–452
  exposure conversion problems, 515
  measurement, 490
Pass box, 291
Pathological conditions, 246–256
  additive conditions, 250–252
  conditions affecting multiple systems, 250, 253
  conditions of abdomen, 252, 253–254
  conditions of chest, 251, 253
  conditions of extremities and skull, 252, 255
  destructive conditions, 253–255
  overview (table), 250
  radiation absorption, 247–250
Pathology, 247
Patient equivalent phantom (PEP), 500
Patient exposure reduction, 161–164
Patient movement, 438
Patient positioning, 209
Patient protection. *See* Protecting patients and personnel
Pattern recognition, 226
Patterson B-2 fluoro screen, 538
PBL devices, 237
P developer, 286
Penalty box, 478
Penetrometer, 295
Penumbra, 433
Peony, 558
PEP, 500
Performance monitoring system. *See* Monitoring equipment performance

Period, 35
Periodic table of elements, 23, 28–31
Permanent magnets, 650
Permeability, 63
Perrier, Carlo, 674
Personnel exposure reduction, 159–161
Personnel monitoring devices, 147–152
Personnel protection. *See* Protecting patients and personnel
Phantom, 552–553
Phantom testing, 490, 491, 496, 502
Phenidone, 286
Phosphor concentration, 436
Phosphorescence, 311
Phosphor layer thickness, 436
Phosphors, 311–312
Phosphor size, 436
Photodisintegration, 199
Photoelectric absorption, 193–196
Photoelectron, 186
Photographic problems, 461
Photomultiplier (PM) tubes, 628
Photon, 35
Photopic vision, 222
Physical contrast, 407
pico-, 17
Picture archiving and communication system (PACS), 363, 478
Pitting, 114
Planck, Max, 35
Planigraphy, 549
Pleural effusions, 251
Plumbicon tube, 541–542
PM tubes, 628
Pneumoconiosis, 251
Pneumonectomy, 251
Pneumonia, 251
Pneumonitis, 251
Pneumothorax, 253
p-n junction semiconductor, 81
Pocket dosimeter, 149
Point spread function (PSF), 425
Positive beam limitation (PBL) devices, 236–237
Positive integer exponents, 7
Positive numbers, 8
Positron, 199
Posteroanterior (PA) chest radiograph, 227
Potassium bromide, 287, 289
Potential difference, 48
Potential energy, 28–31
Potentiometer, 56
Potter, Hollis, 259
Potter-Bucky diaphragm, 263
Power (for x-ray generation), 94–96
Power loss formula, 53
Powers of 10, 7
PQ developer, 287
Precision, 5
Pregnancy, 164
Preservative
  developing, 287
  fixing, 287
Primary barriers, 161
Primary coil, 69
Prime factors, 179
Probability density, 27–28
Problem-solving. *See* Troubleshooting
Procedural factor problems, 463
Processor monitoring, 472
Processor replenishment and circulation system, 289–290
Projection, 164
Protecting patients and personnel, 139–215
  absorbed dose, 145
  activity, 145
  advisory groups, 156
  air kerma, 145
  ALARA, 158–159
  coherent scattering, 196–197
  Compton scattering, 197–198
  digital image receptor systems, 213
  direct square law, 186
  distance, 179–182, 211
  dose limits, 157, 158
  dosimeter, 147–152
  dosimetry reporting, 152
  entrance skin exposure (ESE), 208
  equivalent dose, 145
  exposure, 145

field survey instruments, 147
film/screen image receptor systems, 213
filtration, 162, 171–177 (*See also* Filtration)
gonadal shielding, 163, 212
grids, 162, 213
image receptors, 163–164, 213
immobilization, 209
integral dose, 145
intensifying screens, 213
inverse square law, 185
ionizing radiation, 141–142
kerma, 145
kilovoltage (kVp), 183–188, 209–211
mAs, 179–182, 211
minimizing patient dose, 204–218
pair production, 199
patient exposure reduction, 161–164
patient positioning, 209
15 percent rule, 183
personnel exposure reduction, 159–161
personnel monitoring devices, 147–152
photodisintegration, 199
photoelectric absorption, 193–196
pregnancy, 164–166
prime factors, 178–190
projection, 164
protective barriers, 161
protective devices, 161
regulatory agencies, 156, 158
repeat radiographs, 164
risk-benefit analysis, 214
shielding, 161, 163, 212
subject part density, 213
x-ray interactions, 191–203 (*See also* X-ray interactions)
Protective barriers, 161
Protective devices, 161
Proton, 25, 27
PSF, 425
P-shell, 27–28, 28
P-type materials, 81
Public Law 105-248, 566
Pulmonary edema, 251
Purcell, Edward M., 648
Pyramid problem, 380

Q

Q developer, 286
Q-shell, 27–28
Quad-field intensifiers, 538
Quality factor, 145
Quality management, 467–484
accreditation, 468
definitions, 469
monitoring equipment performance, 470–476 (*See* also Monitoring equipment performance)
purchasing equipment, 469–470
regulation, 468
troubleshooting (*See* Troubleshooting)
Quality management regulations, 468
Quantum mechanics, 24
Quantum mottle, 312–313, 313, 429, 437, 541
Quantum noise, 429
Quark, 24

R

R, 17, 145
Rabelais, Francois, 589
rad, 17, 145
Radiation, 22
Radiation absorption, 247–250. *See also* Pathological conditions
Radiation concepts, 20–37
atomic mass, 27
atomic particles, 25–27
electromagnetic spectrum, 33, 34
energy, 22 (*See also* Energy)
matter, 21–24
orbital electrons, 27–28
particle theory, 35
periodic table of elements, 23, 28–31
wave theory, 34–35
x-ray, discovery of, 35
x-ray properties, 36–37
Radiation dosimetry report, 152
Radiation fog, 198, 410

Radiation protection. *See* Protecting patients and personnel
Radiation therapy
- consultation, 704–706
- historical overview, 704
- image acquisition, 712–715
- image fusion, 708–709
- linear accelerator, 715–720
- proton therapy, 720–721
- stereotactic irradiation, 720–721
- stimulation, 706–708
- TomoTherapy, 721
- treatment, 709–720
- treatment planning, 706–711
- treatment planning systems, 709–711

Radio frequency (RF), 649
Radio frequency subsystem, 651–653
Radiographic cassette, 315
Radiographic duplication unit, 280
Radiographic film, 273–306
- adhesive, 276
- base, 275–276
- coating, 278
- contrast, 301–305
- cross-sectional view, 274
- crystal production, 276–277
- duplication process, 280
- emulsion, 276
- film identification, 281
- film processing, 283–293 (*See also* Film processing)
- film sensitometry, 294–307 (*See also* Film sensitometry)
- Gurney-Mott theory, 278
- latent image formation, 278–279
- latitude, 304
- mixing, 277–278
- resolution, 299
- ripening, 277
- solarization effect, 280
- speed, 299–301
- storage and handling, 280
- supercoat, 276
- types, 279–280

Radiographic film density, 180–182
Radiographic film sizes, 278
Radiographic grid, 162, 258. *See also* Grid
- contrast improvement factor (K), 265
- focused grid, 262
- grid construction, 260–261
- grid errors, 265–269
- grid frequency, 261–262
- grid materials, 259
- grid patterns, 262
- grid performance evaluation, 265
- grid ratio, 260–261
- grid selection/conversions, 264–265
- grid types, 262
- grid uses, 263
- origins, 259
- parallel grids, 263
- purpose, 258
- selectivity, 265
- what is it, 259

Radiographic processing. *See* Film processing
Radiographic table, 92
Radiographic tomography, 548–560
- blur, 551
- circular motions, 555
- CT scan, 617–647 (*See also* Computed tomography (CT))
- curvilinear tomography, 555
- digital tomosynthesis, 556–558
- elliptical motions, 555
- exposure amplitude, 551
- exposure factors, 556–558
- figure eight, 555
- focal plane, 552
- fulcrum, 552
- hypocycloidal motion, 555
- linear tomography, 555
- narrow-angle tomography, 557
- panoramic tomography, 557–558
- performance monitoring, 474–476
- phantoms, 551–552
- quality, 551–554
- section interval, 554
- section thickness, 552–554
- split scan radiography, 557–558
- tomographic amplitude, 551

tomographic principle, 549–551
tomographic procedures, 556–558
trispiral motion, 555
wide-angle tomography, 557
zonography, 557
Radiographic tube rating charts, 123–126
Radiography
anatomically programmed, 490
archaeological, 229
artistic, 227
contact surgical, 280
detail extremity, 280
digital (*See also* Digital radiography)
forensic, 228
mobile, 523–532 (*See also* Mobile radiography)
split scan, 557–558
veterinary, 228
Radon, 25
Radon, J., 619
RAID, 370
Rare earths, 311–312
Raster pattern, 541
Rating charts and cooling curves, 123–126
Rayleigh scattering, 196–197
Reciprocating grid, 264
Reciprocity law failure, 569
Reconstruction software, 638
Recorded detail, 424–441
aliasing, 429
defined, 425
distance, 432–433
ESF, 425
factors to consider, 431
film/screen combinations, 435–437
focal spot size, 433–435
geometry, 432
image receptor, 435–437
LSF, 425
motion, 438
motion unsharpness, 429
MTF, 425, 429
noise, 429
Nyquist criterion, 429
PSF, 425
spatial frequency, 426–429
spatial resolution, 425
Rectification, 81–84
Rectifier, 82
Reducing agents, 284–286
Reduction, 287
Redundant array of independent discs (RAID), 370
Reeve, Christopher, 703
Reformatting, 638
Regulation 10CFR19.12, 165
Regulation 10CFR20, 158
Regulatory agencies, 156, 158–159
Relative speed, 301, 313, 316, 398
Relative speed formula, 516
rem, 17, 145
Repeat image studies, 478–479
Repeat radiographs, 164
Replenishment system, 289–290
Repulsion-attraction law, 40, 41, 63
Resin silver recovery unit, 291
Resistance, 48–50
Resolution, 299, 318–319
Resolution tool, 425
Restrainer, 287
Retentivity, 63
Reversal, 299
Rheostat, 56
Rhodium, 578
Rhodopsin, 223
Right-hand generator rule, 71, 73
Right-hand thumb rule, 66
Ring artifacts, 643, 644
Ripening, 277
Risk-benefit analysis, 214
Rod cell, 222
Roentgen (R), 17, 145
Röntgen, Wilhelm Conrad, 20, 35–36, 39, 121, 129, 514
Roosevelt, Theodore, 275
Rossi, Raymond P., 467
Rotating anode, 113
Rotating anode x-ray tube, 109
Rotor, 76, 118–120
Rounding off, 5
Rutherford, Ernest, 24

S

s, 17
Safelights, 290–291
Saturation current, 113–120
Scale of contrast, 407–409
Scanogram, 632
Scatter control, 234–236
Scattering, 191
Scatter radiation, 121–122, 234–235, 258, 411
Schwartz, Gerhart S., 375
Scientific notation, 7
Scintillation crystal, 628
Scintillation detection devices, 147
Sclerosis, 252
"Scotch Bonnet" (Conklin), 227
Scotopic vision, 223
SCR, 82, 84
Screen film, 280
Screen lag, 311
Secondary barriers, 161
Secondary coil, 69
Secondary radiation, 194
Second-generation CT units, 621
Second law of electromagnetics, 69
Second (s), 17
Section interval, 554
Section thickness, 552–554
Selectivity, 265
Self-induction, 69
Self-rectification, 84
Semiconductor, 46, 47, 83
Sensitivity specks, 277
Sensitometer, 295–297
Sensitometric curve, 298
Sensitometry, 295. *See also* Film sensitometry
Series circuits, 53–56
Shadow shields, 163
Shakespeare, William, 323
Shaped contact shields, 163
Shape distortion, 449–453, 455
Sharpness. *See* Recorded detail
Shell, 27–28
Shell-type transformer, 79
Shielding, 161, 163, 212
Short scale of contrast, 407
SID. *See also* Source-to-image receptor distance (SID)
Siemens, William, 49
Sievert (Sv), 17, 145
Signal-to-noise ratio (S/N), 661–662
Signed numbers, 8–9
Significant digits, 5
Silicon-controlled rectifier (SCR), 83, 84
Silver-bromide crystal production, 276–277
Silver halide crystal, 276–277, 278, 299
Silver iodobromide, 276
Silver recovery systems, 291
Sine wave, 34, 73
Single-phase generators, 99
Single-phase power, 95–96
Sinogram, 632
SI prefixes, 18
SI units, 16–17
SI unit values, 17
Size distortion, 443–448, 454
SMPTE test pattern, 368
SOD. *See also* Source-to-object distance (SOD)
Sodium carbonate, 287
Sodium iodide scintillation crystals, 628
Sodium sulfite, 287
Soft-copy display, 367–369
Soft-copy veiling glare, 368
Solar converters, 46
Solarization, 299
Solarization effect, 280
Solenoid, 66, 68
Solid-state detectors, 630–631
Solid-state detector septal post-patient collimators, 631–632
Solvent
  developing, 287
  fixing, 287
Somatic effects, 142
Sosman, Merrill C., 424
Source-to-image receptor distance (SID). *See also* Distance
  contrast, 418
  density, 394
  mR/mAs charts, 206–207
  recorded detail, 432

resolution, 433
size distortion, 444
Source-to-object distance (SOD)
distortion, 444
entrance skin exposure, 205, 208
recorded detail, 432
Space charge cloud, 83
Space charge effect, 113
Spatial frequency, 426–429
Spatial resolution, 425. *See also* Recorded detail
Special application films, 280
Special imaging systems, 521–700. *See also* individual subject headings
computed tomography, 617–647
fluoroscopy, 533–547
mammography, 561–588
mobile radiography, 523–532
radiographic tomography, 548–560
vascular imaging equipment, 627–640
Specialized diagnostic equipment, 94
Spectral emission, 311
Speed exposure point, 300
Speed point, 300
Spin-echo MRI, 657, 658
Spin magnetic moment, 61
Split scan radiography, 558
Spot filming, 632
Spot imaging systems, 542–543
Staff protection. *See* Protecting patients and personnel
Standby replenishment, 289
Standby switch, 289
Starter solution, 289
Static discharge, 44
Static spot imaging systems, 542–543
Stationary anode, 113
Stationary grids, 264
Stator, 76, 118–119
Step-down transformer, 77, 78
Step in time rule, 390
Stepped variable kVp system, 501
Stepped variable kVp technique chart, 501
Step-up transformer, 77, 78
Step wedge, 295, 304
STIR imaging, 659
Stochastic effects, 156
Storage of film, 370
Stratigraphy, 549
String theory, 25
Structural protective barriers, 161
Subject contrast, 243, 409–411
Subject density, 243
Subject detail, 242–243
Subject distortion, 244
Subject part density, 213
Subject part thickness. *See* Part size (thickness)
Subtraction sign (−), 9
Superadditivity, 287
Supercoat, 276
Superconductor, 46, 47
Sv, 17, 145
Synchronous motors, 76
Système Internationale d'Unites (SI), 16

T

T, 17, 62
Table, 92
Tabletop-to-Bucky tray distance, 432
Talbot, William Fox, 274
Targeting, 638
Target interactions, 130–133
Technical factor problems, 461
Technique chart, 491
Temperature, 33
Temperature control system, 290
10-day rule, 165
tera-, 17
Tesla, Nikola, 62, 649
Tesla (T), 17, 62
Theory of relativity, 22
Thermal energy, 32
Thermionic emission, 83
Thermoluminescent dosimeter (TLD), 149
Third-generation CT units, 621
Thoreaus filter, 173
Three-dimensional CT reconstruction, 633
Three-dimensional thinking, 226–227
Three-phase, 99
Three-phase, six-pulse power, 99
Three-phase generators, 99

Three-phase power, 96
Threshold detection, 224–225
Thyristor, 83
Tilting tables, 92
Time, 17
Timed replenishment, 289
Timer circuit, 98
Tissue density, 411
TLD dosimeter, 149
Toe gradient, 302
Tomographic amplitude, 551
Tomographic blur overlap phantoms, 551–552
Tomographic motions, 554–555
Tomographic principle, 549–551
Tomographic quality, 551–554
Tomography, 549. *See also* Radiographic tomography
Tomography ring artifact, 643, 644
Total brightness gain, 538–539
Total filtration, 175
Total repeat rate, 479–480
Transformer, 76–80
Transformer efficiency, 79
Transformer law, 78
Transport racks, 289
Transport system, 288–289
Transverse angulations, 452
Triple-field intensifiers, 538
Trispiral motion, 555
Troubleshooting, 479–480
  Agfa (*See also* Agfa troubleshooting guide)
  equipment performance monitoring (*See* Monitoring equipment performance)
  Fuji guide (*See also* Fuji troubleshooting guide)
Trough filter, 173
Tube, 108–137. *See also* X-ray tube
Tube angulations, 453
Tube life, 126
Tube rating charts, 123–124, 125
Tuberculosis, 251
Tube suspension systems, 92–93
Tumor, 248, 250
Tungsten, 30
2kVp/cm rule, 515

U

Umbra, 433, 435
Unary minus sign (−), 9
Unary plus sign (+), 9
United States customary system, 16
Units of measurement, 16–18
UNSCEAR, 156
Unsharpness. *See* Recorded detail
Upper gradient, 303
Upright Bucky unit, 93–94
Upside-down grid error, 267

V

v, 17, 48
Vacuum, 45
Valence, 30
Valence energy band, 49
Valve tube, 83
Variable kilovoltage systems, 478, 496–502
  advantages/disadvantages, 496–497
  historical development, 497
  Mayo Clinic (*See also* Mayo Clinic variable kVp system)
  stepped variable kVp system, 501
  variable kVp scales, 497
Variable kVp scales, 500
Variation, 16
Vascular imaging equipment, 627–640
  angiographic tables, 611–612
  C-arm assembly, 610–611
  contrast medium injection devices, 613–615
  digital angiography, 609
  digital cineradiography, 609
  digital image acquisition, 630–632
  digital subtraction angiography (DSA), 609
  generator, 630–631
  historical overview, 628–630
  image intensifier, 631–632
  image post-processing, 610–611
  image processor, 609
  quality control, 615
  x-ray tube, 631

Veil glare, 225
Veterinary radiography, 228
Video camera charge-coupled devices (CCD), 541
Video camera tube, 541–542
Video imaging, 280
Video monitor, 367, 542
Video monitor raster scanning pattern, 368
Vidicon tube, 541–542
View boxes, 477
Viewing distance, 225
Visibility of detail, 404
Visible contrast, 407
Vision and perception, 220–232
  archaeological radiography, 229
  artistic radiography, 227
  art restoration, 228
  biological research, 227
  boundary effect, 224
  edge enhancement, 224
  forensic radiography, 228
  image perception, 221–226
  inefficiency of medical imaging, 223
  Mach effect, 225
  nondestructive testing (NDT), 227
  pattern recognition, 226
  photopic vision, 222
  scotopic vision, 223
  three-dimensional thinking, 226–227
  threshold detection, 224–225
  veterinary radiography, 228
  visual anatomy, 221
  visual physiology, 221–222
Visual acuity, 222
Visual anatomy, 221
Visual physiology, 221–222
Visual purple, 223
Volta, Alessandro, 48
Voltage ripple, 96
Voltage (V), 48
Voltmeter, 78
Volt (v), 17, 48
Volume replenishment, 289
Voluntary accreditation, 468
Voluntary motion, 438

W

W, 17
Washing the film, 288
Watt (W), 17
Wave equation, 35
Wavelength, 34, 35
Wave theory, 34–35
Wb, 17, 62
Weber, Wilhelm, 62
Weber (Wb), 17, 62
Wedge filter, 173
Wet laser film, 366
White snakes, 272
Wide-angle tomography, 557
Wide latitude film, 305–306
Wilde, Oscar, 362
Williams, William A., 500
Williams, William Carlos, 240
Window level, 387
Work, 30

X

x axis, 425
Xenon gas-filled ionization chamber CT detector, 630
Xeromammography, 563, 564
X-Omatic cassette, 316
X-ray, discovery of, 35–37
X-ray circuit, 96–99
  exposure switch, 97–98
  filament circuit, 98
  main circuit, 96
  timer circuit, 98
X-ray emission spectrum, 133–136
X-ray equipment, 90–107
  automatic exposure controls, 104–107
  generator, 99–104
  ionization chambers, 104
  power, 95–96
  specialized diagnostic equipment, 94
  table, 92
  tube, 108–137 (*See also* X-ray tube)
  tube suspension systems, 92–93

X-ray equipment (*continued*)
  upright units, 93–94
  x-ray circuit, 96–99
"X-Ray" (Gilbert), 170
X-Raying the Pharaohs (Harris/Weeks), 229
X-ray interactions, 191–203
  attenuation, 192
  coherent scattering, 196–197
  Compton scattering, 197–198
  effects, 200–202
  pair production, 199
  photodisintegration, 199–200
  photoelectric absorption, 193–196
X-ray production, 129–138
  bremsstrahlung interactions, 130–131
  characteristic interactions, 132–133
  conditions, 130
  emission spectrum, 133–136
  heat production, 130
  target interactions, 130–133
X-ray properties, 36–37
X-ray quality, 179
X-ray quantity, 179
X-ray tube, 108–137
  anode assembly, 113–120
  anode heel effect, 117–118
  cathode assembly, 109–113
  envelope, 120–121
  filament, 110–111
  focusing cup, 112–113
  line-focus principle, 115–117
  off-focus radiation, 122
  rating charts and cooling curves, 123–126
  rotor, 119–120
  stator, 118–119
  tube life, 126
X-ray unit. *See* Mobile radiography
"X-Ray Vision" (Martin et al.), 230

Y

y axis, 425

Z

z axis, 404, 425
Zero exponents, 7
Z number, 26–27
Zonography, 557